The Complete Learning Disabilities Directory

2008

Fourteenth Edition

The Complete Learning Disabilities Directory

Associations • Products • Resources • Magazines
Books • Services • Conferences • Web Sites

A SEDGWICK PRESS Book

Grey House Publishing

PUBLISHER: Leslie Mackenzie
EDITOR: Richard Gottlieb
EDITORIAL DIRECTOR: Laura Mars-Proietti

PRODUCTION MANAGER: Karen Stevens
PRODUCTION ASSISTANTS: Anthony Del Vecchio, Alysia Giglio, Erica Irish
Karynn Kettinq, Erica Schneider, Gerald Simpson
MARKETING DIRECTOR: Jessica Moody

A Sedgwick Press Book
Grey House Publishing, Inc.
185 Millerton Road
Millerton, NY 12546
518.789.8700
FAX 518.789.0545
www.greyhouse.com
e-mail: books @greyhouse.com

First edition published 1993
Fourteenth edition published 2007
Printed in the USA

The complete learning disabilities directory. -- 1994-

v. ; 27.5 cm.
Annual
Continues: Complete directory for people with learning disabilities
Includes index.
1. Learning disabled--Education--United States--Directories. 2. Learning disabilities--United States--Bibliography. 3. Education, Special--United States--Bibliography. 4. Education, Special--United States--Directory. 5. Learning Disorders--rehabilitation--United States--Bibliography. 6. Learning Disorders--rehabilitation--United States--Directory. 7. Rehabilitation Centers--United States--Bibliography. 8. Rehabilitation Centers--United States—Directory.

LC4704.6 .C66
371.9025
ISBN: 978-1-59237-207-2 softcover

Table of Contents

Preface

The National Center for Learning Disabilities (NCLD) is pleased to once again recognize this most recent edition of *The Complete Learning Disabilities Directory.* This fourteenth edition continues to offer a wide range of valuable information to parents, professionals and individuals with LD.

There is a saying 'the more things change, the more they stay the same'. This adage can readily be applied to the field of learning disabilities (LD). Despite more than three decades of progress in understanding how to recognize and best address the needs of individuals with LD across the life span, there is still so much that we do not understand, and the need for helpful information, promising practices and ready access to helpful resources is greater than ever.

And that's where *The Complete Learning Disabilities Directory* can make a difference. By listing organizations and material resources in dozens of categories, it offers thousands of easy-to-access entries for individuals who are searching for information about LD that will help them make informed decisions about school, work, and leisure activities. This newest edition offers an updated and expanded listing of organizations, products, and Web sites that covers the landscape in terms of variety and need, with special attention to an expanded listing of camps and summer programs.

For more than 30 years, NCLD has been addressing these challenges by promoting public awareness and understanding of learning disabilities, dissemination information, conducting educational programs, offering services that advance and disseminate research-based knowledge, and providing national leadership in shaping public policy. We are pleased to have our *Rewards & Roadblocks* report featured in this years Directory, and encourage readers to visit the NCLD Web site at www.LD.org for access to our LDInfoZone, featured newsletters, policy and advocacy updates, and lots more, including a free, online early literacy screening tool (www.GetReadytoRead.org) and a newly launched Parent Center.

Thank you Grey House Publishing for, once again, providing the public with this guide.

Dr. Sheldon H. Horowitz
Director of Professional Services
National Center for Learning Disabilities

Preface

Introduction

Welcome to the fourteenth edition of *The Complete Learning Disabilities Directory*. Published since 1992, it continues to be a comprehensive and sought-after resource for professionals, families and individuals with learning disabilities, which are defined by the Federal Government as a "disorder in one or more of the basic psychological processes involved in understanding or in using spoken or written language, which may manifest itself in an imperfect ability to listen, think, speak, read, write, spell or do mathematical calculations."

According to *"Rewards & Roadblocks: How Special Education Students are Faring Under No Child Left Behind"* by the **National Center for Learning Disabilities**, 6.6 million of our school-age children receive some level of additional support through special education. The complete 24-page report, following this Introduction, details several specific requirements of the NCLB, including Proficiency, Participation, Performance and Accountability, and their impact on students receiving special education supports and services.

This edition of *The Complete Learning Disabilities Directory* includes 7,100 listings – 260 more than last edition. It is designed to provide a comprehensive look at the variety of resources available for the many different types of learning disabilities, including those that occur in spoken language, written language, arithmetic, reasoning and organizational skills. In addition, the material is arranged in subject-specific chapters for quick, effective research.

The Table of Contents is your guide to this database in print form. *The Complete Learning Disabilities Directory's* 7,100 listings are arranged into 21 major chapters and 100 sub chapters, making it easy to pinpoint the exact type of desired reference, including Associations, National/State Programs, Publications, Audio/Video, Web Sites, Products, Conferences, Schools, Learning/Testing Centers, and Summer Programs. Listings provide thousands of valuable contact points, specifically 6,379 fax numbers, 6,492 web sites, and 6,704 key executives, plus descriptions, founding year, designed-for age, and size of LD population.

The Complete Learning Disabilities Directory provides comprehensive and far-reaching coverage not only for individuals with LD, but for parents, teachers and professionals. Users will find answers to legal and advocacy questions, as well as specially-designed computer software and a full range of assistive devices.

This valuable resource includes three indexes: Entry Name Index; Geographic Index; and Subject Index. In addition, a Glossary includes hundreds of definitions and abbreviations for specific disabilities, treatment plans, and legal phrases, such as Auditory Sequencing, FBA (functional behavior assessment) and LRE (least restrictive environment). The Glossary will eliminate guesswork and increase knowledge as you search for listings or network in the LD community.

The Complete Learning Disabilities Directory, *2008*, makes it possible, in this age of information overload, to be confident that this one resource with important LD information is all you need. It assures that this crucial information is readily available at every school and library across the country, not just at state or district level special education resource centers. Now, every special education teacher, student, and parent can have, right at their fingertips, a wealth of information on the critical resources that are available to help individuals achieve in school and in their community. This edition again has been recognized by the **National Center for Learning Disabilities** as a valuable resource for the LD community.

This data is also available as **The Complete Learning Disabilities Directory – Online Database**. Using powerful search and retrieval software, this interactive Online Database searches quickly by dozens of criteria, making it easier than ever to find just the right LD resource.

Starred review:

> *". . . an obvious choice for any parent resource library or professional library serving special education teachers, but its ease of use and the applicable nature of the subject make it suitable for all public libraries."*
>
> Library Journal

User Guide

Descriptive listings in *The Complete Learning Disabilities Directory (LDD)* are organized into 21 chapters and 84 subchapters. You will find the following types of listings throughout the book:

- National Agencies & Associations
- State Agencies & Associations
- Camps & Summer Programs
- Exchange Programs
- Classroom & Computer Resources
- Print & Electronic Media
- Schools & Learning Centers
- Testing & Training Resources
- Conferences & Workshops

Below is a sample listing illustrating the kind of information that is or might be included in an entry. Each numbered item of information is described in the paragraphs on the following page.

1→ 1234

2 → **Association for Children and Youth with Disabilities**

3 → **1704 L Street NW**

Washington, DC 20036

4 → **075-785-0000**

5 → **FAX: 075-785-0001**

6 → **800-075-0002**

7 → **TDY: 075-785-0002**

8 → **info@AGC.com**

9 → **www.AGC.com**

10→ Peter Rancho, Director
Nancy Williams, Information Specialist
Tanya Fitzgerald, Marketing Director
William Alexander, Editor

11→ Advocacy organization that ensures children and youth with learning disabilities receive the best possible education. Services include speaking with an informed specialist, free publications, database searches, and referrals to other organizations.

12→ *$6.99*

13→ *204 pages*

14→ *Paperback*

User Key

1 → **Record Number**: Entries are listed alphabetically within each category and numbered sequentially. The entry numbers, rather than page numbers, are used in the indexes to refer to listings.

2 → **Organization Name**: Formal name of organization. Where organization names are completely capitalized, the listing will appear at the beginning of the alphabetized section. In the case of publications, the title of the publication will appear first, followed by the publisher.

3 → **Address**: Location or permanent address of the organization.

4 → **Phone Number**: The listed phone number is usually for the main office of the organization, but may also be for sales, marketing, or public relations as provided by the organization.

5 → **Fax Number**: This is listed when provided by the organization.

6 → **Toll-Free Number**: This is listed when provided by the organization.

7 → **TDY**: This is listed when provided by the organization. It refers to Telephone Device for the Deaf.

8 → **E-Mail**: This is listed when provided by the organization and is generally the main office e-mail.

9 → **Web Site**: This is listed when provided by the organization and is also referred to as an URL address. These web sites are accessed through the Internet by typing http:// before the URL address.

10 → **Key Personnel**: Name and title of key executives within the organization.

11 → **Organization Description**: This paragraph contains a brief description of the organization and their services.

The following apply if the listing is a publication:

12 → **Price:** The cost of each issue or subscription, often with frequency information. If the listing is a school or program, you will see information on age group served and enrollment size.

13 → **Number of Pages**: Total number of pages for publication.

14 → **Paperback:** The available format of the publication: paperback; hardcover; spiral bound.

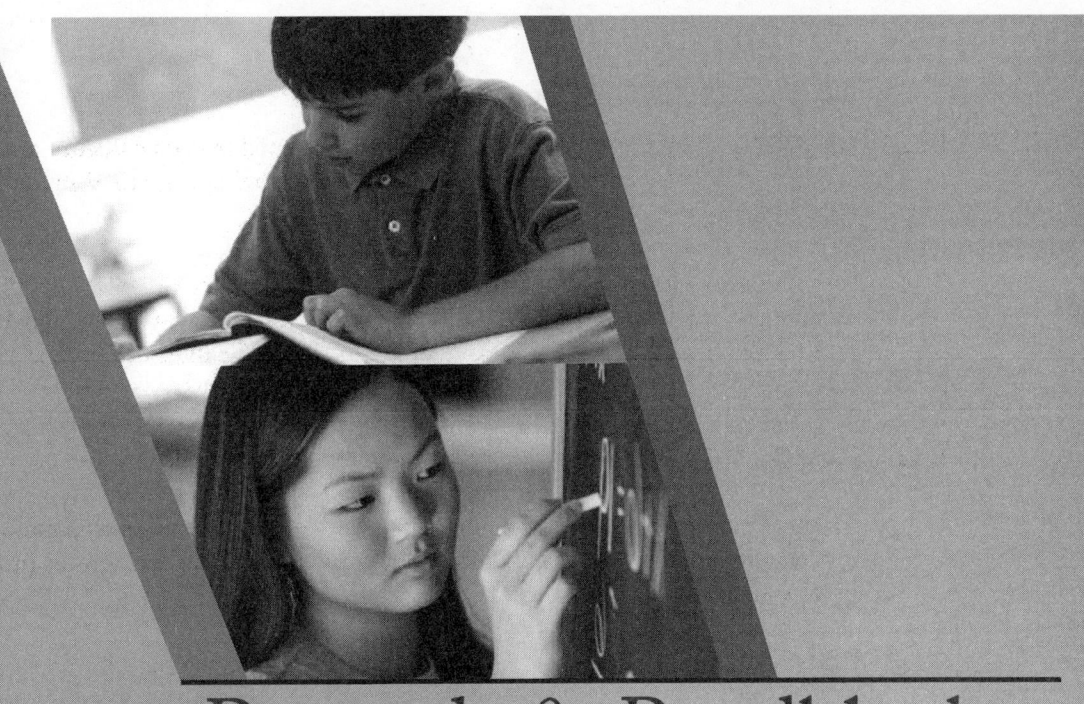

Rewards & Roadblocks:

How Special Education Students are Faring Under No Child Left Behind

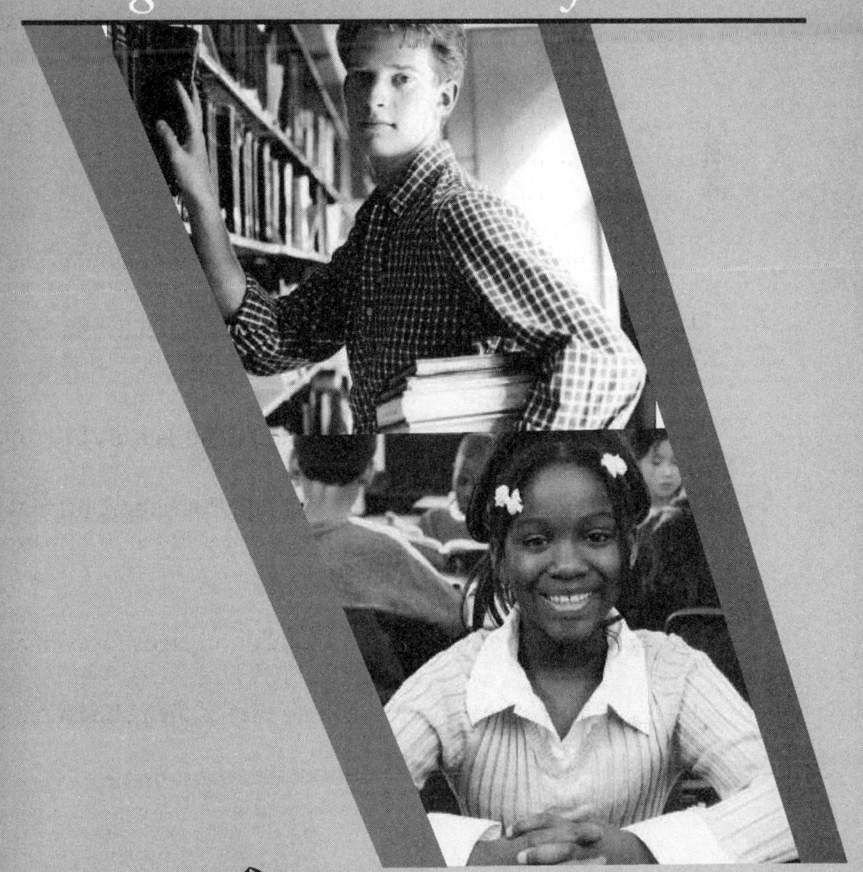

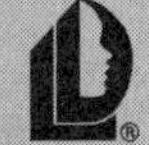

National Center for Learning Disabilities

The power to hope, to learn, and to succeed

Foreword

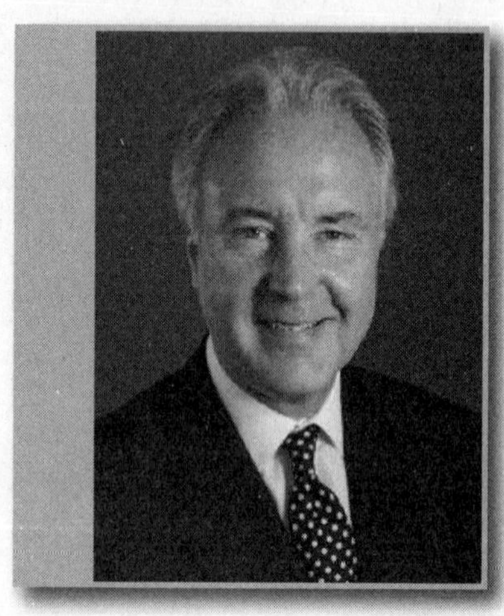

The National Center for Learning Disabilities (NCLD) has a special interest in the reauthorization of No Child Left Behind (NCLB) as the law focuses on improving academic achievement for all children, including improving instructional practice for children who struggle with learning. NCLD has spearheaded activities in support of No Child Left Behind, including the publication of several documents that have been used to educate and inform policy makers, parents and other stakeholders about the positive and meaningful impact the law is having for students with learning disabilities (LD).

While the Individuals with Disabilities Education Act (IDEA) mandates the provision of a free appropriate public education (FAPE) for students with disabilities, it contains no provisions setting high expectations and holding schools accountable for their progress. In fact, in its latest reauthorization of IDEA, Congress once again reminded us that "the implementation of the Act has been impeded by low expectations, and an insufficient focus on applying replicable research on proven methods of teaching and learning" (20 U.S.C. §1400(c)(4). It is NCLB that has provided the long-needed requirement of school accountability and emphasis on doing what works to improve results for students with disabilities.

NCLD is publishing this report to inform the current discussion about gains that students with disabilities have made as a result of NCLB and where further progress must be made to ensure our students are on a pathway to receiving a regular diploma and achieving life success. We offer it with the conviction and hope for a bright and meaningful future for all students, who by definition can achieve and for whom our federal laws are intended to support.

Sincerely,

James H. Wendorf
Executive Director

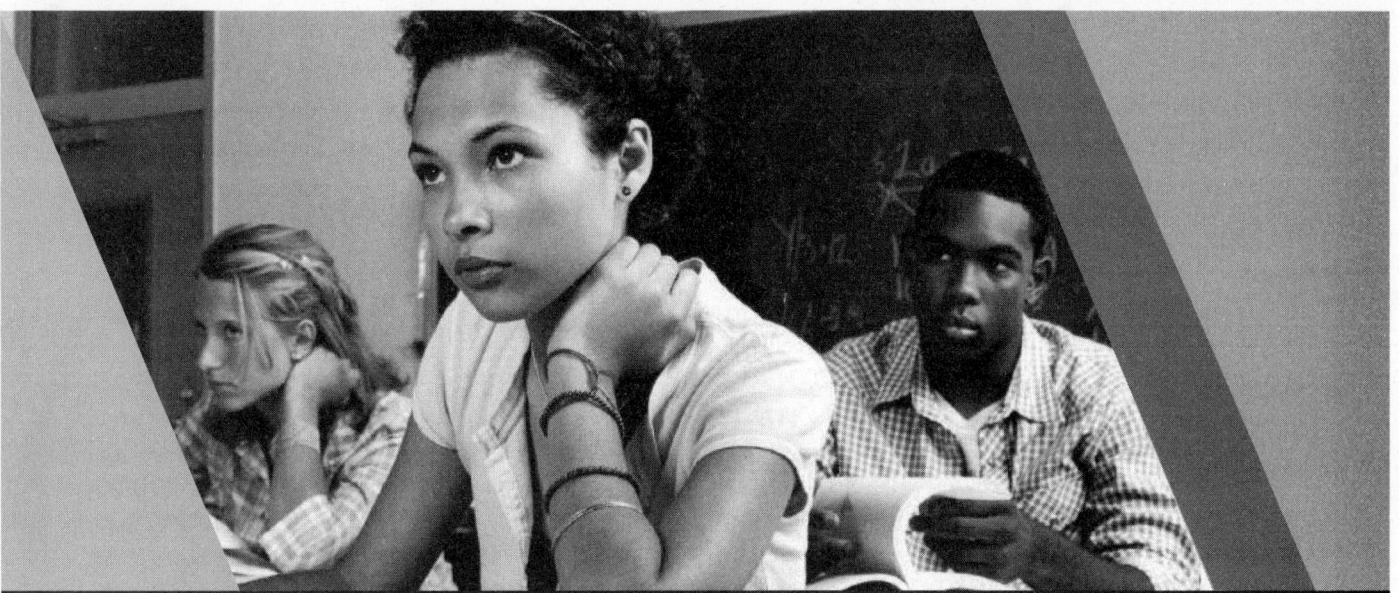

Rewards & Roadblocks:

How Special Education Students are Faring Under No Child Left Behind

The 2001 reauthorization of the Elementary and Secondary Education Act (ESEA), known as No Child Left Behind (NCLB), brought about a dramatic change in the level of attention paid to millions of public school students who historically perform poorly. Its mandate to "close the achievement gap" for specific groups of students – and achieve proficiency for all students in reading and math by 2013-2014 - has provided historic impetus for change.

For one group of students – those who receive special education services – NCLB has provoked discussions that span a wide range of opinions and positions. While much of the impact of NCLB remains to be seen – after all, full implementation only began in the 2005-2006 school year - it's time to take a look at what we know about the rewards and roadblocks for special education students. This report provides a look at several specific requirements of the No Child Left Behind Act (NCLB) and their impact on students receiving special education supports and services.

Who They Are

Almost fourteen percent – some 6.6 million – of this nation's school-age children receive some level of additional support through special education. These children come from all race and ethnic groups and speak many different languages. Significant numbers are served by other school programs, such as Title I and English Language services, in addition to special education.

Many are indistinguishable from students who do not receive special education services. In fact, most spend the vast majority of their school day in general educa-

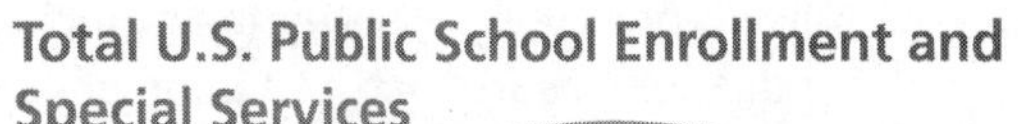

Total U.S. Public School Enrollment and Special Services

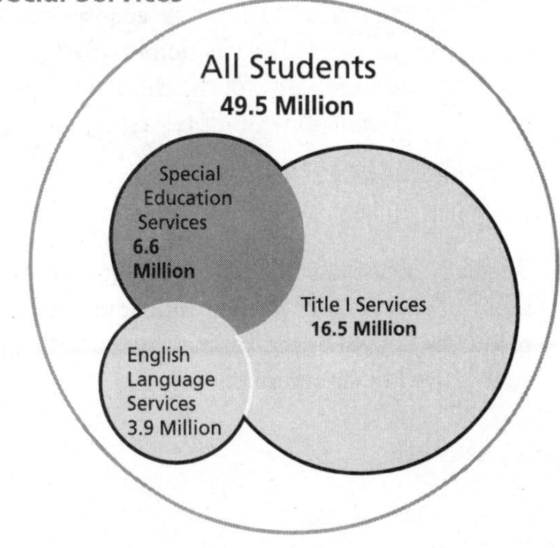

tion classrooms – taught by general education teachers – using the same instructional materials as all other students in the class (see chart). And their parents have the same aspirations for their success in life.

Where Special Education Students Spend Their School Day

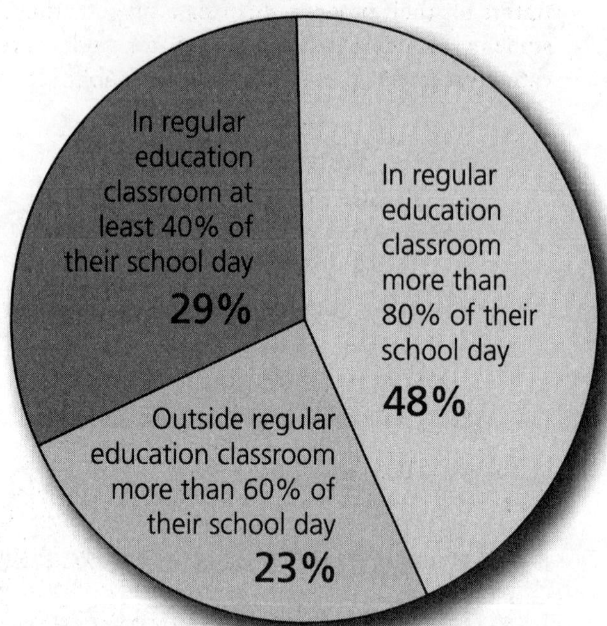

Source: 26th Annual Report to Congress on the Implementation of the Individuals with Disabilities Education Act 2004

It should be noted that vast differences exist across states regarding the percent of students receiving special education services. In the 2003-2004 school year, state rates ranged from a low of 10.5 percent in California to a high of 20.2 percent in Rhode Island. Source: Digest of Education Statistics, 2005, Table 52 [see Appendix A for state-by-state information]

These students – often referred to as "*students with disabilities*" – are afforded a set of important legal protections under the Individuals with Disabilities Education Act (IDEA). Brought about because of a pervasive denial of equal access to public education, the IDEA provides eligible students with special education and related services that allow them to benefit from education just like all other students. IDEA makes locating, identifying and serving students in need of special education the responsibility of all public schools, and, not all students with disabilities are eligible for special education services. Only when the impact of a disability is such that the student requires additional services and supports to benefit from the educational program is special education available.

Defining Special Education

Special education is defined as "*specially designed instruction*, at no cost to parents, to meet the unique needs of a child with a disability, including instruction conducted in the classroom, in the home, in hospitals and institutions, and in other settings ..." [20 U.S.C. §1401 (29)] In turn, *specially designed instruction* is defined as "adapting, as appropriate to the child's needs, the content, methodology, or delivery of instruction to address the unique needs of the child that result from the child's disability; to ensure access of the child to the general education curriculum, so that the child can meet the *educational standards* within the jurisdiction of the public agency that *apply to all children.*" [34 CFR §300.39 (b)(3)]

Special education students are expected to meet the same state educational standards as all other students. The additional assistance of their individualized, specially designed instruction (detailed in an annual commitment of resources known as the Individualized Education Program or IEP) provides the extra support needed to reach such a level of achievement.

Special education classification has too frequently been used to diminish the expectations for the students designated as eligible for such services and to minimize the responsibility of general education teachers and administrators for their progress. Also, data suggests that special education classification is used to segregate minority students, particularly Black boys. Black students represent more than 20 percent of those receiving special education yet make up only 17 percent of public school enrollment.

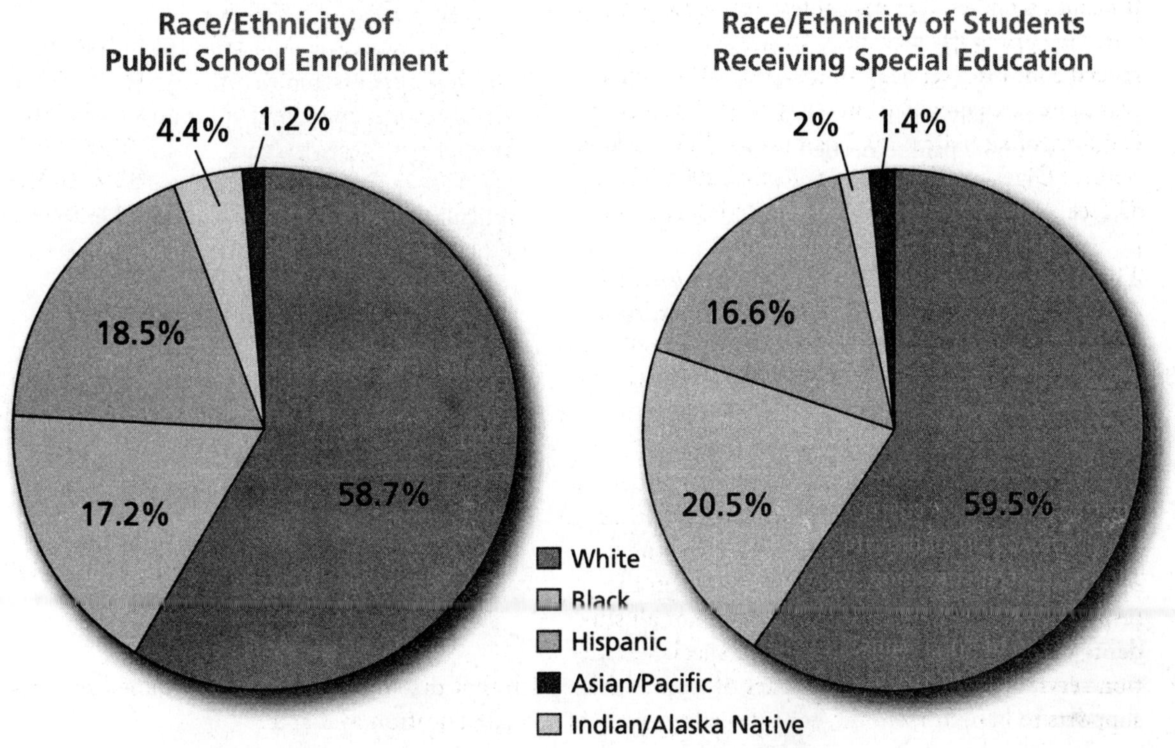

Special education designation also includes a disproportionate number of children in poverty. Data from the Special Education Elementary Longitudinal Study (SEELS) found that the rate of poverty among the households of students with school-identified disabilities is substantially higher than the rate found in the general population. (see box)

"At 24 percent, the rate of poverty among the households of students with disabilities is higher than the 16 percent found in the general population. Despite the fact that parents are about equally likely to be employed, households of students with disabilities are much more likely to have low and very low incomes. The higher rate of poverty among students with disabilities, and factors that can accompany poverty and put children at risk, are particularly evident among children of color, especially African-American children with disabilities. They are significantly more likely to be poor and less likely to be living with two parents than other students with disabilities; their rate of foster care placement is more than three times that of white or Hispanic students with disabilities. Their households average fewer adults and more children. Mothers of African-American children with disabilities are significantly more likely than those of white children to have given birth as teens, to have not completed high school, and to be unemployed."

Source: Overview Of Findings From Wave 1 Of The Special Education Elementary Longitudinal Study (SEELS) June 2004

All in all, there is substantial overlap between students who receive special education and other students who comprise historically low achieving groups - particularly those who are low income and Black. To the extent that overlap exists, these students are those for whom the Elementary and Secondary Education Act was originally enacted and intended to assist.

One aspect of the marginalization of special education students has been the pervasive practice of failing to include these students in the state assessments required of all other students. Despite requirements in both the 1994 version of the ESEA – known as the Improving America's Schools Act – and the 1997 version of the IDEA – that special education students participate in all state assessments and that the results of their participation be publicly reported, massive exclusion prevailed. Without participation, there is no accountability nor will attention be paid to needed improvements in the achievement of these students.

This systematic exclusion from accountability systems is particularly egregious when examined in the context of the characteristics of the disability categories that make up the population of students receiving special education. (see chart)

Students Receiving Special Education Services by Disability Category

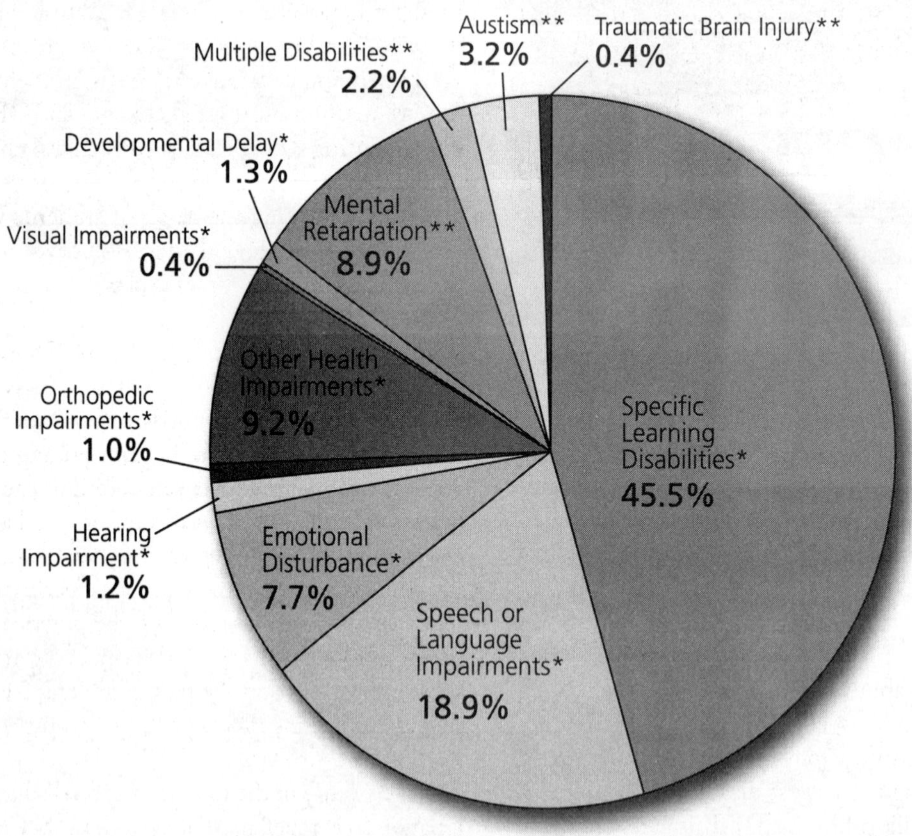

Source: www.IDEAdata.org
Table 1-3: IDEA Part B Child Count (2005), Students ages 6 through 21 served under IDEA, Part B, by disability category and state: Fall 2005

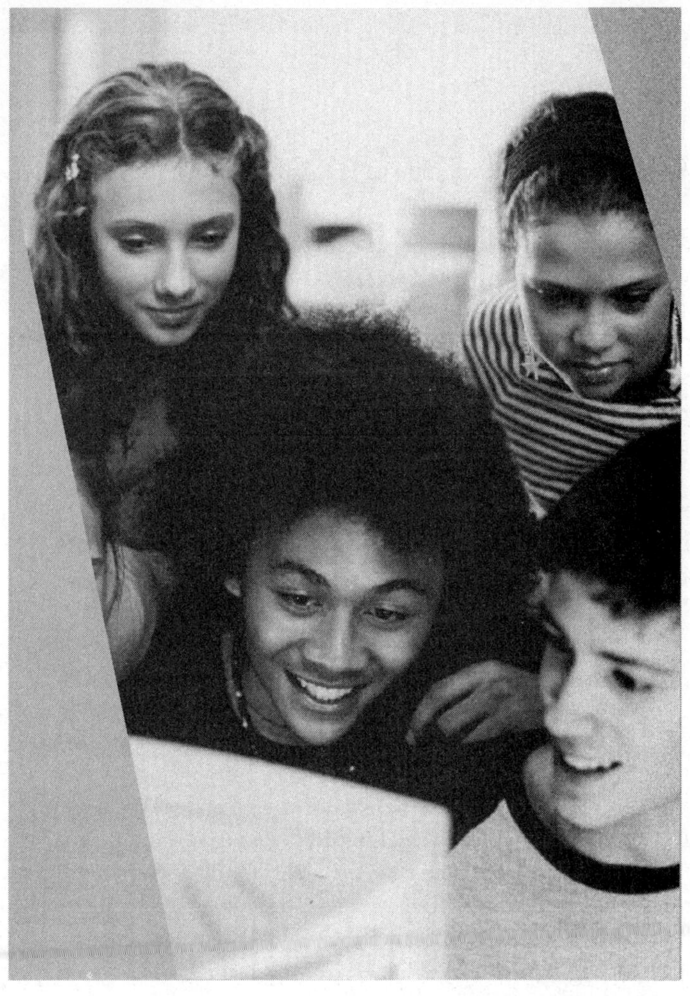

In their often-cited 2001 paper, *Rethinking Learning Disabilities*, a group of prominent researchers posited that:

> "We estimate that the number of children who are typically identified as poor readers and served through either special education or compensatory education programs could be reduced by up to 70 percent through early identification and prevention programs." They went on to state that "From its inception as a category, LD has served as a sociological sponge that attempts to wipe up general education's spills and cleanse its ills."
> *Source: Rethinking Special Education for a New Century, Finn, Rotherham, Hokanson, Jr., 2001*

In fact, the radical growth in the LD category during the 1980's and early 1990's, coupled with mounting skepticism about the method used for its identification, resulted in substantial changes to IDEA and its implementing federal regulations. These changes seek to broaden the role and responsibility of general education in addressing the needs of students who experience difficulty in general education classrooms prior to referring students for special education.

And, in updating the IDEA in 2004, Congress took the unprecedented step of allowing schools to use federal funding intended to assist with the excess cost of special education (IDEA Part B funds) to provide services to students who need additional academic and behavioral support to succeed in a general education classroom without giving them special education status. This new provision – known as "early intervening services" – is aimed at reducing the practice of designating students as in need of special education without substantial efforts on the part of general education to provide robust instruction and early intervention first.

Simply put, the vast majority of students receiving special education in our nation's schools – some 85 percent - are found eligible under a disability category that in no way precludes them from - with appropriate services and supports - functioning at or above grade level or from achieving proficiency on a state's academic content standards in reading and math.*

Our assumptions about the performance potential of students identified for special education is further complicated by positions put forward by leading researchers regarding the largest disability category – specific learning disabilities (LD). This category makes up 45 percent of all special education students – and, more importantly, 48 percent of the special education students in the grades assessed under NCLB.

Given evidence of the misuse of special education designation so compelling that even the U.S. Congress was moved to act, it seems particularly important that students receiving special education services not be further shortchanged in the context of school accountability.

**Note: Reading and math are the only academic areas at stake in NCLB testing requirements.*

Exiting "Program Improvement" by Growing the Proficiency of Students with Disabilities:

Snowline Joint Unified School District

By Jim Canter, Assistant Superintendent, Curriculum

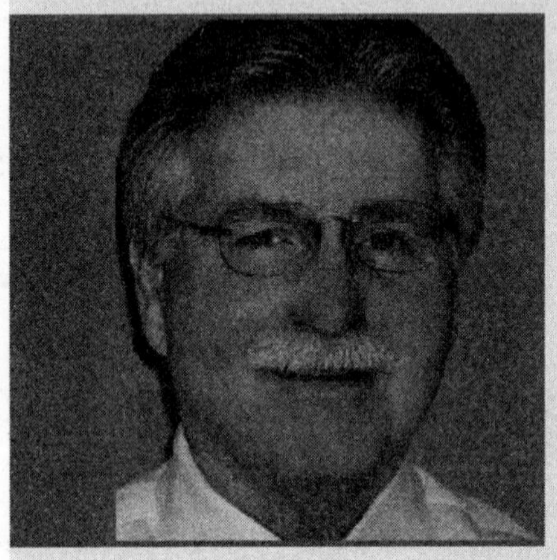

As Assistant Superintendent of Curriculum for Snowline Joint Unified School District in California, I was informed by the California Department of Education that the students with disabilities (SWD) subgroup fell short of the AYP English language arts proficiency rate in 2003 and 2004 and, under new regulations, qualified the district as Program Improvement (PI). The subgroup had increased three percent over the two-year period, but scored overall only ten percent proficient. Within two more years, however, I received gratifying news that Snowline District met all AYP criteria including the SWD proficiency rate and that the district exited PI. The SWD English language arts proficiency rate had tripled since 2003.

Our successful plan of action, developed with input from staff and parents, significantly improved student achievement by implementing a process structured around data and standards. After learning of the PI status, I first realized that I needed to understand the composition of the subgroup, and so I separated the subgroup by specific disability. I found that the subgroup consisted of at least five categories. The largest category, nearly 50% percent of the subgroup, was specific learning disability (SLD), and, of that category, approximately 85% was placed in the Resource Specialist Program. Most students of this category were diagnosed as mildly impaired, yet scored only about seven percent proficient in English language arts. Similarly, I discovered that about 30% of the subgroup was Speech/Language Impaired (SLI), the second largest category, yet these students scored less than 14% proficient. I also found that 60% of SLI was placed for articulation, generally a non-cognitive impairment.

Based on the data, it was obvious that special education needed more involvement in the district's standards-based program. One strategy I used involved special education teachers participating in the district's collaborative process called Structured Teacher Planning Time (STPT). During STPT, district-wide, trained teachers examined state and local data by grade level and course, developed data statements, and made instructional decisions based on the data. Special education teachers were sometimes included in the process, but were now required to attend and encouraged to participate. In addition, I released special education teachers to hold separate STPT meetings by grade span after the regularly held STPT meetings, and the special education teachers soon collaborated about SWD data, teaching strategies, and related issues. To help facilitate STPT, I appointed special education instructors to serve as teacher leaders. Since initiating STPT, teachers have built trust and now readily share best teaching practices.

Another strategy I used helped include SWD in the district standards-based program. As part of our plan, I directed that any student who participated in state assessments take district formative assessments as well. The strategy profoundly effected district instructional practices. It directly influenced teachers to instruct to state standards, and it provided formative data about all students' progress.

As I walk through classrooms, I now observe special education teachers instructing to state standards, and I find that SWD are receiving instruction in regular classes to a greater degree. I am proud that, through our efforts, Snowline District exited PI, but I realize and our administrators and teachers fully understand that we must continue to improve student achievement among SWD and students of other subgroups.

Making Them Matter: Participation

NCLB's requirement that schools, school districts and states test at least 95 percent of all students in the required grades and academic areas (see box) – and at least 95 percent of each required subgroup (see box) – has finally catapulted special education students into the realm of full accountability.

NCLB Testing Requirements

Beginning with the 2005-2006 school year, all students in grades 3 through 8 must be tested in both reading/language arts and math. In addition, high school students must be tested sometime during grades 10-12 in both reading/language arts and math. Beginning in 2008, all students must also be assessed in science once during grades 3-5, once during grades 6-9, and once during grades 10-12. Schools are not held accountable for student performance on science assessments.

NCLB Subgroup Requirements

- Students from major racial/ethnic groups
- Economically disadvantaged students
- Students with limited English proficiency
- Students with disabilities (eligible for services under IDEA)

There is no doubt that this participation requirement – part of the trifecta known as "Adequate Yearly Progress" or, simply, "AYP" – has finally motivated states to begin to fully include all students in state assessments, including students receiving special education services.

The chart below shows the percentages of special education students who participated in the general assessments (with or without accommodations) of several states six years ago in the 2000-2001 school year. Only one state – Kansas – performed at or above the current requirement for at least 95 percent participation.

Participation of Special Education Students in General Assessments in Selected States, 2000-2001

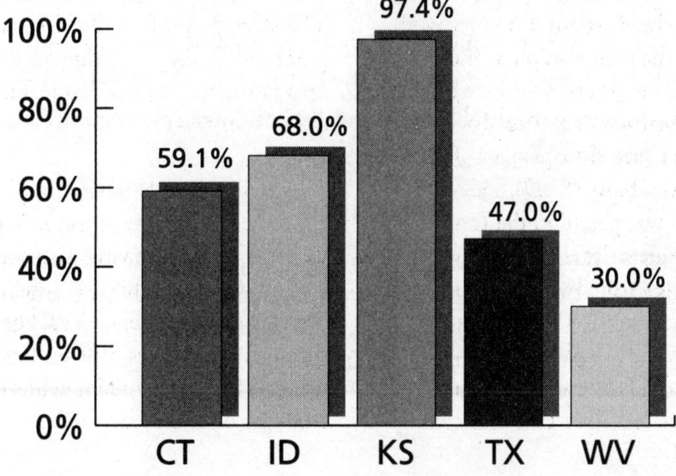

Source: National Center on Educational Outcomes (NCEO)

By contrast, three years later, participation rates showed a marked improvement. The chart below shows the participation rate for 21 states in the 2003-2004 school year (post NCLB implementation) for students receiving special education.

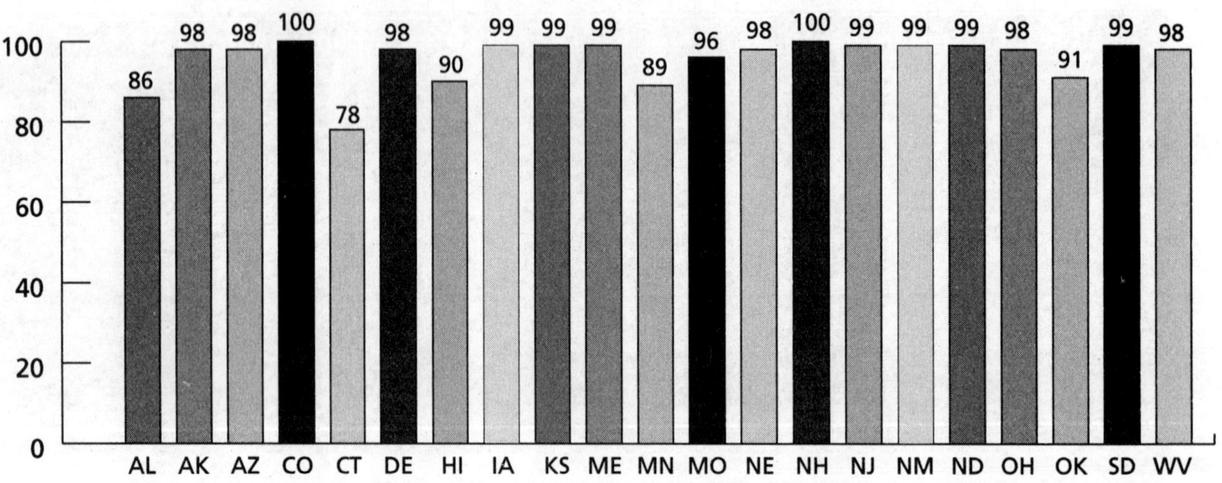

Source: National Center on Educational Outcomes (NCEO)

However, states' ability to fully include all students receiving special education in state assessments continues to be hampered. In its 2006 *National Assessment of Title I Interim Report*, the U.S. Department of Education noted:

> "Most states have met the requirement to annually assess 95 percent or more of their students, including major racial/ethnic groups, students with disabilities, limited English proficient (LEP) students, and low-income students. However, 14 states did not meet the minimum test participation requirement for one or more student subgroups. Ten states assessed fewer than 95 percent of one or more minority student groups (black, Hispanic, and/or Native American), and nine states did not meet the test participation requirement for LEP students.
>
> The lowest participation rates were for students with disabilities. While states missing the test participation requirement for other subgroups often missed by just one or two percentage points, states that failed to assess 95 percent of students with disabilities typically had lower participation rates for those students (as low as 77 percent in one state)."

While participation has seen a dramatic increase due to NCLB's participation requirements, the participation has not always been meaningful. For example, while the percentage of special education students participating in state assessments in Texas increased from 47 percent in 2000-2001 to 99 percent in 2003-2004, more than half of those tested were given an "out of level" test. [see chart]

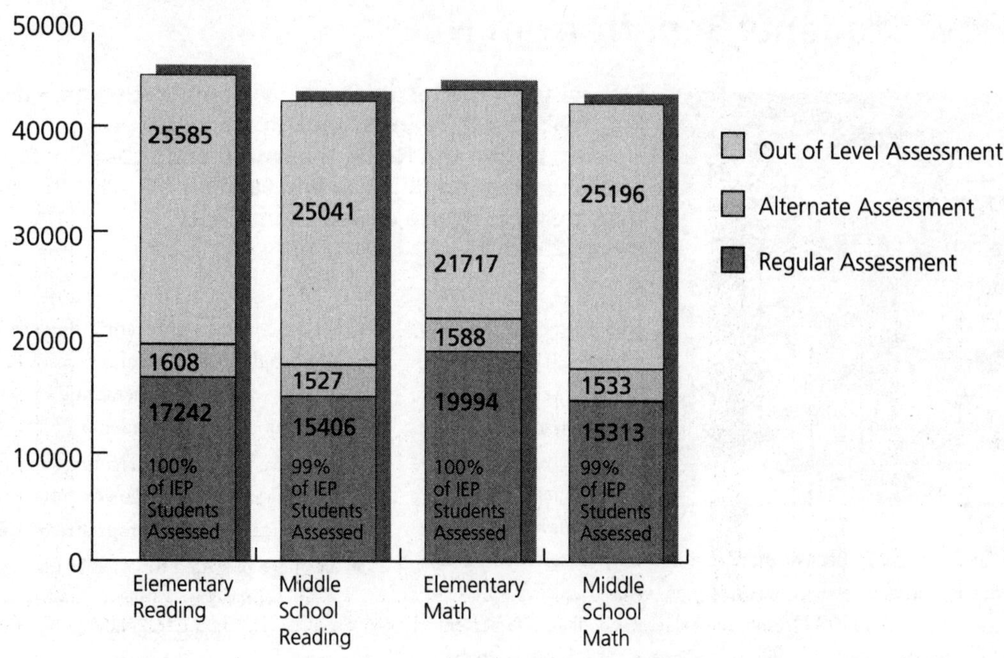

Source: Thurlow, M., Moen, R. & Altman, J. Annual Performance Reports: 2003-2004 State Assessment Data. National Center on Educational Outcomes (NCEO).

Marginal Participation

Out-of-level testing (OOLT) means assessing students enrolled in a specific grade level with tests designed for students at lower grade levels. As such, an OOLT does not measure a student's mastery of grade-level content or achievement standards – a measurement that is key to the school accountability goal of NCLB.

Out-of-level testing is often associated with lower expectations for students receiving special education, tracking these students into lower-level curricula with limited opportunities. It may also limit a student's opportunities for advancing to the next grade or graduating with a regular high school diploma. It also assumes that a student being tested below grade level will automatically recall the content from a past grade. According to the National Center on Educational Outcomes, research does not support the use of out-of-level test scores from state assessments when measuring student proficiency or otherwise on standards for the grade level in which a student is enrolled.

Because an out-of-level assessment fails to measure a student's mastery of grade-level content, states that choose to administer such an assessment must consider it the same as an alternate assessment based on alternate achievement standards for AYP determinations according to NCLB regulations. As such, proficient and advanced scores fall under NCLB's limit of no more than one percent of the scores of all students assessed in the school district or state. This regulatory limitation has provided an important safeguard to what has been an overused assessment practice by states unwilling to develop assessments that can allow students with disabilities to fully demonstrate their knowledge on grade level content.

The O'Hearn School:
How Students Benefit from NCLB

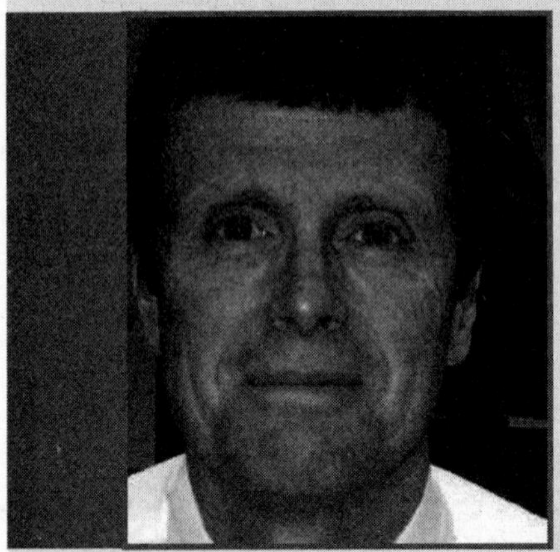

Excerpt from the testimony of William Henderson, Ed.D.
Principal, The O'Hearn School, Boston, MA
Hearing before the House Education and Labor Committee
Subcommittee on Children and Families
United States House of Representatives
March 29, 2007

The O'Hearn is a small, urban elementary school serving 230 children from early childhood through grade five. Approximately 45 percent of our students are African American, 30 percent are Caucasian, and 25 percent are relative new arrivals from many countries around the globe. A majority of our students qualify for free or reduced lunch. The O'Hearn is an inclusive school and 33 percent of our students have a disability. Students who are involved in regular education, students with a range of disabilities, and students considered talented and gifted learn together and from each other. Teachers and support staff collaborate and work as teams to instruct and support all children in fully integrated classrooms. The O'Hearn is a highly selected school under Boston's choice assignment plan. Overall, the performance of O'Hearn students has been strong. In fact, until this past school year, we made all of our AYP goals. However, in 2005-2006, the O'Hearn did not make AYP goals in English / Language Arts.

Our school benefits greatly from the accountability of No Child Left Behind because until its passage, our students receiving special education supports and services would not have been included in our district or state accountability system, nor would they have received full access to the general curriculum in many public schools.

At the O'Hearn, we strive each day to ensure 230 youngsters are provided the following:

- Support from a committed team that strives to collaborate on effective strategies to teach diverse learners and ensure all students learn and succeed.
- Access to universally designed curricula, textbooks and assessments as well as appropriate accommodations — for both instruction and assessment.
- Encouragement, along with their families, to strengthen their artistic, athletic and other talents through music, dance, physical fitness and modern day technology.

All three are critical to the success of my students now and in the future.

NCLB has made a significant difference in how we view the potential of students with disabilities at O'Hearn:

- We have set high expectations and expect proficiency from the majority of our students
- We have targeted our resources to maximize IDEA, Title I, Title II and other dollars to ensure early intervention, early identification and appropriate services are provided
- We have provided top quality teaching and services, by high qualified teachers and staff, including providing extra instructional time before or after school with ample opportunities to participate in the arts.

Our formula allows over 200 students – whose challenges and proficiency scores are spread across a continuum – to learn, blossom and demonstrate what they know.

NCLB could further benefit our school if the following improvements were made:

1. **Require every state to undergo a federal review of assessment accommodations guidelines.**
   It should not be left up to districts and states to decide whether or not students with disabilities can have access to grade level content through universally designed textbooks and assessments as well as receive accommodations to demonstrate the knowledge gained in the classroom. The federal government should provide the safeguards necessary to ensure access to both content and accommodations.
2. **Ensure that a requirement to annually assess student proficiency does not lead to a testing frenzy.**
   Too much testing can work at cross purposes for students and staff. We must strike a balance and continue to explore ways for students to demonstrate success and proficiency. One way that is showing potential to capture that growth is to allow the addition of a growth model to AYP requirements.
3. **Promote family involvement in schools.**
   Students and parents both benefit when opportunities are provided to share the growth and achievements of students in academics, arts, sports, leadership and other activities.

Moving Them Forward: Performance

NCLB's requirement for universal proficiency in reading and math by 2013-2014 has, in the opinion of most, brought about much needed attention to the instruction of students receiving special education. In early 2007, the Commission on No Child Left Behind, a bipartisan, independent commission formed to develop recommendations for the reauthorization of the No Child Left Behind Act, released its final report. In it, the Commission found that

> "Overall, we were left with the strong impression that NCLB has resulted in a much higher awareness of and focus on the achievement of students with disabilities."
> *Source: Beyond NCLB: Fulfilling the Promise to Our Nation's Children, 2007, pg 67*

In fact, given the long-standing practice of excluding students who are receiving special education services from large-scale assessments – or testing them on content far below their age appropriate grade level – these students can be viewed as performing extraordinarily well.

An examination of seven-year trends of the percentage of elementary special education students who achieved proficiency on statewide reading exams across ten states (see table) shows consistent gains in most states.

Seven-Year Trends of the Percentage of Elementary Students with Disabilities who Achieved Proficiency on Statewide Reading Exams

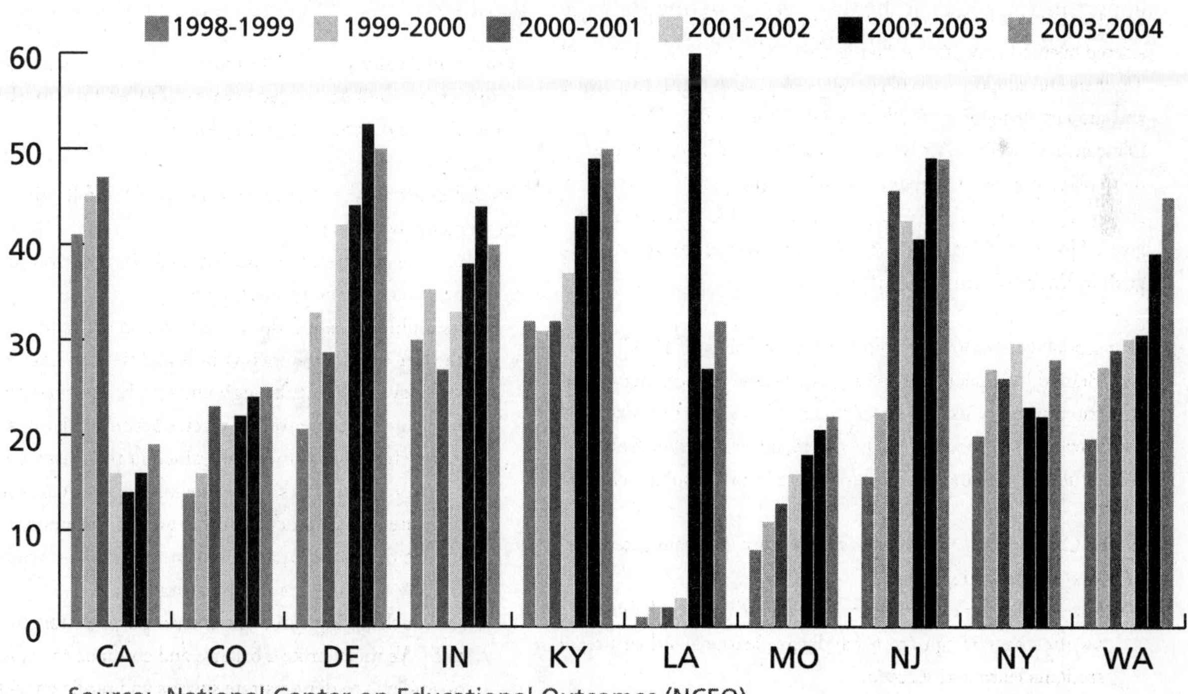

Source: National Center on Educational Outcomes (NCEO).

Further evidence of performance improvement was provided by the U.S. Department of Education in its 2006 National Assessment of Title I Interim Report, which found that from 2000-2001 to 2002-2003, 14 of 20 states experienced an increase in the percentage of 4th-grade special education students performing at or above the state's proficient level in reading and 16 of 20 states experienced an increase in math. This outpaced the improvements experienced for all other student groups.

Closing the Gap

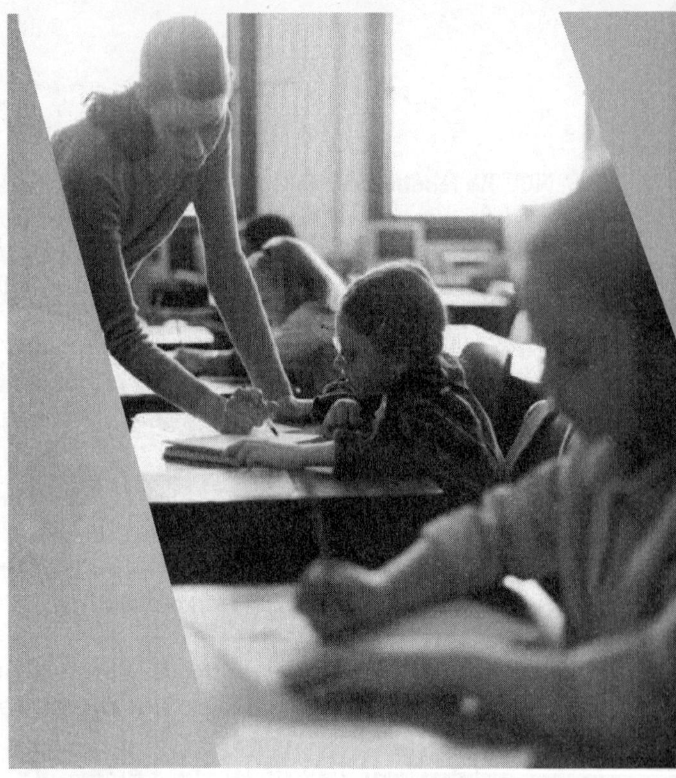

Understanding who receives special education services – as well as how they become eligible by the public school that serves them – is critical to the expectations set for this group. Some would suggest that special education designation – in and of itself – precludes a student from achieving proficiency on state standards. Some recommendations, such as one from the state of Washington, have advocated a complete abandonment of students receiving special education services stating:

> "Students who appropriately meet the eligibility criteria for receipt of special education and related services are, by definition, unable to reach 100% proficiency. If they were able to meet 100% proficiency they would be, by definition, ineligible for special education and related services."
> *Source: Washington State Proposal To Ensure Successful Implementation of No Child Left Behind, Nov. 2003*

If such an assertion is correct, there should be data to support it. Yet, a look at the distribution of one state's 4th graders on its state mathematics test clearly showed that the scores of students with special education status distributed across the performance range (see chart).

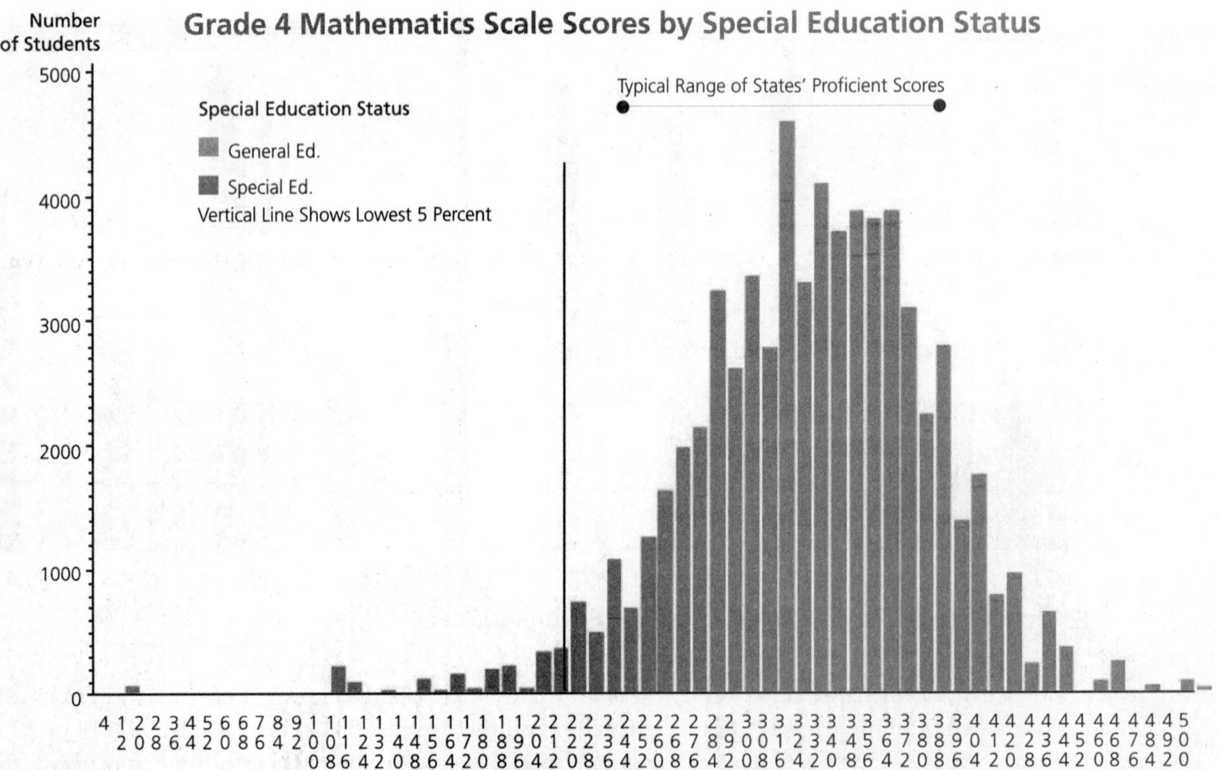

Source: Gong, B. & Simpson, M.A. (2005). "Kids in the Gap?": Academic Performance and Disability Characteristics of Special Education Students. Dover, NH: Center for Assessment. www.nciea.org

Further evidence of improved achievement is provided by extensive analysis done by the National Center on Educational Outcomes (NCEO) – a federally funded center that monitors the participation of special education students in national and state assessments. NCEO analyzed the performance of special education students for 25 states on regular elementary reading assessments for the four years from 2001-2002 through 2004-2005 (see table). In 2001-2002, these states had an average proficiency rate of 34 percent. That proficiency rate improved to 43 percent in 2004-2005. Five states – Alaska, Alabama, Kansas, Maryland, and South Dakota, saw improvements of more than 20 percentage points in the number of special education students achieving proficiency on the state's regular assessment – the same assessment taken by all students.

Four Year Performance Trends for Students with Disabilities on Elementary Reading Assessments (2001-2002 to 2004-2005)

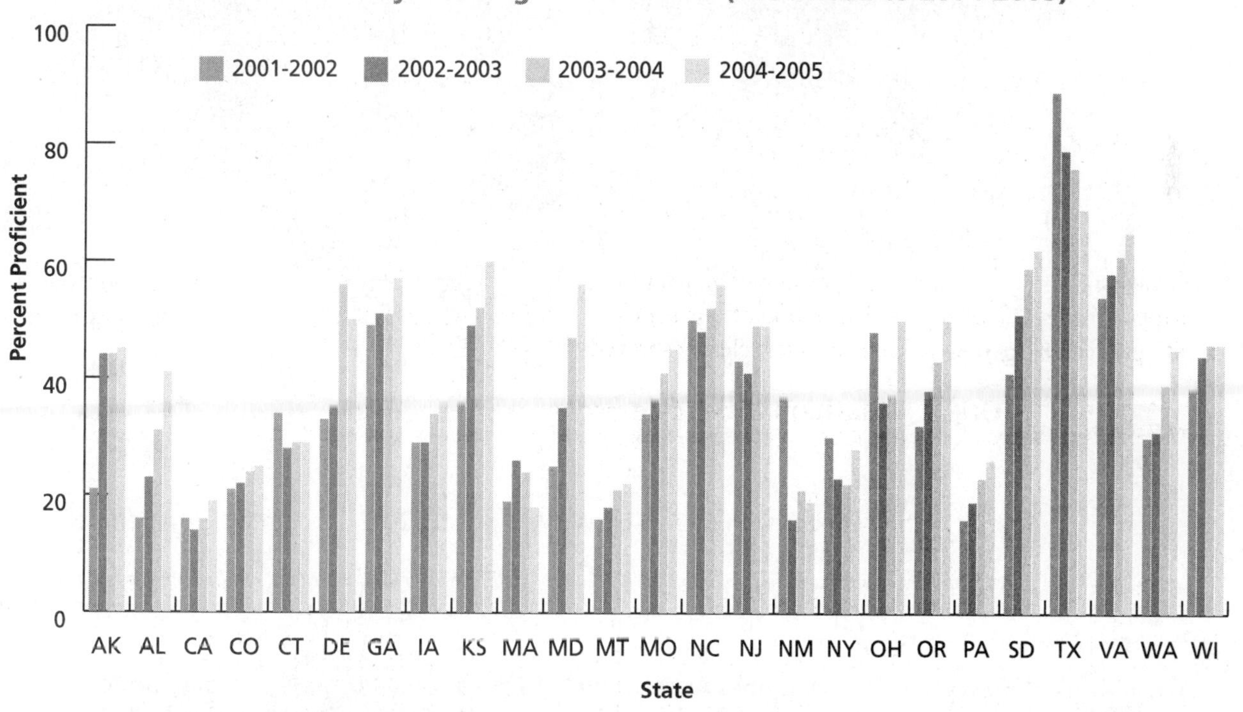

Source: National Center on Educational Outcomes (NCEO)

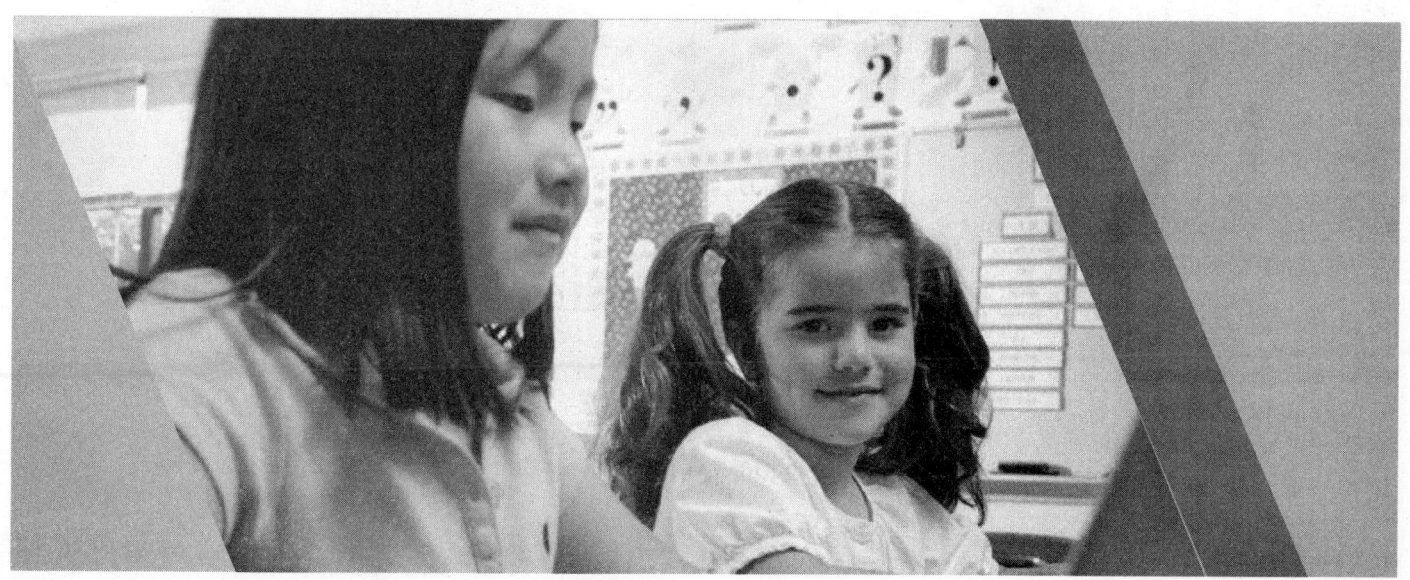

Meaning of Proficient: NAEP vs. State Standards

Improvements in the rate of proficiency on state assessments has been somewhat tempered by reports calling into question the rigor of some state's academic content standards. A recent comparison of the percentage of students scoring proficient or better on each state's reading assessment versus the percentage scoring proficient or better on the reading portion of the National Assessment of Educational Progress (NAEP) revealed remarkable proficiency gaps – some in excess of 60 points. More than half of the states showed a proficiency gap of more than 40 points (see map).

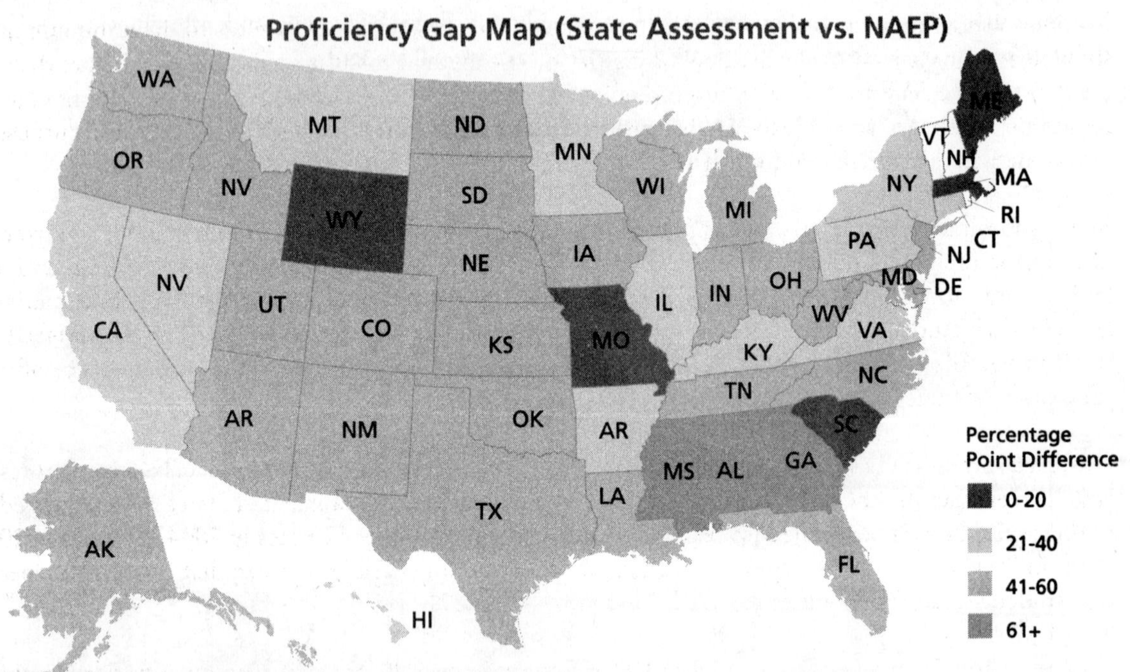

Source: As first appeared in Education Week, April 18, 2007. Reprinted with permission from Editorial Projects in Education.

Notes: If state test results were not available for grade 4, the EPE Research Center used test results from grade 3 or grade 5. No results are reported for New Hampshire, Rhode Island, and Vermont because these states did not test reading in grades 3-5.

Yet, in the face of questionable rigor among many states' academic standards, special education students are posting substantial gains on the NAEP. For example, the scale score for 4th graders in reading increased from 167 in 2000 to 190 in 2005 while the performance of students without special education status showed no significant improvement. (see chart)

National Assessment of Educational Progress Average Scale Scores for Students with and without Disabilities. Reading, Grade 4 1998-2005

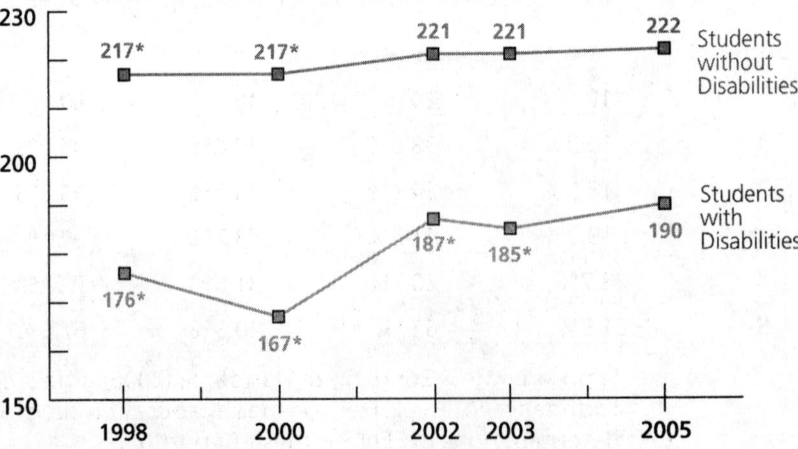

**Significantly different from 2005.*

Source: National Assessment of Educational Progress (NAEP)

Limiting Accountability: Minimum Subgroup Size

While the participation requirements of NCLB have clearly resulted in drastic improvements in the rate at which students receiving special education are included in state assessments, accountability for their proficiency on the assessments is another matter. In many states school accountability for the performance of these students has been greatly compromised by the adoption of a minimum subgroup size that excludes far too many schools from AYP responsibility for the required subgroups.

Minimum subgroup size, frequently called "minimum-n" or simply "N-size", refers to the minimum number of students within each subgroup a school or district must contain across the grades assessed before the requirement to achieve AYP for the subgroup is required. In other words, if a school (or district) does not have the minimum number of students for a subgroup, that subgroup is treated as meeting AYP for the purposes of determining whether the school (or district) met AYP.

States submit a proposed "N-size" as part of their NCLB Accountability Plan to the U.S. Department of Education for approval. Guidelines for establishing the "N-size" are articulated in current NCLB as a number large enough to yield statistically reliable information and protect personally identifiable information about an individual student. Such requirements would suggest that an acceptable "N-size" would, in fact, be quite low. In turn, a low "N-size" would hold most schools in a state accountable for the performance of important subgroups of students.

However, several studies have shown that many states have received approval to use a "N-size" that results in large percentages of schools escaping accountability for student subgroups. Many states have requested increases to their subgroup size over the first years of NCLB implementation – 13 states in 2004, 10 states in 2005, and 4 states in 2006. Some states requested and gained approval for – a subgroup size that is larger for special education students than for the other required subgroups.

"N-sizes"currently in use range from 5 to 100 and the average is 40. Yet a 2005 study of five geographically representative states conducted by the Center for Assessment determined that, once a state's "N-size" reaches 20 or 30 students, significant percentages of special education students are not accounted for as a separate subgroup in AYP determinations.

Percent of special education students excluded from separate subgroup accountability by minimum cell sizes.

State	Minimum Cell Size					
	10	**20**	**30**	**60**	**80**	**100**
1	10.3%	38.5%	49.6%	86.2%	97.7%	97.7%
2	18.5%	54.1%	75.7%	98.6%	98.9%	100.0%
3	10.7%	41.2%	73.7%	99.1%	100.0%	100.0%
4	8.7%	20.7%	31.6%	72.4%	79.7%	87.0%
5	1.5%	6.9%	20.3%	67.5%	79.9%	87.5%

Source: Simpson, M.A., Gong, B., & Marion, S. (2006). Effect of minimum cell sizes and confidence interval sizes for special education subgroups on school-level AYP determinations (NCEO Synthesis Report 61)

A Closer Look: California's "N-Size"

Further evidence of the use of large "N-sizes" to minimize school accountability was uncovered by the Commission on No Child Left Behind. In May 2006 the Commission issued a research report which indicated that only 11 percent of the schools in California - the state that educates a full 10 percent of all public school students in the U.S. – were required to achieve AYP for the subgroup of students with special education status in the 2004-2005 school year.

California has an "N-size" that combines percentages and minimum numbers. Specifically, the "N-size" is 100 students in the grades assessed in a school or 50 students in the grades assessed in a school if the subgroup population is at least 15 percent of the total school enrollment. At this level, it is unlikely that many schools would have enough special education students to be held accountable. In fact, a mere 11 percent of California schools need to achieve AYP for special education students.

In a subsequent report, the Commission calculated the impact of a change in California's "N-size" from its current formula to the Commission's recommended "N-size" of no more than 20 students. The report showed that 38,165 more special education students would be included in the accountability system and 5,574 more schools would be held accountable for the achievement of these students. This is a six-fold increase in the number of schools held accountable for special education students (see charts below).

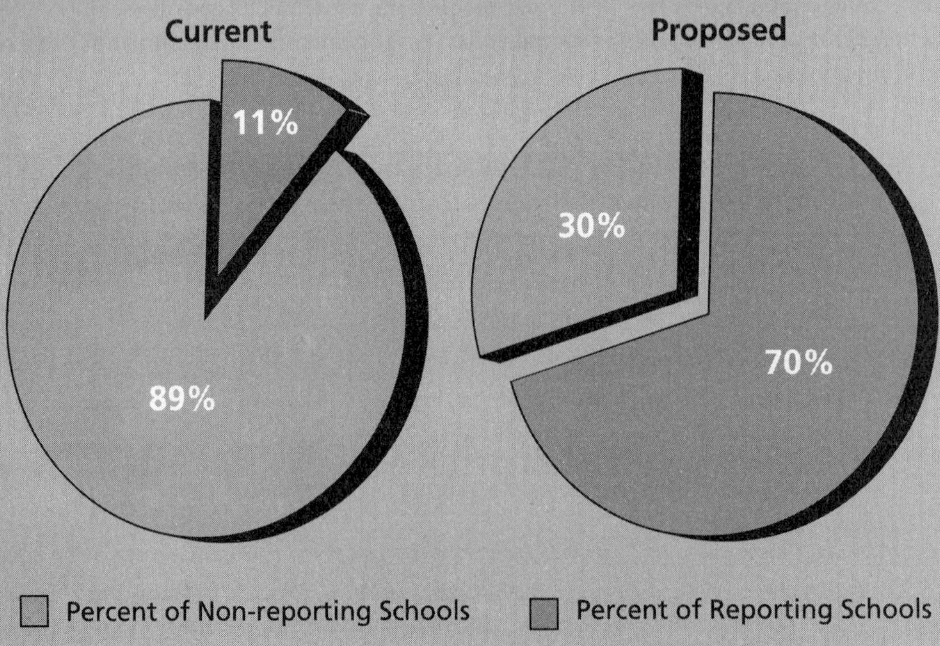

A School District Perspective:

North East Independent School District

By Judith Higgins Moening, Executive Director, Special Education

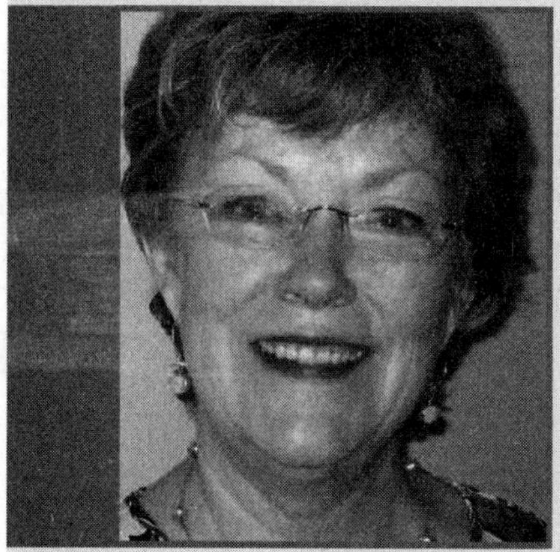

North East Independent School District in San Antonio, Texas is a large (63,000 students) urban/suburban district. We have traditionally been a high performing school district under the state accountability system. Along the path to achieving that high performance, the district placed more and more students in special education and served many/most of those students outside of the general education setting. This path began to change five years ago when the district set out to move students with disabilities back into the general education setting and began to look closely at which students were assigned to special education. The impetus for some of these changes came from the state of Texas looking closely at data and beginning to rate districts on best practice indicators. Parents were a large impetus for change as they began requesting general education placement regardless of the nature or degree of disability of their child.

Our first challenge was addressing instructional placement. Over a two year period through professional development activities, through data reports sent to campus administrators and through hard conversations on campuses we were able to reduce the percentage of students with special needs who were served outside of general education. We changed from a high of 35 percent of students removed from general education — for at least half of the school day — to increasing our inclusion ratio to 78 percent of students served in general education for most of the day. This change occurred over a two year period and has continued for the next three years. Today, 89 percent of IDEA eligible students spend over 60 percent of their school day alongside general education peers. Along with a move toward more inclusive services, we have reduced the percentage of students identified as needing special education from a high of 18 percent of the population to the current 11.5 percent. During this same time period, No Child Left Behind has become part of our accountability picture. The move toward general education instruction has supported our accountability efforts; however, we have struggled with the performance of special needs students. In the school year 2004-05 North East ISD was faced with four campuses which were academically unacceptable under the state accountability system as a result of the performance of students in special education. These four schools, along with six others, also failed to make AYP, again due to the performance of special education students. In 2005-06, we developed a process called "Data Coaching" in which the central office staff worked with each individual school campus to review state test results along with benchmark scores to ensure that students with disabilities, students who were English language learners and any other student at risk of failure received the intervention necessary to insure success. The results for 2005-06 indicated that the process had been successful.

The district was considered "*Recognized*" under the state accountability system and all school campuses made AYP – a rating that requires a minimum of 75 percent proficiency in all subjects tested. Data review for the year found that 98.5 percent of all students were tested on grade level in reading and 98 percent on grade level in math. Special education students posted strong gains on both the alternative tests and the general education tests.

The district is still reviewing data from the 2006-07 accountability report. However, initial review indicates that 99.6 percent of all students were tested on grade level in reading. Special education students again have performed well on both the alternative and general education tests. At this time we believe that all schools will make AYP.

Our district believes that the changes we have made over the past few years have improved services and outcomes for students with disabilities. We have seen school campuses grow both in their belief that students can achieve and in their skills at making that happen. No Child Left Behind has been a positive force for us. It has made a difference for this district.

Road Ahead

While 14 percent of U.S. elementary and secondary public school students are designated eligible for special education, these students are – first and foremost – general education students. As the President's Commission on Excellence in Special Education found in its comprehensive 2002 report, **A NEW ERA**: *Revitalizing Special Education for Children and their Families*

> "Children placed in special education are general education children first. Despite this basic fact, educators and policy-makers think about the two systems as separate and tally the cost of special education as a separate program, not as additional services with resultant add-on expense. In such a system, children with disabilities are often treated, not as children who are members of general education and whose special instructional needs can be met with scientifically based approaches, they are considered separately with unique costs—creating incentives for misidentification and academic isolation—preventing the pooling of all available resources to aid learning. General education and special education share responsibilities for children with disabilities. They are not separable at any level—cost, instruction, or even identification."

As Congress works to update and refine NCLB, great care must be taken to maintain the accountability of special education students so that they may continue to experience rewards. Where roadblocks exist, equitable solutions can be forged. Separate systems serve no purpose, are open to abuse, and achieve less than acceptable results. Unifying and leveraging all available resources and raising expectations for all students can lead to significant improvement and close the achievement gap.

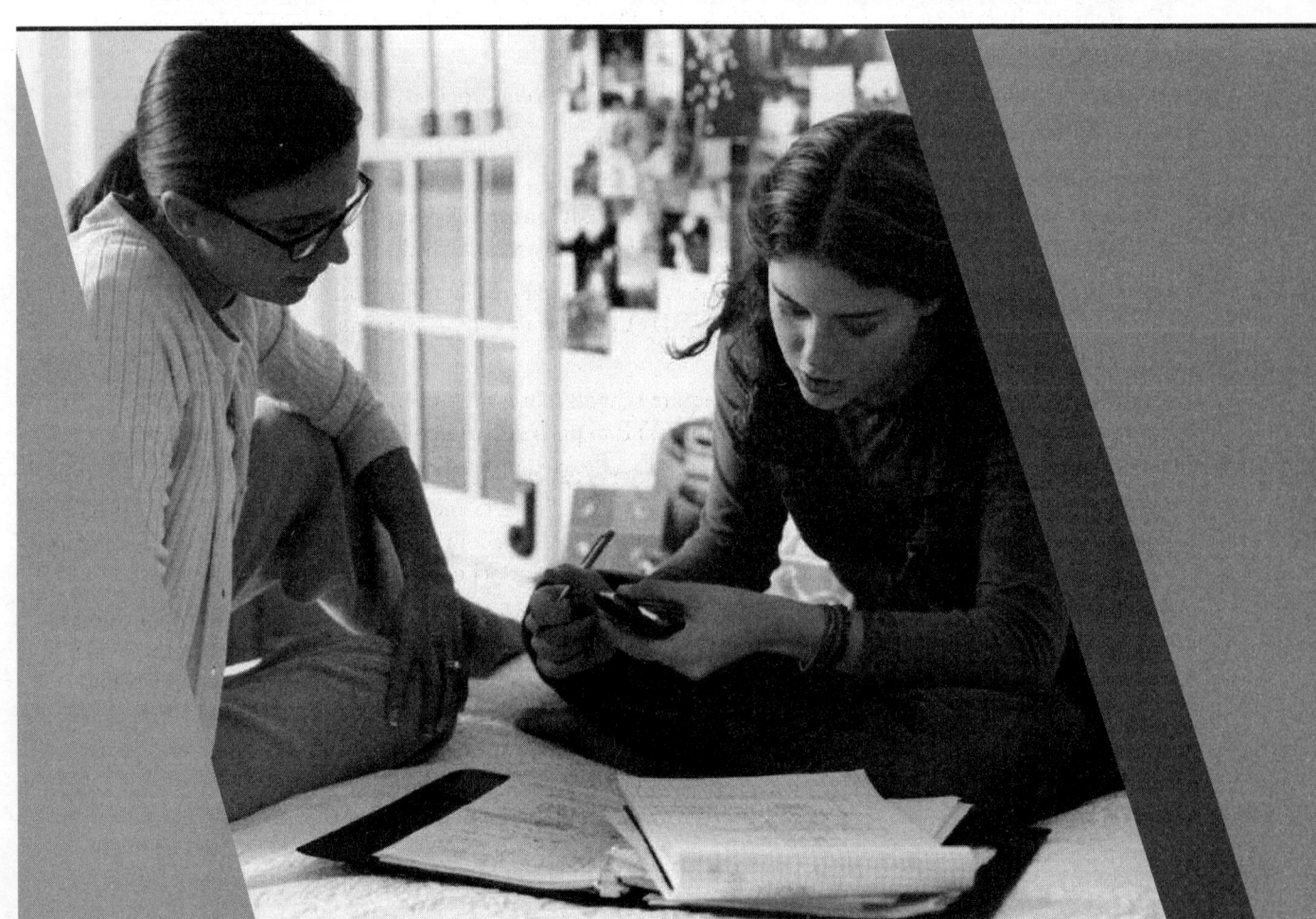

Recommendations to the U.S. Congress

for the Reauthorization of the Elementary and Secondary Education Act of 1965 (ESEA) as amended by No Child Left Behind

The National Center for Learning Disabilities urges Congress to consider the following recommendations in the reauthorization of ESEA:

1. Maintain requirements regarding Adequate Yearly Progress (AYP) for all students.
2. Infuse 'evidence-based intervention models' (commonly referred to as Response to Intervention) throughout ESEA to improve access to early intervention, early identification and improved behavior and academic outcomes for students most at risk.
3. Allow for the addition of a growth model factor to the existing AYP determination procedure for all students.
4. Require states to develop the capacity to build data systems and other infrastructure necessary to include student growth as a part of ESEA accountability.
5. Add a requirement that every state undergo a federal review of assessment accommodations guidelines.
6. Require all states to use an N-size of no greater than 20 for all categories of student groups in AYP determinations.
7. Require all states to use a confidence interval of 99 percent in calculating AYP for all categories of student groups in AYP determinations.
8. Include a provision that confidence intervals shall not be permitted in growth model factors.
9. Do not include any aspects of the ESEA regulations regarding alternate assessment options based on alternate or modified achievement standards.
10. Provide states with incentives to develop alternate assessments aligned to grade-level academic content and achievement standards. Such assessments should be available to all students.
11. Clarify that students to be reported in the student subgroup of "students with disabilities" must be students currently eligible for services under IDEA and have a current Individualized Education Program (IEP) in effect, as required by IDEA.
12. Codify current Title I regulations that require schools to use the student's results from the first administration of the state assessment to determine AYP to prevent repeated re-testing from occurring.
13. Require all states to adopt the National Governors Association (NGA) compact on graduation rate, disaggregate graduation rate and elementary school indicator data and use this disaggregated data for AYP determinations. Additionally, require all states to set goals for improving graduation rates and elementary school indicator by subgroup at the state, school district and school levels.
14. Replace current requirement for Title I schools "in need of improvement" status to provide opportunities for all students to transfer to another school within the district with robust requirements for the implementation of evidence-based school reform activities such as evidence-based intervention models that include positive behavior intervention supports.
15. Maintain requirements in Early Reading First to allow the use of screening assessments to effectively identify preschool age children who may be at risk for reading failure.

Appendix A

Special Education Students, Percent to Total Enrollment and Percent of Change by State

State	Number of Students Receiving Special Education Services (Ages 3-21) 2003-2004	Percent of Total Enrollment Receiving Special Education Services 2003-2004	Percent of Change in Number of Students Receiving Special Education Services 1990-91 to 2003-2004
United States	**6,633,902**	**13.7**	**38.5**
Alabama	93,056	12.7	-1.6
Alaska	17,959	13.4	24.8
Arizona	112,125	11.1	98.0
Arkansas	66,793	14.7	41.5
California	675,763	10.5	44.3
Colorado	82,447	10.9	46.3
Connecticut	73,952	12.8	15.8
Delaware	18,417	15.7	29.6
District of Columbia	13,242	17.0	110.5
Florida	397,758	15.4	69.6
Georgia	190,948	12.5	87.6
Hawaii	23,266	12.7	83.1
Idaho	29,092	11.5	34.0
Illinois	318,111	15.1	34.8
Indiana	171,896	17.0	52.2
Iowa	73,717	15.3	23.3
Kansas	65,139	13.8	45.4
Kentucky	103,783	15.6	31.6
Louisiana	101,933	14.0	40.0
Maine	37,784	18.7	35.0
Maryland	113,865	13.1	29.4
Massachusetts	159,042	16.2	6.2
Michigan	238,292	13.6	43.1
Minnesota	114,193	13.5	44.5
Mississippi	66,848	13.5	9.8
Missouri	143,593	15.9	41.9
Montana	19,435	13.1	14.6
Nebraska	44,561	15.6	37.9

Nevada	45,201	11.7	149.7
New Hampshire	31,311	15.1	64.4
New Jersey	241,272	17.5	34.9
New Mexico	51,814	16.0	43.9
New York	442,665	15.5	44.0
North Carolina	193,956	14.3	57.8
North Dakota	14,044	13.7	14.2
Ohio	253,878	13.8	23.6
Oklahoma	93,045	14.9	42.1
Oregon	76,083	13.8	39.8
Pennsylvania	273,259	15.0	27.5
Rhode Island	32,223	20.2	56.1
South Carolina	111,077	15.9	43.6
South Dakota	17,760	14.1	20.6
Tennessee	122,627	13.1	17.0
Texas	506,771	11.7	47.1
Utah	57,745	11.6	23.9
Vermont	13,670	13.8	12.4
Virginia	172,788	14.5	54.2
Washington	123,673	12.1	48.0
West Virginia	50,772	18.1	19.7
Wisconsin	127,828	14.5	49.2
Wyoming	13,430	15.4	23.8
Bureau of Indian Affairs	8,343	18.2	19.2
Other jurisdictions	**83,948**	**12.7**	**115.3**
American Samoa	1,135	7.1	212.7
Guam	2,460	7.8	40.6
Northern Marianas	669	5.9	62.8
Palau			
Puerto Rico	77,932	13.3	121.8
Virgin Islands	1,752	9.9	31.4

Source: Table 52, NCES Common Core of Data, National Center for Educational Statistics, April 2005.

Our Mission

The National Center for Learning Disabilities works to ensure that the nation's 15 million children, adolescents and adults with learning disabilities have every opportunity to succeed in school, work and life. NCLD provides essential information to parents, professionals and individuals with learning disabilities, promotes research and programs to foster effective learning and advocates for policies to protect and strengthen educational rights and opportunities.

For more information, please visit us on the Web at www.LD.org.

About the Author

Candace Cortiella is Director of The Advocacy Institute (www.AdvocacyInstitute.org) a nonprofit organization dedicated to the development of products, projects and services that work to improve the lives of people with disabilities. She also serves on the Professional Advisory Board of the National Center for Learning Disabilities. The mother of a young adult with learning disabilities, she lives in the Washington, D.C. area.

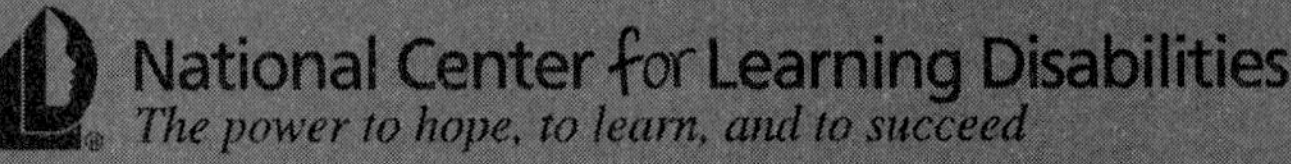

381 Park Avenue South, Suite 1401 New York, NY 10016-8806
Telephone 212.545.7510 Facsimile 212.545.9665

www.LD.org

National

1 **AVKO Dyslexia Research Foundation**
3084 W Willard Road
Clio, MI 48420
810-686-9283
866-285-6612
FAX 810-686-1101
http://www.avko.org
e-mail: avkoemail@aol.com
Devorah Wolf, President
Michael Lane, Vice President
Don Cabe, Research Director
AVKO is a non-profit membership organization that focuses on the development and production of materials and especially techniques to teach reading and spelling, handwriting (manuscript and cursive) and key boarding.

2 **American Association of Collegiate Registrars and Admissions Officers**
One Dupont Circle NW
Washington, DC 20036
202-293-9161
FAX 202-872-8857
http://www.aacrao.org
e-mail: corporateinfo@aacrao.org
Paul Aucoin, President
Paul Wiley, President-Elect
Jerome Sullivan, Executive Director
Provides professional development, guidelines and voluntary standards to be used by higher education officials regarding the best practices in records management, admissions, enrollment management, administrative information technology and student services. It also providees a forum for discussion regarding policy initiation and development, interpretation and implementation at the institutional level and in the global eductional community.
9,500 members

3 **American Association of Health Plans**
American Health Insurance Plan
601 Pennsylvania Avenue NW
Washington, DC 20004
202-778-3200
FAX 202-331-7487
http://www.ahip.org
e-mail: ahip@ahip.org
Karen Ignani, President/CEO
Scott Styles, Senior VP Legislative Affairs

Purpose is to represent the interests of members on legislative and regulatory issues at the federal and state levels, and with the media, consumers, and employers. Provides information and services such as newsletters, publications, a magazine and on-line services. Consucts education, research, and quality assurance programs and engage in a host of other activities to assist members.
1,300 members

4 **American Bar Association Center on Children and the Law: Information Line**
740 15th Street NW
Washington, DC 20005
202-662-1000
FAX 202-662-1032
http://www.abanet.org
e-mail: service@abanet.org
Karen J Mathis, President
William H Neukom, President-Elect
Henry F White Jr, Executive Director
Provides law school accreditation, continuing legal education, information about the law, programs to assist lawyers and judges in their work, and initiatives to improve the legal system for the public. The mission is to be the national representative of the legal profession, serving the public and the profession by promoting justice, professional excellence and respect for the law.
400,000 members

5 **American Camp Association**
5000 State Road 67 N
Martinsville, IN 46151
765-342-8456
FAX 765-342-2065
http://www.acacamps.org
e-mail: acacamps@acacamps.org
Ann Sheets, President
Scott Brody, Vice President
Peg Smith, Executive Director
A community of camp professionals who, for more than 100 years, have joined together to share knowledge and experience and to ensure the quality of camp programs. Just as our membership is diverse and programs distinct, so are the children who com to participate in the camp experience. Through what we teach, the opportunities we offer, and the example we set, children become part of a sharing community.
6,700+ members

6 **American Coaching Association**
PO Box 353
Lafayette Hill, PA 19444
610-825-8542
FAX 610-825-4505
http://www.americoach.org
e-mail: americancoaching@aol.com
Susan Sussman MEd, Director

Founded with the goal of making individualized coaching available to everyone who desirese it. Mission is to: link people who want coaching with people who do coaching; acquaint the general public with the concept of coaching; provide coaches with training, supervision and a professional community.

7 **American College Testing**
500 ACT Drive
Iowa City, IA 52243
319-337-1000
FAX 319-337-1061
http://www.act.org
Richard Ferguson, CEO/Chairman
Cynthia Board Schmeiser, President/COO Education Division
Ann V York, VP Operations
An independent, not-for-profit organization that provides more than a hundred assessment, research, information, and program management services in the broad areas of education and workforce development
1959

8 **American Council of the Blind (ACB)**
1155 15th Street NW
Washington, DC 20005
202-467-5081
800-424-8666
FAX 202-467-5085
http://www.acb.org
e-mail: info@acb.org
Melanie Brunson, Executive Director

Council strives to improve the well-being of all blind and visually impaired people by: serving as a representative national organization of blind people; elevating the social, economic and cultural levels of blind people; improving educational and rehabilitation facilities and opportunities; cooperating with the public and private institutions and organizations concerned with blind services.
1961

9 **American Counseling Association**
5999 Stevenson Avenue NW
Alexandria, VA 22304
800-347-6647
FAX 800-473-2329
http://www.counseling.org
e-mail: aca@counseling.org
Brian Canfield, President
Richard Yep, Executive Director
Brant Heatherington, Director Marketing
A not-for-profit, professional and educational organization that is dedicated to the growth and enhancement of the counseling profession. The largest association exclusively representing professional counselors in various practice settings.
45,000 members 1952

10 **American Dance Therapy Association (ADTA)**
10632 Little Patuxent Parkway
Columbia, MD 21044
410-997-4040
FAX 410-997-4048
http://www.adta.org
e-mail: info@adta.org
Robyn Flaum Cruz, President
Gloria J Farrow, Operations Director

Works to establish and maintain high standards of professional education and competence in the field of dance/movement therapy. ADTA stimulates communication among dance/movement therapists and members of allied professionsl through publication of the ADTA Newsletter, the American Journal of Dance Therapy, monographs, bibliographies, and conference proceedings.
1966

11 American Occupational Therapy Association

4720 Montgomery Lane
Bethesda, MD 20824
301-652-2682
FAX 301-652-7711
http://www.aota.org
e-mail: praota@aota.org

Penelope A Moyers, President
Florence Clark, Vice President
Frederick P Somers, Executive Director

Founded to represent the interests and concerns of occupational therapy practitioners and students of occupational therapy and to improve the quality of occupational therapy services. Advances the quality, availability, use, and support of occupational therapy through standard-setting, advocacy, educationa dnresearch on behalf of its members and the public.
36,000 members 1917

12 American Printing House for the Blind

1839 Frankfort Avenue
Louisville, KY 40206
502-895-2405
800-223-1839
FAX 502-899-2274
http://www.aph.org
e-mail: info@aph.org

Tuck Tinsley, President
Bob Brasher, VP Advisory Services/Research
Tony Grantz, Business Development Manager

Founded in 1858. To promote the independence of blind and visually-impaired persons by providing special media, tools, and materials needed for education and life.

13 American Psychological Association

750 First Street, NE
Washington, DC 20002
202-336-5500
800-374-2721
FAX 202-336-5568
http://www.apa.org
e-mail: psycinfo@apa.org

Sharon Stephens Brehm, President
Alan E Kazdin, President-Elect
Norman Anderson, CEO/Executive VP

A scientific and professional organization that represents psychology in the United States.
148,000 members

14 American Public Human Services Association (APHSA)

810 First Street NE
Washington, DC 20002
202-682-0100
FAX 202-289-6555
http://www.aphsa.org
e-mail: jfriedman@aphsa.org

Jerry Friedman, Executive Director
Elaine Ryan, Dep Exec Dir, Policy/Govt Affair

A nonprofit, bipartisan organization of state and local human service agencies and individuals who work in or are interested in public human service programs. Mission is to develop and promote policies and practices that improve the health and well-being of families, children, and adults
1930

15 American Red Cross

2025 E Street NW
Washington, DC 20006
202-303-4498
http://www.redcross.org
e-mail: info@usa.redcross.org

Bonnie McElveen-Hunter, Chairman
Mark W Everson, President/CEO

Founded in 1881. A humanitarian organization led by volunteers, guided by its Congressional Charter and the fundamental principles of the International Red Cross Movement, will provide relief to victims of disasters and help people prevent, prepare for, and respond to emergencies.

16 American Rehabilitation Counseling Association (ARCA)

5999 Stevenson Avenue
Alexandria, VA 22304
703-823-9800
800-347-6647
FAX 703-461-9260
TDY:937-775-3153
http://www.arcaweb.org

Irmo Marini PhD, President
Patty Nunez, President-Elect

An organization of rehabilitation counseling practitioners, educators, and students who are concerned with improving the lives of people with disabilities. The mission is to enhance the development of people with disabilities throughout their life span and to promote excellence in the rehabilitation counseling profession.

17 American Speech-Language-Hearing Association

10801 Rockville Pike
Rockville, MD 20852
301-897-5700
800-498-2071
FAX 301-571-0457
TDY:301-897-5700
http://www.asha.org
e-mail: actioncenter@asha.org

Arlene Pietranton PhD, Executive Director

Promotes the interests of and provide the highest quality services for professionals in audiology, speech-language pathology, and speech and hearing science, and to advocate for people with communication disabilities
127,000 members 1958

18 Association of Educational Therapists

11300 W Olympic Boulevard
San Francisco, CA 94104
415-982-2389
800-286-4267
FAX 415-982-9204
http://www.aetonline.org
e-mail: aet@aetonline.org

Deborah Doyle MA, President
Risa Graff MA BCET, President-Elect
JaNelle Hasty, Executive Director

A national professional organization dedicated to establishing ethical professional standards, defining the roles and responsibilities of the educational therapist, providing opportunities for professional growth, and to studying techniques and technologies, philosophies and research related to the practice of educational therapy.

19 Association on Higher Education and Disability

107 Commerce Center Drive
Huntersville, NC 28070
704-947-7779
FAX 704-948-7779
http://www.ahead.org
e-mail: ahead@ahead.org

Stephan Smith, Executive Director
Richard Allegra, Director Professional Devel
Tri Do, Operations Manager

The premiere professional association committed to full participation of persons with disabilities in postsecondary education. Since its founding, has delivered quality training to higher education personnel through conferences, workshops, publications and consultation.
1977

20 Attention Deficit Disorder Association

15000 Commerce Pkwy
Mount Laurel, NJ 08054
856-439-9099
FAX 856-439-0525
http://www.add.org
e-mail: adda@ahint.org

Linda S Anderson, President
Mary Jane Johnson PCC ACT, Vice President

Designated as a nonprofit organization by the Internal Revenue Service. Provides information, resources and networking to adults with AD/HD and to the professionals who work with them.

1989

1982

21 **Autism Research Institute**
4182 Adams Avenue
San Diego, CA 92116
619-281-7165
FAX 619-563-6840
http://www.autismresearchinstitute.com
Stephen M Edelson PhD, Director

Founded to conduct and foster scientific research designed to improve methods of diagnosing, treating and preventing autism. ARI also disseminates research findings to parents and others worlwide seeking help.
1967

22 **Autism Society of America**
7910 Woodmont Avenue
Bethesda, MD 20814
301-657-0881
800-328-8476
FAX 301-657-0869
http://www.autism-society.org
e-mail: info@autism-society.org
Lee Grossman, President/CEO
Ann Pulley, Controller/Office Administrator

The leading voice and resource of the entire autism community in education, advocacy, services, research and support. The ASA is committed to meaningful participation and self-determination in all aspects of life for individuals on the autism spectrum and their families.
120,000 members 1965

23 **Autism Treatment Center of America**
2080 S Undermountain Road
Sheffield, MA 01257
413-229-2100
877-766-7473
FAX 413-229-3202
http://www.autismtreatmentcenter.org
Barry Kaufman, Co-Founder
Samahria Lyte Kaufman, Co-Founder
William Hogan, Executive Director Programs
Provides innovative training programs for parents and professionals caring for children challenged by Autism, Autism Spectrum Disorders, Pervasive Developmental Disorder (PDD) and other developmental difficulties. The Son-Rise Program teaches a specific yet comprehensive system of treatment and education designed to help families and caregivers enable their children to dramatically improve in all areas of learning.

24 **Best Buddies International**
100 SE 2nd Street
Miami, FL 33131
305-374-2233
800-892-8339
FAX 305-374-5305
http://www.bestbuddies.org
e-mail: info@bestbuddies.org
Anthony K Shriver, Founder/Chairman

A nonprofit organization dedicated to enhancing the lives of people with intellectual disabilities by providing opportunities for one-to-one friendships and integrated employment. Best Buddies is a vibrant, international organization that has grown from one original chapter to more that 1,300 middle school, high school and college campuses across the country and internationally.
1989

25 **Birth Defect Research for Children (BDRC)**
800 Celebration Ave
Celebration, FL 34747
407-566-8304
FAX 407-566-8341
http://www.birthdefects.org
Betty Mekdeci, Co-Founder
Mike Mekdeci, Co-Founder

A non-profit organization that provides parents and expectant parents with information about birth defects and support services for children. BDRC also has a parent-matching program that links families who have children with similar birth defects

26 **Boy Scouts of America**
Scouting for the Handicapped Services
PO Box 152079
Irving, TX 75015
972-580-2000
FAX 972-580-2502
http://www.scouting.org
Roy Williams, CEO

Provides an educational program for boys and young adults to build character, to train in the responsibilities of participating citizenship, and to develop personal fitness.
1910

27 **Brain Injury Association**
8201 Greensboro Drive
McLean, VA 22102
703-761-0750
800-444-6443
FAX 703-761-0755
http://www.biausa.org
e-mail: info@biausa.org
Susan H Connors, President/CEO
Mary S Reitter, Executive Vice President/COO

A national organization serving and representing individuals, families and professionals who are touched by a life-altering, often devastating, traumatic brain injury.
1980

28 **CASE: Community Alliance for Special Education**
1550 Bryant Street
San Francisco, CA 94103
415-431-2285
FAX 415-431-2289
http://www.caseadvocacy.org
e-mail: case_org@yahoo.com
Joseph Feldman, Director
Laurie Vazquez, CASE Program Assistant

Provides special education advocacy, representation at individual education program (IEP) meetings and due process proceedings, free technical assistance consultations and training throughout the San Francisco Bay area.
1979

29 **Career College Association (CCA)**
1101 Connecticut Avenue NW
Washington, DC 20036
202-336-6700
FAX 202-336-6828
http://www.career.org
e-mail: cca@career.org
Harris Miller, President
Bruce Leftwich, VP Government Relations
Milt Girdner, Chief Financial Officer
CCA has over 1,400 members that educate and support almost two million students each year for employment in over 200 occupational fields.
1,400 members

30 **Career Development & Transition Division of CEC**
Council for Exceptional Children
1110 N Glebe Road
Arlington, VA 05704
703-620-3660
888-232-7733
FAX 703-264-9494
TDY:866-915-5000
http://www.dcdt.org
Kristine Wiest Webb PhD, President
Colleen Thoma, President-Elect
Sherrilyn Fisher, Vice President
Promotes national and international efforts to improve the quality and access to, career/vocational and transition services, increase the participation of education in career development and transition goals and to influence policies affecting career development and transition services for persons with disabilities.

31 **Center for Adult English Language Acquisition (CAELA)**
Washington, DC 20016
202-362-0700
866-845-3378
FAX 202-363-7204
http://www.cal.org/caela
e-mail: caela@cal.org

Joy Peyton, Director
Miriam Burt, Associate Director
Donna Christian, President
A national center focusing on literacy education for adults and out-of-school youth learning English as a second language. CAELA publishes many documents on its website.

32 **Center for Applied Linguistics**
4646 40th Street NW
Washington, DC 20016
202-362-0700
FAX 202-362-3740
e-mail: info@cal.org
Donna Christian, President
Joy Kreeft Peyton, Vice President

A private, nonprofit organization working to omprove communication through better understanding of language and culture. Dedicated to providing a comprehensive range of research-based language tools and resources related to language and culture.
1959

33 **Center for Applied Special Technology (CAST)**
40 Harvard Mills Square
Wakefield, MA 01880
781-245-2212
FAX 978-531-0192
http://www.cast.org
e-mail: cast@cast.org
Anne Meyer, Co-Founder
David H Roseivan, Co-Founder
Ada Sullivan, President
CAST has earned international recognition for its development of innovative, technology-based educational resources and strategies based on the principals of Universal Design for Learning (UDL). The mission is to expand opportunities for all individuals, especially those with disabilities, through the research and development of innovative, technology-based educational resources and strategies.
1984

34 **Closing the Gap**
Computer Technology in Special Education & Rehab.
526 Main Street
Henderson, MN 56044
507-248-3294
FAX 507-248-3810
http://www.closingthegap.com
e-mail: info@closingthegap.com
Dolores Hagan, Co-Founder
Budd Hagan, Co-Founder
Connie Kneip, Vice President/General Manager
An organization that focuses on computer technology for people with special needs through its bi-monthly newsletter, annual international conference and extensive web site.
1983

35 **College Board Services for Students with Disabilities**
PO Box 6336
Princeton, NJ 08541
609-771-7137
FAX 609-771-7944
http://www.collegeboard.org
e-mail: ssd@info.collegeboard.org
Gaston Caperton, President

Founded in 1900. Offers testing accommodations to attempt to minimize the effect of disabilities on test performance. The SAT Program tests eligible students with documented visual, physical, hearing, or learning disabilities who require testing accommodations for SAT.

36 **Commission on Accreditation of Rehabilitation Facilities (CARF)**
4891 E Grant Road
Tucson, AZ 85712
520-325-1044
888-281-6531
FAX 520-318-1129
TDY:888-281-6531
http://www.carf.org
e-mail: feedback@carf.org
Richard Forkosh, Chairman
Brian Boon PhD, President/CEO

An independent, nonprofit accreditor of human service providers in the areas of aging services, behavioral health, child and youth services, DMEPOS, employment anf medical rehabiliation.
1966

37 **Communication Aids: Manufacturers Association**
205 W Randolph Street
Chicago, IL 60606
312-229-5444
800-441-2262
FAX 312-229-5445
TDY:800-441-2262
http://www.aacproducts.org
e-mail: cama@northshore.net
James Neils, President

A nonprofit organization of the world's leading manufacturers of augmentative and alternative communication software and hardware.

38 **Council for Exceptional Children (CEC)**
1110 N Glebe Road
Arlington, VA 22201
703-245-0600
888-232-7733
FAX 703-264-9494
http://www.cec.sped.org
e-mail: cec@cec.sped.org
Bruce Ramirez, Executive Director
Stefani Roth, Program Development Director

An international professional organization dedicated to improving educational outcomes for individuals with exceptionalities, students with disabilities, and/or the gifted. Advocates for appropriate governmental policies, sets professional standards, provides continual professional development, advocates for newly historically underserved individuals with exceptionalities, and helps professionals obtain conditions and resources necessary for effective professional practice.

39 **Council for Learning Disabilities**
11184 Antioch Road
Overland, KS 66210
913-491-1011
FAX 913-491-1012
http://www.cldinternational.org
Linda Higbee Mandlebaum, President
Joseph Boyle, President-Elect
Linda Nease, Executive Director
An international organization concerned about issues related to students with learning disabilities. Working to build a better future for students with LD has been the primary goal of CLD for more than 20 years. Involvement in CLD helps members stary abreast of current issues that are shaping the field, affecting the lives of students, and influencing professional careers.

40 **Council on Rehabilitation Education**
300 N Martingale Road
Schaumburg, IL 60173
847-944-1345
FAX 847-944-1324
http://www.core-rehab.org
e-mail: mkuehn@emporia.edu
Marvin Kuehn, Executive Director
Sue Denys, Administrative Assistant

Seeks to provide effective delivery of rehabilitation services to individuals with disabilities by stimulating and fostering continuing review and improvement of master's degree level rehabilitation counselor education programs.

41 **Culturally & Linguistically Diverse Exceptional Learners Division of CEC**
Council for Exceptional Children
1110 N Glebe Road
Arlington, VA 05704
888-232-7733
FAX 703-264-9494
http://www.cec.sped.org
Beverley Argus-Calvo, President
Sheila Mingo-Jones, President-Elect
Drew Allbritten MD, Executive Director
The official division of the Council for Exceptional Children, that promotes tha advancement and improvement of educationl oportunities for culturally and linguisticall diverse learners with disabilities and/or gifts and talents, their families, and the professionals who serve them.

42 **Disability Rights Education & Defense Fund (DREDF)**
2212 6th Street
Berkeley, CA 94710 510-644-2555
800-466-4232
FAX 510-841-8645
http://www.dredf.org
e-mail: info@dredf.org
Mary Breslin, Senior Policy Advisor
Susan Henderson, Managing Director

A national civil rights law and policy center directed by individuals with disabilities and parents who have children with disabilities. Advances the civil and human rights of people with disabilities through leag advocacy, training, education, and public policy and legislative development.
1979

43 **Disability Support Services**
University of Maryland
0126 Shoemaker Building
College Park, MD 20742 301-314-7682
FAX 301-405-0813
http://www.counseling.umd.edu/dss
Jo Ann Hutchinson RhD, Director
Kimberly Huck, LD/ADD Counselor

Coordinates services that ensure individuals with disabilities equal access to University of Maryland College Park programs.
800 members

44 **Distance Education and Training Council (DETC)**
1601 18th Street NW
Washington, DC 20009 202-234-5100
FAX 202-332-1386
http://www.detc.org
e-mail: rachel@detc.org
Michael Lambert, Executive Director
Rachel Scheer, Information Specialist

A nonprofit educational association thay was founded to promote sound educational standards and ethical business practices within the correspondence field
1926

45 **Dyslexia Research Institute**
5746 Centerville Road
Tallahassee, FL 32309 850-893-2216
FAX 850-893-2440
http://www. dyslexia-add.org
e-mail: dri@dyslexia-add.org
Patricia Hardman Ph.D, Executive Director
Robyn Rennick MS, Assistant Director

The goal is to change the perception of learning differences, specifically in the area of dyslexia and attention deficit disorders (ADD). With proper recognition and intervention, dyslexics and individuals with ADD become successful individuals using their talents and skills to enrich the society.
1975

46 **ED Law Center**
PO Box 817327
Hollywood, FL 33081 954-966-4489
FAX 954-966-8561
http://www.edlaw.net
Provides information on special education law and offers listing of attorneys.

47 **Early Childhood Division of CEC**
27 Ft Missoula Road
Missoula, MT 59804 406-543-0872
FAX 406-543-0887
http://www.dec-sped.org
e-mail: dec@dec-sped.org
Tweety Yates, President
Mark Innocenti, President-Elect
Sarah Mulligan, Executive Director
One of seventeen divisions of the Council for Exceptional Children (CEC), promotes policies and advacnes evidence-based practices that support families and enhance the optimal development of young children who have or are at risk for developmental delays and disabilities.
1973

48 **Easter Seals**
230 W Monroe Street
Chicago, IL 60606 312-726-6800
800-221-6827
FAX 312-726-1494
TDY:312-726-4258
http://www.easterseals.com
e-mail: info@easterseals.com
James Williams Jr, President/CEO
Sara Brewster, VP Communications
Rosemary Garza, Information/Referral Specialist
Easter Seals' mission is to create solutions that change lives for children and adults with disabilities, their families, and their communities. We work to identify the needs of people with disabilities and to provide appropriate developmental and rehabilitation services. Our Easter Seals operate 550 sites that provide services to children and adults with disabilities and their families. All sites provide different services. Call to inquire about Easter Seals in your community.

49 **Educational Equity Center at Academy for Educational Development**
100 Fifth Avenue
New York, NY 10011 212-243-1110
FAX 212-627-0407
http://www.edequity.org
e-mail: information@edequity.org
Merle Froschl, Co-Founder/Co-Director
Barbara Sprung, Co-Founder/Co-Director
Linda Colon, Program Manager
A national not-for-profit organization that promotes bias-free learning through innovative programs and materials. The missions is to decrease discrimination based on gender, race/ethnicity, disability, and level of family income

50 **Edvantia**
PO Box 1348
Charleston, WV 25325 304-347-0400
800 624 9120
FAX 304-347-0487
http://www.edvantia.org
e-mail: info@edvantia.org
Doris Redfield Ph.D, President/CEO

Edvantia is an education research and development not-for-profit corporation.
1966

51 **Families and Advocates Partnership for Education**
PACER Center
8161 Normandale Boulevard
Minneapolis, MN 55437 952-838-9000
888-248-0822
FAX 952-838-0199
http://www.fape.org
e-mail: fape@fape.org
Paula Goldberg, Executive Director

The FAPE project is a strong partnership that aims to improve the educational outcomes for children with disabilities. FAPE links families, advocates, and self-advocates to information about the Individuals with Disabilities Education Act (IDEA). The project represents the needs of seven million children with disabilities.

52 **Federation for Children with Special Needs**
1135 Tremont Street
Roxbury Crossing, MA 02120 617-236-7210
800-331-0688
FAX 617-572-2094
TDY:617-236-7210
http://www.fcsn.org
e-mail: fcsninfo@fcsn.org
Rich Robison, Executive Director
Sarah Miranda, Associate Executive Director
Mary Thompson, Finance Director
The mission of the Federation is to provide information, support and assistance to parents of children with disabilities, their professional partners and their communities. Major services are information and referral and parent and professional training.

1974

53 **Independent Living Research Utilization Program**
Institute of Rehabilitation and Research
2323 S Shepherd Drive
Houston, TX 77019
713-520-0232
FAX 713-520-5785
http://www.ilru.org
e-mail: ilru@ilru.org

Lex Frieden, Director
Laurel Richards, Program Director
Sharon Finney, Info/Communication Specialist
A national center for information, training, research, and technical assistance in independent living. Its goal is to expand the body of knowledge in independent living and to improve utilization of results of research programs and demonstration projects in this field.
1977

54 **Institute for Educational Leadership**
4455 Connecticut Avenue
Washington, DC 20008
202-822-8405
FAX 202-872-4050
http://www.iel.org
e-mail: iel@iel.org

Elizabeth Hale, President
Martin Blank, Community Collaboration Director
Louise Clarke, Chief Administrative Officer
Mission is to improve education and the lives of children and their families through positive and visionary change.

55 **Institutes for the Achievement of Human Potential**
8801 Stenton Avenue
Wyndmoor, PA 19038
215-233-2050
800-736-4663
FAX 215-233-9312
http://www.iahp.org
e-mail: institutes@iahp.org

Glenn Doman, Founder
Janet Doman, Director
Dr Leland Green, Medical Director
Nonprofit educational organization that serves children by introducing parents to the field of child brain development. Parents learn how to enhance significantly the development of their children physically, intellectually and socially in a joyous and sensible way.
1955

56 **International Dyslexia Association**
40 York Road
Baltimore, MD 21206
410-296-0232
800-223-3123
FAX 410-321-5069
http://www.interdys.org
e-mail: info@interdys.org

Emerson Dickman, President
Megan P Cohen MPA CAE, Executive Director
Robert S Hott, Director Development
Nonprofit, scientific and educational organization dedicated to the study and treatment of dyslexia. Focus is educating parents, teachers and professionals in the field of dyslexia in effective teaching methodologies. Programs and services include: information and referral; public awareness; medical and educational research; governmental affairs; conferences and publications.
13,000 members

57 **International Reading Association**
800 Barksdale Road
Newark, DE 19711
302-731-1600
800-336-7323
FAX 302-731-1057
http://www.reading.org
e-mail: pubinfo@reading.org

Linda Gambrell, President
Barbara J Walker, President-Elect
Alan Farstrup, Executive Director
Promotes high levels of literacy for all by improving the quality od reading instruction through studying the reading process and teaching techniques; serving as a clearinghouse for dissemination of reading research through conferences, journals, and other publication; and actively encouraging a lifetime reading habit.

1956

58 **Landmark School Outreach Program**
429 Hale Street
Prides Crossing, MA 01965
978-236-3216
FAX 978-927-7268
http://www.landmarkoutreach.org
e-mail: outreach@landmarkschool.org

Robert J Broudo, President/Headmaster
Chris Murphy, Principal
Kathryn Frye, Administrative Assistant
Offers a comprehensive development program and publications that are based on applied educational research. Seeks to empower children with language-based learning disabilities by offering their teachers an exemplary program of applied research and professional development.
1971Grade Range: 2-12

59 **Learning Disabilities Association of America**
4156 Library Road
Pittsburgh, PA 15234
412-341-1515
FAX 412-344-0224
http://www.ldaamerica.org
e-mail: info@ldaamerica.org

Charlie Giglio, President
Sheila Buckley, Executive Director

Non-profit volunteer organization advocating got individuals with learning disabilities and has over 200 state and local affiliates in 42 state and Puerto Rico
15,000+ members 1964

60 **Learning Resource Network**
1130 Hostetler Drive
Manhattan, KS 66502
785-539-5376
800-678-5376
FAX 785-539-7766
http://www.lern.org
e-mail: rebel@lern.org

William Draves, President
Rebel Rush, Executive Director
Gale Hughes, Fulfillment Specialist
We are an international association of lifelong learning programming, ofering information and resources to providers of lifelong leraning programs.

61 **Legal Services for Children**
Legal Services for Children
1254 Market Street
San Francisco, CA 94102
415-863-3762
FAX 415-863-7708
http://www.lsc-sf.org

Shannan Wilber, Executive Director
Kelli-Ann M Nakayama, Director Development
Helen Jiang, Office Manager
Nonprofit law firm for children and youth. Legal Services for Children provides free legal and social services to children and youth under 18 years old in the San Francisco Bay area.
1975

62 **MATRIX: A Parent Network and Resource Ctr**
94 Galli Drive
Novato, CA 94949
415-884-3535
800-578-2592
FAX 415-884-3555
TDY:415-884-3554
http://www.matrixparents.org
e-mail: info@matrixparents.org

Nora Thompson, Executive Director

Providing families who have children with disabilities and other special needs with the tools they need in order to effectively advocate for themselves.
1983

63 **Marshall University HELP (Higher Educationfor Learning Problems)**
Myers Hall
520 18th Street
Huntington, WV 25755
304-696-6252
FAX 304-696-3231
TDY:202-272-2074
http://www.marshall.edu/help
e-mail: weston@marshall.edu

Lynne Weston, HELP Program Director
Diane Williams, College HELP Coordinator
Barbara Deuyer, Manager
The Marshall Universtiy HELP program is an individualized tutorial and support program for college students, children in the community, medical, and law students. The HELP program offers diagnostic testing to determine it an individual has a Learning Disability, and/or Attention Deficit Disorder.

64 **Menninger Clinic: Center for Learning Disabilities**
PO Box 809045
Houston, TX 77280
713-275-5000
800-351-9058
FAX 713-275-5107
http://www.meninger.clinic.com
e-mail: info@menninger.edu
Ian Aitken, President/CEO
Richard Munich MD, VP/Chief of Staff
James Fox, VP/CFO
The mission of Menninger is to be a national resource providing psychiatric care and treatment of the highest standard, searching for new knowledge and better understanding of mental illness and human behavior, teaching what we know and what we learn, and applying this knowledge in useful ways to promote individual growth and better mental health.
1925Grade Range: All Ages

65 **Miami Lighthouse for the Blind**
601 SW 8th Avenue
Miami, FL 33130
305-856-2288
FAX 305-285-6967
http://www.miamiighthouse.com
e-mail: info@miamilighthouse.org
Virginia Jacko, President/CEO
Sheldon Roy, Deputy Director/Chief Dev. Off.
Roxanne Ortiz, CFO
The oldest and largest private agency in Florida to serve people of all ages who are blind or the visually impaired.

66 **National Admission, Review, Dismissal: Individualized Education Plan Advocates**
PO Box 16111
Sugar Land, TX 77496
281-265-1506
FAX 253-295-9954
http://www.narda.org
e-mail: louis@narda.org
Louis Geigerman, Founder/President

National ARD Advocates is dedicated to obtaining the appropriate educational services for children with special needs.

67 **National Adult Education Professional Development Consortium**
444 N Capitol Street NW
Washington, DC 20001
202-624-5250
FAX 202-624-1497
http://www.naepdc.org
e-mail: lmclendon@naepdc.org
Lennox L McLendon MD, Executive Director
Vonda Lynn Burns, Executive Assistant

Incorporated in 1990 by state and adult education director, provides professional development, policy analysis, and dissemination of information important to state staff in adult education.

68 **National Association for Adults with Special Learning Needs**
c/o Correctional Education Assoc.
Elkridge, MD 21075
888-562-2756
http://www.naasln.org
Robyn Rennick, President
Debra Watkins, Vice President
Richard Cooper PhD, Treasurer
An association for those who serve adults with special learning needs. Members include educators, trainers, wmployers and human service providers

69 **National Association for Child Development**
549 25th Street
Ogden, UT 84401
801-621-8606
FAX 801-621-8389
http://www.nacd.org
e-mail: info@nacd.org
Robert J Domain Jr, Founder/Director
Elizabeth B Severino, MD, Medical Director

Provides neurodevelopmental evaluations and individualized programs for children and adults, updated on a quarterly basis. Stresses parent training and parent implementation of the program.

70 **National Association for Community Mediation**
1527 New Hampshire Avenue NW
Washington, DC 20036
202-667-9700
FAX 202-667-8629
http://www.nafcm.org
e-mail: nafcm@nafcm.org
Joanne Galindo, Senior Director

Supports the maintenance and growth of community-based mediation programs and processes; acts as a resource for mediation information; locates a center to help individuals and groups resolve disputes.

71 **National Association for Gifted Children**
1707 L Street NW
Washington, DC 20036
202-785-4268
FAX 202-785-4248
http://www.nagc.org
e-mail: nacg@nagc.org
Joyce Van Tassel-Baska, President
Del Siegle, President-Elect
Nancy Green CAE, Executive Director
An organization of parents, teachers, educators, other professionals, and community leaders who unite to address the unique needs of children and youth with demonstrated gifts and talents as well as those children who may be able to develop their talent potential with appropriate educational experiences.
8,000+ members

72 **National Association for the Education of Young Children (NAEYC)**
1313 L Street NW
Washington, DC 20005
202-232-8777
800-424-2460
FAX 202-328-1846
http://www.naeyc.org
e-mail: naeyc@naeyc.org
Anne Mitchell, President
Jamilah R Jor'dan, Vice President
Mark Ginsberg, Executive Director
Dedicated to improving the well-being of all young children, with particular focus on the quality of educational and developmental services for all children from birth through age 8. The largest organization working on behalf of young adult children with nearly 100,000 members, a national network of over 300 local, state and regional Affiliates, and a growing global alliance of like-minded organizations.
1926

73 **National Association of Developmental Disabilities Councils (NADDC)**
225 Reinekers Lane
Alexandria, VA 22314
703-739-4400
FAX 703-739-6030
http://www.nacdd.org
e-mail: info@nacdd.org
Becky Harker, President, Iowa
Althea McLuckie, Vice President, New Mexico
Karen Flippo, Executive Director
A national member-driven organization consisting of 55 State and Territorial Councils. PLaces high value on meaningful participation and contribution by Council members and staff of all Member Councils, and we advocate and continually work towards positive system change on hehalf of individuals with developmental disabilities and their families. Founded in 2002.

74 **National Association of Parents With Children in Special Education**
1715 I Street, NW
Washington, DC 20006
800-754-4421
FAX 800-754-4421
http://www.napcse.org
e-mail: contact@napcse.org
Dr George Giuliani, President
Dr Roger Pierangelo, VP

A national membership organization dedicated to rendering all possible support and assistance to parents whose children receive special education services, both in and outside of school. NAPCSE was founded for parents with children with special needs to promote a sense of community and provide a national forum for their ideas.

75 **National Association of Private Special Education Centers**
1522 K Street NW
Washington, DC 20005
202-408-3338
FAX 202-408-3340
http://www.napsec.org
e-mail: napsec@aol.com
Gary Fitzherbert, President
Donald Verleur MD, Vice President
Sherry Kolbe, Executive Director/CEO
A nonprofit association whose mission is to ensure access for individuals to private special education as a vital component of the continuum of appropriate placement and services in American education. The association consists solely of private special education programs that serve both both privately and publicly placed individuals of all ages with disabilities.

76 **National Association of Special Education Teachers (NASET)**
1250 Connecticut Avenue NW
Washington, DC 20036
800-754-4221
FAX 800-754-4221
http://www.naset.org
e-mail: contactus@naset.org
Dr Roger Pierangelo, Co-Executive Director
Dr George Giuliani, Co-Executive Director

A national membership organization dedicated to rendering all possible support and assistance to those preparing for or teaching in the field of special education.

77 **National Association of the Education ofAfrican American Children**
PO Box 09521
Columbus, OH 43209
614-237-6021
FAX 614-238-0929
http://www.charityadvantage.com
e-mail: info@aacld.org
Linda Myers, Chair
Nancy R Tidwell, Founder/President

The NAEAACLD links information and resources provided by an established network of individuals and organizations experienced in minority research and special education with parents, educators and others responsible fo providing an appropriate education for African American students.

78 **National Business and Disability Council**
201 I U Willets Road
Albertson, NY 11507
516-465-1515
FAX 516-465-3730
http://www.nbdc.com
e-mail: lbroder@abilitiesonline.org
Edmund L Cortez, President/CEO
Lynn Broder, Membership Specialist

A leading resource for employers seeking to integrate people with disabilities into the workplace and companies seeking to reach them in the consumer marketplace. The NBDC has played a major role in helping businesses create accessible work conditions for employees accessible products and services for consumers.

79 **National Camp Association**
610 Fifth Avenue
New York, NY 10185
212-645-0653
800-966-2267
http://www.summercamp.org
e-mail: info@summercamp.org
Jeffrey Solomon, Executive Director

Provides a free summer camp referral service online to increase awareness of the benefits that summer camp offers children. NCA is more than a summer camp directory, featuring helpful information to provide personalized guidance and referrals for parents as they research and select a residential sleepawa camp for children.
1983

80 **National Center for Family Literacy**
325 W Main Street
Louisville, KY 40202
502-584-1133
877-FAMLIT-1
FAX 502-584-0172
http://www.famlit.org
e-mail: ncfl@famlit.org
Sharon Darling, President

Mission is to create a literate nation by leveraging the power of family. Family literacy is an intergenerational approach based on the indisputable evidence that low literacy is an unfortunate and debilitating family tradition.
1989

81 **National Center for Learning Disabilities (NCLD)**
381 Park Avenue S
New York, NY 10016
212-545-7510
888-575-7373
FAX 212-545-9665
http://www.ncld.org
e-mail: help@ncld.org
James Wendorf, Executive Director
Jaana Hinkkanen, Asst Dir Corporate/Found Relatio
Marcia Griffith-Pauyo, Exec Assistant Special Projects
Works to ensure that that nation's 15 million children, adolescents and adults with learning disabilities have every opportunity to succees in school, work and life. NCLD also provides essential information to parents, professionals and individuals with learning disabilities, promotes research and programs to foster effective learning and advocates for policies to protect and strengthen educational rights and opportunities.
1977

82 **National Center for Youth Law**
405 14th Street
Oakland, CA 94612
510-835-8098
FAX 510-835-8099
http://www.youthlaw.org
e-mail: info@youthlaw.org
John O'Toole, Director
Patrick Gardner, Deputy Director

Uses the law to improve the lives of poor children. Also works to ensure that low-income children have the resources, support, and opportunities that need for a healthy and productive future. Much of NCYL's work is focused on poor children who are additionally challenged by abuse and neglect, disability, or other disadvantage.

83 **National Center of Higher Education for Learning Problems (HELP)**
Myers Hall
520 18th Street
Huntington, WV 25703
304-696-6313
FAX 304-696-3231
http://www.marshall.edu/help
e-mail: painter@marshall.edu
Lynne Weston, Director
Russell Cook, Development Coordinator
Debbie Painter MA, Coordinator Diagnostics
The HELP Program is committed to providing assistance through individual tutoring, mentoring and support, as well as fair and legal access to educational opportunities for students diagnosed with Learning Disabilities (LD) and related disorders such as ADD/ADHD.

84 **National Council for Support of Disability Issues**
Mountain Road
Haymarket, VA 20169
703-753-9148
http://www.ncsd.org
e-mail: tfink@ncsd.org

Jason Perry, President
Trisha Fink, Executive Director

The goal is to provide a means for sharing information, resources, ideas and support between people with all types of disabilities.

85 **National Council of Juvenile and Family Court Judges (NCJFCJ)**
PO Box 8970
Reno, NV 89507
775-784-6012
FAX 775-784-6628
http://www.ncjfcj.org
e-mail: staff@ncjfcj.org

Judge Dale R Koch, President
Mary Mentaberry, Executive Director

The vision of the NCJFCJ is that every child and young person be reared in a safe, permanent, and nuturing family, where love, self-control, concern for others, and responsibility for the consequences of one's actions are experienced and taught as fundamental values for a successful life. Also seeks a society in which every child and every family in need of judicial oversight has access to fair, effective and timely justice.
1973Grade Range: Professional Ed

86 **National Council on Rehabilitation Education**
2012 W Norwood Drive
Carbondale, IL 62901
618-549-3267
FAX 618-457-3632
http://www.rehabeducators.org
e-mail: sbenshoff@ncre-admin.org

Jorge Garcia, President
David Perry, 1st Vice President
Linda Holloway, 2nd Vice President

A professional organization of educators dedicated to quality services for persons with disabilities through education and research. NCRE advocates-up-to-date education and training and the maintenance of professional standards in the field of rehabilitation
1955

87 **National Data Bank for Disabled Service**
University of Maryland
0126 Shoemaker Building
College Park, MD 20742
301-314-7682
FAX 301-405-0813
http://www.counseling.umd.edu/dss
e-mail: jahutch@umd.edu

Jo Ann Hutchinson RhD, Director
Marja Humphrey, Customer Service Coordinator

Coordinates services that ensure individuals with disabilities equal access to University of Maryland College Park programs.
800 members 1976

88 **National Disabilities Rights Network**
900 2nd Street NE
Washington, DC 20002
202-408-9514
FAX 202-408-9520
TDY:202-408-9521
http://www.napas.org
e-mail: info@ndrn.org

Curtis L Decker JD, Executive Director
Joanna Solkoff, Executive/Public Policy Asst

Nonprofit membership organization for the federally mandated Protection and Advocacy (P&A) Systems and Client Assistance Programs (CAP) for individuals with disabilities. Serves a wide range of individuals with disabilities-including, but not limited to, those with cognitive, mental, sensory, and physical disabilities-by guarding against abuse; advocating for basic rights; and ensuring accountability in health care, education, employment, housing, and transportation.

89 **National Dissemination Center for Children with Disabilities**
NICHCY
PO Box 1492
Washington, DC 20013
202-884-8200
800-695-0285
FAX 202-884-8441
TDY:800-695-0285
http://www.nichcy.org
e-mail: nichcy@aed.org

Susan Ripley, Manager

An information and referral clearinghouse that provides free information on disabilities and disability related issues. Services include speaking with an information specialist, receiving free publications, database searches and referrals to other organizations. Also provides a state resource sheet which identifies resources in each state including state agencies, disability organizations and parent groups.

90 **National Education Association (NEA)**
1201 16th Street NW
Washington, DC 20036
202-833-4000
FAX 202-822-7974
http://www.nea.org

Reg Weaver, President

The nation's largest professional employee organization, is committed to advancing the cause of public education. NEA's members work at every level of education-from pre-school to university graduate programs. Also has affiliate organization in every state and in more than 14,000 communities across the United States.
3.2 million mem

91 **National Federation of the Blind**
1800 Johnson Street
Baltimore, MD 21230
410-659-9314
FAX 410-685-5653
http://www.nfb.org
e-mail: nfb@nfb.org

Marc Maurer, President
Joyce Scanlan, 1st Vice President

The largest and most influential membership organizatoin of blind people in the United States. The NFB improves blind people's lives through advocacy, education, research, technology, and programs encouraging independence and self-confidence. It is also the leading force in the blindness field today and the voice of the nation's blind.
50,000 members 1940

92 **National Institute of Art and Disabilities**
551 23rd Street
Richmond, CA 94804
510-620-0290
FAX 510-620-0326
http://www.niadart.org
e-mail: admin@niadart.org

Patricia Coleman, Executive Director
Gabe Johnson, Art Sales/Exhibitions Director

An innovative visual arts center assisting adults with developmental and other physical disabilities. Provides an art program that promotes creativity, independence, dignity, and community integration for people with developmental and other disabilities.
1982

93 **National Jewish Council for Disabilities Summer Program**
YACHAD East Coast Adventure
11 Broadway
New York, NY 10004
212-613-8369
FAX 212-613-0796
http://www.njcd.org
e-mail: yadbyad@ou.org

Nechama Braun, Administrator

Yachad/NJCD is dedicated to addressing the needs of all individuals with disabilities and including them in the Jewish community. Summer Programs include a variety of summer experiences for youth and adults with developmental disabilities.

94 **National Lekotek Center**
3204 W Armitage Avenue
Chicago, IL 60647
773-276-5164
800-366-7529
FAX 773-276-8644
http://www.lekotek.org
e-mail: lekotek@lekotek.org
Diana Nielander, Executive Director

Uses interactive play experiences, and the learning that results, to promote the inclusion of children with special needs into family and community life.

95 **National Organization for Rare Disorders (NORD)**
55 Kenosia Avenue
Danbury, CT 06813
203-744-0100
800-999-6673
FAX 203-798-2291
TDY:203-797-9590
http://www.rarediseases.org
e-mail: orphan@rarediseases.org
Abbey Meyers, President

A unique federation of voluntary health organizations dedicates to helping people with rare diseases and assisting the organizations that serve them. Committed to the identification, treatment, and cure of rare disorders through programs of education, advocacy, research, and service.
1983

96 **National Organization on Disability (NOD)**
910 16th Street NW
Washington, DC 20006
202-293-5960
FAX 202-293-7999
http://www.nod.org
Tom Ridge, Chairman
Michael Deland, President

The mission of the National Organization on Disability is to expand the participataion and contribution of America's 54 million men, women and children with disabilities in all aspects of life.

97 **National Rehabilitation Association**
633 S Washington Street
Alexandria, VA 22314
703-836-0850
FAX 703-836-0848
TDY:703-836-0849
http://www.nationalrehab.org
e-mail: info@nationalrehab.org
Dr Carl Flowers, President
Dr Raymond Feroz, President-Elect

A membership organization that promotes ethical and state of the art practice in rehabilitation with the goal of the personal and economic independence of persons with disabilities. Members include rehabilitation counselors, physical, speech and occupational therapists, job trainers, consultants, independent living instructors, students in rehabilitation programs, and other professionals involved in the advocacy of programs and services for people with disabilities.

98 **National Rehabilitation Information Center**
8201 Corporate Drive
Lanham, MD 20785
301-459-5900
800-346-2742
FAX 301-459-4263
http://www.naric.com
e-mail: naricinfo@heitechservices.com
Mark Odum, Director

The gateway to an abundance of disability-and rehabilitation-oriented information organized in a variety of formats designed to make it easy for useres to find and use. The mission of the Center is to collect and disseminate the results of research funded by the National Institute in Disability and Rehabilitation Research (NIDRR).

99 **New England ADA and Accessible IT Center**
180-200 Portland Street
Boston, MA 02114
617-695-0085
800-949-4232
FAX 617-482-8099
http://adapteenvironments.org/neada
e-mail: adainfo@newenglandada.org
Oce Harrison, Program Director
Karen Murray, Information Specialist

Provides information and guidance on the Americans with Disabilities Act, Section 508, and accessible information technology to individuals in New England.
1978

100 **Nonverbal Learning Disorders Association**
507 Hopemeadow Street
Simsbury, CT 06070
860-658-5522
FAX 860-658-6688
http://www.nlda.org
e-mail: info@nlda.org
Patricia Carrin, Founder/President
Marcia Rubinstien, Founder/Executive Liaison

A non-profit corporation dedicated to research, education, and advocacy for nonverbal learning disorders.

101 **Parent Advocacy Coalition for EducationalRights (PACER)**
8161 Normandale Boulevard
Minneapolis, MN 55437
952-838-9000
800-537-2237
FAX 952-838-0190
http://www.pacer.org
e-mail: pacer@pacer.org
Paula Goldberg, Executive Director

The mission of PACER Center is to expand opportunities and enhance the quality of life of children and young adults with disabilities and their families, based on the concept of parents helping parents.
1977

102 **Parent Educational Advocacy Training Center (PEATC)**
100 N Washington Street
Falls Church, VA 22046-4523
703-923-0010
800-869-6782
FAX 800-693-3514
http://www.peatc.org
e-mail: partners@peatc.org
Cherie Takemoto, Executive Director
Felicia Kessel-Crawley, Programs/Operations Director
Gail Byrd Ryder, Administrative Coordinator
A non-profit that believes children with disabilities reach their full potential when families and professionals enjoy and equal, respectful partnership. PEATC also provides support education, and training to families, schools and other professionals committed to helping children with disabilities.
1978

103 **Parents Helping Parents, Inc**
3041 Olcott Street
Santa Clara, CA 95054
408-727-5775
866-747-4040
FAX 408-727-0182
http://www.php.com
e-mail: info@php.com
Mary Peterson, CEO
Trudy Marsh Holmes, Community/Family Service Dir

Helping children with special needs receive the resources, love, hope, respect, health care, education and other services they need to achieve their full potential by providing them with strong families and dedicated professionals to serve them.

104 **Promote Real Independence for Disabled & Elderly Foundation**
PO Box 1293
Groton, CT 06340
860-445-7320
800-332-9122
FAX 860-445-1448
http://www.sewtiqueonline.com
e-mail: dresspride@aol.com
Evelyn Kennedy, Owner

Is a nonprofit, tax exempt organization whose main objective is rehabilitation assistance for the disabled and elderly in the areas of home management and independence in dressing and personal grooming. Consulting services are provided to families, agencies, and health organizations dealing with special needs of special persons.
1978

105 **RFB&D Learning Through Listening**
Headquarters
20 Roszel Road
Princeton, NJ 08540
609-452-0606
866-732-3585
FAX 609-987-8116
http://www.rfbd.org
e-mail: custserv@rfbd.org

John Kelly, CEO
Pat Sullivan, Unit Development Director

The nation's educational library for people with print disabilities. We provide educational materials in recorded and computerized formats from kindergarten through postgraduate level.
7,100 members 1948

106 **Rehabilitation Engineering and Assistive Technology Society of North America (RESNA)**
1700 N Moore Street
Arlington, VA 22209
703-524-6686
FAX 703-524-6630
http://www.resna.org
e-mail: info@resna.org

Glenn Hedman, President
Thomas A Gorski, Executive Director

An interdisciplinary association of people with a common interest in technology and disability. The purpose is to improve the potential of people with disabilities to achieve their goals through the use of technology.
1979

107 **Rehabilitation International**
25 E 21st Street
New York, NY 10010
212-420-1500
FAX 212-505-0871
http://www.rehab-international.org
e-mail: ri@riglobal.org

Michael Fox, President/Director
Anne Hawker, President-Elect
Tomas Lagerwall, Secretary General
A global network of people with disabilities, service providers, researchers, government agencies and advocates promoting and implementing the rights and inclusion or people with disabilities

700 members 1922

108 **Research Division of CEC**
Council for Exceptional Children
1110 N Glebe Road
Arlington, VA 22201
703-620-3660
888-232-7733
FAX 703-264-9494
http://www.cecdr.org

Robin McWilliam, President
Frederick Brigham, President-Elect

Devoted to the advancement of research related to the education of individuals with disabilities and/or who are gifted. The goals of CEC-DR include the promotion of equal partnership with practitioners in designing, conducting and interpreting research in special education.

109 **Rural Clearinghouse for Lifelong Education & Development**
Kansas State University
101 College Court
Manhattan, KS 66506
785-532-6879
FAX 913-532-5637
e-mail: abyers@ksuksu.edu

Robert Garcia, Executive Director
Jacqueline Spears, Co-Director

Leads the effort to improve rural access to continued education; provides research, information, and policy recommendations regarding rural adult education to educators and policymakers through special projects, publications, and conferences.

110 **Sertoma International Foundation**
1912 E Meyer Boulevard
Kansas City, MO 64132
816-333-8300
FAX 816-333-4320
http://www.sertoma.org
e-mail: infosertoma@sertoma.org

Steven Murphy, Executive Director
Sheila Reding, Chair
Larry Shealey, President
Activities focus on helping people with speech and hearing problems, but also have programs in the areas of youth, national heritage, drug awareness and community services.

111 **Son-Rise Program®**
Autism Treatment Center of America™
2080 S Undermountain Road
Sheffield, MA 01257
413-229-2100
800-714-2779
FAX 413-229-8931
http://www.autismtreatment.com
e-mail: correspondence@option.org

Raun K Kaufman, CEO
Barry Neil Kaufman, Co-Founder/Co-Creator
Samahria Lyte Kaufman, Co-Founder/Co-Creator
Autism Treatment Center of America has provided innovative training programs for parents and professionals caring for children challenged by Autism, Autism Spectrum Disorders, Pervasive Developmental Disorder (PDD) and other developmental difficulties. The Son-Rise Program teaches a specific yet comprehensive system of treatment and education designed to help families and caregivers enable their children to dramatically improve in all areas of learning.
1983

112 **Stuttering Foundation of America**
3100 Walnut Grove Road
Memphis, TN 38111
901-452-7343
800-992-9392
FAX 901-452-3931
http://www.stutteringhelp.org
e-mail: stutter@stutteringhelp.org

George F Cooley, Founder
Malcolm Fraser, Founder
Jane Fraser, President
Founded with the goal to provide the best and most up-to-date information and help available for the prevention of stuttering in young children and the most effective treatment available for teenagers and adults.
1947

113 **Team of Advocates for Special Kids**
100 W Cerritos Avenue
Anaheim, CA 92805
714-533-8275
FAX 714-533-2533
e-mail: tasca@yahoo.com

Marta Anchondo, Executive Director
Brenda Smith, Deputy Director

TASK's mission is to enable children with disabilities to reach their maximum potential by providing them, their families and the professionals who serve them, with training, support information resources and referrals, and by providing community awareness programs. TASK's TECH Center is a place for children, parents, adult consumers, and professionals to learn about assistive technology by providing hands-on access to computer hardware, software and adaptive equipment.

114 **Technology and Media Division**
Council for Exceptional Children
1110 N Glebe Road
Arlington, VA 22201
703-245-3660
888-232-7733
FAX 703-264-9494
http://www.tamcec.org

Brenda Heiman, President
Tara Jeffs, President-Elect

TAM works to promote the availability and effective use of technology and media for children, birth to 21, with disabilities and/or who are gifted.

115 **Thinking and Learning Connection**
239 Whitclem Court
Palo Alto, CA 94306
650-493-3497
FAX 650-494-3499

Lynne Stietzel, Co-Director
Eric Stietzel, Co-Director

A group of independent associates committed to teaching students to learn new paths of knowledge and understanding. Our primary focus is working with dyslexic and dyscalculia. Individualized educational programs utilize extensive multisensory approaches to teach reading, spelling, handwriting, composition, comprehension, and mathematics. The students are actively involved in learning processes that integrate visual, auditory, and tactile techniques.

116 Very Special Arts
818 Connecticut Avenue NW
Washington, DC 20006
202-628-2800
800-933-8721
FAX 202-429-0868
TDY:202-737-0645
http://www.vsarts.org
e-mail: info@vsarts.org

Jean Kennedy, Founder
Soula Antoniou, President

An international, nonprofit organization founded to create a society where all people with disabilities learn through, participate in and enjoy the arts. VSA arts is committed to driving change - changing perceptions and practice, classroom by classroom, community by community, and ultimatley society
1974

117 Visual Impairments Division of CEC
Council for Exceptional Children
1110 N Glebe Road
Arlington, VA 22201
703-245-3660
888-232-7733
FAX 703-264-9494
http://www.cecdvi.org

Ellyn Ross MD, President
Phyllis T Simmons, President-Elect

An organization whose membership represents a diverse group of individuals committed to the education of students who are blind or visually impaired. DVI attracts members committed to promoting effective educational practices and outcomes through collaborative efforts in partnership with families and colleagues.
1,000 members 1948

118 Washington PAVE: Specialized Training of Military Parents (STOMP)
6316 S 12th Street
Tacoma, WA 98465
253-565-2266
800-572-7368
FAX 253-566-8052
TDY:800-572-7368
http://www.washingtonpave.org
e-mail: stomp@washingtonpave.com

Heather Hebdon, Founder/Program Director
Joanne Butts, Executive Director

STOMP, a parent directed project exists to empower military parents, individuals with disabilities, and service providers with knowledge, skills and resources so that they might access services to create a collaborative environment for a family and professional partnerships without regard to geographic location.
100,000 members 1979

119 World Institute on Disability (WID)
510 16th Street
Oakland, CA 94612
510-763-4100
FAX 510-763-4109
http://www.wid.org
e-mail: wid@wid.org

Martin B Schulter, Chair
Samuel A Simon JD, Vice Chair
Kathy Martinez, Executive Director

A nonprofit public policy center dedicated to promoting independence and full societal inclusion of people with disabilities. Since its founding in 1983 by Ed Roberts, WID has earned a reputation for high quality research and public education on a wide range of issues. Newsletter is published on a regular basis.
1983

120 Young Adult Institute (YAI): National Institute for People with Disabilities
460 W 34th Street
New York, NY 10001
212-273-6100
FAX 212-629-4113
TDY:212-290-2787
http://www.yai.org
e-mail: staff@yai.org

Philip Levy PhD, President/COO
Joe Levy DSW, CEO
Stephen E Freeman CSW, Associate Executive Director

A national leader in the provision of services, education and training in the field of developmental and learning disabilities.
1957

Alabama

121 International Dyslexia Association of Alabama
818 Mountain Gap Court
Huntsville, AL 35803
256-551-1442
FAX 205-942-2688
http://www.interdys.org
e-mail: gibbsdenise@aol.com

Denise P Gibbs, President

ALIDA will provide dyslexic individuals in Alabama with a unified voice to represent their interests to the public, to the educational community, to the legislature, and to others. ALIDA will also serve as a vehicle to increase awareness and understanding of dyslexia in Alabama.

122 Learning Disabilities Association of Alabama
PO Box 11588
Montgomery, AL 36111
334-277-9151
FAX 334-284-9357
http://www.ldaal.org

Mattie Ray, President
Linda Graham, 1st Vice President

A non-profit grassroots organization whose members are individuals with learning disabilities, their families, and the professionals who work with them. LDAA is dedicated to identifying causes and promoting prevention of learning disabilities and to enhance the quality of life for all individuals with learning disabilities and their families by encouraging effective identification and intervention, fostering research, and protecting their rights inder the law.

123 UAB Sparks Center for Developmental and Learning Disorders
University of Alabama at Birmingham
1720 7th Avenue S
Birmingham, AL 35233
205-934-6015
800-UAB-CIRC
FAX 205-975-2380
http://www.circ.uab.com
e-mail: sparksinfo@civmail.circ.uab.edu

Dr Friedlander, Executive Director
Alvin Vogtle, Social Worker

The Sparks Clinics provide an extensive range of interdisciplinary offerings including comprehensive diagnosis, evaluation and treatment of the needs of children and adults with mental retardation and developmental disabilities. Each of the clinics consults with clients in a context that considers the unique needs of individuals and their family members. Additionally, the Sparks Clinics complex is a major site for clinical research.

Alaska

124 Center for Human Development (CHD)
University of Alaska Anchorage
2702 Gambell Street
Anchorage, AK 99503
907-272-8270
800-243-2199
FAX 907-274-4802
http://www.alaskachd.org
e-mail: info@alaskachd.org
Karen Ward PhD, Director
Beverly Tallman, Associate Director

One od 61 University Centers located in every state and territoyr, which attempts to bring together the resources of the university and the community in support of individuals with developmental disabilities.

125 Learning Disabilities Association of Alaska (LDAALaska)
PO Box 243172
Anchorage, AK 99524
907-563-5322
FAX 907-565-1000
http://www.ldaalaska.org
e-mail: info@ldaalaska.org
Matt Wappett, President

A nonprofit organization whose members are individuals with learning disabilities, their families, and the professionals who work with them.

126 Washington State Branch of IDA
PO Box 1247
Mercer Island, WA 98040
206-382-1020
http://www.wabida.org
e-mail: info@wabida.org
Bonnie Meyer, President

The Washington State Branch of the International Dyslexia Association is a 501 (c)(3) non-profit, scientific and educational organization dedicated to the study and treatment of dyslexia. Our all volunteer board of directors seeks to increase public awareness of dyslexia in our branch's area which includes Washington, Alaska, Idaho, and western Montana.

Arizona

127 Arizona Center for Disability Law
100 N Stone Avenue
Tucson, AZ 85701
520-327-9547
800-922-1447
FAX 502-884-0992
http://www.acdl.com
e-mail: center@azdisabilitylaw.org
Peri Jude Radecic, Executive Director

Advocates for the legal rights of persons with disabilities to be free from abuse, neglect and discrimination; and to have access to education, healthcare, housing and jobs, and other services in order to maximize independence and achieve equality.

128 Institute for Human Development: Northern Arizona University
PO Box 5630
Flagstaff, AZ 86011
928-523-4791
FAX 928-523-9127
http://www.nau.edu/ihd/
e-mail: richard.carroll@nau.edu
Richard Carroll PhD, Executive Director

The Institute values and supports the independence, productivity and inclusion of Arizona's citizens with disabilities. Based on the values and beliefs, the Institute conducts training, research and services that further these goal.

129 International Dyslexia Association of Arizona
18647 N 20th Street
Phoenix, AZ 85024
602-867-9660
FAX 602-867-2762
http://www.interdys-az.org
e-mail: willcoxon@cox.net
Marilyn Willcoxon, President

The Arizona Branch of The International Dyslexia Association (AIDA) is a 501 (c)(3) non-profit, scientific organization dedicated to educating the public about the learning disability, dyslexia. The Arizona Branch has four objectives: to increase awareness in the dyslexic and general community; to network with other learning disability groups and legislators in education; to increase membership; to raise funds for future projects that will make a difference in our community.

130 Parent Information Network
Arizona Department of Education
2384 Steves Blvd
Flagstaff, AZ 86004
928-679-8106
800-352-4558
FAX 928-679-8124
http://www.ade.az.gov
e-mail: rkeniso@ade.az.gov
Becky Raabe, Parent Information Network Coord

Provides free training and information to parents on federal and state laws and regulations for special education, parental rights and responsibilities, parent involvement, advocacy, behavior, standards and disability related resources. Provides a clearinghouse of information targeted to parents of children with disabilities. Also assists schools in promoting positive parent/professional/ regional partnerships.

131 Recording for the Blind & Dyslexic: Phoenix Studio
3627 E Indian School Road
Phoenix, AZ 85018
602-468-9144
http://www.rfbd.org/az
Barbara Fenter, Executive Director
Dana Salsbury, Development Director
Pam Bork, Production Director
To create opportunities for individuals, from Kindergarten through Graduate Level, who cannot read standard print because of a visual impairment, learning disability or other physical disability, to succeed in school by providing accessible educational materials.

132 Recording for the Blind & Dyslexic: Sun Cities Studio
9449 N 99th Avenue
Peoria, AZ 85345
623-977-6020
http://www.rfbd.org/az
Michael Kaminer, Production Director
Wendy White, Production Assistant

To create opportunities for individuals, from Kindergarten through Graduate Level, who cannot read standard print because of a visual impairment, learning disability or other physical disability, to succeed in school by providing accessible educational materials.

Arkansas

133 Center for Applied Studies in Education Learning (CASE)
University of Arkansas at Little Rock
2801 S University Avenue
Little Rock, AR 72202
501-569-3422
FAX 501-569-8503
http://www.ualr.edu/CASE
e-mail: rhbradley@ualr.edu
R Bradley, Professor

Improves the quality of education and human services in Arkansas and globally through a number of inter-related activities: conducting research on the effectiveness of programs and practices in education and human services; providing technical assistance in statistics, research design, measurement methodologies, data management, and program evaluation to students, faculty, and external groups and agencies; providing formal and informal consultation, technical assistance and instruction.

134 **International Dyslexia Association of Arkansas**
14070 Proton
Dallas, TX 75244 972-233-9107
FAX 972-490-4219
http://www.dbida.org
Pamela Hudnall Quarterman, President

The Dallas Branch of The International Dyslexia Association is committed to leadership an advocacy for people with dyslexia providing: support for individuals and group internactions; programs to inform and educate; and information for professionals and the general public. This branch also serves the state of Arkansas.

135 **Learning Disabilities Association of Arkansas (LDAA)**
7509 Cantrell Road
Little Rock, AR 72207 501-666-8777
FAX 501-666-4070
http://www.ldaarkansas.org
e-mail: info@lsaarkansas.org
Joe Kelnhofer, President
Stacey Mahurin, President

A nonprofit, volunteer organization of parents and professionals. LDAA is devoted to defining and finding solutions to the broad spectrum of learning disabilities.

California

136 **Berkeley Policy Associates**
4440 Grand Avenue
Oakland, CA 94610 510-465-7884
FAX 510-465-7885
TDY:510-465-4493
http://www.berkeleypolicyassociates.com
e-mail: info@bpacal.com
Hans Bos, CEO
Fannie Tseng PhD, CFO

Conducts social policy research and program evaluations in various topic areas, including disability policy. Although the research typically does not focus on specific disabilities, the reports or other deliverables deriving from the projects may include specific information relating to particular disabilities, and are available for purchase.

137 **California Association of Special Education & Services**
1722 J Street
Sacramento, CA 95814 916-447-7061
FAX 916-447-1320
http://www.capses.com
e-mail: info@capses.com
Wayne K Miyamoto, Public/Govt Affairs Director
Janeth Rodriguez, Communications/Operations Dir

Dedicated to preserving and enhancing the leadership role of the private sector in offering quality alternative services to students with disabilities.
191 members 1973

138 **Client Assistance Program (CAP)California Department of Rehabilitation**
721 Capitol Mall
Sacramento, CA 95814 916-558-5390
800-952-5544
FAX 915-558-5391
http://www.dor.ca.gov
e-mail: capinfo@dor.ca.gov
Sheila Mentkowski, Chief Officer
Tony Sauer, Director

The California Department of Rehabilitation works in partnership with consumers and other stakeholders to provide services and advocacy resulting in employment, independent living and equality for individuals with disabilities.

139 **Dyslexia Awareness and Resource Center**
928 Carpinteria Street
Santa Barbara, CA 93103 805-963-7339
FAX 805-963-6581
http://www.dyslexiacenter.org
e-mail: info@dyslexiacenter.org
Joan Esposito, Founder/Program Director
Leslie V Esposito, Executive/Development Director

Provides direct one-on-one services to adults and children affected with dyslexia, attention disorders and other learning disabilities. Also provides services to families and to parents with children affected with dyslexia, attention disorders and other learning disabilities.
1990

140 **Easter Seals Central California**
9010 Soquel Drive
Aptos, CA 95003 831-684-2166
800-400-0671
FAX 831-684-1018
http://centralcal.easterseals.com
Bruce Hinman, President/CEO
Donna Alvarez, Senior VP/CFO
Tracy Chappell, Chief Development Officer
Create solutions that change lives of children and adults with disabilities or other special needs and their families.

141 **Easter Seals Southern California**
1801 E Edinger Avenue
Santa Ana, CA 92705 714-834-1111
FAX 714-834-1128
http://southerncal.easterseals.com
Provides excpetional services to ensure that all peopel with disabilities or other special needs and their families have equal opportunities to live, learn, work and play in their communities.

142 **International Dyslexia Association of LosAngeles**
PO Box 1808
Studio City, CA 91604 818-506-8866
FAX 818-789-6740
http://www.interdys.org
e-mail: dyslexiala@aol.com
Jennifer Zvi, President

The Los Angeles County Branch of The International Dyslexia Association believes that all individuals have the right to realize their potential, that individual learning abilities can be strengthened, and that language and reading skills can be achieved.

143 **International Dyslexia Association of Northern California**
PO Box 5010
San Mateo, CA 94402 650-328-7667
FAX 650-372-0125
http://www.dyslexia-ncbida.org
e-mail: office@dyslexia-ncbida.org
Leslie Lingas Woodward, President

Formed to increase public awareness of dyslexia in Northern California and Northern Nevada. Have been serving individuals with dyslexia, their families and professionals in the field in this community for 30 years.

144 **International Dyslexia Association of SanDiego**
2515 Camino Del Rio Drive
San Diego, CA 92108 619-685-3722
FAX 760-723-7168
http://www.dyslexiasd.org
e-mail: pph@tfb.com
Jose Cruz, President

A nonprofit scientific and educational organization dedicated to the study and treatment of the learning disability. This branch was informed to increase public awareness of dyslexia.

145 **Learning Disabilities Association of California**
PO Box 601067
Sacramento, CA 95860
916-725-7881
866-532-6322
FAX 916-725-8786
http://www.ldaca.org
e-mail: lda@June.com

Georgia Abi Nader, President
Jo Behm, First Vice President
EunMi Cho, Multicultural Chairs

A non-profit volunteer organization of parents, professionals and adults with learning disabilities. Its purpose is to promote and support the education and general welfare of children and adults of potentially normal intelligence who manifest learning, perceptual, and/or behavioral handicaps.

146 **Lutheran Braille Workerssion**
13471 California Street
Yucaipa, CA 92399
909-795-8977
FAX 909-795-8970
http://www.lbwinc.org
e-mail: lbw@lbwinc.org

Rev. Phillip Pledger, Executive Director

The mission of Lutheran Braille Workers is to provide the message of salvation, through faith in Jesus Christ, to individuals who are blind or visually impaired throughout the world.
1943

147 **Orange County Learning DisabilitiesAssociation**
PO Box 25772
Santa Ana, CA 92799-5772
714-547-4206
http://www.oclda.org
e-mail: oclda@comcast.net

Jim Farell, Board Member

A private, self-help, volunteer, non-profit, charitable organization of parents and professionals who are concerned with the welfare of children and adults who have learning disabilities.
1960

148 **Recording for the Blind & Dyslexic: Los Angeles**
5022 Hollywood Boulevard
Los Angeles, CA 90027
323-664-5525
800-732-8398
FAX 323-664-1881
http://www.rfbd.org/la
e-mail: los_angeles@rfbd.org

Carol Smith, Executive Director
Melissa MacRae, Development Director
Diane Kelber, Director Communications

A nonprofit organization that serves individuals who cannot read standard print because of a vision, physical or learning disability, by providing them with educational materials in accessible formats.

149 **Recording for the Blind & Dyslexic: Northern California**
488 W Charleston Road
Palo Alto, CA 94306
650-493-3717
866-493-3717
FAX 650-493-5513
http://www.rfbd.org

Matt Ward, Production Director
Valley Brown, Educational Outreach Director
Lynne Van Tilburg, Development Director

Our territory covers nine counteis including San Francisco, San Mateo, Santa Clara, Santa Cruz, Monterey, Alameda, Contra Costa, Marin, and Sonoma. We have 3 field educational outreach offices in San Francisio, the South Bay, and the East Bay serving individual students and 160 schools in those local areas.
4,500 members 1967

150 **Recording for the Blind & Dyslexic: SantaBarbara**
5638 Hollister Ave
Santa Barbara, CA 93110
805-681-0531
FAX 805-681-0532
http://www.rfbd.org

Tim Owens, Executive Director
David Hardin, Production Coordinator

Our mission is to create opportunities for individual success by providing, and promoting the effective use of, accessible educational materials.

151 **Recording for the Blind and Dyslexic: Inland Empire-Orange County Unit**
Inland Empire Studio
1844 W 11th Street
Upland, CA 91786
909-949-4316
FAX 909-981-8457
http://www.rfbd.org
e-mail: mdavis@rfbd.org

Sherry Weekes, Production Director
Michael Davis, Executive Director

Volunteers record textbooks on computer disks for the visually, physically and perceptually disabled.

Colorado

152 **Easter Seals Colorado**
PO Box 115
Empire, CO 80438
303-569-2333
http://co.easterseals.com

Lynn Robinso, President/CEO

Provides services to children and adults with disabilities and other special needs, and support to their families.

153 **Internatational Dyslexia Association of Colorado**
PO Box 46-1010
Glendale, CO 80246
303-721-9425
http://www.dyslexia-rmbida.org
e-mail: ida_rmb@yahoo.com

Elenn Steinberg, President

300+ members 1949

154 **Learning Disabilities Association of Colorado**
4400 E Iliff Avenue
Denver, CO 80222
303-894-0992
http://www.ldacolorado.com
e-mail: info@ldacolorado.com

Nina Healy, President

The Learning Disabilities Association of Colorado is committed to supporting the potential of individuals with learning and attention disabilities through accurate identification, advocacy, and education.

155 **PEAK Parent Center**
611 N Weber Street
Colorado Springs, CO 80903
719-531-9400
800-284-0251
FAX 719-531-9452
http://www.peakparent.org
e-mail: info@peakparent.org

Barbara Bushwell, Executive Director
Kent Willis, 207sident, Board of Directors

A federally-designated Parent Traning and Information Center (PTI). As a PTI, PEAK supports and empowers parents, providing them with information and strategies to use when advocating for their children with disabilities by expanding knowledge of special education and offering new strategies for success.

156 **Recording for the Blind & Dyslexic: Colorado-Rocky Mountain Unit**
1355 S Colorado Boulevard
Denver, CO 80222
303-757-0787
http://www.rfbd.org
e-mail: bboudreau@rfbd.org

Betsy Boudreau, Executive Director

Produces the textbooks that students and professionals with print impairments need for the academic and career success that lead to lifelong self-sufficiency and self-fulfillment. Also provide and educational outreach program to schools to help them use and understand the program and our services.

157 **Rocky Mountain Disability and Business Technical Assistance Center**
3630 Sinton Road
Colorado Springs, CO 80907
719-444-0268
800-949-4232
FAX 719-444-0269
http://www.adainformation.org
e-mail: rmdbtac@mtc-inc.com
Randy Dipner, Senior Advisor
Patrick Going, Project Director
Cristi Harris, Information Specialist
Provides information on the Americans with Disabilities Act to Colorado, Utah, Montana, Wyoming, North Dakota and South Dakota.

Connecticut

158 **Connecticut Association for Children and Adults with Learning Disabilities**
25 Van Zant Street
Norwalk, CT 06855
203-838-5010
FAX 203-866-6108
http://www.cacld.org
e-mail: cacld@optonline.net
Beryl Kaufman, Executive Director
Ida Kubaryth, Office Manager

A regional, non-profit organization that supports individuals, families and professionals by providing information, education, and consultation while promoting public awareness and understanding. CACLD's goal is to ensure access to the resources needed to help children and adults with learning disabilities and attention deficit disorders achieve their full potential.
1963

159 **Connecticut Association of Private Special Education Facilities (CAPSEF)**
330 Main Street
Hartford, CT 06106
860-525-1318
FAX 860-541-6484
http://www.capsef.org
e-mail: info@capsef.org
Alan Deckman, Executive Director
Allyson Deckman, Assistant Executive Director

A voluntary association of provate schools which provides quality, cost effective, special education and related services to the special needs of children and adolescents (birth to 21 years) of Connecticut. The focus of these education services is social and vocation programs designed to enable students to succeed in the least restrictive environment
2,500 members 1974

160 **Connecticut Capitol Region Educational Council**
Administrator Capitol Education Council
111 Charter Oak Avenue
Hartford, CT 06106
860-247-2732
877-850-2832
FAX 860-246-3304
http://www.crec.org
e-mail: bdouglas@crec.org
Bruce Douglas Ph.D, Executive Director
Colleen A Palmer, Deputy Executive Director
Donald Walsh, Asst Executive Dir Finance/Ops
Will promote cooperation and collaboration with local school districts and other organizations committed to the improved quality of public education; provide cost-effective services to member districts and other clients; listen and respond to client needs for the improved quality of public education; and provide leadership in the region through the quality of its services and its ability to identify and share quality services of its member districts and other organizations to public education.
1966

161 **International Dyslexia Association of Connecticut**
69 Hillsport Road
Westport, CT 06880
203-865-6163
http://www.connbida.net
e-mail: mbgillis@aol.com
Margie Bussman Gillis, President

162 **Learning Disabilities Association of Conneecticut**
999 Asylum Avenue
Hartford, CT 06105
860-560-1711
FAX 860-560-1750
http://www.ldact/org
e-mail: ldact@idact.org
William Bossi, President

LDA of Connecticut is a non-profit organization of parents, professionals, and persons with learning disabilities. We are dedicated to promoting a better understanding of learning disabilities, securing appropriate educational and employment opportunities for children and adults with learning disabilities and improving the quality of life for this population.

163 **Nonverbal Learning Disorders Association**
2446 Albany Avenue
West Hartford, CT 06117
860-570-0217
FAX 860-570-0218
http://www.nlda.org
e-mail: info@nlda.org
Patricia Carrin, Founder/President
Marcia Rubinstien, Founder, Executive Liasion

A non-profit corporation dedicated to research, education and advocacy for nonverbal learning disorders.

164 **Parent-to-Parent Network of Connecticut**
Family Center Dept of CT Children's Medical Center
282 Washington Street
Hartford, CT 06106
860-566-5298
FAX 860-545-9201
http://www.ccmckids.org
e-mail: mcole@ccmckids.org
Loreen Canter, Manager
Mary Ann Meade, Network Coordinator

A group of trained parent volunteers who help other parents who are seeking professional information and emotional support. Parent volunteers attend a series of training workshops designed to prepare them to provide support and information to other parents.

165 **Recording for the Blind & Dyslexic: Connecticut**
209 Orange Street
New Haven, CT 06510
203-624-4334
FAX 203-865-0203
http://www.rfbd.org
e-mail: connecticut@rfbd.org
Anne Fortunato, State Director

Provides textbooks on tape and computer disks to individuals who cannot read standard print because of a visual, perceptual or physical disability. Books span the entire educational spectrum from kindergarten through post graduate work and professional support. Master Tape Library contains almost 80,000 books on tape including a wide variety of science and technology books.
1959

166 **State Education Resources Center of Connecticut**
25 Industrial Park Road
Middletown, CT 06457
860-632-1485
FAX 860-632-8870
http://www.ctserc.org
e-mail: info@ctserc.org
Marianne Kirner, Executive Director
Sarah Barzee, Associate Director

A nonprofit agency primarily funded by the Connecticut State Department of Education. SERC provides professional development and information dissemination in the latest research and best practices to educators, services providers, and families throughout the state, as well as job-embedded technical assistance and training within schools, programs and districts.

1969

Delaware

167 **Easter Seals Delaware & Maryland's Eastern Shore**
61 Corporate Circle
New Castle, DE 19720
302-324-4444
800-677-3800
FAX 302-324-4441
TDY:302-324-4442
http://de.easterseals.com
Provides exceptional services to ensure that all people with disabilities or special needs and their families have equal opportunities to live, learn, work and play in their communities.

168 **Parent Information Center of Delware**
5570 Kirkwood Highway
Wilmington, DE 19808
302-999-7394
FAX 302-999-7637
http://www.picofdel.org
e-mail: picofdel@picofdel.org
A statewide non-profit organization dedicated to providing information, education and support, to families and caregivers of children with disabilites or special needs from birth to age 26. We strive to promote partnerships among families, educators, policy makers and the greater Delaware Community.

District of Columbia

169 **Center for Child and Human Development**
Georgetown University
PO Box 571485
Washington, DC 20057
202-687-5000
FAX 202-687-8899
http://www.gucchd.georgetown.edu
e-mail: gucdc@georgetown.edu
Phyllis Magrab PhD, Executive Director
Vernicy Thompson, Administrative Officer

Established over four decades ago to improve the quality of life for all children and youth, especially those with, or at risk for, special needs and their families. Brings together policy, research and clincal practice for the betterment of individuals and families, especially childre, youth and those with special needs including: developmental disabilities and special health care needs, mental health needs, young children and those in the child welfare system.

170 **Easter Seals Greater Washington BaltimoreRegion**
4041 Powder Mill Road
Calverton, MD 20705
301-931-8700
800-886-3771
FAX 301-931-8690
http://gwbr.easterseals.com
Lisa Reeves, President/CEO
Patricia Rohrer, Senior VP Programs

Provides exceptional services to ensure that all people with disabilities or special needs and their families have equal opportunities to live, learn, work and play in their communities. Proudly servinf Washington-Baltimore Region and the surrounding communities in Maryland, Northern Virginia and West Virginia.

171 **International Dyslexia Association of theDistrict of Columbia**
5914 Reservior Heights Avenue
Alexandria, VA 22311
703-827-9019
http://www.interdys.org
Ruth T Tifford, MEd, LCSW, President

The D.C. Capital Area Branch of the International Dyslexia Association provides support for individuals with dyslexia and their families in the Washington, DC metropolitan area, including parts of Maryland, Virginia and West Virginia. Our conferences, book sales and online information resources are designed to further the understanding of dyslexia and encourage the use of systematic, multisensory teaching methods enabling children and adults to reach their educational potential.

172 **Learning Disabilities Association of the District of Columbia**
PO Box 73275
Washington, DC 20015
202-387-1772
e-mail: ldaofdc@gmail.com
Connie Bumbaugh, Executive Director

LDA's mission is to create opportunities for success for all individuals affected by learning disabilities and to reduce the incidence of learning disabilities in future generations.

173 **Recording for the Blind & Dyslexic of Metropolitan Washington**
5225 Wisconsin Avenue NW
Washington, DC 20015
202-244-8990
FAX 202-244-1346
http://www.rfbd.org
e-mail: washingtondc@rfbd.org
Betsy Paul O'Connell, Executive Director
Courtney Arnold, Program Director
Toni Thomas, Outreach Director
Provides unlimited numbers of recorded textbooks to students with documented learning disability. Serves students in the District of Columbia, Montgomery and Prince Georges counties Maryland, and Northern Virginia.

174 **University Legal Services: Client Assistance Program**
University Legal Services
2201 Street NE
Washington, DC 20002
202-547-0198
877-221-4638
FAX 202-547-2662
http://www.uls-dc.org
e-mail: jcooney@uls-dc.org

Joe Cooney, Executive Director
William Findlan, Administrative Assistant

The goal of CAP is to identify, explain, and resolve the problems residents of the District of Columbia may be having with the rehabilitation program as quickly as possible.
1973

Florida

175 **Florida Advocacy Center for Persons with Disabilities**
2728 Centerview Drive
Tallahassee, FL 32301
850-488-9071
800-342-0823
FAX 850-488-8640
TDY:800-346-4127
http://www.advocacycenter.org
e-mail: webmaster@advocacycenter.org
Gary Weston, Executive Director

The Advocacy Center for Persons with Disabilities is a nonprofit organization providing protection and advocacy services in the State of Florida. Our mission is to advance the dignity, equality, self-determination and expressed choices of individuals with disabilities.

176 **Florida Bureau of Instructional Support &Community Services**
325 W Gaines Street
Tallahassee, FL 32399
850-488-1570
FAX 850-921-8246
Kate Kemker, Bureau Chief

The bureau has a broad range of responsibilities in the outgoing examination of state and federal laws, rules and regulations affecting public education and coordinating among other agencies, the delivery of services to public school students in Florida.

177 **International Dyslexia Association of Florida**
108 Lakeshore Drive
North Palm Beach, FL 33408
http://www.idafla.org
e-mail: jwsida@aol.com
Jean Walsh Schmidt, President

A non-profit, scientific and educational organization, which was formed to increase public awareness of dyslexia in Florida.
1949

178 **Learning Disabilities Association of Florida**
331 E Henry Street
Punta Gorda, FL 33950
941-637-8957
FAX 941-637-0617
http://www.lda-fl.org
e-mail: ldaf00@sunline.net
Jacky Egli, President
Alan Smolowe, Director
Kathy Shatlock, Executive Vice President
A nonprofit volunteer organization of parents, professionals, and LD adults. It is devoted to defining and finding solutions to the broad spectrum of learning issues.

179 **Mailman Center for Child Development: University of Miami Department of Pediatrics**
University of Miami School of Medicine
PO Box 1820
Miami, FL 33283
305-243-5790
FAX 305-326-7594
http://www.pediatrics.med.miami.edu
e-mail: reuben@miami.edu
Ruben Garcia, Asst Director Database Systems
Ana M Matias, Staff Associate
Neil Pilier, Communications Tech
The mission is to enhance the lives of individuals with developmental disabilities and their families by supporting personal and family relationships and facilitating independence, productivity, integration and inclusion.

180 **Recording for the Blind & Dyslexic: MiamiStudio**
6704 SW 80th Street
Miami, FL 33143
305-666-0552
http://www.rfbd.org
e-mail: cmccarthy@rfbd.org
Christine McCarthy, Executive Director
Kathleen Fisler, Studio Director

Georgia

181 **Easter Seals North Georgia**
1200 Lake Hearn Drive
Atlanta, GA 30319
404-943-1070
http://northgeorgia.easterseals.com
Donna Davidson, President/CEO

Provides information and referral, physical, occupational, and speech therapy, child care, Head Start and teacher training.

182 **Easter Seals Southern Georgia**
1906 Palmyra Road
Albany, GA 31701
229-439-7061
Creates solutions that change the lives of children, adults and families with disabilities or special needs by offering a variety of programs and services that enable individuals to lead lives of equality, dignity and independence.

183 **International Dyslexia Association of Geor**
1951 Greystone Road NW
Atlanta, GA 30318
404-256-1232
http://www.idaga.org
e-mail: info@midaga.org
Deborah Knight, President

Formed to increase public awareness about dyslexia in the State of Georgia. The Branch encourages teachers to train in multisensory language instruction. Provides a network for individuals with dyslexia, their families and professionals in the educational and medical fields.
300 members

184 **Learning Disabilities Association of Georg**
2566 Shallowford Road
Atlanta, GA 30345
404-303-7774
FAX 404-467-0190
http://www.ldag.org
e-mail: office@ldga.org
Joan Teach, PhD, President
Beth Martin, Secretary

One of 50 volunteer state organizations which comprise the Learning Disabilities Association of America. For over 30 years, LDAG has been enhancing the quality of life for individuals of all ages with Learning Disabilities and/or Attention Deficit and Hyperactivity Disorders.

185 **Recording for the Blind & Dyslexic: Georgi**
120 Florida Avenue
Athens, GA 30605
706-549-1313
FAX 706-227-6161
http://www.rfbd.org
e-mail: lmartin@rfbd.org
Lenore Martin, Executive Director
Fred Smith, Production Director
Bill Pass, Educational Outreach Director
A nonprofit volunteer organization, is the nation's educational library serving people who cannot effectively read standard print because of visual impairment, dyslexia and other physical disability. Our mission is to create opportunities for individual success by providing and, in the state of Georgia, promoting the effective use of, accessible educational materials.

Hawaii

186 **Aloha Special Technology Access Center**
710 Green Street
Honolulu, IH 96813
808-523-5547
FAX 808-536-3765
http://www.alohastac.org
e-mail: astachi@yahoo.com
Ali Sildert, President

Provide individuals with disabilities and their families access to computers, peripheral tools, and appropriate software. Aloha Stac aims to increase awareness, understanding, and implementation of microcomputer technology by establishing a program of activities and events to educate the community about what computers make possible for persons with disabilities.
1988

187 **Assistive Technology Resource Centers ofHawaii (ATRC)**
414 Kuwili Street
Honolulu, IH 96817
808-532-7110
800-645-3007
FAX 808-532-7120
http://www.atrc.org
e-mail: atrc-info@atrc.org
Barbara Fischlowitz-Leong, Executive Director

A statewide, non-profit organization committed to ensuring access to assistive technology for persons with disabilities. ATRC links individuals with technology so all people can participate in every aspect of community life. Also empowers individuals to maintain dignity and control their lives by promoting technology thorough, advocacy, training, information, and education.

188 **Easter Seals Hawaii**
710 Green Street
Honolulu, HI 96813
808-536-1015
FAX 808-536-3765
http://hawaii.easterseals.com

Norman Kawakami, Senior VP Operations

Provide exceptional services to ensure that all people with disabilities of special needs and their families have equal opportunities to live, learn, work and play in their communities.

189 **International Dyslexia Association of Hawaii**
PO Box 61610
Honolulu, HI 96839
808-538-7007
FAX 808-538-7009
http://www.dyslexia-hawaii.org
e-mail: hida@dyslexia-hawaii.org
Sue , President

HIDA's mission is to increase awareness of dyslexia in the community, provide support for parents and teachers, and promote teacher training. We also provide tutoring and testing referrals and information about other resources in Hawaii.
1986

190 **Learning Disabilities Association of Hawaii (LDAH)**
200 N Vineyard Boulevard
Honolulu, HI 96817
808-536-9684
FAX 808-5376780
http://www.ldahawaii.org
e-mail: ldah@ldaHawaii.org
Steven , President
Michael L , Executive Director
Tayne , Treasurer/Secretary
A non-profit organization founded in 1968 by parents of children with learning disabilities.
1968

Idaho

191 **Comprehensive Advocacy of Idaho**
1177 Emerald Street
Boise, ID 83706
208-336-5353
866-262-3462
FAX 208-336-5396
TDY:208-336-5353
http://www.users.moscow.com/co-ad
e-mail: coadinc@cableone.net
James R Baugh, Executive Director

The designated Protection and Advocacy System for Idaho provides advocacy for people with disabilities who have been abused/neglected; denied services or benefits; have experienced rights violations or discrimination because of their disability, or have voting accessibility problems. Also provides information & referral; negotiation & mediation; short term & technical assistance; legal advice/representation.
1977

192 **High Reachers Arc**
140 E 2nd N
Mountain Home, ID 83647
208-587-5804
800-559-5804
TDY:208-343-2950
http://www.thearcinc.org
Steve Patterson, President
Sharon Hubler, Vice President
Robert Brannam, Treasurer
Our mission is to secure for people with disabilities the opportunity to choose and realize their goals of where and how they learn, liver, work and play; to foster the development of programs on their behalf; to support families in the solution of their problems; to develop a better public understanding of mental retardation; to cooperate with public, private, religious, and professional groups in the furtherance of these efforts.
1956

193 **International Dyslexia Association of Idah**
PO Box 1247
Mercer Island, WA 98040
206-382-1020
http://www.wabida.org
e-mail: info@wabida.org
Bonnie Meyer, President

The Washington State Branch of the International Dyslexia Association is a 501 (c)(3) non-profit, scientific and educational organization dedicated to the study and treatment of dyslexia. This banch serves individuals in Washington, Alaska, Idaho, and western Montana.

194 **Learning Disabilities Association of America: Idaho**
9797 N Circle Drive
Hayden, ID 83835
208-762-2316
http://www.ldanatl.org
e-mail: connect4kids@imbris.com
Ginny , Contact

To create opportunities for success for all individuals affected by learning disabilities and to reduce the incidence of learning disabilities in tfuture generations.

Illinois

195 **Child Care Association of Illinois**
300 E Monroe Street
Springfield, IL 62701
217-528-4409
FAX 217-528-6498
http://www.cca-il.org
e-mail: ilccamb@aol.com

A voluntary, not-for-profit organization dedicated to improving the delivery of social services to the abused, neglected, and troubled children, youth and families of Illinois.
1964

196 **Easter Seals Metropolitan Chicago**
14 E Jackson Boulevard
Chicago, IL 60604
312-939-5115
FAX 312-939-0283
http://chicago.easterseals.com
F Timothy , President/CEO

Provides comprehensive services for individuals with disabilities or other special needs and their families to improve quality of life and maximize independence.

197 **Guild for the Blind**
180 N Michigan Avenue
Chicago, IL 60601
312-236-8569
FAX 312-236-8128
http://www.guildfortheblind.org
e-mail: info@guildfortheblind.org
David , Executive Director
Kathy , Operations Director

Support and information for families and individuals with visual disabilities.

198 **Illinois Protection & Advocacy Agency: Equip for Equality**
20 N Michigan Avenue
Chicago, IL 60602
312-341-0022
800-537-2632
FAX 312-341-0295
http://www.equipforequality.org
e-mail: hn6177@handsnet.org
Michael A , Chairperson
Zena , President/CEO

Advances the human and civil rights of children and adults with physical and mental disabilities in Illinois. The only statewide, cross-disability, comprehensive advocacy organization providing self-advocacy assistance, legal services, and disability rights education while also engaging in public policy and legislative advocacy and conducting abuse investigations and other oversight activities.
1985

199 **International Dyslexia Association of Illinois/Missouri**
751 Roosevelt Road
Glen Ellyn, IL 60137
630-469-6900
FAX 630-469-6810
http://www.readibida.org
e-mail: info@readibida.org

Kathleen L Wagner, Executive Director
Jo Ann Paldo, President
Formed to increase public awareness of dyslexia in Illinois and Eastern Missouri. We have been serving individuals with dyslexia, their families, and professionals for 25 years. One of our primary objectives is to increase early intervention efforts.

200 **Jewish Child & Family Services**
216 W Jackson Boulevard
Chicago, IL 60606
312-444-2090
FAX 312-855-3754
http://www.jcfs.org
e-mail: robertbloom@jcbchicago.org
Robert Bloom PhD, Manager

Provides a range of comprehensive programs designed to enable individuals and families to grow and develop positively throughout their lives.

201 **Learning Disabilities Association of Illinois**
10101 S Roberts Road
Palos Hills, IL 60465
708-430-7532
FAX 708-430-7592
http://www.ldaamerica.org
e-mail: ldaofil@ameritech.net
Ernie Florence, President
Sharon Schussler, Manager

A nonprofit organization dedicated to the advancement of the education and general welfare of children and youth of normal or potentially normal intelligence who have learning disabilities of a perceptual, conceptual or coordinative nature or related problems. Publishes quarterly newsletter.

202 **Recording for the Blind & Dyslexic: Chicago Loop Studio**
180 N Michigan Avenue
Chicago, IL 60603
312-236-8715
FAX 312-236-8719
http://www.rfbd.org/Illinois_unit
e-mail: jmilkovich@rfvd.org
Janet Milkovich, State Director
Nate Meyer, Production Director
Doug Hagman, Outreach Director

203 **Recording for the Blind & Dyslexic: Lois C Klein Studio**

9612C W 143rd Street
Orland Park, IL 60462
708-349-9356
http://www.rfbd.org
e-mail: selhenicky@rfbd.org
Sandy Elhenicky, Studio Director

204 **Recording for the Blind & Dyslexic: Naperville**
1266 E Chicago Avenue
Naperville, IL 60540
630-420-0722
FAX 630-420-8975
http://www.rfbd.org
e-mail: nleone@rfbd.org
Nina Leone, Production Director

Indiana

205 **Bridgepointe Services & Goodwill of Southern Indiana**
1329 Applegate Lane
Clarksville, IN 47131
812-283-7908
800-660-3355
FAX 812-288-8127
TDY:812-283-7908
e-mail: cmarshall@bridgepointe.org
Caren Marshall, Executive Director
Candice Barksdale, VP Development

Children's Academy is an inclusive early childhood center and preschool program ages 6 weeks to 5 years.

206 **Easter Seal Arc of Northeast Indiana**
4919 Coldwater Road
Fort Wayne, IN 46825
260-456-4534
800-234-7811
FAX 260-745-5200
http://neindiana.easterseals.com

207 **Indiana Vocational Rehabilitation Services**
1452 Vaxter Avenue
Clarksville, IN 47129
877-228-1967
FAX 812-282-7048
Delbert Hayden, Supervisor

Purpose is to assist the community by providing services which allow individuals to maximize their potential and to participate in work, family and the community. To do this we will provide rehabilitation, education and training.

208 **International Dyslexia Association of Indiana**
2511 E 46th Street
Indianapolis, IN 46205
FAX 317-705-2067
http://www.inbofida.org
e-mail: inbofida@hotmail.com
Mary Ian McAteer, President

A non-profit organization dedicatedt to helping individuals with dyslexia, their families and the communities that support them. Promotes and disseminates researched-based knowledge for early identification, effective teaching approaches and intervention strategies for dyslexics.
1971

209 **Learning Disabilities Association of India**
508 E 86th Street
Indianapolis, IN 46240
317-872-4331
800-284-2519
FAX 574-272-3058
http://www.ldaofindiana.org
Sharla Griffith, Owner
Sharon Harris, President
Dawn Lytle, Vice President
A non-profit, volunteer organization of parents, educators, and other individuals who are committed to promoting awareness, knowledge and acceptance of individuals with learning disabilities and associated disorders such as attention deficit/hyperactivity disorders.
1972

210 **Southwestern Indiana Easter Seal**
Rehabilitation Center
3701 Bellemeade Avenue
Evansville, IN 47714
812-479-1411
FAX 812-437-2634
http://www.easterasealswindiana.com
Ray Rasior, President

The Easter Seals Rehabilitation Center in Evansville, IN provides services to children and adults with disabilities and other special needs and support to their families.

Iowa

211 **Center for Disabilities and Developemnt**
University of Iowa Children's Hospital
100 Hawkins Drive
Iowa City, IA 52242
319-353-6900
877-686-0031
FAX 319-356-8284
http://www.uihealthcare.com/cdd
e-mail: cdd-scheduling@uiowa.edu
Elayne O Sexsmith MA, Adminstrator
Stacy McConkey MD, Medical Director

Improve the health and independence of people with disabilities and advance the community systems on which they rely.

1947

212 **International Dyslexia Association of Iowa**
PO Box 11188
Cedar Rapids, IA 52410 319-377-8371
http://www.ida-ia.org
Terri Petersen, President

Provides workshops, hands-on simulations, and resources to incease public awareness of dyslexia.

213 **Iowa Program for Assistive Technology**
Center for Disabilities and Development
100 Hawkins Drive
Iowa City, IA 52242 319-353-6900
800-331-3027
FAX 319-384-5139
TDY:877-686-0032
http://www.uiowa.edu/infotech/
e-mail: jane-gay@uiowa.edu
Jane Gay, Director
Amy Mikelson, Outreach Coordinator
Mark Moser, Administrator
IPAT's goals are to promote and create systems change in the state with regards to assistive technology (AT) and it's use. IPAT works with consumers and family members, service providers, and state and local agencies/organizations to promote assistive technology through awareness, training, and policy work. IPAT accomplishes this through five specifi goal areas: education, employment, health, community living and recreation, telecommunication and information technology.

214 **Learning Disabilities Association of Iowa**
321 E 6th Street
Cedar Falls, IA 50309 515-280-8558
888-690-5324
FAX 515-243-1902
http://www.lda-ia.org
e-mail: kahtylda@askresource.org
Richard Owens, President
Kathy Specketer, State Coordinator

Kansas

215 **Capper Foundation Easter Seals**
3500 SW 10th Avenue
Topeka, KS 66604 785-272-4060
FAX 785-272-7912
http://capper.easterseals.com
Jim Leiker, President/CEO
Debby O'Neill, VP Programs/Services
Pam Walstrom, VP Development
A community resource providing services to enhance the independence of people with disabilities, primarily children.

216 **Disability Rights Center of Kansas (DRC)**
635 SW Harrison Street
Topeka, KS 66603 785-273-9661
877-776-1541
FAX 785-273-9414
http://www.drckansas.org
e-mail: info@ksadv.org
Rocky Nichols MPA, Executive Director
Kirk Lowry, Litigation Director
Timothy Voth JD, Advocacy Director
Formerly Kansas Advocacy & Protection Services, a public interest legal advocacy agency empowered by federal law to advocate for the civil and legal rights of Kansans with disabilities.

217 **Goodwill Industries Easter Seals of Kansas**
3636 N Oliver
Wichita, KS 67208 316-744-9291
http://goodwillkansas.easterseals.com
Emily Compton, President/CEO
Gayle Goetz, VP Development

Provides education, training and employment for people with disabilities and other barriers to employment.

218 **International Dyslexia Association of Kansas/Missouri**
430 E Blue Ridge Boulevard
Topeka, KS 64145 816-838-7323
http://www.ksmoida.org
e-mail: info@ksmoida.org
Billie Calvery, President
Susan Long, Treasurer

Focuses efforts on Kansas and Western Missouri. By hosting events and establishing a presence, the leaders have begun to work with parents, schools and teachers to help children with dyslexia. Maintains a list of individuals who have specialized training and who are available for remediation of reading, writing and spelling problems. Provides information for parents and teachers, an annual spring conference, quarterly newsletter dealing with local issues, and teacher training.
1949

219 **Learning Disabilities Association of Kansas**
PO Box 4424
Topeka, KS 66604 785-273-4505
FAX 785-228-9527
http://www.ldakansas.org
e-mail: marciasu@aol.com
Diane Miller, President
Cindy Swarner, Vice President
Andrea Blair, Secretary
LDAK is a nonprofit, volunteer organization whose purpose is to advance the education and general well-being of children and adults with learning disabilities.

Kentucky

220 **International Dyslexia Association of Kentucky: Ohio Valley Branch**
317 E 5th Street
Cincinati, OH 45202 513-651-4747
http://www.cincinnatidyslexia.org
Martha Chiodi, President

A non-profit, scientific and educational organization dedicated to the study and treatment of the learning disability, dyslexia. This Branch was formed to increase public awareness of dyslexia on the Southern Ohio, Southeast Indiana, Kentucky and Huntington, West Virginia areas.

221 **International Dyslexia Association:Kentucky**
3508 Hackworth Road
Knoxville, TN 37931 877-836-6432
FAX 865-693-3656
http://www.tn-interdys.org
e-mail: Tennessee_IDA@hotmail.com
Martie Wood, President

The Tennessee Branch of the International Dyslexia Association (TN-IDA) was formed to increase awareness about Dyslexia in the state of Tennessee. TN-IDA supports efforts to provide information regarding appropriate language arts instruction to those involved with language-based learning differences and to encourage the identity of these individuals at-risk for such disorders as soon as possible. This branch also serves individuals in the state of Kentucky.

222 **Learning Disabilities Association of Kentuucky**
2210 Goldsmith Lane
Louisville, KY 40218 502-473-1256
877-587-1256
FAX 502-473-4695
http://www.ldaofky.org
e-mail: ldaofky@yahoo.com
Catherine Senn, President
Tim Woods, Executive Director

A non-profit organization of individuals with learning differences and attention difficulties, their parents, educators, and other service providers.

223 **Recording for the Blind & Dyslexic: Kentucky**

240 Haldeman Avenue
Louisville, KY 40206
502-895-9068
FAX 502-897-1145
http://www.rfbd.org
e-mail: strester@rfbd.org

Sarah , Executive Director
Joel , Production Director

Utilizes volunteers in multiple areas of operation including board and committee, membership, ausio production, educational outreach, public information and fundraising.

Louisiana

224 **Baton Rouge Advocacy Center**

8225 Florida Blvd
Baton Rouge, LA 70806
225-925-8884
800-711-1696
FAX 225-925-9625
http://www.advocacyla.org

Sharia , Intake Specialist

Protects and advocates for the human and legal rights of persons living in Louisiana who are elderly or disabled.

225 **Easter Seals Louisiana**

1010 Common Street
New Orleans, LA 70112
504-523-7325
800-695-7325
FAX 504-523-3465
http://louisiana.easterseals.com

A non-profit, community-based health agency whose mission is to help children and adults with disabilities achieve independence through a variety of programs and services.
1951

226 **International Dyslexia Association of Louisiana**

149 Jefferson Oaks Drive
Ruston, LA 71270
985-414-2575
http://www.labida.org
e-mail: alicehigginbotham@hotmail.com

Alice Higginbotham, President

Provides infomraiton and resources to parents, educators, students and the community in a way that creates a clear and psoitive understanding of dyslexia and related language learning needs so that every individual has the opportunity to lead a productive and fulfilling life for the benefit of the society.

227 **Lafayette Advocacy Center**

600 Jefferson Street
Lafayette, LA 70501
337-237-7380
800-822-0210
FAX 337-237-0486
http://www.advocacyla.org

Christy Lamas, CAP Client Advocate

Protects and advocates for the human and legal rights of persons living in Louisiana who are elderly or disabled.

228 **New Orleans Advocacy Center**

1010 Common Street
New Orleans, LA 70112
504-522-2337
800-960-7705
FAX 504-522-5507
http://www.advocacyla.org
e-mail: advocacycenter@advocacyla.org

Lois Simpson, Executive Director
Susan Bushnell, Advocacy Services Director

Protects and advocates for the human and legal rights of persons living in Louisiana who are elderly or disabled.

229 **Shreveport Advocacy Center**

2620 Centenary Boulevard
Shreveport, LA 71104
318-227-6186
800-839-7688
FAX 318-227-1841
http://www.advocacyla.org

Jackolyn Sanchez, Intake Specialist Coordinator
Diane Mirvis, Client Asst Program Director

Protects and advocates for the human and legal rights of persons living in Louisiana who are elderly or disabled.

Maine

230 **Easter Seals Maine**

125 Presumpscot Street
Portland, ME 04103
207-828-0754
FAX 207-828-5355
http://maine.easterseals.com

Todd Mosher, Chairman

Creates solutions that change lives of children and adults with disabilities or other special needs and their families.

231 **International Dyslexia Association of Maine**

PO Box 3724
Concord, NH 03302
603-229-7355
http://www.nhida.org
e-mail: information@nhida.org

Colleen Silva, President

The New Hampshire Branch of The International Dyslexia Association (NH/IDA) is a 501(c)(3) non-profit, scientific and educational organization dedicated to the study and treatment of the learning disability, dyslexia. The New Hampshire Branch was formed in 2002 to increase public awareness of dyslexia. The New Hampshire Branch serves New Hampshire, Maine and Vermont.

232 **Learning Disabilities Association of Maine (LDA)**

97 Rocky Shore Lane
Oakland, ME 04963
207-465-7700
FAX 207-465-4844
http://www.ldame.org
e-mail: info@ldame.org

Kim LeClair, President
Brenda Bennett, Executive Director

Dedicated to assisting individuals with learning and attention disabilities through support, education and advocacy.

233 **Maine Parent Federation**

12 Shuman Ave, Ste 7
Augusta, ME 04338
207-623-2144
800-870-7746
FAX 207-623-2148
http://www.mpf.org
e-mail: parentconnnect@mpf.org

Janice LaChance, Executive Director

The Maine Parent Federation is a statewide organiztion that provides information, advocacy, education, and training to benefit all children. We promote individual aspirations and community inclusion for people with disabilities.
1984

Maryland

234 **Association for Childhood Education International (ACEI)**

17904 Georgia Avenue
Olney, MD 20832
301-570-2111
800-423-3563
FAX 301-570-2212
http://www.acei.org
e-mail: headquarters@acei.org

Karen Liu, President
Gerald C Odland, Executive Director

Mission is to promote and support in global community the optimal education and development of children, from birth through early adolescence, and to influence the professional growth of educators and the efforts of others who are committed to the needs of children in a changing society.

235 Federation of Families for Children'sMental Health
9605 Medical Center Drive
Rockville, MD 20850
240-403-1901
FAX 240-403-1909
http://www.ffcmh.org
e-mail: ffcmh@ffcmh.org
Sandra Spencer, Executive Director
Ashwanda Fleming, COO

Dedicated exclusively to helping children with mental health needs and their families achieve a better quality of life.

236 International Dyslexia Association of Maryland
PO Box 792
Brooklandville, MD 21022
410-825-2881
http://www.interdys.org
e-mail: mbida4@hotmail.com
Lucinda Draine, President

Believes that all individuals have the right to achieve their full potential and that individual learning abilities can be strengthen. MBIDA will promote and organize classes and workshops to provide informtion and training for dyslexic individuals, educators, parents and others.

237 Learning Disabilities Association of Maryland
PO Box 268
Huntingtown, MD 20639
888-265-6459
http://www.ldamaryland.org
e-mail: ldamaryland@aol.com
Diane Chesley, President

Dedicated to enhancing the quality of life for all individuals with learning disabilities and their families through awareness, advocacy, education, service and collaborative efforts.

238 Maryland Association of University Centers on Disabilities
1010 Wayne Avenue
Silver Spring, MD 20910
301-588-8252
FAX 301-588-2842
http://www.aucd.org
e-mail: gjesien@aucd.org
Royal P Walker Jr, JD, President
George Jesien, Executive Director

The mission of AUCD is to advance policy and practice for and with people living with developmental and other disabilities, their families, and communities by supporting our members to engage in research, education, and service activities that achieve our vision

Massachusetts

239 Access to Design Professions
Adaptive Environments
374 Congress Street
Boston, MA 02210
617-695-1225
800-949-4232
FAX 617-482-8099
http://www.adaptiveenvironments.org
e-mail: info@adaptiveenvironments.org
Valerie Fletcher, Executive Director
Ana Julian, Design & Communications Coord

This project wil find ways that people with disabilities can enter and sustain themselves in the professions of architecture, industrial design, interior design, and landscape architecure.

240 Adaptive Environments
180-200 Portland St
Boston, MA 02114
617-695-1225
FAX 617-482-8099
http://www.adaptiveenvironments.org
e-mail: info@adaptiveenvironments.org
Valerie Fletcher, Executive Director
Ana Julian, Design & Communications Coord

Committed to advancing the role of design in expanding opportunity and enhancing experience for people of all ages and abiliites.
1978

241 Easter Seals Massachusetts
484 Main Street
Worcester, MA 01608
800-922-8290
FAX 508-831-9768
http://ma.easterseals.com
e-mail: info@eastersealsma.com
John S Cleary, Chairman

Provides services to ensure that children and adults with disabilities have equal opportunities to live, learn, work and play.

242 International Dyslexia Association of Massachusetts
PO Box 662
Lincoln, MA 01773
617-650-0011
http://www.interdys.org
e-mail: mabida@comcast.net
Isabel Wesley, President

The Massachusetts Branch of The International Dyslexia Association (MABIDA) is a 501(c)(3) non-profit, scientific and educational organization dedicated to the study and treatment of dyslexia. This Branch was formed to increase public awareness of dyslexia in Massachusetts.

243 Learning Disabilities Worldwide (LDW)
PO Box 142
Weston, MA 02493
781-890-5399
FAX 781-647-5141
http://www.ldam.org
Robin Welch, President
Georgios Sideridis, Vice President
Teresa Allissa Citro, Executive Director
Formerly the Learning Disabilities Association of Massachusetts, works to enhance the lives of individuals with learning disabilities, with a specail emphasis on the underserved. The purpose is to identify and support the unrecognized strengths and capabilities of a person with learning disabilities. We strive to increase awareness and understanding of learning disabilities through our multilingual media productions and publications that serve populations across cultures and nations.
15,000 members 1965

244 Massachusetts Association of 766 ApprovedPrivate Schools (MAAPS)
591 N Avenue
Wakefield, MA 01880
781-245-1220
FAX 781-245-5294
http://www.spedschools.com
e-mail: info@maaps.org
James Major, Manager
Rita Greenberg, Business Manager

Nonprofit association of Chapter 766 approved private schools dedicated to providing educational programs and services to students with special needs throughout Massachusetts. Concerned that children with special needs have appropriate, quality education and that they and their families know the rights, policies, procedures and options that make the education process a productive reality for special needs children.

245 Recording for the Blind & Dyslexic: Berkshire/Williamstown
622A Main Street
Williamstown, MA 01267
413-458-3641
800-221-4792
http://www.rfbd.org
e-mail: berkshire@rfbd.org
Jeff Owens, Executive Director
Cristina Osorio, Studio Director

The Berkshire United Way operates recording studios in both Lenox and Williamstown. The studios offer information on recordings of books on audio cassette and computer disk, and provides outreach to: four western counties of Massachusetts; Albany, Columbia, Rensselaer, Saratoga, Schenectady and Washington counties in New York; Bennington County in Vermont; Litchfield County in Connecticut.

246 **Recording for the Blind & Dyslexic: Boston**
58 Charles Street
Cambridge, MA 02141 617-577-1111
http://www.rfbd.org
Christina Raimo, Executive Director
Jennifer Dougherty, Outreach Coordinator
Jeanne Guiney, Educational Outreach Director
A nonprofit volunteer organization and educational library serving people who cannot effectively read standard print because of visual impairment, dyslexia or other physical disability. We strive to create opportunities for individual success by providing accessible educational material. Comprehensive source of recorded textbooks and other educational printed matter. One-time registration fee of $50.00 plus a $25.00 annual fee. School memberships are available.

247 **Recording for the Blind & Dyslexic:Berkshire/Lenox**
55 Pittsfield-Lenox Road
Lenox, MA 01240 413-637-0889
http://www.rfbd.org
e-mail: berkshire@rfbd.org
The Berkshire United Way operates recording studios in both Lenox and Williamstown. The studios offer information on recordings of books on audio cassette and computer disk, and provides outreach to: four western counties of Massachusetts; Albany, Columbia, Rensselaer, Saratoga, Schenectady and Washington counties in New York; Bennington County in Vermont; Litchfield County in Connecticut.

Michigan

248 **Easter Seals Michigan**
1105 N Telegraph Road
Waterford, MI 48328 248-451-2900
FAX 248-338-0095
http://mi.easterseals.com
Creates solutions that change lives of children and adults with disabilities or other special needs and their families.

249 **International Dyslexia Association of Michigan**
983 Spaulding Avenue SE
Ada, MI 49301 616-717-2984
http://www.idamib.org
e-mail: postmaster@idamib.org
Michael Ryan PhD, President

The purpose of the Michigan Branch of the International Dyslexia Association is to develop awareness and provide information about Dyslexia.

250 **Learning Disabilities Association of Michigan (LDA)**
200 Museum Drive
Lansing, MI 48933 517-485-8160
888-597-7809
FAX 517-485-8462
http://www.ldaofmichigan.org
e-mail: info@ldaofmichigan.org

Ed Schlitt, President
Flo Curtis, Manager

A nonprofit, volunteer association that is dedicated to enhancing the quality of life for all individuals with learning disabilities and their families through advocacy, education, training, services and support of research. Our goal is to see LD understood and addressed and the individuals with learning disabilities will thrive and participate fully in society.
1,200 Members

251 **Michigan Citizens Alliance to Uphold Special Education (CAUSE)**
6412 Centurion Drive
Lansing, MI 48917 517-886-9167
800-221-9105
FAX 517-886-9366
TDY:888-814-4013
http://www.causeonline.org
e-mail: info@causeonline.org
Mary Suurmeyer, Executive Director
Frances Spring, Assistant Program Director
CAUSE shall provide a collaborative forum where consumers and providers can actively support an individualized Free Appropriate Public Education (FAPE) that enables all students to maximize their options in the world community. Our priority is to protect and advocate for all the educational rights of students with disabilities.
1970

252 **Recording for the Blind & Dyslexic Learning**
5600 Rochester Road
Troy, MI 48085 248-879-0101
FAX 248-879-9927
http://www.rfbd.org
e-mail: creeb@rfbd.org

Carla Reeb, Executive Director
Don Haffner, Studio Director

Recording for the Blind & Dyslexic is the nation's educational library serving people who cannot effectively read standard print because of visual impairment, dyslexia or other physical disability. We provide textbooks, educational and professional materials in an audio format. The Michigan Unit's outreach volunteers offer students and their parents training sessions at the studio by appointment.
1958

Minnesota

253 **International Dyslexia Association of Minnesota**
5021 Vernon Avenue S
Minneapolis, MN 55436 651-450-7589
http://www.umbida.org
e-mail: info@umbida.org
Claire Eckley, President

254 **Learning Disabilities Association of Minnesota**
5354 Parkdale Drive
St Louis Park, MN 55416 952-922-8374
FAX 952-922-8102
http://www.ldaminnesota.org
e-mail: info@ldaminnesota.org
Kitty Christiansen, Executive Director

255 **Minnesota Access Services**
3131 19th Avenue S
Minneapolis, MN 55407 612-668-4326
FAX 612-668-4310
http://www.mplscommunityed.com
e-mail: jean.dutcher@mpls.k12.mn.us
Jack Tamble, Director

Minneapolis Commuity Education exists to support the learning and participation of adults and children so they can improve their lives and their community.

256 **Minnesota Disability Protection & Advocacy Agency**
430 1st Avenue N
Minneapolis, MN 55401 612-334-5784
800-292-4150
FAX 612-334-5755
TDY:612-332-4668
http://www.mndlc.org
e-mail: mndlc@midmnlegal.org

Pamela Hoopes, Manager
Brenda Jursik, Administrator

Mission is to advance the dignity, self-determination and equality of individuals with disabilities.

257 **Technical Assistance Alliance for ParentCenters**
8161 Normandale Boulevard
Minneapolis, MN 55437 952-838-9000
888-248-0822
FAX 952-838-0199
http://www.taalliance.org
e-mail: alliance@taalliance.org

Paula F Goldberg, Co-Director
Sue Folger, Project Co-Director
Sharman Davis Barren, Project Co-Director
An innovative project that supports a unified technical assistance system for the purpose of developing, assisting and coordinating Parent Training Information Projects and Community Parent Resource Centers.

Mississippi

258 Learning Disabilities Association of Mississippi
4080 Old Canton Road
Jackson, MS 39216
601-362-1667
FAX 301-362-9180
http://www.ldams.org
e-mail: ldams@bellsouth.net
Martha Kabbes Burns, Contact

A non-profit, volunteer organization that is an informational Support Center for parents of children with learning disabilities, adults with learning disabilities, and professionals providing services related to learning disabilities.

Missouri

259 Easter Seals Missouri
13975 Manchester Road
Manchester, MO 63011
636-227-6030
800-664-5025
FAX 636-779-2270
http://mo.easterseals.com
e-mail: mail@mo.easterseals.com
Craig Byrd, President/CEO
Kathleen Fagin, COO

Provides exceptional services to ensure all people with disabilities have equal opportunities to live, learn, work and play in their communities.

260 Learning Disabilities Association of Missouri
1942 E Meadowmere #104
Springfield, MO 65808
417-864-5110
FAX 417-864-7290
http://www.ldamo.org
Donna Blevins, President
Eileen Hunt, First VP

261 Learning Disabilities Association of the Ozarks
PO Box 4362
Springfield, MO 65808
417-882-2008
http://www.ldaozarks.org
e-mail: info@ldaozarks.org
Kim Nye, President
Sara Hester, Vice President

A non-profit, volunteer organization committed to children and adults who have learning disabilities. Founded by parents of children with learning disabilities, they saw the need to provide support and guidance to other families experiencing this challenge.
1967

262 Missouri Protection & Advocacy Servicesn Inc
925 S Country Club Drive
Jefferson, MO 65109
573-893-3333
800-392-8667
FAX 573-893-4231
http://www.moadvocacy.org
e-mail: mopasjc@earthlink.net
Cynthia Keele, Chair
Patricia Flood, Secretar/Treasurer

A federally mandated system in the state which provides protection of the rights of persons with disabilities through leagally-based advocacy. The mission is to protect the rights of individuals with disabilities by providing advocacy and legal services.
1977

263 St. Louis Learning Disabilities Association Inc
13537 Barrett Parkway Drive
Ballwin, MO 63021
314-966-3088
FAX 314-966-1806
http://www.ldastl.org
e-mail: info@ldastl.org
Pam Kortum, Executive Director
Anna Rich, Educational Consultant/Prog. Dir

A non-profit organization dedicated to enhancing the understanding and acceptance of learning disabilities. Education, support, and consultation are provided to children, parents, and professionals to help reach their full potential.
1993

Montana

264 International Dyslexia Association of Montana
PO Box 1247
Mercer Island, WA 98040
206-382-1020
http://www.wabida.org
e-mail: info@wabida.org
Bonnie Meyer, President

The Washington State Branch of the International Dyslexia Association is a 501 (c)(3) non-profit, scientific and educational organization dedicated to the study and treatment of dyslexia. Our all volunteer board of directors seeks to increase public awareness of dyslexia in our branch's area which includes Washington, Alaska, Idaho, and western Montana.

265 Learning Disabilities Association of Montana
3544 Toboggan Road
Billings, MT 59101
406-259-3110
http://www.ldaofmt.org
e-mail: info@ldaofmt.org
Marl Taylor, President

The Learning Disabilities Association of Montana assists individuals with learning disabilities through information, advocacy and support.

266 Montana Advocacy Program (MAP)
400 N Park, 2nd Floor
Helena, MT 59624
406-449-2344
800-245-4743
FAX 406-449-2418
http://www.mtadv.org
e-mail: advocate@mtadv.org
Bernadette Franks-Ongoy, Executive Director
Liesl Beck, Advocacy Specialist

A non-profit coporatoin that administers eight Protection and Advocacy programs and one private program that advocates the rights of Montanans with disabilities. Protect and advocate the human, legal, and civil rights of Montanans with disabilities while advancing dignity, equality, and self-determination.

267 Montana Parents, Let's Unite for Kids (PLUK)
516 N 32nd Street
Billings, MT 59101
406-255-0540
800-222-7585
FAX 406-255-0523
http://www.pluk.org/
e-mail: plukinfo@pluk.org
Bill O'Connor, President
Dave Rye, VP

PLUK is a private, nonprofit organization formed by parents of children with disabilities and chronic illnesses. Its purpose is to provide information, support, training and assistance to aid parents with their children at home, in school and as adults. We keep current on best practices in education, medicine, law, human services, rehabilitation, and technology to insure families with disabilites have access to high quality services.

1984

Nebraska

268 Easter Seals Nebraska
638 N 109th Plaza
Omaha, NE 68154
402-345-2500
800-650-9880
Provides exceptional services to help ensure all people with disabilities have an equal opportunity to live, learn, work and play.

269 International Dyslexia Association of Nebraska
5921 Sunrise Road
Lincoln, NE 68510
402-488-7920
FAX 410-321-5069
http://www.ne-ida.com
e-mail: carolyn.brandl@ne-ida.com
Carolyn Brandle, President

Nebraska Branch works to enhance the public's perception and understanding of dyslexia and related language/learning disabilities.
1984

270 Learning Disabilities Association of Nebraska
3135 N 93rd Street
Ohama, NE 68134
402-348-1567
FAX 402-934-1479
http://www.ldanebraska.org
e-mail: ldaofneb@yahoo.com
Stephanie Cain, President

Support groups for parents and teachers, information for school and the community about ADHD and LD children/adults. Offers book and video library, educational seminars and conferences, parent panels. Quarterly newsletter.
1984

Nevada

271 Easter Seals Southern Nevada
6200 W Oakey Boulevard
Las Vegas, NV 89146
702-870-7050
http://sn.easterseals.com
Provides services to children and adults with disabilities and other special needs, and support to their families.

272 International Dyslexia Association of Arizona
18647 N 20th Street
Phoenix, AZ 85024
602-867-9660
FAX 602-867-2762
http://www.dyslexia-az.org
e-mail: willcoxon@cox.net
Marilyn Willcoxon, President

The Arizona Branch of The International Dyslexia Association (AIDA) is a 501 (c)(3) non-profit, scientific organization dedicated to educating the public about the learning disability, dyslexia. The Arizona Branch has four objectives: to increase awareness in the dyslexic and general community; to network with other learning disability groups and legislators in education; to increase membership; to raise funds for future projects that will make a difference in our community. Serves Arizona.

273 International Dyslexia Association of Central California

28847 Ave 176
Porterville, CA 93257
559-781-8505
FAX 559-781-8505
http://www.interdys.org
e-mail: gailjrider@aol.com

Gail Januska, President

We are a non-profit organization, that disseminates information concerning the work of the late Dr. Samuel T Orton in the field of reading, writing, spelling and speech disabilities and associated disorders. We provide referral services (tutors, testers, schools, etc.), workshops, speakers, fact sheets, answer questions etc. about studies, research, diagnosis, treatment, acdemic difficulties, facilities for help with training. Serves individuals in the state of Nevada.

274 International Dyslexia Association of Nevada: Inland Empire Branch
5225 Canyon Crest Drive
Riverside, CA 92507
951-686-9837
http://www.dyslexia-ca.org
e-mail: dyslexiainfo@gmail.com
Regina G Richards, President

We are a volunteer organization of parents and professionals who care about literacy. Our focus is to benefit individuals, adults, students, families, educators, and professionals dealing with dyslexia and learning disabilities. Serves individuals in the state of Nevada.

275 Learning Disabilities Association of Nevada
1944 Sioux City Court
Henderson, NV 89052
http://www.ldaamerica.org
e-mail: adhdservices@cox.net
Rose Moore, Contact

To create opportunities for success for all individuals affected by learning disabilities and to reduce the incidence of learning disabilities in future generations.

New Hampshire

276 Easter Seals New Hampshire
555 Auburn Street
Manchester, NH 03103
603-623-8863
800-870-8728
FAX 603-625-1148
http://www.eastersealsnh.org
Larry Gammon, President
Christine M McMahon, Senior VP/COO
Elin A Treanor, SVP/CFO
Easter Seals New Hampshire is one of the most comprehensive affiliates in the nation, assisting more than 18,000 children and adults with disabilities through a network of more than a dozen service sites around the state and in Vermont. Each center provides top-quality, family-focused and innovative services tailored to meet the specific needs of the particular community it serves.
1936

277 International Dyslexia Association of NewHampshire
PO Box 3724
Concord, NH 03302
603-229-7355
http://http://www.nhida.org
e-mail: information@nhida.org
Colleen Sliva, President

The New Hampshire Branch of The International Dyslexia Association (NH/IDA) is a 501(c)(3) non-profit, scientific and educational organization dedicated to the study and treatment of the learning disability, dyslexia. The New Hampshire Branch was formed in 2002 to increase public awareness of dyslexia. The New Hampshire Branch serves New Hampshire, Maine and Vermont

278 Learning Disabilities Association of New Hampshire
PO Box 127
Concord, NH 03302
603-424-6667
http://www.ldanh.org
e-mail: information@ldanh.org
Carol Schapira, President
Gale Cossette, Vice President
Susan Frenette, Treasurer
Resources for people with learning disabilities.

279 **New Hampshire Disabilities Rights Center (DRC)**
18 Low Avenue
Concord, NH 03302
603-228-0432
800-834-1721
FAX 603-225-2077
TDY:603-228-0432
http://www.drcnh.org
e-mail: advocacy@drcnh.org
Richard Cohen, Executive Director

A statewide organization that is independent from state government or service providers and is dedicated to the full and equal enjoyment of civil and other legal rights by people with disabilities. The DRC is New Hampshire's designated Protection and Advocacy agency and authorized by federal statute to pursue legal, administrative and other appropriate remedies on behalf of individuals with disabilities.
1978

280 **New Hampshire-ATEC Services**
67 Communication Drive
Laconia, NH 03246
603-528-3060
800-932-5837
FAX 603-524-0702
http://www.nhassistivetechnology.org
e-mail: lorraineh@atechservices.org
Lorraine Halton, MA, Clinical Director
Therese Wilkhomm, Executive Director
Donna Furlong, BS, Administrative Assistant
ATECH Services is a non-profit organization providing local, state, national and international assistive technology information and services to individuals affected by injuries, illnesses, disabling conditions or the aging process. Services provided include: assistive technology evaluation and consultation; reuse of donated equipment; assistive technology exploration and training information and referral.

281 **Parent to Parent of New Hampshire**
Upper Valley Support Group
12 Flynn Street
Lebanon, NH 03766
603-448-6311
800-698-LINK
http://www.p2pnh.org
Philip Eller, Executive Director

If you are a parent of a child with special challenges and you would like to speak to a parent whose child has similar needs - someone who will understand, Parent to Parent is a network of families willing to share experiences. Should you call a Supporting Parent will contact you by phone or visit within 24 hours. All information will be kept confidential and there is no cost for the service.

New Jersey

282 **ASPEN Asperger Syndrome Education Network**
9 Aspen Circle
Edison, NJ 08820
732-321-0880
http://www.aspennj.org
Lori Shery, President
Claudia Loomis, Executive Vice President

Provides families and individuals whose lives are affected by Autism Spectrum Disorders (Asperger Syndrome, Pervasive Developmental Disorder-NOS, High Functioning Autism), and Nonverbal Learning Disabilities with education, support and advocacy.

283 **American Self-Help Clearinghouse of New Jersey**
Saint Clare's Health Services
100 E Hanover Avenue
Cedar Knolls, NJ 07927
973-326-6789
800-367-6274
FAX 973-326-6789
http://www.njgroups.org
Ed Madara, Executive Director
Howard Lerner, Office Assistant

Puts callers in touch with any of several hundred national and international self-help groups covering a wide range of illnesses, disabilities, addictions, bereavement and stressful life situations.

284 **Easter Seals New Jersey**
1 Kimberly Road
East Brunswick, NJ 08816
732-257-6662
FAX 732-257-7373
TDY:732-257-6662
http://nj.easterseals.com
e-mail: essnj@nj.easter-seals.org
Helping people and families with disabilities and special needs live, work and play in their communities with equality, dignity and independence.

285 **Family Support Center of New Jersey**
2516 Route 35 N
Manasquan, NJ 08736
723-262-8020
800-372-6510
FAX 732-262-4373
TDY:800-852-7899
http://www.fsnj.org
Jacqueline Moskowitz, Executive Director
Ramona Carmeci, Senior Resource Coordinator

The clearinghouse on information and referral for families and individuals with developmental disabilities and chronic or serious illnesses in New Jersey.

286 **International Dyslexia Association of NewJersey**
PO Box 32
Long Valley, NJ 07853
908-879-1179
FAX 908-876-3621
http://www.interdys.org
e-mail: riegpainting@msn.com
Susan Tramaglini, President

An international nonprofit, scientific and educational organization dedicated to the study of dyslexia. We offer tutoring and testing referrals, as well as support teacher education and hold outreach programs. Teacher Scholarships are offered to our Annual Fall Conferences, Wilson Reading Overviews and Project Read programs. Newsletter published bi-annually.
700 members

287 **Learning Disabilities Association of New Jersey**
PO Box 492
Towaco, NJ 07082
973-265-4303
http://www.ldaamerica.org
e-mail: ldanj@optonline.net
Terry Cavanaugh, State President

To create opportunities for success in all individuals affected by learning disabilities and to reduce the incidence of learning disabilities in future generations.

288 **New Jersey Family Resource Associates**
35 Haddon Avenue
Shrewsbury, NJ 07702
732-747-5310
FAX 732-747-1896
http://www.frainc.org
e-mail: info@frainc.org
Bill Sheeser, President
Nancy Phalanukorn, Executive Director
Sue Levine, Early Intervention/Programs
A non-profit agency with the mission of helping children, adolescents and people of all ages with disabilities to reach their fullest potenttial. Provides home-based early intervention for infants, therapeutic recreation programs and assistive technology services, along with family and sibling support groups.

289 **New Jersey Protection and Advocacy (NJP&A)**
210 S Broad Street
Trenton, NJ 08608
609-292-9742
800-922-7233
FAX 609-777-0187
http://www.njpanda.org
e-mail: advocate@njpanda.org
Sarah Mitchell, Executive Director
Joseph Young, Deputy Director
Marie Davis, Office Manager
NJP&A is a private nonprofit consumer driven organization established to advocate for and protect the civil, human, and legal rights of citizens of New Jersey with disabilities.

New Mexico

290 Easter Seals Santa Maria El Mirador
PO Box 39
Alcalde, NM 87511 505-852-4243
FAX 505-852-4138
http://smem.easterseals.com
Provides an array of quality supports for individuals with developmental disabilities in community integrated environments centered on personl choice, self value, and dignity.

291 International Dyslexia Association of NewMexico
3915 Carlisle Boulevard NE
Albuquerque, NM 87107 505-255-8234
http://www.southwestida.com
e-mail: swida@southwestlda.com
Martha Steger, President

Deeply committed to the training of teachers, speech pathologists, parents, literacy volunteers, and other professionals in appropriate instructional methods for individuals with dyslexia. IDA's Southwest Branch encourages the use of Orton-Gilligham multisensory structured language based (MSL-based) methodology, which has proven to be the most effective way to teach individuals with dyslexia and related learning disabilities.
1985

292 Learning Disabilities Association of NewMexico: Albuquerque
6301 Menaul Boulevard NE
Albuquerque, NM 87110 505-851-2545
http://www.vivanewmexico.com/nm/nmlda
e-mail: bp@peavler.org
Penny White, President

A nonprofit volunteer organization affiliated with the Learning Disabilities Association of America (LDAA). LDAA gives support and information to persons with learning disabilities, parents, teachers, and other professionals through 50 state affiliates and 800 local units.

293 Learning Disabilities Association of New Mexico: Las Cruces
PO Box 20001/3SPE
Las Cruces, NM 88003 505-882-6221
FAX 505-867-3398
http://www.education.nmsu.edu/projects/NMLDA
e-mail: epoel@nmsu.edu
Elisa Wolf Poel PhD, President
Pam Gough, Vice-President
Selma Nevarez, Treasurer
LDA is a non-profit organization of volunteers including individuals with learning disabilities, their families and professionals. LDA is dedicated to identifying causes and promoting prevention of learning disabilities and to enhancing the quality of life for all individuals with learning disabilities and their families by encouraging effective identification and intervention, fostering research, and protecting their rights under the law.

New York

294 Advocates for Children of New York
151 W 30th Street
New York, NY 10001 212-947-9779
FAX 212-947-9790
http://www.advocatesforchildren.org
e-mail: info@advocatesforchildren.org
Jamie A Levitt, President
Barry Ford, Treasurer

Works on behalf of children from infancy to age 21 who are at greatest risk for school-based discrimination and/or academic failure. AFC provides a full range of services: free individual case advocacy, technical assistance, and training for parents, students, and professionals about children's educational entitlements and due process rights in New York City.

295 International Dyslexia Association of NewYork
71 W 23rd Street
New York, NY 10010 212-691-1930
FAX 212-633-1620
http://www.nybida.org
e-mail: info@nybida.org
Eileen Marzola, President
Linda Selvin, Executive Director

This is a nonprofit organization whose mission is to provide continuing education in appropriate diagnostic remedial approaches and to support the rights of people with dyslexia in order that they may lead fulfilling lives. To this end, the NYB-IDA disseminates information, publishes a quarterly newsletter, and provides information and referral services, teacher training, conferences, adult support groups, and workshops for parents. Annual teen conference.

296 International Dyslexia Association of Suffolk County
728 Route 25A
Northport, NY 11768 631-261-7441
FAX 631-261-7834
http://www.lidyslexia.org
e-mail: kleo@optonline.net
Kerry Leo, President

Our objectives are to increase awareness of dyslexia in the community; provide support for parents and teachers; promote teacher training. We offer a telephone message system for information requests; sponsor an annual conference and four topic workshops as well as a summer Orton-Gillingham course. We have a network of local school officials, parents, attorneys and other professionals to help parents navigate the channels of the school system.

297 International Dyslexia Association of Western New York
c/o Gow School
South Wales, NY 14139 716-687-2030
http://www.interdys.org
e-mail: bufida@gow.org
Timothy Madigan, President

Strives to be a resource for information and services that address the full scope of dyslexia in a way that builds cooperation, partnership and understanding among professional communities and dyslexic individuals so that everyone is valued and has the opportunity to be productive and fulfilled in life. Newsletter and teacher training scholarships.

298 Learning Disabilities Association of Central New York
722 W Manlius Street
East Syracuse, NY 13057 315-432-0665
FAX 315-431-0606
http://www.ldacny.org
e-mail: LDACNY@LDACYN.org
Aggie Glavin, Co-Exec Director/Programs
Paulette Purdy, Co-Exec Director/Finance

Enhances the quality of life for children and adults with learning disabilities by providing advocacy, programs and educational resources. Serving the counties of Cayuga, Cortland, Madison, Onondaga and Owsego.

299 Learning Disabilities Association of NewYork City
27 W 20th Street
New York, NY 10011 212-645-6730
FAX 212-924-8896
http://www.ldanyc.com
e-mail: ldanyc@verizon.net
Martha Bernard, President
Stephen Baldwin, Executive Director

Serves the counties of Brooklyn, Bronx, Manhattan, Queens and Staten Island. Facilitates access to needed services for all New Yorkers with Learning Disabilities, especially those in the more disadvantaged communities, and provides support to those individuals and their families.

1989

300 Learning Disabilities Association of Western New York
2555 Elmwood Avenue
Kenmore, NY 14217 716-874-7200
FAX 716-874-7205
http:// www.ldaoswny.org
e-mail: information@ldaoswny.org
Mike Helman, Executive Director
Brenda Frazier, Executive Assistant

To create conditions under which persons with learning disabilities, neurological impairments, and developmental disabilities are given opportunities to make choices and develop and achieve independence. The association also addresses each individual's health, future, participation in the community, and personal relationships. LDA Southern Fredonia Tier branch can be reached at 716-679-1601.

301 Learning Disabilities Association of theCapital District
2995 Curry Road Extension
Schenectady, NY 12303 518-356-6410
FAX 518-356-3603
http://www.ldaofwny.org
Serves the counties of Albany, Columbia, Fulton, Greene, Montgomery, Rensselaer, Saratoga, Schenectady, Schoharie and Washington

302 Learning Disabilities of the Genesee Valley
339 E Avenue
Rochester, NY 14604 585-263-3323
FAX 585-263-2461
http://www.ldagvi.org
e-mail: info@ldagvi.org
Timothy McNamara, President
Peggy Beaty, VP

A non-profit agency that partners with individuals who seek hlep in learning, so that they can succeed in school, work, and community life. The primaty constituents include people who are working to overcome cognitive or developmental barriers to learning. Also serve as a resource to people who are involved in the lives of these individuals, such as family members, employers, teachers and health care professionals.

303 New York Easter Seal Society
29 W 36th Street
New York, NY 10018 212-244-6053
FAX 212-244-6059
http://www.ny.easterseals.com
John W McGrath, VP Organizational Development
Rita Stella, SCSEP Project Director

Provides programs and services to children and adults with disabilities and other special needs, and their families. The goal is to help individuals with special needs gain dignity, equality and independence. Also provide the highest quality services in the most caring and cost-effective manner.
1922

304 Recording for the Blind & Dyslexic
545 Fifth Avenue
New York, NY 10017 212-557-5720
http://www.rfbd.org
e-mail: dcrupain@rfbd.org
Diane Crupain, Executive Director
John Fernandes, Production Director
Gretchen McGarry, Development Director
Serves New Yorkers who are blind, visually impaired, physically disabled or have a learning disability.

305 Resources for Children with Special Needs
116 E 16th Street
New York, NY 10003 212-677-4650
FAX 212-254-4070
http://www.resourcesnyc.org
e-mail: info@resourcesnyc.org
Karen Thoreson Schlesinger, Executive Director
Helene Craner, Associate Director

An information, referral, advocacy, tranining and support center for NYC parents/professionals looking for services for children-birth to 26 with learning, developmental, emotional of physical disabilities. Publications available on website.

306 Strong Center for Developmental Disabilities
Golisano Children's Hospital at Strong
601 Elmwood Avenue
Rochester, NY 14642 585-275-0355
FAX 585-275-3366
http://www.urmc.rochester.edu/gchas/div/scdd
e-mail: scdd@cc.urmc.rochester.edu
Philip Davidson PhD, Chief Director

A University Center of Excellence for Developmental Disabilities, Education, Research and Service. Provides services, advocacy, education, technical assistance, and research to ensure full inclusion of persons with developmental disabilities in their communities and to maximize their potentional for leading independent and productive lives.

307 Westchester Institute for Human Development
Westchester Medical Center
Cedarwood Hall
Valhalla, NY 10595 914-493-8202
FAX 914-493-1973
http://www.wihd.org
e-mail: wihd@wihd.org
Ansley Bacon, PhD, President/CEO
Daniel Tillotson, COO
David O'Hara PhD, VP Development
WIHD advances policies and practices that foster the healthy development and ensure the safety of all children, strenghten families and communities, and promote health and well-being among people of all ages with disabilities and special health care needs.
1950

North Carolina

308 All Kinds of Minds of North Carolina
1450 Raleigh Road
Chapel Hill, NC 27517 919-933-8082
888-956-4637
FAX 919-843-9955
http://www.allkindsofminds.org
Dr Mel Levine, Co-Chair/Co-Founder

A non-profit Institute that helps students who struggle with learning measurably improve their success in school and life by providing programs that integrate educational, scientific, and clinical expertise. The primary goal is to educate teachers, parents, educational specialists, psychologists, pediatricians, and students about differences in learning, so that children who are struggling in school because of the way their brains are wierd are no longer misunderstood.

309 International Dyslexia Association of North Carolina
1829 E Franklin Street
Chapel Hill, NC 27514 919-933-8880
FAX 828-963-1883
http://www.nc-ida.org
e-mail: edutherapy@earthlink.com
Susan Lowell, MA, BCET, President

The North Carolina Branch of The International Dyslexia Association (NCIDA) is a 501 (c)(3) non-profit, scientific and organization dedicated to educating the public about the learning disability, dyslexia. The North Carolina Branch has four objectives: to increase awareness in the dyslexic and general community; to network with other learning disability groups and legislators in education; to increase membership and provide services that will strengthen members presence in their communities.

310 Learning Disabilities Association of North Carolina (LDANC)
9650 Strickland Road
Raleigh, NC 27615 919-493-5362
FAX 919-489-0788
http://www.ldanc.org
e-mail: idanc@mindspring.com
Jonathan Jones, Co-President
Pat Lillie, Co-President

Promotes awareness of the multifaceted nature of learning disabilities. We support equitable opportunities for people with learning disabilities to participate in life's experiences. LDANC seeks to accomplish this through education, support, advocacy, collaboration and the encouragement of ongoing research.

North Dakota

311 International Dyslexia Association of theUpper Midwest Branch

5021 Vernon Avenue
Minneapolis, MN 55436 621-450-7589
http://http://www.umbida.org
e-mail: infi@umbida.org

Claire Eckley, President

UMBIDA-the Upper Midwest Branch of the International Dyslexia Association (IDA-serves the residents of Minnesota, North Dakota, South Dakota, and Winnipeg, Canada and offers: local educational conferences about dyslexia and related subjects; Orton-Gillingham training for teachers, tutors, and parents; quarterly speaker series; quarterly newsletter; member discounts on conferences; information line; and tutor referral.

Ohio

312 Easter Seals: Youngstown

299 Edwards Street
Youngstown, OH 44502 330-743-1168
FAX 330-743-1616
http://www.mtc.easterseals.org

Ken Sklenar, CEO

Physical Therapy, Speech Therapy, Occupational Therapy, Aquatic Therapy, Child Care, Preschool for Children with Special Needs and In-Home Respite Care are offered.

313 International Dyslexia Association of Central Ohio

PO Box 16216
Columbus, OH 43216 614-899-5711
http://www.interdys.org
e-mail: cyndischultz@columbus.rr.com

Cyndi Schultz, President

Increases awareness of dyslexia and related learning disabilities; assist professionals, dyslexics and their families; promote use of effective teaching methods; and disseminate research-based knowledge. Serves Central Ohio and parts of West Virginia.

314 International Dyslexia Association of Northern Ohio

7597 Herrick Park Drive
Hudson, OH 44236 216-556-0883
http://www.dyslexia-nohio.org

A non-profit, scientific and educational organization dedicated to the study and treatment of the language-based reading disability, dyselxia.

315 International Dyslexia Association of theOhio Valley

317 E 5th Street
Cincinnati, OH 45202 513-651-4747
http://www.cincinnatidyslexia.org

Martha Chiodi, President

The local Ohio Valley Branch is an all volunteer organization that was founded in 1978. The branch provides workshops for parents and professionals, training opportunities for regular and special education teachers, support groups, and referral assistance for adults and parents of dyslexic children.

316 Learning Disabilities Association of Ohio

PO Box 784
Springfield, OH 43085 937-325-1923
e-mail: memartin@glasscity.net

Mary Ellen Martin, Contact

A nonproft organization whose members are individuals with learnin disabilities, their families, and the professionals who work with them.

Oklahoma

317 Center for Learning & Leadership (UAP)

University of Oklahoma Health Sciences Center
PO Box 26901
Oklahoma City, OK 73190 405-271-4500
800-627-6827
FAX 405-271-1459
TDY:405-271-1464
http://www.ouhsc.edu
e-mail: valerie-williams@ouhscd.edu

Valerie Williams, Director

The UAP is a federally designated organization dedicated to promoting the independence, productivity and inclusion of people with disabilities in the life of the community. The core value of the UAP is to build an accepting, respectful and accessible environment for all.

318 Easter Seals Oklahoma

701 NE 13th Street
Oklahoma City, OK 73104 405-239-2525
http://ok.easterseals.com

Provides services to children and adults with disabilities and other special needs, and support to their families.

319 International Dyslexia Association of Oklahoma: Dallas Branch

14070 Proton
Dalas, TX 75244 972-233-9107
FAX 972-490-4219
http://www.dbia.org

Pamela Hundall Quarterman, President

The Dallas Branch of The International Dyslexia Association is committed to leadership and advocacy for people with dyslexia by providing: support for individuals and group interactions; programs to inform and educate; information for professionals and the general public. Serves individuals in the state og Oklahoma.

320 International Dyslexia Association: Oklahoma-Kansas/Missouri Branch

430 East Blue Ridge Boulevard
Kansas City, MO 64145 816-838-7323
http://www.ksmoida.org
e-mail: info@ksmoida.org

IDA members in Kansas and Missouri work to establish and maintain a presence for IDA with parents, schools, and teachers in order to help individuals with dyslexia. Serves individuals in the state of Oklahoma.

321 Learning Disabilities Association of Oklahoma

PO Box 1134
Jenks, OK 74037 918-298-1600
http://www.ldao.org
e-mail: lda2002@sbcglobal.net

Joy Modenbach, President
Joyce Lackey, First Vice President
Vicky Foster, Second Vice President

A nonprofit organization committed to enhancing the lives of individuals with learning disabilities and their families through education, advocacy, research, and service

Oregon

322 Easter Seals Oregon

5757 SW Macadam Ave
Portland, OR 97239 503-228-5108
800-556-6020
FAX 503-228-1352
http://or.easterseals.com

Provides services to children and adults with disabilities and other special needs, helping them to live with equality, dignity and independence.

323 **International Dyslexia Association of Oregon**

2525 NW Lovejoy Street
Portland, OR 97210-2865
800-530-2234
FAX 503-228-3152
http://www.orbida.org
e-mail: info@orbida.org

Judith L Wright, President

The Oregon Branch of the International Dyslexia Association (ORBIDA) focuses on increasing public awareness of how dyslexia affects both children and adults.

324 **Learning Disabilities Association of Oregon**

PO Box 1221
Beaverton, OR 97008 503-641-3768
http://www.ldaor.org
e-mail: mtsoule@ix.netcom.com

Myrna Soule, President
Larry Bruseau, Vice President
Kim Barton, Treasurer

Works to promote the welfare of children and adults with learning disabilities. A non-profit organization that serves as a resource, referral, and information center for adults with learning disabilities, parents of children with learning disabilities, and profesionals working in the field of learning disabilities.

325 **Oregon Disabilities Commission**

500 Summer Street NE
Salem, OR 97301 503-378-3142
800-358-3117
FAX 503-378-3142
http://www.odc.state.or.us
e-mail: odc@state.or.us

Danielle Knight, Executive Director
Wendy Leedle, Executive Assistant
Georgia Ortiz, Manager

The Oregon Disabilities Commission provides information and referral services to advise persons with disabilities on services, rights and employment. They serve as the state's ADA coordinator and building code advisor which mandates the Commission to encourage and facilitate ADA and structural code compliance by local governments, private entities, businesses, and employers.

326 **University of Oregon for Excellence in Developmental Disabilities**

Center on Human Development, College of Education
5252 University of Oregon
Eugene, OR 97403 541-346-3591
FAX 541-346-2594
http://http://ucedd.uoregon.edu
e-mail: uocedd@uoregon.edu

Hill Walker PhD, Director
Jane Squires PhD, Associate Director

The mission of our UCEDD in Developmental Disabilities is to be of assistance in improving the quality of life for Oregonians and all persons with developmental disabilities and their families. To accomplish this mission, we provide training, technical assistance, interdisciplinary training, dissemination, networking and model development that responds effectively, and in a culturally competent fashion, to the multiple needs of individuals and their families.

Pennsylvania

327 **AAC Institute**

1000 Killarney Drive
Pittsburgh, PA 15234 413-523-6424
http://www.aacinstitute.org
e-mail: khill@aacinstitute.org

Katya Hill PhD, Executive Director

Established in 2000, a resource for all who are interested in enhancing the communication of people who rely on AAC. A not-for-profit charitable organization, offers information and provides services worldwide.

328 **Adult Basic Educational Development Programs for Blind, Visually Impaired & Print Handicapped**

Philadelphia Library for the Blind (LBPH)
919 Walnut Street
Philadelphia, PA 19107 215-683-3213
800-222-1754
FAX 215-683-3211
e-mail: flpblind@library.thila.gov

Vickie L Collins, Manager
Jill Gross, Program Coordinator
Renee Snouten, LBPH Liaison

Adult basic education, GED classes and GED testing for the print handicapped, blind and visually impaired.

329 **Easter Seals Society of Western Pennsylvana: Fayette**

2525 Railroad Street
Pittsburgh, PA 15222 412-281-7244
800-587-3257
FAX 412-281-9333
http://www.westernpa.easterseals.com

Lawrence Rager, CEO
Tina Outrich, VP Programs/Services

Speech, language, learning disabilities and hearing evaluations and therapy for all ages. PA licensed preschool on the premises. Open five days per week; 12 months. Call for an appointment or information on the programs provided.

1934

330 **Huntingdon County PRIDE**

1301 Mt Vernon Ave
Huntingdon, PA 16652 814-643-5724
FAX 814-643-6085
http://www.huntingdonpride.org
e-mail: pride@huntingdon.net

Sandra Bair, Executive Director
Kathleen Renninger, Service Development Coordinator
Adam Pfingstl, Social Recreation Director

Provide programs which enable people who are developmentally and/or physically disabled to function at their optimal level of performance.

331 **International Dyslexia Association of Pennsylvania**

PO Box 251
Bryn Mawr, PA 19010 610-527-1548
FAX 610-527-5011
http://www.pbida.org
e-mail: dyslexia@pbida.org

John T Rogers JD, President

The Pennsylvania Branch of the International Dyslexia Association (PBIDA), serving Pennsylvania and Delaware provides support and information for individuals, families and educational professionals concerned with the issues of dyslexia and learning differences.

332 **Learning Disabilities Association of Pennsylvania**

Toomey Building
Uwchland, PA 19480 610-458-8193
http://www.ldapa.org

Debbie Rodes, President
Sister Marie Gayda, Vice President
Kristina Smith, Treasurer

A nonprofit organization dedicated to serving Pennsylvania residents by providing accurate, up-to-date information regarding learning disabilities as well as support.

333 **Pennsylvania Center for Disability Law and Policy**

1617 JFK Boulevard
Philadelphia, PA 19103 215-557-7112
888-745-CDLP
FAX 215-557-7602
TDY:215-557-7112
http://www.equalemployment.org
e-mail: info@equalemployment.org

Stephen S Pennington, Executive Director
Jamie Ray, Assistant Director
Margaret Passio McKenna, Senior Advocate

An advocacy program for people with disabilities administered by the Center for Disability Law & Policy. CAP helps people who are seeking services from the Office of Vocational Rehabilitation, Blindness and Visual Services, Centers for Independent Living and other progrmas funded under federal law. Hep is provided to you at no charge, regardless of income. Dedicated to ensuring that the rehabilitation system in Pennsylvania is open and responsive to your needs.

334 **Public Interest Law Center of Philadelphia**
125 S Ninth Street
Philadelphia, PA 19107
215-627-7100
FAX 215-627-3183
TDY:215-627-7300
http://www.pilcop.org
e-mail: pubint@aol.com
Jennifer R Clarke, Executive Director
Michael Churchill, Co-Chief Counsel
Thomas K Gilhool, Co-Chief Counsel
Founded by the Philadelphia Bar Association and is one of eight local affiliates of the Lawyers' Committee fot Civil Rights Under Law. Dedicated to advancing the Constitutional promise of equal citizenship to all persons irrespective of race, ethnicity, national origin, disability, gender or poverty.
1974

335 **Recording for the Blind & Dyslexic**
215 W Church Road
King of Prussia, PA 19406
610-265-8090
http://www.rfbd.org
e-mail: mgollapalli@rfbd.org
Michelle S Gollapalli CFRE, Interim Exec Dir/Development Dir
Mary McDermott, Studio Director

Rhode Island

336 **International Dyslexia Association of Rhode Island**
16 Houston Avenue
Newport, RI 02840
401-521-0020
FAX 401-847-6720
e-mail: ribida@yahoo.com
Dawn Cronin Pigott, President

South Carolina

337 **Easter Seals South Carolina**
PO Box 5715
Columbia, SC 29250
803-256-0735
800-951-4090
FAX 803-738-1934
http://sc.easterseals.com
Provides services to children and adults with disabilities and other special needs, and support to their families.

338 **International Dyslexia Association of South Carolina**
Camperdown Academy
Greenville, NC 29615
864-244-8899
http://www.interdys.org
e-mail: kchickvary@camperdown.org
Karin Chickvary, President

The South Carolina Branch provides general information about dyslexia and makes referrals to various professionals and schools serving individuals with learning disabilities.
130 members

339 **Laurence County Literacy Council**
221 W Laurens Street
Laurens, SC 29360
864-984-0466
FAX 864-984-2920
e-mail: rhenderson@backroads.net
Rita Henderson, Manager

Promotes literacy for people of all ages in Laurence County.

South Dakota

340 **Division of Rehabilitation Services and Childrens Rehabilitation Services**
3800 E Highway 34
Pierre, SD 57501
605-773-3195
800-264-9684
FAX 605-773-5483
TDY:605-773-5990
Grady Kickul, Executive Director

Our mission is to assist individuals with disabilities to obtain employment, economic self-sufficiency, personal idependence and full inclusion in society.

341 **International Dyslexia Association of South Dakota**
5201 Vernon Avenue
Minneapolis, MN 55436
651-450-7589
http://www.umbida.org
e-mail: info@umbida.org
Claire Eckley, President

UMBIDA-the Upper Midwest Branch of the International Dyslexia Association (IDA-serves the residents of Minnesota, North Dakota, South Dakota, and Winnipeg, Canada and offers: local educational conferences about dyslexia and related subjects; Orton-Gillingham training for teachers, tutors, and parents; quarterly speaker series; quarterly newsletter; member discounts on conferences; information line; and tutor referral.

342 **Learning Disabilities Association of South Dakota**
PO Box 9760
Rapid City, SD 57709
605-388-9291
888-388-5553
FAX 605-787-7848
http://www.geocities.com/athens/ithaca/8835
e-mail: dthom@rapidnet.com
Dee Thompson, Executive Director

The Association conducts workshops and conferences, assists local communities, collaborates with other organizations with similar missions and concerns, and provides 1-on-1 assistance to individuals and families. Most visible among its efforts is the Association's statewide annual conference.
1996

343 **South Dakota Center for Disabilities**
Sanford School of Medicine, USD
1400 W 22nd Street
Sioux Falls, SD 57105
605-357-1439
800-658-3080
FAX 605-357-1438
TDY:800-658-3080
http://www.usd.edu/cd
e-mail: cd@usd.edu
Judy Struck, Executive Director
Kristen Blaschke, Director of Development

A division of the Department of Pediatrics at the Sanford School pf Medicine at the University of South Dakota. The Center for Disabilities is South Dakota's University Center for Excellence in Developmental Disabilities Education, Research and Service sometimes referred to as University Centers for Excellence in Developmental Disabilities.

Tennessee

344 **Easter Seals Tennessee**
2001 Woodmont Boulevard
Nashville, TN 37215
615-292-6640
800-264-0078
FAX 615-292-7206
http://tn.easterseals.com
Susan Armiger, President/CEO
Rita Baumgartner, VP Development

Creates solutions that change the lives of children and adults with disabilities or other special needs and their families.

345 **International Dyslexia Association of Tennessee**
3508 Hackworth Road
Knoxville, TN 37931
877-836-6432
FAX 865-693-3656
http://www.tn-interdys.org
e-mail: tennessee_ida@hotmail.com
Martie Wood, President

Formed to increase awareness about Dyslexia in the state of Tennessee. Supports efforts to provide information regarding appropriate language arts instruction to those involved with language-based learning differences and to encourage the identity of these indivduals at-risk for such disorders as soon as possible.
1989

346 **Learning Disabilities Association of Tennessee**
PO Box 40562
Memphis, TN 38174
http://www.learningdisabilities-tn.org
e-mail: info@learningdisabilities-tn.org
Joy Sue Marsh, President

The Learning Disabilities Association of Tennessee has a mission to provide information concerning awareness, advocacy, parent information, and community education to maximize the quality of life for individuals and families affected by Learning Disabilities and related disorders in the state of Tennessee.

347 **Recording for the Blind & Dyslexic: Tennessee**
205 Badger Road
Oak Ridge, TN 37830
865-482-3496
FAX 865-483-9934
http://www.rfbd.org
e-mail: kperry@rfbd.org
Brian Jenkins, Executive Director
Karen Perry, Outreach Director

Part of the national, nonprofit organization which records educational and career-related materials for print impaired students and professionals. The special focus is educational books. Blind and other print impaired students at every level, from elementary through graduate school, depend on RFBD tapes for the texts they need.
1952

Texas

348 **Easter Seals of Central Texas**
1611 Headway Circle
Austin, TX 78754
512-478-2581
FAX 512-476-1638
http://www.centraltx.easterseals.com
Brently Weber, Chairperson
Kevin T Coleman, President/CEO

Easter Seals Central Texas provides exceptional services so people with disabilities and their families can fully participate in their communities.

349 **Easter Seals of North Texas**
4443 N Josey Lane
Carrollton, TX 75010
972-394-8900
800-580-4718
FAX 972-394-6266
http://www.ntx.easterseals.com
e-mail: info@easterseals.com
Monica Prather, President
Jennifer Friesen, Vice President, Clinical Service

Created by the merger of Easter Seals of Greater Dallas and Easter Seals Greater Northwest Texas. Creates opportunities that advance the independence of individuals with disabilities and other special needs.

350 **International Dyslexia Association of Austin**
PO Box 92604
Austin, TX 78709
512-452-7658
http://www.austinida.org
Sharon McMichael, President

The Austin Area Branch of the International Dyslexia Association is a 501(c)(3) non profit organization dedicated to promoting reading excellence for all children through early identification of dyslexia, effective literacy education for adults and children with dyslexia, and teacher training.

351 **International Dyslexia Association of Dallas**
14070 Proton
Dallas, TX 75244
972-233-9107
FAX 972-490-4219
http://www.dbida.org/
Pamela Hudnall Quarterman, President

The Dallas Branch of The International Dyslexia Association is committed to leadership and advocacy for people with dyslexia by providing: support for individuals and group interactions; programs to inform and educate; information for professionals and the general public.

352 **International Dyslexia Association of Houston**
PO Box 540504
Houston, TX 77254
832-282-7154
FAX 972-490-4219
http://www.houstonida.org
e-mail: president@houstonida.org
Cathy Lorino, President

A non-profit organization dedicated to helping individuals with dyslexia and related learning disorders, their families and the communities that support them.

353 **Learning Disabilities Association of Texas**
1011 W 31st Street
Austin, TX 78705
512-458-8234
800-604-7500
FAX 512-458-3826
http://www.ldat.org
e-mail: contact@ldat.org
Jean Kueker, President
Ann Robinson, State Coordinator

Promotes the educational and general welfare of individuals with learning disabilities.
1963

354 **Learning Disabilities Association: El Paso**
8929 Viscount Boulevard
El Paso, TX 79925
915-591-8080
FAX 915-591-8150
e-mail: eplda@elpn.com
Lina Monroy, Executive Director

Non-profit organization of parents and professionals working together to provide assistance to learning disabled persons and their families. Services range from support and information for parents, counseling, and advocacy and in services to agencies and professionals.

355 **North Texas Rehabilitation Center**
1005 Midwestern Parkway
Wichita Falls, TX 76302
940-322-0771
800-861-1322
FAX 940-766-4943
http://www.ntrehab.org
Mike Castles, President
Lesa Enlow, Director of Programs

A not-for-profit organization providing nationally accredited outpatient medical, academic, and developmental rehabilitation to North Texas and Southern Oklahoma. From the Early Childhood Intervention program to the Aquatics programs, these services are designed to help our patients acheive their highest level of independence.

1948

356 **Recording for the Blind & Dyslexic**
1314 W 45th Street
Austin, TX 78756
512-323-9390
877-246-7321
FAX 512-323-9399
http://www.rfbd.org
e-mail: lil@rfbdtexas.org
Lil Serafine, Regional Executive Director
Ginger Dillard Cleveland, Regional Program Director
Laurie Born, Regional Development Director

Utah

357 **International Dyslexia Association of Utah**
PO Box 783
American Fork, UT 84003
801-319-8079
http://www.ubida.org
e-mail: jane@theriches.org
Jane Rich, Chair

Dedicated to ensuring that every student with the learning difference of Dyslexia will receive scientifically based instruction and services consistent with his/her needs.

358 **Learning Disabilities Asssociation of Utah**
PO Box 900726
Sandy, UT 84090
801-553-9156
http://www.ldau.org
e-mail: info@ldauinfo.org
A non-profit volunteer organization supporting people with learning disabilities and their families. Our mission is to create opportunities for individuals with learning abilities to succeed and for their families to participate in their success.

Vermont

359 **International Dyslexia Association of Vermont**
PO Box 3724
Concord, NH 03302
603-229-7355
http://www.nhida.org
e-mail: information@nhida.org
Colleen Sliva, President

The New Hampshire Branch of The International Dyslexia Association (NH/IDA) is a 501(c)(3) non-profit, scientific and educational organization dedicated to the study and treatment of the learning disability, dyslexia. The New Hampshire Branch was formed in 2002 to increase public awareness of dyslexia. The New Hampshire Branch serves New Hampshire, Maine and Vermont

360 **Vermont Protection & Advocacy**
141 Main Street
Montpelier, VT 05602
802-229-1355
800-834-7890
FAX 802-229-1359
http://www.vtpa.org
e-mail: info@vtpa.org
Ed Paquin, Executive Director
Marshe Bancroft, Intake Paralegal

Dedicated to addressing problems, questions and complaints brought to it by Vermonters with disabilities. VP&A's mission is to promote the equality, dignity, and self-determination of people with disabilities. VP&A provides infomraion, referral and advocacy services, including leagl representation when appropriate, to individuals with disabilities throughout Vermont.

Virginia

361 **Easter Seals Virginia**
8003 Franklin Farms Drive
Richmond, VA 23229
804-287-1007
866-874-4153
FAX 804-287-1008
http://va.easterseals.com
Tom Haake, Chairman
Tara Hazelbaker, President/CEO

Provides exceptional services to ensure that all people with disabilities or special needs and their families have equal opportunities to live, learn, work and play in their communities.

362 **International Dyslexia Association of Virginia**
PO Box 17605
Richmond, VA 23226
804-272-2881
FAX 804-272-0277
http://bida.org
e-mail: info@vbida.org
Debra Farrar, President

363 **Learning Disabilities Association of Virginia**
4324 Fordham Road
Richmond, VA 23236
804-745-9325
FAX 804-346-8383
http://www.ldavirginia.org
e-mail: info@ldavirginia.org
Anna Johnson, President
Justine Maloney, Representative

Our organization focuses on enhancing educational and vocational services for individuals with learning disabilities who live in Virginia while supporting the efforts of LDA at the national level.

Washington

364 **Disability Rights Washington**
315 5th Avenue S
Seattle, WA 98104
206-324-1521
800-562-2702
FAX 206-957-0729
http://www.disabilityrightswa.org
Mark Stroh, Executive Director
Jessica McDaneld, Administrative Assistant

Is a private, non-profit organization that has been protecting the rights of people with disabilities.
1974

365 **Easter Seals Washington**
157 Roy Streey
Seattle, WA 98109-4111
206-281-5700
800-678-5708
FAX 206-284-0938
http://wa.easterseals.com
Provides exceptional services to ensure that people living with autism and other disabilities have equal opportunities to live, learn, work and play.

366 **International Dyslexia Association of Washington**
PO Box 1247
Mercer Island, WA 98040
206-382-1020
http://www.wabida.org
e-mail: info@wabida.org
Bonnie Meyer, President

The Washington State Branch of the International Dyslexia Association is a 501 (c)(3) non-profit, scientific and educational organization dedicated to the study and treatment of dyslexia. Our all volunteer board of directors seeks to increase public awareness of dyslexia in our branch's area which includes Washington, Alaska, Idaho, and western Montana.

367 Learning Disabilities Association of Washington
Family Resource Center Campus
16315 NE 87th Street
Redmond, WA 98052
425-882-0820
800-536-2343
FAX 425-861-4642
http://www.ldawa.org
e-mail: dsiegel@ldawa.org
Lee Kueckelhan, President
Tom Chatriand, Vice President
Cyd Imel, Executive Director
Promotes and provides services and support to improve the quality of life for individuals and families affected by learning and attentional disabilities
1965

368 Washington Parent Training Project: PAVE
6316 S 12th Street
Tacoma, WA 98465
253-565-2266
800-572-7368
FAX 253-566-8052
TDY:800-572-7368
http://www.washingtonpave.org
e-mail: wapave9@washingtonpave.com
Joanne Butts, Executive Director
Karen Anderson, Program Coordinator
Heather M Hebdon, Compliance Officer
PAVE, a parent directed organization, exists to increase independence, empowerment, future opportunities and choices for consumers with special needs, their families and communities, through training, information, referral and support.
1979

West Virginia

369 Easter Seals West Virginia
Rehabilitation Center
1305 National Road
Wheeling, WV 26003
304-242-1390
800-677-1390
FAX 304-243-5880
http://wv.easterseals.com
The Rehabilitaiton Center primary service area includes Ohio, Marshal, Wetzel, Tyler, Brooke and Hancock counties in West Virginia and Belmont, Monroe, Jefferson and Harrison Counties in Ohio.

Wisconsin

370 Easter Seals of Southeast Wisconsin
3090 N 53rd Street
Milwaukee, WI 53210
414-449-4444
FAX 414-449-4447
http://www.eastersealskindcare.com
Robert Glowacki, President

Provides exceptional services to ensure that all people with disabilities or special needs and their families have equal opportunities to live, learn, work and play in their communities

371 International Dyslexia Association of Wisconsin
WBIDA
Baraboo, WI 53913
608-355-0811
FAX 608-355-0911
http://www.wis-dys.org
e-mail: loral@centurytel.com
Lorinda L Clary, President

We believe all individuals have the right to achieve their potential, that individual learning abilities can be strengthened and that social, educaitonal, and cultural barriers to language acquisition and use must be removed.

372 Learning Disabilities Association of Wisconsin
PO Box 14690
Madison, WI 53908
414-299-9002
866-532-9472
http://www.ldawisconsin.com
e-mail: info@ldawisconsin.com
Diane Sixel, President

The Learning Disabilities Association of Wisconsin is dedicated to providing support to children and adults with learning disabilities through advocacy, education, information and research.

National Programs

373 **Attention Deficit Disorder Association**
15000 Commerce Parkway
Mount Laurel, NJ 08054
856-439-9099
FAX 856-439-0525
http://www.add.org
e-mail: adda@ahint.com
Linda S Anderson MA/MCC, President
Evelyn Polk Green MS.Ed, Vice President
Mary Jane Johnson PCC/ACT, Vice President
The mission of ADDA is to provide information, resources and networking to adults with ADD/ADHD and to the professionals who work with them. In doing so, ADDA generates hope, awareness, empowerment and connections worldwide in the field of ADD/ADHD.
1989

374 **Attention Deficit Disorder Warehouse**
300 Northwest 70th Avenue
Plantation, FL 33317
954-792-8100
800-233-9273
FAX 954-792-8545
http://www.addwarehouse.com
e-mail: websales@addwarehouse.com
Roberta Parker, Co-Founder/Owner/Manager
Harvey Parker PhD, Co-Founder/Owner/Manager

A comprehensive resource for the understanding and treatment of all developmental disorders, including ADHD and related problems, the ADD Warehouse provides a vast collection of ADHD-related books, videos, training programs, games, professional texts and assessment products.
1990

375 **Children and Adults with Attention Deficit Hyperactivity Disorder (CHADD)**
8181 Professional Place
Landover, MD 20785
301-306-7070
800-233-4050
FAX 301-306-7090
http://www.chadd.org
e-mail: national@chadd.org
E Clark Ross, Chief Executive Officer
Paul Seifert, Director Public Policy
Russell L Shipley Jr, Chief Development Officer
Children and Adults with Attention-Deficit/Hyperactivity Disorder (CHADD), is a national non-profit, tax-exempt (Section 501) organization providing education, advocacy and support for individuals with AD/HD. In addition to an informative Web site, CHADD also publishes a variety of printed materials to keep members and professionals current on research advances, medications and treatments affecting individuals with AD/HD.
16,000 members 1987

376 **Council for Exceptional Children (CEC)**
1110 North Glebe Road
Arlington, VA 22201
703-620-3660
FAX 703-264-9494
http://www.cec.sped.org
e-mail: service@cec.sped.org
Bruce Ramirez, Executive Director
Lynda Van Kuren, Communications Director
Elizabeth Turnbull, Administrator
The Council for Exceptional Children (CEC) is an international organization dedicated to improving educational outcomes for individuals with exceptionalities, students with disabilities, and/or the gifted. CEC advocates for appropriate governmental policies, sets professional standards, provides continual professional development, advocates for newly and historically underserved individuals with exceptionalities, and helps professionals obtain resources necessary for professionsl practice.

377 **Council for Learning Disabilities CLD)**
11184 Antioch Road
Overland, KS 66210
913-491-1011
FAX 913-491-1012
http://www.cldinternational.org/
e-mail: lnease@cldinternational.org
Linda Higbee Mandlebaum, President Board of Director
Mary Provost, Conference Director
Linda Nease, Executive Director
The mission of the Council for Learning Disabilities/CLD is to enhance the education and life span development of individuals with learning disabilities. CLD establishes standards of excellence and promotes innovative strategies on research and practice through interdisciplinary collegiality, collaboration, and advocacy. CLD's publication, Learning Disability Quarterly, focuses on the latest research in the field of learning disabilities with an applied focus.

378 **Dyslexia Research Institute**
5746 Centerville Road
Tallahassee, FL 32309
850-893-2216
FAX 850-893-2440
http://www.dyslexia-add.org
e-mail: dri@dyslexia-add.org
Patricia K Hardman PhD, Director
Robyn A Rennick MS, Director

Addresses academic, social and self-concept issues for dyslexic and ADD children and adults. College prep courses, study skills, advocacy, diagnostic testing, seminars, teacher training, day school, tutoring and an adult literacy and life skills program is available using an accredited MSLE approach.

379 **LD Online**
c/o WETA Public Television
Arlington, VA 22206
703-998-3290
FAX 703-998-0206
http://www.ldonline.org
Noel Gunther, Executive Driector
Kelly Andrews, Project Coordinator
Dale Brown, Senior Manager
LD OnLine seeks to help children and adults reach their full potential by providing accurate and up-to-date information and advice about learning disabilities and ADHD. The site features hundreds of helpful articles, monthly columns by noted experts, first person essays, children's writing and artwork, a comprehensive resource guide, very active forums, and a Yellow Pages referral directory of professionals, schools, and products.

380 **Learning Disabilities Association of America**
Learning Disabilities Association of America
4156 Library Road
Pittsburgh, PA 15234
412-341-1515
888-300-6710
FAX 412-344-0224
http://www.ldaamerica.org
e-mail: info@ldaamerica.org
Sheila Buckley, Executive Director
Sharon Tanner, Development Coordinator
Andrea Turkheimer, Referral Specialist
An information and referral center for parents and professionals dealing with Attention Deficit Disorders, and other learning disabilities. Free materials and referral service to nearest chapter.

381 **National Alliance on Mental Illness (NAMI)**
2107 Wilson Boulevard
Arlington, VA 22201-3042
703-524-7600
888-999-6264
FAX 703-524-9094
TDY:703-516-7227
http://www.nami.org
e-mail: info@nami.org
Michael J Fitzpatrick, Executive Director
Lynn Borton, Chief Operating Officer
Ken Duckworth, Medical Director
NAMI/National Alliance on Mental Illness is a mental health organization dedicated to improving the lives of persons living with serious mental illness and their families. NAMI members, leaders, and friends work across all levels to meet a shared NAMI mission of support, education, advocacy, and research for people living with mental illness.

382 **National Center for Learning Disabilities(NCLD)**
381 Park Avenue South
Suite 1401
New York, NY 10016
212-545-7510
888-575-7373
FAX 212-545-9665
http://://www.ld.org
e-mail: mg@ncld.org

James J Wendorf, Executive Direcotr
Karen Golembeski, Assistant Director
Laura Kaloi, Director Public Policy
NCLD develops and delivers programs and promote research to improve instruction, assessment and support services for individuals with learning disabilities. They create and disseminate essential information for parents and educators, providing help and hope.

383 National Clearinghouse of RehabilitationTraining Materials (NCRTM)
Utah State Univerity
6524 Old Main Hill
Logan, UT 84322 405-744-2000
866-821-5355
FAX 435-797-7537
TDY:405-744-2002
http://www.nchrtm.okstate.edu
e-mail: ncrtm@cc.us.edu
Michael Millington PhD, Director
Jared Schultz, Principal Investigator

The mission of the NCRTM is to advocate for the advancement of best practice in rehabilitation counseling through the development, collection, dissemination, and utilization of professional information, knowledge and skill.

384 National Dissemination Center for Children with Disabilities
P.O. Box 1492
Washington, DC 20013 202-884-0285
FAX 202-884-8441
http://www.nichcy.org
e-mail: nichcy@aed.org
Stephen F Moseley, President/CEO
Jack Downey, SVP/COO
Judy L Shanley Ph.D, Project Officer OSEP
National Dissemination Center for Children with Disabilities is a central source of information on: disabilities in infants, toddlers, children, and youth; IDEA, which is the law authorizing special education; No Child Left Behind (as it relates to children with disabilities); and research-based information on effective educational practices.

385 National Institute of Mental Health (NIMH)National Institute of Neurological Disorders and Stroke
(NINDS)
6001 Executive Boulevard
Bethesda, MD 20892 301-443-4513
FAX 301-443-4279
http://www.nimh.nih.gov
e-mail: nimhinfo@nih.gov
Story C Landis Ph.D, Director NINDS
Walter J Koroshetz M.D., Deputy Director NINDS
Paul Scott Ph.D, Director Office Science Pol/Plng
NINDS is part of the National Institutes of Health several components of which support research on developmental disorders such as ADHD. Research programs of the NINDS, the National Institute of Mental Health (NIMH), and the National Institute of Child Health and Human Development (NICHD) seek to address unanswered questions about the causes of ADHD, as well as to improve diagnosis and treatment.

386 National Resource Center on AD/HD
CHADD
8181 Professional Drive
Landover, MD 20785 301-306-7070
800-233-4050
FAX 301-306-7090
http://www.help4adhd.org/
Timothy J MacGeorge MSW, Director
Micole Roder MSW, Operations Manager
E Clarke Ross, CEO/CHADD
The National Resource Center on AD/HD (NRC): A Program of CHADD (Children and Adults with Attention-Deficit/Hyperactivity Disorder), was established in 2002 to be the national clearinghouse for the latest evidence-based information on AD/HD. The NRC provides comprehensive information and support to individuals with AD/HD, their families and friends, and the professionals involved in their lives.

387 U.S. Department of Health & Human ServicesAdministration on Developmental Disabilities
370 L'Enfant Promenade SW
Washington, DC 20447 202-690-6590
FAX 202-690-6904
http://www.acf.hhs.gov/programs/add/
e-mail: fmccormick@acf.hhs.gov
Patricia A Morrissey Ph.D, Commissioner
Faith McCormick, Director
Carla Thomas, Management Analyst
The Administration on Developmental Disabilities ensures that individuals with developmental disabilities and their families participate in the design of and have access to culturally competent services, supports, and other assistance and opportunities that promotes independence, productivity, and integration and inclusion into the community.

Publications

388 A New Look at ADHD: Inhibition, Time, andSelf-Control
Guilford Publications
72 Spring Street
New York, NY 10012 212-431-9800
800-365-7006
FAX 212-966-6708
http://www.guilford.com
e-mail: info@guilford.com
Russell A Barkley Ph.D, Author
Robert Matloff, President
Seymour Weingarten, Editor-in-Chief
Marian Robinson, Marketing Director
This video provides an accessible introduction to Russell A. Barkley's influential theory of the nature and origins of ADHD. The companion manual reviews and amplifies key ideas and contains helpful suggestions for further reading. The package also includes a leader's guide, providing tips on the optimal use of the video with a variety of audiences. *$99.00*
Video & Manual
ISBN 1-593854-21-8

389 AD/HD For Dummies
American Psychiatric Publishing, Inc (APPI)
1000 Wilson Boulevard
Arlington, VA 22209 703-907-7322
800-368-5777
FAX 703-907-1091
http://www.appi.org
e-mail: appi@psych.org
Jeff Strong and Michael O Flanagan, Author
Robert E Hales MD, Editor-in-Chief
Robert S Pursell, Marketing Director
Karen Fraley, International Translation Rights
This book provides answers for parents of children who may have either condition, as well as for adult sufferers. Written in a friendly, easy-to-understand style, it helps people recognize and understand ADD and ADHD symptoms and offers an authoritative, balanced overview of both drug and non-drug therapies. *$29.95*
Paperback
ISBN 0-764537-12-7

390 ADD and Creativity: Tapping Your Inner Muse
Taylor Publishing
1550 W Mockingbird Lane
Dallas, TX 75235 214-637-2800
800-677-2800
FAX 214-819-8580
http://www.taylorpublishing.com
e-mail: brosser@taylorpublishing.com
Lynn Weiss, PhD, Author
Don Percenti, CEO
Boyd Rosser, Human Resources Director
Stacy Young, Office Manager
Raises and answers questions about the dynamic between the two components and shows how they can be a wonderful gift but also a painful liability if not properly handled. Real-life stories and inspirational affirmations throughout.

216 pages Paperback
ISBN 0-878339-60-4

391 **ADD and Romance: Finding Fulfillment in Love, Sex and Relationships**
Taylor Publishing
1550 W Mockingbird Lane
Dallas, TX 75235
214-637-2800
800-677-2800
FAX 214-819-8580
http://www.taylorpublishing.com
e-mail: brosser@taylorpublishing.com
Jonathan Scott Halverstadt, Author
Don Percenti, CEO
Charles Kass, Assistant Director
Boyd Rosser, Human Resources Director
A look at how attention deficit disorder can damage romantic relationships when partners do not take time, or do not know how to address this problem. This book provides the tools needed to build and sustain a more satisfying relationship.
240 pages Paperback
ISBN 0-878332-09-X

392 **ADD and Success**
Taylor Publishing
1550 W Mockingbird Lane
Dallas, TX 75235
214-637-2800
800-677-2800
FAX 214-819-8580
http://www.taylorpublishing.com
e-mail: brosser@taylorpublishing.com
Lynn Weiss, PhD, Author
Don Percenti, CEO
Charles Kass, Assistant Director
Boyd Rosser, Human Resources Director
Presents the stories of 13 individuals and their experiences and challenges of living with adult attention disorder and achieving success.
224 pages Paperback
ISBN 0-878339-94-9

393 **ADD in Adults**
Taylor Publishing
1550 W Mockingbird Lane
Dallas, TX 75235
214-637-2800
800-677-2800
FAX 214-819-8580
http://www.taylorpublishing.com
e-mail: brosser@taylorpublishing.com
Lynn Weiss, PhD, Author
Don Percenti, CEO
Charles Kass, Assistant Director
Boyd Rosser, Human Resources Director
Updated version of this best-selling book on the topic of ADD helps others to understand and live with the issues related to ADD. *$17.95*
192 pages Paperback
ISBN 0-878338-50-0

394 **ADD/ADHD Behavior-Change Resource Kit: Ready-to-Use Strategies & Activities for Helping Children**
With Attention Deficit Disorder
American Psychiatric Publishing
Arlington, VA 22209
703-907-7322
800-368-5777
FAX 703-907-1091
http://www.appi.org
e-mail: appi@psych.org
Grad L Flick Ph.D, Author
Robert E Hales MD, Editor-in-Chief
Robert S Pursell, Marketing Director
Karen Fraley, International Translation Rights
For teachers, counselors and parents, this comprehensive new resource is filled with up-to-date information and practical strategies to help kids with attention deficits learn to control and change their own behaviors and build the academic, social, and personal skills necessary for success in school and in life. The Kit first explains ADD/ADHD behavior, its biological bases and basic characteristics and describes procedures used for diagnosis and various treatment options. *$29.95*
Paperback
ISBN 0-876281-44-4

395 **ADHD**
Learning Disabilities Association of America
4156 Library Road
Pittsburgh, PA 15234
412-341-1515
FAX 412-344-0224
http://www.ldaamerica.org
e-mail: info@ldaamerica.org
Larry B Silver, MD, Author
Sheila Buckley, President
Sharon Tanner, Development Coordinator

A booklet for parents offering information on Attention Deficit-Hyperactivity Disorders and learning disabilities. *$3.95*

396 **ADHD - What Can We Do?**
Guilford Publications
72 Spring Street
New York, NY 10012
212-431-9800
800-365-7006
FAX 212-966-6708
http://www.guilford.com
e-mail: info@guilford.com
Russell A Barkley Ph.D, Author
Robert Matloff, President
Seymour Weingarten, Editor-in-Chief
Marian Robinson, Marketing Director
This program introduces viewers to a variety of the most effective techniques for managing ADHD in the classroom, at home, and on family outings. Illustrated are ways that parents, teachers, and other professionals can work together to implement specific strategies that help children with the disorder improve their school performance and behavior. Informative interviews, demonstrations of techniques, and commentary from Dr. Barkley illuminate the significant difference that treatment can make. *$99.00*
Manual-DVD/VHS
ISBN 1-593854-25-0

397 **ADHD - What Do We Know?**
Guilford Publications
72 Spring Street
New York, NY 10012
212-431-9800
800-365-7006
FAX 212-966-6708
http://www.guilford.com
e-mail: info@guilford.com
Russell A Barkley Ph.D, Author
Robert Matloff, President
Seymour Weingarten, Editor-in-Chief
Marian Robinson, Marketing Director
Covering all the basic issues surrounding ADHD, this program is highly instructive. Through commentary from Dr. Barkley and interviews with parents, teachers, and children, viewers gain an understanding of: the causes and prevalence of ADHD; effects on children's learning and behavior; other conditions that may accompany ADHD, and, long-term prospects for children with the disorder. *$99.00*
Manual-DVD/VHS
ISBN 1-593854-17-X

398 **ADHD Challenge Newsletter**
PO Box 2277
Peabody, MA 01960
800-233-2322
FAX 978-535-3276
http://www.dyslexiacenter.org/ar/000039.shtml/
e-mail: info@dyslexiacenter.org
Joan T Esposito, Founder/Program Director

National newsletter on ADD/ADHD that presents interviews with nationally-known scientists, as well as physicians, psychologists, social workers, educators, and other practitioners in the field of ADHD. *$35.00*
Bimonthly

399 **ADHD Report**
Guilford Publications
72 Spring Street
New York, NY 10012
212-431-9800
800-365-7006
FAX 212-966-6708
http://www.guilford.com
e-mail: info@guilford.com

Russell A Barkley PhD, Author
Robert Matloff, President
Seymour Weingarten, Editor-in-Chief

Presents the most up-to-date information on the evaluation, diagnosis and management of ADHD in children, adolescents and adults. This important newsletter is an invaluable resource for all professionals interested in ADHD. *$79.00*

16 pages Bimonthly
ISSN 1065-8025

400 ADHD and the Nature of Self-Control

Guilford Publications
72 Spring Street
New York, NY 10012
212-431-9800
800-365-7006
FAX 212-966-6708
http://www.guilford.com
e-mail: info@guilford.com

Russell A Barkley Ph.D, Author
Robert Matloff, President
Seymour Weingarten, Editor-in-Chief
Marian Robinson, Marketing Director

This instructive program integrates information about ADHD with the experiences of adults from different walks of life who suffer from the disorder. Including interviews with these individuals, their family members, and the clinicians who treat them, the program addresses such important topics as the symptoms and behaviors that are characteristic of the disorder, how adult ADHD differs from the childhood form, the effects of ADHD on the family, and successful coping strategies. *$55.00*

Hardcover
ISBN 1-593853-89-0

401 ADHD in Adolescents: Diagnosis and Treatment

Guilford Publications
72 Spring Street
New York, NY 10012
212-431-9800
800-365-7006
FAX 212-966-6708
http://www.guilford.com
e-mail: info@guilford.com

Arthur L Robin, forward by Russell A Barkley Ph.D, Author
Robert Matloff, President
Seymour Weingarten, Editor-in-Chief
Marian Robinson, Marketing Director

This highly practical guide presents an empirically based approach to understanding, diagnosing, and treating ADHD in adolescents. Practitioners learn to conduct effective assessments and formulate goals that teenagers can comprehend, accept, and achieve. Educational, medical, and family components of treatment are described in depth, illustrated with detailed case material. Included are numerous reproducible handouts and forms. *$32.00*

Paperback
ISBN 1-572305-45-2

402 ADHD in Adults: What the Science Says

Guilford Publications
72 Spring Street
New York, NY 10012
212-431-9800
800-365-7006
FAX 212-966-6708
http://www.guilford.com
e-mail: info@guilford.com

Russell Barkley, Kevin Murphy, Mariellen Fischer, Author
Robert Matloff, President
Seymour Weingarten, Editor-in-Chief
Marian Robinson, Marketing Director

Providing a new perspective on ADHD in adults, this book analyzes findings from two major studies directed by leading authority Russell A. Barkley. Information is presented on the significant impairments produced by the disorder across major functional domains and life activities, including educational outcomes, work, relationships, health behaviors, and mental health. Accessible tables, figures, and sidebars encapsulate the study results and offer detailed descriptions of the methods. *$50.00*

Hardcover
ISBN 1-593855-86-9

403 ADHD in the Schools: Assessment and Intervention Strategies

Guilford Publications
72 Spring Street
New York, NY 10012
212-431-9800
800-365-7006
FAX 212-966-6708
http://www.guilford.com
e-mail: info@guilford.com

George J DuPaul and Gary Stoner, Author
Robert Matloff, President
Seymour Weingarten, Editor-in-Chief
Marian Robinson, Marketing Director

This popular reference and text provides essential guidance for school-based professionals meeting the challenges of ADHD at any grade level. Comprehensive and practical, the book includes several reproducible assessment tools and handouts. A team-based approach to intervention is emphasized in chapters offering research-based guidelines for identifying and assessing children with ADHD and those at risk. *$29.00*

Paperback
ISBN 1-593850-89-1

404 ADHD/Hyperactivity: A Consumer's Guide For Parents and Teachers

GSI Publications
Dewitt, NY 13214
315-446-4849
800-550-2343
FAX 315-446-2012
http://www.gsi-add.com
e-mail: info@gsi-add.com

Michael Gordon Ph.D, President/Founder

The publication is designed to assist parents and teachers in understanding ADHD/Hyperactivity, providing guidance in the selection of educational programs, effective evaluations, and offers suggestions for choosing medications. Dr. Gordon discusses 30 easy-to-understand principles that will help parents, teachers, and clinicians avoid the many pitfalls along the path to effective diagnosis and treatment. *$14.95*

405 ADHD: Attention Deficit Hyperactivity Disorder in Children, Adolescents, and Adults

Oxford University Press
198 Madison Avenue
New York, NY 10016
212-726-6000
FAX 212-726-6453
http://www.oup.com/us
e-mail: intlsales.us@oup.com OR patrick.lynch@oup.com

Paul H Wender, Author
Timothy Barton, President
Ellen Taus, Chief Financial Officer
Patrick Lynch, Psychology Dept Editor

ADHD provides parents and adults whose lives have been touched by this disorder an indispensable source of help, hope, and understanding. Explains the vital importance of drug therapy in treating ADHD; provides practical and extensive instructions for parents of ADHD sufferers; includes personal accounts of ADHD children, adolescents, and adults; and, offers valuable advice on where to find help. *$13.95*

ISBN 0-195113-49-7

406 Assessing ADHD in the Schools

Guilford Publications
72 Spring Street
New York, NY 10012
212-431-9800
800-365-7006
FAX 212-966-6708
http://www.guilford.com
e-mail: info@guilford.com

George J DuPaul and Gary Stoner, Author
Robert Matloff, President
Seymour Weingarten, Editor-in-Chief
Marian Robinson, Marketing Director

This dynamic program demonstrates an innovative model for assessing ADHD in the schools. In a departure from other approaches, DuPaul and Stoner depict assessment as a collaborative, problem-solving process that is inextricably linked to the planning of individualized interventions. A range of crucial assessment techniques are considered, including parent interviews, behavior and academic performance rating scales, and direct observation. *$99.00*

Manual-DVD/VHS
ISBN 1-572304-14-6

407 Attention Deficit Disorder in Adults Workbook
Taylor Publishing
1550 W Mockingbird Lane
Dallas, TX 75235
214-637-2800
800-677-2800
FAX 214-819-8580
http://www.taylorpublishing.com
e-mail: brosser@taylorpublishing.com
Lynn Weiss, Author
Don Percenti, CEO
Charles Kass, Assistant Director
Boyd Rosser, Human Resources Director
Dr. Lynn Weiss's best-selling Attention Deficit Disorder In Adults has sold over 125,000 copies since its publication in 1991. This updated volume still contains all the original information — how to tell if you have ADD, ways to master distraction, ADD's impact on the family, and more—plus the newest treatments available. *$17.99*
192 pages Paperback
ISBN 0-878338-50-0

408 Attention Deficit Disorder: A Concise Source of Information for Parents
Temeron Books
PO Box 896
Bellingham, WA 98227
360-738-4016
FAX 360-738-4016
http://www.temerondetselig.com
e-mail: temeron@telusplanet.net
H Moghadam, MD and Joel Fagan, MD, Author

The authors travel from a brief historical review of ADD, through a description of symptoms and consequences, to a discussion of treatment. *$12.95*
128 pages Paperback
ISBN 1-550590-82-0

409 Attention Deficit Hyperactivity Disorder: Handbook for Diagnosis & Treatment
Guilford Publications
72 Spring Street
New York, NY 10012
212-431-9800
800-365-7006
FAX 212-966-6708
http://www.guilford.com
e-mail: info@guilford.com
Russell A Barkley, PhD, Author
Robert Matloff, President
Seymour Weingarten, Editor-in-Chief

This second edition helps clinicians diagnose and treat Attention Deficit Hyperactivity Disorder. Written by an internationally recognized authority in the field, it covers the history of ADHD, its primary symptoms, associated conditions, developmental course and outcome, and family context. A workbook companion manual is also available.
700 pages Hardcover

410 Attention Deficit/Hyperactivity DisorderFact Sheet
National Dissemination Center for Children with Disabilities
Washington, DC 20013
202-884-0285
FAX 202-884-8441
http://www.nichcy.org/pubs/factshe/fs19txt.htm
e-mail: nichcy@aed.org
Stephen F Moseley, President/CEO
Jack Downey, SVP/COO
Judy L Shanley Ph.D, Project Officer OSEP
An 8 page informational fact sheet, a publication of the National Dissemination Center for Children with Disabilities, that provides information on attention deficit/hyperactivity disorder in infants, toddlers, children, and youth. The brochure provides suggestions and tips for parents and teachers in addition to providing links to organizations where individuals can obtain further details on ADHD.

411 Attention-Deficit Disorders and Comorbidities in Children, Adolescents, and Adults
American Psychiatric Publishing, Inc (APPI)
1000 Wilson Boulevard
Arlington, VA 22209
703-907-7322
800-368-5777
FAX 703-907-1091
http://www.appi.org
e-mail: appi@psych.org
Thomas Brown, Author
Robert E Hales MD, Editor-in-Chief
Robert S Pursell, Marketing Director
Karen Fraley, International Translation Rights
Book provides in-depth discussion of both ADD/Attention Deficit Disorders and that of ADHD/Attention Deficit-Hyperactivity Disorders, providing readers with information that focuses on several perspectives including learning disorders in children and adolescents; cognitive therapy for adults with ADHD; educational interventions for students with ADDs; tailoring treatments for individuals with ADHD; clinical and research perspectives, etc. *$82.00*
Hardcover
ISBN 0-880487-11-9

412 Attention-Deficit Hyperactivity Disorder:A Clinical Workbook
Guilford Publications
72 Spring Street
New York, NY 10012
212-431-9800
800-365-7006
FAX 212-966-6708
http://www.guilford.com
e-mail: info@guilford.com
Russell A Barkley and Kevin R Murphy, Author
Robert Matloff, President
Seymour Weingarten, Editor-in-Chief
Marian Robinson, Marketing Director
The revised and expanded third edition of this user-friendly workbook provides a master set of the assessment and treatment forms, questionnaires, and handouts recommended by Barkley in the third edition of the Handbook. Formatted for easy photocopying, many of these materials are available from no other source. Includes interview forms and rating scales for use with parents, teachers, and adult clients; checklists and fact sheets; daily school report cards for monitoring academic progress. *$34.00*
Paperback
ISBN 1-593852-27-4

413 Attention-Deficit/Hyperactivity Disorder: A Clinical Guide To Diagnosis and Treatment
American Psychiatric Publishing, Inc (APPI)
1000 Wilson Boulevard
Arlington, VA 22209
703-907-7322
800-368-5777
FAX 703-907-1091
http://www.appi.org
e-mail: appi@psych.org
Larry B Silver, Author
Robert E Hales MD, Editor-in-Chief
Robert S Pursell, Marketing Director
Karen Fraley, International Translation Rights
This new edition of Dr. Larry Silver's groundbreaking clinical book incorporates recent research findings on attention-deficit/hyperactivity disorder (ADHD), covering the latest information on diagnosis, associated disorders, and treatment, as well as ADHD in adults. The publication thoroughly reviews disorders often found to be comorbid with ADHD, including specific learning disorders, anxiety disorders, depression, anger regulation problems, obsessive-compulsive disorder, and tic disorders. *$36.95*
Paperback
ISBN 1-585621-31-5

414 CHADD Educators Manual
CHADD
8181 Professional Place
Landover, MD 20785
301-306-7070
800-233-4050
FAX 301-306-7090
http://www.chadd.org
e-mail: national@chadd.org
Anne Teeter-Ellison MD, Author
Chris Dendy, Editor
Marsha Bokman, Manager
Paul Seifart, Public Policy

An in-depth look at Attention Deficit Disorders from an educational perspective. *$10.00*

415 Children with ADD: A Shared Responsibility
Council for Exceptional Children
1110 N Glebe Road
Arlington, VA 22201
703-620-3660
888-232-7733
FAX 703-264-9494
TDY:866-915-5000
http://www.cec.sped.org
e-mail: service@cec.sped.org
Suzanne Martin, President
Bruce Ramirez, Executive Director
Doug Faulke, Senior Director
This book represents a consensus of what professionals and parents believe ADD is all about and how children with ADD may best be served. Reviews the evaluation process under IDEA and 504 and presents effective classroom strategies.
35 pages
ISBN 0-865862-33-8

416 Classroom Interventions for ADHD
Guilford Publications
72 Spring Street
New York, NY 10012
212-431-9800
800-365-7006
FAX 212-966-6708
http://www.guilford.com
e-mail: info@guilford.com
George J DuPaul and Gary Stoner, Author
Robert Matloff, President
Seymour Weingarten, Editor-in-Chief
Marian Robinson, Marketing Director
This informative video provides an overview of intervention approaches that can be used to help students with ADHD enhance their school performance while keeping the classroom functioning smoothly. The video features an illuminating discussion among DuPaul, Stoner, and Russell A. Barkley, addressing provocative questions on the benefits of proactive, preventive measures, on the one hand, and reactive techniques, on the other. *$99.00*
Manual-DVD/VHS
ISBN 1-572304-15-4

417 Coping: Attention Deficit Disorder: A Guide for Parents and Teachers
Temeron Books
PO Box 896
Bellingham, WA 98227
360-738-4016
FAX 360-738-4016
http://www.temerondetselig.com
e-mail: temeron@telusplanet.net
Mary Ellen Beugin, Author

The author investigates medical and behavioral interventions that can be tried with ADD children and gives suggestions on coping with these children at home and at school. *$15.95*
173 pages Paperback 1990
ISBN 1-550590-13-8

418 Driven to Distraction: Attention Deficit Disorder from Childhood Through Adulthood
Hallowell Center
142 North Road
Sudbury, MA 01776
978-287-0810
FAX 978-287-5566
http://www.drhallowell.com/hallowell_center/
e-mail: drhallowell@gmail.com
Edward Hallowell, John Ratey, Author
Edward M Hallowell, Founder/President

Through vivid stories of the experience of their patients, Drs. Hallowell and Ratey show the varied forms ADD takes — from the hyperactive search for high stimulation to the floating inattention of daydreaming — and the transforming impact of precise diagnosis and treatment. *$10.40*
336 pages 1995
ISBN 0-684801-28-0

419 E-ssential Guide: A Parent's Guide to AD/HD Basics
Schwab Learning
1650 S Amphlett Boulevard
San Mateo, CA 94402
650-655-2410
FAX 650-655-2411
http://www.schwablearning.org
e-mail: marketing@schwablearning.org
Marcelle White, Managing Editor
Linda Broatch, Editor/Writer
Scott Moore Sr, Online Community Manager
This guide covers the fundamental facts about Attention-Deficit/Hyperactivity Disorder (AD/HD) that will provide a better understanding of AD/HD. Included is: A general overview of AD/HD and helpful strategies for managing your child's AD/HD at home and at school.

420 Fact Sheet-Attention Deficit Hyperactivity Disorder
Attention Deficit Disorder Association
15000 Commerce Parkway
Mount Laurel, NJ 08054
856-439-9099
FAX 856-439-0525
http://www.add.org/articles/factsheet.html
e-mail: DrJaksa@aol.com
Linda S Anderson, President Board of Directors
Evelyn Polk Green, VP/Board of Directors
Mary Jane Johnson, VP/Board of Directors
A pamphlet offering factual information on ADHD. *$10.00*

421 Family Therapy for ADHD - Treating Children, Adolescents, and Adults
Guilford Publications
72 Spring Street
New York, NY 10012
212-431-9800
800-365-7006
FAX 212-966-6708
http://www.guilford.com
e-mail: info@guilford.com
Craig A Everett and Sandra Volgy Everett, Author
Robert Matloff, President
Seymour Weingarten, Editor-in-Chief
Marian Robinson, Marketing Director
Presents an innovative approach to assessing and treating ADHD in the family context. Readers learn strategies for diagnosing the disorder and evaluating its impact not only on affected young persons but also on their parents and siblings. From expert family therapists, the volume outlines how professionals can help families mobilize their resources to manage ADHD symptoms; improve functioning in school and work settings; and develop more effective coping strategies. *$ 29.00*
Paperback
ISBN 1-572307-08-0

422 Focus Magazine
Attention Deficit Disorder Association
15000 Commerce Parkway
Mount Laurel, NJ 08054
856-439-9099
FAX 856-439-0525
http://www.add.org
e-mail: mail@add.org
Linda Anderson, President/Board of Directors
Evelyn Polk Green, VP/Board of Directors

The National Attention Deficit Disorder Association is an organization focused on the needs of adults and young adults with ADD/ADHD, and their children and families. We seek to serve individuals with ADD, as well as those who love, live with, teach, counsel and treat them. Free with membership.
Quarterly

423 Getting a Grip on ADD: A Kid's Guide to Understanding & Coping with ADD
Educational Media Corporation
4256 Central Avenue NE
Minneapolis, MN 55421
818-708-0962
800-966-3382
FAX 763-781-7753
http://www.educationalmedia.com
e-mail: emedia@educationalmedia.com
Kim Frank EdS, Susan Smith Rex EdD, Author
William Meisel, President
Susan Smith, Author

Help your elementary and middle school students cope more effectively with Attention Deficit Disorders. *$9.95*

64 pages Paperback 1994

ISBN 0-932796-60-5

424 How to Reach & Teach Teenagers With ADHD

John Wiley & Sons Inc
111 River Street
Hoboken, NJ 07030-5774
201-748-6000
800-225-5945
FAX 201-748-6088
http://www.wiley.com
e-mail: info@wiley.com

Grad L Flick Ph.D, Author
Peter B Wiley, Chairman
William J Pesce, President/CEO
Warren C Fristensky, SVP/Chief Information Officer

This comprehensive resource is pack with tested, up-to-date information and techniques to help teachers, counselors and parents understand and manage adolescents with attention deficit disorder, including step-by-step procedures for behavioral intervention at school and home and reproducible handouts, checklists and record-keeping forms. *$29.00*

ISBN 0-130320-21-6

425 Hyperactive Child Book

St. Martin's Press
175 5th Avenue
New York, NY 10010
212-674-5151
800-321-9299
FAX 212-674-6132
http://www.stmartins.com
e-mail: george.witte@stmartins.com

Patricia Kennedy, Lief G Terdal, Author
John Sargent, CEO
George Witte, President

The Hyperactive Child Book contains a comprehensive review of information about raising, treating, and educating a child with Attention Deficit-Hyperactivity Disorder. The book will be useful to parents, teachers, and health care professionals in their efforts to provide for the ADHD child. *$12.95*

288 pages 1994

ISBN 0-312112-86-6

426 Hyperactive Child, Adolescent and Adult

Oxford University Press
198 Madison Avenue
New York, NY 10016
212-726-6000
800-451-7556
FAX 212-726-6440
http://www.oup.com/us
e-mail: custserv.us@oup.com

Paul H Wender MD, Author
Laura Brown, CEO
Terry Dickerson, Office Manager

How does one know if a youngster is hyperactive? How do you know if you are hyperactive yourself? The answers may lie in this easy-to-read and comprehensive volume written by one of the leading researchers in the field. *$27.00*

172 pages Hardcover 1987

ISBN 0-195042-91-3

427 Hyperactive Children Grown Up: ADHD in Children, Adolescents, and Adults

Guilford Publications
72 Spring Street
New York, NY 10012
212-431-9800
800-365-7006
FAX 212-966-6708
http://www.guilford.com
e-mail: info@guilford.com

Gabrielle Weiss and Lily Trokenberg Hechtman, Author
Robert Matloff, President
Seymour Weingarten, Editor-in-Chief
Marian Robinson, Marketing Director

Based on the McGill prospective studies, research that now spans more than 30 years, the volume reports findings on the etiology, treatment, and outcome of attention deficits and hyperactivity at all stages of development. This second edition includes entirely new chapters that describes new developments in Attention Deficit Hyperactivity Disorder (ADHD) in addition to the assessment, diagnosis, and treatment of ADHD adults. *$35.00*

Paperback

ISBN 0-898625-96-3

428 I Would if I Could: A Teenager's Guide ToADHD/Hyperactivity

GSI Publications
Dewitt, NY 13214
315-446-4849
800-550-2343
FAX 315-446-2012
http://www.gsi-add.com
e-mail: info@gsi-add.com

Michael Gordon Ph.D, President/Founder

Provides youngsters with straightforward information about the disorder in addition to exploring its impact on family relationships, self-esteem, and friendships. Dr. Gordon uses humor and candor to educate and encourage teenagers who too often find themselves confused and frustrated, providing youngsters with straightforward information about the disorder and exploring its impact on family relationships, self-esteem, and friendships. *$12.50*

429 I'd Rather Be With a Real Mom Who Loves Me: A Story for Foster Children

GSI Publications
Dewitt, NY 13214
315-446-4849
800-550-2343
FAX 315-446-2012
http://www.gsi-add.com
e-mail: info@gsi-add.com

Michael Gordon Ph.D, President/Founder

This book tells the story of a young boy who's lived most of his life away from his birth parents. It's an honest, realistic account of the frustrations and heartache he endures. This fully illustrated book sensitively but forthrightly deals with the entire range of concerns that confront foster children with ADHD/Hyperactivity disorder. *$12.00*

430 Identifying and Treating Attention Deficit Hyperactivity Disorder: A Resource for School and Home

U S Department of Education/Special Ed-Rehab Srvcs
Education Publications Center
Jessup, MD 20794
800-872-5327
FAX 301-470-1244
http://www.ed.gov/rschstat/research/pubs/adhd
e-mail: edpubs@inet.ed.gov

Alexa Posny, Director Special Ed Programs
Louis Danielson, Director Research Division
Kelly Henderson, Technical Representative

Publication from the U S Department of Education that provides comprehensive information on attention deficit hyperactivity disorders, including causes, medical evaluation and treatment options in addition to helpful hints and tips for both the home and school environments. *$6.00*

431 International Reading Association Newspaper: Reading Today

International Reading Association
800 Barksdale Road
Newark, DE 19711
302-731-1600
800-336-7323
FAX 302-731-1057
http://www.reading.org
e-mail: pubinfo@reading.org

Timothy Shanahan, President
Linda Gambrell, President-Elect
Alan Farstrup, Executive Director

Reading Today, the Association's bimonthly newspaper, is the first choice of IRA members for news and information on all these topics and more. It is available in print exclusively as an IRA membership benefit.

Bimonthly

432 Jumpin' Johnny

GSI Publications
Dewitt, NY 13214
315-446-4849
800-550-2343
FAX 315-446-2012
http://www.gsi-add.com
e-mail: info@gsi-add.com

Michael Gordon Ph.D, President/Founder

This entertaining and informative book will help children understand the basic ideas about the evaluation of ADHD/Hyperactivity. Jumpin' Johnny tells what it is like to be inattentive and impulsive, and how his family and school work with him to make life easier. Children find this book amusing, educational, and accurate in its depiction of the challenges that confront them daily. *$11.00*

433 LD Child and the ADHD Child

John F Blair, Publisher
1406 Plaza Drive
Winston Salem, NC 27103
336-768-1374
800-222-9796
FAX 336-768-9194
http://www.blairpub.com
e-mail: blairpub@blairpub.com
Suzanne H Stevens, Author
Carolyn Sakowski, President
Steve Kirk, Editor-in-Chief

It is a brief, upbeat, always realistic look at what learning disabilities are and what problems LD children and parents face at home and at school. It contains a wealth of valuable suggestions, and its tempered optimism may dimish one's sense of futility and helplessness. *$12.95*

261 pages Paperback
ISBN 0-895871-42-4

434 Learning Times

Learning Disabilities Association of Georgia
2566 Shallowford Road
Atlanta, GA 30345
404-303-7774
FAX 404-467-0190
http://www.ldag.org
e-mail: services@ldag.org
Joan Teach Ph.D, President
Beth Martin, Board of Directors Secretary
Debra Wathen, Treasurer

Information and helpful articles on learning disabilities. *$40.00*

Bimonthly

435 Making the System Work for Your Child with ADHD

Guilford Publications
72 Spring Street
New York, NY 10012
212-431-9800
800-365-7006
FAX 212-966-6708
http://www.guilford.com
e-mail: info@guilford.com
Peter S Jensen, Author
Robert Matloff, President
Seymour Weingarten, Editor-in-Chief
Marian Robinson, Marketing Director

Child psychiatrist Dr. Peter Jensen guides parents over the rough patches and around the hairpin curves in this empowering, highly informative book. Readers learn the whats, whys, and how-tos of making the system work and in getting their money's worth from the healthcare system, cutting through red tape at school, and making the most of fleeting time with doctors and therapists. *$17.95*

Paperback
ISBN 1-572308-70-2

436 Managing Attention Deficit Hyperactivity Disorder: A Guide for Practitioners

John Wiley & Sons Inc
111 River Street
Hoboken, NJ 07030-5774
201-748-6000
800-225-5945
FAX 201-748-6088
http://www.wiley.com
e-mail: info@wiley.com
Sam Goldstein and Michael Goldstein, Author
Peter B Wiley, Chairman
William J Pesce, President/CEO
Warren C Fristensky, SVP/Chief Information Officer

A valuable working resource for practitioners who manage children with ADHD, Managing Attention Deficit Hyperactivity in Children, Second Edition features: in-depth reviews of the latest research into the etiology and development of ADHD; Step-by-step guidelines on evaluating ADHD-medically, at home, and in school; a multidisciplinary approach to treating ADHD that combines medical, family, cognitive, behavioral, and school interventions; and critical discussions of controversial new treatments. *$130.00*

Hardcover
ISBN 0-471121-58-9

437 Mastering Your Adult ADHD: A CognitiveBehavioral Treatment Program Therapist Guide

Oxford University Press
198 Madison Avenue
New York, NY 10016
212-726-6000
FAX 212-726-6453
http://www.oup.com/us
e-mail: intlsales.us@oup.com OR patrick.lynch@oup.com
Steven A Safren, Author
Timothy Barton, President
Ellen Taus, Chief Financial Officer
Patrick Lynch, Psychology Dept Editor

Used in conjunction with the corresponding client workbook, this therapist guide offers effective treatment strategies that follow an empirically-supported treatment approach. It provides clinicians with effective means of teaching clients skills that have been scientifically tested and shown to help adults cope with ADHD. *$35.00*

ISBN 0-195188-18-7

438 Mastering Your Adult ADHD: A Cognitive Behavioral Treatment Program Client Workbook

Oxford University Press
198 Madison Avenue
New York, NY 10016
212-726-6000
FAX 212-726-6453
http://www.oup.com/us
e-mail: intlsales.us@oup.com OR patrick.lynch@oup.com
Steven A Safren, Author
Timothy Barton, President
Ellen Taus, Chief Financial Officer
Patrick Lynch, Psychology Dept Editor

The intervention described in this client workbook contains all of the necessary information for participating in a practical, tested, and effective cognitive-behavioral intervention for adults with ADHD and residual symptoms not full treated by medications alone. *$29.95*

ISBN 0-195188-19-5

439 Maybe You Know My Kid: A Parent's Guide to Identifying ADHD

Kensington Publishing
Citadel Books
New York, NY 10022
888-345-2665
FAX 201-866-1886
http://www.kensingtonbooks.com/
e-mail: customerservice@kensingtonbooks.com
Mary Cahill Fowler, Author
Steven Zacharius, President

A guide for parents of children diagnosed with ADD discusses the recent changes in the education of these children and offers practical guidelines for improving educational performance. *$14.95*

260 pages Paperback
ISBN 1-559724-90-0

440 Meeting the ADD Challenge

Research Press
PO Box 9177
Champaign, IL 61826
217-352-3273
800-519-2707
FAX 217-352-1221
http://www.researchpress.com
e-mail: rp@researchpress.com
Steven B Gordon MD, Michael J Asher MD, Author
Russell Pence, President

Provides educators with accurate up-to-date information about the needs and treatment of children and adolescents with ADD. Case examples are utilized throughout to illustrate the diversity of problems experienced by children diagnosed with ADD and to point out defining characteristics of the disorder. *$21.95*

196 pages Paperback
ISBN 0-878223-45-2

441 **Meeting the ADD Challenge: A PracticalGuide for Teachers**
Research Press
PO Box 9177
Champaign, IL 61826
217-352-3273
800-519-2707
FAX 217-352-1221
http://www.researchpress.com
e-mail: rp@researchpress.com
Steve B Gordon MD & Michael J Asher MD, Author
Russell Pence, President
Susan Allen, Office Manager

Provides educators with practical information about the needs and treatment of children and adolescents with ADD. The book addresses the defining characteristics of ADD, common treatment approaches, myths about ADD, matching intervention to student, use of behavior-rating scales and checklists evaluating interventions, regular verses, special class placement, helps students regulate their own behavior and more. Case examples are used throughout. *$17.95*
196 pages
ISBN 0-878223-45-2

442 **My Brother is a World Class Pain: A Sibling's Guide to ADHD/Hyperactivity**
GSI Publications
Dewitt, NY 13214
315-446-4849
800-550-2343
FAX 315-446-2012
http://www.gsi-add.com
e-mail: info@gsi-add.com
Michael Gordon Ph.D, President/Founder

A book for the often forgotten group of those affected by ADHD, the brothers and sisters of ADHD children, this story about an older sister's efforts to deal with her active and impulsive brother sends the clear message to siblings of the ADHD child that they can play an important role in a family's quest for change. *$11.00*

443 **NINDS Attention Deficit-Hyperactivity Disorder Information Fact Sheet**
National Institutes of Health
6001 Executive Boulevard
Bethesda, MD 20892
301-443-4513
FAX 301-443-4279
http://www.nimh.nih.gov
e-mail: nimhinfo@nih.gov
Story C Landis Ph.D, Director NINDS
Walter J Koroshetz M.D., Deputy Director NINDS
Paul Scott Ph.D, Director Office Science Pol/Plng
NINDS (National Institute of Neurological Disorders and Stroke) is part of the National Institutes of Health several components of which support research on developmental disorders such as ADHD. Informational fact sheet provides data relative to research, symptons and diagnosis, in addition to links for organizational resources relative to the disorder.

444 **National Alliance on Mental Illness (NAMI) Attention-Deficit/Hyperactivity Disorder Fact Sheet**
2107 Wilson Boulevard
Arlington, VA 22201-3042
703-524-7600
888-999-6264
FAX 703-524-9094
TDY:703-516-7227
http://www.nami.org
e-mail: info@nami.org
Michael J Fitzpatrick, Executive Director
Lynn Borton, Chief Operating Officer
Ken Duckworth, Medical Director
NAMI/National Alliance on Mental Illness is a mental health organization dedicated to improving the lives of persons living with serious mental illness and their families. ADHD fact sheet provides information on attention-deficit/hyperactivity disorder through NAMI's mission of support, education, advocacy, and research for people living with mental illness.

445 **Natural Therapies for Attention Deficit Hyperactivity Disorder**
Comprehensive Psychiatric Resources/CPR
Sterling Medical Building
Waltham, MA 02453
781-647-6657
FAX 781-647-6133
http://www.natualadd.com
e-mail: cpr@naturaladd.com
James M Greenblatt MD, Founder/Medical Director
Justine Blanc, Manager

A full day workshop professionally recorded on six audiotapes featuring Dr. James M. Greenblatt, M.D., neuropsychiatrist. Dr. Greenblatt explores updated research on nutrition and ADD, food additives, food allergies, fatty acids and more, provides practical treatment strategies and helps you make informed choices between effective and worthless therapies. *$59.95*

446 **Nutritional Treatment for Attention Deficit Hyperactivity Disorder**
Comprehensive Psychiatric Resources/CPR
Sterling Medical Building
Waltham, MA 02453
781-647-6657
FAX 781-647-6133
http://www.naturaladd.com
e-mail: cpr@naturaladd.com
James M Greenblatt MD, Founder/Medical Director
Justine Blanc, Manager

A full day workshop professionally recorded on six audiotapes featuring Dr. James M. Greenblatt, M.D., neuropsychiatrist. Dr. Greenblatt explores updated research on nutrition and ADD, food additives, food allergies, fatty acids and more, provides practical treatment strategies and helps you make informed choices between effective and worthless therapies.

447 **Power Parenting for Children with ADD/ADHD A Practical Parent's Guide for Managing Difficult Beha**
viors
John Wiley & Sons Inc
Hoboken, NJ 07030-5774
201-748-6000
800-225-5945
FAX 201-748-6088
http://www.wiley.com
e-mail: info@wiley.com
Grad L Flick Ph.D, Author
Peter B Wiley, Chairman
William J Pesce, President/CEO
Warren C Fristensky, SVP/Chief Information Officer
A Practical Parent's Guide for Managing Difficult Behaviors. Written in clear, non-technical language, this much-needed guide provides practical, real-life techniques and activities to help parents. *$19.95*

ISBN 0-876288-77-1

448 **Putting on the BrakesYoung People's Guide to Understanding Attention Deficit**
American Psychological Association/APA
APA Service Center/Magination Press
Washington, DC 20002
202-336-5500
800-374-2721
FAX 202-336-5502
TDY:202-336-6123
http://www.maginationpress.com/4414576.html
e-mail: magination@apa.org
Patricia O Quinn MD, Judith M Stern, Author
Norman Anderson, CEO

This book allows children to put their understanding of ADHD into action. Using pictures, puzzles, and other techniques to assist in the learning of a range of skills, this book helps teach problem solving, organizing, setting priorities, planning, maintaining control — all of those hard-to-learn skills that make everyday life just a little more manageable. *$14.95*
1988Grade Range: Ages 8-13
ISBN 0-945354-57-6

449 **Rethinking Attention Deficit Disorders**
Brookline Books
34 University Road
Cambridge, MA 02238
617-734-6772
FAX 617-734-3952
http://www.brooklinebooks.com
e-mail: brooklinebks@delphi.com

Miriam Cherkes-Julkowski, Author, Author
Susan Sharp, Author
Jonathan Stolzenberg, Author
Milt Budoff, Founder/President
This ground-breaking work argues that the two behavioral manifestations of attention deficit disorder—hyperactivity and impulsivity—represent a person's attempts at self-regulation. The authors view Attention Deficit Disorder as a problem with control and fluency of attention; people with ADD have sustaining focus when faced with novel and/or intense stimulae. *$27.95*

272 pages 1997
ISBN 1-571290-37-0

450 Ritalin Is Not The Answer: A Drug-Free Practical Program for Children Diagnosed With ADD or ADHD
John Wiley & Sons Inc
111 River Street
Hoboken, NJ 07030-5774
201-748-6000
800-225-5945
FAX 201-748-6088
http://www.wiley.com
e-mail: info@wiley.com
David P Stein Ph.D, Author
Peter B Wiley, Chairman
William J Pesce, President/CEO
Warren C Fristensky, SVP/Chief Information Officer
Ritalin Is Not the Answer confronts and challenges what has become common practice and teaches parents and educators a healthy, comprehensive behavioral program that really works as an alternative to the epidemic use of medication-without teaching children to use drugs in order to handle their behavioral and emotional problems. *$15.00*
Paperback
ISBN 0-787945-14-5

451 Shelley, the Hyperactive Turtle
Woodbine House
6510 Bells Mill Road
Bethesda, MD 20817
301-897-3570
800-843-7323
FAX 301-897-5838
http://www.woodbinehouse.com
e-mail: info@woodbinehouse.com
Deborah M Moss, Author
Nancy Gray Paul, Acquisitions Editor

Shelley the turtle has a very hard time sitting still, even for short periods of time. During a visit to the doctor, Shelley learns that he is hyperactive, and that he can take medicine every day to control his wiggly feeling. *$ 14.95*
20 pages Hardcover
ISBN 1-890627-75-5

452 Stimulant Drugs and ADHD Basic and Clinical Neuroscience
Oxford University Press
198 Madison Avenue
New York, NY 10016
212-726-6000
FAX 212-726-6453
http://www.oup.com/us
e-mail: intlsales.us@oup.com OR patrick.lynch@oup.com
Ed.: Mary Solanto/Amy Arnsten/F. Xavier Castellano, Author
Timothy Barton, President
Ellen Taus, Chief Financial Officer
Patrick Lynch, Psychology Dept Editor
This volume is the first to integrate advances in the basic and clinical neurosciences in order to shed new light on this important question. The chapter topics span basic research into the neuroanatomy, neurophysiology and neuropsychology of catecholamines, animal models of ADHD, and clinical studies of neuroimaging, genetics, pharmacokinetics and pharmacodynamics, and the cognitive pharmacology of stimulants. *$81.50*

ISBN 0-195133-71-4

453 The ADD/ADHD Checklist
American Psychiatric Publishing, Inc (APPI)
1000 Wilson Boulevard
Arlington, VA 22209
703-907-7322
800-368-5777
FAX 703-907-1091
http://www.appi.org
e-mail: appi@psych.org
Sandra F Rief MA, Author
Robert E Hales MD, Editor-in-Chief
Robert S Pursell, Marketing Director
Karen Fraley, International Translation Rights
Written by a nationally known educator with two decades of experience in working with ADD/ADHD students. This unique resource is packed with up-to-date facts, findings, and proven strategies and techniques for understanding and helping children and adolescents with attention deficit problems and hyperactivity- all in a handy list format. *$12.95*
Paperback
ISBN 0-137623-95-2

454 The ADHD Book of Lists: A Practical Guidefor Helping Children and Teens With ADD
American Psychiatric Publishing, Inc (APPI)
1000 Wilson Boulevard
Arlington, VA 22209
703-907-7322
800-368-5777
FAX 703-907-1091
http://www.appi.org
e-mail: appi@psych.org
Sandra F Rief MA, Author
Robert E Hales MD, Editor-in-Chief
Robert S Pursell, Marketing Director
Karen Fraley, International Translation Rights
The ADHD Book of Lists is a comprehensive, reliable source of answers, practical strategies, and tools written in a convenient list format. Created for teachers (K-12), parents, school psychologists, medical and mental health professionals, counselors, and other school personnel, this important resource contains the most current information about Attention Deficit/Hyperactivity Disorder (ADHD). *$29.95*
Paperback
ISBN 0-787965-91-4

455 The Down & Dirty Guide to Adult ADD
GSI Publications
Dewitt, NY 13214
315-446-4849
800-550-2343
FAX 315-446-2012
http://www.gsi-add.com
e-mail: info@gsi-add.com
Michael Gordon Ph.D, President/Founder

A book about Adult ADD that is informative, and uncomplicated. Drs. Gordon and McClure spare no effort or humor in clearly describing concepts essential to understanding how this disorder is best identified and treated. You'll find a refreshing absence of jargon and an abundance of common sense, practical advice, and healthy skepticism. This fine brew of scientific evidence and clinical wisdom is so cleverly presented that even the most inattentive reader will breeze through its pages. *$16.95*

456 The Hidden Disorder: A Clinician's Guide to Attention Deficit Hyperactivity Disorder in Adults
American Psychological Association (APA)
APA Service Center
Washington, DC 20002
202-336-5510
800-374-2721
FAX 202-336-5502
TDY:202-336-6123
http://www.apa.org/publications
e-mail: order@apa.org
Robert J Resnick Ph.D, Author
Sharon Stephens Brehm Ph.D, President Board of Directors
Norman B Anderson Ph.D, EVP/Chief Executive Officer
Carol D Goodheart Ed.D, Treasurer
Through accessible writing and engaging case studies, Robert J. Resnick, PhD, provides expert clinical guidance on etiology, differential diagnosis, assessment, and treatment. Adults with ADHD often require intermittent treatment at different points in their lives. This book provides various treatment interventions over the livespan. Also covered are the various co-morbid and look alike disorders that can confound diagnosis and lead to unsuccessful treatment. *$34.95*

Hardcover
ISBN 1-557987-24-2

457 **Treating Huckleberry Finn: A New Narrative Approach to Working With Kids Diagnosed ADD/ADHD**
John Wiley & Sons Inc
111 River Street
Hoboken, NJ 07030-5774
201-748-6000
800-225-5945
FAX 201-748-6088
http://www.wiley.com
e-mail: info@wiley.com

David Nylund, Author
Peter B Wiley, Chairman
William J Pesce, President/CEO
Warren C Fristensky, SVP/Chief Information Officer
Ritalin Is Not the Answer confronts and challenges what has become common practice and teaches parents and educators a healthy, comprehensive behavioral program that really works as an alternative to the epidemic use of medication-without teaching children to use drugs in order to handle their behavioral and emotional problems. *$32.00*
Paperback
ISBN 0-787961-20-6

458 **Understanding and Teaching Children With Autism**
John Wiley & Sons Inc
111 River Street
Hoboken, NJ 07030
201-748-6645
800-825-7550
FAX 201-748-6021
http://www.wiley.com
e-mail: subinfo@wiley.com

Rita Jordan, Stuart Powell, Author
William J Pesce, President/CEO
Ellis E Cousens, EVP/CFO & COO
Warren Fristensky, SVP/Chief Information Officer
The triad of impairment: social, language and communication and thought behavior aspects of development discussed. Difficulties in interacting, transfer of learning and bizarre behaviors are part of syndrome. Many LD are associated with autism. *$65.00*
188 pages Paperback 1995
ISBN 0-471957-14-3

459 **Understanding and Treating Adults With Attention Deficit Hyperactivity Disorder**
American Psychiatric Publishing, Inc (APPI)
1000 Wilson Boulevard
Arlington, VA 22209
703-907-7322
800-368-5777
FAX 703-907-1091
http://www.appi.org
e-mail: appi@psych.org

Brian B Doyle MD, Author
Robert E Hales MD, Editor-in-Chief
Robert S Pursell, Marketing Director
Karen Fraley, International Translation Rights
Understanding the evolution of the concept and treatment of ADHD in children illuminates current thinking about the disorder in adults. Dr. Doyle presents guidelines for establishing a valid diagnosis, including clinical interviews and standardized rating scales. He covers genetic and biochemical bases of the disorder. He also addresses the special challenges of forming a therapeutic alliance-working with coach caregivers; cultural, ethnic, and racial issues; and legal considerations. *$52.00*
Paperback
ISBN 1-585622-21-4

460 **What Causes ADHD?: Understanding What Goes Wrong and Why**
Guilford Publications
72 Spring Street
New York, NY 10012
212-431-9800
800-365-7006
FAX 212-966-6708
http://www.guilford.com
e-mail: info@guilford.com

Joel T Nigg, Author
Robert Matloff, President
Seymour Weingarten, Editor-in-Chief
Marian Robinson, Marketing Director

This book focuses on the multiple pathways by which attention-deficit/ hyperactivity disorder (ADHD) develops. Joel T. Nigg discusses the processes taking place within the symptomatic child's brain and the reasoning for such activity, tracing intersecting causal influences of genetic, neural, and environmental factors. Specific suggestions are provided for studies that might further refine the conceptualization of the disorder, with significant potential benefits for treatment and prevention. *$44.00*
Hardcover
ISBN 1-593852-67-3

461 **Why Can't My Child Behave?**
Feingold Association of the United States
554 East Main Street
Riverhead, NY 11901
631-369-9340
800-321-3287
FAX 631-369-2988
http://www.feingold.org/book.html
e-mail: help@feingold.org OR janefaus@aol.com
Jane Hersey, Author
Lynn Murphy, President
Jane Hersey, Director

This book shows how foods and food additives can trigger learning and behavior problems in sensitive people. It provides practical guidance on using a simple diet to uncover the causes of ADD and ADHD. *$22.00*
473 pages Paperback 1996Grade Range: All grades
ISBN 0-965110-50-8

462 **You Mean I'm Not Lazy, Stupid or Crazy?**
Simon & Schuster
1230 Avenue of the Americas
New York, NY 10020
212-698-7000
800-622-6611
FAX 212-698-7007
http://www.simonsays.com

Peggy Ramundo, Author
Kate Kelly, Author

This new book is the first written by ADD adults for other ADD adults. A comprehensive guide, it provides accurate information, practical how-to's, and moral support. Among other issues, readers will get information on: unique differences in ADD adults; the impact on their lives; up-to-date research findings; treatment options available for adults; and much more. *$16.00*
464 pages
ISBN 0-743264-48-7

Web Sites

463 **www.add.org**
Attention Deficit Disorder Association

The National Attention Deficit Disorder Association is an organization focused on the needs of adults and young adults with ADD/ADHD, and their children and families. We seek to serve individuals with ADD, as well as those who love, live with, teach, counsel and treat them.

464 **www.addhelpline.org**
ADD Helpline for Help with ADD

A site dedicated to providing information and support to all parents, regardless of their choice of treatment, belief or approach toward ADD/ADHD.

465 **www.additudemag.com**
Attitude Magazine

Information and inspiration for adults and children with attention deficit disorder.

466 **www.addvance.com**
ADDvance Online Newsletter

A resource for girls and women with ADD. Site has books, tapes, support groups, chat and links.

467 **www.addwarehouse.com**
ADD Warehouse

The world's largest collection of ADHD-related books, videos, training programs, games, professional texts and assessment products.

468 **www.adhdnews.com/ssi.htm**

Guidance in applying for Social Security disability benefits on behalf of a child who has ADHD.

469 **www.cec.sped.org**
Council for Exceptional Children

Dedicated to improving educational outcomes for individuals with exceptionalities, students with disabilities, and/or the gifted.

470 **www.chadd.org**
National Resource Center on AD/HD

CHADD works to improve the lives of people affected by AD/HD.

471 **www.childdevelopmentinfo.com**
Child Development Institute

Online information on child development, child psychology, parenting, learning, health and safety as well as childhood disorders such as attention deficit disorder, dyslexia and autism. Provides comprehensive resources and practical suggestions for parents.

472 **www.dyslexia.com**
Davis Dyslexia Association International

Links to internet resources for learning. Includes dyslexia, Autism and Asperger's Syndrome, ADD/ADHD and other learning disabilities.

473 **www.my.webmd.com**
Web MD Health

Medical website with information which includes learning disabilities, ADD/ADHD, etc.

474 **www.ncgiadd.org**
National Center for Gender Issues and AD/HD

Offers knowledge and understanding of girls and women with ADHD to improve their lives.

475 **www.nichcy.org**
Nat'l Dissemination Center for Children Disabiliti

Provides information on disabilties in children and youth and programs and services.

476 **www.oneaddplace.com**
One A D D Place

A virtual neighborhood of information and resources relating to ADD, ADHD and learning disorders.

477 **www.therapistfinder.net**

Locate psychologists, psychiatrists, social workers, family counselors, and more specializing in all disorders.

478 **www.webmd.com**
Web MD Health

Medical website with information which includes learning disabilities, ADD/ADHD, etc.

Publications

479 **Directory of Summer Camps for Children with Learning Disabilities**
Learning Disabilities Association of America
4156 Library Road
Pittsburgh, PA 15234
412-341-1515
FAX 412-344-0224
http://www.ldaamerica.org
e-mail: info@ldaamerica.org
Sheila Buckley, Executive Director
Sharon Tanner, Development Coordinator
Andrea Turkheimer, Information/Referral Specialist
Offers a full range of listings for the learning disabled. *$4.00*

480 **Guide to ACA Accredited Camps**
American Camping Association
5000 State Road 67 N
Martinsville, IN 46151
765-342-8456
800-428-2267
FAX 765-349-2065
TDY:765-342-8456
http://www.acacamps.org
e-mail: bookstore@acacamps.org OR hlowe@ACAcamps.org

Peg Smith, Chief Executive Officer
Harriet Gamble Lowe, Director of Communications
Kat Shreve, Director of Education
A national listing of accredited camping programs. Listed by activity, special clientele, camp name, and specific disabilities. *$14.95*
285 pages Annually
ISBN 0-876031-66-1

481 **Guide to Summer Camps and Summer Schools**
Porter Sargent Publishers
11 Beacon Street
Boston, MA 02108
617-523-1670
800-342-7470
FAX 617-523-1021
http://www.portersargent.com
e-mail: info@portersargent.com
Dan McKeever, Senior Editor
John Yonce, Manager
Leslie A Weston, Production Manager
Covers a broad spectrum of recreational and educational summer opportunities in the US and abroad. Current facts from 1750 camps and schools, as well as programs for those with special needs and disabilities. *$27.00*
960 pages Biannual/Paper 1924Grade Range: K-12
ISBN 9-780875-58-7

482 **Resources for Children with Special Needs**
Publications/Department B
116 E 16th Street
New York, NY 10003
212-677-4650
FAX 212-254-4070
http://www.resourcesnyc.org/rcsn.htm
e-mail: info@resourcesnyc.org
Karen Thoreson-Schlesinger, Executive Director
Dianne Littwin, Publishing Director
Linda Lew, Director of Information Services
The 23rd edition of Resources for Children with Special Needs' Camp Guide, Camps 2007, includes more than two dozen new camps, expanding both the range of special needs camps beyond the New York area and the northeast, and the types of disabilities served. It provides up-to-date information on more than 300 camps and programs that provide a wide range of summer activities for children with emotional, developmental, learning and physical disabilities and special needs.

483 **Summer Camps for Children with Disabilities**
National Dissemination Center for Children with Di sabilities (NICHY)
Washington, DC 20013
202-884-8200
800-695-0285
FAX 202-884-8441
http://www.nichcy.org/pubs/genresc/camps.htm
e-mail: nichcy@aed.org
Stephen F Moseley, President/CEO
Jack Downey, SVP/Chief Operating Officer
Judy L Shanley Ph.D, OSHP Project Officer
Extensive listing of resources available providing information on a variety of summer camps for children with disabilities. Address and contact info in addition to Website links are included.

Alabama

484 **Camp ASCCA**
Easter Seals of Alabama
5278 Camp ASCCA Drive
Jacksons Gap, AL 36861
256-825-9226
800-843-2267
FAX 256-825-8332
http://http://alabama.easterseals.com/
e-mail: info@campascca.org
Matt Rickman, Camp Director
John Stevenson, Administrator
Dana Rickman, Public Affairs Director
Helps children and adults with disabilities achieve equality, dignity and maximum independence. This is to be accomplished through a safe and quality program of camping, recreation and education in a year-round barrier-free environment. Founded 1976.

485 **Easter Seals Gulf Coast**
2448 Gordon Smith Drive
Mobile, AL 36617
251-471-1581
800-411-0068
FAX 251-476-4303
http://www.alabama.easterseals.com
e-mail: esmob@zebra.net
Frank Harkins, CEO
Loretta Yound, Office Manager

Easter Seals camping and recreation programs serve children, adults and families of all abilities. Various programs are available with the united purpose of giving disabled individuals a fun and safe camping or recreational experience. Camperships are available.

Alaska

486 **Trailside Discovery Camp: Alaskan Quest 1Day Program (Ages 6-7)**
Alaska Center for the Environment
Anchorage, AK 99501
907-274-3621
FAX 907-274-8733
http://www.akcenter.org/about_ace/
e-mail: ace@akcenter.org
Thomas Burek, Trailside Discovery Director
Clare Stockert, Assistant Director
Dwayne Lee, Financial Director
Stimulating day programs are designed to encourage young adventurers to use all of their senses while exploring the outdoors. Games, stories, and hands on activities encourage students to interact with their environment and with each other. At Alaskan Quest 1, the wild country beckons, introducing young adventurers to the joys of outdoor skills. Explorers learn about low-impact camping, safety in the outdoors, orienteering and wilderness survival. Day Programs Ages 6-7.

487 **Trailside Discovery Camp: Alaskan Quest IIDay Program (Ages 8-9)**
Alaska Center for the Environment
Anchorage, AK 99501
907-274-3621
FAX 907-274-8733
http://www.akcenter.org/about_ace/
e-mail: ace@akcenter.org
Thomas Burek, Trailside Discovery Director
Clare Stockert, Assistant Director
Dwayne Lee, Financial Director
Stimulating day programs are designed to encourage young adventurers to use all of their senses while exploring the outdoors. During Alaskan Quest II, the wild country beckons as young adventurers learn about the joys of camping. Explorers learn about low-impact camping, safety in the outdoors, and other techniques that will help them survive a Wednesday through Friday camp out in Eklutna Lake (Chugach State Park).

488 Trailside Discovery Camp: Alaskan Quest IV Cellular One Reach High Day Program (Ages 12-14)

Alaska Center for the Environment
Anchorage, AK 99501
907-274-3621
FAX 907-274-8733
http://www.akcenter.org/about_ace/
e-mail: ace@akcenter.org
Thomas Burek, Trailside Discovery Director
Clare Stockert, Assistant Director
Dwayne Lee, Financial Director

Alaskan Quest IV trips for teens combine backcountry skills with scientific studies for a fun week of adventure in Alaska's wild areas. Campers spend the first day preparing for their adventure by checking gear, reviewing equipment use, safety, and honing skills. Learn basic climbing safety and techniques in a safe environment. Improve your climbing skills, reach high to gain the summit of an outside climbing wall, and experience group building activities that develop your leadership potential.

489 Trailside Discovery Camp: Alpine TrekkersAlaskan Quest III (Ages 10-11)

Alaska Center for the Environment
Anchorage, AK 99501
907-274-3621
FAX 907-274-8733
http://www.akcenter.org/about_ace/
e-mail: ace@akcenter.org
Thomas Burek, Trailside Discovery Director
Clare Stockert, Assistant Director
Dwayne Lee, Financial Director

During Alpine Trekkers Alaskan Quest III, the wild country beckons young adventurers to the joys of backpacking. Trekkers prepare for two days learning low impact camping skills and safety in the outdoors, then backpack for three days in the wilderness of Chugach.

490 Trailside Discovery Camp: Amazing AnimalsDay Program (Ages 6-7)

Alaska Center for the Environment
Anchorage, AK 99501
907-274-3621
FAX 907-274-8733
http://www.akcenter.org/about_ace/
e-mail: ace@akcenter.org
Thomas Burek, Trailside Discovery Director
Clare Stockert, Assistant Director
Dwayne Lee, Financial Director

Stimulating day programs are designed to encourage young adventurers to use all of their senses while exploring the outdoors. Games, stories, and hands on activities encourage students to interact with their environment and with each other. Students will become a predator in a game of survival of the fittest, track creatures, and return home with proof of your journey. Hold the vital link to an entire food web in your hands and create a mural that tells the story of your week-long adventure.

491 Trailside Discovery Camp: Arctic Adaptions Day Program (Ages 8-9)

Alaska Center for the Environment
Anchorage, AK 99501
907-274-3621
FAX 907-274-8733
http://www.akcenter.org/about_ace/
e-mail: ace@akcenter.org
Thomas Burek, Trailside Discovery Director
Clare Stockert, Assistant Director
Dwayne Lee, Financial Director

During the Arctic Adaptions Day Program, students will learn how animals and plants rely on their bodies and brains to keep warm, find shelter and feed themselves in the harsh climate and rugged terrain of Alaska. In addition, campers will also learn all about why and how animals, plants, and even insects undergo adaptations while playing Adaptations Park Ranger, dissecting a plant, and designing the Ultimate Alaskan Animal.

492 Trailside Discovery Camp: Birds of a Feather Day Program (Ages 6-7)

Alaska Center for the Environment
Anchorage, AK 99501
907-274-3621
FAX 907-274-8733
http://www.akcenter.org/about_ace/
e-mail: ace@akcenter.org
Thomas Burek, Trailside Discovery Director
Clare Stockert, Assistant Director
Dwayne Lee, Financial Director

Stimulating day programs are designed to encourage young adventurers to use all of their senses while exploring the outdoors. Games, stories, and hands on activities encourage students to interact with their environment and with each other. From the point of their beaks to the tip of their feathers, birds are fascinating creatures. Students will explore the things that make our feathered friends so special, and be transformed into a loon for a day.

493 Trailside Discovery Camp: Campbell Creek Expedition Day Program (Ages 8-9)

Alaska Center for the Environment
Anchorage, AK 99501
907-274-3621
FAX 907-274-8733
http://www.akcenter.org/about_ace/
e-mail: ace@akcenter.org
Thomas Burek, Trailside Discovery Director
Clare Stockert, Assistant Director
Dwayne Lee, Financial Director

Stimulating day programs are designed to encourage young adventurers to use all of their senses while exploring the outdoors. Games, stories, and hands on activities encourage students to interact with their environment and with each other. The Campbell Creek watershed is a connected web of plants, animals, and people. As a team of explorers on a scientific expedition, students will gather clues to help determine the health of this web.

494 Trailside Discovery Camp: Canoe VoyagerAlaskan Quest III (Ages 10-11)

Alaska Center for the Environment
Anchorage, AK 99501
907-274-3621
FAX 907-274-8733
http://www.akcenter.org/about_ace/
e-mail: ace@akcenter.org
Thomas Burek, Trailside Discovery Director
Clare Stockert, Assistant Director
Dwayne Lee, Financial Director

Canoe Voyager is a program that will introduce students to the joys of canoeing, water safety, and low-impact camping skills. Students spend the first two days preparing for their adventure by checking gear, reviewing equipment use, and learning basic paddling skills. On Wednesday, the group will head to Nancy Lake State Park for three days of paddling, portaging, team building, wetland study, and outdoor survival.

495 Trailside Discovery Camp: Caterpillar Creations Day Program (Ages 8-9)

Alaska Center for the Environment
Anchorage, AK 99501
907-274-3621
FAX 907-274-8733
http://www.akcenter.org/about_ace/
e-mail: ace@akcenter.org
Thomas Burek, Trailside Discovery Director
Clare Stockert, Assistant Director
Dwayne Lee, Financial Director

Stimulating day programs are designed to encourage young adventurers to use all of their senses while exploring the outdoors. Games, stories, and hands on activities encourage students to interact with their environment and with each other. During Caterpillar Creations Day Program, students discover, imagine, and create fun, hands-on projects using natural materials. Encounter sand art, crafts, pottery, beading, and Alaskan art in addition to enhancing self-confidence and creative skills.

496 Trailside Discovery Camp: Cellular One Reach High Day Program - Alaskan Quest III (Ages 10-11)

Alaska Center for the Environment
Anchorage, AK 99501
907-274-3621
FAX 907-274-8733
http://www.akcenter.org/about_ace/
e-mail: ace@akcenter.org
Thomas Burek, Trailside Discovery Director
Clare Stockert, Assistant Director
Dwayne Lee, Financial Director

During Cellular One Reach High, students will learn basic climbing safety and techniques in a safe environment. Improve your climbing skills, reach high to gain the summit of an outside climbing wall, and experience group building activities that will develop your leadership potential. Get in shape, and have lots of fun.

497 Trailside Discovery Camp: Climate Connection Day Program (Ages 6-7)
Alaska Center for the Environment
Anchorage, AK 99501
907-274-3621
FAX 907-274-8733
http://www.akcenter.org/about_ace/
e-mail: ace@akcenter.org
Thomas Burek, Trailside Discovery Director
Clare Stockert, Assistant Director
Dwayne Lee, Financial Director
Stimulating day programs are designed to encourage young adventurers to use all of their senses while exploring the outdoors. Games, stories, and hands on activities encourage students to interact with their environment and with each other. Students will be monitoring the weather, learning about energy and the atmosphere, discovering the secrets to Earth's rising temperatures, the impacts climate change has on Alaska and the ways in which it influences forest fires, polar bears and sea ice.

498 Trailside Discovery Camp: Creek Seekers Day Program (Ages 6-7)
Alaska Center for the Environment
Anchorage, AK 99501
907-274-3621
FAX 907-274-8733
http://www.akcenter.org/about_ace/
e-mail: ace@akcenter.org
Thomas Burek, Trailside Discovery Director
Clare Stockert, Assistant Director
Dwayne Lee, Financial Director
Stimulating day programs are designed to encourage young adventurers to use all their senses while exploring the outdoors. Games, stories, and hands on activities encourage students to interact with their environment and with each other. Students will use a microscope to observe tiny water creatures and build their own beaver lodge and make their way through the life of a water droplet and be ready to manage a river plot. Don't forget your rubber boots because this week will be a splash!

499 Trailside Discovery Camp: Creepy CrawlersPreschool Program (Ages 4-5)
Alaska Center for the Environment
Anchorage, AK 99501
907-274-3621
FAX 907-274-8733
http://www.akcenter.org/about_ace/
e-mail: ace@akcenter.org
Thomas Burek, Trailside Discovery Director
Clare Stockert, Assistant Director
Dwayne Lee, Financial Director
Stimulating day programs are designed to encourage young adventurers to use all of their senses while exploring the outdoors. Children hike through forests and discover creeks while investigating the creatures that live in them. Games, stories, and hands on activities encourage students to interact with their environment and with each other. Creepy Crawlers Camp is a preschool program ages 4-5. Creepy Crawlers students will catch and study insects to discover how they live.

500 Trailside Discovery Camp: Day Programs (Ages 6-13)
Alaska Center for the Environment
Anchorage, AK 99501
907-274-3621
FAX 907-274-8733
http://www.akcenter.org/about_ace/
e-mail: ace@akcenter.org
Thomas Burek, Trailside Discovery Director
Clare Stockert, Assistant Director
Dwayne Lee, Financial Director
All programs are designed to be both fun and informative. Naturalists lead small groups teaching natural history and the natural sciences, nature craft, social growth, as well as leadership and outdoor skills. Programs emphasize interactive, enjoyable, hands-on outdoor experiences. Participants slog through bogs, explore forests, and tread gently across trails and beaches learning about nature while immersed in it. Join us for a fun-filled summer in the great outdoors!

501 Trailside Discovery Camp: Earth and Sky Day Program (Ages 10-13)
Alaska Center for the Environment
Anchorage, AK 99501
907-274-3621
FAX 907-274-8733
http://www.akcenter.org/about_ace/
e-mail: ace@akcenter.org
Thomas Burek, Trailside Discovery Director
Clare Stockert, Assistant Director
Dwayne Lee, Financial Director
Stimulating day programs are designed to encourage young adventurers to use all of their senses while exploring the outdoors. Games, stories, and hands on activities encourage students to interact with their environment and with each other. During the Earth and Sky Day Program, students will seek knowledge and insight into the forces that connect us with the Earth and distant atmosphere. Dig up the past in Archeology, read the Alaskan skies with meteorology.

502 Trailside Discovery Camp: Energy Sleuth Day Program (Ages 8-9)
Alaska Center for the Environment
Anchorage, AK 99501
907-274-3621
FAX 907-274-8733
http://www.akcenter.org/about_ace/
e-mail: ace@akcenter.org
Thomas Burek, Trailside Discovery Director
Clare Stockert, Assistant Director
Dwayne Lee, Financial Director
During the Energy Sleuth Day Program, students will get the buzz on what's new with energy and natural resources. Create models and discover through experiments how wind, water, and sunlight are used to produce usable energy. Find out how technology, smart shopping, worms, and daily choices can reduce pollution and waste. Games and field visits are guaranteed to get you charged up about energy!

503 Trailside Discovery Camp: Fat Tire BikeAlaskan Quest III (Ages 10-11)
Alaska Center for the Environment
Anchorage, AK 99501
907-274-3621
FAX 907-274-8733
http://www.akcenter.org/about_ace/
e-mail: ace@akcenter.org
Thomas Burek, Trailside Discovery Director
Clare Stockert, Assistant Director
Dwayne Lee, Financial Director
This unique program will introduce students to mountain biking and to appreciate the valuable trails we have in Alaska. Students spend the first two days preparing for the adventure by checking gear, reviewing equipment use, and learning basic mountain biking skills. On Wednesday, the group will head to Kenai for three days of pedaling, low-impact camping, outdoor survival, and local ecology. All participants must have their own mountain bike. (Wednesday through Friday campout).

504 Trailside Discovery Camp: Fat Tire Bike-Johnson Pass Alaskan Quest IV (Ages 12-14)
Alaska Center for the Environment
Anchorage, AK 99501
907-274-3621
FAX 907-274-8733
http://www.akcenter.org/about_ace/
e-mail: ace@akcenter.org
Thomas Burek, Trailside Discovery Director
Clare Stockert, Assistant Director
Dwayne Lee, Financial Director
Alaskan Quest IV trips for teens combine backcountry skills with scientific studies for a fun week of adventure in Alaska's wild areas. Campers spend the first day preparing for their adventure by checking gear, reviewing equipment use, safety, and honing skills. This program lets campers appreciate the scenic and unique Johnson Pass Trail. The group will head to the pass for four days of biking, team-building, and leadership skills. All campers must have their own mountain bike and panniers.

505 Trailside Discovery Camp: Flying Friends Preschool Program (Ages 4-5)
Alaska Center for the Environment
Anchorage, AK 99501
907-274-3621
FAX 907-274-8733
http://www.akcenter.org/about_ace/
e-mail: ace@akcenter.org
Thomas Burek, Trailside Discovery Director
Clare Stockert, Assistant Director
Dwayne Lee, Financial Director

Stimulating day programs are designed to encourage young adventurers to use all of their senses while exploring the outdoors. Children hike through forests and discover creeks while investigating the creatures that live in them. Games, stories, and hands on activities encourage students to interact with their environment and with each other. Flying Friends Camp is a preschool program ages 4-5. Flying Friends students will study songbirds and birds of prey and how they adapt to their environment.

506 Trailside Discovery Camp: Forest ProwlersPreschool Program (Ages 4-5)

Alaska Center for the Environment
Anchorage, AK 99501
907-274-3621
FAX 907-274-8733
http://www.akcenter.org/about_ace/
e-mail: ace@akcenter.org

Thomas Burek, Trailside Discovery Director
Clare Stockert, Assistant Director
Dwayne Lee, Financial Director

Stimulating day programs are designed to encourage young adventurers to use all of their senses while exploring the outdoors. Children hike through forests and discover creeks while investigating the creatures that live in them. Games, stories, and hands on activities encourage students to interact with their environment and with each other. Forest Prowlers Camp is a preschool program ages 4-5. Forest Prowlers students will investigate how predators and prey interact to create healthy forests.

507 Trailside Discovery Camp: Geology Surveyors Day Program (Ages 8-9)

Alaska Center for the Environment
Anchorage, AK 99501
907-274-3621
FAX 907-274-8733
http://www.akcenter.org/about_ace/
e-mail: ace@akcenter.org

Thomas Burek, Trailside Discovery Director
Clare Stockert, Assistant Director
Dwayne Lee, Financial Director

Stimulating day programs are designed to encourage young adventurers to use all of their senses while exploring the outdoors. Campers will discover that Geology Rocks when they dive into 4.6 billion years of Earth history with a team of surveyors! Discover how fossils help scientists understand the Earth's mysterious past. Build an erupting volcano, study how a glacier moves, and watch a river cut through new land.

508 Trailside Discovery Camp: Habitat HuntersPreschool Program (Ages 4-5)

Alaska Center for the Environment
Anchorage, AK 99501
907-274-3621
FAX 907-274-8733
http://www.akcenter.org/about_ace/
e-mail: ace@akcenter.org

Thomas Burek, Trailside Discovery Director
Clare Stockert, Assistant Director
Dwayne Lee, Financial Director

Stimulating day programs are designed to encourage young adventurers to use all of their senses while exploring the outdoors. Children hike through forests and discover creeks while investigating the creatures that live in them. Games, stories, and hands on activities encourage students to interact with their environment and with each other. Habitat Hunters Camp is a preschool program ages 4-5. Habitat Hunters students will study animals and the environments within which they live.

509 Trailside Discovery Camp: Kayak Kachemak Bay Alaskan Quest V (Ages 14-16)

Alaska Center for the Environment
Anchorage, AK 99501
907-274-3621
FAX 907-274-8733
http://www.akcenter.org/about_ace/
e-mail: ace@akcenter.org

Thomas Burek, Trailside Discovery Director
Clare Stockert, Assistant Director
Dwayne Lee, Financial Director

Alaskan Quest V trips for teens combining backcountry skills with scientific studies for a fun week of adventure in Alaska's wild areas. This trip is designed for those students who want to spend more time on the water using their paddling skills. This trip will begin with a day of preparations. Campers will then head to Homer for a week of paddling, leadership, team building, marine science, and outdoor survival. A valuable experience for those wanting to have fun while building new skills.

510 Trailside Discovery Camp: Kayak ScoutAlaskan Quest III (Ages 10-11)

Alaska Center for the Environment
Anchorage, AK 99501
907-274-3621
FAX 907-274-8733
http://www.akcenter.org/about_ace/
e-mail: ace@akcenter.org

Thomas Burek, Trailside Discovery Director
Clare Stockert, Assistant Director
Dwayne Lee, Financial Director

This program will introduce students to kayaking skills, water safety, and low-impact camping skills. Students spend the first two days preparing for their adventure by checking gear, reviewing equipment use, and learning basic paddling skills. On Wednesday, the group will head to Kenai Lake for three days of paddling, team building, outdoor survival, glaciers, and lake study. (Wednesday through Friday campout).

511 Trailside Discovery Camp: Marine Encounter Alaskan Quest III (Ages 10-11)

Alaska Center for the Environment
Anchorage, AK 99501
907-274-3621
FAX 907-274-8733
http://www.akcenter.org/about_ace/
e-mail: ace@akcenter.org

Thomas Burek, Trailside Discovery Director
Clare Stockert, Assistant Director
Dwayne Lee, Financial Director

Scramble around tide pools and pebble beaches stalking colorful sunflower stars, baby king crab, and spiny Sea Urchins. We will spend three days camping at Caines Head State Park, visit the Alaska Sea Life Center, and will be part of the Pinniped Picnic. Learn how seals and sea lions are trained and get the skinny on pinniped fat. (Wednesday through Friday campout).

512 Trailside Discovery Camp: Ocean CommotionDay Program (Ages 10-13)

Alaska Center for the Environment
Anchorage, AK 99501
907-274-3621
FAX 907-274-8733
http://www.akcenter.org/about_ace/
e-mail: ace@akcenter.org

Thomas Burek, Trailside Discovery Director
Clare Stockert, Assistant Director
Dwayne Lee, Financial Director

During the Ocean Commotion Day Program, young adventurers will investigate the mysteries of the Pacific Ocean: tides, waves, and even some remarkable looking deep sea inhabitants and find out the truth behind the myths you have heard, and get the real scoop on mermaids. Become a marine expert while doing some beach combing at several sites around the Anchorage area. Don't forget the sunscreen, because most of the week will be spent at the beach!

513 Trailside Discovery Camp: Outdoor OdysseyDay Program (Ages 10-13)

Alaska Center for the Environment
Anchorage, AK 99501
907-274-3621
FAX 907-274-8733
http://www.akcenter.org/about_ace/
e-mail: ace@akcenter.org

Thomas Burek, Trailside Discovery Director
Clare Stockert, Assistant Director
Dwayne Lee, Financial Director

During Outdoor Odyssey, young adventurers will experience a variety of natural encounters in an array of outdoor adventures. Get the inside buzz on bee-keeping, tackle oil spill simulation on Goose Lake, band birds on the Campbell Tract, pan for gold in the Alaska wilderness, and greet raptors from Bird TLC. Bring plenty of energy for this odyssey!

514 Trailside Discovery Camp: Plant Power DayProgram (Ages 6-7)

Alaska Center for the Environment
Anchorage, AK 99501
907-274-3621
FAX 907-274-8733
http://www.akcenter.org/about_ace/
e-mail: ace@akcenter.org

Thomas Burek, Trailside Discovery Director
Clare Stockert, Assistant Director
Dwayne Lee, Financial Director

Stimulating day programs are designed to encourage young adventurers to use all their senses while exploring the outdoors. Games, stories, and hands on activities encourage students to interact with their environment and with each other. As members of the Trailside Planet Power crew, students will spend the week giving back to the environment by planting trees on the Campbell Tract, creating art projects using recycled materials, and getting others involved by creating a mural to inspire change.

515 Trailside Discovery Camp: River Run Adventure Alaskan Quest IV (Ages 12-14)
Alaska Center for the Environment
Anchorage, AK 99501 907-274-3621
FAX 907-274-8733
http://www.akcenter.org/about_ace/
e-mail: ace@akcenter.org
Thomas Burek, Trailside Discovery Director
Clare Stockert, Assistant Director
Dwayne Lee, Financial Director
Alaskan Quest IV trips for teens combine backcountry skills with scientific studies for a fun week of adventure in Alaska's wild areas. Campers spend the first day preparing for their adventure by checking gear, reviewing equipment use, safety, and honing skills. This adventure will take campers down to the Kenai Peninsula to experience backpacking as well as a river raft trip. The group will head to the Kenai for four days of backpacking, river rafting, low-impact camping and outdoor survival.

516 Trailside Discovery Camp: Rocks, Ice, Volcanoes, Quakes Day Program (Ages 10-13)
Alaska Center for the Environment
Anchorage, AK 99501 907-274-3621
FAX 907-274-8733
http://www.akcenter.org/about_ace/
e-mail: ace@akcenter.org
Thomas Burek, Trailside Discovery Director
Clare Stockert, Assistant Director
Dwayne Lee, Financial Director
During the Rocks, Ice, Volcanoes, Quakes Day Program, young adventurers will visit with different professionals in the Earth Sciences. We will explore the natural forces that shape southcentral Alaska. We also will explore the effects of these forces on our natural and built environment. Our travels may take us to Portage Glacier, Earthquake Park, and Wishbone Hill.

517 Trailside Discovery Camp: Seward Kayak Trip Alaskan Quest IV (Ages 12-14)
Alaska Center for the Environment
Anchorage, AK 99501 907-274-3621
FAX 907-274-8733
http://www.akcenter.org/about_ace/
e-mail: ace@akcenter.org
Thomas Burek, Trailside Discovery Director
Clare Stockert, Assistant Director
Dwayne Lee, Financial Director
Alaskan Quest IV trips for teens combine backcountry skills with scientific studies for a fun week of adventure in Alaska's wild areas. Campers spend the first day preparing for their adventure by checking gear, reviewing equipment use, safety, and honing skills. Campers will paddle along the shores of Caines Head State Park. The group will head for Seward for four days of paddling, teambuilding, marine science, and outdoor survival.

518 Trailside Discovery Camp: Spirit KeepersPreschool Program (Ages 4-5)
Alaska Center for the Environment
Anchorage, AK 99501 907-274-3621
FAX 907-274-8733
http://www.akcenter.org/about_ace/
e-mail: ace@akcenter.org
Thomas Burek, Trailside Discovery Director
Clare Stockert, Assistant Director
Dwayne Lee, Financial Director
Stimulating day programs are designed to encourage young adventurers to use all of their senses while exploring the outdoors. Spirit Keepers Camp is a preschool program ages 4-5. Spirit Keepers students will experience the ways of Native Alaskans by making traditional crafts, listening to stories from master storytellers, and performing exciting dances. Preschoolers will get a special look into Native culture through art, music, and dance.

519 Trailside Discovery Camp: Spirit Keepers Day Program (Ages 6-7)
Alaska Center for the Environment
Anchorage, AK 99501 907-274-3621
FAX 907-274-8733
http://www.akcenter.org/about_ace/
e-mail: ace@akcenter.org
Thomas Burek, Trailside Discovery Director
Clare Stockert, Assistant Director
Dwayne Lee, Financial Director
During the Spirit Keepers Day Program, Native Alaskans share their knowledge and traditional ways of living. This program emphasizes native arts and culture while teaching respect for the natural world. Activities may include making a clan emblem, dance fans, and learning different dances. Program will hold a potlatch to culminate the week and parents will be invited. (July 2,3,5,6 only).

520 Trailside Discovery Camp: Spirit Keepers-Day Program (Ages 8-9)
Alaska Center for the Environment
Anchorage, AK 99501 907-274-3621
FAX 907-274-8733
http://www.akcenter.org/about_ace/
e-mail: ace@akcenter.org
Thomas Burek, Trailside Discovery Director
Clare Stockert, Assistant Director
Dwayne Lee, Financial Director
During the Spirit Keepers Day Program for those ages 8-9, Native Alaskans share their knowledge and traditional ways of living. This program emphasizes native arts and culture while teaching respect for the natural world. Activities may include making a clan emblem, dance fans, and learning different dances. Program will hold a potlatch and parents will be invited. (July 2,3,5,6 only).

521 Trailside Discovery Camp: Sunship Earth Day Program (Ages 10-13)
Alaska Center for the Environment
Anchorage, AK 99501 907-274-3621
FAX 907-274-8733
http://www.akcenter.org/about_ace/
e-mail: ace@akcenter.org
Thomas Burek, Trailside Discovery Director
Clare Stockert, Assistant Director
Dwayne Lee, Financial Director
During the Sunship Earth Day Program, students will learn that we are all passengers riding a fragile globe through space powered by energetic rays from the sun. Participants are led on a wild and wonderful tour of the natural world, seeking knowledge in Mario's Pizza Parlor, the place in solarville where the true cost of pizza becomes clear.

522 Trailside Discovery Camp: Survival Challenge Day Program (Ages 8-9)
Alaska Center for the Environment
Anchorage, AK 99501 907-274-3621
FAX 907-274-8733
http://www.akcenter.org/about_ace/
e-mail: ace@akcenter.org
Thomas Burek, Trailside Discovery Director
Clare Stockert, Assistant Director
Dwayne Lee, Financial Director
During the Survival Challenge Day Program, campers will experience the way people lived long ago! Nature provides the supplies, and the staff provides the knowledge to guide campers through a week of adventure that includes animal tracking, building shelters, identifying and taste testing wild edible plants, and back-country first aid and healing. Campers will even get to make tools and containers that can help them survive in the woods.

523 Trailside Discovery Camp: Swanson Lakes Canoe Alaskan Quest IV (Ages 12-14)
Alaska Center for the Environment
Anchorage, AK 99501 907-274-3621
FAX 907-274-8733
http://www.akcenter.org/about_ace/
e-mail: ace@akcenter.org
Thomas Burek, Trailside Discovery Director
Clare Stockert, Assistant Director
Dwayne Lee, Financial Director

Alaskan Quest IV trips for teens combine backcountry skills with scientific studies for a fun week of adventure in Alaska's wild areas. Campers spend the first day preparing for their adventure by checking gear, reviewing equipment use, safety, and honing skills. Campers will paddle in the Swanson Lake system and then head to the Kenai for four days of paddling, teambuilding, local ecology, and outdoor survival.

524 **Trailside Discovery Camp: Tidelands to Tundra Day Program (Ages 10-13)**

Alaska Center for the Environment
Anchorage, AK 99501
907-274-3621
FAX 907-274-8733
http://www.akcenter.org/about_ace/
e-mail: ace@akcenter.org

Thomas Burek, Trailside Discovery Director
Clare Stockert, Assistant Director
Dwayne Lee, Financial Director

During the Tidelands to Tundra Day Program, students will travel from Anchorage's coastal tidelands to the tundra. Participants are led on a wild and wonderful tour of the natural world, seeking knowledge in Mario's Piazza Parlor, the place in solarville where the true cost of pizza becomes clear.

525 **Trailside Discovery Camp: Venture Bound Alaskan Quest IV Day Program (Ages 12-14)**

Alaska Center for the Environment
Anchorage, AK 99501
907-274-3621
FAX 907-274-8733
http://www.akcenter.org/about_ace/
e-mail: ace@akcenter.org

Thomas Burek, Trailside Discovery Director
Clare Stockert, Assistant Director
Dwayne Lee, Financial Director

Alaskan Quest IV trips for teens combine backcountry skills with scientific studies for a fun week of adventure in Alaska's wild areas. Campers spend the first day preparing for their adventure by checking gear, reviewing equipment use, safety, and honing skills. This is a preparation program for our Alaskan Quest IV Trips which will introduce students to different skills including hiking, canoeing, mountain biking, and kayaking. In addition, campers will learn wilderness safety and GPS.

526 **Trailside Discovery Camp: Venture Bound Day Program - Alaskan Quest III (Ages 10-11)**

Alaska Center for the Environment
Anchorage, AK 99501
907-274-3621
FAX 907-274-8733
http://www.akcenter.org/about_ace/
e-mail: ace@akcenter.org

Thomas Burek, Trailside Discovery Director
Clare Stockert, Assistant Director
Dwayne Lee, Financial Director

This is a preparation program for our Alaskan Quest III. Each day we will introduce students to different skills. We will explore hiking, canoeing, mountain biking, and kayaking. In addition, we will cover low-impact camping skills, wilderness safety, and learn about GPS.

527 **Trailside Discovery Camp: Water Wonders Preschool Program (Ages 4-5)**

Alaska Center for the Environment
Anchorage, AK 99501
907-274-3621
FAX 907-274-8733
http://www.akcenter.org/about_ace/
e-mail: ace@akcenter.org

Thomas Burek, Trailside Discovery Director
Clare Stockert, Assistant Director
Dwayne Lee, Financial Director

Stimulating day programs are designed to encourage young adventurers to use all of their senses while exploring the outdoors. Children hike through forests and discover creeks while investigating the creatures that live in them. Games, stories, and hands on activities encourage students to interact with their environment and with each other. Water Wonders Camp is a preschool program ages 4-5. Students hike to Campbell Creek or the forest to study how animals and plants depend on water to live.

528 **Trailside Discovery Camp: Whale and SalmonTales Day Program (Ages 6-7)**

Alaska Center for the Environment
Anchorage, AK 99501
907-274-3621
FAX 907-274-8733
http://www.akcenter.org/about_ace/
e-mail: ace@akcenter.org

Thomas Burek, Trailside Discovery Director
Clare Stockert, Assistant Director
Dwayne Lee, Financial Director

Stimulating day programs are designed to encourage young adventurers to use all of their senses while exploring the outdoors. During the Whale and Salmon Tales Day Program, students will experience the lives of these sensational swimmers as they explore the aquatic adventures of these famous Alaskan inhabitants. Search for salmon in Campbell Creek and learn the wonders of whales from experts while creating incredible works of art.

529 **Trailside Discovery Camp: Wild Country Explorers Day Program (Ages 8-9)**

Alaska Center for the Environment
Anchorage, AK 99501
907-274-3621
FAX 907-274-8733
http://www.akcenter.org/about_ace/
e-mail: ace@akcenter.org

Thomas Burek, Trailside Discovery Director
Clare Stockert, Assistant Director
Dwayne Lee, Financial Director

Wild Country Explorers Day Program is a preparation for the Alaskan Quest II camping program. Each day campers will be introduced to different skills including hiking, canoeing, mountain biking and orienteering. In addition, the program will cover low-impact camping skills, wilderness safety, and teach campers about GPS. Games, stories, and hands on activities encourage students to interact with their environment and with each other.

530 **Trailside Discovery Camp: Willow Winds Day Program (Ages 10-13)**

Alaska Center for the Environment
Anchorage, AK 99501
907-274-3621
FAX 907-274-8733
http://www.akcenter.org/about_ace/
e-mail: ace@akcenter.org

Thomas Burek, Trailside Discovery Director
Clare Stockert, Assistant Director
Dwayne Lee, Financial Director

During Willow Winds Day Program, students will learn the traditional skills of our ancestors; use a bow and drill to make a fire; discover trees and plants that hide their fire within; create a container from tree bark and roots; learn to remove bark without destroying the tree; use fire as a tool to make spoons and other camp utensils, and learn to process plants and bark into useful twine or bowstring. (July 2,3,5,6 only).

531 **Trailside Discovery Camp: Woodland WizardsDay Program (Ages 6-7)**

Alaska Center for the Environment
Anchorage, AK 99501
907-274-3621
FAX 907-274-8733
http://www.akcenter.org/about_ace/
e-mail: ace@akcenter.org

Thomas Burek, Trailside Discovery Director
Clare Stockert, Assistant Director
Dwayne Lee, Financial Director

Stimulating day programs are designed to encourage young adventurers to use all of their senses while exploring the outdoors. Games, stories, and hands on activities encourage students to interact with their environment and with each other. During the Woodland Wizards Day Program, students will unlock the secrets held within a rotting log and discover wildflowers as they hunt for mushrooms and edible plants while walking through the forest. Program includes a trip to the Botanical Gardens.

Arizona

532 **Lions Camp Tatiyee**
5283 White Mountain Boulevard
Lakeside, AZ 85929 480-380-4254
http://www.ArizonaLionsCamp.org
e-mail: ArizonaLionsCamp@cox.net
Joan Williamson, Lions Club Board Chairman
Barbara Russell, Lions Club Board Secretary

The Mission of Lions Camp Tatiyee is to provide a camping experience for challenged individuals, among their peers, that encourages independence and self-confidence. Camp Tatiyee is operated by the Lions Clubs International Multiple District 21. Lions Camp Tatiyee facilities includes 4 dormitories, a large dining hall with lounge area, a recreation hall with recreation area, sound room, stage and craft room, an indoor swimming pool and a fishing pond.

533 **Montlure Presbyterian Camp**
County Road 1121
Greer, AZ 85927 928-735-7534
888-514-3230
FAX 928-735-7816
http://www.montlure.org
e-mail: montlure@wmonline.com
Weslee Kenney, Director
Peter Flynn, President
Kristy Gropel, Camp Manager
The primary emphasis of this ministry is to offer a Christian experience through a carefully developed curriculum and competent directors and counselors who staff the camp each week. Summer camping sessions are held for groups from grade 4 through High School seniors. Over 550 young people benefit from the Montlure camping experience each summer.

534 **Reality Ranch Military Camp**
PO Box 340
Ft Thomas, AZ 85536 928-337-4500
877-273-7427
FAX 866-387-5027
http://www.realityranchcamp.com
e-mail: base@campcommo.com
Jeremy M Denton Sr, Executive Director

Reality Ranch Military Camp offers plenty of structure and challenging activities that will benefit nearly everyone, and will provide campers with activities designed to bring out their full potential. Campers will learn the value of teamwork and leadership while competing against the opposing platoon in various activities and camp missions. Responsibility and timeliness are skills that your child will learn through experience and education at Reality Ranch.

Arkansas

535 **Easter Seals Adult Services Center**
Easter Seals Adult Services Center
11801 Fairview Road
Little Rock, AR 72212 501-221-1063
877-533-3600
FAX 501-227-7180
http://www.ar.easterseals.com
e-mail: mail@easter-seals.org
Sharon Moone-Jochums, President/CEO
Johnny Baldwin, Vice President
Lauren Zilk, Administrator
Easter Seals camping and recreation programs serve children, adults and families of all abilities. Various programs are available with the united purpose of giving disabled individuals a fun and safe camping or recreational experience.

California

536 **Camp Costanoan**
2851 Park Avenue
Santa Clara, CA 95050 408-243-7861
FAX 408-243-0452
http://www.viaservices.org
e-mail: camp@viaservices.org
Richard Frazier, Camp Director
Kathleen Tucker, Volunteer Coordinator
Leslie Leger, Operations Director
Camp Costanoan is a residential, respite and recreational camp for children and adults, ages 5 and older, with physical and/or developmental disabilities. Camp Costanoan enhances camper self-esteem, improves socialization skills and provide hands-on learning and therapeutic recreation opportunities. Additionally, Camp provides respite for families of individuals with disabilities.

537 **Camp Krem - Camping Unlimited**
4610 Whitesands Court
El Sobrante, CA 94803 510-222-6662
FAX 510-223-3046
http://www.campingunlimited.com
e-mail: campkrem@campingunlimited.com
Teresa Tucker, Camp Director

Camping Unlimited provides recreational activities and summer camping for children and adults with developmental disabilities. Each season Camp Krem provides summer camp for more than 500 children and adults with developmental disabilities. Camp Krem has ten rustic cabins, an arts and crafts center, specially designed swimming pool, campfire arena, a playground, miles of hiking trails and outdoor camping areas.

538 **Camp ReCreation**
2110 Broadway
Sacramento, CA 95818 916-733-0136
FAX 916-733-0195
http://www.camprec.org
e-mail: mail@camprec.org
Vicky Flaig MEd RD, Camp Director

Camp ReCreation is a residential summer camp program for persons with developmental disabilities, offering participants opportunities for fun, social interaction, and spiritual growth while providing valuable respite for parents and care givers. Camp ReCreation is held at Camp Ronald McDonald at Eagle Lake, owned and operated by Ronald McDonald House Charities Northern California and is sponsored by the Catholic Diocese of Sacramento.

539 **Camp Ronald McDonald at Eagle Lake**
c/o Ronald McDonald House Charities
Sacramento, CA 95817 916-734-4230
FAX 916-734-4238
http://www.campronald.org
e-mail: vicky@campronald.org
Vicky Flaig MEd RD, Camp Director

Camp Ronald McDonald at Eagle Lake is a fully accessible residential summer camp for children who are at-risk with a variety of special medical needs, economic hardship and/or emotional, developmental or physical disabilities. Traditional camping activities include arts & crafts, hikes, fishing, canoeing, sports, swimming, talent show and campfires.

540 **Camp-A-Lot**
The Arc of San Diego
3030 Market Street
San Diego, CA 92102 619-685-1175
FAX 619-234-3759
http://http://arc-sd.com/Recreation.htm
e-mail: pals@arc-sd.com
Lin Taylor, Camp Director
Anthony DeSalis, Operations Director ARC
C E Skip Covell, Executive Director ARC

The Arc of San Diego's traditional summer resident camp for children, teens and adults, offers you a relaxing week in the local San Diego Mountains. The days are filled with swimming, hiking, sports, field trips, sing-a-longs, talent shows, dances, carnivals and camp crafts. Campers can also sign up for specialty classes - cooking, candle, jewelry and soap making, and T-shirt art are just a few of the choices.

541 **Easter Seals Bay Area: San Jose**

Easter Seals Bay Area
730 Empey Way
San Jose, CA 95128
408-295-0228
FAX 408-275-9858
http://http://bayarea.easterseals.com
e-mail: info@easterseals.com.

Peter Olson, Manager

Easter Seals camping and recreation programs serve children, adults and families of all abilities. Various programs are available with the united purpose of giving disabled individuals a fun and safe camping or recreational experience.

542 **Easter Seals Bay Area: Tri-Valley Campus**

7425 Larkdale Avenue
Dublin, CA 94568
925-828-8857
FAX 925-828-5245
http://http//bayarea.easterseals.com
e-mail: info@easterseals.com

Bryant Potts, Service Supervisor
Ron Halog, Program Manager

Easter Seals camping and recreation programs serve children, adults and families of all abilities. Various programs are available with the united purpose of giving disabled individuals a fun and safe camping or recreational experience.

543 **Easter Seals Central California: Camp Harmon**

9010 Soquel Drive
Aptos, CA 95003
831-684-2166
FAX 831-684-1018
http://www.centralcal.easterseals.com
e-mail: jennifer@es-cc.org OR info@easterseals.com.

Bruce Hinman, President
Donna Alvarez, Finance/Service VP

The following are camping and recreational services offered: Easter Seals own and operated camps and residential camping programs.

544 **Easter Seals Eureka**

3289 Edgewood Road
Eureka, CA 95501
707-445-8841
800-675-7325
FAX 707-445-3106
http://http://noca.easterseals.com
e-mail: info@easterseals.com

Helen Gale, Manager

Easter Seals camping and recreation programs serve children, adults and families of all abilities. Various programs are available with the united purpose of giving disabled individuals a fun and safe camping or recreational experience. Camperships are available.

545 **Easter Seals Northern California**

20 Pimentel Court
Novato, CA 94949
415-382-7450
800-234-7325
FAX 415-382-6052
http://www.noca.easter-seals.com
e-mail: cking@noca.easterseals.com

Jaclyn Reinhardt, Chief Executive Officer
Janet Clarke, Administrative Assistant

Easter Seals camping and recreation programs serve children, adults and families of all abilities. arious programs are available with the united purpose of giving disabled individuals a fun and safe camping or recreational experience. The following are camping and recreational services offered: camp respite for adults, camperships, recreational services for adults and recreational services for children. Speech and language therapy and occupational therapy for children ages 0-3.

546 **Easter Seals Northern California: RohnertPark**

501-B N Main Street
Rohnert Park, CA 94928
707-584-1443
800-234-7325
FAX 707-584-3438
TDY:707-584-1889
http://www.noca.easterseals.com
e-mail: skreuzer@ca-no.easter-seals.org

Susanne Kreuzer, Vice President
Jackie Rainheadt, Senior President

Easter Seals camping and recreation programs serve children, adults and families of all abilities. Various programs are available with the united purpose of giving disabled individuals a fun and safe camping or recreational experience. The folllowing are camping and recreational services offered: Camp respite for adults, camperships, day camping for children, recreational services for children and residential camping programs.

547 **Easter Seals Superior California**

3205 Hurley Way
Sacramento, CA 95864
916-485-6711
888-877-3257
FAX 916-485-2653
http://www.easterseals-superiorca.org
e-mail: info@easterseals-superiorca.org

Gary Kasai, President
Joanna Budd, Manager

Easter Seals camping and recreation programs serve children, adults and families of all abilities. Various programs are available with the united purpose of giving disabled individuals a fun and safe camping or recreational experience. Camping and recreational services offered are swim programs.

548 **Easter Seals Superior California: Stockton**

102 W Bianchi Road
Stockton, CA 95207
209-957-3625
FAX 209-957-6031
http://superiorca.easterseals.com
e-mail: info@easterseals.com

Gary Kasai, President/CEO
Joanna Budd, Manager

Easter Seals camping and recreation programs serve children, adults and families of all abilities. Various programs are available with the united purpose of giving disabled individuals a fun and safe camping or recreational experience. Camping and recreational services offered are: Swim programs.

549 **Easter Seals Tri-Counties California**

National Organization of Easter Seals
10730 Henderson Road
Ventura, CA 93004
805-647-1141
FAX 805-647-1148
http://http://centralcal.easterseals.com
e-mail: info@easterseals.com

Jamie Polis, Assistant Aquatic Director

Easter Seals camping and recreation programs serve children, adults and families of all abilities. Various programs are available with the united purpose of giving disabled individuals a fun and safe camping or recreational experience. Camping and recreational services offered are: Camperships and swim programs.

550 **Lazy J Ranch Camp**

12220 Cotharin Road
Malibu, CA 90265
310-457-5572
FAX 310-457-8882
http://www.lazyjranchcamp.com
e-mail: crazzycraig@earthlink.net

Craig Johnson, Camp Director

At the Lazy J Ranch Camp children 5-13 may participate in activities such as horseback riding, ocean kayaking, tennis, swimming, fencing, archery, and many others. A special event is enjoyed b the entire camp family daily. Trophies, ribbons and an assortment of awards are earned by each camper.

551 **Los Angeles School of Gymnastics Day Camp**

8450 Higuera Street
Culver City, CA 90232
310-204-1980
888-849-6627
FAX 310-204-6864
http://www.lagymnastics.com
e-mail: info@lagymnastics.com

Alla Svirsky, Executive Director
Tanya Barber, General Manager

Runs summer and winter camps for boys and girls. Founded 1975.

552 **Quest Camp: Huntington Beach**

2333 San Ramon Valley Boulevard
San Ramon, CA 94583
714-841-5534
FAX 714-841-5104
http://www.netwest2.com/quest/index.html
e-mail: quest@netwest2.com

Linda Sanicola Ph.D, Executive Director

Quest's therapeutic program uniquely combines behavioral methods, group therapy, recreational activities and instructional athletics to assist each child in developing new skills and eliminating those actions which create difficulties for them. Issues are presented to the child in a positive manner, helping the child to see the problem and possible positive solutions. Structured program activities include instructional athletics, games, arts and crafts, swimming, special guests and field trips.

553 **Quest Therapeutic Camps: San Ramon**

2333 San Ramon Valley Boulevard
San Ramon, CA 94583
925-743-1370
FAX 925-743-1937
http://www.questcamps.com
e-mail: questcamps@mac.com

Robert Field Ph.D, Executive Director
Debra Forrester Field MA, Administrative Director
Zack Oelerich MA, Assistant Director

Through camp activities, children learn to have more fun while counselors assist them to solve problems and increase confidence. Daily sports, games, arts and crafts and Fabulous Fridays provide activities to enjoy and learn from. Art, drama, music and nature programs will provide more creative programming. Campers may choose to go on an extended hike, create art projects, movies and plays, or play one of their favorite games for a two to three hour period.

554 **Wasewagan Camp**

42121 Seven Oaks Road
Angelus Oaks, CA 92305
909-794-2910
FAX 310-457-8882
http://lazyjranchcamp.com/html/wasewagan.html
e-mail: crazzycraig@earthlink.net

Craig Johnson, Camp Director

Wasewagan Camp offers a wide variety of camping options. Summer camp offers kids 5-17 years of age numerous activities such as archery, volleyball, swimming, hiking, fishing, arts and crafts, kayaking and canoeing. Wasewagen Camp is located within the beautiful Angelus forest amongst the reaching pines.

Colorado

555 **Camp Paha Rise Above**

City of Lakewood
12100 W Alameda Parkway
Lakewood, CO 80228
303-987-4869
FAX 303-987-4863
http://www.lakewood.org
e-mail: shawri@lakewood.org

Shane Wright, Camp Director
Jo Burns, Assistant Camp Director

Camp Paha is a day camp for children ages 6-17 and young adults ages 18-25 with disabilities. Camp Paha offers safe, quality, fun and challenging activities. Camp provides campers and opportunity to participate in aquatics, sports, games, nature, music, drama, hiking, arts and crafts, and field trips into the community.

556 **Easter Seals Camp Rocky Mountain Village**

2644 Alvarado Road
Empire, CO 80438
303-569-2333
FAX 303-569-3857
http://http://co.easterseals.com
e-mail: campinfo@eastersealscolorado.org

Roman Krafczyk, Camp Director

Camping and recreational services are: Adventure, camp respite for adults, camp respite for children, camperships, conference rental, family retreats, recreational services for adults, recreational services for children, residential camping programs, swim programs and therapeutic horseback riding.

557 **Easter Seals Colorado**

Steve Vestal Center
Lakewood, CO 80226
303-233-1666
FAX 303-233-1028
http://http://co.easterseals.com
e-mail: info@eastersealscolorado.org

Lynn Robinson, CEO

Easter Seals camping and recreation programs serve children, adults and families of all abilities. Various programs are available with the united purpose of giving disabled individuals a fun and safe camping or recreational experience. Camping and recreational services offered are: Swim programs.

558 **Easter Seals Southern Colorado**

225 S Academy Boulevard
Colorado Springs, CO 80910
719-574-9002
FAX 719-574-1330
http://www.co-so.easterseals.com
e-mail: info@easterseals.com

Kathyrn M Salt, President
John Schmidt, CEO

Easter Seals camping and recreation programs serve children, adults and families of all abilities. Various programs are available with the united purpose of giving disabled individuals a fun and safe camping or recreational experience. Camping and recreational services offered: Summer camp opportunities for children and adults; some financial aid provided based on income. Respite services offered year round.

559 **The Learning Camp**

PO Box 1146
Vail, CO 81658
970-524-2706
FAX 970-524-4178
http://www.learningcamp.com
e-mail: information@learningcamp.com

Ann Cathcart, Founder/Director
Tom Macht, Director
Kay Cochran, Art Program Director

Summer camp that focuses on helping children with learning disabilities, such as dyslexia, ADD, ADHD and other learning challenges. The Learning Camp provides adventurous summer camp fun for boys and girls ages 7 - 14 combined with carefully designed academic programs. Camp activities include swimming, horseback riding, backpacking, archery, arts and crafts, fishing, canoeing, board games, and Colorado River rafting.

Connecticut

560 **Artists in the Country**

52 County Road
West Woodstock, CT 06281
860-455-0103
http://http://www.artistsinthecountry.com
e-mail: achuk@mindspring.com

Ann Chuk, Founder/President/Director

A family-owned non profit that sponsors an outdoor Art Show and Sales in conjunction with Eden's Institute's Camp for children with Autism. Held in September in West Woodstock Connecticut.

561 **CREC Summer School**
Capitol Region Education Council
111 Charter Oak Avenue
Hartford, CT 06106
860-247-2732
FAX 860-246-3304
http://www.crec.org
e-mail: info@crec.org
Bruce E Douglas PhD, Executive Director
Roger L LaFleur, Operations Director
Dwight F Blint, Communications Director
Offers an educationally oriented program with recreational opportunities, strong behavior management and highly structured groupings.
1966Grade Range: Ages 4-21

562 **Camp Chase Specialty Camps: Creative ArtsCamp**
Farmington Valley YMCA
Granby, CT 06035
860-653-5524
FAX 860-844-8074
http://www.ghymca.org/camppage.htm
e-mail: camp.chase@ghymca.org
Neil Domer Shank, Camp Director
Jake Rosengrant, Onsite Director
Reed Domer Shank, Program Director
Go beyond arts and crafts! Special emphasis on the exploration of individual talents and interests in many areas, including painting, drawing, photography, and other fine arts. Swimming and other camp activities complete the camper's experience. Session 2 and 4 - Grades 3, 4, 5, 6. Camp Chase features a 85 acre wooded site with nature trails, streams for nature exploration, four pavilions for nature classes, arts & crafts, and two recreation halls for rainy day activities.

563 **Camp Chase Specialty Camps: Girl Power Camp**
Farmington Valley YMCA
Granby, CT 06035
860-653-5524
FAX 860-844-8074
http://www.ghymca.org/camppage.htm
e-mail: camp.chase@ghymca.org
Neil Domer Shank, Camp Director
Jake Rosengrant, Onsite Director
Reed Domer Shank, Program Director
Campers will focus on activities designed to bolster self-esteem, self-confidence and activate young imaginations. Swimming and other camp activities complete the camper's experience Camp Chase features a 85 acre wooded site with nature trails, streams for nature exploration, four pavilions for nature classes, arts & crafts, and two recreation halls for rainy day activities. Session 1 & 3 - Grades 5, 6, 7, 8.

564 **Camp Chase Specialty Camps: Media Camp**
Farmington Valley YMCA
Granby, CT 06035
860-653-5524
FAX 860-844-8074
http://www.ghymca.org/camppage.htm
e-mail: camp.chase@ghymca.org
Neil Domer Shank, Camp Director
Jake Rosengrant, Onsite Director
Reed Domer Shank, Program Director
Capture nature through photography, take photos of fellow campers and post to a web site each day. Create a DVD of your Camp Chase experience. Swimming and other camp activities complete the camper's experience. Camp Chase features a 85 acre wooded site with nature trails, streams for nature exploration, four pavilions for nature classes, arts & crafts, and two recreation halls for rainy day activities. Session 1, 2, 3, 4 - Grades 5, 6, 7, 8.

565 **Camp Chase Specialty Camps: Outdoor Adventure Camp**
Farmington Valley YMCA
Granby, CT 06035
860-653-5524
FAX 860-844-8074
http://www.ghymca.org/camppage.htm
e-mail: camp.chase@ghymca.org
Neil Domer Shank, Camp Director
Jake Rosengrant, Onsite Director
Reed Domer Shank, Program Director
Exciting outdoor experiences as campers take day trips to hike, kayak, and rock climb. Safety and proper trip preparedness are emphasized through pre-trip activities at Camp Chase. Each day is a new adventure. Camp Chase features a 85 acre wooded site with nature trails, streams for nature exploration, four pavilions for nature classes, arts & crafts, and two recreation halls for rainy day activities. Session 1, 2, 4 - Grades 6, 7, 8, and, Session 3 - Grades 9,10,11.

566 **Camp Chase Specialty Camps: Performing Arts Camp**
Farmington Valley YMCA
Granby, CT 06035
860-653-5524
FAX 860-844-8074
http://www.ghymca.org/camppage.htm
e-mail: camp.chase@ghymca.org
Neil Domer Shank, Camp Director
Jake Rosengrant, Onsite Director
Reed Domer Shank, Program Director
Learn role playing, set design, acting, theatre direction, improvisation, and perform in a play presentation. Swimming and other camp activities complete the camper's experience. Camp Chase features a 85 acre wooded site with nature trails, streams for nature exploration, four pavilions for nature classes, arts & crafts, and two recreation halls for rainy day activities. Session 1 and 3 - Grades 3, 4, 5, 6.

567 **Camp Chase Specialty Camps: Rescue 911 Camp**
Farmington Valley YMCA
Granby, CT 06035
860-653-5524
FAX 860-844-8074
http://www.ghymca.org/camppage.htm
e-mail: camp.chase@ghymca.org
Neil Domer Shank, Camp Director
Jake Rosengrant, Onsite Director
Reed Domer Shank, Program Director
What little camper isn't fascinated by firemen, policemen, and ambulance professionals? Sign your child up for a unique camping opportunity that combines elements of traditional camp with the excitement of rescue workers' experiences. Camp Chase features a 85 acre wooded site with nature trails, streams for nature exploration, four pavilions for nature classes, arts & crafts, and two recreation halls for rainy day activities. Session 5 Grades 1, 2, 3.

568 **Camp Chase Specialty Camps: Sports Camp**
Farmington Valley YMCA
Granby, CT 06035
860-653-5524
FAX 860-844-8074
http://www.ghymca.org/camppage.htm
e-mail: camp.chase@ghymca.org
Neil Domer Shank, Camp Director
Jake Rosengrant, Onsite Director
Reed Domer Shank, Program Director
Learn sport skills, fair play and teamwork. Experienced instructors will lead warm-ups, technique drills, and introduce strategies to each skill level group. Swimming and other camp activities complete the camper's experience. Basketball - Session 1 - Grades 3, 4, 5; Multi-Sport - Session 2 - Grades 4, 5, 6; Basketball - Session 3 - Grades 6, 7, 8; Soccer - Session 4 - Grades 3, 4, 5, 6; Baseball Camp - Session 5; Grades 3, 4, 5, 6.

569 **Camp Chase Specialty Camps: Wee WanderersCamp**
Farmington Valley YMCA
Granby, CT 06035
860-653-5524
FAX 860-844-8074
http://www.ghymca.org/camppage.htm
e-mail: camp.chase@ghymca.org
Neil Domer Shank, Camp Director
Jake Rosengrant, Onsite Director
Reed Domer Shank, Program Director
At Wee Wanderers, campers will have new and exciting adventures daily learning and having fun with nature. Swimming and other camp activities complete the camper's experience. Camp Chase features a 85 acre wooded site with nature trails, streams for nature exploration, four pavilions for nature classes, arts & crafts, and two recreation halls for rainy day activities. Session 3 - Grades 1, 2, 3.

570 **Camp Chase Specialty Camps: Wildlife Explorers Camp**
Farmington Valley YMCA
Granby, CT 06035
860-653-5524
FAX 860-844-8074
http://www.ghymca.org/camppage.htm
e-mail: camp.chase@ghymca.org

Neil Domer Shank, Camp Director
Jake Rosengrant, Onsite Director
Reed Domer Shank, Program Director
Join our nature expert for field trips, animal tracking, plant identification, and environmental study. Learn the secrets of nature through daily projects, hands on activities, eye witness investigation, and enjoy ecological field trips. Camp Chase features a 85 acre wooded site with nature trails, streams for nature exploration, four pavilions for nature classes, arts & crafts, and two recreation halls for rainy day activities. Session 1, 2, 3, 4 - Grades 4,5,6.

571 Camp Downtown
YMCA of Greater Hartford
Hartford, CT 06103
860-522-4183
FAX 860-724-9858
http://http://ghymca.org
e-mail: comments@ghymca.org
Kevin Washington, Executive Director

The YMCA Camp Downtown offers a variety of Specialty Camps. These camps are fantastic weeks of exploring special interest areas. Specialty Camps are a great way for children to exhibit their talents or learn about something new and interesting. Each week campers will participate in activities that are novel and bursting with creativity and excitement. All activities are supervised by the YMCA staff that is well trained in each special interest area.

572 Camp Hemlocks Easter Seals
85 Jones Street
Hebron, CT 06248
860-228-9496
800-832-4409
FAX 860-228-2091
http://www.ct.easterseals.com
e-mail: info@eastersealscamphemlocks.org
John Quinn, President
Sunny Ku, Director Camping

Offers an environment that allows campers with disabilities optimal independence. Camping and recreational services are: Aquatics, Family Camp, Recreational Services for Adults and Children, Residential Camping Programs, Adventure/Traveling Program.

573 Camp Horizons
127 Babcock Hill Road
South Windham, CT 06266
860-456-1032
FAX 860-456-4721
http://www.camphorizons.org
e-mail: staffpage@camphorizons.org
Chris Naboe, Executive Director
Janice Chamberlain, Associate Director
Lauren Perrotti, Operations Director
To provide high quality residential, recreational, support and work programs for people who are developmentally disabled or who have other challenging social and emotional needs.

574 Camp Indian Valley Specialty Camps: AnimalAdventures Preschool Camp
Indian Valley YMCA
Vernon, CT 06066
860-872-7329
FAX 860-875-5245
http://www.ghymca.org/camppage.htm
e-mail: indian.valleyymca@ghymca.org
Suzanne M Appleton, Branch Executive
Howard Pitkin, Branch Board Co-Chair
Mark Summers, Branch Board Co-Chair
This half-day preschool camp is for all animal lovers. Campers will enjoy lots of fun and furry activities including live animal visits, and animal arts and crafts. Above all, campers will make new friends and have a great YMCA experience. Session 6: Age 3 - 5 years old.

575 Camp Indian Valley Specialty Camps: Community Hero Preschool Camp
Indian Valley YMCA
Vernon, CT 06066
860-872-7329
FAX 860-875-5245
http://www.ghymca.org/camppage.htm
e-mail: indian.valleyymca@ghymca.org
Suzanne M Appleton, Branch Executive
Howard Pitkin, Branch Board Co-Chair
Mark Summers, Branch Board Co-Chair
This camp is a fun summer camp experience that will help preschoolers to build their sense of community. A community hero will visit each day. Children will meet a real live policeman, fireman, postman, and crossing guard. Children will also enjoy theme-related art, and play activities! Session 7: Age 3 - 5 years old.

576 Camp Indian Valley Specialty Camps: Dinosaur Preschool Camp
Indian Valley YMCA
Vernon, CT 06066
860-872-7329
FAX 860-875-5245
http://www.ghymca.org/camppage.htm
e-mail: indian.valleyymca@ghymca.org
Suzanne M Appleton, Branch Executive
Howard Pitkin, Branch Board Co-Chair
Mark Summers, Branch Board Co-Chair
Preschoolers will enter the prehistoric world of Dinosaurs as they participate in many fun dinosaur theme activities. Campers will learn the different types of dinosaurs, dig for dinosaur bones, go on a dinosaur hunt, create their own dinosaurs, and sing some popular purple dinosaur songs. Session 8: Age 3 - 5 years old.

577 Camp Indian Valley Specialty Camps: Escapades Camp

Indian Valley YMCA
Vernon, CT 06066
860-872-7329
FAX 860-875-5245
http://www.ghymca.org/camppage.htm
e-mail: indian.valleyymca@ghymca.org
Suzanne M Appleton, Branch Executive
Howard Pitkin, Branch Board Co-Chair
Mark Summers, Branch Board Co-Chair
Escapade campers get to do something fun every day. Highlights of the week will include a trip to the beach, Connecticut Golf land, Camp Woodstock, bowling, and some trampoline fun! Campers will have the opportunity to spend their summer vacation visiting some of their favorite places with their camp friends! Session 5 - Grades 6,7,8; and Session 6 - Grades 6,7,8.

578 Camp Indian Valley Specialty Camps: Extreme Aqua Camp
Indian Valley YMCA
Vernon, CT 06066
860-872-7329
FAX 860-875-5245
http://www.ghymca.org/camppage.htm
e-mail: indian.valleyymca@ghymca.org
Suzanne M Appleton, Branch Executive
Howard Pitkin, Branch Board Co-Chair
Mark Summers, Branch Board Co-Chair
Swimming, fun, and friends is what Camp Indian Valley is all about. At Camp Indian Valley campers have a great camp experience right at the Indian Valley YMCA. You will need a bathing suit, towel, and sunscreen each day as you brave the waves and waterslides! Each day will include a trip to a water adventure. Highlights include tubing down the Farmington River, riding the waves at Misquamicut, and a trip to the water park at Lake Compounce. Session 6 - Grades 5, 6, 7, 8, and 9.

579 Camp Indian Valley Specialty Camps: FairyTale Preschool Camp
Indian Valley YMCA
Vernon, CT 06066
860-872-7329
FAX 860-875-5245
http://www.ghymca.org/camppage.htm
e-mail: indian.valleyymca@ghymca.org
Suzanne M Appleton, Branch Executive
Howard Pitkin, Branch Board Co-Chair
Mark Summers, Branch Board Co-Chair
Preschoolers will delve in to the wonderful world of Peter Pan, Cinderella, Snow White and the Seven Dwarfs, Sleeping Beauty, and Goldilocks as they read about the character's fun adventures. There will also be theme-related art and of course lots of dress up and dramatic play. Session 2: Age 3 - 5 years old.

580 Camp Indian Valley Specialty Camps: Family Night Camp
Indian Valley YMCA
Vernon, CT 06066
860-872-7329
FAX 860-875-5245
http://www.ghymca.org/camppage.htm
e-mail: indian.valleyymca@ghymca.org

Suzanne M Appleton, Branch Executive
Howard Pitkin, Branch Board Co-Chair
Mark Summers, Branch Board Co-Chair
Swimming, fun, and friends is what Camp Indian Valley is all about. Two family nights will be held during the summer at our Yankee Trails Camp. It's a great time for campers, parents, and staff to get together for some camp fun.

581 Camp Indian Valley Specialty Camps: GirlsJust Want to Have Fun Camp
Indian Valley YMCA
Vernon, CT 06066
860-872-7329
FAX 860-875-5245
http://www.ghymca.org/camppage.htm
e-mail: indian.valleyymca@ghymca.org
Suzanne M Appleton, Branch Executive
Howard Pitkin, Branch Board Co-Chair
Mark Summers, Branch Board Co-Chair
This camp celebrates the fun of being a girl! This week is full of relaxed fun, enjoying activities that many girls like. Girls will get tips on fashion and makeup and will be pampered with a professional manicure. They will participate in a self-defense workshop and will spend a fun day at the beach! Girls will also spend time scrap booking. Session 4 - Grades 6, 7, and 8.

582 Camp Indian Valley Specialty Camps: Horsing Around Camp
Indian Valley YMCA
Vernon, CT 06066
860-872-7329
FAX 860-875-5245
http://www.ghymca.org/camppage.htm
e-mail: indian.valleyymca@ghymca.org
Suzanne M Appleton, Branch Executive
Howard Pitkin, Branch Board Co-Chair
Mark Summers, Branch Board Co-Chair
At Camp Indian Valley campers have a great camp experience right at the Indian Valley YMCA. This camp is for horse lovers! Trips will include a visit to a local barn, a veterinarian, and lots of horsing around activities. We will end the week with horseback riding. Session 3 - Grades 8, 9, 10, 11, 12.

583 Camp Indian Valley Specialty Camps: New Games Sports Explosion Preschool Camp
Indian Valley YMCA
Vernon, CT 06066
860-872-7329
FAX 860-875-5245
http://www.ghymca.org/camppage.htm
e-mail: indian.valleyymca@ghymca.org
Suzanne M Appleton, Branch Executive
Howard Pitkin, Branch Board Co-Chair
Mark Summers, Branch Board Co-Chair
Sports of all sorts! The focus is on learning the concepts and fundamentals of a variety of games. Physical activities incorporate teamwork, trust, and skills needed to have fun as well as the basics of traditional and nontraditional games. Pre Camp Session: Age 3 - 5 years old.

584 Camp Indian Valley Specialty Camps: Tumble Bugs Preschool Camp
Indian Valley YMCA
Vernon, CT 06066
860-872-7329
FAX 860-875-5245
http://www.ghymca.org/camppage.htm
e-mail: indian.valleyymca@ghymca.org
Suzanne M Appleton, Branch Executive
Howard Pitkin, Branch Board Co-Chair
Mark Summers, Branch Board Co-Chair
Preschoolers will enjoy spending each morning in the air-conditioned YMCA mini gym jumping, climbing, tumbling, and sliding. Children will have fun moving to music, singing, playing with soft balls, and puppets. Children will even get a chance to climb the new preschool rock wall. Session 5: Age 3 - 5 years old.

585 Camp Jewell YMCA
6 Prock Road
Colebrook, CT 06021
860-379-2782
888-412-2267
FAX 860-379-8715
http://ghymca.org/branches/jewell/jwelcom.htm
e-mail: camp.jewell@ghymca.org
Brian Rupe, Executive Director
Eric Tucker, Associate Executive Director
Ray Zetye, Summer Camp Director
Located on a picturesque 540 acre site surrounding Triangle Lake in Colebrook, Connecticut, Camp Jewell YMCA hosts a day camp program for local residents in Colebrook and surrounding towns. This program serves youth in kindergarten through 5th grade. Day camp is a great way for area youth to enjoy the facilities, programs and special spirit at Camp Jewell.

586 Camp Lark
Litchfield County Association for Retarded Citizen
314 Main Street
Torrington, CT 06790
860-482-9364
FAX 860-489-2492
TDY:860-496-4049
http://www.litchfieldarc.org/camp_larc.htm
e-mail: larc@litchfieldarc.org
Larry Cassella, Executive Director
Katherine Marchand-Beyer, Community Services Director

Program offers arts and crafts, swimming, field sports, archery, outdoor education, music, drama and adventure courses. Once a week overnights are offered and the program runs in conjunction with the Torrington YMCA camp, Northwest YMCA, Camp Torymca. Additional staff supports are available when needed.

587 Camp Tepee
204 Stanley Road
Monroe, CT 06468
203-261-2566
FAX 203-261-3146
http://www.cccymca.org
Dawn Dalryntle, Executive Director
Meg Ballard, Manager

Each summer, over 1,700 campers experience exciting thrills and make memories that last a lifetime. We are a fully modernized facility located on 47 beautiful acres nestled in the Stephney section of Monroe, CT. We pride ourselves on providing a safe and nurturing environment in which children of all ages conquer new challenges, make new friends, and share in the unique and wonderful experience that is day camp.

588 Camp Woodstock YMCA
42 Camp Road
Woodstock, CT 06282
860-379-2782
800-782-2344
FAX 860-379-8715
http://www.ghymca.org/camppage.htm
e-mail: camp.woodstockymca@ghymca.org
Michael Sherman, Executive Director
Kevin Washington, President/CEO Central Office
Art Snyder, Branch Board Chairman
Kids come to Camp Woodstock to have fun and make friends. In the process they also acquirc values, learn skills, develop self-reliance, and build character. At this camp these life skills lie behind every laugh, hug, splash, or song. A boy or girl can leave behind the pressures of the day and just be a kid in a community for kids.

589 Cyber Launch Pad
Learning Incentive
139 N Main Street
West Hartford, CT 06107
860-236-5807
FAX 860-233-9945
http://www.learningincentive.com/TLI_Intr.html
e-mail: Inquire@learningincentive.com
Aileen Stan-Spence MD, Executive Director
Cythnia Cordes MA, Study Skills Services Director
Susan Sharp Ph.D, Education Director
Half days camp where children and their parents learn to use Cyberslate which is learning keyboarding, word processing, programming and remedial sessions in reading, writing and arithmetic for learning disabled children.

590 Eagle Hill Southport School
214 Main Street
Southport, CT 06890
203-254-2044
FAX 203-255-4052
http://www.eaglehillsouthport.org
e-mail: info@eaglehillsouthport.org
Leonard Tavormina, Principal
Dede Warner, Administrative Assistant
Lea Sylvestro, Patient Liaison
The summer program at Eagle Hill is designed to help students 6 to 13 years old maintain their academic progress.

591 **Eagle Hill Summer Program**
45 Glenville Road
Greenwich, CT 06831
203-622-9240
FAX 203-622-0914
http://www.eaglehillschool.org
e-mail: info@eaglehillschool.org
Mark Griffin, Director
Abby Hanrahan, Teacher Camp
Nelson Dorta, Manager
Designed for children experiencing academic difficulty. Open to boys and girls ages 5-11.

592 **East Hartford Special Education Camp**
East Hartford Park and Recreation Department
50 Chapman Place
East Hartford, CT 06108
860-528-1458
FAX 860-282-8239
http://www.ci.east-hartford.ct.us
e-mail: dmailloux@ci.east-hartford.ct.us
C Roger Moss, CPRP, Director
Jim Uhrij, CPRP/CPSI, Assistant Director
Diane Mailloux, CPRP, Recreation Supervisor
For East Hartford residents only. A day camp offering swimming, sports, arts and crafts, projects, music and field trips.

593 **Haddam-Killingworth Recreation Department**
95 Little City Road
Higganum, CT 06441
860-345-8334
FAX 860-345-8252
http://www.hkrec.com
e-mail: frank@hkrec.com
Frank Sparks, Executive Director
Robyne Brennan, Assistant Director
Jennifer Saglio, Director of Childcare
Programs offered include arts and crafts, games, sports workshops, field trips, movies, special events and a carnival.

594 **Marvelwood Summer**
Marvelwood School
PO Box 3001
Kent, CT 06757
860-927-0047
800-440-9107
FAX 860-927-0021
http://www.themarvelwoodschool.com
e-mail: summer@marvelwood.org
Anne Scott, Principal
Scott E Pottbecker, Headmaster
Katherine Almquist, Summer Admissions Director
A coeducational boarding and day school enrolling 150 students in grades 9-12. Provides an environment in which young people of varying abilities and learning needs can prepare for success in college and in life. In a nurturing, structured community, students who have not thrived academically in traditional settings are guided and motivated to reach and exceed their personal potential.

595 **Middletown Summer Day Programs**
Middletown Parks and Recreation Department
100 Riverview Center
Middletown, CT 06457
860-343-6620
FAX 860-344-3319
http://www.cityofmiddletown.com
e-mail: john.milardo@cityofmiddletown.com
John Milardo, Superintendent of Parks
Ray Jacobs, Superintendent of Recreation
Raymond Santostefano, Director Parks & Recreation
These camps offer a variety of recreational and social activities. Each camp will be integrated with at least 12% population of children with disabilities. Campers must be Middletown residents.

596 **Milford Recreation Department Camp Happiness**
70 W River Street
Milford, CT 06460
203-783-3280
FAX 203-783-3284
http://www.ci.milford.ct.us/
e-mail: bmccarthy@ci.milford.ct.us
William Carthy, Recreation Director
Marelene Sanchez, Summer Camp Director
Paul Piscitelli, Recreation Supervisor
A camp specifically designed for learning disabled children from the Milford area.

597 **Norwalk Public Schools: Special Education Summer Programs**
125 East Avenue
Norwalk, CT 06852
203-854-4001
FAX 203-854-4125
http://www.norwalkpublicschools.org/cont.html
e-mail: corda@norwalkpublicschool.net
Salvador Corda, Superintendent
Barbara Sacks, Assistant
Sheri L McCready, Public Affairs Officer
Offers pre-school/elementary students developmental and remedial academics summer programs.

598 **Our Victory Day Camp**
Stamford, CT 06902
203-329-3394
800-329-3394
FAX 203-329-3394
http://www.ourvictory.com/
e-mail: ourvictory@aol.com
Fred Tunick, Executive Director

Our Victory Day Camp is a 7-week day camping program for children from 5 to 12 years of age. It is oriented toward children with learning disabilities and/or attention deficit disorder. The program is designed to expose each camper to a wide variety of activities. The goal is to create an opportunity for each camper to achieve success, whatever the camper's ability. Activities include arts and crafts, drama, music, nature, dancing, hiking, jewelry making, swimming, and sports.

599 **Shriver Summer Developmental Program**
Nathan Hale School
5 Taylor Road
Enfield, CT 06082
860-763-8899
FAX 860-763-8897
http://www.enfieldschools.org
e-mail: leann.beaulieu@ensieldschool.org
LeAnn Beaulieu, Principal
Kathi Steinert, Assistant Principal
Bethany Holland, Guidance Counselor
Academic/recreational program including instructional swimming for the learning disabled.

600 **Timber Trails Camps**
Connecticut Valley Girl Scout Council
340 Washington Street
Hartford, CT 06106
860-522-0163
FAX 860-548-0325
http://www.girlscouts-ct.org/camp.htm
e-mail: info@girlscouts-ct.org
Janet Kissin, Acting Director
Terry Terrell, Manager
Theresa Miller, Camp Director
All girls age 6 to 17 who can function in a group in a mainstream environment are welcome, including those with chronic illnesses, learning disabilities, and physical or emotional needs.

601 **Valley-Shore YMCA**
201 Spencer Plains Road
Westbrook, CT 06498
860-399-9622
FAX 860-399-8349
http://www.vsymca.org
e-mail: vsymca@vsymca.org
Paul Mohabir, Chief Executive Officer
Richard Ward, Program Development Director
Dana Duncan, Health & Wellness Coordinator
Family Play Dates, an adaptive recreation program designed for special language need children ages 3-7 years. (Pervasive Developmental Disorder and high functioning Autism, Asperger's, Down Syndrome). Daycamp with swimming, hiking, sports, games, nature study, archery and low ropes course.

602 **Wheeler Regional Family YMCA**
149 Farmington Avenue
Plainville, CT 06062
860-793-3500
800-793-3588
FAX 860-793-3520
TDY:860-792-9631
http://www.ghymca.org
e-mail: kevin.washington@ghymca.org
Kevin Washington, President & CEO
Hyacinth Douglas-Bailey, VP/Child Care & Camping Services
Joseph Weist, VP/Finance & CFO
The Wheeler Regional Family YMCA is a non-profit charitable community organization. The YMCA provides a wide variety of programs for all ages. The YMCA's main programs include Child Care, Aquatic Programs, Day Camp, Teen programs, Wellness and Fitness Programs. The Wheeler Regional Family YMCA serves Plainville, Bristol, Farmington, Burlington and Plymouth.

603 **Winston Prep School Summer Program**
Norwalk, CT 06851
203-229-0465
http://www.winstonprep.edu/Welcome.html
e-mail: bsugerman@winstonprep.edu.
Beth Sugarman, Operations & Research Director
Elizabeth Tauber, Focus Program Director
Courtney DeHoff, Admissions Director
For 6th through 12th grade students with learning differences such as dyslexia, nonverbal learning disabilities, expressive or receptive language disorders and attention deficit problems. The Summer Enrichment Program at their New York City branch school is designed to enhance academic skills. Students from area parochial, public and private schools attend the program every year. They receive daily one-on-one instruction in addition to attending class in the courses they have selected.

Delaware

604 **Cedars Academy**
PO Box 103
Bridgeville, DE 19933
302-337-3200
866-339-0165
FAX 302-337-8496
http://www.cedarsacademy.com
John Singleton, Executive Director
Dottie Kopple-Lank, Admissions Director
Tara Drayton, Operations Director
A seven week program which encourages positive feelings of self worth and increased interpersonal skills. Activities include camping, sailing and art.

District of Columbia

605 **Summer Adventure Program**
Trinity University
125 Michigan Avenue NE
Washington, DC 20017
202-884-9000
FAX 202-244-8065
http://www.trinitydc.edu/news_events/2006/camps
e-mail: mcewene@trinitydc.edu
Lynne Israel, Director
Elle McEwen, Camp Coordinator

A six week day camp to enhance sensory motor development. Activities include tactile activity, gross and fine motor skills, swimming instruction, music, language and visualization skills.

606 **Summer Camp for Children who are Deaf or Hard of Hearing**
Laurent Clerc National Deaf Education Center
Gallaudet University
Washington, DC 20002
202-651-5300
FAX 202-651-5477
http://http://infotogo.gallaudet.edu/142.html
e-mail: infotech.services@gallaudet.edu
Erving Jordan, President
Paul Kelly, Vice President

To serve as a comprehensive, multipurpose facility of higher education for deaf and hard of hearing.

Florida

607 **3D Learner Program**
State Land of Learning Disability Association
580 Riverside Drive
Coral Springs, FL 33071
954-341-2578
866-411-2578
FAX 954-796-3883
http://www.3dlearner.com
e-mail: success@3dlearner.com
Mark Halpert, Executive Director
Mira Halpert, Educational Director

3D Learner Program, a one-week program for struggling students who learn best when they see and experience information. We have had students from all over the US. We address attention, self-esteem and reading with a natural and effective method. Our students make immediate gains and often see significant gains with 3 months. Free learning survey and 10 minute consult. Also speak toparents and professionals.

608 **ALERT-US**
Coalition for Independent Living
6800 Forest Hill Boulevard
Greenacres, FL 33413
561-966-4288
800-683-7337
FAX 561-641-6619
http://www.cilo.org
Shelly Gottsagen, Executive Director
Linda Kirtley, Administrative Assistant
Sharon D'Eusanio, President
Promotes the independence of people with disabilties by offering programs and a network of support.

609 **Camp Challenge**
Easter Seals Florida: Central Florida
31600 Camp Challenge Road
Sorrento, FL 32776
352-383-4711
800-377-3257
FAX 321-383-0744
http://www.campchallengefl.com
e-mail: camp@fl.easter-seals.org
Susan Ventura, President
Melissa Guinta, Center Director
John K Hazelton, Director of Camping/Recreation
At Easter Seals Camp Challenge, campers participate in arts & crafts, nature activities, a universal high and low ropes course, music and dancing, outside entertainers, farm animals and other camp activities.

610 **Camp WorldLight**
1230 Hendricks Avenue
Jacksonville, FL 32207
904-396-2351
800-226-8584
FAX 904-396-0271
http://www.campworldlight.org
e-mail: awilson@flbaptist.org
Anne Wilson, Camp Director
Donald Hepburn, Public Relations Director
Stephens Baumgardner, Business Services Director
Camp WorldLight is a Florida camp for girls designed to be explored, enjoyed and filled with expectations, providing a week of fun-filled, life-changing experiences. Activities include crafts, music, drama, swimming, canoeing and recreation in addition to making new friend and meeting missionaries. CampWorld Light is located in the Florida Panhandle at Blue Springs Conference Center in Marianna and in Central Florida at Lake Yale Conference Center in Leesburg.

611 **Dimensions Kids Camp: Aquatics Program Camp**
20700 W Dixie Highway
Aventura, FL 33180
305-933-5887
FAX 305-933-8991
http://www.dimensionstherapy.com
e-mail: dimensions@bellsouth.net

Robin Bersson, Executive Director
Amber Reid, Camp Director
Jane Burrows, Equestrian Center Director
During Aquatics Program Camp the campers will develop water safety skills and will learn and/or improve their swimming abilities while enhancing their peer relationships in a state-of-the-art water environment. The camp experience will be fun, educational and will continue to promote the child's overall development.

612 Dimensions Kids Camp: Arts and Crafts Camp

20700 W Dixie Highway
Aventura, FL 33180
305-933-5887
FAX 305-933-8991
http://www.dimensionstherapy.com
e-mail: dimensions@bellsouth.net
Robin Bersson, Executive Director
Amber Reid, Camp Director
Jane Burrows, Equestrian Center Director
During Arts and Crafts Camp the campers will participate in a variety of activities to increase in-hand manipulation, dexterity, hand strength, visual motor skills and overall fine motor development. The camp experience will be fun, educational and will continue to promote the child's overall development.

613 Dimensions Kids Camp: Community Experiences Camp

20700 W Dixie Highway
Aventura, FL 33180
305-933-5887
FAX 305-933-8991
http://www.dimensionstherapy.com
e-mail: dimensions@bellsouth.net
Robin Bersson, Executive Director
Amber Reid, Camp Director
Jane Burrows, Equestrian Center Director
During Community Experiences Camp the campers will venture out on a weekly field trip to age appropriate places to encourage carryover of skills into a real world setting. The camp experience will be fun, educational and will continue to promote the child's overall development.

614 Dimensions Kids Camp: Cooking Camp

20700 W Dixie Highway
Aventura, FL 33180
305-933-5887
FAX 305-933-8991
http://www.dimensionstherapy.com
e-mail: dimensions@bellsouth.net
Robin Bersson, Executive Director
Amber Reid, Camp Director
Jane Burrows, Equestrian Center Director
During Cooking Camp the campers will make fun foods to learn about taste, color, texture, and use of kitchen utensils in a highly social and safe environment. The camp experience will be fun, educational and will continue to promote the child's overall development.

615 Dimensions Kids Camp: Creative Movement Camp

20700 W Dixie Highway
Aventura, FL 33180
305-933-5887
FAX 305-933-8991
http://www.dimensionstherapy.com
e-mail: dimensions@bellsouth.net
Robin Bersson, Executive Director
Amber Reid, Camp Director
Jane Burrows, Equestrian Center Director
During Creative Movement Camp the campers will engage in musical experiences to enhance fine and gross motor skills, compliance, attention and behavior, imitation of movement and rhythmic patterns, various ball activities and development of peer relations. The camp experience will be fun, educational and will continue to promote the child's overall development.

616 Dimensions Kids Camp: Equine/Horse Assisted Activities Camp

20700 W Dixie Highway
Aventura, FL 33180
305-933-5887
FAX 305-933-8991
http://www.dimensionstherapy.com
e-mail: dimensions@bellsouth.net
Robin Bersson, Executive Director
Amber Reid, Camp Director
Jane Burrows, Equestrian Center Director
During Equine (Horse) Assisted Activities Camp the campers will engage in horseback riding and horse related activities in a fun and safe environment that promotes self accomplishment, social interaction, balance, core strength, coordination, motor planning and animal care responsibility. The camp experience will be fun, educational and will continue to promote the child's overall development.

617 Dimensions Kids Camp: Indoor Rock Climbing and Vertical Playground Camp

20700 W Dixie Highway
Aventura, FL 33180
305-933-5887
FAX 305-933-8991
http://www.dimensionstherapy.com
e-mail: dimensions@bellsouth.net
Robin Bersson, Executive Director
Amber Reid, Camp Director
Jane Burrows, Equestrian Center Director
During Indoor Rock Climbing/Vertical Playground Camp the campers will be challenged to achieve the heights by the bouldering wall, climbing tower and overhead trails while developing higher aspirations, expanding gross motor skills and improving decision-making skills. The camp experience will be fun, educational and will continue to promote the child's overall development.

618 Dimensions Kids Camp: Life Skills Group Camp

20700 W Dixie Highway
Aventura, FL 33180
305-933-5887
FAX 305-933-8991
http://www.dimensionstherapy.com
e-mail: dimensions@bellsouth.net
Robin Bersson, Executive Director
Amber Reid, Camp Director
Jane Burrows, Equestrian Center Director
During Life Skills Group Camp the campers will have an opportunity to engage in activities to increase overall independence to encourage carryover of skills into community settings. The camp experience will be fun, educational and will continue to promote the child's overall development.

619 Dimensions Kids Camp: Occupational Therapy Group Camp

20700 W Dixie Highway
Aventura, FL 33180
305-933-5887
FAX 305-933-8991
http://www.dimensionstherapy.com
e-mail: dimensions@bellsouth.net
Robin Bersson, Executive Director
Amber Reid, Camp Director
Jane Burrows, Equestrian Center Director
Dimensions Kids Camp is a day camp for children, adolescents and young adults with special needs of all ages and backgrounds. Occupational Therapy Group Camp provides the opportunity for campers to enjoy an environment that is developmentally appropriate, stimulating and provides the just right challenge to encourage socialization and motor skills, to challenge their minds and to explore and discover new skills through play.

620 Dimensions Kids Camp: Speech/Language Therapy Group Camp

20700 W Dixie Highway
Aventura, FL 33180
305-933-5887
FAX 305-933-8991
http://www.dimensionstherapy.com
e-mail: dimensions@bellsouth.net
Robin Bersson, Executive Director
Amber Reid, Camp Director
Jane Burrows, Equestrian Center Director
During Speech/Language Therapy Group Camp, the campers will participate in an environment that is developmentally appropriate, stimulating and fun. Groups are interactive and facilitate social language skills, vocabulary, on-task behavior and emotions, and will be themed to interface traditional and social language goals with exploration of feelings. The camp experience will be fun, educational and will continue to promote the child's overall development.

621 Dimensions Kids Camp: Yoga-Pilates Group Camp

20700 W Dixie Highway
Aventura, FL 33180
305-933-5887
FAX 305-933-8991
http://www.dimensionstherapy.com
e-mail: dimensions@bellsouth.net

Robin Bersson, Executive Director
Amber Reid, Camp Director
Jane Burrows, Equestrian Center Director

During Yoga-Pilates Group Camp the campers will engage in a comprehensive group that will promote improved strength, flexibility, coordination, posture, relaxation, body awareness, attention and self-esteem. The camp experience will be fun, educational and will continue to promote the child's overall development.

622 Easter Seals Volusia and Flagler Counties

Easter Seals Volusia & Flagler Counties of Chicago
1219 Dunn Avenue
Daytona Beach, FL 32114
386-255-4568
877-255-4568
FAX 386-258-7677
TDY:877-255-4568
http://fl-vf.easterseals.com
e-mail: info@fl-vf.easter-seals.org

Lynn Sinnott, President
Catherine Colwell, Vice President
Kathy Catron, Media

Easter Seals camping and recreation programs serve children, adults and families of all abilities. Various programs are available with the united purpose of giving disabled individuals a fun and safe camping or recreational experience. Camping and recreational services are: Day camping for children.

623 Eckerd Family Youth Alternatives

PO Box 7450
Clearwater, FL 33758
727-461-2990
FAX 727-442-5911
http://www.eckerd.org
e-mail: admissions@eckerd.org

Karen Waddell, President
Richard Nedelkoff, Chief Operation Officer

Designed to combine the wilderness living experience with the reality treatment perspective, the psychology perspective and behavior modification techniques. Founded 1968

624 Frontier Travel Camp

1000 Quayside Terrace
Miami Shores, FL 33138
305-895-1123
866-750-2267
FAX 305-893-4169
http://www.frontiertravelcamp.com
e-mail: info@frontiertravelcamp.com

Scott Fineman MSW, Camp Director
Deborah D'Annunzio, Assistant Camp Director
Martha Calero, Head Counselor

Frontier Travel Camp was established in 1997 as a summer camp alternative for individuals with special needs. Frontier travelers are high functioning individuals ranging in age from 15 to 35 years. They have varying learning disabilities, developmental disabilities, and/or other difficulties requiring more supervision and guidance than the mainstream camper. Frontier Travel Camp facilitates independence, improved social skills, and increased self-esteem in a secure and exciting environment.

625 YMCA: Lakeland

3620 Cleveland Heights Boulevard
Lakeland, FL 33803
863-644-3528
FAX 863-644-2517
http://www.ymcawcs.org
e-mail: leonard.speed@ymcawcf.org

Alice Collins, CEO
Leonard Speed, Executive Director

Camp runs June through July, and is coed, ages 12-16.

Georgia

626 Easter Seals Southern Georgia

1906 Palmyra Road
Albany, GA 31701
229-439-7061
800-365-4583
FAX 229-435-6278
http://www.southerngeorgia.easterseals.com
e-mail: benglish@swga-easterseals.org

Lynda Hammond, President
Carol Holloman, Secretary

Easter Seals camping and recreation programs serve children, adults and families of all abilities. Various programs are available with the united purpose of giving disabled individuals a fun and safe camping or recreational experience. Camping and recreational services offered are: Camp respite for adults, camp respite for children, day camping for children and therapeutic horseback riding.

627 Squirrel Hollow

Bedford School Organization
5665 Milam Road
Fairburn, GA 30213
770-774-8001
FAX 770-774-8005
http://www.thebedfordschool.org
e-mail: bbox@thebedfordschool.org

Betsy Box, Executive Director
Bonnie Sides, Secretary
Anne Miller, Development Director

A remedial summer program for children with academic needs held on the campus of The Bedford School in Fairburn, Georgia. It is a five week Day Camp held from June 19 to July 21 and serves children ages 6-16. For more information contact Betsy Box at (770) 774-8001.

Hawaii

628 Easter Seals Hawaii: Oahu Service Center

710 Green Street
Honolulu, HI 96813
808-536-1015
888-241-7450
FAX 808-536-3765
http://www.eastersealshawaii.org
e-mail: nicole@eastersealshawaii.org

John Howell, President
Norman Kawakami, SVP/Operations

Easter Seals camping and recreation programs serve children, adults and families of all abilities. Various programs are available with the united purpose of giving disabled individuals a fun and safe camping or recreational experience. Camping and recreational services offered are: Residential camping programs.

Idaho

629 SUWS Troubled Teen Wilderness Programs

911 Preacher Creek Road
Shoshone, ID 83352
888-879-7897
FAX 208-886-2153
http://www.suws.com

Kathy Rex, Executive Director
Cliff Stockton, Program Director

Specializes in helping troubled teens and defiant teens with behaviioral and emotional problems. Assist in helping young people to identify and work through internal conflicts and emotional obstacles that have kept them from responding to parental efforts, schools and treatment.

Illinois

630 Camp Algonquin
1889 Cary Road
Algonquin, IL 60102
847-658-8212
FAX 847-658-8431
http://www.campalgonquin.org
e-mail: info@campalgonquin.org
Tabatha Endres Cruz, Program Director
Lynda Blacker, Assistant Program Director

To inspire, educate and strengthen individuals, families and groups toward growth, achievement, positive community and environmental stewardship through education, experiential and recreational opportunities.

631 Camp Discovery
241 US Highway 45
Indian Creek, IL 60061
847-367-2267
FAX 847-367-4202
http://www.campdiscovery.com
e-mail: director@campdiscovery.com
Karen Schwartzwald, Camp Coordinator
Emily Schwartzwald, Camp Coordinator
Mitchell Schwartzwald, Camp Coordinator
Camp Discovery is a small nurturing camp where your child receives individualized attention. Campers are grouped in small age appropriate groups where they receive individualized attention while participating in: swimming (twice daily), fine arts, sports, nature, ropes course and special events. The young people are challenged to try new skills that are taught in a non-competitive atmosphere as they form memorable relationships with their group and group leaders.

632 Camp Little Giant: Touch of Nature Environmental Center
Southern Illinois University
1208 Touch of Nature Road
Carbondale, IL 62901
618-453-5348
FAX 618-453-1188
http://www.tonec.siu.edu/?littlegiant
e-mail: camplittlegiant99@yahoo.com
Randy Osborn, Program Coordinator
Arron Stearn, Manager
Chiland Lanlessna, Registrar
A residential camp program designed to meet the recreational needs of adults and children with disabilities.

633 Camp Red Leaf Respite Weekends
JCYS/Jewish Council for Youth Services
PO Box 297
Ingleside, IL 60041
847-740-5010
FAX 847-740-5014
http://www.jcys.org/redleaf/index.html
e-mail: awarner@jcys.org
Anthony Warner, Director JCYS Camp Red Leaf
Martin Oliff Ph.D, Executive Director JCYS Central
Lisa Kudish, Development & Communications
The Camp Red Leaf Respite program is designed to serve young people with developmental disabilites. Participants enjoy trying new recreational activities and developing a variety of social and physical skills in a community setting. Activities are adaptable and encourage participation. Our staff are highly qualified and will provide your children with a safe and fun environment. The program fee will cover food, housing at camp and community outings.

634 Camp Red Leaf Summer Camp
JCYS/Jewish Council for Youth Services
PO Box 297
Ingleside, IL 60041
847-740-5010
FAX 847-740-5014
http://www.jcys.org/redleaf/index.html
e-mail: awarner@jcys.org
Anthony Warner, Director JCYS Camp Red Leaf
Martin Oliff Ph.D, Executive Director JCYS Central
Lisa Kudish, Development & Communications

Camp Red Leaf is designed to serve youth and adults with developmental disabilities, emotional and behavioral needs for ages 9 and upward. The highly adaptable summer programs at Camp Red Leaf strive to increase self-esteem, promote interaction, improve social skills and encourage independence in a natural environment. Some featured activities include: swimming, arts and crafts, sports, games, boating, expressive arts, dances, talent shows, camp fires, fishing, and musical activities.

635 Easter Seals Camping and Recreation List
National Easter Seals Society
230 W Monroe Street
Chicago, IL 60606
312-726-6200
800-221-6827
FAX 312-726-1494
http://http://joliet.easterseals.com
e-mail: info@easter-seals.com
Jim Williams, Jr, CEO
Rosemary Garza, Interim Specialist

Various programs with the united purpose of giving disabled children a fun and safe camping or recreational experience. Call for information on activities in your state.

636 Easter Seals Central Illinois
2715 N 27th Street
Decatur, IL 62526
217-429-1052
FAX 217-423-7605
http://www.easterseals-ci.org
e-mail: info@easterseals-ci.org
Jan Kelsheimer, President
Margie Malone, Office Manager

Easter Seals camping and recreation programs serve children, adults and families of all abilities. Various programs are available with the united purpose of giving disabled individuals a fun and safe camping or recreational experience. The following are Camping and Recreational services offered: Recreational services for adults and recreational services for children.

637 Easter Seals Jayne Shover Center
National Easter Seals Society
799 S McLean Boulevard
Elgin, IL 60123
847-742-3264
FAX 847-742-9436
http://www.il-js.easterseals.com
e-mail: admin@il-js.easterseals.com
Susan Dilley, Chief Executive Officer

Easter Seals camping and recreation programs serve children, adults and families of all abilities. Various programs are available with the united purpose of giving disabled individuals a fun and safe camping or recreational experience. The following are Camping and Recreational services offered: Recreational services for adult and recreational services for children.

638 Easter Seals Joliet
National Easter Seals Society
212 Barney Drive
Joliet, IL 60435
815-725-2194
FAX 815-725-5150
http://www.joliet.easterseals.com
e-mail: dcondotti@il-wg.easter-seals.org
Debra Condotti, President
Carol Baces, Human Resource Director

Easter Seals camping and recreation programs serve children, adults and families of all abilities. Various programs are available with the united purpose of giving disabled individuals a fun and safe camping or recreational experience. The following are camping and recreational services offered: Camperships.

639 Easter Seals Missouri
602 E 3rd Street
Alton, IL 62002
618-462-7325
FAX 618-462-8170
http://www.mo.easterseals.org
e-mail: mail@mo-easter-seals.org
Craig Byrd, CEO
Lynn Stonecipher, Manager
Susan Gunning, Development Therapist
Easter Seals camping and recreation programs serve children, adults and families of all abilities. Various programs are available with the united purpose of giving disabled individuals a fun and safe camping or recreational experience. The following are camping and recreational services offered: Camperships.

640 **Easter Seals UCP: Peoria**
Easter Seals of Peoria Bloomington
20 Timber Pointe Drive
Hudson, IL 61748
309-365-8021
FAX 309-365-8934
e-mail: kpodeszwa@easterseals.com
Steve Thompson, President/CEO
Andrew M Morgan, Medical Director

Easter Seals camping and recreation programs serve children, adults and families of all abilities. Various programs are available with the united purpose of giving disabled individuals a fun and safe camping or recreational experience. The following are Camping and Recreational services offered: Recreational services for adults and recreational services for children.

641 **JCYS Adventure Education: Hyde Park Academy and Camp Henry Horner**
JCYS/Jewish Council for Youth Services
Chicago, IL 60614
312-482-9517
FAX 312-482-6413
http://www.jcys.org/lakeview/adventure.html
e-mail: lashe@jcys.org
Elisabeth Ashe, Director Adventure Education
Martin Oliff Ph.D, Executive Director JCYS Central
Lisa Kudish, Development & Communications
JCYS Adventure Education employs the principles of experiential and adventure education to engage students in their own learning and creating an environment where participants challenge themselves and expand their comfort zones to learn and grow - as people and as students. The program culminates with a two-day overnight trip to JCYS Camp Henry Horner for further challenge and growth experiences at the High Sierra Adventure Center's high and low ropes course.

642 **JCYS Adventure Education: Mather Public High School and Camp Henry Horner**
JCYS/Jewish Council for Youth Services
Chicago, IL 60614
312-482-9517
FAX 312-482-6413
http://www.jcys.org/lakeview/adventure.html
e-mail: lashe@jcys.org
Elisabeth Ashe, Director Adventure Education
Martin Oliff Ph.D, Executive Director JCYS Central
Lisa Kudish, Development & Communications
JCYS Adventure Education employs the principles of experiential and adventure education to engage students in their own learning and creating an environment where participants challenge themselves and expand their comfort zones to learn and grow - as people and as students. The program culminates with a two-day overnight trip to JCYS Camp Henry Horner for further challenge and growth experiences at the High Sierra Adventure Center's high and low ropes course.

643 **JCYS Adventure Education: Sullivan PublicHigh School and Camp Henry Horner**
JCYS/Jewish Council for Youth Services
Chicago, IL 60614
312-482-9517
FAX 312-482-6413
http://www.jcys.org/lakeview/adventure.html
e-mail: lashe@jcys.org
Elisabeth Ashe, Director Adventure Education
Martin Oliff Ph.D, Executive Director JCYS Central
Lisa Kudish, Development & Communications
JCYS Adventure Education employs the principles of experiential and adventure education to engage students in their own learning and creating an environment where participants challenge themselves and expand their comfort zones to learn and grow - as people and as students. The program culminates with a two-day overnight trip to JCYS Camp Henry Horner for further challenge and growth experiences at the High Sierra Adventure Center's high and low ropes course.

644 **Western Du Page Special Recreation Association**
116 N Schmale Road
Carol Stream, IL 60188
630-681-0962
FAX 630-681-1262
TDY:630-681-0962
http://www.wdsra.com
e-mail: info@wdsra.com
Jane Hodgkinson, Executive Director
Nancy Miner, Recreation Superintendent

Offers year-round recreational services and programs to special residents of its nine member communities.

Indiana

645 **Bradford Woods Summer Camp**
Indiana University Outdoor Center
Martinsville, IN 46151
765-342-2915
FAX 765-349-1086
http://www.indiana.edu/~bradwood
e-mail: bradwood@indiana.edu
Shay Dawson, Camping/Retreats Center Director
Zeena Brillantes, Challenge Education Ctr Director
Shane Gibson, Environmental Resource Ctr Drtcr
Bradford Woods Summer Camp offers both single-day and overnight programs and events for children with special health care needs and their families. Overnight programs have been fulfilling the recreational and therapeutic requirements of both children and adults with disabilities and chronic illnesses for over forty years. Canoeing, archery, and swimming are a few of the fun activities children take part in.

646 **Camp Brosend Ministries**
7599 Brosend Road
Newburgh, IN 47630
812-853-3466
FAX 812-853-5585
http://www.campbrosend.org
e-mail: info@campbrosend.org
Kevin Heil, Executive Director

Campers enjoy a wide variety of program activities while building confidence.

647 **Camp Nexus Summer Camp**
City of Bloomington Parks & Recreation
401 N Morton Street
Bloomington, IN 47404
812-349-3700
FAX 812-349-3705
http://http://bloomington.in.gov/parks/
e-mail: parks@bloomington.in.gov
Pamela Dunscombe, Youth Services Specialist
Dave Fox, Operations Superintendent
Daren Eads, Facility/Program Coordinator
Inspired by the Rhino's after-school programs, Camp Nexus provides an introduction to the multimedia world of video, radio, publication and art. Campers will learn from expert staff and create pieces for broadcast, production, publication or display. In addition, on Friday afternoons, campers will have the opportunity to share their best work during the Nexus Gallery.

648 **Easter Seals ARC of Northeast Indiana**
4919 Coldwater Road
Fort Wayne, IN 46825
260-456-4534
800-234-7811
FAX 260-745-5200
http://http://neindiana.easterseals.com
e-mail: damstutz@esarc.org
Steve Hinkle, Chief Executive Officer
Darlene Amstutz, Annual Gifts Coordinator

Easter Seals camping and recreation programs serve children, adults and families of all abilities. Various programs are available with the united purpose of giving disabled individuals a fun and safe camping or recreational experience. The following are camping and recreational services offered: Recreational services for adults and camp respite for adults and children.

649 **Easter Seals Crossroads**
4740 Kingsway Drive
Indianapolis, IN 46205
317-466-1000
FAX 317-466-2000
http://www.eastersealscrossroads.org
e-mail: info@easterseals.org
James J Vento, President/CEO
Janine S Sheppard MD, Medical Director
David S Brandt, Chairman
Easter Seals camping and recreation programs serve children, adults and families of all abilities. Various programs are available with the united purpose of giving disabled individuals a fun and safe camping or recreational experience. The following are camping and recreational services offered: Camperships and recreational services for children.

650 Englishton Park Academic Remediation &Training Center
Englishton Park Prebyterian Ministries Inc
PO Box 228
Lexington, IN 47138 812-889-2046
http://www.englishtonpark.org
e-mail: tbarnet@venus.net
Thomas Barnett, Co-Director
Lisa Barnett, Co-Director

To improve academic skills, change attitudes toward learning, modify behavior interferring with learning in the classroom. Founded 1968

651 Indy Parks Summer Camps: Brookside Park Gather on the Move Day Camp
c/o Indy Parks & Recreation Customer Service
Indianapolis, IN 46202 317-327-7275
FAX 317-327-7090
http://www.indygov.org/eGov/City/DPR/Programs
e-mail: indyparkscs@indygov.org
Joenne Pope, Manager Outreach Summer Programs
Paula Hartzer, Camp Coordinator

Indy Parks' traditional day camps are age-specific (kids entering kindergarten through 6th grade) offering a variety of activities that revolve around weekly themes, giving every week of summer camp its own distinct flavor. The Gather on the Move experience is for youth ages 13-21 with physical and/or intellectual disabilities. Campers enjoy a fun, structured day of swimming, fitness, crafts, field trips and multi-sensory activities.

652 Indy Parks Summer Camps: Carnivore Day Camp
c/o Indy Parks & Recreation Customer Service
Indianapolis, IN 46202 317-327-7275
FAX 317-327-7090
http://www.indygov.org/eGov/City/DPR/Programs
e-mail: indyparkscs@indygov.org
Joenne Pope, Manager Outreach Summer Programs
Paula Hartzer, Camp Coordinator

Indy Parks' traditional day camps are age-specific (kids entering kindergarten to 6th grade) offering a variety of activities that revolve around weekly themes, giving every week of summer camp its own distinct flavor. During Carnivore Camp week at Holliday Park, campers will study skulls, hike the trails, watch some of the nature center animals eat, and many more hands-on activities! Come prepared to get messy and have fun! There will be no camp on July 4th. July 2 - 6 9:00 a.m.- 4:00 p.m. $72.

653 Indy Parks Summer Camps: Critter Day Camp
c/o Indy Parks & Recreation Customer Service
Indianapolis, IN 46202 317-327-7275
FAX 317-327-7090
http://www.indygov.org/eGov/City/DPR/Programs
e-mail: indyparkscs@indygov.org
Joenne Pope, Manager Outreach Summer Programs
Paula Hartzer, Camp Coordinator

Indy Parks' traditional day camps are age-specific (kids entering kindergarten to 6th grade) offering a variety of activities that revolve around weekly themes, giving every week of summer camp its own distinct flavor. Come explore Holliday Park and discover the many different animals, insects, and spiders living there. Campers will get a chance to watch different critters in their natural habitat as well as feed and touch some of the nature center animals. June 18 - 22 9:00 a.m.-4:00 p.m. $90.

654 Indy Parks Summer Camps: Day Camp Holliday Habitats II
c/o Indy Parks & Recreation Customer Service
Indianapolis, IN 46202 317-327-7275
FAX 317-327-7090
http://www.indygov.org/eGov/City/DPR/Programs
e-mail: indyparkscs@indygov.org
Joenne Pope, Manager Outreach Summer Programs
Paula Hartzer, Camp Coordinator

Indy Parks' traditional day camps are age-specific (kids entering kindergarten through 6th grade) offering a variety of activities that revolve around weekly themes, giving every week of summer camp its own distinct flavor. Join us in exploring the habitats of Holliday Park! We will be discovering prairies, forest, and wetlands and the animals and plants that call those habitats home. So dress for the weather and come prepared to get messy! June 11 - 15 10:30 a.m.-12:30 p.m. $40.

655 Indy Parks Summer Camps: Eagle Creek ParkDay Camp
c/o Indy Parks & Recreation Customer Service
Indianapolis, IN 46202 317-327-7275
FAX 317-327-7090
http://www.indygov.org/eGov/City/DPR/Programs
e-mail: indyparkscs@indygov.org
Joenne Pope, Manager Outreach Summer Programs
Paula Hartzer, Camp Coordinator

Indy Parks' traditional day camps are age-specific (kids entering kindergarten through 6th grade) offering a variety of activities that revolve around weekly themes, giving every week of summer camp its own distinct flavor. Do you want your child to experience the great outdoors? Campers will spend time hiking, getting dirty and exploring the different habitats at the park. Wear comfortable shoes, bring a water bottle, bathing suit, sunscreen and rain gear for this summer outdoor adventure.

656 Indy Parks Summer Camps: Earth Explorers Day Camp
c/o Indy Parks & Recreation Customer Service
Indianapolis, IN 46202 317-327-7275
FAX 317-327-7090
http://www.indygov.org/eGov/City/DPR/Programs
e-mail: indyparkscs@indygov.org
Joenne Pope, Manager Outreach Summer Programs
Paula Hartzer, Camp Coordinator

Indy Parks' traditional day camps are age-specific (kids entering kindergarten to 6th grade) offering a variety of activities that revolve around weekly themes, giving every week of summer camp its own distinct flavor. Explore our forest, prairie and pond through nature camp by hiking, playing games and investigating different habitats each day. Have fun catching insects in our prairie, exploring a creek bed and hiking in the forest at night. June 18-22 and July 23-27, 9:00 a.m.-3:00 p.m. $90.

657 Indy Parks Summer Camps: Garden Buds Day Camp
c/o Indy Parks & Recreation Customer Service
Indianapolis, IN 46202 317-327-7275
FAX 317-327-7090
http://www.indygov.org/eGov/City/DPR/Programs
e-mail: indyparkscs@indygov.org
Joenne Pope, Manager Outreach Summer Programs
Paula Hartzer, Camp Coordinator

Indy Parks' traditional day camps are age-specific (kids entering kindergarten to 6th grade) offering a variety of activities that revolve around weekly themes, giving every week of summer camp its own distinct flavor. Children discover the wonder of gardening during camp planting vegetables and herbs in Holliday Park's children's garden, learning about gardening as they dig around observing plants, insects, soil, and all the things that help the garden grow. July 9-13 10:30 a.m.-12:30 p.m. $25.

658 Indy Parks Summer Camps: Garden Sprouts Day Camp
c/o Indy Parks & Recreation Customer Service
Indianapolis, IN 46202 317-327-7275
FAX 317-327-7090
http://www.indygov.org/eGov/City/DPR/Programs
e-mail: indyparkscs@indygov.org
Joenne Pope, Manager Outreach Summer Programs
Paula Hartzer, Camp Coordinator

Indy Parks' traditional day camps are age-specific (kids entering kindergarten to 6th grade) offering a variety of activities that revolve around weekly themes, giving every week of summer camp its own distinct flavor. Children discover the wonders of gardening planting vegetables and herbs in Holliday Park's children's garden! Campers learn about gardening as they dig around observing plants, insects, soil, and all things that help the children's garden grow! June 4-8 9:00 a.m.- 4:00 p.m. $90.

659 Indy Parks Summer Camps: Holliday Habitats I Day Camp
c/o Indy Parks & Recreation Customer Service
Indianapolis, IN 46202 317-327-7275
FAX 317-327-7090
http://www.indygov.org/eGov/City/DPR/Programs
e-mail: indyparkscs@indygov.org
Joenne Pope, Manager Outreach Summer Programs
Paula Hartzer, Camp Coordinator

Indy Parks' traditional day camps are age-specific (kids entering kindergarten through 6th grade) offering a variety of activities that revolve around weekly themes, giving every week of summer camp its own distinct flavor. Join us in exploring the habitats of Holliday Park! During this week, we will be discovering animals and plants in different habitats, so dress for the weather! An adult is required to stay only if the camper is not yet potty-trained. June 11 - 15 9:00-10:00 a.m. $25.

660 **Indy Parks Summer Camps: Krannert Park Day Camp**
c/o Indy Parks & Recreation Customer Service
Indianapolis, IN 46202 317-327-7275
FAX 317-327-7090
http://www.indygov.org/eGov/City/DPR/Programs
e-mail: indyparkscs@indygov.org
Joenne Pope, Manager Outreach Summer Programs
Paula Hartzer, Camp Coordinator

Indy Parks' traditional day camps are age-specific (kids entering kindergarten through 6th grade) offering a variety of activities that revolve around weekly themes, giving every week of summer camp its own distinct flavor. Great adventures is what summer vacation is all about at Krannert! Enjoy a knock your socks off themed summer line up featuring games, field trips, sports, environmental education, arts/crafts and swimming.

661 **Indy Parks Summer Camps: Little Acorns Day Camp**
c/o Indy Parks & Recreation Customer Service
Indianapolis, IN 46202 317-327-7275
FAX 317-327-7090
http://www.indygov.org/eGov/City/DPR/Programs
e-mail: indyparkscs@indygov.org
Joenne Pope, Manager Outreach Summer Programs
Paula Hartzer, Camp Coordinator

Indy Parks' traditional day camps are age-specific (kids entering kindergarten to 6th grade) offering a variety of activities that revolve around weekly themes, giving every week of summer camp its own distinct flavor. Bring your little nut for a bushel of fun! We will be playing games, reading stories, singing songs and exploring the great outdoors. Parents are welcome to stay for the fun! Children must be potty-trained. June 11-15 9:00 a.m.-4:00 p.m. and 2:00 p.m.-4:00 p.m. $40 each session.

662 **Indy Parks Summer Camps: Outdoor Adventures Retreat Day Camp**
c/o Indy Parks & Recreation Customer Service
Indianapolis, IN 46202 317-327-7275
FAX 317-327-7090
http://www.indygov.org/eGov/City/DPR/Programs
e-mail: indyparkscs@indygov.org
Joenne Pope, Manager Outreach Summer Programs
Paula Hartzer, Camp Coordinator

Indy Parks' traditional day camps are age-specific (kids entering kindergarten to 6th grade) offering a variety of activities that revolve around weekly themes, giving every week of summer camp its own distinct flavor. During Outdoor Adventures Retreat Day Camp the campers will go on several trips learning basic outdoor living skills. Campers will learn how to build a shelter, cook over a fire, work a Coleman stove, and paddle a canoe and more! July 9 - 13 9:00 a.m.- 4:00 p.m. $105.

663 **Indy Parks Summer Camps: Rhodius Park Gather Day Camp**
c/o Indy Parks & Recreation Customer Service
Indianapolis, IN 46202 317-327-7275
FAX 317-327-7090
http://www.indygov.org/eGov/City/DPR/Programs
e-mail: indyparkscs@indygov.org
Joenne Pope, Manager Outreach Summer Programs
Paula Hartzer, Camp Coordinator

Indy Parks' traditional day camps are age-specific (kids entering kindergarten through 6th grade) offering a variety of activities that revolve around weekly themes, giving every week of summer camp its own distinct flavor. The Camp Gather experience is for children ages 6-12 with physical and/or intellectual disabilities. Campers are engaged and stimulated daily with swimming, crafts, and multi-sensory activities. Weekly pet therapy, science exploration, and reading educational field trips.

664 **Indy Parks Summer Camps: Riverside Park Day Camp**
c/o Indy Parks & Recreation Customer Service
Indianapolis, IN 46202 317-327-7275
FAX 317-327-7090
http://www.indygov.org/eGov/City/DPR/Programs
e-mail: indyparkscs@indygov.org
Joenne Pope, Manager Outreach Summer Programs
Paula Hartzer, Camp Coordinator

Indy Parks' traditional day camps are age-specific (kids entering kindergarten through 6th grade) offering a variety of activities that revolve around weekly themes, giving every week of summer camp its own distinct flavor. Riverside Park offers your child a safe, fun filled and quality summer experience. The camp includes sports, arts/crafts, cultural enrichment programs, field trips, swimming, special events and a colorful T-shirt.

665 **Indy Parks Summer Camps: Rowdy Rascals Day Camp**

c/o Indy Parks & Recreation Customer Service
Indianapolis, IN 46202 317-327-7275
FAX 317-327-7090
http://www.indygov.org/eGov/City/DPR/Programs
e-mail: indyparkscs@indygov.org
Joenne Pope, Manager Outreach Summer Programs
Paula Hartzer, Camp Coordinator

Indy Parks' traditional day camps are age-specific (kids entering kindergarten to 6th grade) offering a variety of activities that revolve around weekly themes, giving every week of summer camp its own distinct flavor. Does your child like to explore the outdoors, get dirty, catch bugs and play with water? If so, this is the camp for them! We will be exploring our world hands-on! July 30 - August 3 9:00 a.m.-4:00 p.m. $90.

666 **Indy Parks Summer Camps: Slugs Hugs & Other Bugs II Day Camp**
c/o Indy Parks & Recreation Customer Service
Indianapolis, IN 46202 317-327-7275
FAX 317-327-7090
http://www.indygov.org/eGov/City/DPR/Programs
e-mail: indyparkscs@indygov.org
Joenne Pope, Manager Outreach Summer Programs
Paula Hartzer, Camp Coordinator

Indy Parks' traditional day camps are age-specific (kids entering kindergarten through 6th grade) offering a variety of activities that revolve around weekly themes, giving every week of summer camp its own distinct flavor. Come and explore some creepy crawlies and beautiful bugs. We will learn about beetles, dragonflies, and other wonderful winged creatures and their favorite habitats. This is nature up close! June 25 - 29 10:30 a.m.-12:30 p.m. $40.

667 **Indy Parks Summer Camps: Slugs Hugs and Other Bugs I Day Camp**
c/o Indy Parks & Recreation Customer Service
Indianapolis, IN 46202 317-327-7275
FAX 317-327-7090
http://www.indygov.org/eGov/City/DPR/Programs
e-mail: indyparkscs@indygov.org
Joenne Pope, Manager Outreach Summer Programs
Paula Hartzer, Camp Coordinator

Indy Parks' traditional day camps are age-specific (kids entering kindergarten through 6th grade) offering a variety of activities that revolve around weekly themes, giving every week of summer camp its own distinct flavor. Come explore some creepy crawlies and beautiful bugs. We will examine everything from butterflies to worms, and take a closer look at the habitats some of our invertebrates call home. An adult is required to stay if the camper is not potty-trained. June 25-29 9:00-10:00 $25.

668 **Indy Parks Summer Camps: Survivor I Day Camp**
c/o Indy Parks & Recreation Customer Service
Indianapolis, IN 46202 317-327-7275
FAX 317-327-7090
http://www.indygov.org/eGov/City/DPR/Programs
e-mail: indyparkscs@indygov.org
Joenne Pope, Manager Outreach Summer Programs
Paula Hartzer, Camp Coordinator

Indy Parks' traditional day camps are age-specific (kids entering kindergarten to 6th grade) offering a variety of activities that revolve around weekly themes, giving every week of summer camp its own distinct flavor. Campers learn survival techniques such as pitching a tent, building a campfire, and foraging for food. Bring your camper at 7 p.m. on Friday night for a sleep-over at Holliday Park. Pick up at 8 a.m. Saturday. July 16 - 20 9:00 - 4:00 p.m. $90.

669 Indy Parks Summer Camps: Trail Kickers Day Camp

c/o Indy Parks & Recreation Customer Service
Indianapolis, IN 46202
317-327-7275
FAX 317-327-7090
http://www.indygov.org/eGov/City/DPR/Programs
e-mail: indyparkscs@indygov.org
Joenne Pope, Manager Outreach Summer Programs
Paula Hartzer, Camp Coordinator

Indy Parks' traditional day camps are age-specific (kids entering kindergarten through 6th grade) offering a variety of activities that revolve around weekly themes, giving every week of summer camp its own distinct flavor. Experience a fun week that highlights the natural world around us. We have packed each day with fun things kids love to do - games, stories, hands-on activities, and of course, some trail fun! An adult is required to stay. July 30 - August 3 2:00-2:45 p.m. $25.

670 Indy Parks Summer Camps: Trail Stompers Day Camp

c/o Indy Parks & Recreation Customer Service
Indianapolis, IN 46202
317-327-7275
FAX 317-327-7090
http://www.indygov.org/eGov/City/DPR/Programs
e-mail: indyparkscs@indygov.org
Joenne Pope, Manager Outreach Summer Programs
Paula Hartzer, Camp Coordinator

Indy Parks' traditional day camps are age-specific (kids entering kindergarten through 6th grade) offering a variety of activities that revolve around weekly themes, giving every week of summer camp its own distinct flavor. Bring your little trail goers for a roaring good time! We will be expanding our knowledge of native species, doing crafts, singing songs, and of course, hiking the trails! An adult is required to stay only if camper is not yet potty-trained. July 9 - 13 9:00-10:00 a.m. $25.

671 Indy Parks Summer Camps: Wilderness Wonders Day Camp

c/o Indy Parks & Recreation Customer Service
Indianapolis, IN 46202
317-327-7275
FAX 317-327-7090
http://www.indygov.org/eGov/City/DPR/Programs
e-mail: indyparkscs@indygov.org
Joenne Pope, Manager Outreach Summer Programs
Paula Hartzer, Camp Coordinator

Indy Parks' traditional day camps are age-specific (kids entering kindergarten to 6th grade) offering a variety of activities that revolve around weekly themes, giving every week of summer camp its own distinct flavor. This camp is designed to stimulate the natural interest young children have in the world around them. Spend a funfilled week wandering the trails of Holliday Park and meeting some of the animals that live here! July 9 - 13 1:00-4:00 p.m. $50.

672 Indy Parks Summer Camps: Wonders in the Water Day Camp

c/o Indy Parks & Recreation Customer Service
Indianapolis, IN 46202
317-327-7275
FAX 317-327-7090
http://www.indygov.org/eGov/City/DPR/Programs
e-mail: indyparkscs@indygov.org
Joenne Pope, Manager Outreach Summer Programs
Paula Hartzer, Camp Coordinator

Indy Parks' traditional day camps are age-specific (kids entering kindergarten to 6th grade) offering a variety of activities that revolve around weekly themes, giving every week of summer camp its own distinct flavor. Let's go to the wetlands! Wet places are wonderful areas to discover amazing animals and plants. Make sure to send a change of clothes with your camper each day and prepare for them to be messy! July 30 - August 3 9:00 a.m.-1:00 p.m. $60.

673 Isanogel Center Summer Camp

7601 W Isanogel Road
Muncie, IN 47304
765-288-1073
FAX 765-288-3103
http://www.isanogelcenter.org/day_camp.htm
e-mail: isanogel@comcast.net
Karen Kovac, Camp Director

The Isanogel Center is a one or two week summer residential camp program for children and adults with disabilities for ages 8-Adult. The primary objective of Camp Isanogel is to promote the emotional and physical well being of each camper. All programs are designed to enhance spiritual, social, intellectual and physical growth. In turn, campers develop a positive self-esteem, improve independent skills, make new friends and have a great time.

674 Kid City Original Summer Camp

City of Bloomington Parks & Recreation
401 N Morton Street
Bloomington, IN 47404
812-349-3700
FAX 812-349-3705
http://http://bloomington.in.gov/parks/
e-mail: parks@bloomington.in.gov
Pamela Dunscombe, Youth Services Specialist
Dave Fox, Operations Superintendent
Daren Eads, Facility/Program Coordinator

During Kid City Original, campers will explore the world around them with field trips and special events. Daily programs give campers the chance to try specialized activities in the areas of nature and the outdoors, sports and games, and arts and media. The unique weekly themes provide something fun for everyone giving every child a summer to remember.

675 Kid City Quest Summer Camp

City of Bloomington Parks & Recreation
401 N Morton Street
Bloomington, IN 47404
812-349-3700
FAX 812-349-3705
http://http://bloomington.in.gov/parks/
e-mail: parks@bloomington.in.gov
Pamela Dunscombe, Youth Services Specialist
Dave Fox, Operations Superintendent
Daren Eads, Facility/Program Coordinator

Kid City Quest campers design their own program experience through Choice Exploration periods (activity options that differ from the usual camp fare). In addition, campers experience field trips, splash the summer away swimming and learn more about themselves and their friends while team building.

676 Myron S Goldman Union Camp Institute (GUCI)

9349 Moore Road
Zionsville, IN 46077
317-873-3361
FAX 317-873-3742
http://www.guci.bunk1.com
e-mail: Gucioffice@aol.com
Ron Klotz, Rabbi, Camp Director

Singing songs around a campfire, spending time with cabin-mates and counselors, playing on the athletic field, swimming and learning about our heritage are just a few of the activities that help our campers have an experience that they will never forget. GUCI is a place where children experience what it's like to live, learn and grow with other Jewish children which is enhanced by being a part of a community that includes rabbis, rabbinic students and young people working at the camp.

677 Teen Extreme Summer Camp

City of Bloomington Parks & Recreation
401 N Morton Street
Bloomington, IN 47404
812-349-3700
FAX 812-349-3705
http://http://bloomington.in.gov/parks/
e-mail: parks@bloomington.in.gov
Pamela Dunscombe, Youth Services Specialist
Dave Fox, Operations Superintendent
Daren Eads, Facility/Program Coordinator

During Teen Extreme, campers with an adventurous spirit will pick the weeks that match their interests, trying something brand new. Each session participants will have the opportunity to use the Low Ropes Challenge Course or participate in team-building activities.

678 Teen X-Treme Travel Summer Camp
City of Bloomington Parks & Recreation
401 N Morton Street
Bloomington, IN 47404
812-349-3700
FAX 812-349-3705
http://http://bloomington.in.gov/parks/
e-mail: parks@bloomington.in.gov
Pamela Dunscombe, Youth Services Specialist
Dave Fox, Operations Superintendent
Daren Eads, Facility/Program Coordinator
During Teen X-Treme Travel, campers will spend five days exploring the state parks, adventure sites and natural areas of Indiana and surrounding states. These overnight camping excursions each have a different focus and destination, but they all provide an incredible experience. Teen X-treme Travel campers return with new freinds, new skills and a backpack of memories!

Iowa

679 Camp Albrecht Acres
PO Box 50
Sherill, IA 52073
563-552-1771
FAX 563-552-2732
http://www.albrechtacres.org
e-mail: dking@albrechtacres.org
Daniel King, Camp Director
Karen Fox, Office Manager

Camp Albrecht Acres provides a camping experience to individuals with special needs and is located on 40 acres of wooded land, providing a camper to counselor ratio of 3 to 1, and when needed, 1 to 1. Activities include crafts, fishing, swimming, cookouts, dances, awards ceremony, camping in an authentic teepee, exploring the woods on almost two miles of paved trails, hay wagon rides, volleyball, ping pong and pool tables.

680 Camp Courageous of Iowa
12007 190th Street
Monticello, IA 52310-0418
319-465-5916
FAX 319-465-5919
http://www.campcourageous.org
e-mail: info@campcourageous.org
Jeanne Muellerleile, Camp Director
Sharon Poe, Respite Care Volunteer Director
Becky Melchert, Camp Visitors Center Coordinator
Camp Courageous of Iowa is a year-round recreational and respite care facility for individuals of all ages with disabilities. The camp provides opportunities for social and personal growth within a supportive environment. Campers learn to try a variety of creative and challenging activities and experience success. Campers develop enhanced self-esteem which carries over to work, home, or school environments.

681 Easter Seals Camp Sunnyside
401 NE 66th Avenue
Des Moines, IA 50313
515-289-1933
FAX 515-274-6434
http://http://ia.easterseals.com
e-mail: info@eastersealsia.org
Donna Elbrecht, President
Claire Lecroy, Director
Sherrie Nielsen, Administrator
Easter Seals camping and recreation programs serve children, adults and families of all abilities. Various programs are available with the united purpose of giving disabled individuals a fun and safe camping or recreational experience. The following are Camping and Recreational services offered: Adventure, camp respite for children, day camping for children, easter seals own and operated camps and residential camping programs.

Kentucky

682 Bethel Mennonite Camp
2773 Bethel Church Road
Clayhole, KY 41317
606-666-4911
FAX 606-666-4216
http://www.bethelcamp.org
e-mail: grow@bethelcamp.org
Roger Voth, Camp Director
Mark Driskill, Summer Camp Pastor
Mary Driskill, Summer Camp Pastor
A camp with an emphasis on bible study. Founded 1957

683 Easter Seals Camp KYSOC
Alpenglow Adventures
1902 Easter Day Road
Carrollton, KY 41008
502-732-5333
866-357-4712
FAX 502-732-0783
http://www.alpenglowadventures.org/about.htm
e-mail: info@AlpenglowAdventures.org
Jim Edert, Alpenglow Director
Bob Crosno, Easter Seals Chairman

Easter Seals camping and recreation programs serve children, adults and families of all abilities. Various programs are available with the united purpose of giving disabled individuals a fun and safe camping or recreational experience. The following are camping and recreational services offered: Camp respite for adults, camp respite for children, camperships, canoeing, day camping for children and family retreats.

Louisiana

684 Camp Ruth Lee
4874 Constitution Avenue
Baton Rouge, LA 70808
225-924-2267
FAX 225-924-1774
http://campfirebr.org/explore.cfm/campruthlee/
e-mail: campruthlee@campfirebr.org
Paula Braud, Youth Program Director
Jim Phillips, Camp Ranger
Susan Brown, Executive Director
Campers experience a variety of activities designed to help them explore new interests and develop new skills. Cabinmates not only live together, but they learn to make decisions together and to divide responsibilities. Campers also learn to work as part of the larger community by planning and participating in programs and all camp events. Camp activities can include swimming, canoeing, fishing, hiking, arts and crafts, in addition to various sports and games such as baseball and football.

685 Easter Seals Louisiana
New Orleans Corporate Office
1010 Common Street
New Orleans, LA 70112
504-523-7325
800-695-7325
FAX 504-523-3465
http://http://louisiana.easterseals.com
e-mail: info@easterseals.org
Mark Stafford, Corporate Program Director
Daniel Underwood, Chief Executive Officer

Easter Seals camping and recreation programs serve children, adults and families of all abilities. Various programs are available with the united purpose of giving disabled individuals a fun and safe camping or recreational experience. The following are camping and recreational services offered: Camperships.

686 Med-Camps of Louisiana
102 Thomas Road
West Monroe, LA 71291
318-329-8405
FAX 318-329-8407
http://www.medcamps.com
e-mail: caledseney@medcamps.com
Caled Seney, Executive Director
Gabriel Davison, Vice President

Regardless of special needs this camp offers participants a sense of well being, belonging, accomplishment and self worth.

Maine

687 Camp Waban
Waban's Projects
5 Dunaway Drive
Sanford, ME 04073
207-324-7955
FAX 207-324-6050
http://www.waban.org/admin.html
e-mail: waban@waban.org
Neal Meltzer, Executive Director
Gervaise Flynn, Director Residential Services
Cynthia Caron-Wilcox, Director Day Services
This program provides campers from a wide geograhic area a chance to enjoy the outdoors in a theraputic recreational setting.

Maryland

688 ABC Care Summer Camp
100 E Main Street
Westminster, MD 21157
410-751-3700
FAX 410-751-3702
http://www.abccareinc.com
e-mail: abccare@abccareinc.com
Susan Holmes, Co-Director
Shannon Howell, Co-Director

ABC Care, a nonprofit corporation, intends for our school-age childcare centers to provide a safe, secure, fun recreational and educational experience and in providing an exceptional childcare program for children of varying ages, kindergarten through the eighth grade.

689 Access Adventures
Melwood's Recreation & Travel Service
9035 Ironsides Road
Nanjemoy, MD 20662
301-870-3215
FAX 301-870-2620
http://www.melwood.org/CAMP/INDEX.HTM
e-mail: accessadventures@melwood.org
Janice Frey Angel, President/CEO
Donald Pollock, VP/External Relations
Ron Stubblefield, Chief Financial Officer
Access Adventures' mission is to provide year round, community based, affordable vacations to persons with disabilities. Travelers are supported by dedicated staff who provide a safe and caring atmosphere. Travelers have opportunities to explore exciting new experiences, make friends and try a variety of age appropriate activities.

690 Camp Fairlee Manor
Easter Seals Fairlee Manor Recreation/Education
22242 Bay Shore Road
Chestertown, MD 21620
410-778-0566
FAX 410-778-0567
http://www.de.easterseals.com
e-mail: fairlee@dmv.com
Sandra Tuttle, President
Bill Morgan, Director Camping/Recreation

Sessions offer a wide range of activities including arts and crafts, sports and games, nature walks, swimming, fishing, high/low ropes courses and canoeing. Sessions are divided according to age and ability.
1954

691 Camp JCC
JCC of Greater Washington
Rockville, MD 20852
301-230-3759
FAX 301-881-6549
http://http://www.jccgw.org/camp_jcc/
e-mail: jcccamp@jccgw.org
Sara Portmann Milner, Camp Director
Oshrat Schaffer, Assistant Camp Director
Eva Cowen, Special Needs Director
JCC's comprehensive camp includes traditional day camp programs for children age 4-13, as well as specialty programs in art, theater, sports, teen trips, and a self-contained program for teens and young adults with special needs. Activities in the general camp units include sports, arts and crafts, nature/science, movement, computers, music, recreational and instructional swim, and guest performers. Campers also enjoy age-appropriate overnights, late stays, day trips, and weekly special events.

692 Camp Odyssey Specialty Camp: ArtologySecret House Expeditions Camp
6279 Hobbs Road
Salisbury, MD 21804
410-742-4464
FAX 410-546-2310
http://www.campodyssey.org/spec_camp.cfm
e-mail: harlan@campodyssey.org
Harlan Eagle, Executive Director
Chris Atkins, Day Camp Director
Jamey Landon, Assistant Day Camp Director
Secret House Expeditions allows campers the chance to explore their interests in-depth, in a relaxed, fun, safe and supportive atmosphere. Secret House is a world of imagination and adventure within 260 acres on the Tangier Sound. Learn techniques for creating masterpieces inspired by the big sky beauty of the Chesapeake Bay. The adventure includes such activities as making and decorating pottery, painting and drawing, and other creative activities. Ages: 7 to 10.

693 Camp Odyssey Specialty Camp: Chesapeake Discovery Camp
6279 Hobbs Road
Salisbury, MD 21804
410-742-4464
FAX 410-546-2310
http://www.campodyssey.org/spec_camp.cfm
e-mail: harlan@campodyssey.org
Harlan Eagle, Executive Director
Chris Atkins, Day Camp Director
Jamey Landon, Assistant Day Camp Director
Spend a day on the Chesapeake Bay crabbing with Captain Fred Pomeroy, who has more than 30 years of experience on the water. Campers should bring sunscreen, lunch, plenty to drink and a thirst for adventure. Participants have the opportunity to interact with qualified professionals in small groups that ensure ample individual attention and quality instruction. Two days: July 10 and August 7 (Week 5: Tuesday; Week 9: Tuesday). Ages: 10 to 13 (Maximum: 6 campers/day).

694 Camp Odyssey Specialty Camp: Cool Kids Creations Camp
6279 Hobbs Road
Salisbury, MD 21804
410-742-4464
FAX 410-546-2310
http://www.campodyssey.org/spec_camp.cfm
e-mail: harlan@campodyssey.org
Harlan Eagle, Executive Director
Chris Atkins, Day Camp Director
Jamey Landon, Assistant Day Camp Director
Play indoors and out, exploring nature and discovering your artistic talents. Music, art, nature and cooking are all part of the adventure. Different themes each week. Pat McKenzie, certified teacher (Westside Primary Kindergarten), parent and veteran camp counselor, orchestrates the fun. Meet at The Salisbury School Upper School Room 1. Ages: 4 to 8 (Maximum: 12 campers per week). Four weeks.

695 Camp Odyssey Specialty Camp: Delmarva Cross Country Camp
6279 Hobbs Road
Salisbury, MD 21804
410-742-4464
FAX 410-546-2310
http://www.campodyssey.org/spec_camp.cfm
e-mail: harlan@campodyssey.org
Harlan Eagle, Executive Director
Chris Atkins, Day Camp Director
Jamey Landon, Assistant Day Camp Director
Runners will learn how to prepare for the upcoming season, racing strategies, conditioning, strength and flexibility training. Each day consists of a training session and classroom session. The week concludes on Saturday with participation in a 5K (3.1 mile) race at Winter Place Park in Salisbury. This camp is designed for the novice as well as the advanced runner striving to reach higher levels. One week: Aug. 6 to 10 (Week 9: Monday thru Friday evenings, 6:30 to 8:30 p.m.). Ages: 11 to Adult.

696 **Camp Odyssey Specialty Camp: Earth Treks Explorations Camp**
6279 Hobbs Road
Salisbury, MD 21804
410-742-4464
FAX 410-546-2310
http://www.campodyssey.org/spec_camp.cfm
e-mail: harlan@campodyssey.org
Harlan Eagle, Executive Director
Chris Atkins, Day Camp Director
Jamey Landon, Assistant Day Camp Director
Campers will tackle rock-climbing at Earth Treks in Columbia, Maryland. The week also includes ropes course, geo-caching (an adventure treasure hunt with a GPS device), beach and water park trips. Participants have the opportunity to interact with qualified professionals in small groups that ensure ample individual attention and quality instruction. One week: July 16 to July 20 (Week 6: Monday thru Friday) Ages: 10 to 14.

697 **Camp Odyssey Specialty Camp: Eastern Shore Lacrosse Camp**
6279 Hobbs Road
Salisbury, MD 21804
410-742-4464
FAX 410-546-2310
http://www.campodyssey.org/spec_camp.cfm
e-mail: harlan@campodyssey.org
Harlan Eagle, Executive Director
Chris Atkins, Day Camp Director
Jamey Landon, Assistant Day Camp Director
The Eastern Shore Lax Camp offers each camper a fun, exciting and instructional experience. Dynamic coaching staff will provide both fundamental and advanced skills to help players in all stages of development. Morning sessions will focus on individual skill development - footwork, dodging, cutting, feeding, defensive positioning and more - while afternoon sessions will be devoted to team practice with a focus on the transition game, team play and specialty situations.

698 **Camp Odyssey Specialty Camp: Eco-Aqua Adventures Camp**
6279 Hobbs Road
Salisbury, MD 21804
410-742-4464
FAX 410-546-2310
http://www.campodyssey.org/spec_camp.cfm
e-mail: harlan@campodyssey.org
Harlan Eagle, Executive Director
Chris Atkins, Day Camp Director
Jamey Landon, Assistant Day Camp Director
Specialty camps allow kids, teens and adults a chance to explore their interests in-depth, in a relaxed, fun, safe and supportive atmosphere. Participants have the opportunity to interact with qualified professionals in small groups that ensure ample individual attention and quality instruction. Campers will go fishing, spend two days at a water park, relax for a day at the beach and go canoeing. One week: August 13 to 17 (Week 10: Monday thru Friday) Ages: 10 to 14.

699 **Camp Odyssey Specialty Camp: Enviro Enforcers Camp**
6279 Hobbs Road
Salisbury, MD 21804
410-742-4464
FAX 410-546-2310
http://www.campodyssey.org/spec_camp.cfm
e-mail: harlan@campodyssey.org
Harlan Eagle, Executive Director
Chris Atkins, Day Camp Director
Jamey Landon, Assistant Day Camp Director
Taking care and pride in our natural resources is increasingly important in today's world. Science teacher Alvin Kruger takes this to the next level with our new Environmental Enforcers program. Campers will work in an outdoor setting to explore and cultivate our own wilderness lab. One Week: July 9 to 13 (Week 5: Monday thru Friday mornings, 8:30 a.m. to noon). Ages 10 to 13.

700 **Camp Odyssey Specialty Camp: Greenbriar State Park Adventure Camp**
6279 Hobbs Road
Salisbury, MD 21804
410-742-4464
FAX 410-546-2310
http://www.campodyssey.org/spec_camp.cfm
e-mail: harlan@campodyssey.org
Harlan Eagle, Executive Director
Chris Atkins, Day Camp Director
Jamey Landon, Assistant Day Camp Director
Travel with veteran leader and teacher Barb Farrell to Greenbriar State Park, located three hours away in Boonsboro, Maryland. Barb and her highly qualified staff will lead campers through a week of awesome hiking, swimming, biking, white-water rafting and day trips to Harper's Ferry and Cunningham Falls. Food, tents and camping gear will be provided. One week: July 30 to August 3 (Week 8: Monday thru Friday) Ages: 11 to 14.

701 **Camp Odyssey Specialty Camp: Guitar StarsWorkshop Camp**
6279 Hobbs Road
Salisbury, MD 21804
410-742-4464
FAX 410-546-2310
http://www.campodyssey.org/spec_camp.cfm
e-mail: harlan@campodyssey.org
Harlan Eagle, Executive Director
Chris Atkins, Day Camp Director
Jamey Landon, Assistant Day Camp Director
Weekly Guitar Stars Workshops led by Jimmy Rowbottom. Sessions held in the Lower School Music Room. Specialty camps allow kids, teens and adults a chance to explore their interests in-depth, in a relaxed, fun, safe and supportive atmosphere. Participants have the opportunity to interact with qualified professionals in small groups that ensure ample individual attention and quality instruction. Ten weeks: June 11 to August 17. (Weeks 1 thru 10, Tuesdays 12 to 1 p.m). Ages: All.

702 **Camp Odyssey Specialty Camp: Jessie BrownGirls Basketball Camp**
6279 Hobbs Road
Salisbury, MD 21804
410-742-4464
FAX 410-546-2310
http://www.campodyssey.org/spec_camp.cfm
e-mail: harlan@campodyssey.org
Harlan Eagle, Executive Director
Chris Atkins, Day Camp Director
Jamey Landon, Assistant Day Camp Director
Girls will develop their basic skills and learn to love the game. Jessie Brown is a former Bayside Conference Player of the Year at Bennett High School, an All- Conference Team Captain and star player for UMBC. Meets at The Salisbury School Lower School Gym. One week. August 13 to 17. (Week 10. Monday thru Friday Mornings, 9:30 to 11:30 a.m.) Ages: 6 to 9. Maximum 15 participants.

703 **Camp Odyssey Specialty Camp: Jimmy BrownCoed Basketball Camp**
6279 Hobbs Road
Salisbury, MD 21804
410-742-4464
FAX 410-546-2310
http://www.campodyssey.org/spec_camp.cfm
e-mail: harlan@campodyssey.org
Harlan Eagle, Executive Director
Chris Atkins, Day Camp Director
Jamey Landon, Assistant Day Camp Director
Join Jimmy Brown for a week of skill improvement and development. Meets at The Salisbury School Upper School Gym. Participants have the opportunity to interact with qualified professionals in small groups that ensure ample individual attention and quality instruction. One week: July 30 to August 3 (Week 8: Monday thru Friday Mornings, 8:30 a.m. to Noon). Ages: 10+.

704 **Camp Odyssey Specialty Camp: Little Players Camp**
6279 Hobbs Road
Salisbury, MD 21804
410-742-4464
FAX 410-546-2310
http://www.campodyssey.org/spec_camp.cfm
e-mail: harlan@campodyssey.org
Harlan Eagle, Executive Director
Chris Atkins, Day Camp Director
Jamey Landon, Assistant Day Camp Director
Learn about performing and participate in a fun theatrical production under the fantastic direction of veteran theater director Susan Rogers. Young actors will start out on Monday and take the stage on Friday at The Salisbury School Lower School Theater. One week: August 13 to 17 (Week 10: Monday thru Friday mornings: 10 a.m. to 11:30 a.m.) Ages: 5 to 8.

705 **Camp Odyssey Specialty Camp: Math Magic Camp**
6279 Hobbs Road
Salisbury, MD 21804 410-742-4464
FAX 410-546-2310
http://www.campodyssey.org/spec_camp.cfm
e-mail: harlan@campodyssey.org
Harlan Eagle, Executive Director
Chris Atkins, Day Camp Director
Jamey Landon, Assistant Day Camp Director
Young math magicians challenge themselves by applying math skills like probability and geometry in hands-on activities like making potions and working with Bertie Bott's Every Flavour Beans. Discover the fun of chess, too. Teacher Flo Terrill leads the way at The Salisbury School Lower School. One week: July 30 to August 3 (Week 8: Monday thru Friday mornings, 8:30 a.m. to noon). Ages: Entering 2nd or 3rd grade.

706 **Camp Odyssey Specialty Camp: Microscopic Discovery and Science Fun Camp**
6279 Hobbs Road
Salisbury, MD 21804 410-742-4464
FAX 410-546-2310
http://www.campodyssey.org/spec_camp.cfm
e-mail: harlan@campodyssey.org
Harlan Eagle, Executive Director
Chris Atkins, Day Camp Director
Jamey Landon, Assistant Day Camp Director
Younger scientists learn dissection techniques viewing nature under microscopes, studying insects and many more natural wonders. Program includes science crafts and experimental designs for the creative minds of younger children. Instructor Michelle Thomas, a middle school teacher at Sussex Academy of Arts & Sciences, will introduce and familiarize students with basic science methods in a fun atmosphere that nurtures a budding interest in science. Ages: 8 to 10 (Maximum 10 campers). Two weeks.

707 **Camp Odyssey Specialty Camp: Morning Swimming Lessons Camp**
6279 Hobbs Road
Salisbury, MD 21804 410-742-4464
FAX 410-546-2310
http://www.campodyssey.org/spec_camp.cfm
e-mail: harlan@campodyssey.org
Harlan Eagle, Executive Director
Chris Atkins, Day Camp Director
Jamey Landon, Assistant Day Camp Director
Specialized swimming instruction tailored to each child's abilities. Swimming instruction provided by Cora Miles, an experienced and dynamic teacher and her crew of talented assistants. Campers are transported to the Elks Club pool from camp for a half hour morning lesson, then are returned to their groups. Six weeks: June 19 thru July 27 (Weeks 2 thru 7: Tuesday thru Friday mornings). Ages: 5 to 13.

708 **Camp Odyssey Specialty Camp: Musical Theater Camp**
6279 Hobbs Road
Salisbury, MD 21804 410-742-4464
FAX 410-546-2310
http://www.campodyssey.org/spec_camp.cfm
e-mail: harlan@campodyssey.org
Harlan Eagle, Executive Director
Chris Atkins, Day Camp Director
Jamey Landon, Assistant Day Camp Director
Aspiring actors, dancers and singers will take the stage under the direction of veteran theater director Susan Rogers to create a musical theatrical production. They begin warm-ups and rehearsals on Monday and present their performance on Friday, all in The Salisbury School Lower School Theater. One week: August 6 to 10 (Week 9: Monday thru Friday mornings: 8:30 a.m. to noon). Ages: 9 to 12.

709 **Camp Odyssey Specialty Camp: Nature Explorers Camp**
6279 Hobbs Road
Salisbury, MD 21804 410-742-4464
FAX 410-546-2310
http://www.campodyssey.org/spec_camp.cfm
e-mail: harlan@campodyssey.org
Harlan Eagle, Executive Director
Chris Atkins, Day Camp Director
Jamey Landon, Assistant Day Camp Director
Join resident science expert and Salisbury School teacher Alvin Kruger for a week of discoveries in the great outdoors. Campers will learn about our natural surroundings as well as work together to preserve its beauty. One Week: July 16 to 20 (Week 6: Monday thru Friday mornings, 8:30 a.m. to noon). Ages: 7 to 9.

710 **Camp Odyssey Specialty Camp: Piano Lessons Camp**
6279 Hobbs Road
Salisbury, MD 21804 410-742-4464
FAX 410-546-2310
http://www.campodyssey.org/spec_camp.cfm
e-mail: harlan@campodyssey.org
Harlan Eagle, Executive Director
Chris Atkins, Day Camp Director
Jamey Landon, Assistant Day Camp Director
Lessons will cover note-reading and keyboard geography with campers choosing repertoire of their preference: Classical, Jazz, Oldies Rock & Roll, Folk, Patriotic, Children's Songs, Disney, Movie/TV Themes and more! Individual 30-minute lessons led by Susan Boone, a piano guild member who is certified by the American College of Musicians. Ages four and up are welcome, beginners to advanced. 9 weeks: June 11 to July 6, July 16 to August 18 (Weeks 1 to 4 and 6 to 10, Mondays thru Wednesdays).

711 **Camp Odyssey Specialty Camp: Sail the Local Waterways Camp**
6279 Hobbs Road
Salisbury, MD 21804 410-742-4464
FAX 410-546-2310
http://www.campodyssey.org/spec_camp.cfm
e-mail: harlan@campodyssey.org
Harlan Eagle, Executive Director
Chris Atkins, Day Camp Director
Jamey Landon, Assistant Day Camp Director
Sailors will meet at Camp Odyssey and depart by van for Somers Cove Marina (located in Crisfield, MD). Instructors are certified by US Sailing and will teach beginning campers in a safe and comfortable environment, using Optimist class single-handed boats. Two Weeks: July 9 to 12 and July 16 to 19 (Weeks 5 and 6: Monday thru Thursday) Depart from camp at 7 a.m. and return by 1 p.m. Ages: 8 to 13 (Maximum: 5 campers; Must be able to swim).

712 **Camp Odyssey Specialty Camp: Surf Camp**
6279 Hobbs Road
Salisbury, MD 21804 410-742-4464
FAX 410-546-2310
http://www.campodyssey.org/spec_camp.cfm
e-mail: harlan@campodyssey.org
Harlan Eagle, Executive Director
Chris Atkins, Day Camp Director
Jamey Landon, Assistant Day Camp Director
Experienced surf instructor Oliver Johnson will help a group of strong swimmers discover their inner surfer, while learning to respect and safely enjoy the ocean. Surfers will meet before sunrise at Camp Odyssey and depart by van for an Ocean City beach. A lifeguard will be with this group. For beginner to advanced surfers. One week: July 23 to 27 (Week 7: Monday thru Friday mornings) depart from camp by 6:30 a.m. and return by noon. Ages: 12 and up (Maximum 10 campers; Must be able to swim).

713 **Camp Odyssey Specialty Camp: SurvivorSecret House Expeditions Camp**
6279 Hobbs Road
Salisbury, MD 21804 410-742-4464
FAX 410-546-2310
http://www.campodyssey.org/spec_camp.cfm
e-mail: harlan@campodyssey.org
Harlan Eagle, Executive Director
Chris Atkins, Day Camp Director
Jamey Landon, Assistant Day Camp Director
Secret House Expeditions allows campers the chance to explore their interests in-depth, in a relaxed, fun, safe and supportive atmosphere. Secret House is a world of imagination and adventure within 260 acres on the Tangier Sound. During the Survivor Expedition, campers explore fun challenges and compete in creative games. Two weeks: June 25 to 29 (Week 3: Monday thru Friday). Ages: 7 to 10.

714 **Camp Odyssey Specialty Camp: Survivor IISecret House Expeditions Camp**

6279 Hobbs Road
Salisbury, MD 21804 410-742-4464
FAX 410-546-2310
http://www.campodyssey.org/spec_camp.cfm
e-mail: harlan@campodyssey.org

Harlan Eagle, Executive Director
Chris Atkins, Day Camp Director
Jamey Landon, Assistant Day Camp Director

Secret House Expeditions allows campers the chance to explore their interests in-depth, in a relaxed, fun, safe and supportive atmosphere. Secret House is a world of imagination and adventure within 260 acres on the Tangier Sound. During the Survivor Expedition, campers explore fun challenges and compete in creative games. Survivor II includes an overnight on Thursday. Two weeks: July 23 to 27 (Weeks 7: Monday thru Friday). Ages: 9 to 12.

715 **Jemicy Community Outreach**

Jemicy Community Outreach
11 Celadon Road
Owings Mills, MD 21117 410-653-2700
FAX 410-653-1972
http://www.jemicyschool.org
e-mail: bshifrin@jemicyschool.org

Ben Shifrin, Headmaster
Jane Evans, Director of Development
LuJean Hall, Director of Finance

Two special camps for dyslexic children that blends fun camp activities which includes swimming and nature experiences.

716 **Kamp A-Kom-plish**

9035 Ironsides Road
Nanjemoy, MD 20662 301-870-3226
FAX 301-934-3590
http://www.kampakomplish.org
e-mail: kampakomplish@melwood.com

Heidi Aldous Fick, Director

A sleep-away camp for for children and teens aged 8 to 16 years old. Located on 108 acres there are air-conditioned cabins, fish ing, boating and trails for hiking. We welcome children with a variety of disabilities, such as developmental, physical and emotional however we are not able to support children with extreme behavioral issues or intense medical needs.

1968

717 **League for People with Disabilities Summer Camp**

1111 E Cold Spring Lane
Baltimore, MD 21239 410-323-0500
FAX 410-323-3298
http://www.leagueforpeople.org
e-mail: leaguelink@leagueforpeople.org

David Greenburg, Chief Executive Officer
Emily H Mann, Director Marketing & Development
Stephen Freeman, Employment & Wellness Center

Campers sleep in tents, cook over a fire and explore the outdoors. Travel Camp allows campers to travel to local points of interest during the summer. Travel campers will spend their nights in hotels and their days sight seeing and discovering the area.

718 **Mar-Lu-Ridge Summer Camps: Adult Camp**

Conference and Educational Center
Jefferson, MD 21755 301-874-5544
800-238-9974
FAX 301-874-5545
http://www.mar-lu-ridge.org
e-mail: mlr@mar-lu-ridge.org

Rod Pearce, Executive Administrator
Thomas Semeta, Associate Director
Tom Waskiewicz, Food Service Manager

Enjoy a week of fellowship, crafts, Bible study, evening programs, an off-site excursion. Relax with a cup of coffee while watching the sunrise, campfire, indoor and outdoor games, and cross-generational sharing. Accommodations will be in the Ridge Inn - our high-comfort motel-style facility that has individual air-conditioning units in each room. The only requirement is that you must be at least 55 years of age.

719 **Mar-Lu-Ridge Summer Camps: Day Camp**

Conference and Educational Center
Jefferson, MD 21755 301-874-5544
800-238-9974
FAX 301-874-5545
http://www.mar-lu-ridge.org
e-mail: mlr@mar-lu-ridge.org

Rod Pearce, Executive Administrator
Thomas Semeta, Associate Director
Tom Waskiewicz, Food Service Manager

Day-long programs for those who have completed Kindergarten through 5th grade. Campers spend the day playing games, singing, hiking, swimming, participating in Bible study, and having a campfire. A hot lunch and afternoon snack are provided. Campers can choose between several different kinds of lodging accommodations - including arks, cabins, teepees, and hammocks. Full and parital camperships are available through churces and from the camp for those in need of them.

720 **Mar-Lu-Ridge Summer Camps: Junior/Jr HighCamp**

Conference and Educational Center
Jefferson, MD 21755 301-874-5544
800-238-9974
FAX 301-874-5545
http://www.mar-lu-ridge.org
e-mail: mlr@mar-lu-ridge.org

Rod Pearce, Executive Administrator
Thomas Semeta, Associate Director
Tom Waskiewicz, Food Service Manager

Junior and Jr. High week offers campers a variety of special themes and activities. All Junior and Jr. High programs include: archery, worship, Bible study, hiking, swimming, campfires, arts and crafts, cookouts, singing, games and making new friends. Campers can choose between several different kinds of lodging accommodations - including arks, cabins, teepees, and hammocks. Full and parital camperships are available through churces and from the camp for those in need of them.

721 **Mar-Lu-Ridge Summer Camps: Mid-Drift Camp**

Conference and Educational Center
Jefferson, MD 21755 301-874-5544
800-238-9974
FAX 301-874-5545
http://www.mar-lu-ridge.org
e-mail: mlr@mar-lu-ridge.org

Rod Pearce, Executive Administrator
Thomas Semeta, Associate Director
Tom Waskiewicz, Food Service Manager

A chance for friends ages 9-12 to spend a week at camp together. Experience worship, Bible studies, archery, hiking, swimming, camfires, arts and crafts, cookouts, singing and lots of games. Campers can choose between several different kinds of lodging accommodations - including arks, cabins, teepees, and hammocks. Full and parital camperships are available through churces and from the camp for those in need of them.

722 **Mar-Lu-Ridge Summer Camps: Mini Camp**

Conference and Educational Center
Jefferson, MD 21755 301-874-5544
800-238-9974
FAX 301-874-5545
http://www.mar-lu-ridge.org
e-mail: mlr@mar-lu-ridge.org

Rod Pearce, Executive Administrator
Thomas Semeta, Associate Director
Tom Waskiewicz, Food Service Manager

The Mini Camp program is an excellent opportunity to get a taste of overnight camp experience. Camp activities includes swimming, games, arts and crafts, hiking, singing, and more. Campers can choose between several different kinds of lodging accommodations - including arks, cabins, teepees, and hammocks. Full and parital camperships are available through churces and from the camp for those in need of them.

723 **Mar-Lu-Ridge Summer Camps: Senior High Camp**

Conference and Educational Center
Jefferson, MD 21755 301-874-5544
800-238-9974
FAX 301-874-5545
http://www.mar-lu-ridge.org
e-mail: mlr@mar-lu-ridge.org

Rod Pearce, Executive Administrator
Thomas Semeta, Associate Director
Tom Waskiewicz, Food Service Manager

Get connected, strengthen your faith, explore and rejuvenate. Senior High week has it all - including the late-night games, high ropes, rock climbing, great fellowship, talent show, and small group discussions about the issues that face Senior High youth today. Lots of other special events are in the works. Experience a different type of camp and have a great week at Mar-Lu-Ridge.

724 The League at Camp Greentop

1111 E Cold Spring Lane
Baltimore, MD 21239
410-323-0500
FAX 410-323-2398
http://www.campgreentop.org
e-mail: jrondeau@leagueforpeople.org

Jonathan Rondeau, Camp Director
Emily Carmichael, Camping Program Specialist
Bill Morgan, Community Recreation Specialist

The League at Camp Greentop is a traditional summer camp for youth and adults with disabilities in Thurmont, Maryland. Campers enjoy swimming, horseback riding, arts & crafts, sports and other social activities. Campers sleep in tents, cook over a fire and explore the outdoors. The League's year round Camping & Therapeutic Recreation program provides joyful, life-changing experiences in a safe environment and builds meaningful relationships in the lives of youth and adults.

Massachusetts

725 Abilities Unlimited Kamp for Kids

754 Russell Road
Westfield, MA 01085
413-562-5678
FAX 413-562-1239
http://http://abilitiesunlimited.org
e-mail: info@abilitiesunlimited.org

C David Scanlin Ph.D, Executive Director

Kamp for Kids is located on the grounds of Western Mass Hospital in Westfield and provides recreational summer day camp activities for able-bodied and disabled children and young adults ages 3-22. The Kamp runs two-week sessions in July and August, during which campers are offered activities such as: swimming, arts and crafts, recreational games, nature walks, and, challenge education.

726 Boston Nature Center Day Camp

208 S Great Road
Lincoln, MA 01773
617-983-8500
FAX 617-983-8012
http://www.massaudubon.org
e-mail: gvcardoza@massaudubon.org

Gloria Villegas Cardoza, Camp Director

Boston Nature Center Summer Camp provides an environment where the diversity of the participants is encouraged and celebrated and a safe environment where campers can learn firsthand about the natural world. Trained, qualified teachers/naturalists and staff will provide campers with an enjoyable, educational and noncompetitive camp experience, age appropriate activities for small group nature studies, gardening, nature arts, and cooperative games, and a great experience.

727 Camp Half Moon for Boys & Girls

PO Box 188
Great Barrington, MA 01230
413-528-0940
FAX 413-528-0941
http://www.camphalfmoon.com
e-mail: info@camphalfmoon.com

Til Mann, Director/Owner
Gretchen Mann-Fitch, Director/Owner
Ric Fritch, Director/Owner

The philosophy is based on six principles: structure, social values, sound learning skills, spirit, guidance and individuality. Half Moon provides a safe orderly environment that stresses skill improvement rather than high competition.

728 Camp Howe

4H Camp Howe
Goshen, MA 01032
413-549-3969
FAX 413-268-8206
http://www.camphowe.com
e-mail: info@camphowe.com

Terrie Campbell, Camp Director

This program is for children ages 7-12 or campers in the ECHO Program who are not ready for an overnight experience. They will be placed in a cabin and spend the day with their cabin group going to all the great activities ncluding, but not limited, climbing tower, low challenge course, waterfront activities, arts and crafts, sports and farm life.

729 Camp Joy

Boston Centers for Youth & Families
1483 Tremont Street
Boston, MA 02120
617-635-4920
FAX 617-635-5074
http://www.cityofboston.gov/bcyf
e-mail: michaeltriant@ci.boston.ma.us

Robert Lewis, Executive Director
Michael Triant, Program Manager
Kevin Stanton, After/Out School Services Dir.

A therapeutic recreational program for special needs children and adults. Currently serving over 700 participants with a professionally qualified staff of 290 at 15 sites throughout the city. Serves the physically and cognitively challenged, multi-handicapped, behaviorally involved, legally blind/visually impaired, deaf/hearing impaired, learning disabled, and pre-school special needs children.

730 Camp Lapham

731 South Road
Ashby, MA 01431
978-386-5633
FAX 978-386-0128
http://www.crossroads4kids.org/lapham.html
e-mail: office@crossroads4kids.org

Allyson Burley, Director
Joanne Fay, Program Development Director
Sue Bradford, Communications Director

Designed to meet the needs of children who thrive in a small, structured environment. The program emphasis includes anger and behavior management, along with strong self-image building all in a fun, noncompetitive camp atmosphere. With a maximum of 50 children enrolled per session and a low camper to counselor ratio of 1 to 4, the campers experience success in a more family-like atmosphere which enables each child to focus on personal goals and nonviolent methods of interaction.

731 Camp Polywog

Malden YMCA
99 Dartmouth Street
Malden, MA 02148
781-324-7680
FAX 781-324-7856
TDY:781-324-7680
http://www.ymcamalden.org

Darryl Bullock, Camp Director
Beth Cameron, Associate Executive Director
Susan Hogan, Program Director

Offers a gym, swimming, city tours and more. Structured recreation that teaches.

732 Camp Ramah

35 Highland Circle
Needham, MA 02494
781-449-7090
FAX 781-449-6331
http://www.campramahne.org
e-mail: sallyr@campramahne.org

Sally Rosensield, Director
Erica Silverman, Assistant Business Manager
Ethan Linden, Assistant Director

Young people have fun while developing skills, strong friendships and a Jewish conciousness that lasts a lifetime through a variety of experiences such as sports, nature, music, arts and crafts, boating, study, Shabbat and Judaica. Campers have developmental disabilities. Some campers with LD are included in typical divisions.

733 Carroll School Summer Camp

25 Baker Bridge Road
Lincoln, MA 01773
781-259-8342
FAX 781-259-8361
http://www.carrollschool.org
e-mail: summer@carrollschool.org

Steve Wilkins, Headmaster
Philip Burling, Chairman
Sam Foster, Co-Treasurer

Summer at Carroll is designed to offer academic intervention and remediation to children diagnosed with primary language learning difficulties, such as dyslexia. Small group teaching, individualized instruction and attention to the needs of goals of the students are what Carroll prides themselves on.

734 Crossroads for Kids

119 Myrtle Street
Duxbury, MA 02332
781-834-2700
888-543-7284
FAX 781-834-2701
http://www.crossroads4kids.org
e-mail: office@crossroads4kids.org

Allyson Burley, Director
Sue Bradford, Communications & Development
Joanne Fay, Program Development

The daily programs provide a good balance between active and quiet, sport, cultural, group and individual activities. We place campers into smaller, age appropriate groups so they receive the extra support, care and encouragement they need to feel at home here at camp.

735 Easter Seals Massachusetts

484 Main Street
Worcester, MA 01608
508-757-2756
800-922-8290
FAX 508-831-9768
http://www.eastersealsma.org
e-mail: maryd@eastersealsma.org

Kirk Joslyn, Chief Executive Officer
Mary D'Antonino, Resource Disability Manager
Susan Caracciolo, Manager

The following are camping and recreational services offered: Camp respite for adults, camp respite for children, canoeing, computer camp, computer program, day camping for children, residential camping programs, sailing, swim programs, therapeutic horseback riding and water skiing.

736 Handi Kids Camp

470 Pine Street
Bridgewater, MA 02324
508-697-7557
FAX 508-697-1529
http://www.handikids.org
e-mail: handi7557@aol.com

Ginny Pitts, Executive Director
Mary Gallant, Program Director
Jane Pariseau, Therapeutic Riding Director

Handi Kids is a non-profit, recreational facility for children and young adults with physical and cognitive disabilities. Handi Kids provides therapeutic recreation to hundreds of individuals on a year-round basis, the goal of which is to benefit each child emotionally, physically and socially while helping those who require individualized attention and guidance enjoy and participate in recreational activities.

737 Handi Kids Camp: Expressive Arts Therapy Camp Program

470 Pine Street
Bridgewater, MA 02324
508-697-7557
FAX 508-697-1529
http://www.handikids.org
e-mail: handi7557@aol.com

Ginny Pitts, Executive Director
Mary Gallant, Program Director
Jane Pariseau, Therapeutic Riding Director

Handi Kids is a non-profit, recreational facility for children and young adults with physical and cognitive disabilities. The Expressive Arts Therapy Program provides a safe, confidential and caring space for children to express feelings and concerns through art materials, sandplay, music, drama, storytelling and play.

738 Handi Kids Camp: Hippotherapy Camp Program

470 Pine Street
Bridgewater, MA 02324
508-697-7557
FAX 508-697-1529
http://www.handikids.org
e-mail: handi7557@aol.com

Ginny Pitts, Executive Director
Mary Gallant, Program Director
Jane Pariseau, Therapeutic Riding Director

Handi Kids is a non-profit, recreational facility for children and young adults with physical and cognitive disabilities. The Hippotherapy Camp Program provides campers with physical, occupational and speech treatment therapy by utilizing equine (horse) movement. Working with the movements of a horse, therapists provide treatment to individuals with a variety of physical, developmental, and cognitive disabilities.

739 Handi Kids Camp: Karate Camp Program

470 Pine Street
Bridgewater, MA 02324
508-697-7557
FAX 508-697-1529
http://www.handikids.org
e-mail: handi7557@aol.com

Ginny Pitts, Executive Director
Mary Gallant, Program Director
Jane Pariseau, Therapeutic Riding Director

Handi Kids is a non-profit, recreational facility for children and young adults with physical and cognitive disabilities. The goal is to benefit each child emotionally, physically and socially while helping those who require individualized attention and guidance enjoy and participate in recreational activities. The Karate Camp Program is a unique children's program that teaches well-being and health through praise, encouragement and positive reinforcement.

740 Handi Kids Camp: Music Therapy Camp Program

470 Pine Street
Bridgewater, MA 02324
508-697-7557
FAX 508-697-1529
http://www.handikids.org
e-mail: handi7557@aol.com

Ginny Pitts, Executive Director
Mary Gallant, Program Director
Jane Pariseau, Therapeutic Riding Director

Handi Kids is a non-profit, recreational facility for children and young adults with physical and cognitive disabilities. The Music Therapy Program is used to address physical, emotional, cognitive and social needs through creating, singing, moving and/or listening to music. This form of therapy also provides avenues of communication for those who find it difficult to express themselves in words.

741 Hillside School Summer Program

404 Robin Hill Road
Marlborough, MA 01752-1099
508-485-2824
FAX 508-485-4420
http://www.hillsideschool.net/about.htm
e-mail: admissions@hillsideschool.net

David Z Beecher, Headmaster
Chuck Redepenning, President Board of Trustees

Hillside School is an independent boarding and day school for boys, grades 5-9. Hillside provides educational and residential services to boys needing to develop their academic and social skills while building self-confidence and maturity. The 200-acre school is located in a rural section of Marlborough and includes a working farm. Hillside accommodates both traditional learners who want a more personalized education, and those boys with learning difficulties and/or attention problems.

742 Kolburne School

Kolburne School
343 NM Southfield Road
New Marlborough, MA 01230
413-229-8787
FAX 413-229-4165
http://www.kolburne.net
e-mail: info@kolburne.net

Jeane K Weinstein, Executive Director
James Stevens, Operations Director
John Sandillo, Quality Assurance Director

A family operated residential treatment center located in the Berkshire Hills of Massachusetts. Through integrated treatment services, effective behavioral management, recreational programming, and positive staff relationships, our students develop the emotional stability, interpersonal skills and academic/vocational background necessary to return home with success.

743 Landmark School Summer Programs: Exploration and Recreation
429 Hale Street
Prides Crossing, MA 01965
978-236-3000
FAX 978-927-7268
http://www.landmarkschool.org
e-mail: admission@landmarkschool.org
Robert Broudo, Headmaster
Maureen Flores, Development Director
David Seiter, Facilities Director
For students in grades 3-6, Landmark's Exploration Program provides the opportunity to combine a half-day of academic classes with a half-day Marine Science/Adventure Ropes experience. Students entering grades 1-5 may choose the Recreation Program which combines a half-day of academics with an afternoon of recreational activities. Both programs provide intensive academic study for students with language-based learning disabilities, and daily one-to-one tutorials.

744 Landmark Summer Program: Marine Science
429 Hale Street
Prides Crossing, MA 01965
978-236-3000
FAX 978-927-7268
http://www.landmarkschool.org
e-mail: admission@landmakrschool.org
Robert Broudo, Headmaster
Maureen Flores, Development Director
David Seiter, Facilities Director
Landmark's Marine Science Summer Program enrolls students in grades 7-12, who have been diagnosed with a language-based learning disability, and are interested in marine studies. Students spend half the day exploring local coastal ecosystems, working on research teams and collecting data. The other half of the day is spent developing their language skills in an academic classroom setting and in one-to-one tutorial sessions.

745 Landmark Summer Program: Musical Theater
429 Hale Street
Prides Crossing, MA 01965
978-236-3000
FAX 978-927-7268
http://www.landmarkschool.org
e-mail: admission@landmarkschool.org
Robert Broudo, Headmaster
Maureen Flores, Development Director
David Seiter, Facilities Director
Landmark's new Musical Theater program gives students the opportunity to perform on stage or develop technical theater skills behind-the-scenes. The class culminates in a full-scale theatrical production at the end of six weeks. On-stage performers learn to act, dance, and sing as part of a musical company. Technical theater students try their hand at set-design and building, sound and lighting, and produce the summer's musical production.

746 Linden Hill School Summer Program
154 South Mountain Road
Northfield, MA 01360
413-498-2906
FAX 413-498-2908
http://www.lindenhs.org/
e-mail: office@lindenhs.org
James McDaniel, Headmaster
Walter Sanieski, Assistant Headmaster
Jason Russell, Athletic Director
The Linden Hill Summer Program provides a balance of academic work and traditional camp experiences. Support and remdiation is offered through a multi-sensory approach to language training based in the renowned and clinically-proven Orton-Gillingham method. Honesty, integrity and pride in their success are goals for each of our participants. Linden Hill has hundreds of acres of fields, woods, ponds and streams, as well as a comfortable dormitory lodging and healthy, delicious home-cooked meals.

747 Moose Hill Nature Day Camp
208 S Great Road
Lincoln, MA 01773
617-983-8500
FAX 617-983-8012
http://www.massaudubon.org
e-mail: gvcardoza@massaudubon.org
Kay Andberg, Camp Director
Nature Day Camp is a welcoming environment with fewer than one hundred campers in each weekly session. The goal is to educate children and enrich their lives through outdoor exploration, focused activities, games, hikes, and crafts. Most weeks include special visitors and camp-wide theme days. The camp day runs from 9 a.m. to 3 p.m. with before and after camp programs available. The camp uses the Nature Center of Moose Hill Wildlife Sanctuary as its base.

748 Patriots' Trail Girl Scout Council SummerCamp
95 Berkeley Street
Boston, MA 02116
617-482-1078
800-882-1662
FAX 617-482-9045
TDY:800-882-1662
http://www.ptgirlscouts.org/properties_camps/
e-mail: info@ptgirlscouts.org
Shannon O'Brien, Chief Executive Officer
Leah McLean, Chief of Staff
Barbara Fortier, Chief Operating Officer
Canoeing, swimming, windsurfing, life-saving, sailing, biking and trips.

749 The Drama Play Connection, Inc.
298 Crescent Street
Waltham, MA 02453
781-899-1160
FAX 781-899-1180
http://www.dramaplayconnection.org
e-mail: info@dramaplayconnection.org
Liana Pena Morgens Ph.D, President & Director
Andrew Dietz Morgens, Vice President

The Summer Pragmatic Language Drama Program serves primarily children and adolescents with Asperger's Disorder, Nonverbal Learning Disabilities, and those with related social pragmatic difficulties. The pragmatic program is designed to help children acquire the skills necessary to function more competently with their peers. The program includes drama curriculum that focuses on teaching nonverbal language skills through the use of improvisation and other drama techniques.

750 Valleyhead
79 Reservoir Road
Lenox, MA 01240
413-637-3635
FAX 413-637-3501
http://www.valleyhead.org
e-mail: cmacbeth@valleyhead.org
M Christine Macbeth, Executive Director
Terrry Owens Gilbert, Director of Admissions
Matthew J Merritt Jr, President
A residential school for girls nestled in the scenic Berkshire Hills of Lenox, Massachusetts that provides a home and education for girls ages 12-22 with emotional needs. Most of the girls come from abusive and traumatic backgrounds. Many do not have intact families.

Michigan

751 Adventure Learning Center at Eagle Village
4507 170th Avenue
Hersey, MI 49639
231-832-2234
800-748-0061
FAX 231-832-0385
http://www.eaglevillage.org
e-mail: info@eaglevillage.org
Gary Bennett, President/CEO
Tamara McLeod, Executive Director
Craig Weidner, Development & Marketing Director
Adventure Learning Center at Eagle Village offers a variety of fun camp experiences for any child, including those with emotional and/or behavioral impairments. Challenging activities make the camps rewarding experiences.

1968

752 Easter Seals Genesee CountyGreater Flint Therapy Center

1420 W 3rd Avenue
Flint, MI 48504
810-238-0475
FAX 810-238-9270
http://http://mi.easterseals.com
e-mail: kwright@essmichigan.org

Kindra Wright, Manager
Rosemary Parnow, Office Manager

Children and adults with mental and physical disabilities and other special needs have access to services designed to meet their individual needs. Health professionals from a variety of disciplines work with each person to overcome obstacles to independence, and to reach his/her personal goals through person centered planning. The following are camping and recreational services offered: Recreational services for adults and children, residential camping programs, therapeutic horseback riding.

753 Easter Seals Grand RapidsWest Michigan Therapy Center

4065 Saladin Drive SE
Grand Rapids, MI 49546
616-942-2081
800-757-3257
FAX 616-942-5932
TDY:248-338-1188
http://http://mi.easterseals.com

John Kersten, President
John Collison, Chairman
Julie Dorcey, Regional Manager

Children and adults with mental and physical disabilities and other special have access to services designed to meet their individual needs. Health professionals from a variety of disciplines work with each person to overcome obstacles to independence, and to reach his/her personal goals through person centered planning. The following are camping and recreational services offered: Camperships.

754 Easter Seals SaginawSaginaw Valley Therapy Center

1401 N Michigan Avenue
Saginaw, MI 48602
989-753-4773
800-753-4773
FAX 989-753-4795
http://http://mi.easterseals.com
e-mail: esofmi@aol.comesfmichigan.org

Julie Dorcey, Regional Manager
Sue Combs, Administrative Assistant

Children and adults with mental and physical disabilities and other special needs have access to services designed to meet their individual needs. Health professionals from a variety of disciplines work with each person to overcome obstacles to independence, and to reach his/her personal goals through person centered planning. The following are camping and recreational services offered: Camperships.

755 Fowler Center Summer Camp

2315 Harmon Lake Road
Mayville, MI 48744
989-673-2050
FAX 989-673-6355
http://www.thefowlercenter.org
e-mail: info@thefowlercenter.org

John Fowler, Chairman/Founder
Tom Hussnann, Executive Director

The Fowler Center is an outdoor recreation and education facility that provides programs with particular emphasis on people with developmental and physical disabilities. The Center has programs for children, teens and adults. Each program has been created to accommodate each person's needs. Campers at Camp Fowler have always enjoyed the security and comfort in knowing that four counselors sleep in the same cabin as they do. Counselors are available around the clock to comfort special needs.

756 Kids All Together/KAT: All Star Basketball Camp with Coach Shoe JCC Summer Sports Camp

Jewish Community Center of Metropolitan Detroit
D Dan & Betty Kahn Building
West Bloomfield, MI 48322
248-432-5578
FAX 248-432-5552
http://www.jccdet.org/specialtyprograms/
e-mail: apatronik@jccdet.org

Forest Levy, JCC Executive Camp Director
Michael Sandweiss, JCC Sports Camps Director
Ann Patronik, Special Needs Programs Director

The mission of KAT is to include children ages 3-14 with a disability into general youth programming at the Center. KAT provides staff training, extra staff support as needed and program accommodations so children with disabilities can be successfully included in Center programming. All Star Basketball Camp with Coach Shoe takes place June 25-29, July 9-13, July 16-20, and August 6-10. Please provide the following for your child: basketball or gym shoes. Wear shorts.

757 Kids All Together/KAT: Archery Camp at the Detroit Archers Club JCC Summer Sports Camp

Jewish Community Center of Metropolitan Detroit
D Dan & Betty Kahn Building
West Bloomfield, MI 48322
248-432-5578
FAX 248-432-5552
http://www.jccdet.org/specialtyprograms/
e-mail: apatronik@jccdet.org

Forest Levy, JCC Executive Camp Director
Michael Sandweiss, JCC Sports Camps Director
Ann Patronik, Special Needs Programs Director

The mission of KAT is to include children ages 3-14 with a disability into general youth programming at the Center. KAT provides staff training, extra staff support as needed and program accommodations so children with disabilities can be successfully included in Center programming. Archery Camp at the Detroit Archers Club will take place June 18-22, and July 9-13. Please provide the following for your child: insect repellent, sunscreen, and close toed shoes. All archery equipment is provided.

758 Kids All Together/KAT: Baseball Camp at Total Sports JCC Summer Sports Camp

Jewish Community Center of Metropolitan Detroit
D Dan & Betty Kahn Building
West Bloomfield, MI 48322
248-432-5578
FAX 248-432-5552
http://www.jccdet.org/specialtyprograms/
e-mail: apatronik@jccdet.org

Forest Levy, JCC Executive Camp Director
Michael Sandweiss, JCC Sports Camps Director
Ann Patronik, Special Needs Programs Director

The mission of KAT is to include children ages 3-14 with a disability into general youth programming at the Center. KAT provides staff training, extra staff support as needed and program accommodations so children with disabilities can be successfully included in Center programming. Baseball Camp at Total Sports takes place July 9-13, and July 30-August 3. Please provide the following for your child: bring a baseball glove and baseball shoes. All other baseball equipment is provided.

759 Kids All Together/KAT: Camp Hollywood Stars & Stripes Gymnastics Academy JCC Summer Sports Camp

Jewish Community Center of Metropolitan Detroit
D Dan & Betty Kahn Building
West Bloomfield, MI 48322
248-432-5578
FAX 248-432-5552
http://www.jccdet.org/specialtyprograms/
e-mail: apatronik@jccdet.org

Forest Levy, JCC Executive Camp Director
Michael Sandweiss, JCC Sports Camps Director
Ann Patronik, Special Needs Programs Director

The mission of KAT is to include children ages 3-14 with a disability into general youth programming at the Center. KAT provides staff training, extra staff support as needed and program accommodations so children with disabilities can be successfully included in Center programming. Camp Hollywood at Stars & Stripes Gymnastics Academy takes place July 30-August 3. All equipment will be provided.

760 Kids All Together/KAT: Camp of the Ars Te'atron JCC Summer Camp

Jewish Community Center of Metropolitan Detroit
D Dan & Betty Kahn Building
West Bloomfield, MI 48322
248-432-5578
FAX 248-432-5552
http://www.jccdet.org/specialtyprograms/
e-mail: apatronik@jccdet.org

Forest Levy, JCC Executive Camp Director
Greg Trzaskoma, JCC Arts & Theatre Camp Director
Ann Patronik, Special Needs Programs Director

The mission of KAT is to include children ages 3-14 with a disability into general youth programming at the Center. KAT provides staff training, extra staff support as needed and program accommodations so children with disabilities can be successfully included in Center programming. Camp of the Arts Te'atron campers will learn about theatre, acting, singing, dancing, improv, costumes and scenery and create and rehearse a variety shows that will be performed for other camps, friends and family.

761 Kids All Together/KAT: Cheer Tumble at Stars & Stripes Gymnastics Academy JCC Summer Sports Camp
Jewish Community Center of Metropolitan Detroit
D Dan & Betty Kahn Building
West Bloomfield, MI 48322 248-432-5578
FAX 248-432-5552
http://www.jccdet.org/specialtyprograms/
e-mail: apatronik@jccdet.org
Forest Levy, JCC Executive Camp Director
Michael Sandweiss, JCC Sports Camps Director
Ann Patronik, Special Needs Programs Director
The mission of KAT is to include children ages 3-14 with a disability into general youth programming at the Center. KAT provides staff training, extra staff support as needed and program accommodations so children with disabilities can be successfully included in Center programming. Cheer Tumble at Stars & Stripes Gymnastics Academy takes place July 16-20. Please provide: proper gymnastics attire (leotards for girls or shorts and a tee shirt). All other gymnastics equipment will be provided.

762 Kids All Together/KAT: Co-Ed Volleyball JCC Summer Sports Camp
Jewish Community Center of Metropolitan Detroit
D Dan & Betty Kahn Building
West Bloomfield, MI 48322 248-432-5578
FAX 248-432-5552
http://www.jccdet.org/specialtyprograms/
e-mail: apatronik@jccdet.org
Forest Levy, JCC Executive Camp Director
Michael Sandweiss, JCC Sports Camps Director
Ann Patronik, Special Needs Programs Director
The mission of KAT is to include children ages 3-14 with a disability into general youth programming at the Center. KAT provides staff training, extra staff support as needed and program accommodations so children with disabilities can be successfully included in Center programming. Co-Ed Volleyball takes place July 2-6. Please provide the following for your child: shorts and gym shoes, knee pads (optional),

763 Kids All Together/KAT: Coach G's Star Soccer JCC Summer Sports Camp
Jewish Community Center of Metropolitan Detroit
D Dan & Betty Kahn Building
West Bloomfield, MI 48322 248-432-5578
FAX 248-432-5552
http://www.jccdet.org/specialtyprograms/
e-mail: apatronik@jccdet.org
Forest Levy, JCC Executive Camp Director
Michael Sandweiss, JCC Sports Camps Director
Ann Patronik, Special Needs Programs Director
The mission of KAT is to include children ages 3-14 with a disability into general youth programming at the Center. KAT provides staff training, extra staff support as needed and program accommodations so children with disabilities can be successfully included in Center programming. Coach G's Star Soccer Camp will take place June 25-29, and July 9-13. Campers should wear shorts and soccer shoes and bring shin guards.

764 Kids All Together/KAT: Girl Power Camp JCC Summer Sports Camp
Jewish Community Center of Metropolitan Detroit
D Dan & Betty Kahn Building
West Bloomfield, MI 48322 248-432-5578
FAX 248-432-5552
http://www.jccdet.org/specialtyprograms/
e-mail: apatronik@jccdet.org
Forest Levy, JCC Executive Camp Director
Michael Sandweiss, JCC Sports Camps Director
Ann Patronik, Special Needs Programs Director
The mission of KAT is to include children ages 3-14 with a disability into general youth programming at the Center. KAT provides staff training, extra staff support as needed and program accommodations so children with disabilities can be successfully included in Center programming. Girl Power Camp takes place July 23-27. Please provide the following for your child: bring workout clothes.

765 Kids All Together/KAT: Girls Fitness at the JCC Summer Sports Camp
Jewish Community Center of Metropolitan Detroit
D Dan & Betty Kahn Building
West Bloomfield, MI 48322 248-432-5578
FAX 248-432-5552
http://www.jccdet.org/specialtyprograms/
e-mail: apatronik@jccdet.org
Forest Levy, JCC Executive Camp Director
Michael Sandweiss, JCC Sports Camps Director
Ann Patronik, Special Needs Programs Director
The mission of KAT is to include children ages 3-14 with a disability into general youth programming at the Center. KAT provides staff training, extra staff support as needed and program accommodations so children with disabilities can be successfully included in Center programming. Girls Fitness at the JCC takes place July 16-20. Please provide the following for your child: bring workout clothes.

766 Kids All Together/KAT: Gold Medal Swimming JCC Summer Sports Camp
Jewish Community Center of Metropolitan Detroit
D Dan & Betty Kahn Building
West Bloomfield, MI 48322 248-432-5578
FAX 248-432-5552
http://www.jccdet.org/specialtyprograms/
e-mail: apatronik@jccdet.org
Forest Levy, JCC Executive Camp Director
Michael Sandweiss, JCC Sports Camps Director
Ann Patronik, Special Needs Programs Director
The mission of KAT is to include children ages 3-14 with a disability into general youth programming at the Center. KAT provides staff training, extra staff support as needed and program accommodations so children with disabilities can be successfully included in Center programming. Gold Medal Swimming will take place July 2-6, and July 30-August 3. Please provide the following for your child: Earplugs if needed, swimming cap.

767 Kids All Together/KAT: Golf Camp at OasisGolf Center JCC Summer Sports Camp
Jewish Community Center of Metropolitan Detroit
D Dan & Betty Kahn Building
West Bloomfield, MI 48322 248-432-5578
FAX 248-432-5552
http://www.jccdet.org/specialtyprograms/
e-mail: apatronik@jccdet.org
Forest Levy, JCC Executive Camp Director
Michael Sandweiss, JCC Sports Camps Director
Ann Patronik, Special Needs Programs Director
The mission of KAT is to include children ages 3-14 with a disability into general youth programming at the Center. KAT provides staff training, extra staff support as needed and program accommodations so children with disabilities can be successfully included in Center programming. Golf Camp at Oasis Golf Center takes place July 9-13, and July 23-27; Advanced Golf takes place July 23-27. Provide the following for your child: must bring your own clubs; signed waiver needed for participation.

768 Kids All Together/KAT: Gymnastics Camp Stars & Stripes Gymnastics Academy JCC Summer Sports Camp
Jewish Community Center of Metropolitan Detroit
D Dan & Betty Kahn Building
West Bloomfield, MI 48322 248-432-5578
FAX 248-432-5552
http://www.jccdet.org/specialtyprograms/
e-mail: apatronik@jccdet.org
Forest Levy, JCC Executive Camp Director
Michael Sandweiss, JCC Sports Camps Director
Ann Patronik, Special Needs Programs Director

The mission of KAT is to include children ages 3-14 with a disability into general youth programming at the Center. KAT provides staff training, extra staff support as needed and program accommodations so children with disabilities can be successfully included in Center programming. Gymnastics Camp takes place August 20-24. Please provide the following for your child: Proper gymnastics attire (leotards for girls or shorts and a tee shirt). All other gymnastics equipment will be provided.

769 Kids All Together/KAT: Gymnastics Camp atOakland Gymnastics JCC Summer Sports Camp
Jewish Community Center of Metropolitan Detroit
D Dan & Betty Kahn Building
West Bloomfield, MI 48322 248-432-5578
FAX 248-432-5552
http://www.jccdet.org/specialtyprograms/
e-mail: apatronik@jccdet.org
Forest Levy, JCC Executive Camp Director
Michael Sandweiss, JCC Sports Camps Director
Ann Patronik, Special Needs Programs Director
The mission of KAT is to include children ages 3-14 with a disability into general youth programming at the Center. KAT provides staff training, extra staff support as needed and program accommodations so children with disabilities can be successfully included in Center programming. Gymnastics Camp at Oakland takes place June 25-29, and August 6-10. Provide the following: proper gymnastics attire (leotards for girls or shorts and a tee shirt). All other gymnastics equipment will be provided.

770 Kids All Together/KAT: Hip-Hop Dance CampJCC Summer Sports Camp
Jewish Community Center of Metropolitan Detroit
D Dan & Betty Kahn Building
West Bloomfield, MI 48322 248-432-5578
FAX 248-432-5552
http://www.jccdet.org/specialtyprograms/
e-mail: apatronik@jccdet.org
Forest Levy, JCC Executive Camp Director
Michael Sandweiss, JCC Sports Camps Director
Ann Patronik, Special Needs Programs Director
The mission of KAT is to include children ages 3-14 with a disability into general youth programming at the Center. KAT provides staff training, extra staff support as needed and program accommodations so children with disabilities can be successfully included in Center programming. Hip-Hop Dance Camp will take place at the Neu Wixom Dance Studio from June 18-22, and August 13-17. Bring comfortable clothes and shoes for dancing.

771 Kids All Together/KAT: Horseback Riding Camp at Windmill Farms JCC Summer Sports Camp
Jewish Community Center of Metropolitan Detroit
D Dan & Betty Kahn Building
West Bloomfield, MI 48322 248-432-5578
FAX 248-432-5552
http://www.jccdet.org/specialtyprograms/
e-mail: apatronik@jccdet.org
Forest Levy, JCC Executive Camp Director
Michael Sandweiss, JCC Sports Camps Director
Ann Patronik, Special Needs Programs Director
The mission of KAT is to include children ages 3-14 with a disability into general youth programming at the Center. KAT provides staff training, extra staff support as needed and program accommodations so children with disabilities can be successfully included in Center programming. Horseback Riding Camp will take place June 18-22, July 23-27, and August 20-24. Please provide: pants below the knees, close tied shoes, insect repellent and sunscreen, signed waiver. Must be 8 years old, 4'2" tall.

772 Kids All Together/KAT: Imagitivity JCC Summer Camp
Jewish Community Center of Metropolitan Detroit
D Dan & Betty Kahn Building
West Bloomfield, MI 48322 248-432-5578
FAX 248-432-5552
http://www.jccdet.org/specialtyprograms/
e-mail: apatronik@jccdet.org
Forest Levy, JCC Executive Camp Director
Elisabeth A Rogers, Imagitivity Camp Director
Ann Patronik, Special Needs Programs Director
The mission of KAT is to include children ages 3-14 with a disability into youth programs at the Center. Extra staff support and program accommodations are provided so children with disabilities can be included in Center activities. Imagitivity Camp at the Jimmy Prentis Morris Building is designed to spark imagination and creativity within your child, focusing on the arts and sciences. Young campers will spend part of his/her summer involved in exciting activities filled with hands-on fun!

773 Kids All Together/KAT: In-Line Hockey Camp at the IHC JCC Summer Sports Camp
Jewish Community Center of Metropolitan Detroit
D Dan & Betty Kahn Building
West Bloomfield, MI 48322 248-432-5578
FAX 248-432-5552
http://www.jccdet.org/specialtyprograms/
e-mail: apatronik@jccdet.org
Forest Levy, JCC Executive Camp Director
Michael Sandweiss, JCC Sports Camps Director
Ann Patronik, Special Needs Programs Director
The mission of KAT is to include children ages 3-14 with a disability into general youth programming at the Center. KAT provides staff training, extra staff support as needed and program accommodations so children with disabilities can be successfully included in Center programming. In-Line Hockey Camp takes place June 18-22, July 2-6, and July 23-27. Please provide: skates, shin guards, elbow pads, gloves, HECC approved helmet and stick. Equipment is not provided.

774 Kids All Together/KAT: Junior Olympics with Coach Shoe JCC Summer Sports Camp
Jewish Community Center of Metropolitan Detroit
D Dan & Betty Kahn Building
West Bloomfield, MI 48322 248-432-5578
FAX 248-432-5552
http://www.jccdet.org/specialtyprograms/
e-mail: apatronik@jccdet.org
Forest Levy, JCC Executive Camp Director
Michael Sandweiss, JCC Sports Camps Director
Ann Patronik, Special Needs Programs Director
The mission of KAT is to include children ages 3-14 with a disability into general youth programming at the Center. KAT provides staff training, extra staff support as needed and program accommodations so children with disabilities can be successfully included in Center programming. Junior Olympics with Coach Shoe takes place June 25-29. Please provide the following for your child: comfortable clothes, gym shoes, sunscreen, water bottle.

775 Kids All Together/KAT: K'Ton Ton Camp JCCSummer Camp
Jewish Community Center of Metropolitan Detroit
D Dan & Betty Kahn Building
West Bloomfield, MI 48322 248-432-5578
FAX 248-432-5552
http://www.jccdet.org/specialtyprograms/
e-mail: apatronik@jccdet.org
Forest Levy, JCC Executive Camp Director
Michael Sandweiss, JCC Sports Camps Director
Ann Patronik, Special Needs Programs Director
The mission of KAT is to include children ages 3-14 with a disability into general youth programming at the Center. KAT provides staff training, extra staff support as needed and program accommodations so children with disabilities can be successfully included in Center programming. K'Ton Ton provides young campers with a variety of fun activities that includes daily swimming in the morning and using the Berlin playground. A kosher-dairy lunch is provided for all full-day preschool campers.

776 Kids All Together/KAT: Kidz Choice JCC Summer Camp
Jewish Community Center of Metropolitan Detroit
D Dan & Betty Kahn Building
West Bloomfield, MI 48322 248-432-5578
FAX 248-432-5552
http://www.jccdet.org/specialtyprograms/
e-mail: apatronik@jccdet.org
Forest Levy, JCC Executive Camp Director
Ann Patronik, Special Needs Programs Director
Brenda Hiltz, Camp Registrar

The mission of KAT is to include children ages 3-14 with a disability into general youth programming at the Center. KAT provides staff training, extra staff support as needed and program accommodations so children with disabilities can be successfully included in Center programming. Kidz Choice campers participate in a variety of activities including swimming, sports, arts and crafts, R.O.P.E.S., mini golf, volleyball and more. Drop-off and pick-up area is in the Southeast Event Rooms.

777 **Kids All Together/KAT: Lacrosse JCC Summer Sports Camp**
Jewish Community Center of Metropolitan Detroit
D Dan & Betty Kahn Building
West Bloomfield, MI 48322 248-432-5578
FAX 248-432-5552
http://www.jccdet.org/specialtyprograms/
e-mail: apatronik@jccdet.org
Forest Levy, JCC Executive Camp Director
Michael Sandweiss, JCC Sports Camps Director
Ann Patronik, Special Needs Programs Director
The mission of KAT is to include children ages 3-14 with a disability into general youth programming at the Center. KAT provides staff training, extra staff support as needed and program accommodations so children with disabilities can be successfully included in Center programming. Lacrosse will take place June 25-29, and August 6-10. Please provide the following for your child: gym shoes; wear shorts; bring water bottle and sunscreen; all lacrosse equipment provided.

778 **Kids All Together/KAT: Martial Arts at the JCC Summer Sports Camp**
Jewish Community Center of Metropolitan Detroit
D Dan & Betty Kahn Building
West Bloomfield, MI 48322 248-432-5578
FAX 248-432-5552
http://www.jccdet.org/specialtyprograms/
e-mail: apatronik@jccdet.org
Forest Levy, JCC Executive Camp Director
Michael Sandweiss, JCC Sports Camps Director
Ann Patronik, Special Needs Programs Director
The mission of KAT is to include children ages 3-14 with a disability into general youth programming at the Center. KAT provides staff training, extra staff support as needed and program accommodations so children with disabilities can be successfully included in Center programming. Martial Arts at the JCC will take place July 16-20, and July 30-August 3. Please provide the following for your child: comfortable clothes (uniforms will be available for purchase).

779 **Kids All Together/KAT: Mini Camp JCC Summer Camp**
Jewish Community Center of Metropolitan Detroit
D Dan & Betty Kahn Building
West Bloomfield, MI 48322 248-432-5578
FAX 248-432-5552
http://www.jccdet.org/specialtyprograms/
e-mail: apatronik@jccdet.org
Forest Levy, JCC Executive Camp Director
Ann Patronik, Special Needs Programs Director
Brenda Hiltz, Camp Registrar
The mission of KAT is to include children ages 3-14 with a disability into general youth programming at the Center. KAT provides staff training, extra staff support as needed and program accommodations so children with disabilities can be successfully included in Center programming. Mini Camp campers participate in a variety of activities including swimming, sports, arts/crafts, R.O.P.E.S., mini golf, volleyball and more. Drop-off and pick-up area is in the Southeast Event Rooms. 9:30 a.m.-3:30.

780 **Kids All Together/KAT: Multi Sports with Coach Shoe JCC Summer Sports Camp**
Jewish Community Center of Metropolitan Detroit
D Dan & Betty Kahn Building
West Bloomfield, MI 48322 248-432-5578
FAX 248-432-5552
http://www.jccdet.org/specialtyprograms/
e-mail: apatronik@jccdet.org
Forest Levy, JCC Executive Camp Director
Michael Sandweiss, JCC Sports Camps Director
Ann Patronik, Special Needs Programs Director
The mission of KAT is to include children ages 3-14 with a disability into general youth programming at the Center. KAT provides staff training, extra staff support as needed and program accommodations so children with disabilities can be successfully included in Center programming. Multi-Sports with Coach Shoe takes place June 18-June 22. Please provide the following for your child: comfortable clothes, gym shoes, swimsuit and towel, sunscreen and water bottle.

781 **Kids All Together/KAT: NFL Flag Football Camp JCC Summer Sports Camp**
Jewish Community Center of Metropolitan Detroit
D Dan & Betty Kahn Building
West Bloomfield, MI 48322 248-432-5578
FAX 248-432-5552
http://www.jccdet.org/specialtyprograms/
e-mail: apatronik@jccdet.org
Forest Levy, JCC Executive Camp Director
Michael Sandweiss, JCC Sports Camps Director
Ann Patronik, Special Needs Programs Director
The mission of KAT is to include children ages 3-14 with a disability into general youth programming at the Center. KAT provides staff training, extra staff support as needed and program accommodations so children with disabilities can be successfully included in Center programming. NFL Flag Football Camp takes place June 18-22, July 16-20, August 13-17. Provide the following: gym shoes preferred, water bottle, sunscreen. Signed waiver is required for participation. Football equipment provided.

782 **Kids All Together/KAT: Outdoor Adventure Camp JCC Summer Sports Camp**
Jewish Community Center of Metropolitan Detroit
D Dan & Betty Kahn Building
West Bloomfield, MI 48322 248-432-5578
FAX 248-432-5552
http://www.jccdet.org/specialtyprograms/
e-mail: apatronik@jccdet.org
Forest Levy, JCC Executive Camp Director
Michael Sandweiss, JCC Sports Camps Director
Ann Patronik, Special Needs Programs Director
The mission of KAT is to include children ages 3-14 with a disability into general youth programming at the Center. KAT provides staff training, extra staff support as needed and program accommodations so children with disabilities can be successfully included in Center programming. Outdoor Adventure Camp takes place July 2-6. Provide the following: close toed shoes; light weight long sleeve shirt; long light weight pants or zip offs; bandanna/sunglasses; bug spray/sunscreen; bottle of water.

783 **Kids All Together/KAT: PK-5 Extended CareJCC Summer Camp**
Jewish Community Center of Metropolitan Detroit
D Dan & Betty Kahn Building
West Bloomfield, MI 48322 248-432-5578
FAX 248-432-5552
http://www.jccdet.org/specialtyprograms/
e-mail: apatronik@jccdet.org
Forest Levy, JCC Executive Camp Director
Ann Patronik, Special Needs Programs Director
Brenda Hiltz, Camp Registrar
The mission of KAT is to include children ages 3-14 with a disability into general youth programming at the Center. KAT provides staff training, extra staff support as needed and program accommodations so children with disabilities can be successfully included in Center programming. Extended Care campers can choose from daily activities such as swimming, gym, playground, arts and crafts and other fun organized activities. Drop-off and pick-up area is in the Southeast Event Rooms.

784 **Kids All Together/KAT: RAH Cheer Camp JCCSummer Sports Camp**
Jewish Community Center of Metropolitan Detroit
D Dan & Betty Kahn Building
West Bloomfield, MI 48322 248-432-5578
FAX 248-432-5552
http://www.jccdet.org/specialtyprograms/
e-mail: apatronik@jccdet.org
Forest Levy, JCC Executive Camp Director
Michael Sandweiss, JCC Sports Camps Director
Ann Patronik, Special Needs Programs Director

The mission of KAT is to include children ages 3-14 with a disability into general youth programming at the Center. KAT provides staff training, extra staff support as needed and program accommodations so children with disabilities can be successfully included in Center programming. RAH Cheer Camp takes place July 9-13. Please provide the following for your child: comfortable clothes and gym shoes.

785 Kids All Together/KAT: Renaissance Fencing Camp JCC Summer Sports Camp

Jewish Community Center of Metropolitan Detroit
D Dan & Betty Kahn Building
West Bloomfield, MI 48322 248-432-5578
FAX 248-432-5552
http://www.jccdet.org/specialtyprograms/
e-mail: apatronik@jccdet.org
Forest Levy, JCC Executive Camp Director
Michael Sandweiss, JCC Sports Camps Director
Ann Patronik, Special Needs Programs Director

The mission of KAT is to include children ages 3-14 with a disability into general youth programming at the Center. KAT provides staff training, extra staff support as needed and program accommodations so children with disabilities can be successfully included in Center programming. Renaissance Fencing Camp takes place July 9-13, and July 16-20. All fencing equipment will be provided.

786 Kids All Together/KAT: Rock Climbing at Planet Rock JCC Summer Sports Camp

Jewish Community Center of Metropolitan Detroit
D Dan & Betty Kahn Building
West Bloomfield, MI 48322 248-432-5578
FAX 248-432-5552
http://www.jccdet.org/specialtyprograms/
e-mail: apatronik@jccdet.org
Forest Levy, JCC Executive Camp Director
Michael Sandweiss, JCC Sports Camps Director
Ann Patronik, Special Needs Programs Director

The mission of KAT is to include children ages 3-14 with a disability into general youth programming at the Center. KAT provides staff training, extra staff support as needed and program accommodations so children with disabilities can be successfully included in Center programming. Rock Climbing At Planet Rock will take place June 18-22, July 23-27, and August 6-10. Please provide the following for your child: gym shoes preferred and signed waiver. All rock climbing equipment will be provided.

787 Kids All Together/KAT: Splash Point Adventure JCC Summer Camp

Jewish Community Center of Metropolitan Detroit
D Dan & Betty Kahn Building
West Bloomfield, MI 48322 248-432-5578
FAX 248-432-5552
http://www.jccdet.org/specialtyprograms/
e-mail: apatronik@jccdet.org
Forest Levy, JCC Executive Camp Director
Ann Patronik, Special Needs Programs Director
Brenda Hiltz, Camp Registrar

The mission of KAT is to include children ages 3-14 with a disability into youth programs at the Center. Extra staff support and program accommodations are provided so children with disabilities can be included in Center activities. Splash Adventure Camp is a fun and exciting week of riding waterslides, floating down lazy rivers and swimming amongst the waves. Campers will visit several water parks including Waterford Oaks Water Park, Red Oaks Water Park, and Rolling Oaks Water Park.

788 Skyline Camp and Conference Center:Camp for Me

5650 Sandhill Road
Almont, MI 48003 810-798-8240
FAX 810-798-3680
http://www.campskyline.org
e-mail: cskyline@hotmail.com
Mary Cupples, Camp Director

Two separate weeks of camp experiences for adults who are differently-abled. Campers will discover the gifts that they have to share, as they participate in experiences of giving back to the community. During a week of fun, outdoor activities, campers learn responsibility, develop self-confidence, self-worth, and build lifelong friendships. June 10 to June 14, and June 24 to June 28.

789 Skyline Camp and Conference Center: Camp Far Far Out

5650 Sandhill Road
Almont, MI 48003 810-798-8240
FAX 810-798-3680
http://www.campskyline.org
e-mail: cskyline@hotmail.com
Mary Cupples, Camp Director

A camp experience for youth with special needs, in partnership with the Variety FAR Conservatory. Campers will discover the gifts that they have to share, as they participate in experiences of giving back to the community. During a week of fun, outdoor activities, campers learn responsibility, develop self-confidence, self-worth, and build lifelong friendships. June 17 to June 22.

790 Skyline Camp and Conference Center: Camp Joy

5650 Sandhill Road
Almont, MI 48003 810-798-8240
FAX 810-798-3680
http://www.campskyline.org
e-mail: cskyline@hotmail.com
Mary Cupples, Camp Director

Two separate weeks of camp experiences for adults who are differently-abled. Campers will discover the gifts that they have to share, as they participate in experiences of giving back to the community. During a week of fun, outdoor activities, campers learn responsibility, develop self-confidence, self-worth, and build lifelong friendships. June 10 to June 14, and June 24 to June 28.

791 Skyline Camp and Conference Center: Discover Camp

5650 Sandhill Road
Almont, MI 48003 810-798-8240
FAX 810-798-3680
http://www.campskyline.org
e-mail: cskyline@hotmail.com
Mary Cupples, Camp Director

This week at Skyline is designed for campers (from Oakland County Youth Assistance Programs) to discover new things. Discover who you are and what that means. Discover new things about yourself. Participate in activities including: arts & crafts, swimming, fishing, hiking, archery, drumming, canoeing, Challenge Program, and much more. July 22 to July 27.

792 Skyline Camp and Conference Center: Mini Camp

5650 Sandhill Road
Almont, MI 48003 810-798-8240
FAX 810-798-3680
http://www.campskyline.org
e-mail: cskyline@hotmail.com
Mary Cupples, Camp Director

Enjoy 3 days/2 nights of camp. An introduction to camp or a chance for those who prefer a shorter session. Campers will participate in all the traditional camp activities including faith exploration, swimming, canoeing, arts & crafts, daily devotions, hiking, drum circles, singing, Challenge Program, worship, nightly campfires, and much more! July 15-July 17. Entering 1st through 4th grade.

793 Skyline Camp and Conference Center: NightOwls Camp for Senior High and Mid-High Campers

5650 Sandhill Road
Almont, MI 48003 810-798-8240
FAX 810-798-3680
http://www.campskyline.org
e-mail: cskyline@hotmail.com
Mary Cupples, Camp Director

Do you like to stay up late? Do you want to experience camp after the sun goes down? If yes, then this is the camp for you! Everything that Traditional Camp has to offer but with the excitement of camp at night. Learn about night time animals, have a late night cook out, and play glow-in-the-dark games. July 8-July 13. Entering grades 6-8.

794 Skyline Camp and Conference Center: Senior High and Mid-High Traditional Camp

5650 Sandhill Road
Almont, MI 48003
810-798-8240
FAX 810-798-3680
http://www.campskyline.org
e-mail: cskyline@hotmail.com
Mary Cupples, Camp Director

Campers enjoy a full week of activities designed to provide a fun filled camp experience. Camp also helps young people grow in their faith and develop personal and social skills that will benefit them throughout their lives. Campers participate in faith exploration, swimming, canoeing, fishing, archery, drum circles, arts & crafts, daily devotions, hiking, singing, Challenge Program, worship, nightly campfires, and much more! July 8-July 13. Entering grades 6-8.

795 Skyline Camp and Conference Center: Traditional Camp Elementary Campers

5650 Sandhill Road
Almont, MI 48003
810-798-8240
FAX 810-798-3680
http://www.campskyline.org
e-mail: cskyline@hotmail.com
Mary Cupples, Camp Director

Skyline provides a traditional camp experience for campers to practice outdoor living skills while encountering nature and having lots of fun. During a week of fun, outdoor activities, field games, arts and crafts, nature hikes, fishing, swimming and canoeing, campers learn responsibility, develop self-confidence and self-worth, and build lifelong friendships. July 1-July 6 and July 15-July 20. Grades 2-5.

796 Spring Hill Camps: Cooper Country Adventure Challenge Camp

7717 95th Avenue
Evart, MI 49631
231-734-2616
FAX 866-332-5572
http://www.springhillcamps.com/MI/summercamp/
e-mail: register@springhillcamps.com
Todd Leinberger, Camp Director
Mike Krick, Facility Rental Coordinator
Danae Faber, Volunteer Coordinator

Spring Hill Camps is a youth camp program that offers extreme sports, exhilarating activities, and outdoor adventures. Spring Hill has specially trained staff, adaptive transportation, and housing solutions ready to accommodate children with special needs. Cooper Country Camps are for youth grades 4-6. Adventure Challenge will explore the High Adventure courses and eco-challenges of camp. Activities include the zipline, teams' course, climbing tower, high ropes, and river exploration.

797 Spring Hill Camps: Cooper Country Art Camp

7717 95th Avenue
Evart, MI 49631
231-734-2616
FAX 866-332-5572
http://www.springhillcamps.com/MI/summercamp/
e-mail: register@springhillcamps.com
Todd Leinberger, Camp Director
Mike Krick, Facility Rental Coordinator
Danae Faber, Volunteer Coordinator

Spring Hill Camps is a youth camp program that offers extreme sports, exhilarating activities, and outdoor adventures. Spring Hill has specially trained staff, adaptive transportation, and housing solutions ready to accommodate children with special needs. Cooper Country Camps are for youth grades 4-6. Art Camp activities include drawing, clay, watercolor, mosaics and painting. Girls only for now. Program is two to three hours daily.

798 Spring Hill Camps: Cooper Country BMX Camp

7717 95th Avenue
Evart, MI 49631
231-734-2616
FAX 866-332-5572
http://www.springhillcamps.com/MI/summercamp/
e-mail: register@springhillcamps.com
Todd Leinberger, Camp Director
Mike Krick, Facility Rental Coordinator
Danae Faber, Volunteer Coordinator

Spring Hill Camps is a youth camp program that offers extreme sports, exhilarating activities, and outdoor adventures. Spring Hill has specially trained staff, adaptive transportation, and housing solutions ready to accommodate children with special needs. Cooper Country Camps are for youth grades 4-6. BMX camp includes jumping, tricks, competition techniques, tabletops, step-ups, step-downs, beams, rollers, rhythm jumps, bike maintenance and safety. Pads, bikes and helmets provided. Boys only.

799 Spring Hill Camps: Cooper Country Basketball Camp

7717 95th Avenue
Evart, MI 49631
231-734-2616
FAX 866-332-5572
http://www.springhillcamps.com/MI/summercamp/
e-mail: register@springhillcamps.com
Todd Leinberger, Camp Director
Mike Krick, Facility Rental Coordinator
Danae Faber, Volunteer Coordinator

Spring Hill Camps is a youth camp program that offers extreme sports, exhilarating activities, and outdoor adventures. Spring Hill has specially trained staff, adaptive transportation, and housing solutions ready to accommodate children with special needs. Cooper Country Camps are for youth grades 4-6. Basketball Camp is for both beginners and seasoned veterans that will learn the fundamentals, drills and strategies and get an overview of the rules.

800 Spring Hill Camps: Cooper Country Camp Classic

7717 95th Avenue
Evart, MI 49631
231-734-2616
FAX 866-332-5572
http://www.springhillcamps.com/MI/summercamp/
e-mail: register@springhillcamps.com
Todd Leinberger, Camp Director
Mike Krick, Facility Rental Coordinator
Danae Faber, Volunteer Coordinator

Spring Hill Camps is a youth camp program that offers extreme sports, exhilarating activities, and outdoor adventures. Spring Hill has specially trained staff, adaptive transportation, and housing solutions ready to accommodate children with special needs. Cooper Country Camps are for youth grades 4-6. Camp Classic includes lots of activities such as the zipline, crafts, swimming, waterslide, horseback riding and nature exploration - you can't beat that variety!

801 Spring Hill Camps: Cooper Country Cheerleading Camp

7717 95th Avenue
Evart, MI 49631
231-734-2616
FAX 866-332-5572
http://www.springhillcamps.com/MI/summercamp/
e-mail: register@springhillcamps.com
Todd Leinberger, Camp Director
Mike Krick, Facility Rental Coordinator
Danae Faber, Volunteer Coordinator

Spring Hill Camps is a youth camp program that offers extreme sports, exhilarating activities, and outdoor adventures. Spring Hill has specially trained staff, adaptive transportation, and housing solutions ready to accommodate children with special needs. Cooper Country Camps are for youth grades 4-6. Cheerleading Camp is for individuals with spirt that love to show it! Campers will learn cheer technique, jumps, basic stunting, tumbling, routines and dances. Girls only.

802 Spring Hill Camps: Cooper Country Construction Camp

7717 95th Avenue
Evart, MI 49631
231-734-2616
FAX 866-332-5572
http://www.springhillcamps.com/MI/summercamp/
e-mail: register@springhillcamps.com
Todd Leinberger, Camp Director
Mike Krick, Facility Rental Coordinator
Danae Faber, Volunteer Coordinator

Spring Hill Camps is a youth camp program that offers extreme sports, exhilarating activities, and outdoor adventures. Spring Hill has specially trained staff, adaptive transportation, and housing solutions ready to accommodate children with special needs. Cooper Country Camps are for youth grades 4-6. Construction Campers build a real shed or mobile pavilion from start to finish, learn work site safety, basic building skills, hand tool use, blueprint reading and painting. Boys only.

803 Spring Hill Camps: Cooper Country CreativeDrama Camp
7717 95th Avenue
Evart, MI 49631
231-734-2616
FAX 866-332-5572
http://www.springhillcamps.com/MI/summercamp/
e-mail: register@springhillcamps.com
Todd Leinberger, Camp Director
Mike Krick, Facility Rental Coordinator
Danae Faber, Volunteer Coordinator
Spring Hill Camps is a youth camp program that offers extreme sports, exhilarating activities, and outdoor adventures. Spring Hill has specially trained staff, adaptive transportation, and housing solutions ready to accommodate children with special needs. Cooper Country Camps are for youth grades 4-6. Creative Drama Campers experience real costume changes, interaction with other actors, improv sketches with props, clowning, miming and skit writing. Week concludes with a special performance.

804 Spring Hill Camps: Cooper Country Dance Camp
7717 95th Avenue
Evart, MI 49631
231-734-2616
FAX 866-332-5572
http://www.springhillcamps.com/MI/summercamp/
e-mail: register@springhillcamps.com
Todd Leinberger, Camp Director
Mike Krick, Facility Rental Coordinator
Danae Faber, Volunteer Coordinator
Spring Hill Camps is a youth camp program that offers extreme sports, exhilarating activities, and outdoor adventures. Spring Hill has specially trained staff, adaptive transportation, and housing solutions ready to accommodate children with special needs. Cooper Country Camps are for youth grades 4-6. Dance Campers will spin, twirl, boogie and rock their way through dance routines, learn techniques and fundamentals, along with jazz, hip-hop line dancing and other fun dances! Girls only for now.

805 Spring Hill Camps: Cooper Country ExtremeSports Camp
7717 95th Avenue
Evart, MI 49631
231-734-2616
FAX 866-332-5572
http://www.springhillcamps.com/MI/summercamp/
e-mail: register@springhillcamps.com
Todd Leinberger, Camp Director
Mike Krick, Facility Rental Coordinator
Danae Faber, Volunteer Coordinator
Spring Hill Camps is a youth camp program that offers extreme sports, exhilarating activities, and outdoor adventures. Spring Hill has specially trained staff, adaptive transportation, and housing solutions ready to accommodate children with special needs. Cooper Country Camps are for youth grades 4-6. Extreme Sports Campers will experience hours of skating (boards or blades), increasing their skills on half-pipes, fly boxes, rhythm sections and verts. Pads, equipment and helmets provided.

806 Spring Hill Camps: Cooper Country Horse Camp (Grades 4-6)
7717 95th Avenue
Evart, MI 49631
231-734-2616
FAX 866-332-5572
http://www.springhillcamps.com/MI/summercamp/
e-mail: register@springhillcamps.com
Todd Leinberger, Camp Director
Mike Krick, Facility Rental Coordinator
Danae Faber, Volunteer Coordinator
Spring Hill Camps is a youth camp program that offers extreme sports, exhilarating activities, and outdoor adventures. Spring Hill has specially trained staff, adaptive transportation, and housing solutions ready to accommodate children with special needs. Cooper Country Horse Camp provides both veteran riders and rookies alike the opportunity to be totally involved in the riding experience, improving their techniques on trail rides and arena, learning horse care, feeding and grooming.

807 Spring Hill Camps: Cooper Country Water Sports Camp
7717 95th Avenue
Evart, MI 49631
231-734-2616
FAX 866-332-5572
http://www.springhillcamps.com/MI/summercamp/
e-mail: register@springhillcamps.com
Todd Leinberger, Camp Director
Mike Krick, Facility Rental Coordinator
Danae Faber, Volunteer Coordinator
Spring Hill Camps is a youth camp program that offers extreme sports, exhilarating activities, and outdoor adventures. Spring Hill has specially trained staff, adaptive transportation, and housing solutions ready to accommodate children with special needs. Cooper Country Camps are for youth grades 4-6. Water Sports Campers will head out to Rose Lake, a nearby 370-acre lake and learn the basic fundamentals of water sports where they will go tubing, wakeboarding, water skiing and kneeboarding.

808 Spring Hill Camps: New Frontiers Adventure Challenge Camp
7717 95th Avenue
Evart, MI 49631
231-734-2616
FAX 866-332-5572
http://www.springhillcamps.com/MI/summercamp/
e-mail: register@springhillcamps.com
Todd Leinberger, Camp Director
Mike Krick, Facility Rental Coordinator
Danae Faber, Volunteer Coordinator
Spring Hill Camps is a youth camp program that offers extreme sports, exhilarating activities, and outdoor adventures. Spring Hill has specially trained staff, adaptive transportation, and housing solutions ready to accommodate children with special needs. New Frontiers Camps are for youth grades 6-9. Adventure Challenge will explore the High Adventure courses and eco-challenges of camp. Activities include the zipline, teams' course, climbing tower, high ropes, and river exploration.

809 Spring Hill Camps: New Frontiers All StarSports Camp
7717 95th Avenue
Evart, MI 49631
231-734-2616
FAX 866-332-5572
http://www.springhillcamps.com/MI/summercamp/
e-mail: register@springhillcamps.com
Todd Leinberger, Camp Director
Mike Krick, Facility Rental Coordinator
Danae Faber, Volunteer Coordinator
Spring Hill Camps is a youth camp program that offers extreme sports, exhilarating activities, and outdoor adventures. Spring Hill has specially trained staff, adaptive transportation, and housing solutions ready to accommodate children with special needs. New Frontiers Camps are for youth grades 6-9. All Star Sports Campers play basketball, lacrosse, soccer, volleyball and hockey. All Star Sports includes basic level instruction, sport overviews, game fundamentals, skill drills and scrimmages.

810 Spring Hill Camps: New Frontiers English Horsemanship Camp
7717 95th Avenue
Evart, MI 49631
231-734-2616
FAX 866-332-5572
http://www.springhillcamps.com/MI/summercamp/
e-mail: register@springhillcamps.com
Todd Leinberger, Camp Director
Mike Krick, Facility Rental Coordinator
Danae Faber, Volunteer Coordinator
Spring Hill Camps is a youth camp program that offers extreme sports, exhilarating activities, and outdoor adventures. Spring Hill has specially trained staff, adaptive transportation, and housing solutions ready to accommodate children with special needs. New Frontiers Camps are for youth grades 6-9. English Horsemanship Campers will learn the basics on horse training, riding safety, grooming and more. Girls only. English Horsemanship requires horseback riding experience.

811 Spring Hill Camps: New Frontiers Golf Camp
7717 95th Avenue
Evart, MI 49631
231-734-2616
FAX 866-332-5572
http://www.springhillcamps.com/MI/summercamp/
e-mail: register@springhillcamps.com
Todd Leinberger, Camp Director
Mike Krick, Facility Rental Coordinator
Danae Faber, Volunteer Coordinator
Spring Hill Camps is a youth camp program that offers extreme sports, exhilarating activities, and outdoor adventures. Spring Hill has specially trained staff, adaptive transportation, and housing solutions ready to accommodate children with special needs. New Frontiers Camps are for youth grades 6-9. New Frontiers Golf Campers will get individual coaching while putting their skills to the test on the course in some real matches. Campers should bring their own clubs. Boys only.

812 **Spring Hill Camps: New Frontiers Outdoor Sportsman Camp**

7717 95th Avenue
Evart, MI 49631
231-734-2616
FAX 866-332-5572
http://www.springhillcamps.com/MI/summercamp/
e-mail: register@springhillcamps.com
Todd Leinberger, Camp Director
Mike Krick, Facility Rental Coordinator
Danae Faber, Volunteer Coordinator

Spring Hill Camps is a youth camp program that offers extreme sports, exhilarating activities, and outdoor adventures. Spring Hill has specially trained staff, adaptive transportation, and housing solutions ready to accommodate children with special needs. New Frontiers Camps are for youth grades 6-9. Outdoor Sportsman Campers will have the opportunity to try fly fishing, trap shooting, archery and riflery. Boys only.

813 **Spring Hill Camps: New Frontiers Paintball Camp**

7717 95th Avenue
Evart, MI 49631
231-734-2616
FAX 866-332-5572
http://www.springhillcamps.com/MI/summercamp/
e-mail: register@springhillcamps.com
Todd Leinberger, Camp Director
Mike Krick, Facility Rental Coordinator
Danae Faber, Volunteer Coordinator

Spring Hill Camps is a youth camp program that offers extreme sports, exhilarating activities, and outdoor adventures. Spring Hill has specially trained staff, adaptive transportation, and housing solutions ready to accommodate children with special needs. New Frontiers Camps are for youth grades 6-9. Paintball Campers will have their knowledge of paintball challenged, becoming part of a team and learning how communication, strategy and team work can take their paintball game to the extreme.

814 **Spring Hill Camps: New Frontiers Roller Hockey Camp**

7717 95th Avenue
Evart, MI 49631
231-734-2616
FAX 866-332-5572
http://www.springhillcamps.com/MI/summercamp/
e-mail: register@springhillcamps.com
Todd Leinberger, Camp Director
Mike Krick, Facility Rental Coordinator
Danae Faber, Volunteer Coordinator

Spring Hill Camps is a youth camp program that offers extreme sports, exhilarating activities, and outdoor adventures. Spring Hill has specially trained staff, adaptive transportation, and housing solutions ready to accommodate children with special needs. New Frontiers Camps are for youth grades 6-9. Roller Hockey Campers will brush up on their skills and learn some new ones while covering the game rules, learning strategy and competing in scrimmages and mini competitions.

815 **Spring Hill Camps: New Frontiers Tennis Camp**

7717 95th Avenue
Evart, MI 49631
231-734-2616
FAX 866-332-5572
http://www.springhillcamps.com/MI/summercamp/
e-mail: register@springhillcamps.com
Todd Leinberger, Camp Director
Mike Krick, Facility Rental Coordinator
Danae Faber, Volunteer Coordinator

Spring Hill Camps is a youth camp program that offers extreme sports, exhilarating activities, and outdoor adventures. Spring Hill has specially trained staff, adaptive transportation, and housing solutions ready to accommodate children with special needs. New Frontiers Camps are for youth grades 6-9. Tennis Campers learn performance strategies, get game fundamentals, learn to serve and do drills. Then through scrimmages, both doubles and singles games, campers play in competition. Girls only.

816 **Spring Hill Camps: New Frontiers The EdgeCamp**

7717 95th Avenue
Evart, MI 49631
231-734-2616
FAX 866-332-5572
http://www.springhillcamps.com/MI/summercamp/
e-mail: register@springhillcamps.com
Todd Leinberger, Camp Director
Mike Krick, Facility Rental Coordinator
Danae Faber, Volunteer Coordinator

Spring Hill Camps is a youth camp program that offers extreme sports, exhilarating activities, and outdoor adventures. Spring Hill has specially trained staff, adaptive transportation, and housing solutions ready to accommodate children with special needs. New Frontiers Camps are for youth grades 6-9. The Edge Campers get involved in group competitions, coed activities, solo time, evening events, live music, real live skits and much more! Additional activities include water skiing and kayaking.

817 **Spring Hill Camps: New Frontiers Volleyball Camp**

7717 95th Avenue
Evart, MI 49631
231-734-2616
FAX 866-332-5572
http://www.springhillcamps.com/MI/summercamp/
e-mail: register@springhillcamps.com
Todd Leinberger, Camp Director
Mike Krick, Facility Rental Coordinator
Danae Faber, Volunteer Coordinator

Spring Hill Camps is a youth camp program that offers extreme sports, exhilarating activities, and outdoor adventures. Spring Hill has specially trained staff, adaptive transportation, and housing solutions ready to accommodate children with special needs. New Frontiers Camps are for youth grades 6-9. Volleyball Campers will brush up their volleyball skills during the week at camp where they will learn the fundamentals and participate in friendly competition on the volleyball court. Girls only.

818 **Spring Hill Camps: New Frontiers Water Sports Camp**

7717 95th Avenue
Evart, MI 49631
231-734-2616
FAX 866-332-5572
http://www.springhillcamps.com/MI/summercamp/
e-mail: register@springhillcamps.com
Todd Leinberger, Camp Director
Mike Krick, Facility Rental Coordinator
Danae Faber, Volunteer Coordinator

Spring Hill Camps is a youth camp program that offers extreme sports, exhilarating activities, and outdoor adventures. Spring Hill has specially trained staff, adaptive transportation, and housing solutions ready to accommodate children with special needs. New Frontiers Camps are for youth grades 6-9. Water Sports Campers will water ski, tube, wakeboard, slalom ski and kneeboard their way through the week.

819 **Spring Hill Camps: Storybrook 1 Hour Horse Camp (Grades 1-3)**

7717 95th Avenue
Evart, MI 49631
231-734-2616
FAX 866-332-5572
http://www.springhillcamps.com/MI/summercamp/
e-mail: register@springhillcamps.com
Todd Leinberger, Camp Director
Mike Krick, Facility Rental Coordinator
Danae Faber, Volunteer Coordinator

Spring Hill Camps is a youth camp program that offers extreme sports, exhilarating activities, and outdoor adventures. Spring Hill has specially trained staff, adaptive transportation, and housing solutions ready to accommodate children with special needs. Storybrook 1 Hour Sport Horse Camp provides both veteran riders and rookies alike the opportunity to be totally involved in the riding experience, improving their techniques on trail rides and arena, learning horse care, feeding and grooming.

820 **Spring Hill Camps: Storybrook 1 Hour Sport Camp (Grades 1-3)**

7717 95th Avenue
Evart, MI 49631
231-734-2616
FAX 866-332-5572
http://www.springhillcamps.com/MI/summercamp/
e-mail: register@springhillcamps.com
Todd Leinberger, Camp Director
Mike Krick, Facility Rental Coordinator
Danae Faber, Volunteer Coordinator

Spring Hill Camps is a youth camp program that offers extreme sports, exhilarating activities, and outdoor adventures. Spring Hill has specially trained staff, adaptive transportation, and housing solutions ready to accommodate children with special needs. Storybrook Campers that register for the 1 Hour Sport Camp will have basic level instruction, sport overviews, game fundamentals, skill drills and scrimmages in addition to basketball, lacrosse, flag football, soccer, and hockey.

821 **Spring Hill Camps: Storybrook Explorer Camp**
7717 95th Avenue
Evart, MI 49631
231-734-2616
FAX 866-332-5572
http://www.springhillcamps.com/MI/summercamp/
e-mail: register@springhillcamps.com
Todd Leinberger, Camp Director
Mike Krick, Facility Rental Coordinator
Danae Faber, Volunteer Coordinator
Spring Hill Camps is a youth camp program that offers extreme sports, exhilarating activities, and outdoor adventures. Spring Hill has specially trained staff, adaptive transportation, and housing solutions ready to accommodate children with special needs. Storybrook Explorer Camp is for youngsters grades 1-3. Camp activities include boating, crafts, nature, and swimming.

822 **Spring Hill Camps: Storybrook Junior Explorer Camp**
7717 95th Avenue
Evart, MI 49631
231-734-2616
FAX 866-332-5572
http://www.springhillcamps.com/MI/summercamp/
e-mail: register@springhillcamps.com
Todd Leinberger, Camp Director
Mike Krick, Facility Rental Coordinator
Danae Faber, Volunteer Coordinator
Spring Hill Camps is a youth camp program that offers extreme sports, exhilarating activities, and outdoor adventures. Spring Hill has specially trained staff, adaptive transportation, and housing solutions ready to accommodate children with special needs. Storybrook Junior Explorer Camp is for youngsters grades 1-3. Junior Explorers will experience the fun of camp through skits and evening events in addition to boating, crafts, nature, and swimming.

Minnesota

823 **Camp Buckskin**
PO Box 389
Ely, MN 55731
218-365-2121
FAX 218-365-2880
http://www.campbuckskin.com
e-mail: buckskin@spacestar.net
Tom Bauer, Director

Buckskin operates a therapeutic summer program for youth with ADD/ADHD and related difficulties. We have two 32-day sessions which utilize a combination of traditional camp activities and academics (reading, writing, environmental education) to allow multiple successes which develop self-confidence and improves self-esteem. High staff to camper ratio provides individualized instruction. The program is supportive, yet provides adequate structure to improve social skills and peer relations.
1959Grade Range: Ages 6-18

824 **Camp Chi RhoChi Rho Center**
4842 Nicollet S
Minneapolis, MN 55419
612-827-7123
FAX 612-827-0574
http://www.chirhocenter.org
e-mail: sjchirho@aol.com
Jim Greenlee, Executive Director
Doug Johnson, Camp Manager
Morgan Hale, President/Board of Directors
A year round ecumenical retreat and conference center available for rental.

825 **Camp Confidence**
1620 Mary Fawcett Memorial Drive
East Gull Lake, MN 56401
218-828-2344
FAX 218-828-2618
http://www.campconfidence.com
e-mail: info@campconfidence.com
Jeff Olson, Executive Director
Shelli Fairone, Office Manager

A year-round center for persons with developmental disabilities specializing in recreation and outdoor education. Aimed at promoting self confidence and self esteem and the necessary skills to become full, contributing members of society.

826 **Camp Eden Wood**
Friendship Ventures
6350 Indian Chief Road
Eden Prairie, MN 55346
952-852-0101
800-450-8376
FAX 952-852-0123
http://www.friendshipventures.org
e-mail: fv@frientshipventures.org
Georgann Rumsey, President/CEO
John Kokula, Chair/Friendship Foundation
Ed Stracke, President/Friendship Foundation
Eden Wood is operated by Friendship Ventrues, a private non-profit agency that provides short-term, direct care services for children and adults with cognitive and other developmental disabilities. Traditional/specialty resident camp sessions, year round respite care for persons with or without disabilities. Beautiful 20-acre site on Birch Island Lake in Minnesota. Accessible modern cabins and dormitory housing, dining and welcome lodge, ropes challenge course indoor/outdoor recreation areas.

827 **Camp Friendship**
Friendship Ventures
10509 108th Street NW
Annandale, MN 55302
952-852-0101
800-450-8376
FAX 952-852-0123
http://www.friendshipventures.org
e-mail: fv@friendshipventures.org
Georgann Rumsey, President
John Kokula, Chair/Friendship Foundation
Ed Stracke, President/Friendship Foundation
A summer resident camp that is open to anyone five or older who has developmental and/or physical disabilities.

828 **Camp New Hope**
Friendship Ventures
53035 Lake Avenue
McGregor, MN 55760
952-852-0101
800-450-8376
FAX 952-852-0123
http://www.friendshipventures.org
e-mail: fv@friendshipventures.org
Georgann Rumsey, President
John Kokula, Chair/Friendship Foundation
Ed Stracke, President/Friendship Foundation
A summer resident camp that is open to anyone five or older who has developmental and/or physical disabilities.

829 **Camp Winnebago**
19708 Camp Winnebago Road
Caledonia, MN 55921
507-724-2351
FAX 507-724-3786
http://www.campwinnebago.org
e-mail: director@CampWinnebago.org
Theresa Burroughs, Executive Director
Cathy Greeley, Director
Al Fravert, Executive Commitee President
Individuals with developmental disabilities, six years of age and older, are eligable to attend Camp Winnebago. A variety of traditional summer camp activities abound: swimming, cooking over a fire, games, arts and crafts, hay-wagon rides, dancing and more. Activities are adapted to the age and ability of each camper to ensure maximum participation.

Missouri

830 **Wonderland Camp**
18591 Miller Circle
Rocky Mount, MO 65072
573-392-3605
FAX 573-392-3605
http://www.wonderlandcamp.org
e-mail: Info@wonderlandcamp.org
Marcella Trujillo, Program Director
Allen Moore, Chief Executive Officer
Ray Garrett, Maintenance Director

Wonderland Camp offers programs for campers of all ages and disabilities. Specialized events are planned for campers each week. All mentally and physically challenged individuals are encouraged to come and join the summer fun. At Wonderland Camp, campers will participate in various different activities such as swimming, boating, fishing, arts and crafts, recreation, nature, music and different games. Evening activities include dances, karaoke, pool parties, carnivals and various other events.

831 YMCA Camp Discovery

YMCA of Greater St. Louis
St. Louis, MO 63103 314-436-1177
FAX 314-436-1901
http://www.ymcastlouis.org/carondelet/daycamp
e-mail: metro@ymcastlouis.org

Kelly Grillo, Program Coordinator
Caroline Mitchell, Literacy Council
Debbie Redmond, Habilitation Council

Camp Discovery June 11 - August 17 at the Carondelet YMCA offers everything a summer needs - leadership, friendship, learning and fun. Including swimming, arts & crafts, sports, games and field trips there's something for everyone. There is a 1:12 counselor to camper ratio.

Nebraska

832 Camp Kitaki YMCA

6000 Cornhusker Highway
Lincoln, NE 68507 402-434-9225
FAX 402-434-9226
http://www.ymcalincoln.org/kitaki/
e-mail: campkitaki@ymcalincoln.org

Chris Klingenberg, District Executive Director
Russ Koos, Senior Program Director
Jason Smith, Associate Executive Director

A Christian camp for children with ADD and other disabilities. Archery, climbing, horseback riding, fishing and aquatic activities are some of the activities.

833 Easter Seals Nebraska

638 North 109th Plaza
Omaha, NE 68154 402-345-2200
800-650-9880
FAX 402-345-2500
http://http://ne.easterseals.com
e-mail: mtufte@ne.easter-seals.com

Mike Tufte, Camp Director/Coordinator
Joanne Schulte, Product Support

The following are camping and recreational services offered: Camp respite for adults, camp respite for children, camperships, recreational services for children and residential camping programs.

New Hampshire

834 Camp Calumet Lutheran Ministries

1090 Ossipee Lake Road
West Ossipee, NH 03890 603-539-4773
FAX 603-539-5343
http://www.calumet.org/contact.htm
e-mail: Nancy@Calumet.org

Nancy Hess, Executive Director
Karl Ogren, Director Children/Youth Programs
Paul Lindahl, Director Family/Adult Programs

Camp Calumet is for kids, adults, seniors, singles, church groups, families and the developmentally disabled.

835 Camp Kaleidoscope

City of Lebanon, NH
Lebanon, NH 03766 603-448-5121
FAX 603-448-1496
http://www.lebcity.com
e-mail: recreation@lebcity.com

Cindy Heath, Camp Director
Kevin Talcott, Assistant Camp Director
Paul Coats, Program Coordinator

Basic Camp is designed for ages 5-11. Arts & crafts, games/sports, trips to State parks and area attractions, environmental education and swimming lessons. Guaranteed fun with a qualified and enthusiastic staff. Leadership Camp is is designed for 12-13 years olds. Learn games leadership, communication skills, CPR/First Aid, and enjoy field trips and other fun camp activities. Team building through outdoor adventure, art and community service activities will be offered.

836 Camp Runels

Girl Scouts of Spar & Spindle Council
270 Gage Hill Road
Pelham, NH 03076 603-635-1662
FAX 603-635-2366
http://www.ssgsc.org/for_girls/camp_runels.html
e-mail: info@ssgsc.org

Judith Wise, Chief Executive Officer
Bonnie Batchelor, Chief Operating Officer
Jennifer VanBuren, Outdoor Program Specialist

General camping, aquatics, arts, drama, hiking, sailing and more.

837 Easter Seals New Hempshire

555 Auburn Street
Manchester, NH 03103 603-623-8863
800-870-8728
FAX 603-625-1148
http://www.eastersealsnh.org
e-mail: Eastersealsnh@eastersealsnh.org

Larry Gammon, President
Christine M McMahon, SVP/Chief Operating Officer
Elin A Treanor, SVP/Development & Communication

Easter Seals camping and recreation programs serve children, adults and families of all abilities. Various programs are available with the united purpose of giving disabled individuals a fun and safe camping or recreational experience. The following are camping and recreational services offered: Camp respite for adults, camperships, day camping for children, recreational services for children and residential camping programs.

New Jersey

838 Alpine Scout Camp

Boy Scout of America
441 Route 9W
Alpine, NJ 07620 201-768-1910
FAX 201-784-1663
http://www.alpinescoutcamp.org/#top
e-mail: bmadsen@alpinescoutcamp.org

Bob Madsen, Camp Director
Ken Hager, Region Chief
Randy Cline, Region Chairman

The Alpine Scout Camp is the primary site for all Cub Scout camping in the Greater New York area and is the location of the John E Reeves Cub World, Learning for Life Day Camp and also host the only Scout camp built for children with disabilities called Camp Kalikow.

839 Camp Excel

4041 Squankum Road
Allenwood, NJ 08720 732-281-0275
FAX 732-281-2363
http://www.campexcel.com
e-mail: info@campexcel.com

Kathleen M Cable, Camp Director

Camp Excel is a comprehensive program that includes academics to promote growth and avoid regression over the summer months, therapeutic activities to assist in making friends and keeping friends, sports to develop skills and build self-esteem and recreational activities just for fun. Throughout the day, staff members provide encouragement and guidance in using appropriate social skills, giving the children the opportunity to experience in the moment learning, learning that stays with them.

840 **Camp Tikvah**
Jewish Community Center on the Palisades
411 E Clinton Avenue
Tenafly, NJ 07670
201-569-7900
FAX 201-569-7448
http://www.jcconthepalisades.org
e-mail: info@jccotp.org
Avi A Lewinson, Executive Director
Sue Gelsey, Chief Operating Officer
Carol Lesley, Programming Director
Camp Tikvah is designed to meet the special needs of children and adolescents who have been classified with mild neurological and/or perceptual impairment.

841 **Easter Seals Camp Merry Heart**
21 O'Brien Road
Hackettstown, NJ 07840
908-852-3896
FAX 908-852-9263
http://www.eastersealnj
e-mail: ahumanick@nj.easter-seals.org
Alexander Humanick, Executive Director
Mary Simpson, Office Manager

Easter Seals camping and recreation programs serve children, adults and families of all abilities. Various programs are available with the united purpose of giving disabled individuals a fun and safe camping or recreational experience. The following are camping and recreational services offered: Camp respite for adults, camperships, canoeing, day camping for children, recreational services for adults and residential camping programs.

842 **Elks Camp Moore**
New Jersey Elks Association
PO Box 375
Pompton Lakes, NJ 07442
973-835-1542
FAX 973-835-4125
TDY:609-271-0138
http://www.njelks.org/index.php
e-mail: elkscampmoore@aol.com
Todd Garmer, Manager
Laurie Miller, Assistant Director
Anthony Alfonso, Facilities Director
Elks Camp Moore offers a fun filled vacation away from home for children with special needs. A week at Elks Camp Moore is a remarkable experience not soon to be fogotten. The primary goal of the camp is to further develop the recreational and social skills of each child. In a relaxed and accepting atmosphere, each camper experiences new adventures, lasting friendships, and opportunities that promote independence and greater self-confidence.

843 **Fairview Lake YMCA Camp**
1035 Lakeview Road
Newton, NJ 07860
973-383-9282
FAX 973-383-6386
http:////metroymcas.org/html/fairview_lake.cfm
e-mail: fairviewlake@metroymcas.org
Ellie Daingerfield, Executive Director
Marc Koch, Summer Camp Director
Steven Michaelis, Facility Manager
Fairview Lake YMCA Camps is committed to providing the most fun, safe, positive experience, possible for everyone. In addition to having a great time, the goal is to develop leadership, bridge racial gaps, develop an appreciation for the outdoors, promote physical fitness, foster teamwork, and develop techniques for resolving conflict. The Fairview Lake Experience gives birth to life-long friendships, self-discovery, and a home away from home.

844 **Harbor Haven Camp**
1155 W Chestnut Street
Union, NJ 07083
908-964-5411
FAX 908-964-0511
http://www.harborhaven.com
e-mail: info@harborhaven.com
Robyn Tanne, Executive Director
Skip Vichness, Executive Director

Harbor Haven Camp is a 7 week co-ed summer program for 3-15 year olds with mild to moderate special needs. Harbor Haven provides continuous opportunities for each child to grow, explore, develop new skills and form friendships, all within a safe, nurturing and accepting environment. Harbor Haven serves as a bridge between one school year and the next, offering a valuable way to prevent regression in children with learning issues.

845 **Harbor Hills Day Camp**
75 Doby Road
Mount Freedom, NJ 07970
973-895-3200
FAX 973-895-7239
http://www.hhdc.com
e-mail: info@hhdc.com
Herb Tanaenbaum, President
Robyn Tanny, Executive Director
Chris Marangon, Assistant Director
A seven-week, co-ed day camp for children ages 5-15 with special needs. Provides a nurturing and supportive summer. The camp is oriented towards youngsters with learning disabilities and/or attention deficit disorders. It may also be appropriate for children with other types of learning challenges.

846 **Round Lake Camp**
21 Plymouth Street
Fairfield, NJ 07004
973-575-3333
FAX 973-575-4188
http://www.roundlakecamp.org/
e-mail: rlc@njycamps.org
David Friedman, Camp Director

A camp for children who have been identified with ADD, and/or mild social disorders.

New Mexico

847 **Easter Seals New Mexico**
Cousins Road
Vanderwagen, NM 87326
707-480-8154
800-279-5261
http://www.campisfun.org/newmexico/index.html
e-mail: janecarres@aol.com
Jane Carr, Camp Director

Camp Easter Seals New Mexico provides fun for children and adults with disabilities. Its unique combination of comfortable accessible facilities and energetic, outgoing staff offers a fun, exciting, summer experience with memories to last a lifetime. Camp Easter Seals is held at Kamp Kiwanis' site, located in Vanderwagen, New Mexico.

New York

848 **Camp Dunnabeck at Kildonan School**
425 Morse Hill Road
Amenia, NY 12501
845-373-8111
FAX 845-373-2004
http://www.kildonan.org
e-mail: admissions@kildonan.org
Ronald Wilson, Principal
Bonnie Wilson, Admissions Director
Robert Lane, Academic Dean
Specializes in helping intelligent children with specific reading, writing and spelling disabilities. Provides Orton-Gillingham tutoring with camp activities, including swimming, sailing, waterskiing, horseback riding, ceramics, tennis and woodworking.

849 **Camp HASC**
5902 14th Avenue
Brooklyn, NY 11219
718-686-5930
FAX 718-686-5935
http://www.camphasc.org/
e-mail: office@camphasc.org
Rabbi Stern, Executive Director
Avi Sacks, Program Director
Chaya Miller, Camp Administrator
Provides over 300 mentally and physcially handicapped children and adults with the opportunity to enjoy a seven week sleep away camp experience.

1964

850 **Camp Huntington**

56 Bruceville Road
High Falls, NY 12440
845-687-7840
FAX 845-687-7211
http://www.camphuntington.com/
e-mail: dfalk@camphuntington.com

Bruria Bodek Falik Ph.D, Executive Director Emeritus
Daniel Falk, Executive Director
Harvey Goodman, Operations/Program Supervisor

For boys and girls with learning disabilities and developmental disabilities, ADD and PDD.

851 **Camp Jened**

Cerebral Palsy Association of NY
New York, NY 10001
845-434-2220
FAX 845-434-2253
http://www.campjened.org
e-mail: campjened@pronetisp.net

Sue Ann Minister, Camp Director
Thomas Mandelkow, EVP/CAO/CFO NY Cerebral Palsy
Duane Schielke, EVP/COO NY Cerebral Palsy

Jened Recreation Village (JRV) is an outdoor camping and recreation facility located in the Catskill Mountains near Rock Hill, New York. It offers a variety of residential camping or travel options to adults with developmental and physical disabilities including those with moderate to severe disabilities. Growth through self-awareness is stressed along with active participation in numerous leisure activities such as swimming and aquatic therapy, crafts, music, and sports.

852 **Camp Kehilla**

Sid Jacobson Jewish Community Center
300 Forest Drive
Greenvale, NY 11548
516-484-1545
FAX 516-484-7354
http://http://sfysummercamps.org/kehilla.htm
e-mail: MPlotkin@sfy.org

David Slotnick MSW, Camp Director
Marisa Plotkin, Camp Coordinator
Paul Isserles, Program Coordinator

A summer day camp for high functioning children and teens with minimal learning disabilities, speech and language delays and ADHD.

853 **Camp Northwood**

132 State Route 365
Remsen, NY 13438
315-831-3621
FAX 315-831-5867
http://www.nwood.com
e-mail: northwoodprograms@hotmail.com

Gordon Felt, Camp Director/President/Co-Owner
Donna Felt, Co-Director/Co-Owner

Camp Northwood provides programming to a coed population of 165 children in need of structure and individualization, ranging in age from 8-18 that experience difficulties in social and academic settings due to a variety of types of learning challenges.

854 **Camp Pa-Qua-Tuck**

PO Box 677
Center Moriches, NY 11934
631-878-1070
FAX 631-878-2596
http://www.camppaquatuck.com
e-mail: camppaquatuck@optonline.net

Gary Nagle PhD, Camp Director
Thomas Chieffo, President/Board of Directors
Kevin Spellman, VP/Board of Directors

Handicapped children experience the joys of boating, fishing, campfires and more. In a supportive, enriching environment they are encouraged to reach beyond the limits of their handicaps and join with their fellow campers in activities designed to enhance their lives.

855 **Camp Sunshine-Camp Elan**

Mosholu-Montefiore Community Center
3450 Dekalb Avenue
Bronx, NY 10467
718-882-4000
FAX 718-882-6369
http://www.mmcc.org/daycamp.html
e-mail: daycamp@mmcc.org OR info@mmcc.org

Donald Bluestone, Executive Director
Lee Sheiman, Operations Director
Mike Halpern, Country Day Camp Director

Serves children who are intellectually limited, emotionally impaired and/or demonstrate special learning disabilities.

856 **Clover Patch Camp**

Glenville, NY 12302
518-384-3080
FAX 518-384-3001
http://www.cloverpatchcamp.org
e-mail: cloverpatchcamp@cfdsny.org

Laura Taylor, Camp Director
Christopher Schelin, Camp Program Administrator

Clover Patch is a summer camp for individuals with disabilities where each camper is encouraged to reach his or her fullest potential. Since 1965, Clover Patch Camp has provided individuals with disabilities opportunities to make new friends, create everlasting memories, and experience a genuine camp setting. Camp activities include arts and crafts, music and drama, sports and recreation, parades and magicians.

857 **Coda's Day Camp**

Community Opportunity Development Agency
564 Thomas S Boyland Street
Brooklyn, NY 11212
718-345-4779

Emil DeLoache MD, Executive Director

858 **Cross Island YMCA Day Camp**

238-10 Hillside Avenue
Bellerose, NY 11426
718-479-0505
FAX 718-465-1665
http://www.ymcanyc.org
e-mail: kjohnson@ymcanyc.org

Karen Johnson-Radigan, Camp Coordinator
Pat Matos, Camp Coordinator/Early Childhood

Day camp offers opportunity to improve self esteem through age appropriate, structured activities and trips.

859 **Easter Seals Albany**

Easter Seals New York
292 Washington Avenue Extension
Albany, NY 12203
518-456-4880
800-727-8785
FAX 518-456-5094
http://http://ny.easterseals.com
e-mail: info@ny.easter-seals.org

Carrie Taylor, Development Director
John W McGrath, VP/Organizational Development

Easter Seals camping and recreation programs serve children, adults and families of all abilities. Various programs are available with the united purpose of giving disabled individuals a fun and safe camping or recreational experience. The following are camping and recreational services offered: Camp respite for children, camperships, day camping for children and recreational services for children.

860 **Easter Seals East Rochester**

International Easter Seals
349 W Commercial Street
East Rochester, NY 14445
585-264-9550
800-727-8785
FAX 585-264-9547
http://www.ny.easterseals.com
e-mail: info@ny.easter-seals.org

Larry Gammon, President
Michael Donneloy, Vice President
Lori Venderhoof, Executive Director

Easter Seals camping and recreation programs serve children, adults and families of all abilities. Various programs are available with the united purpose of giving disabled individuals a fun and safe camping or recreational experience. The following are camping and recreational services offered: Recreational services for children.

861 **GAP Summer Program**

Syosset/Woodbury Community Park
977 Hicksville Road
Massapequa, NY 11758
516-797-7900
FAX 516-797-7919
http://www.oysterbaytown.com

Mary Ryan, Director
Mary Hurst, Assistant Director
Bruce Foley, Manager
A program for children with mental and learning disabilities.

862 GOW Summer Programs
2491 Emery Road
South Wales, NY 14139
716-652-3450
FAX 716-652-3457
http://www.gow.org
e-mail: summer@gow.org
David Mendlewski, Summer Program Director
Gayle Hutton, Director of Development
Robert Garcia, Admissions Director
For boys and girls who have experienced past academic difficulties and have learning differences but possess the potential for success. The five week co-educational Gow School Summer Program (GSSP) serves students ages 8-16. Academic classes are combined with traditional camp activities and weekend trips.

863 Harlem Branch YWCA Summer Day Camp
Harlem YMCA/Jackie Robinson Youth Center
181 West 135th Street
New York, NY 10030
212-283-8570
FAX 212-283-2809
http://www.ymcanyc.org/harlem
e-mail: adharris@ymcanyc.org
Elaine Edmonds, Sr Executive Director
A D Harris, Summer Camp Director

The Harlem YMCA offers an array of activities designed to give campers the opportunity to improve their skills and develop new ones. The Y camping curriculum includes an emphasis on values, sportsmanship, teamwork and friendship. Campers can participate in activities designed to challenge their skills and expand their knowledge. In addition to traditional sports, campers can learn newsletter publishing, dance, computer technology, ecology, fitness and sports.

864 Hillside Summer Camp: Adventure Camp
400 Doansburg Road
Brewster, NY 10509
845-279-2995
FAX 845-279-3077
http://www.hillsidesummercamp.org
e-mail: bkorson@greenchimneys.org
Beth Korson, Camp Director
Duncan Lester, Director Educational Services

The Adventure Camp is committed to providing young people with a fun, safe and positive outdoor program where they can learn about themselves, others and the environment. The design of each program is based on the belief that learning comes most naturally in a fun, supportive, and noncompetitive environment. The program focus is on adventure challenges to create personal growth and development of skills that are useful throughout the camper's life. Girls and boys ages 10 - 15 yrs.

865 Hillside Summer Camp: Blazers Camp
400 Doansburg Road
Brewster, NY 10509
845-279-2995
FAX 845-279-3077
http://www.hillsidesummercamp.org
e-mail: bkorson@greenchimneys.org
Beth Korson, Camp Director
Duncan Lester, Director Educational Services

The Blazers Camp Program is designed as a place to learn, grow, make friends and have fun, offering the child many positive and rewarding experiences. Blazers Camp provides an opportunity to develop activity-oriented and interpersonal skills while offering children a chance to become more responsible and independent. A variety of activities are available including environmental awareness, horticulture, playground, pony rides, swim lessons, and special events. Girls and boys ages 8 - 10 yrs.

866 Hillside Summer Camp: Trackers Camp
400 Doansburg Road
Brewster, NY 10509
845-279-2995
FAX 845-279-3077
http://www.hillsidesummercamp.org
e-mail: bkorson@greenchimneys.org
Beth Korson, Camp Director
Duncan Lester, Director Educational Services

The Trackers Camp Program is designed as a place to learn, grow, make friends and have fun, offering the child many positive and rewarding experiences. Trackers Camp provides an opportunity to develop activity-oriented and interpersonal skills while offering children a chance to become more responsible and independent. A variety of activities are available including archery, arts and crafts, canoeing, ceramics, hiking, music, water adventures and wood crafts. Girls and boys ages 11 - 15 yrs.

867 Hillside Summer Camp: Trailblazers Camp
400 Doansburg Road
Brewster, NY 10509
845-279-2995
FAX 845-279-3077
http://www.hillsidesummercamp.org
e-mail: bkorson@greenchimneys.org
Beth Korson, Camp Director
Duncan Lester, Director Educational Services

The Trailblazers Camp Program is designed as a place to learn, grow, make friends and have fun, offering the child many positive and rewarding experiences. Trailblazers Camp provides an opportunity to develop activity-oriented and interpersonal skills while offering children a chance to become more responsible and independent. A variety of activities are available including grandparents luncheon, mini adventures, Native American culture, sand castles and story time. Girls and boys ages 5 - 8.

868 Jimmy Vejar Day Camp
United Cerebral Palsy of Westchester
David G Osterer Center
Rye Brook, NY 10573
914-937-3800
FAX 914-937-0967
http://www.cpwestchester.org/agencyservices.asp
e-mail: Jimmy.Vejardc@cpwestchester.org
Annabelle Strozza, Director of Children Services
Linda Kuck, Executive Director
Judy Katzen, Associate Executive Director
The camp is open to children and young adults with disabilities ages 4 to 21, and to children without disabilities, ages 4 to 7. Campers are grouped by age so they can fully enjoy age-appropiate activities and an enriching summer camp experience.

869 Kamp Kiwanis
NY District Kiwanis Foundation
9020 Kiwanis Road
Taberg, NY 13471
315-336-4568
FAX 315-336-3845
http://www.kiwanis-ny.org/kamp
e-mail: kamp@kiwanis-ny.org
Nelson Tucker, Kiwanis International President
Rebecca Lopez, Executive Director

Serves youths with many forms of disabilities to include ADD, autism, and learning disabilities.

870 MAC Mainstreaming at Camp
Frost Valley YMCA
460 W 34th Street
New York, NY 10001
212-273-6298
FAX 212-273-6161
http://www.frostvalley.org/ www.yai.org/
e-mail: campdirector@frostvalley.org jmedler@yai.org
Joe Medler, Camp Director

MAC is designed to serve children with developmental disabilities and to promote inclusion into the broader camp community.

871 Maplebrook School
5142 Route 22
Amenia, NY 12501
845-373-8191
FAX 845-373-7029
http://www.maplebrookschool.org
e-mail: admissions@maplebrookschool.org
Roger Fazzone, President/CEO
Jennifer Scully, Admissions Director
Lori Hale, Director of Development
Academic instruction is given in the morning hours of each weekday and afternoon hours are filled with culturally enriching classes in drama, dance and art.

872 Mid Island Y JCC Summer Camps: Camp Junior Plus

45 Manetto Hill Road
Plainview, NY
516-822-3535
FAX 516-822-3288
http://www.miyjcc.org
e-mail: miyjcc.org@aol.com

Sheryl Kirschenbaum, Camp Director
Laurie Guttenberg, Camp Unit Leader

The Mid Island Y JCC offers a wide variety of social, cultural, recreational and educational activities for people of all ages. Camp Junior Plus is for children with special needs, ages kindergarten through 4th grade. A typical camp day with a camper/counselor ratio of 3:1. Full Session (6/28-8/17). Session I (6/28-7/24) or Session II (7/25-8/17).

873 New Country Day Camp

Educational Alliance
197 E Broadway
New York, NY 10002
212-533-0078
FAX 212-979-1225
http://www.edalliance.org
e-mail: info@edalliance.org

Jessica Wolf, Director
Miriam Matowitz, Chief Operating Officer
Lynn Appelbaum, Chief Program Officer

Clients must be toilet trained. A special program for teens and young adults emphasizes independent living skills and prevocational training.

874 Parkside School

48 W 74th Street
New York, NY 10023
212-721-8888
FAX 212-721-1547
http://www.parksideschool.org/flash.html
e-mail: parksideschool@parksideschool.org

Alison Lankenau, Program & Placement Director
Christine Hayden, Director of Development
Thomas Casey, Facility Manager

A New York State chartered, not-for-profit school established in 1986 for children with language-based learning problems in the New York City area. An educational setting that promotes active participation in learning.

875 Pioneer Camp and Retreat Center

9324 Lakeshore Road
Angola, NY 14006
716-549-1420
FAX 716-549-6018
http://www.pioneercamp.org
e-mail: info@pioneercamp.org

Jeff Blair, Operations Director
Beth Niermann, Camp Director
Suan Brese, Chairman

Offers a variety of activities for growing in faith and in service towards one another. Children, teens, adults and seniors are welcome all summer.

876 Queens Camp Smile (REACH)

80-30 Parkland Q Gardens
Kew Gardens, NY 11415
718-699-4213
FAX 718-699-4243
TDY:718-699-4213
http://www.nycgovparks.org
e-mail: alwilliams@nyc.gov/parks

Dorothy Lewandowski, Borough Commissioner
Al Williams, Director
Iris Rodriguez Rosa, Chief of Recreation

Parks runs summer camp programs in recreation centers citywide from early July through late August for children ages 5-13 (age range varies at each site). Programs include arts & crafts, sports, computers, field trips and more.

877 Samuel Field/Bay Terrace YM & YWHA Special Services

58-20 Little Neck Parkway
Little Neck, NY 11362
718-225-6750
FAX 718-423-8276
http://http://sfysummercamps.org/special.htm
e-mail: SamFieldY@aol.com

David Slotnick MSW, Camp Director
Marisa Plotkin CSW, Camp Coordinator

Day camps specialize in serving children who have developmental disabilities 5-21 years old. Younger campers enjoy the center-based Childhood Program where they swim, play in the gym, cook, dance, as well as share arts and crafts activities and music. Activities for older campers include swimming, nature fun, an overnight at the Little Neck Site, community field trips, as well as a wide variety of specialty activities, such as drama, music, sports and arts and crafts.

878 School Vacation Camps: Youth with Developmental Disabilities

YWCA of White Plains-Central Westchester
515 N Street
White Plains, NY 10605
914-949-6227
FAX 914-949-8903
http://www.ywca.whiteplains.org
e-mail: jkrentsa@ywcawhiteplains.com

Amy Kohn, Chief Executive Officer
Jeff Krentsa, Facilities Director
Jim Adasek, Information Services Director

Camp for people with developmental disabilities.

879 Shield Summer Play Program

Shield Institute
14461 Roosevelt Avenue
Flushing, NY 11354
718-939-8700
FAX 718-961-7669
http://www.shield.org
e-mail: webmaster@shield.org ecohen@shield.org

Helen Berman, Director
Susan Provenzanao, Administrator
Eileen Cohen, Principal

The School Program provides a school for children, adolescents, and young adults, ages 6 to 21, who have been diagnosed with either mental retardation or other developmental disabilities. The program provides special education and related services based on each student's skills and potential for independence. Instruction focuses on developing and enhancing skills in community, recreational, and vocational settings. Year-round services are available.

880 Summit Camp

Summit Travel
18 E 41st Street
New York, NY 10017
212-689-3880
800-323-9908
FAX 212-689-4347
http://www.summitcamp.com
e-mail: info@summitcamp.com

Mayer Stiskin, Executive Director
Ninette Stiskin, Assistant to Executive Director
Eugene Bell, Associate Director

Summit offers co-ed 4 week and 8 week programs, along with a 10 day Mini-Camp, providing many camp activities that feature a heated swimming pool, complete lake activities, climbing wall, go-karts, computer labs, adventure programs, field trips, etc. The programs and staffing are tailored to the needs of the children dealing with social/emotional challenges, Aspergers, Tourette's, Non-verbal LD, Bipolar Disorder. The camp serves 300 children and provides a staff of 270.

881 Trailblazers at JCC Camp Discovery

RR 129
Croton on Hudson, NY 10520
914-741-0333
FAX 914-741-6150
http://www.rosenthaljcc.org
e-mail: tom@rosenthaljcc.org

Tom Naviglia, Camp Director
Audrey Ronis-Tobin, Communications & Marketing
Ellie Aronowitz Witke, Administrative Director

Located on 19 acres of scenic woodland, the Trailblazers program at Camp Discovery offers swimming, sports, arts and crafts, music, drama and Jewish culture for children with special needs in an integrated environment.

882 Willow Hill Farm Camp

75 Cassidy Road
Keeseville, NY 12944
518-834-9746
FAX 518-834-9746
http://www.willowhillfarm.com
e-mail: julie@willowhillfarm.com

Julie Edwards, Co-Director
Gerald Edwards, Co-Director

Come to Willow Hill to experience a complete immersion into the world of Horses. From dawn to dusk, horses come first. Experience all the joys and fantasies of horse lovers including learning to post and canter, galloping in the field over jumps, riding the mountain trails, and competing in horse shows. Camp Willow is situated on 500 acres in the beautiful AuSable River Valley in the Adirondacks of upstate New York. Accepts 32 resident campers and 5 day campers per session.

883 Winston Prep School Summer Program

New York, NY 10011
646-638-2705
FAX 646-638-2706
http://www.winstonprep.edu/Welcome.html
e-mail: bsugerman@winstonprep.edu.

Beth Sugarman, Operations & Research Director
Elizabeth Tauber, Focus Program Director
Courtney DeHoff, Admissions Director

For 6th through 12th grade students with learning differences such as dyslexia, nonverbal learning disabilities, expressive or receptive language disorders and attention deficit problems. The Summer Enrichment Program at their New York City branch school is designed to enhance academic skills. Students from area parochial, public and private schools attend the program every year. They receive daily one-on-one instruction in addition to attending class in the courses they have selected.

884 YAI/Rockland County Association for the Learning Disabled (YAI/RCALD)

2 Crosfield Avenue
West Nyack, NY 10994
845-353-4344
FAX 845-358-6119
http://www.yai.org/
e-mail: nsilverman@yai.org

Melissa Yu, MD, Chief Executive Officer
Norman Silverman, Deputy Director
Trish Austin, Communications Specialist

YAI/RCALD conducts a wide variety of programs, supervised by experienced and professional staff, designed to build life skills, promote self-esteem, provide information exchange and offer other support services for individuals with learning and other developmental disabilities. The programs include, vocational evaluation and placements, recreational, residential, camping, service coordination and support groups.

North Carolina

885 Discovery Camp

Talisman Programs
Zirconia, NC 28790
828-697-6313
888-458-8226
FAX 828-697-6249
http://www.talismancamps.com/discovery.html
e-mail: info@talismancamps.com

Linda Tatsapauagh, Camp Director
Aaron McGinley, Base Camp Program Manager
Pete Weiss, Program Manager

Discovery Camp is a 2-week program designed for children ages 8-11, who may have ADD, learning disabilities, or experiencing some social anxiety. The activity packed schedule and 1:2.5 staff-camper ratio allows campers to have a positive experience at camp. In a nurturing yet structured environment, campers are challenged to become more independent and outgoing within the emotionally and physically safe setting that small group living provides. A good introduction to camp for younger kids.

886 Explorers Camp

Talisman Programs
Zirconia, NC 28790
828-697-6313
888-458-8226
FAX 828-697-6249
http://www.talismancamps.com/jrTrek.html
e-mail: info@talismancamps.com

Linda Tatsapauagh, Camp Director
Aaron McGinley, Base Camp Program Manager
Pete Weiss, Program Manager

Explorers Camp is for younger teens, ages 12-14, who are looking for an off-campus challenge. Explorers learn the value of self and group-reliance as they build the skills to accomplish their journey. This translates to increased self-confidence and independence. The targeted goal of completing the hike promotes advancement in focus, goal-setting and completion, and internal motivation.

887 Foundations Camp

Talisman Programs
Zirconia, NC 28790
828-697-6313
888-458-8226
FAX 828-697-6249
http://www.talismancamps.com/baseCamp.html
e-mail: info@talismancamps.com

Linda Tatsapauagh, Camp Director
Aaron McGinley, Base Camp Program Manager
Pete Weiss, Program Manager

Foundations Camp is co-educational accepting children ages 9-13 who have been diagnosed with LD, ADD, ADHD, and mild behavior issues. Participants live on campus in rustic cabins participating in a variety of activities designed to promote better communication and cooperation skills. Limited enrollment helps to facilitate an extended-family environment. The 2.5 to 1 camper-to-staff ratio ensures that no child is lost in the crowd and that each camper receives the attention he or she deserves.

888 SOAR Camp

226 Soar Lane
Balsam, NC 28707
828-456-3435
FAX 828-456-3449
http://www.soarnc.org
e-mail: admissions@soarnc.org

Jonathan Jones, Executive Director
John Wilson, Director
Ed Parker, Admissions Director

Features success-oriented, high-adventure programs for learning disabled and ADD preteens, teens and adults. Emphasis is placed on developing self-confidence, social skills, problem-solving techniques, a willingness to attempt new challenges and the motivation that comes through successful goal orientation.

889 Talisman Summer Camp

64 Gap Creek Road
Zirconia, NC 28790
828-669-8639
888-458-8226
http://www.talismanprograms.com
e-mail: info@talismancamps.com

Linda Tatsapaugh Director
Pete Weiss, Program Manager
Aaron McGinley, Base Camp Manager

Includes three programs for children with learning disabilities, high functioning Autism and Asperger's Snydrome.

890 Wilderness Experience

Ashe County 4-H
134 Government Circle
Jefferson, NC 28640
336-219-2650
FAX 336-229-2682
http://www.nc4h.org/centers/
e-mail: vickie_moore@ncsu.edu

Julie Landry, Executive Director
Vickie Moore, Assistant Director

The type of 4-H Camp program operating in North Carolina offers campers a greater chance to learn, develop life skills and form attitudes that will help them to become self-directing and productive members of society. At camp, youth focus on subjects that might be difficult to handle at home due to need for special equipment. Camp then becomes a learning laboratory that allows youth to apply their new knowledge to real-life situations.

Ohio

891 Akron Rotary Camp

4460 Rex Lake Drive
Akron, OH 44319
330-644-4512
FAX 330-644-1013
http://www.akronymca.org
e-mail: rotarycamp@akronymca.org

Dan Reynolds, Camp Director
Melissa Roddy, YMCA Executive Director

Rotary Camp was founded in 1924 with the purpose of providing children with special needs a place to spend their summers - a place where disabilities and limits do not hold kids back. Children ages 6-17 and who have physical or developmental disabilities are eligible to participate in this fun-filled camping experience.

892 **Camp Allyn**
1414 Camp Allyn Road
Batavia, OH 45103
513-831-4660
FAX 513-831-5918
http:////steppingstonescenter.org/services.htm
e-mail: ssc@steppingstonescenter.org
Chris Brockman, Camp Director
Sam Browne, Personnel Director

Weekend residential programming, sponsored by Stepping Stones Center, suitable for children, teens, and adults with disabilities, offered twice a month, providing a respite for both camper and family as well as a place to spend time with friends, play games, participate in arts and crafts projects, attend cookouts and campfires and outdoor exploration under the supervision of a qualified and dedicated staff.

893 **Camp Campbell Gard**
4803 Augspurger Road
Hamilton, OH 45011
513-867-0600
877-224-9622
FAX 513-867-0127
http://www.ccgymca.org/Special_Needs.html
e-mail: sexstone@gmvYMCA.org
Jim Sexstone, Executive Director
Tom Dearth, Facilities Director
Luke Ogonek, Outdoor Program Director
Camp Campbell Gard ofers a program for those campers ages 6-18 with special needs. These sessions are designed to give campers with a wide variety of special needs an opportunity to participate in summer camp activities alongside their peers. Campers select morning activities together with the Junior Explorer and Senior Camper programs at camp while participating in cabin-centered activities in the afternoon. Camp activities include hiking, swimming, crafts, sports, and horseback riding.

894 **Camp Cheerful: Achievement Center for Children**
15000 Cheerful Lane
Strongsville, OH 44136
440-238-6200
FAX 440-238-1858
http://www.achievementcenters.org
e-mail: tim.fox@achievementctrs.org
Tim Fox, Executive Director
Sally Farwell, Program Coordinator

Children ages 5 and older with and without special needs can enjoy all that Camp Cheerful has to offer in a day camp setting. Cheerful Day Camp includes all the activities of the traditional camp sessions, including swimming, horseback riding, archery, nature study, sports, canoeing and much more.

895 **Camp Echoing Hills**
Echoing Hills Village
Warsaw, OH 43844
740-327-2311
800-419-6513
FAX 740-327-6371
http://www.echoinghillsvillage.org/new/home.php
e-mail: ckuhns@echoinghillsvillage.org
Christy Kuhns, Camp Program Director
Larry Stitt, Camp Administrator
Lauren Samuel, Camp Activities Coordinator
Camp Echoing Hills is a ministry of Echoing Hills Village, which specializes in providing various programs for individuals with developmental disabilities in six locations across Ohio and Ghana West Africa. Camp Echoing Hills provides a safe and encouraging residential camping experience where campers develop friendships, skills and life-long memories.

896 **Camp Happiness at Corde Campus**
Catholic Charities Disability Services
7911 Detroit Avenue
Cleveland, OH 44102
216-334-2945
FAX 216-334-2905
http://www.clevelandcatholiccharities.org/
e-mail: contactus@clevelandcatholiccharities.org
Dennis McNulty, Director
Marilyn Scott, Program Administrator

A summer camp program for persons with developmental disabilities, Camp Happiness is a six-week day camp offered at several sites throughout the Diocese of Cleveland that provides educational, social and recreational services to children and adults with developmental disabilities during the summer months. See Website for detailed information at: http://www.clevelandcatholiccharities.org/ccpcm/happiness.htm.

897 **Camp Happiness at St. Augustine**
Catholic Charities Disability Services
7911 Detroit Avenue
Cleveland, OH 44102
216-334-2945
FAX 216-334-2905
http://www.clevelandcatholiccharities.org/
e-mail: contactus@clevelandcatholiccharities.org
Dennis McNulty, Director
Marilyn Scott, Program Administrator

A summer camp program for persons with developmental disabilities, Camp Happiness is a six-week day camp offered at several sites throughout the Diocese of Cleveland that provides educational, social and recreational services to children and adults with developmental disabilities during the summer months. See Website for additional information at: http://www.clevelandcatholiccharities.org/ccpcm/happiness.htm.

898 **Camp Happiness at St. Joseph Center**
Catholic Charities Disability Services
7911 Detroit Avenue
Cleveland, OH 44102
216-334-2945
FAX 216-334-2905
http://www.clevelandcatholiccharities.org/
e-mail: contactus@clevelandcatholiccharities.org
Dennis McNulty, Director
Marilyn Scott, Program Administrator

A summer camp program for persons with developmental disabilities, Camp Happiness is a six-week day camp offered at several sites throughout the Diocese of Cleveland that provides educational, social and recreational services to children and adults with developmental disabilities during the summer months. See Website for additional information at: http://www.clevelandcatholiccharities.org/ccpcm/happiness.htm.

899 **Camp Nuhop**
404 Hillcrest Drive
Ashland, OH 44805
419-289-2227
FAX 419-289-2227
http://www.campnuhop.org
e-mail: campnuhop@zoominternet.net
Jerry Dunlap, Co-Executive Director
Terrie Dunlap, Co-Executive Director
Trevor Dunlap, Associate Executive Director
A residential camp for all children with learning disabilities, attention deficit disorders and behavior disorders.

900 **Camp O'BannonCenter for Service Learning at Denison Community Assoc.**
Neward, OH 43055
740-345-8295
FAX 740-349-5093
http://denison.edu/campuslife/servicelearning/
Ted Cobb, Camp Director
Roberta Larson, Community Service Director
Jenny Orten, Big Brothers & Big Sisters
Camp O'Bannon provides a summer residential camp experience free of charge to referred children from Licking County. The majority of the children come from disadvantaged and/or at-risk homes. Summer camp starts the second week in June and continues for 10 weeks. For children aged 9-13, there are four 2-week sessions and two 1-week sessions in the regular camp. For teens 14-16 there are five 2-week sessions at Outpost, a separate camp. Activities include art, music, drama, and nature lore.

901 Camp Oty Okwa: Special Care Camp
Big Brothers Big Sisters of Central Ohio
1855 E Dublin Granville Road
Columbus, OH 43229 614-839-2447
FAX 614-839-5437
http://www.campotyokwalodging.com
e-mail: dschirner@bbbscentralohio.org
David Schirner, Camp Director

Special Care Camp is designed for children who have learning disabilities, ADD, and ADHD, behavior disorders or a combination of disabilities. In some cases, they may be children who have had a difficult start and just need more attention. Facilities include three lodges, dining hall, shelter house, medical building, activity center, rustic summer cabins/platform tents, swimming pool, campfire ring, indoor/outdoor basketball courts, sand volleyball court, seven-acre field,and laundry facilities.

902 Camp Robin Rogers
The Arc of Allen County
Lima, OH 45805 419-225-6285
FAX 419-228-7770
http://www.arcallencounty.org/camp.htm
e-mail: arc@wcoil.com
Joshua R Ebling MSW/LISW, Executive Director
Sherry Kunz, Camp Director
Kathy Shockency, Property Manager
The camp sits on 38 partially wooded acres which surrounds a two acre pond and has a lodge hall which can seat up to 200 people. Available activities at the camp include an in-ground pool, sand volleyball courts, basketball/tennis courts, nature trails, horseshoe pits, a baseball diamond, and a playground area for children.

903 Camp-I-Can
Children's Home of Cincinnati, The
5050 Madison Road
Cincinnati, OH 45227 513-272-2800
800-639-4965
FAX 513-272-2807
http://www.thechildrenshomecinti.org
e-mail: wyoung@thechildrenshomecinti.org
Ellen Katz Johnson, President/CEO
Wesley Young, Vice President

A summer day camp that enhances creativity and promotes positive social skills.

904 Easter Seals Broadview Heights
Easter Seals North East Ohio
1929 E Royalton Road
Broadview Heights, OH 44147 440-838-0990
888-325-8532
FAX 440-838-8440
http://http://neohio.easterseals.com/
e-mail: spowers@eastersealsneo.org
Sheila Dunn, Chief Executive Officer
Susan Powers, Rehabilitation Services Director

The following are camping and recreational services offered: Camperships and day camping for children. Through our summer campership program, funding is available to children and adults with disabilities so they can select a summer day or residential camp of their choice. The program provides individuals with the opportunity to attend a camp specifically designed for their special needs and optimal enjoyment.s

905 Easter Seals Central and Southeast Ohio
565 Childrens Drive W
Columbus, OH 43205 614-228-5523
FAX 614-443-1848
http://http://centralohio.easterseals.com
e-mail: tshiverd@easterseals-cseohio.org
Karin A Zuckerman, Chief Executive Officer
John Bitler, Development Director
Benedicta Enrile MD, Medical Director
The following are camping and recreational services offered: Aquatics. Summer Day Camp is open to toddlers, ages 18 months to 2 years, and preschoolers and young school-aged children from 3-8 years of age with and without disabilities.

906 Easter Seals Cincinnati
2901 Gilbert Avenue
Cincinnati, OH 45215 513-281-2316
800-288-1123
FAX 513-475-6787
http://http://swohio.easterseals.com
e-mail: twatson@oh-sw.easter-seals.com
Tamara Watson, Executive Director
Lisa Fitz Gibbon, President/CEO
Kelly Ulman, Volunteer Program Coordinator
Easter Seals camping and recreation programs serve children, adults and families of all abilities. Various programs are available with the united purpose of giving disabled individuals a fun and safe camping or recreational experience. The following are camping and recreational services offered: Adventure.

907 Easter Seals Lorain
Easter Seals Lorain
1909 N Ridge Road E
Lorain, OH 44055 440-277-7337
888-723-5602
FAX 440-277-7339
http://www.eastersealsnwohio.org/
e-mail: pfisher@eastersealsnwohio.org
Kevin Walter, Chief Executive Officer
Stephanie Engle, Billing Specialist
Phil Fisher, Camp Coordinator
Easter Seals camping and recreation programs serve children, adults and families of all abilities. Various programs are available with the united purpose of giving disabled individuals a fun and safe camping or recreational experience. The following are camping and recreational services offered: Camperships and day camping for children.

908 Easter Seals Marietta
Easter Seals
River Cities Office/609 Putnam St
Marietta, OH 45750 740-374-8876
800-860-5523
FAX 740-374-4501
http://www.eastersealscentralohio.org
e-mail: info@easterseals.com
Karin A Zuckerman, Chief Executive Officer
John Bitler, Director of Development
Benedicta Enrile MD, Medical Director
Easter Seals camping and recreation programs serve children, adults and families of all abilities. Various programs are available with the united purpose of giving disabled individuals a fun and safe camping or recreational experience. The following are camping and recreational services offered: Camp respite for children and therapeutic horseback riding.

909 Easter Seals Northeast Ohio
3085 W Market Street
Akron, OH 44333 330-836-9741
800-589-6834
FAX 330-836-4967
http://http://neohio.easterseals.com/
e-mail: susan@eastersealsneo.org
Susan Powers, Rehabilitation Services Director
Jenny Mason, Manager

Easter Seals camping and recreation programs serve children, adults and families of all abilities. Various programs are available with the united purpose of giving disabled individuals a fun and safe camping or recreational experience. The following are camping and recreational services offered: Swim programs.

910 Easter Seals Youngstown
299 Edwards Street
Youngstown, OH 44502 330-743-1168
FAX 330-743-1616
http://http://mtc.easterseals.com
e-mail: jwalston@mtc.easter-seals.com
Ken Sklenar, Chief Executive Officer
Vickie Villano, Director
Janet Walston, Pediatric Services Manager
Easter Seals camping and recreation programs serve children, adults and families of all abilities. Various programs are available with the united purpose of giving disabled individuals a fun and safe camping or recreational experience. The following are camping and recreational services offered: Recreationsl/Day care for Ages 6-12.

911 **Leo Yassenoff JCC/Jewish Community CenterSummer Camp**

1125 College Avenue
Columbus, OH 43209
614-231-2731
FAX 614-231-8222
http://www.columbusjcc.org/summercamps/
e-mail: rfox@columbusjcc.org

Rachel Fox, Camp Services Director
Carol Folkerth, JCC Executive Director
Jeanna Brownlee, Recreation Director

The Leo Yassenoff Jewish Community Center serves individuals and families in three locations in Central Ohio. Its primary mission is to sersve the Jewish and general community in a wide variety of programs including summer camp programs for individuals ages 3-25 with disabilities. Camp activities include canoeing, arts and crafts, archery, field trips and hiking, swimming, nature and environmental studies, dance and drama.

912 **Marburn Academy Summer Programs**

1860 Walden Drive
Columbus, OH
614-433-0822
FAX 614-433-0812
http://www.marburnacademy.org/summer.html
e-mail: marburnadmission@marburnacademy.org

Earl B Oremus, Headmaster
Donna Klein, Director of Education
Scott Burton, Director of Admission

A four program academic day camp for children with LD and dyslexia, offering remediation in reading, math, phonemic awareness, or writing.

913 **Pilgrim Hills CampOhio Conference / United Church of Christ**

33833 Township Road 20
Brinkhaven, OH 43006
740-599-6314
800-282-0740
FAX 740-599-9790
http://www.ocucc.org/
e-mail: campregistrar@ocucc.org

Jeff Thompson, Regional Manager
Cynthia Speller, Camp Director
Helen Schultz, Outdoor Ministries Registrar

Many camp programs for all children including learning disabled. Pilgrim Hills Camp is located on 375 acres of woodlands, meadows, ponds and trails. The facilities includes a large dining hall and full kitchen to feed up to 300 with full food service and menu options available. For additional information visit Website at: http://www.ocucc.org/OutdoorMin/PilgrimHills/Pilgrimhills.htm

914 **Recreation Unlimited Farm and FunRecreation Unlimited Foundation**

7700 Piper Road
Ashley, OH 43003
740-548-7006
FAX 740-747-3139
http://www.recreationunlimited.org
e-mail: info@recreationunlimited.org

Paul Huttlin, Executive Director/CEO
David D Hudler, Business Development Coordinator

A not-for-profit organization providing programs in sports, recreation and education for individuals with physical and developmental disabilities on an accessible 165-acre campus in a safe, fun and challenging environment.

Oklahoma

915 **Camp Classen YMCA**

Route 1
Davis, OK 73030
580-369-2272
FAX 580-369-2284
http://www.ymcaokc.org/campclassen.html
e-mail: rburris@ymcaokc.org

Albert McWhorter, Executive Director
Rick Burris, Associate Executive Director
Lyn Cooper, Camping & Conference Director

The YMCA's resident camp, Camp Classen, is located on 2,400 acres of forest, open meadows, lakes, ponds, streams and a wide variety of protected wildlife in the Arbuckle Mountains near Davis, Oklahoma. One and two week sessions are available throughout the summer for young people ages 8 through 17.

916 **Camp Fire USA**

National Camp Fire USA
706 S Boston Avenue
Tulsa, OK 74119
918-592-2267
888-553-2267
FAX 918-592-3473
http://www.tulsacampfire.org/tulsacampfire/
e-mail: vproctor@Tulsacampfire.org

Bobbie Henderson, Executive Director
Vicki Proctor, Camp Services Director
Mary A Ahlgren, Program Director

Camp Fire USA builds caring, confident youth and future leaders. Founded in 1910, Camp Fire USA's outcome-based programs include youth leadership, self-reliance, after school groups, camping and environmental education. Camp Fire Girls were in Tulsa as early as 1912. Green Country Council received its charter in 1938 and today serves girls and boys in 22 counties in Northeast Oklahoma.

917 **Central Christian Camp & Conference Center**

One Twin Cedar Lane
Guthrie, OK 73044
405-282-2811
800-299-2811
FAX 405-282-1367
http://www.centralchristiancamp.org
e-mail: james@centralchristiancamp.org

Spencer Bowen, Executive Director
James Wheeler, Program Director
Susan Shields, Operations Director

Central Christian Camp & Conference Center, established in 1955, is a year-round camp, conference, retreat and program center of the Christian Church in Oklahoma that offers settings for everyone's comfort and enjoyment, including the elderly and disabled. The camp also hosts Make Promises Happen, one of the nation's largest camping and outdoor recreational programs for persons with disabilities and serious illnesses.

918 **Easter Seals Oklahoma**

701 NE 13th Street
Oklahoma City, OK 73104
405-239-2525
FAX 405-239-2278
http://http://ok.easterseals.com
e-mail: info@easterseals.org OR esok1@coxinet.net

Patricia Filer, President
Linda Maisch, Administrative Assistant

Easter Seals camping and recreation programs serve children, adults and families of all abilities. Various programs are available with the united purpose of giving disabled individuals a fun and safe camping or recreational experience. The following are camping and recreational services offered: Camperships.

Oregon

919 **Easter Seals Medford**

711 E Main Street
Medford, OR 97504
541-842-2199
800-244-5289
FAX 541-842-4048
http://www.or.easterseals.com
e-mail: info@or.easterseals.com

J David Cheveallier, President/CEO
Katie Shepard, Manager
Diane Mathews, Program Coordinator

Programs offered in Medford include summer day camp, Recreation & Respite, and the popular First Saturday dance and social event. Programs are held at various community centers in Medford.

920 **Easter Seals Oregon**
Easter Seals National
5757 SW Macadam Avenue
Portland, OR 97239
503-228-5108
800-556-6020
FAX 503-228-1352
http://www.or.easterseals.com
e-mail: info@or.easter-seals.com

J David Cheveallier, President/CEO
Debbie Seymour, Office Manager

Easter Seals camping and recreation programs serve children, adults and families of all abilities. Various programs are available with the united purpose of giving disabled individuals a fun and safe camping or recreational experience. The following are camping and recreational services offered: Residential camping programs. In addition, the Portland program center hosts a warm water aquatic facility.

921 **Mobility International USA**
132 E Broadway
Eugene, OR 97401
541-343-1284
FAX 541-343-6812
http://www.miusa.org
e-mail: info@miusa.org

Susan Sygall, Co-Founder/CEO
Cindy Lewis, Program Director
Cerise Roth Vinson, Director of Administration
A nonprofit organization founded in 1981 to empower people with disabilities around the world through international exchange promoting cross-cultural understanding and providing leadership and disability rights training to people with disabilities. We also provide consultation, publications, resources and technical assistance promoting the full participation of people with disabilities in international exchange opportunities and at all levels of the international development process.

922 **Mt. Hood Kiwanis Camp: Canoeing at Trillium Lake Camp**
9320 SW Barbur Boulevard
Portland, OR 97219
503-452-7416
FAX 503-452-0062
http://www.mhkc.org/
e-mail: info@mhkc.org

Dianne Zellner, President
Marilee Payne, VP Program
Glenn Fudge, VP Site & Facilities
Mt. Hood Kiwanis Camp offers a great time to campers with disabilities with a variety of activities to choose from. Campers may have one or more physical, emotional or intellectual disabilities. Canoeing campers spend the week at pristine Trillium Lake Campground. Activities include canoeing, fishing, swimming, hiking, huckleberry picking and crafts. Campers stay in tents, traveling to Kiwanis Camp for the Wednesday evening dance, Thursday evening campfire and horseback riding. Ages 15 to 35.

923 **Mt. Hood Kiwanis Camp: Main Camp**
9320 SW Barbur Boulevard
Portland, OR 97219
503-452-7416
FAX 503-452-0062
http://www.mhkc.org/
e-mail: info@mhkc.org

Dianne Zellner, President
Marilee Payne, VP Program
Glenn Fudge, VP Site & Facilities
Mt. Hood Kiwanis Camp offers children and adults with disabilities a great time with a variety of camp activities to choose from. Campers may have one or more physical, emotional or intellectual disabilities. Activities include the challenge ropes course, horseback riding, fishing, hiking, arts and crafts, swimming, a dance and a campfire program at the main camp, as well as canoeing, and fishing at Trillium Lake. Eight sessions for ages ranging from 9 to 35 years old.

924 **Mt. Hood Kiwanis Camp: Trip and Travel Camp**
9320 SW Barbur Boulevard
Portland, OR 97219
503-452-7416
FAX 503-452-0062
http://www.mhkc.org/
e-mail: info@mhkc.org

Dianne Zellner, President
Marilee Payne, VP Program
Glenn Fudge, VP Site & Facilities

Trip and Travel campers enjoy day-long excursions as well as regular activities at Mt. Hood Kiwanis Camp. Campers experience additional challenges on the ropes course, spend a day river-rafting on the Deschutes, tour Wildwood Recreation Area, and go to Skibowl Adventure Park. There is one counselor for every two campers. Outings are active and rigorous. Ages 13-35.

925 **Oregon Trails**
Talisman Programs
Zirconia, NC 28790
828-697-6313
888-458-8226
FAX 828-697-6249
http://www.talismancamps.com/baseCamp.html
e-mail: info@talismancamps.com

Linda Tatsapauagh, Camp Director
Aaron McGinley, Base Camp Program Manager
Pete Weiss, Program Manager
Foundations Camp is co-educational accepting children ages 9-13 who have been diagnosed with LD, ADD, ADHD, and mild behavior issues. Participants live on campus in rustic cabins participating in a variety of activities designed to promote better communication and cooperation skills. Limited enrollment helps to facilitate an extended-family environment. The 2.5 to 1 camper-to-staff ratio ensures that no child is lost in the crowd and that each camper receives the attention he or she deserves.

926 **Upward Bound Camp for Special Needs**
PO Box C
Stayton, OR 97383
503-897-2447
FAX 503-897-4116
http://www.upwardboundcamp.org/home.html
e-mail: ubc@open.org

Jerry Pierce, Co-Director
Laura Pierce, Co-Director

The purpose of Upward Bound Camp is to provide on-going Christian based recreational and educational camp experiences for persons with disabilities, twelve years of age and over in an environment that presents opportunities for growth outside the individual's usual routine or habitat. Activities include fishing, hiking, swimming, arts and crafts, archery, Bible study, nature explorations, campfires, games, basketball, volleyball, horseshoes and badminton. Founded 1978.

Pennsylvania

927 **Camp Arc Spencer**
500 Market Street
Bridgewater, PA 15009
724-775-1602
FAX 724-775-2905
http://www.achieva.info
e-mail: mgrivna@achieva.info

Marc Grivna, Camp Director
Mary Haider, Respite Coordinator
Rochelle Tyler, Respite Coordinator
Camp Arc Spencer provides a fun and enjoyable environment where individuals with disabilities can gain insight into their own unique abilities. A camp setting promotes motivational, emotional, and social benefits. It helps campers develop acceptable group living skills, maintain or enhance personal health, and enhance self-worth and self-esteem by assuming a meaningful role in a camp community.

928 **Camp Hebron**
957 Camp Hebron Road
Halifax, PA 17032
717-896-3441
800-864-7747
FAX 717-896-3391
http://www.camphebron.org
e-mail: hebron@camphebron.org

Lanny Millette, Executive Director
Curtis Louder, Program Director
Ron Prohaska, Food Service Director
A place where people connect with God, nature and each other. This is accomplished through the creation of a Christ-centered sanctuary where people find renewal and growth through recreation, teaching and fellowship in God's creation.

929 Camp Horsin' Around

Wyndhaven Farms Inc
McDonald, PA 15057 412-292-4977
http://www.wyndhavenfarms.com/camp.htm
e-mail: horsecamp@verizon.net

Kim Radinick, Camp Director/Owner
Dana Fleming, Instructor
Beth Hopta, Instructor

Camp Horsin' Around provides campers with the opportunity to ride and work around horses, in addition to: greatly enhancing motor skills; teaching responsibility; creating a sense of accomplishment; teaching focus and concentration; and, helping to develop a greater sense of balance. Planned activities at camp includes: horse grooming, horse safety, care of horse and tack, games, worksheets, basic horse knowledge, and, arts and crafts.

930 Camp Joy

3325 Swamp Creek Road
Schwenksville, PA 19473 610-754-6878
FAX 610-754-7880
http://www.campjoy.com
e-mail: campjoy@fast.net

Angus Murray, Camp Director

A camp for kids and adults with developmental disabilities, mental retardation, autism, brain injury and neurological disorders. Activities include swimming, horseback riding, music, dancing, arts & crafts, drama and field trips.

931 Camp Lee Mar

805 Redgate Road
Dresher, PA 19025 215-658-1708
FAX 215-658-1710
http://www.leemar.com
e-mail: gtour400@aol.com

Ari Segal, Camp Co-Director
Lee Morrone, Camp Co-Director

Camp Lee Mar is a private residential special needs camp for children and young adults with mild to moderate learning and developmental challenges. A structured environment, individual attention and guidance are emphasized at all times. Campers enjoy traditional camp and recreation activities plus academics, speech and language therapy, music and art therapy, daily living skills, sensory-motor-perceptual training, and computers, in addition to therapeutic horseback riding and overnight trips.

932 Camp Poyntelle Lewis Village

State Road 4031
Poyntelle, PA 18454 570-448-2161
FAX 570-448-2117
http://www.poyntelle.com
e-mail: Debby@poyntelle.com

Debbie Shriber LMSW, Executive Director
Matt Dorter, Assistant Director
Amy Feigenbaum, Creative Programming Director

Camp Poyntelle Lewis Village provides a warm, friendly, fun and safe Jewish environment for your child. Children leave for camp looking to have a good time, and return home from camp with a sense of independence, a greater respect towards others, a healthy attitude towards competition, and a lifetime full of memories and friendships. For boys and girls entering second grade through seventh grade, and for teens entering eighth grade through eleventh grade.

933 Capital Camps & Retreat Center

12750 Buchanan Trail East
Waynesboro, PA 17298 717-794-2177
FAX 717-794-5789
http://www.capitalcamps.org
e-mail: info@capitalcamps.org

Jon Shapiro, Camp Director
Karen Bernstein, Assistant Camp Director
Penny Hartzman, Camp Registrar

Offers four village programs on their 267 acre facility serving campers entering grades 3 through 10. In addition, the LIT/Leaders in Training and CIT/Counselors in Training programs train young adults to be future staff and community leadership within their camp programs. The goal is to offer Jewish camping to anyone who wishes to participate. To achieve this Capital Camps operates an inclusive special needs program.

934 Easter Seals BethlehemLehigh Valley Division

2200 Industrial Drive
Bethlehem, PA 18017 610-866-8092
FAX 610-866-3450
http://http://esep.easterseals.com
e-mail: barbara.carlson@easterseals-easternpa.org

Barbara Carlson, VP/Program Services
Frank Malone, Office Manager
Nancy L Teichman, CEO

Easter Seals camping and recreation programs serve children, adults and families of all abilities. Various programs are available with the united purpose of giving disabled individuals a fun and safe camping or recreational experience. The following are camping and recreational services offered: Recreational services for children and day camp for children.

935 Easter Seals Central Pennsylvania

501 Valley View Boulevard
Altoona, PA 16602 814-944-5014
888-463-3093
FAX 814-944-6500
http://www.centralpa.easterseals.com
e-mail: jhanlin@eastersealscentralpa.org

David Bateman, President/CEO

Easter Seals camping and recreation programs serve children, adults and families of all abilities. Various programs are available with the united purpose of giving disabled individuals a fun and safe camping or recreational experience. The following are camping and recreational services offered: Day camping for children, recreational services for children and therapeutic horseback riding.

936 Easter Seals Downingtown

797 E Lancaster Avenue
Downingtown, PA 19335 610-873-3990
FAX 610-873-3992
http://www.easterseals-sepa.org
e-mail: dkeiths@easterseals-sepa.org

Donna Keiths, Executive Director
April Williams, Secretary

Easter Seals camping and recreation programs serve children, adults and families of all abilities. Various programs are available with the united purpose of giving disabled individuals a fun and safe camping or recreational experience. The following are camping and recreational services offered: Day camping for children, recreational services for children.

937 Easter Seals Eastern Pennsylvania

1040 Liggett Avenue
Reading, PA 19611 610-775-1431
FAX 610-796-1954
http://http://esep.easterseals.com/
e-mail: info@easterseals.com

Heidi Goss, Vice President
Anna Mountz, Office Manager

Easter Seals camping and recreation programs serve children, adults and families of all abilities. Various programs are available with the united purpose of giving disabled individuals a fun and safe camping or recreational experience. The following are camping and recreational services offered: Camperships, day camping for children and recreational services for children.

938 Easter Seals FranklinVenango Division Office

Easter Seals
200 12th Street
Franklin, PA 16323 814-437-3071
FAX 814-432-2269
http://www.westernpa.easter-seals.com
e-mail: dgriffith@pa-ws.easter-seals.org

Donna Griffith, Executive Director
Lyn Cross, Division Secretary
Rory Cooper, Board of Directors Chairman

Easter Seals camping and recreation programs serve children, adults and families of all abilities. Various programs are available with the united purpose of giving disabled individuals a fun and safe camping or recreational experience. The following are camping and recreational services offered: Day camping for children, recreational services for children.

939 Easter Seals KulpsvilleTucker & Perry Gresh Center
1161 Forty Foot Road
Kulpsville, PA 19443 215-368-7000
FAX 216-368-1199
http://http://sepa.easterseals.com/
e-mail: bstrasser@easterseals-sepa.org
Betsi Strasser, Executive Director

Easter Seals camping and recreation programs serve children, adults and families of all abilities. Various programs are available with the united purpose of giving disabled individuals a fun and safe camping or recreational experience. The following are camping and recreational services offered: Day camping for children, recreational services for children.

940 Easter Seals Levittown
2400 Trenton Road
Levittown, PA 19056 215-945-7200
FAX 215-945-4073
http://http://sepa.easterseals.com
e-mail: lremick@easterseals-sepa.org
Adrienne Young, Manager
Pat Van, Administrative Assistant

Easter Seals camping and recreation programs serve children, adults and families of all abilities. Various programs are available with the united purpose of giving disabled individuals a fun and safe camping or recreational experience. The following are camping and recreational services offered: Day camping for children, recreational services for children.

941 Easter Seals Media
468 N Middletown Road
Media, PA 19063 610-565-2353
FAX 610-565-5256
http://http://sepa.easterseals.com
e-mail: jwright@easterseals-sepa.org
Donna Keiths, Executive Director

Easter Seals camping and recreation programs serve children, adults and families of all abilities. Various programs are available with the united purpose of giving disabled individuals a fun and safe camping or recreational experience. The following are camping and recreational services offered: Day camping for children, recreational services for children.

942 Easter Seals South Central Pennsylvania
2201 S Queen Street
York, PA 17402 717-741-3891
888-372-7280
FAX 717-741-5359
http://www.centralpa.easterseals.com
e-mail: info@easterseals.com
Debbie Noel, President
Matt Ernst, Therapeutic Recreation Director

The following are camping and recreational services offered: Adventure, day camping for children, recreational services for adults, recreational services for children, sports camp, swim programs, therapeutic horseback riding, water skiing and snow skiing.

943 Easter Seals of Southeastern Pennsylvania
3975 Conshohocken Avenue
Philadelphia, PA 19131 215-879-1000
FAX 215-879-8424
http://http://sepa.easterseals.com
e-mail: jpodgajny@easterseals-sepa.org
Carl Webster, Executive Director
John Podgajny, Division Director
Sandy Miller, Administrative Assistant
Easter Seals camping and recreation programs serve children, adults and families of all abilities. Various programs are available with the united purpose of giving disabled individuals a fun and safe camping or recreational experience. The following are camping and recreational services offered: Day camping for children, recreational services for adults and recreational services for children.

944 Outside In School Expedition Camp
303 Center Avenue
Greensburg, PA 724-837-1518
FAX 724-837-0801
http://www.outsideinschool.com/NewPath.htm
e-mail: administration@outsideinschool.com
Michael C Henkel, Camp Director

Expedition Camp presents stressful but stimulating opportunities that are highly structured and engineered for success to increase the students' motivation to change behaviorally, spiritually and emotionally; thus increasing self efficacy assisting them with managing the pressures of society. Students must actively engage the environment with their peers and instructors as a team to successfully complete the expedition.

945 Summit Camp Program
Summit Camp Program New York Office
18 E 41st Street
New York, NY 10017 212-689-3880
800-323-9908
FAX 212-689-4347
http://www.summitcamp.com
e-mail: info@summitcamp.com
Mayer Stiskin, Director
Ninette Stiskin, Assistant Director
Eugene Bell, Associate Director
Summit camp in Honsdales Pennsylvania serves boys and girls diagnosed with Attention Deficit Disorders, Asperger Snydrome and learning disabilities.

946 Wesley Woods
PO Box 155A
Grand Valley, PA 16420 814-436-7802
800-295-0420
FAX 814-436-7669
http://www.wesleywoods.com
e-mail: camp@wesleywoods.com
Herbert West, Executive Director
Doug Beichner, Maintenance Director
Rick Brown, Food Services Director
The mission is to meet spiritual needs of children, youth, and adults in a Christian camp and retreat setting.

Rhode Island

947 Camp Aldersgate: Adventure Camp
1043 Snake Hill Road
North Scituate, RI 02857 401-568-4350
FAX 401-568-1840
http://www.campaldersgate.com/
e-mail: info@campaldersgate.com
Jennifer L B Carpenter, Executive Director

Adventure Camp provides a week of tenting, cooking, and sharpening camping skills as we enjoy the great outdoors. Stretch yourself physically, emotionally, and spiritually. Includes ropes course, group challenges, and other activities. Summer program provides special experiences for children with a variety of special needs, giving them the chance to grow in exciting and different ways. Junior High Camps Program - completed grades 6-8.

948 Camp Aldersgate: Adventure Week Day Camp
1043 Snake Hill Road
North Scituate, RI 02857 401-568-4350
FAX 401-568-1840
http://www.campaldersgate.com/
e-mail: info@campaldersgate.com
Jennifer L B Carpenter, Executive Director

During Adventure Week Intermediate Day Camp for ages 10-12 camp activities include using the low ropes, group initiatives and high ropes (optional) where campers will learn lots about others and even more about themselves. Weekly session from August 6 to August 10.

949 Camp Aldersgate: Basketball Camp

1043 Snake Hill Road
North Scituate, RI 02857
401-568-4350
FAX 401-568-1840
http://www.campaldersgate.com/
e-mail: info@campaldersgate.com
Jennifer L B Carpenter, Executive Director

Basketball Camp will help girls and boys learn plays, improve skills, and play hoops, completing the week with fun camp activities. Summer program provides special experiences for children with a variety of special needs, giving them the chance to grow in exciting and different ways. Junior High Camps Program - completed grades 6-8.

950 Camp Aldersgate: Cabin Camp

1043 Snake Hill Road
North Scituate, RI 02857
401-568-4350
FAX 401-568-1840
http://www.campaldersgate.com/
e-mail: info@campaldersgate.com
Jennifer L B Carpenter, Executive Director

Sample a bit of everything camp has to offer, with a daily theme. Campers grades 5 through 7 will stay in the waterfront cabins. Summer program provides special experiences for children with a variety of special needs, giving them the chance to grow in exciting and different ways.

951 Camp Aldersgate: Camper's Choice Week DayCamp

1043 Snake Hill Road
North Scituate, RI 02857
401-568-4350
FAX 401-568-1840
http://www.campaldersgate.com/
e-mail: info@campaldersgate.com
Jennifer L B Carpenter, Executive Director

During Camper's Choice Week Intermediate Day Camp for ages 10-12 the schedule is wide open upon arrival where fellow campers will be able to decide the camp activities for the week. Weekly session from August 13 to August 17.

952 Camp Aldersgate: Campers' Choice

1043 Snake Hill Road
North Scituate, RI 02857
401-568-4350
FAX 401-568-1840
http://www.campaldersgate.com/
e-mail: info@campaldersgate.com
Jennifer L B Carpenter, Executive Director

The schedule is wide open when you get to camp, you and your fellow campers will be able to decide the camp activities for the week. Enjoy freedom and fun! Summer program provides special experiences for children with a variety of special needs, giving them the chance to grow in exciting and different ways. Junior High Camps Program - completed grades 6-8.

953 Camp Aldersgate: Classic Camp

1043 Snake Hill Road
North Scituate, RI 02857
401-568-4350
FAX 401-568-1840
http://www.campaldersgate.com/
e-mail: info@campaldersgate.com
Jennifer L B Carpenter, Executive Director

Campers will make new friends, have campfires, go swimming, do cookouts, play all camp games, and much more. Summer program provides special experiences for children with a variety of special needs, giving them the chance to grow in exciting and different ways. Elementary Camps - completed grades 3-5; and Junior High Camps - completed grades 6-8.

954 Camp Aldersgate: Classics Week Day Camp

1043 Snake Hill Road
North Scituate, RI 02857
401-568-4350
FAX 401-568-1840
http://www.campaldersgate.com/
e-mail: info@campaldersgate.com
Jennifer L B Carpenter, Executive Director

Classics Week Intermediate Day Camp for ages 10-12 provides campers with a variety of activities where they can sample a bit of everything that camp has to offer, making new friends, going swimming, playing camp games, and much more. Weekly session during June 25 to June 29.

955 Camp Aldersgate: Cooking Week Day Camp

1043 Snake Hill Road
North Scituate, RI 02857
401-568-4350
FAX 401-568-1840
http://www.campaldersgate.com/
e-mail: info@campaldersgate.com
Jennifer L B Carpenter, Executive Director

Cooking Week Intermediate Day Camp for ages 10-12 provides campers with a variety of activities where they will spend the week exploring the kitchen and learning which ingredients work well together. Weekly session during July 2 to July 6.

956 Camp Aldersgate: Day Camp

1043 Snake Hill Road
North Scituate, RI 02857
401-568-4350
FAX 401-568-1840
http://www.campaldersgate.com/
e-mail: info@campaldersgate.com
Jennifer L B Carpenter, Executive Director

Day Camp for campers that are 6-9 years old focuses on the basic camping experiences that includes a variety of activities such as exploring the wilderness of Camp Aldersgate and learning about the different types of plants and animals that live there. Additional activities include arts and crafts and daily swimming.

957 Camp Aldersgate: Discovery Camp

1043 Snake Hill Road
North Scituate, RI 02857
401-568-4350
FAX 401-568-1840
http://www.campaldersgate.com/
e-mail: info@campaldersgate.com
Jennifer L B Carpenter, Executive Director

Discover camp is for veteran campers (ages 13-15) or new campers who want to grow in a fun atmosphere. Learn new leadership skills, do summer reading, build self-confidence and self-esteem by helping young campers and having fun with peers. Lead games, read to campers, accompany campers to various locations around camp, assist with program activities and more. Have fun with swimming, boating, sports, relaxation time and special rewards from camp to say thanks for helping out.

958 Camp Aldersgate: Early Explorers Camp

1043 Snake Hill Road
North Scituate, RI 02857
401-568-4350
FAX 401-568-1840
http://www.campaldersgate.com/
e-mail: info@campaldersgate.com
Jennifer L B Carpenter, Executive Director

Campers spend a full week at Aldersgate and will stay in the Native American Village and explore all of the great adventures of camping. Summer program provides special experiences for children with a variety of special needs, giving them the chance to grow in exciting and different ways. Early Elementary Program - ages 7 & 8.

959 Camp Aldersgate: Elementary Fishing Camp

1043 Snake Hill Road
North Scituate, RI 02857
401-568-4350
FAX 401-568-1840
http://www.campaldersgate.com/
e-mail: info@campaldersgate.com
Jennifer L B Carpenter, Executive Director

Campers who love to fish will learn more about the great world of fishing - baiting the hook, casting, and removing the fish. Girls and boys will discover where and when to fish as well as the importance of water safety. Summer program provides special experiences for children with a variety of special needs, giving them the chance to grow in exciting and different ways. Elementary Camps Program - completed grades 3-5.

960 **Camp Aldersgate: Elementary Horse Riding Camp**

1043 Snake Hill Road
North Scituate, RI 02857 401-568-4350
FAX 401-568-1840
http://www.campaldersgate.com/
e-mail: info@campaldersgate.com
Jennifer L B Carpenter, Executive Director

Elementaty Horse Riding Camp features English (balance seat) horseback riding lessons. Horse riders attend stables each day. Summer program provides special experiences for children with a variety of special needs, giving them the chance to grow in exciting and different ways. Elementary Camps Program - completed grades 3-5.

961 **Camp Aldersgate: Expedition Camp**

1043 Snake Hill Road
North Scituate, RI 02857 401-568-4350
FAX 401-568-1840
http://www.campaldersgate.com/
e-mail: info@campaldersgate.com
Jennifer L B Carpenter, Executive Director

Campers stay in the great outdoors while pushing their physical limits during the day, exploring the high ropes and taking day trips that will include hiking, rock climbing, etc. Summer program provides special experiences for children with a variety of special needs, giving them the chance to grow in exciting and different ways. Senior High Camps - completed grades 9-12.

962 **Camp Aldersgate: Family Camp**

1043 Snake Hill Road
North Scituate, RI 02857 401-568-4350
FAX 401-568-1840
http://www.campaldersgate.com/
e-mail: info@campaldersgate.com
Jennifer L B Carpenter, Executive Director

Family Camp is a great chance to spend time together as a family while enjoying all camp has to offer. Family Camp is priced by the week for the cabin in addition to separate weekly pricing per person for the available food service. Children 3 and under receive half-price food.

963 **Camp Aldersgate: Finders Sleepers Camp**

1043 Snake Hill Road
North Scituate, RI 02857 401-568-4350
FAX 401-568-1840
http://www.campaldersgate.com/
e-mail: info@campaldersgate.com
Jennifer L B Carpenter, Executive Director

Campers will figure out where they will sleep using clues as they move from the woods to the fields while enjoying the traditional fun camp activities. Summer program provides special experiences for children with a variety of special needs, giving them the chance to grow in exciting and different ways. Elementary Camps Program - completed grades 3-5.

964 **Camp Aldersgate: Freshwater Fishing Camp**

1043 Snake Hill Road
North Scituate, RI 02857 401-568-4350
FAX 401-568-1840
http://www.campaldersgate.com/
e-mail: info@campaldersgate.com
Jennifer L B Carpenter, Executive Director

Junior High Freshwater Fishing is for campers who love to fish where they will learn more about the great world of fishing - baiting the hook, casting, and removing the fish. Girls and boys will discover where and when to fish. Summer program provides special experiences for children with a variety of special needs, giving them the chance to grow in exciting and different ways. Junior High Camps Program - completed grades 6-8.

965 **Camp Aldersgate: Gals & Pals Camp**

1043 Snake Hill Road
North Scituate, RI 02857 401-568-4350
FAX 401-568-1840
http://www.campaldersgate.com/
e-mail: info@campaldersgate.com
Jennifer L B Carpenter, Executive Director

Gals & Pals Camp is like a weeklong slumber party where campers can meet and make new friends. Campers can challenge themselves on the ropes course, enjoy arts & crafts, and canoe and swim beautiful Aldersgate Lake. Summer program provides special experiences for children with a variety of special needs, giving them the chance to grow in exciting and different ways. Elementary Camps - completed grades 3-5; and Junior High Camps - completed grades 6-8.

966 **Camp Aldersgate: Grandparent & Me Camp**

1043 Snake Hill Road
North Scituate, RI 02857 401-568-4350
FAX 401-568-1840
http://www.campaldersgate.com/
e-mail: info@campaldersgate.com
Jennifer L B Carpenter, Executive Director

Campers spend quality time during the summer together with their grandparent(s) while sharing their camping experiences with each other you. Program is a half-week in length and pricing includes both grandparent and child, with a discounted price for each additional grandparent and child that would like to attend the program.

967 **Camp Aldersgate: Hogan Camp**

1043 Snake Hill Road
North Scituate, RI 02857 401-568-4350
FAX 401-568-1840
http://www.campaldersgate.com/
e-mail: info@campaldersgate.com
Jennifer L B Carpenter, Executive Director

Campers live in Hogans - platform tents that hold five campers and a counselor. Each site consists of a small family group with two Hogans and a campfire circle. Campers spend the week sharing crafts, swimming, boating, nature study, outdoor living skills, and many more activities. Summer program provides special experiences for children with a variety of special needs, giving them the chance to grow in exciting and different ways. Elementary Camps Program - completed grades 3-5.

968 **Camp Aldersgate: Junior/Senior Horseriding Camp**

1043 Snake Hill Road
North Scituate, RI 02857 401-568-4350
FAX 401-568-1840
http://www.campaldersgate.com/
e-mail: info@campaldersgate.com
Jennifer L B Carpenter, Executive Director

Junior/Senior Horse Riding Camp features Western style horseback riding lessons. Daily trips to the stable include basic horse care followed by trail riding. All of the traditional camp fun will round out the week. Summer program provides special experiences for children with a variety of special needs, giving them the chance to grow in exciting and different ways. Junior High Camps Program - completed grades 6-8.

969 **Camp Aldersgate: Leadership Camp**

1043 Snake Hill Road
North Scituate, RI 02857 401-568-4350
FAX 401-568-1840
http://www.campaldersgate.com/
e-mail: info@campaldersgate.com
Jennifer L B Carpenter, Executive Director

Leadership Camp will help campers recognize special abilities and talents as a potential leader and how those skills can be used at church, school, and camp. Some campers will be asked back to counsel during the summer or at other times during the year. Must be 16 or have completed 10th grade. Summer program provides special experiences for children with a variety of special needs, giving them the chance to grow in exciting and different ways.

970 **Camp Aldersgate: Living Arts Camp**

1043 Snake Hill Road
North Scituate, RI 02857 401-568-4350
FAX 401-568-1840
http://www.campaldersgate.com/
e-mail: info@campaldersgate.com
Jennifer L B Carpenter, Executive Director

Campers spend the week painting, dancing, performing, crafting, and making music, ending the week with a performance for parents and campers. Summer program provides special experiences for children with a variety of special needs, giving them the chance to grow in exciting and different ways. Elementary Camps - completed grades 3-5; Junior High Camps - completed grades 6-8; and Senior High Camps - completed grades 9-12.

971 **Camp Aldersgate: Living Arts Week Day Camp**

1043 Snake Hill Road
North Scituate, RI 02857
401-568-4350
FAX 401-568-1840
http://www.campaldersgate.com/
e-mail: info@campaldersgate.com
Jennifer L B Carpenter, Executive Director

During Living Arts Week Intermediate Day Camp for ages 10-12 campers can bring their own musical instrument if they play one. Activities include singing, special crafts, writing, art and other artistic expression. Weekly session from July 30 to August 3.

972 **Camp Aldersgate: Mission Camp**

1043 Snake Hill Road
North Scituate, RI 02857
401-568-4350
FAX 401-568-1840
http://www.campaldersgate.com/
e-mail: info@campaldersgate.com
Jennifer L B Carpenter, Executive Director

Campers will work alongside friends making the world a better place and serve with other youth from all over New England and the U.S. Evening programs include concerts, fun, and all camp games. Register as a youth group, or as an individual. Cost includes supplies, food, housing, and transportation. Summer program provides special experiences for children with a variety of special needs, giving them the chance to grow in exciting and different ways. Senior High Camps - completed grades 9-12.

973 **Camp Aldersgate: Music Week Day Camp**

1043 Snake Hill Road
North Scituate, RI 02857
401-568-4350
FAX 401-568-1840
http://www.campaldersgate.com/
e-mail: info@campaldersgate.com
Jennifer L B Carpenter, Executive Director

During Music Week Intermediate Day Camp for ages 10-12 campers will jam with the Aldersgate Band. Campers will bring their own musical instruments - traditional, unique, or make their own. No experience necessary. Weekly session during July 9 to July 13.

974 **Camp Aldersgate: Nature/Environmental Week Day Camp**

1043 Snake Hill Road
North Scituate, RI 02857
401-568-4350
FAX 401-568-1840
http://www.campaldersgate.com/
e-mail: info@campaldersgate.com
Jennifer L B Carpenter, Executive Director

During Nature/Environmental Week Intermediate Day Camp for ages 10-12 campers will explore the world around them and look at ways to conserve, restore and increase awareness of how one can live in harmony with the beauty of nature around us. Weekly session from July 16 to July 20.

975 **Camp Aldersgate: Night Camp**

1043 Snake Hill Road
North Scituate, RI 02857
401-568-4350
FAX 401-568-1840
http://www.campaldersgate.com/
e-mail: info@campaldersgate.com
Jennifer L B Carpenter, Executive Director

Night Camp campers stay up late as they hoot with the owls at night! Campers will go to sleep later every night as they go for the all-nighter and then reverse the process. Summer program provides special experiences for children with a variety of special needs, giving them the chance to grow in exciting and different ways. Junior High Camps Program - completed grades 6-8.

976 **Camp Aldersgate: Sailing Camp**

1043 Snake Hill Road
North Scituate, RI 02857
401-568-4350
FAX 401-568-1840
http://www.campaldersgate.com/
e-mail: info@campaldersgate.com
Jennifer L B Carpenter, Executive Director

Young sailors will learn using a small sailboat on the lake, along with all of the fun camp activities. Emphasis will be on learning skills and safety. Summer program provides special experiences for children with a variety of special needs, giving them the chance to grow in exciting and different ways. Elementary Camps Program - completed grades 3-5.

977 **Camp Aldersgate: Shoot for the Stars Camp**

1043 Snake Hill Road
North Scituate, RI 02857
401-568-4350
FAX 401-568-1840
http://www.campaldersgate.com/
e-mail: info@campaldersgate.com
Jennifer L B Carpenter, Executive Director

Campers spend the days building and flying their own rockets, and the nights learning about the stars while looking through telescopes. Summer program provides special experiences for children with a variety of special needs, giving them the chance to grow in exciting and different ways. Elementary Camps Program - completed grades 3-5.

978 **Camp Aldersgate: Single Parent Weekend Camp**

1043 Snake Hill Road
North Scituate, RI 02857
401-568-4350
FAX 401-568-1840
http://www.campaldersgate.com/
e-mail: info@campaldersgate.com
Jennifer L B Carpenter, Executive Director

At the Single Parent Weekend Camp single parents and guardians can bring their children for a great weekend of fun, spending time together with their kids while swimming, biking, canoeing, taking nature walks, and making crafts. Campers can meet other single parents while their kids make new friends.

979 **Camp Aldersgate: Special Needs Camp**

1043 Snake Hill Road
North Scituate, RI 02857
401-568-4350
FAX 401-568-1840
http://www.campaldersgate.com/
e-mail: info@campaldersgate.com
Jennifer L B Carpenter, Executive Director

Special Needs Camp provides a week of fun, friendship, and caring. Open to mentally disabled persons age 21 and older who have self-help skills. Participants accepted based on required skills and abilities. Family groups will participate in all camp programs including swimming, boating, nature hikes, crafts, games, campfires, singing, and special events.

980 **Camp Aldersgate: Sports Camp**

1043 Snake Hill Road
North Scituate, RI 02857
401-568-4350
FAX 401-568-1840
http://www.campaldersgate.com/
e-mail: info@campaldersgate.com
Jennifer L B Carpenter, Executive Director

Campers play a variety of sports games including softball, basketball, touch rugby, tennis, kickball, and others. Campers will vote on their activities and be able to enjoy the traditional camp activities. Summer program provides special experiences for children with a variety of special needs, giving them the chance to grow in exciting and different ways. Elementary Camps - completed grades 3-5; Junior High Camps - completed grades 6-8; and Senior High Camps - completed grades 9-12.

981 **Camp Aldersgate: Teddy Bears Camp**

1043 Snake Hill Road
North Scituate, RI 02857
401-568-4350
FAX 401-568-1840
http://www.campaldersgate.com/
e-mail: info@campaldersgate.com
Jennifer L B Carpenter, Executive Director

Campers come for a half week of camp where they can bring their own teddy bear or make one there. Designed for 7 and 8 year olds, Teddy Bear campers will stay in main camp and sample a bit of everything that camp has to offer. Summer program provides special experiences for children with a variety of special needs, giving them the chance to grow in exciting and different ways.

982 Camp Aldersgate: Unplugged Camp
1043 Snake Hill Road
North Scituate, RI 02857 401-568-4350
FAX 401-568-1840
http://www.campaldersgate.com/
e-mail: info@campaldersgate.com
Jennifer L B Carpenter, Executive Director

Unplugged campers will jam with the band, bringing their own instruments - traditional, unique, or make their own, and then put on a performance for fellow campers. Other camp activities including swimming or canoeing in the lake. Summer program provides special experiences for children with a variety of special needs, giving them the chance to grow in exciting and different ways. Junior High Camps Program - completed grades 6-8; and Senior High Camps - completed grades 9-1.

983 Camp Aldersgate: Vacation Camp
1043 Snake Hill Road
North Scituate, RI 02857 401-568-4350
FAX 401-568-1840
http://www.campaldersgate.com/
e-mail: info@campaldersgate.com
Jennifer L B Carpenter, Executive Director

Campers will visit the beach, an amusement park, travel to a local major city, catch a movie, and do other fun activities while making new friends. Summer program provides special experiences for children with a variety of special needs, giving them the chance to grow in exciting and different ways. Senior High Camps - completed grades 9-12.

984 Camp Aldersgate: Water Week Day Camp
1043 Snake Hill Road
North Scituate, RI 02857 401-568-4350
FAX 401-568-1840
http://www.campaldersgate.com/
e-mail: info@campaldersgate.com
Jennifer L B Carpenter, Executive Director

During Water Week Intermediate Day Camp for ages 10-12 campers will learn to sail small sailboats and canoe on Lake Aldersgate, along with all of the fun camp activities. The week will also include a lot of fun water activities throughout each day. Weekly session from July 23 to July 27.

985 Camp Aldersgate: Waterskills Camp
1043 Snake Hill Road
North Scituate, RI 02857 401-568-4350
FAX 401-568-1840
http://www.campaldersgate.com/
e-mail: info@campaldersgate.com
Jennifer L B Carpenter, Executive Director

Campers will learn and improve their boating and swimming skills while enjoying swim lessons and free swim time with basic canoe and rowing lessons. Summer program provides special experiences for children with a variety of special needs, giving them the chance to grow in exciting and different ways. Elementary Camps Program - completed grades 3-5.

986 Camp Aldersgate: White Water Rafting Camp
1043 Snake Hill Road
North Scituate, RI 02857 401-568-4350
FAX 401-568-1840
http://www.campaldersgate.com/
e-mail: info@campaldersgate.com
Jennifer L B Carpenter, Executive Director

White Water Rafting campers will travel to the white waters of Maine after a few days at camp. Summer program provides special experiences for children with a variety of special needs, giving them the chance to grow in exciting and different ways. Senior High Camps - completed grades 9-12.

987 Camp Aldersgate: Young Voyagers Camp
1043 Snake Hill Road
North Scituate, RI 02857 401-568-4350
FAX 401-568-1840
http://www.campaldersgate.com/
e-mail: info@campaldersgate.com
Jennifer L B Carpenter, Executive Director

Young Voyagers Camp is for the beginner who wants to explore new outdoor skills like camp site selection and preparation, safe use of fire, and knot tying. Summer program provides special experiences for children with a variety of special needs, giving them the chance to grow in exciting and different ways. Elementary Camps Program - completed grades 3-5.

988 Camp Ruggles
113 Stone Dam Road
North Scituate, RI 02857 401-647-5508
George M Jacques, Camp Director

Camp Ruggles located in Glocester, Rhode Island, is a summer day camp for emotionally handicapped children. It offers a six-week co-ed summer session for sixty children ages 6-12. Special education teachers, a psychologist, and a nurse oversee the program. Camp Ruggles offers a three campers to one counselor ratio and is accredited through the American Camping Association.

South Carolina

989 Clemson Outdoor Lab: Camp Again
Clemson University Outdoor Laboratory
Lehotsky Hall
Clemson, SC 29634 864-646-7502
FAX 864-646-3620
http://www.clemson.edu/outdoorlab/camps.html
e-mail: cuolcamps-L@clemson.edu
Leslie Conrad, Camp Director
Norman A McGee Jr, Executive Director
Janay Whitesel, Camp Reservations Coordinator
This program is open to all active older adults with special needs. The cost includes meals, lodging and activities for 5 days and 4 nights of adventure. Activities include but are not limited to, trips to scenic areas, fishing, boating, crafts, historical tours, nature walks, hayrides, apple picking and many more special events. Evening activities include campfires, musical entertainment, talent shows and other fun-filled programs.

990 Clemson Outdoor Lab: Camp Hope
Clemson University Outdoor Laboratory
Lehotsky Hall
Clemson, SC 29634 864-646-7502
FAX 864-646-3620
http://www.clemson.edu/outdoorlab/camps.html
e-mail: cuolcamps-L@clemson.edu
Leslie Conrad, Camp Director
Norman A McGee Jr, Executive Director
Janay Whitesel, Camp Reservations Coordinator
Jaycee Camp Hope is a statewide residential camp for mentally challenged citizens. Its purposes are to give the camper helpful experiences in an outdoor environment, develop the ability to work and play as a group, and provide new experiences unique to a camp setting. The SC Junior Chamber of Commerce has provided financial support for every camper attending Jaycee Camp Hope since 1969. Individuals participating in Camp Hope are ages 8 and older.

991 Clemson Outdoor Lab: Camp Odyssey
Clemson University Outdoor Laboratory
Lehotsky Hall
Clemson, SC 29634 864-646-7502
FAX 864-646-3620
http://www.clemson.edu/outdoorlab/camps.html
e-mail: cuolcamps-L@clemson.edu
Leslie Conrad, Camp Director
Norman A McGee Jr, Executive Director
Janay Whitesel, Camp Reservations Coordinator

Camp Odyssey is a one week program serving children with special needs between the ages of 6-12. The camp begins on Sunday afternoon and ends on Saturday morning. Our unique setting offers opportunity for many exciting activities, including (but not limited to): hiking, fishing, canoeing, instructional swimming, boat rides, arts and crafts, campfire programs and overnight camping trips.

992 **Clemson Outdoor Lab: Camp Sertoma**
Clemson University Outdoor Laboratory
Lehotsky Hall
Clemson, SC 29634
864-646-7502
FAX 864-646-3620
http://www.clemson.edu/outdoorlab/camps.html
e-mail: cuolcamps-L@clemson.edu
Leslie Conrad, Camp Director
Norman A McGee Jr, Executive Director
Janay Whitesel, Camp Reservations Coordinator
Sponsored by the Sertoma clubs of South Carolina, this program serves children between the ages of 7-13 who are either underprivileged or who have speech/hearing impairments. The program offers opportunities for fun, skills development and education in an outdoor environment. Because of the support of Sertoma Clubs across the state, there is no fee to attend. Children are placed in groups with seven other children according to age and previous camp experience.

993 **Clemson Outdoor Lab: Camp Sunshine**
Clemson University Outdoor Laboratory
Lehotsky Hall
Clemson, SC 29634
864-646-7502
FAX 864-646-3620
http://www.clemson.edu/outdoorlab/camps.html
e-mail: cuolcamps-L@clemson.edu
Leslie Conrad, Camp Director
Norman A McGee Jr, Executive Director
Janay Whitesel, Camp Reservations Coordinator
This weekend camp programs serves children and adults who have severe and profound special needs. Designed to provide a respite to the caregivers and families, participants also benefit from the program designed to offer fun and fellowship. Camp Sunshine is funded through the Sunshine Lady Foundation and is offered six weekends throughout the fall and spring. Campers enjoy pontoon boat rides, archery, crafts, campfire programs, hayrides and many other special events throughout the weekend.

994 **Easter Seals Greenville**
Easter Seals South Carolina
1122 Rutherford Road
Greenville, SC 29609
864-232-4185
800-951-4090
FAX 864-232-8161
http://www.sc.easter-seals.org
e-mail: deanna.lewis@eastersc.org
Barbara Jardno, Executive Director
Patti Reins, Assistant Director
Deanna Lewis, President/CEO Easter Seals SC
Easter Seals camping and recreation programs serve children, adults and families of all abilities. Various programs are available with the united purpose of giving disabled individuals a fun and safe camping or recreational experience. The following are camping and recreational services offered: Residential camping program.

South Dakota

995 **Easter Seals Pierre**
1351 N Harrison Avenue
Pierre, SD 57501
605-224-5879
800-592-1852
FAX 605-224-1033
http://www.sd.easterseals.com
e-mail: abush@sd.easterseals.com
Ann Bush, Executive Director

Easter Seals camping and recreation programs serve children, adults and families of all abilities. Various programs are available with the united purpose of giving disabled individuals a fun and safe camping or recreational experience. The following are camping and recreational services offered: Day camping for children.

Tennessee

996 **Camp Discovery Tennessee Jaycees**
400 Camp Discovery Lane
Gainesboro, TN 38562
931-268-0239
FAX 931-268-6737
http://www.jayceecamp.org/
e-mail: director@jayceecamp.org
Dawn Hickman, Executive Director
Ronnie Petty, Camp Caretaker
Paula Petty, Camp Caretaker
Provides summer camp for people with special needs.

997 **Easter Seals Camp**
Easter Seal Camp
6333 Benders Ferry Road
Mount Juliet, TN 37122
615-444-2829
FAX 615-444-8576
TDY:615-385-3485
http://http://tn.easterseals.com
e-mail: camp@eastersealstn.com
Leslie Sohl, Camp Director
Mary Gardner, Program Operations
Rita Baumgartner, VP/Development
Easter Seals camping and recreation programs serve children, adults and families of all abilities. Various programs are available with the united purpose of giving disabled individuals a fun and safe camping or recreational experience. The following are camping and recreational services offered: Camp respite for adults, camp respite for children, camperships and residential camping programs.

998 **River's Way Outdoor Adventure Center**
889 Stoney Hollow Road
Bluff City, TN 37618
423-538-0405
FAX 423-538-8183
http://www.riversway.org
e-mail: tom@riversway.org
Tom Hanlon, Executive Director
Carson G Rivers, Adventures Program Director
Adam Combs, Assc Adventures Program Director
Providing opportunities for youth of all abilities to work, learn and have fun together in educational and outdoor adventure settings. Founded 1993

Texas

999 **ADD Summer Camp**
River Oaks Academy
10600 Richmond Avenue
Houston, TX 77042
713-783-7200
FAX 713-783-7286
http://www.riveroaksacademy.com/summer-camp
e-mail: info@riveroaksacademy.com
Luis Valdes MD, Program Director
Brenda Gardner-Valdes MD, School Director

A specialized summer camp for children and adolescents with ADHD or conduct disorder.

1000 **Camp Aranzazu**
PO Box 1059
Rockport, TX 78381
361-727-0800
FAX 361-727-0818
http://www.camparanzazu.org
e-mail: info@camparanzazu.org
Tammie Shelton, Camp Director
Glenna Buck, Facilities Manager
Judy Simon, Development Director
Camp Aranzazu is a year-round camp facility specially designed to serve the needs of people with chronic illnesses or disabilities where they may enjoy the independence, fellowship, and adventure that a camping experience provides. Through their interactions with the environment, physically challenging activities, and spiritual awareness, the campers gain an increased level of confidence and enhanced self-esteem, thus providing them with emotional healing.

1001 **Camp C.A.M.P.**
Children's Association for Maximum Potential
515 Skyline Drive
Center Point, TX 78010
210-292-3566
FAX 210-292-3577
http://www.campcamp.org
e-mail: campmail@campcamp.org
Hope DeLamos, Camp Director
Ben Elble, Associate Camp Director
T Paul Furukawa Ph.D/LMSW, Executive Director
CAMP, or Children's Association for Maximum Potential, enables children with disabilities to thrive in a recreational environment where safety and nurturing are primary. Camp CAMP is a series of five-day summer camp sessions for children with special needs who may not be eligible to attend other camps due to the severity of their disability or medical condition. We also include activities for campers' siblings without disabilities.

1002 **Camp Funtastic**
City of Carrollton, Texas
4220 N Josey Lane
Carrollton, TX 75011
972-466-3080
FAX 972-466-4722
http://www.cityofcarrollton.com/
e-mail: sharilyn.rabb@cityofcarrollton.com
Sharilyn Rabb, Camp Coordinator
Ana Rivera, Camp Coordinator

Camp Funtastics provides youth with disabilities an enriching, educational and purposeful summer recreation and leisure experience in a safe and fun environment that is supportive of independence. Camper independence is promoted by facilitating the development of new life skills. (ages 8-21 years).

1003 **Camp SummerScapes**
City of Carrollton, Texas
4220 N Josey Lane
Carrollton, TX 75011
972-466-3080
FAX 972-466-4722
http://www.cityofcarrollton.com/
e-mail: sharilyn.rabb@cityofcarrollton.com
Sharilyn Rabb, Camp Coordinator
Ana Rivera, Camp Coordinator

Camp Funtastics provides youth with disabilities an enriching, educational and purposeful summer recreation and leisure experience in a safe and fun environment that is supportive of independence. Camper independence is promoted by facilitating the development of new life skills. (ages 6-8 years).

1004 **Charis Hills Summer Camp**
149 Camp Scenic Loop
Ingram, TX 78025
830-367-4868
888-681-2173
FAX 830-367-2814
http://www.charishills.org/dayatcamp.htm
e-mail: info@charishills.org
Rand Southard, President/Executive Director
Paul Brouse, Camp Program Director
Tim Brown, Assistant Director
Charis Hills is a Christian Summer Camp for kids with learning and social difficulties such as ADD, AD/HD, and Asperger's disorder. Charis Hills is dedicated to the development of kids who have average to above average intelligence, but who have an inability to process information in traditional ways. Campers receive academic reinforcement each day while participating in a traditional summer camping program geared to encourage success and reward positive behavior consistently.

1005 **Easter Seals Central Texas**
1611 Headway Circle
Austin, TX 78754
512-478-2581
FAX 512-476-1638
http://http://centraltx.easterseals.com/
e-mail: info@easterseals.com
Kevin Coleman, President/CEO
Miriam Nisenbaum, Manager
Derrick Chubbs, Chairman
Easter Seals camping and recreation programs serve children, adults and families of all abilities. Various programs are available with the united purpose of giving disabled individuals a fun and safe camping or recreational experience. The following are camping and recreational services offered: Day camping for children.

1006 **El Paso LDA Vacation AdventureEl Paso Learning Disability Association**
8929 Viscount Boulevard
El Paso, TX 79925
915-591-8080
FAX 915-591-8150
http://http://ww2.ldaelpaso.org:8060/
e-mail: webmaster@ldaelpaso.org
Barbara Monroy, Director
Lina Monroy, Executive Director

Summer developmental learning program for children currently placed in Special Education or section 504 programs.

1007 **Girl Scout Camp La Jita**
Girls Scout of America
10443 Gulfdale Street
San Antonio, TX 78216
210-349-2404
877-543-1188
FAX 210-349-2666
http://www.sagirlscouts.org
e-mail: camp@sagirlscouts.org
Kathy Gratham, Executive Director
Jean Larose, Administrative Assistant
Becky Jennings, Outdoor Program Manager
The resident camp experience gives girls the self-confidence and skills they need to succeed in the future. Outdoor and experiential education activities build not only confidence in girls, but also teach the importance of setting and working towards goals, as well as enhance communication skills. All campers will help plan their own daily activities, giving them the chance to express their opinions and to contribute to the decision-making process as much as possible.

1008 **Kamp Kidscope**
City of Carrollton, Texas
4220 N Josey Lane
Carrollton, TX 75011
972-466-3080
FAX 972-466-4722
http://www.cityofcarrollton.com/
e-mail: sharilyn.rabb@cityofcarrollton.com
Sharilyn Rabb, Camp Coordinator
Ana Rivera, Camp Coordinator

Camp Funtastics provides youth with disabilities an enriching, educational and purposeful summer recreation and leisure experience in a safe and fun environment that is supportive of independence. Camper independence is promoted by facilitating the development of new life skills. (ages 9-12 years).

1009 **Rocking L Guest Ranch**
240 Van Zandt County Road
Wills Point, TX 75169
903-560-0246
866-841-1137
FAX 972-495-1131
http://www.rockinglranch.com
e-mail: bradlarsen@rockinglranch.com
Brad Larsen, Owner
Alicia Larsen, Owner

Campers benefit mentally, physically and socially from the camp experience. Additional activities include canoeing, fishing, volleyball, basketball and swimming.

1010 **Teen Cool Connections Summer Camp**
City of Carrollton, Texas
4220 N Josey Lane
Carrollton, TX 75011
972-466-3080
FAX 972-466-4722
http://www.cityofcarrollton.com/
e-mail: sharilyn.rabb@cityofcarrollton.com
Sharilyn Rabb, Camp Coordinator
Ana Rivera, Camp Coordinator

This camp provides opportunities to explore, establish and appreciate participants' unique contributions to serving the needs of their community, while simultaneously learning to utilize resources to best fulfill their needs. (ages 13-15 years).

1011 **Texas Elks Summer Youth Camp**

Texas Elks Children's Services Inc
Gonzales, TX 78629 830-875-2425
FAX 830-875-5455
http://www.texaselks.org/tecsi_camp.html
e-mail: txelks@gvec.net

Mike Cropps, Chairman Board of Directors
Don Pepper, President
Orville Weiss, Secretary

Texas Elks Camp provides special needs children with an opportunity to try new things and to make new friends. Any child with a special need, between the ages of 7 and 15, who is a resident of the state of Texas, is eligible for admission to Texas Elks Camp. Activities include swimming, fishing, hiking, field trips, bowling, dancing, arts and crafts, cookouts, and horseback riding.

Utah

1012 **Camp Kostopulos**

2500 Emigration Canyon
Salt Lake City, UT 84108 801-582-0700
FAX 801-583-5176
http://www.campk.org
e-mail: gethington@campk.org

Gary Ethington, Camp Director
Jan Murphy, Development Director
Mike Divricean, Operations Manager

The Kostopulos Dream Foundation is an agency dedicated to improving the lives of people with disabilities. Our longest running program, Camp Kostopulos, is a residential summer camp where kids, teens, and adults with disabilities are able to engage in a variety of activities. During a week-long stay, campers go fishing, ride horses, camp out, sing songs, work on arts and crafts projects, challenge themselves on the ropes course, make new friends, and renew old friendships.

1013 **Reid Ranch**

3310 S 2700 E
Salt Lake City, UT 84109 801-486-5083
800-468-3274
FAX 801-466—421
http://www.reidschool.com/ranch.html
e-mail: ereid@xmission.com

Gardner Reid, Owner
Ethna R Reid Ph.D, Executive Director

Provides students, ages 8-18, with an opportunity to receive small group and tutorial instruction in reading and language skills development. The program operates three weeks during the summer.

Vermont

1014 **Camp Betsy Cox**

140 Betsey Cox Lane
Pittsford, VT 05763 802-483-6611
888-345-9193
http://www.campbetseycox.com
e-mail: betcoxvt@aol.com

Lorrie Byrom, Camp Director
Devri Byrom, Winter Office Director

Summer camp for girls only, ages 9 to 15, that offers a wide variety of activities including aquatics, horseback riding, outdoor skills, creative arts, sports, farm and garden activities in addition to special events. Campers become deeply involved in the activites and develop good decision-making skills. Every girl learns at her own pace, at her own level of interest.

1015 **Camp Thorpe**

680 Capen Hill Road
Goshen, VT 05733 802-247-6611
FAX 802-247-6611
http://www.campthorpe.org
e-mail: cthorpe@sover.net

Lyle Jepson, Camp Director
Ralph O'Hathoway, Board of Trustees
Peter Lynch, Board of Trustees

Camp Thorpe gives our special campers a chance to succeed through activities including swimming, boating, theater, nature study, music, art, and sports. The program is designed to meet the individual needs of each camper. Particular emphasis is placed upon skill development, socialization, exercise, and emotional growth.

1016 **Easter Seals Vermont**

641 Comstock Road
Berlin, VT 05602 802-223-4744
888-372-2636
http://http://nh.easterseals.com
e-mail: info@easterseals.com

Larry J Gammon, President
Christine M McMahon, SVP/COO
Karen Van Der Beken, SVP/Development & Communication

Easter Seals camping and recreation programs serve children, adults and families of all abilities. Various programs are available with the united purpose of giving disabled individuals a fun and safe camping or recreational experience. The following are camping and recreational services offered: Camp respite for children, camperships.

1017 **Partners in Adventure Day Camp**

Shelburne, VT 05482 802-425-2638
FAX 802-425-2638
http://www.partnersinadventure.org/
e-mail: dlamden@gmavt.net

Deborah Lamden, Executive Director
Sue Minter, Administrative Coordinator
Liz Robitaille, VP Board of Directors

Partners in Adventure Day Camp offers programs for young people with and without disabilities, activities of which include swimming, boating, playing tennis, wall climbing, archery, gymnastics, cooking, exploring arts, crafts, science and nature, playing games, dancing, making music and immersing themselves in the outdoors. All adaptive equipment programs are taught by trained instructors. Each session will include field trips to a variety of locations. Ages 12-21.

1018 **Pine Ridge School Summer Programs**

Williston, VT 05495 802-434-2161
FAX 802-434-5512
http://www.pineridgeschool.com/ProgramsFr.php
e-mail: dblackhurst@pineridgeschool.com

Dana Blackhurst, Head of School
John Kaufman, Dean of Students
Pamela Blum, Business Manager

Pine Ridge School is an educational community committed to empowering students with learning disabilities to define and achieve success throughout their lives. The School offers a residential program in the summer for learning disabled students ages nine to eighteen. The students spend six weeks improving language processing skills by attending two one-to-one Orton-Gillingham tutorials per day. In addition, they enjoy a full range of outdoor sports and regular camp activities.

1019 **Silver Towers Camp**

125 Goshen Road
Ripton, VT 05766
800-385-8524
http://www.silvertowerscamp.org
e-mail: earlc@svcable.net

Carolyn Ravenna, Director
Beverly Bearor, Head Women's Counselor
Noah Heloo, Head Men's Counselor

A one-week residential camp for exceptional people six years old and up to enjoy varied opportunities for personal enrichment and development of social skills, including swimming, arts and crafts, sing alongs, music, dancing and bowling

Virginia

1020 **Camp Baker**

Richmond ARC
Chesterfield, VA 23838 804-748-4789
FAX 804-796-6880
http://www.richmondarc.org/camp.html
e-mail: campbaker@richmondarc.org

Charles Sutherland, Camp Director
Collen Kraft, Medical Director
Joe & April Niamtu, Honorary ARC Spokescouple
Camp Baker supports children from age six through adulthood with mental retardation and similar developmental disabilities. Campers receive care and supervision in a safe, nurturing environment. Beyond assistance with personal hygiene, meals, toileting and medication management, campers participate in therapeutic, recreational and social activities both at the camp and in the community. A 1:3 staff-to-camper ratio is maintained.

1021 Civitan Acres Summer Camp
Civitan Acres Vacation Services
Chesapeake, VA 23323 757-487-6062
FAX 757-487-4143
http://egglestonservices.org/programs_ca.html
e-mail: civitan@egglestonservices.org
Meghan Hurt, Camp Director
Jeffrey Parker, Chairman Board of Directors
Pam Wright, Treasurer Board of Directors
Civitan Acres offers summer camps for adult and children with disabilities. Participants can choose from day or overnight packages. With swimming, cabins, soccer and baseball fields, playground facilities, and a variety of community outings, participants have many opportunities to enjoy themselves and develop a variety of skills.

1022 Civitan Acres Summer Camp: Explore Hampton Roads Camp
Civitan Acres Vacation Services
Chesapeake, VA 23323 757-487-6062
FAX 757-487-4143
http://egglestonservices.org/programs_ca.html
e-mail: civitan@egglestonservices.org
Meghan Hurt, Camp Director
Jeffrey Parker, Chairman Board of Directors
Pam Wright, Treasurer Board of Directors
At Explore Hampton Roads campers enjoy a week of different museums, including the Living Museum and the Mariner's Museum in addition to arts and crafts, a talent show, games, and many more fun and exciting events. Adults only, $399, overnight only. Week 1: June 25-29.

1023 Civitan Acres Summer Camp: Fun in the SunCamp
Civitan Acres Vacation Services
Chesapeake, VA 23323 757-487-6062
FAX 757-487-4143
http://egglestonservices.org/programs_ca.html
e-mail: civitan@egglestonservices.org
Meghan Hurt, Camp Director
Jeffrey Parker, Chairman Board of Directors
Pam Wright, Treasurer Board of Directors
During Fun in the Sun Week campers will enjoy numerous activities including a trip to the Virginia Zoo, lunch and a movie at Cinema Cafe, and much more. Kids only, $399 overnight, $350 day camp. Week 7: August 6-10.

1024 Civitan Acres Summer Camp: Outdoor Adventure Camp
Civitan Acres Vacation Services
Chesapeake, VA 23323 757-487-6062
FAX 757-487-4143
http://egglestonservices.org/programs_ca.html
e-mail: civitan@egglestonservices.org
Meghan Hurt, Camp Director
Jeffrey Parker, Chairman Board of Directors
Pam Wright, Treasurer Board of Directors
Outdoor Adventure Camp is a new program for 2007. This is a day camp only week. Campers will enjoy fun packed days in the great outdoors where they will visit local parks, go fishing, and attend a Norfolk Tides Game. Camp open from 8a.m.-5p.m. Adults only, $425 day camp only. Week 4: July 16-20.

1025 Civitan Acres Summer Camp: Rollercoaster Mania Camp
Civitan Acres Vacation Services
Chesapeake, VA 23323 757-487-6062
FAX 757-487-4143
http://egglestonservices.org/programs_ca.html
e-mail: civitan@egglestonservices.org
Meghan Hurt, Camp Director
Jeffrey Parker, Chairman Board of Directors
Pam Wright, Treasurer Board of Directors
During Rollercoaster Mania Camp activities include a visit to Busch Gardens Europe for fun and adventure. Campers will enjoy rides and rollercoasters or entertaining shows in addition to visting Northwest River Park for a full day of adventure. Adults only, $499, overnight only. Week 5: July 23-27.

1026 Civitan Acres Summer Camp: Take a Break Camp Part 1 Week
Civitan Acres Vacation Services
Chesapeake, VA 23323 757-487-6062
FAX 757-487-4143
http://egglestonservices.org/programs_ca.html
e-mail: civitan@egglestonservices.org
Meghan Hurt, Camp Director
Jeffrey Parker, Chairman Board of Directors
Pam Wright, Treasurer Board of Directors
At Take a Break campers will enjoy an exciting week that includes a trip to the bowling alley and seeing a movie at Cinema Cafe. Additional activities include watching fireworks in celebration of 4th of July. Adults only, $399, overnight only. Week 2: July 2-6.

1027 Civitan Acres Summer Camp: Take a Break Part 2 Week Camp
Civitan Acres Vacation Services
Chesapeake, VA 23323 757-487-6062
FAX 757-487-4143
http://egglestonservices.org/programs_ca.html
e-mail: civitan@egglestonservices.org
Meghan Hurt, Camp Director
Jeffrey Parker, Chairman Board of Directors
Pam Wright, Treasurer Board of Directors
Part 2 of Take a Break Camp provides another week of relaxation. Activities includes arts and crafts, beads and music in addition to a trip to a restaurant to enjoy lunch and live entertainment. Also, there will be a full night of dancing and partying. Adults only, $399, overnight only. Week 3: July 9-13.

1028 Civitan Acres Summer Camp: Wet & Wild FunCamp
Civitan Acres Vacation Services
Chesapeake, VA 23323 757-487-6062
FAX 757-487-4143
http://egglestonservices.org/programs_ca.html
e-mail: civitan@egglestonservices.org
Meghan Hurt, Camp Director
Jeffrey Parker, Chairman Board of Directors
Pam Wright, Treasurer Board of Directors
At Wet & Wild Fun Camp adventures include a trip to Ocean Breeze Water Park. Campers will also enjoy water balloons, swimming, and a trip to the Virginia Aquarium and much more in this fun filled week. Adults only, $399, overnight only. Week 6: July 30-August 3.

1029 Easter Seals Virginia
8003 Franklin Farms Drive
Richmond, VA 23229 804-287-1007
866-874-4153
FAX 804-287-1008
http://www.va.easterseals.com
e-mail: thazelbaker@va.easterseals.com
Tara Hazelbaker, President/CEO
Sarah Hutchinson, Camp Director

Easter Seals camping and recreation programs serve children, adults and families of all abilities. Various programs are available with the united purpose of giving disabled individuals a fun and safe camping or recreational experience. The following are camping and recreational services offered: Family retreats and Residential Family Programs.

1030 Fairfax County Community and Recreation
12011 Government Center Parkway
Fairfax, VA 22035 703-324-4386
FAX 703-222-9722
TDY:703-222-9693
http://www.fairfaxcounty.gov/rec/
Patricia Franckewitz, Executive Director
Sara Mumsord, Branch Manager

Therapeutic recreation services summer activities for children with disabilities to include LD and ADHA.

1031 Makemie Woods Summer Camp
3700 Ropers Church Road
Lanexa, VA 23089
757-566-1496
800-566-1496
FAX 757-566-8803
http://www.makwoods.org
e-mail: makwoods@makwoods.org
Mike Burcher, Reverend, Camp Director
Jenny McDevitt, Program Director
Karen Broughman, Office Administrator
For over 40 years, Makemie Woods has been changing lives by providing a high-quality, fun! and safe Christian summer camp for youth. Established in 1964, Makemie Woods offers a chance for campers to try new things, learn new skills, make new friends, and develop and nurture their faith in Jesus Christ. Camp activities includes swimming, canoeing, music and drama, horseback riding, scuba diving, and high ropes adventure.

1032 Oakland School Summer Programs
Boyd Tavern
Keswick, VA 22947
434-293-9059
FAX 434-296-8930
http://www.oaklandschool.net/summer_program
e-mail: OaklandSchool@earthlink.net
Carol Smieciuch, School Director
Donna Darden, Assistant Director
Kelly Oakes, Development Director
Oakland School is a small co-ed boarding and day school that enables children who have dyslexia, learning disabilities, or organizational and study skills difficulties to reach their academic and personal potential. The summer program at Oakland is a wonderful balance of academic and traditional camp classes. Recreational activities include swimming, tennis, archery, arts and crafts, nature study, team sports in soccer, volleyball, and basketball, in addition to horseback riding.

1033 Sensational Explorers Day Camp
PO Box 10693
Burke, VA 22009
703-978-6532
e-mail: SensoryCamp@hotmail.com
Joanne Kennedy, Clinical Director
Susan Miller, Administrative Director

A camp for high functioning children with sensory integration needs. The camp is run by sensory integration clinicians.

1034 Shady Grove Family YMCA Summer Camps
Glen Allen, VA 23059
804-270-3866
FAX 804-270-0478
http://www.ymcarichmond.org
e-mail: oneillm@ymcarichmond.org
Megan O'Neill, Executive Director
Anne Finnegan, Youth & Adult Sports Director
Clay Mottley, Fine Arts & Adventure Director
Whether it's through singing or swimming, nature hikes or computer classes, counselors at YMCA camps lead kids in developing good values and having fun every summer. Each YMCA is structured to meet the needs of the children and community is serves, providing the same outcome. YMCA camps fully utilize their natural setting, teaching youth about the wonders of the world around them. In addition, special sessions on academics, sports, arts, or teen adventure or leadership may be offered.

Washington

1035 Camp Easter Seals West
17809 S Vaughn Road KPN
Vaughn, WA 98394
253-884-2722
FAX 253-884-0200
http://http://www.wa.easterseals.com
e-mail: eastersealare@seals.org
Mary McIntyre, Office Manager
Mike Mooney, Summer Camp Director
Lori Hall, Respite Coordinator
The camp offers six day sessions geared to the age, level of ability and needs of the camper. Includes a wide range of activities including horseback riding, dancing and waterfront activities.

1036 Camp Killoqua/Camp Fire USA
Snohomish County Council
4312 Rucker Avenue
Everett, WA 98203
425-258-5437
FAX 452-252-2267
http://www.campfireusasnohomish.org/killoqua
e-mail: Killoqua@campfireusasnohomish.org
Dave Surface, Executive Director
Carol Johnson, Assistant Director

Provides a unique outdoor experience for youth and adults offering a full range of options and opportunities.

1037 Camp Sweyolakan
524 N Mullan Road
Spokane Valley, WA 99206
509-747-6191
800-386-2324
FAX 509-747-4913
http://www.campfireinc.org/camp/sweyolakan/
e-mail: sweyolakan@campfireinc.org
Lee Taylor, Executive Director
Peggy Clark, Camp Director
Judy Lippman, Special Programs
Both resident and day camp on 300 wooded acres is open to all boys, girls, adults, those with special needs and families.

1038 Camp Volasuca
Volasuca Volunteers of America
Everett, WA 98201
360-793-0646
FAX 360-793-0646
http://www.voaww.org/camp
e-mail: camp@voaww.org
Dave Wood, Camp Director
Tom Robinson, President/CEO
Blair Marshall, Information Services Director
Camp Volasuca provides a unique, safe atmosphere for at-risk youth and adults with developmental disabilities; individuals who might not otherwise have the opportunity to experience summer camp. Camp is situated at the foothills of the Cascade Mountains and lies nestled in a wooded area of the Skykomish Valley. An array of activities captures the imagination of the campers and is an powerful experience that can contribute to each participant's well-being and can create a lifetime of memories.

1039 Easter Seals Spokane
Easter Seals
606 W Sharp Avenue
Spokane, WA 99201
509-326-8292
FAX 509-326-2261
http://http://wa.easterseals.com
e-mail: gperkins@wa.easter-seals.org
Ginette Perkins, Executive Director
Stefanie Butlar, Assistant Director

Easter Seals camping and recreation programs serve children, adults and families of all abilities. Various programs are available with the united purpose of giving disabled individuals a fun and safe camping or recreational experience. The following are camping and recreational services offered: Recreational services for children and residential camping programs.

1040 Trek Northwest
c/o Talisman Programs
Zirconia, NC 28790
828-697-6313
888-458-8226
FAX 828-697-6249
http://www.talismancamps.com/trek.html
e-mail: info@talismancamps.com
Linda Tatsapauagh, Camp Director
Aaron McGinley, Base Camp Program Manager
Pete Weiss, Program Manager
Campers ages 13-17 with ADHD, Asperger's, NLD, and other social skills needs, participate in this 2 week long backpacking program. Working in small groups with highly trained staff, campers hone their social skills, develop self-confidence and learn the value of accountability. Campers backpack through the scenic Olympic National Forest, then whitewater raft on the beautiful and exciting Elwha River.

West Virginia

1041 **Easter Seals Rehabilitation Center**
1305 National Road
Wheeling, WV 26003
304-242-1390
800-677-1390
FAX 304-243-5880
TDY:304-242-1390
http://www.wv.easterseals.com
e-mail: ateaster@stargate.net

Lorie Untch, President/CEO
Denise Knouse Snyder, Chairman of the Board

Easter Seals camping and recreation programs serve children, adults and families of all abilities. Various programs are available with the united purpose of giving disabled individuals a fun and safe camping or recreational experience. Offers camps for adults and children, camperships, computer programs, family retreats, residential camping programs, and swimming programs.

1042 **Mountain Milestones**
Stepping Stones
400 Mylan Park Lane
Morgantown, WV 26501
304-296-0150
800-982-8799
FAX 304-296-0194
http://www.steppingstonecenter.net
e-mail: abilitywv@hotmail.com

Susan Fox, Director
Jack Porter, President
Bob Pirner, Manager
People with disabilities of all ages can take part in a variety of recreation programs that include adventures, team sports, special events and camps.

Wisconsin

1043 **Beginning Adventures Camp**
Stevens Point Area YMCA
Stevens Point, WI 54481
715-342-2980
FAX 715-342-2987
http://www.glacierhollow.com/Resident-Camp.html
e-mail: pmatthai@spymca.org
Pete Matthai, Camp Director

Beginning Adventurers, a 4-day session for younger and first-time campers, is a great intermediate progression point from day camp to the full 7-day resident camp. Campers will experience hands-on camp activities like canoe lessons, fishing, archery and more. Special attention will be given to helping campers feel comfortable in new surroundings. Enthusiastic counselors will guide young campers in discovering the wonders of nature and camping, while building confidence and independence.

1044 **Camp Tekawitha**
W5248 Lake Drive
Shawano, WI 54166
715-526-2316
FAX 715-526-6448
http://gbdioc.org/pg/dioceseCampTekawitha.tpl
e-mail: camptekawitha@gbdioc.org
Mary Piezker, Camp Director
Tom Long Fr, Vocations Director

Camp Tekawitha provides a positive summer experience where Christian ideals are integrated into daily activities. In addition to our new chapel, camp facilities include a main lodge, a recreation hall with a stage and large stone fireplace, craft area, kitchen, spacious dining room, 8 sleeping cabins, modern shower building, trading post, health care and office. Two qualified counselors are assigned to each cabin and ensure that your children have the chance to explore the world around them.

1045 **Camp Wise Spirits**
Stevens Point Area YMCA
Stevens Point, WI 54481
715-342-2980
FAX 715-342-2987
http://www.glacierhollow.com/Resident-Camp.html
e-mail: pmatthai@spymca.org
Pete Matthai, Camp Director

YMCA Resident Camps offer youth a safe environment in which positive values, personal growth, lifelong friendships, environmental awareness, and outrageous fun are key elements. The YMCA has been operating resident camps and teen trips since 1997. Camp Wise Spirits is just for girls. This camp is all about learning who you are and learning to believe in yourself. You'll share traditional camp activities, outdoor adventures, learn new skills, make meaningful friendships and have lots of fun.

1046 **Easter Seals Camp Wawbeek**
1450 State Highway 13
Wisconsin Dells, WI 53965
608-277-8031
800-422-2324
FAX 608-277-8333
TDY:608-277-8031
http://www.wi-easterseals.org
e-mail: Wawbeek@wi-easterseals.org
Valerie Croissant, Director
Mel Drake, Camp Program Coordinator
Christine Fessler, CEO
Easter Seals camping and recreation programs serve children, adults and families of all abilities. Various programs are available with the united purpose of giving disabled individuals a fun and safe camping or recreational experience.The following are camping and recreational services offered: Adventure, camperships, canoeing, conference rental, day camping for children, family retreats, residential camping programs and swim programs.

1047 **Easter Seals Southeastern Wisconsin**
3090 N 53rd Street
Milwaukee, WI 53210
414-449-4444
FAX 414-449-4447
http://http://wi.easterseals.com
e-mail: agency@easterseals-sewi.org
Bob Glowacki, Executive Director
Sheolia Underwoods, Office Manager

Easter Seals camping and recreation programs serve children, adults and families of all abilities. Various programs are available with the united purpose of giving disabled individuals a fun and safe camping or recreational experience. The following are camping and recreational services offered: Before/After school program for Ages 6 through 18.

1048 **Holiday Home Camp**
Lake Geneva Fresh Air Association
Williams Bay, WI 53191
262-245-5161
FAX 262-245-6518
http://www.holidayhomecamp.org
e-mail: gail@holidayhomecamp.org
Gail Tumidajewicz, Camp Director

Holiday Home Camp, owned and operated by the Lake Geneva Fresh Air Association, provides campers with a variety of activities the program focus of which is designed to help them to develop living skills. Included are daily activities such as arts and crafts, rope course, swimming and fishing, sailing, archery, canoeing, computers, and basketball.

1049 **Nature Quest Camp**
Stevens Point Area YMCA
Stevens Point, WI 54481
715-342-2980
FAX 715-342-2987
http://www.glacierhollow.com/Resident-Camp.html
e-mail: pmatthai@spymca.org
Pete Matthai, Camp Director

YMCA Resident Camps offer youth a safe environment in which positive values, personal growth, lifelong friendships, environmental awareness, and outrageous fun are key elements. Nature Quest Camp participants will enjoy a mix of traditional camp activities with special attention on outdoor living skills and environmental education. In addition, through evening campfires, group games and activities, campers will laugh and create new memories and friends.

1050 Timbertop Nature Adventure Camp
Stevens Point Area YMCA
1000 Division Street
Stevens Point, WI 54481
715-342-2980
FAX 715-342-2987
http://www.glacierhollow.com
e-mail: pmatthai@spymca.org
Dave Morgan, Executive Director
Jackie Clussman, Special Needs Director
Peter Matthai, Camp Director
For youth identified by their school districts as needing extra help for a learning disability. Combines traditional camp activities focused on dealing with learning disabilities in a structured daily setting. Special attention is paid to peer relations, building self-confidence and learning new skills.

1051 Wisconsin Badger Camp
PO Box 723
Plattesville, WI 53818
608-348-9689
FAX 608-348-9737
http://www.badgercamp.org
e-mail: wiscbadgercamp@centurytel.net
Brent Bowers, Camp Director

Wisconsin Badger Camp's mission is to provide a positive natural environment where individuals with developmental challenges can learn about their surroundings and realize their full potential. Through a group living experience, campers develop friendships and expand their social skills. Everyone, regardless of the severity of their disability, are welcome at Badger Camp. Activities inclue swimming, arts and crafts, recreation, nature, overnight camping, fishing, hay rides and dances.

1052 Wisconsin Elk/Easter Seals Respite Camp
1550 Waubeek Road
Wisconsin Dells, WI 53965
608-254-2502
800-422-2342
FAX 608-277-8333
TDY:608-277-8031
http://http://wi.easterseals.com
e-mail: respite1@wi-easterseals.org
Valerie Croissant, Director
Nance Roepke, Executive Vice President
Christine Fessler, CEO
The following are camping and recreational services offered: Camp respite for adults, camp respite for children, canoeing, family retreats, residential camping programs and swim programs.

1053 YMCA Camp Matawa: Adventure Camp Program
YMCA of Metropolitan Milwaukee
Campbellsport, WI 53010
262-626-2149
FAX 262-626-8189
http://www.matawa.org
e-mail: jfeltz@ymcamke.org
Jennifer S Feltz, Camp Director
Wendy Mieske, Program Director
Jerry Carman, Camp Registrar
The Camp Matawa experience is a fun, educational and exciting adventure! With more than 130 acres of pines, open fields and 30,000 acres of adjacent state forest, YMCA Camp Matawa has since 1996 offered a wide variety of activities that challenge and inspire campers of all ages. Adventure programs include mountain biking, arts and crafts, nature study, archery, skateboarding, canoeing, swimming and nature study. Ages 7-15.

1054 YMCA Camp Matawa: Equestrian Summer Camp
YMCA of Metropolitan Milwaukee
Campbellsport, WI 53010
262-626-2149
FAX 262-626-8189
http://www.matawa.org
e-mail: jfeltz@ymcamke.org
Jennifer S Feltz, Camp Director
Wendy Mieske, Program Director
Jerry Carman, Camp Registrar
Horses and horseback riding are a perennial favorite for campers of all ages and abilities. Campers work with our equestrian instructors during three equestrian activity periods each day, allowing campers to have more riding time and hone their new skills. Equestrian campers also participate in our regular camp programs such as canoeing, arts and crafts and more. Campers are placed in a riding class appropriate to their skill level. Western or English riding instruction is offered.

1055 YMCA Camp Matawa: Extend Your Stay SummerCamp
YMCA of Metropolitan Milwaukee
Campbellsport, WI 53010
262-626-2149
FAX 262-626-8189
http://www.matawa.org
e-mail: jfeltz@ymcamke.org
Jennifer S Feltz, Camp Director
Wendy Mieske, Program Director
Jerry Carman, Camp Registrar
With more than 130 acres of pines, open fields and 30,000 acres of adjacent state forest, YMCA Camp Matawa has since 1996 offered a wide variety of activities that challenge and inspire campers of all ages. One week not enough? Can't seem to leave your second home? Why not take advantage of our Extend Your Stay option? Offered at the conclusion of sessions 1,3 and 5, campers choosing this option will participate in activities as part of our Stay Program, checking out of camp Sunday at 11:00 a.m.

1056 YMCA Camp Matawa: Frontier Village Program
YMCA of Metropolitan Milwaukee
Campbellsport, WI 53010
262-626-2149
FAX 262-626-8189
http://www.matawa.org
e-mail: jfeltz@ymcamke.org
Jennifer S Feltz, Camp Director
Wendy Mieske, Program Director
Jerry Carman, Camp Registrar
The Camp Matawa experience is a fun, educational and exciting adventure! With more than 130 acres of pines, open fields and 30,000 acres of adjacent state forest, YMCA Camp Matawa has since 1996 offered a wide variety of activities that challenge and inspire campers of all ages. The Frontier Village Program is for campers ages 10-12. Activities include mountain biking and climbing wall. Main Camp campout.

1057 YMCA Camp Matawa: Gone Fishin Camp
YMCA of Metropolitan Milwaukee
Campbellsport, WI 53010
262-626-2149
FAX 262-626-8189
http://www.matawa.org
e-mail: jfeltz@ymcamke.org
Jennifer S Feltz, Camp Director
Wendy Mieske, Program Director
Jerry Carman, Camp Registrar
If you love to fish but also enjoy swimming, climbing, archery, sports and more, then this is the camp for you. There is plenty of fishing for pike, bass, walleye and panfish and even a half-day charter on Lake Michigan angling for giant salmon, steelhead and lake trout. Additional fishing spots to include Mauthe Lake and Lake Winnebago. Campers bring their tackle and we supply the bait and instructions. Ages 11-15.

1058 YMCA Camp Matawa: Halloween Camp
YMCA of Metropolitan Milwaukee
Campbellsport, WI 53010
262-626-2149
FAX 262-626-8189
http://www.matawa.org
e-mail: jfeltz@ymcamke.org
Jennifer S Feltz, Camp Director
Wendy Mieske, Program Director
Jerry Carman, Camp Registrar
The Camp Matawa experience is a fun, educational and exciting adventure with more than 130 acres of pines, open fields and 30,000 acres of adjacent state forest. Campers can sip hot cider and munch on fresh roasted pumpkin seeds while spending Halloween in the perfect autumn spot! Pleasure Valley Farms, llama shows, corn maze, hayrides, costume contest, stories around the campfire and a pumpkin carving contest are just some of the activities campers will enjoy throughout their stay. Ages 7-16.

1059 YMCA Camp Matawa: Mini Session Summer Camp (Ages 7-12)
YMCA of Metropolitan Milwaukee
Campbellsport, WI 53010
262-626-2149
FAX 262-626-8189
http://www.matawa.org
e-mail: jfeltz@ymcamke.org
Jennifer S Feltz, Camp Director
Wendy Mieske, Program Director
Jerry Carman, Camp Registrar

The Camp Matawa experience is a fun, educational and exciting adventure! With more than 130 acres of pines, open fields and 30,000 acres of adjacent state forest, YMCA Camp Matawa has since 1996 offered a wide variety of activities that challenge and inspire campers of all ages. This 4 day, 3 night program is an introduction to resident camping with lots of individual attention. Activities include arts & crafts, new games, hiking, campfires, swimming and horseback riding. Ages 7-12.

1060 YMCA Camp Matawa: Pioneer Village Program

YMCA of Metropolitan Milwaukee
Campbellsport, WI 53010
262-626-2149
FAX 262-626-8189
http://www.matawa.org
e-mail: jfeltz@ymcamke.org

Jennifer S Feltz, Camp Director
Wendy Mieske, Program Director
Jerry Carman, Camp Registrar

The Camp Matawa experience is a fun, educational and exciting adventure! With more than 130 acres of pines, open fields and 30,000 acres of adjacent state forest, YMCA Camp Matawa has since 1996 offered a wide variety of activities that challenge and inspire campers of all ages. The Pioneer Village Program is for campers ages 7-9, activities of which include an evening cookout and swim lessons in addition to a low staff-camper ratio.

1061 YMCA Camp Matawa: Pony Club Summer Camp Program

YMCA of Metropolitan Milwaukee
Campbellsport, WI 53010
262-626-2149
FAX 262-626-8189
http://www.matawa.org
e-mail: jfeltz@ymcamke.org

Jennifer S Feltz, Camp Director
Wendy Mieske, Program Director
Jerry Carman, Camp Registrar

Our Pony Club is perfect for campers who would like to add a horse experience to their week of camp, but aren't ready to jump into Equestrian Camp. Campers will spend one activity session per day at the barn, learning about horse care, tack and general horsemanship, culminating in a trail ride at the end of the week. Perfect for campers who would like to see if Equestrian Camp might be right for them next year!

1062 YMCA Camp Matawa: Ropes Challenge Camp

YMCA of Metropolitan Milwaukee
Campbellsport, WI 53010
262-626-2149
FAX 262-626-8189
http://www.matawa.org
e-mail: jfeltz@ymcamke.org

Jennifer S Feltz, Camp Director
Wendy Mieske, Program Director
Jerry Carman, Camp Registrar

In our Ropes Challenge Camp, campers use the Alpine Tower, indoor climbing wall and our Low Ropes Confidence Course to learn climbing and team work skills. Each day the camper will spend two periods in these fun and exciting ropes activities that will include learning knots, how to belay, climbing techniques, proper use and care of equipment such as rope, helmets and carabiners, and how to work together as a team. Safety training and procedures are emphasized in each activity. Ages 10-15.

1063 YMCA Camp Matawa: Stayover Weekends Summer Camp

YMCA of Metropolitan Milwaukee
Campbellsport, WI 53010
262-626-2149
FAX 262-626-8189
http://www.matawa.org
e-mail: jfeltz@ymcamke.org

Jennifer S Feltz, Camp Director
Wendy Mieske, Program Director
Jerry Carman, Camp Registrar

With more than 130 acres of pines, open fields and 30,000 acres of adjacent state forest, YMCA Camp Matawa has since 1996 offered a wide variety of activities that challenge and inspire campers of all ages. Campers who register for the two-week sessions will enjoy a special weekend of programming including horseback riding, outdoor cooking, their own special pool party and other fun activities. The second week allows campers to maximize the opportunity to make new friends and try new activities.

1064 YMCA Camp Matawa: Summer Adventure Camp

YMCA of Metropolitan Milwaukee
Campbellsport, WI 53010
262-626-2149
FAX 262-626-8189
http://www.matawa.org
e-mail: jfeltz@ymcamke.org

Jennifer S Feltz, Camp Director
Wendy Mieske, Program Director
Jerry Carman, Camp Registrar

The Camp Matawa experience is a fun, educational and exciting adventure! With more than 130 acres of pines, open fields and 30,000 acres of adjacent state forest, YMCA Camp Matawa has since 1996 offered a wide variety of activities that challenge and inspire campers of all ages. Adventure programs include mountain biking, arts and crafts, nature study, archery, skateboarding, canoeing, swimming and nature study. Ages 7-15.

1065 YMCA Camp Matawa: Teen Extreme Summer Camp Program (Ages 13-15)

YMCA of Metropolitan Milwaukee
Campbellsport, WI 53010
262-626-2149
FAX 262-626-8189
http://www.matawa.org
e-mail: jfeltz@ymcamke.org

Jennifer S Feltz, Camp Director
Wendy Mieske, Program Director
Jerry Carman, Camp Registrar

In this very exciting program, campers will spend two weeks participating in traditional camping activities and several offsite adventures. Week one is filled with all the thrills and excitement you have come to expect from Camp Matawa. During the second week, campers will travel to Devil's Lake for an overnight campout and a thrilling day of rock climbing. Teen Extreme campers will also head into the Kettle Moraine State Forest for a backpacking and mountain biking excursion. Go extreme!

1066 YMCA Camp Matawa: Teen Weekend Camp

YMCA of Metropolitan Milwaukee
Campbellsport, WI 53010
262-626-2149
FAX 262-626-8189
http://www.matawa.org
e-mail: jfeltz@ymcamke.org

Jennifer S Feltz, Camp Director
Wendy Mieske, Program Director
Jerry Carman, Camp Registrar

The Camp Matawa experience is a fun, educational and exciting adventure! With more than 130 acres of pines, open fields and 30,000 acres of adjacent state forest, YMCA Camp Matawa has since 1996 offered a wide variety of activities that challenge and inspire campers of all ages. Teen Weekend campers will enjoy a variety of their favorite camp activities such as rock climbing, archery, arts and crafts as well as some new teen favorites! Ages 13-16.

1067 YMCA Camp Matawa: Toolin' It Camp

YMCA of Metropolitan Milwaukee
Campbellsport, WI 53010
262-626-2149
FAX 262-626-8189
http://www.matawa.org
e-mail: jfeltz@ymcamke.org

Jennifer S Feltz, Camp Director
Wendy Mieske, Program Director
Jerry Carman, Camp Registrar

A five-day manufacturing camp experience designed for young women and men. Each day campers will travel to Moraine Park Technical College's state-of-the-art Applied Manufacturing Technology Center where they will get hands-on experience designing and producing a product from start to finish. Attendees will explore 3-D design, computer numerical control programming, welding, machining, engines and more, all while emphasizing problem solving and team building skills. Ages 13-17.

1068 YMCA Camp Matawa: Trekker Village Program

YMCA of Metropolitan Milwaukee
Campbellsport, WI 53010
262-626-2149
FAX 262-626-8189
http://www.matawa.org
e-mail: jfeltz@ymcamke.org

Jennifer S Feltz, Camp Director
Wendy Mieske, Program Director
Jerry Carman, Camp Registrar

The Camp Matawa experience is a fun, educational and exciting adventure! With more than 130 acres of pines, open fields and 30,000 acres of adjacent state forest, YMCA Camp Matawa has since 1996 offered a wide variety of activities that challenge and inspire campers of all ages. Trekker Village Program is for ages 13-15, activities of which include the 50 foot Alpine Tower and offsite trips. Wilderness campout.

1069 YMCA Camp Matawa: Winter Camp

YMCA of Metropolitan Milwaukee
Campbellsport, WI 53010
262-626-2149
FAX 262-626-8189
http://www.matawa.org
e-mail: jfeltz@ymcamke.org

Jennifer S Feltz, Camp Director
Wendy Mieske, Program Director
Jerry Carman, Camp Registrar

The Camp Matawa experience is a fun, educational and exciting adventure with more than 130 acres of pines, open fields and 30,000 acres of adjacent state forest. Come and see Camp Matawa in all of its winter beauty! Winter camp is a great time for returning summer campers, new campers and their friends to get together over Christmas vacation. Join us for great indoor and outdoor activities including rock climbing, archery, campfires, snow tubing and much more. Ages 7-16.

Language Arts

1070 100% Concepts: Intermediate
LinguiSystems
3100 4th Avenue
East Moline, IL 61244
309-755-2300
800-776-4332
FAX 309-755-2377
TDY:800-933-8331
http://www.linguisystems.com
e-mail: service@linguisystems.com
LinguiSystems Staff, Author
Linda Bowers, Co-Owners/Co-Founder
Rosemary Huisingh, Co-Owners/Co-Founders

Concepts learning doesn't stop in the early grades. Your older students with language disorders need to understand the terms they hear in the classroom. These terrific activities will help. Teach higher level concepts, including location and direction, quality or condition, comparison, time and occurrence, and relationship. *$37.95*
174 pages Ages 10-14

1071 100% Concepts: Primary
LinguiSystems
3100 4th Avenue
East Moline, IL 61244
309-755-2300
800-776-4332
FAX 309-755-2377
TDY:800-933-8331
http://www.linguisystems.com
e-mail: service@linguisystems.com
LinguiSystems Staff, Author
Linda Bowers, Co-Owner/Co-Founder
Rosemary Huisingh, Co-Owner/Co-Founder

Concepts are the building blocks of language. This approach gives students practice with familiar concepts in different formats for strong language comprehension skills. You'll teach tons of concepts, including following directions, grouping, association, math, and time. *$37.95*
157 pages Ages 5-9

1072 100% Grammar
LinguiSystems
3100 4th Avenue
East Moline, IL 61244
309-755-2300
800-776-4332
FAX 309-755-2377
TDY:800-933-8331
http://www.linguisystems.com
e-mail: service@linguisystems.com
Mike LoGiudice, Carolyn LoGiudice, Author
Linda Bowers, Co-Owner/Co-Founder
Rosemary Huisingh, Co-Owner/Co-Founder

Make the link between grammar and communication skills with this incredible resource. You'll get relevant, fun activities to develop clear, accurate, excellent communication skills. Covers all the essential grammar areas including nouns, pronouns, complements, verbals, clauses, and fine points. *$37.95*
174 pages Ages 9-14

1073 100% Grammar LITE
LinguiSystems
3100 4th Avenue
East Moline, IL 61244
309-755-2300
800-776-4332
FAX 309-755-2377
TDY:800-933-8331
http://www.linguisystems.com
e-mail: service@linguisystems.com
Mike LoGiudice, Carolyn LoGiudice, Author
Linda Bowers, Co-Owner/Co-Founder
Rosemary Huisingh, Co-Owner/Co-Founder

Teach one grammar concept at a time. Compared to 100% Grammar, this resource is lighter in the amount of content per page and contextual demands of the practice items. The fun art and light approach will appeal to your hardest-to-teach students. The book is divided into two sections covering parts of speech and sentence structures. *$37.95*
178 pages Ages 9-14

1074 100% Vocabulary: Intermediate
LinguiSystems
3100 4th Avenue
East Moline, IL 61244
309-755-2300
800-776-4332
FAX 309-755-2377
TDY:800-933-8331
http://www.linguisystems.com
e-mail: service@linguisystems.com
Vicki Rothstein, Rhoda Zacker, Author
Linda Bowers, Co-Owner/Co-Founder
Rosemary Huisingh, Co-Owner/Co-Founder

Teach vocabulary through an organized, systematic approach that works. These challenging semantic exercises teach word flexibility and verbal reasoning skills. You'll teach strategies for understanding word relationships with activities for classification, absurdities, comparisons, exclusion and more. *$37.95*
188 pages Ages 9-14

1075 100% Vocabulary: Primary
LinguiSystems
3100 4th Avenue
East Moline, IL 61244
309-755-2300
800-776-4332
FAX 309-755-2377
TDY:800-933-8331
http://www.linguisystems.com
e-mail: service@linguisystems.com
Vicki Rothstein, Rhoda Zacker, Author
Linda Bowers, Co-Owner/Co-Founder
Rosemary Huisingh, Co-Owner/Co-Founder

Help younger students begin to understand complex word relationships with these outstanding exercises. Students work through a hierarchy of task complexity based on how we think about words. Students will recognize answers with yes/no or true/false, choose answers from alternatives, and infer answers when information isn't directly stated. *$37.95*
187 pages Ages 6-9

1076 125 Vocabulary Builders
LinguiSystems
3100 4th Avenue
East Moline, IL 61244
309-755-2300
800-776-4332
FAX 309-755-2377
TDY:800-933-8331
http://www.linguisystems.com
e-mail: service@linguisystems.com
LinguiSystems Staff, Author
Linda Bowers, Co-Owner/Co-Founder
Rosemary Huisingh, Co-Owner/Co-Founder

This resource goes beyond teaching words by teaching students how to recognize, learn, and integrate new words into their daily vocabulary. Gives students strategies for connecting new vocabulary words to each other, to curriculum and to their prior experience. Your students will learn and remember sets of words because they're used in meaningful ways. *$35.95*
158 pages Ages 10-15

1077 American Heritage Children's Dictionary
Sunburst Technology
1550 Executive Drive
Elgin, IL 60123
800-321-7511
FAX 88-800-3028
http://http://store.sunburst.com/Home.aspx
e-mail: service@sunburst.com
Michael Guillory, Sunburst Channel Sales/Mktg Mgr

This multimedia dictionary uses sound, color illustrations and animations to demonstrate the spelling, definition and pronunciation of 13,000 words. Three additional word games enhance the students' language usage and vocabulary levels. Available formats in MAC CD-ROM, Win CD-ROM. *$99.95*

1078 Analogies 1, 2 & 3
Educators Publishing Service
PO Box 9031
Cambridge, MA 02139
617-547-6706
800-435-7728
FAX 888-440-2665
http://www.epsbooks.com
e-mail: eps@epsbooks.com
Alana Trisler, Alexandra Bigelow, Ann Staman, Author

Studying analogies helps students to sharpen reasoning ability, develop critical thinking, understand relationships between words and ideas, learn new vocabulary, and prepare for the SAT's and for standardized tests.

1079 Artic 1-2-3 Combo: CD
Abilitations Speech Bin
PO Box 922668
Norcross, GA 30010
770-449-5700
800-850-8602
FAX 770-510-7290
http://www.speechbin.com
e-mail: info@speechbin.com
Tobi Isaacs, Catalog Director

Combo - Articulation I (22 Consonant Phonemes) and Articulation II (Clusters) and Articulation III (Vowels + [r], [r] Clusters). Item #L176. *$279.00*

1080 Artic Shuffle
LinguiSystems
3100 4th Avenue
East Moline, IL 61244
309-755-2300
800-776-4332
FAX 309-755-2377
TDY:800-933-8331
http://www.linguisystems.com
e-mail: service@linguisystems.com
Tobie Nan Kaufman, Author
Linda Bowers, Co-Owner/Co-Founder
Rosemary Huisingh, Co-Owner/Co-Founder

Your students can play Go Fish, Crazy Eights, or Concentration while they practice their target sounds. Use them for vocabulary drills or naming practice. *$89.95*
Ages 5-Adult

1081 Artic-Pic
Abilitations Speech Bin
PO Box 922668
Norcross, GA 30010
770-449-5700
800-850-8602
FAX 770-510-7290
http://www.speechbin.com
e-mail: info@speechbin.com
Tobi Isaacs, Catalog Director

You're just going to love this topsy-turvy upside-down book! Artic-Pic is a clever book that gives you delightful interactive practice materials for those troublesome r and s sounds. You get twenty story poems for each phoneme, each with Artic-Pic answer choices featuring the target sound in varying co-articulatory contexts. Item number 1513. *$21.95*

1082 ArticBURST Articulation Practice for S, R, Ch, and Sh
LinguiSystems
3100 4th Avenue
East Moline, IL 61244
309-755-2300
800-776-4332
FAX 309-755-2377
TDY:800-933-8331
http://www.linguisystems.com
e-mail: service@linguisystems.com
LinguiSystems Staff, Author
Linda Bowers, Co-Owner/Co-Founder
Rosemary Huisingh, Co-Owner/Co-Founder

Here's a fun quick thinking game for your older students and clients who continue to need articulation therapy. You'll get a set of cards for each of the toughest sounds. Players have to think of a word with their target sound in these four areas: rhyming, compounds, antonyms, and synonyms. *$37.95*
Ages 10-Adult

1083 AtoZap!
Sunburst Technology
1550 Executive Drive
Elgin, IL 60123
800-321-7511
FAX 888-800-3028
http://http://store.sunburst.com/Home.aspx
e-mail: service@sunburst.com
Michael Guillory, Channel Sales/Marketing Manager

A whimsical world of magical talking alphabet blocks and energetic playful characters this program provides young children with exciting opportunities to explore new concepts through open-ended activities and games. Mac/Win CD-ROM

1084 Autism & PPD: Concept Development
LinguiSystems
3100 4th Avenue
East Moline, IL 61244
309-755-2300
800-776-4332
FAX 309-755-2377
TDY:800-933-8331
http://www.linguisystems.com
e-mail: service@linguisystems.com
Pam Britton Reese, Nena Challenner, Author
Linda Bowers, Co-Owner/Co-Founder
Rosemary Huisingh, Co-Owner/Co-Founder

This great program teaches a variety of concepts grouped by themes. The simple, realistic artwork provides the visual clues so many students need. As students work through each concept-building program, they'll also develop important language skills such as naming, attributes, categorizing, and giving descriptions. *$155.70*
Ages 3-8

1085 Autism & PPD: Pictured Stories and Language Activities
LinguiSystems
3100 4th Avenue
East Moline, IL 61244
309-755-2300
800-776-4332
FAX 309-755-2377
TDY:800-933-8331
http://www.linguisystems.com
e-mail: service@linguisystems.com
Patricia Snair Koski, Author
Linda Bowers, Co-Owner/Co-Founder
Rosemary Huisingh, Co-Owner/Co-Founder

These sequential picture stories focus on simple, easy-to-follow elements. The repetition, structure, and routine make this a great program for students with autism, PPD, or delayed language development. It's a field tested program that works. *$149.75*
Ages 3-8

1086 Basic Signing Vocabulary Cards
Harris Communications
15155 Technology Drive
Eden Prairie, MN 55344
952-906-1180
800-825-6758
FAX 952-906-1099
http://www.harriscomm.com
e-mail: info@harriscomm.com
Robert Harris, Owner

Designed to build signed English vocabulary at a beginners level. Two sets. *$6.95*
100 cards/set

1087 Basic Words for Children: Software
Abilitations Speech Bin
PO Box 922668
Norcross, GA 30010
770-449-5700
800-850-8602
FAX 770-510-7290
http://www.speechbin.com
e-mail: info@speechbin.com
Tobi Isaacs, Catalog Director

This exciting software uses beautiful full color photos and action videos to teach 100 basic words essential for the young child's vocabulary. Item number L197: English, Item number L174: Spanish. *$99.00*

1088 **Blonigen Fluency Program**
Abilitations Speech Bin
PO Box 922668
Norcross, GA 30010
770-449-5700
800-850-8602
FAX 770-510-7290
http://www.speechbin.com
e-mail: info@speechbin.com
Tobi Isaacs, Catalog Director

The Blonigen Fluency Program is a systematic approach to teaching the stuttering modification technique of prolongation to treat stuttering in 7-17 year olds. It features easy-to-follow step-by-step directions and exercises to identify and alter disfluency patterns and gain control over the moment of stuttering. Item #1492. *$24.95*

1089 **Bubbleland Word Discovery**
Sunburst Technology
1550 Executive Drive
Elgin, IL 60123
800-321-7511
FAX 888-800-3028
http://http://store.sunburst.com/Home.aspx
e-mail: service@sunburst.com
Michael Guillory, Channel Sales/Marketing Manager

Build and sharpen language arts skills with this multimedia dictionary. Students explore ten familiar locations that include a pet shop, zoo, toy store, hospital, playground, beach and airport where they engage in 40 activities that build word recognition, pronunciation and spelling skills.

1090 **Carolina Picture Vocabulary Test (CPVT): For Deaf and Hearing Impaired Children**
Pro-Ed
8700 Shoal Creek Boulevard
Austin, TX 78757
512-451-3246
800-897-3202
FAX 800-397-7633
http://www.proedinc.com
e-mail: info@proedinc.com
Matt Synatschk, Permissions Editor

A norm-referenced, validated, receptive sign vocabulary test for deaf and hearing-impaired children. *$133.00*

1091 **Central Auditory Processing Kit**
LinguiSystems
3100 4th Avenue
East Moline, IL 61244
309-755-2300
800-776-4332
FAX 309-755-2377
TDY:800-933-8331
http://www.linguisystems.com
e-mail: service@linguisystems.com
Mary Ann Mokhemar, Author
Linda Bowers, Co-Owner/Co-Founder
Rosemary Huisingh, Co-Owner/Co-Founder

This unique, comprehensive program addresses auditory processing skills with a direct focus on academics including decoding, following directions, and more. Three books cover a wide range of skills including auditory memory, discrimination, closure, synthesis, figure ground, cohesion, and compensatory strategies. *$89.95*
180 pages Ages 6-13

1092 **Complete Oral-Motor Program for Articulation: Book Only**
LinguiSystems
3100 4th Avenue
East Moline, IL 61244
309-755-2300
800-776-4332
FAX 309-755-2377
TDY:800-933-8331
http://www.linguisystems.com
e-mail: service@linguisystems.com
Harriet Pehde, Ann Geller, Bonnie Lechner, Author
Linda Bowers, Co-Owner/Co-Founder
Rosemary Huisingh, Co-Owner/Co-Founder

Manual guides you through oral-motor lessons with clear instructions for exercise. Students will increase oral-motor awareness, strength and tone. There's even a specific sound remediation program for S, Z, Sh, Ch, J, and R. *$ 39.95*
159 pages Ages 3-12

1093 **Complete Oral-Motor Program for Articulation**
LinguiSystems
3100 4th Avenue
East Moline, IL 61244
309-755-2300
800-776-4332
FAX 309-755-2377
TDY:800-933-8331
http://www.linguisystems.com
e-mail: service@linguisystems.com
Harriet Pehde, Ann Geller, Bonnie Lechner, Author
Linda Bowers, Co-Owner/Co-Founder
Rosemary Huisingh, Co-Owner/Co-Founder

These authors have pooled their years of experience to create this big, best selling kit. You'll get everything you need to help students increase awareness, strength and tone of oral musculature, associate oral-motor function to speech sound musculature, associate oral-motor function to speech sound production, and improve overall articulation skills. *$119.95*
159 pages Ages 3-12

1094 **Complete Oral-Motor Program for Articulation: Refill Kit**
LinguiSystems
3100 4th Avenue
East Moline, IL 61244
309-755-2300
800-776-4332
FAX 309-755-2377
TDY:800-933-8331
http://www.linguisystems.com
e-mail: service@linguisystems.com
Harriet Pehde, Ann Geller, Bonnie Lechner, Author
Linda Bowers, Co-Owner/Co-Founder
Rosemary Huisingh, Co-Owner/Co-Founder

Refill kit for Complete Oral-Motor Program for Articulation. *$54.95*
Ages 3-12

1095 **Curious George Pre-K ABCs**
Sunburst Technology
1550 Executive Drive
Elgin, IL 60123
800-321-7511
FAX 888-800-3028
http://http://store.sunburst.com/Home.aspx
e-mail: service@sunburst.com
Michael Guillory, Channel Sales/Marketing Manager

Children go on a lively adventure with Curious George visiting six multi level activities that provide an animated introduction to letters and their sounds. Students discover letter names and shapes, initial letter sounds, letter pronunciations, the order of the alphabet and new vocabulary words during the fun exursions with Curious George. Mac/Win CD-ROM

1096 **Curriculum Vocabulary Game**
LinguiSystems
3100 4th Avenue
East Moline, IL 61244
309-755-2300
800-776-4332
FAX 309-755-2377
TDY:800-933-8331
http://www.linguisystems.com
e-mail: service@linguisystems.com
Paul Johnson, Stephen Johnson, Author
Linda Bowers, Co-Owner/Co-Founder
Rosemary Huisingh, Co-Owner/Co-Founder

The organized lessons teach the classroom vocabulary your students need to know. Each lesson is curricular, flexible, and comprehensive. You'll tap all the learning styles in your case-load. Activities work through a hierarchy from introducing the concepts, to hands-on activities, to writing and take home practice. *$44.95*

Ages 9-13

1097 **Daily Starters: Quote of the Day**
LinguiSystems
3100 4th Avenue
East Moline, IL 61244
309-755-2300
800-776-4332
FAX 309-755-2377
TDY:800-933-8331
http://www.linguisystems.com
e-mail: service@linguisystems.com
Dave Wisniewski, Author
Linda Bowers, Co-Owner/Co-Founder
Rosemary Huisingh, Co-Owner/Co-Founder

Get your students off to a focused start in therapy or in the classroom. These quick activities help older students integrate several language arts skills at once including writing, thinking, grammar, punctuation, vocabulary, and more. *$21.95*
142 pages Ages 12-18

1098 **Dyslexia: An Introduction to the Orton-Gillingham Approach**
Educators Publishing Service
PO Box 9031
Cambridge, MA 02139
617-547-6706
800-225-5750
FAX 888-440-2665
http://www.epsbooks.com
e-mail: eps@epsbooks.com
Gunnar Voltz, President

This ten-lesson, online course provides an introduction to the Orton-Gillingham approach to teaching students with dyslexia. Topics include: the nature of the individual with dyslexia; principles of the Orton-Gillingham approach; multisensory instruction and the brain; and the phonology, structure, and history of the English language.

1099 **Early Communication Skills**
Therapro
225 Arlington Street
Framingham, MA 01702
508-872-9494
800-257-5376
FAX 508-875-2062
http://www.theraproducts.com
e-mail: info@theraproducts.com
Libby Kumin PhD, Author
Karen Conrad, Owner

Provides professional expertise in understandable terms. Parents and professionals learn how their skills are evaluated by professionals, and what activities they can practice with a child immediately to encouarge a childs's communication skill development. *$19.95*
368 pages Ages Birth-K

1100 **Early Listening Skills**
Therapro
225 Arlington Street
Framingham, MA 01702
508-872-9494
800-257-5376
FAX 508-875-2062
http://www.theraproducts.com
e-mail: info@theraproducts.com
Diana Williams, Author
Karen Conrad, Owner

Two hundred activities designed to be photocopied for classroom or home. Includes materials on auditory detection, discrimination, recognition, sequencing and memory. Describes listening projects and topics for the curriculum. Activity sheets for parents are included. A practical, comprehensive and effective manual for professionals working with preschool children or the older child with special needs. *$55.00*

1101 **Earobics Step 2: Home Version**
Abilitations Speech Bin
PO Box 922668
Norcross, GA 30010
770-449-5700
800-850-8602
FAX 770-510-7290
http://www.speechbin.com
e-mail: info@speechbin.com
Tobi Isaacs, Catalog Director

Step 2 teaches critical language comprehension skills and trains the critical auditory skills children need for success in learning. It offers hundreds of levels of play, appealing graphics, and entertaining music to train the critical auditory skills young children need for success in learning. Item number C483. *$58.99*

1102 **Earobics Step 2: Specialist/Clinician Version**
Abilitations Speech Bin
PO Box 922668
Norcross, GA 30010
770-449-5700
800-850-8602
FAX 770-510-7290
http://www.speechbin.com
e-mail: info@speechbin.com
Tobi Isaacs, Catalog Director

Earobics features: tasks and level counter with real time display; adaptive training technology for individualized programs; and reporting to track and evaluate each individual's progress. Step 2 teaches critical language comprehension skills and trains the critical auditory skills children need for success in learning. Item number C484. *$298.99*

1103 **Easy Does It for Fluency: Intermediate**
LinguiSystems
3100 4th Avenue
East Moline, IL 61244
309-755-2300
800-776-4332
FAX 309-755-2377
TDY:800-933-8331
http://www.linguisystems.com
e-mail: service@linguisystems.com
Barbara Roseman, Karin Johnson, Author
Linda Bowers, Co-Owner/Co-Founder
Rosemary Huisingh, Co-Owner/Co-Founder

This program addresses the motor, linguistic, and psychosocial components of stuttering as students work toward fluent speech. This updated and revised version of an old favorite will help your students become fluent. *$49.95*
165 pages Ages 6-11

1104 **Easy Does It for Fluency: Preschool/Primary**
LinguiSystems
3100 4th Avenue
East Moline, IL 61244
309-755-2300
800-776-4332
FAX 309-755-2377
TDY:800-933-8331
http://www.linguisystems.com
e-mail: service@linguisystems.com
Barbara Roseman, Karin Johnson, Author
Linda Bowers, Co-Owner/Co-Founder
Rosemary Huisingh, Co-Owner/Co-Founder

This systematic program of fluency shaping uses slow, easy speech for the youngest stutterers. The therapy manual contains step-by-step activities with goals and objectives. There are also sample lesson plans for individualizing therapy, strategies and materials to involve care givers. *$49.95*
117 pages Ages 2-6

1105 **Elementary Spelling Ace ES-90**
Franklin Electronic Publishers
One Franklin Plaza
Burlington, NJ 08016
800-266-5626
FAX 609-239-5948
http://www.franklin.com
e-mail: service@franklin.com
Barry Lipsky, CEO
John Applegate, Director
Bettie Albertson, Executive Assistant
Designed for elementary children, provides them with spelling correction for over 80,000 words. Accompanied by Webster's Elementary Dictionary. *$34.95*

1106 **Every Child a Reader**
Sunburst Technology
1550 Executive Drive
Elgin, IL 60123
800-321-7511
FAX 888-800-3028
http://http://store.sunburst.com/Home.aspx
e-mail: service@sunburst.com

Michael Guillory, Channel Sales/Marketing Manager

Traditional reading strategies in a rich literary context. Designed to promote independent reading and develop oral and written language expression.

1107 Explode the Code: Wall Chart
Educators Publishing Service
PO Box 9031
Cambridge, MA 02139
617-547-6706
800-225-5750
FAX 888-440-2665
http://www.epsbooks.com
e-mail: eps@epsbooks.com
Nancy M Hall, Rena Price, Author
Gunnar Voltz, President

Learning sounds is exciting with the new Explode The Code alphabet chart! Each letter is represented by a colorful character from the series and is stored inside a felt pocket embroidered with the letter's name.

1108 Expressive Language Kit
LinguiSystems
3100 4th Avenue
East Moline, IL 61244
309-755-2300
800-776-4332
FAX 309-755-2377
TDY:800-933-8331
http://www.linguisystems.com
e-mail: service@linguisystems.com
Linda Bowers, Rosemary Huisingh, Carolyn LoGiudice, Author
Linda Bowers, Co-Owner/Co-Founder
Rosemary Huisingh, Co-Owner/Co-Founder

It's our biggest language therapy kit ever. The focus is on strengthening expressive language skills so your students will become effective communicators. A combination of colorful photographs, picture cards, and activity sheets work together to create an outstanding expressive language program. A comprehension therapy manual is included to help you direct this incredibly wide variety of language activities. *$149.95*
250 pages Ages 5-11

1109 First Phonics
Sunburst Technology
1550 Executive Drive
Elgin, IL 60123
800-321-7511
FAX 888-800-3028
http://http://store.sunburst.com/Home.aspx
e-mail: service@sunburst.com
Michael Guillory, Channel Sales/Marketing Manager

Targets the phonics skills that all children need to develop, sounding out the first letter of a word. This program offers four different engaging activities that you can customize to match each child's specific need.

1110 Follow Me! 2
LinguiSystems
3100 4th Avenue
East Moline, IL 61244
309-755-2300
800-776-4332
FAX 309-775-2377
TDY:800-933-8331
http://www.linguisystems.com
e-mail: service@linguisystems.com
Grace Frank, Author
Linda Bowers, Co-Owner/Co-Founder
Rosemary Huisingh, Co-Owner/Co-Founder

These activities are relevant to classroom listening demands. The directions relate specifically to an accompanying worksheet. It's a pick-up-and-use-now resource to teach the vocabulary of language arts, math, social studies and more. *$34.95*
201 pages Ages 7-11

1111 Fun with Language: Book 1
Therapro
225 Arlington Street
Framingham, MA 01702
508-872-9494
800-257-5376
FAX 508-875-2062
http://www.theraproducts.com
e-mail: info@theraproducts.com
Kathleen Yardley, Author
Karen Conrad, Owner

A wonderful reproducible workbook of thinking and language skill exercises for children ages 4-8. Perfect when you need something on a moment's notice. Over 100 beautifully illustrated exercises in the following categories: Spatial Relationships; Opposites; Categorizing; Following Directions; Temporal Concepts; Syntax & Morphology; Same and Different; Plurals; Memory; Reasoning; Storytelling; and Describing. Targets both receptive and expressive language as well as problem- solving skills. *$55.00*

1112 Goldman-Fristoe Test of Articulation: 2nd Edition
Abilitations Speech Bin
PO Box 922668
Norcross, GA 30010
770-449-5700
800-850-8602
FAX 770-510-7290
http://www.speechbin.com
e-mail: info@speechbin.com
Ronald Goldman, Macalyne Fristoe, Author
Tobi Isaacs, Catalog Director

It systematically measures a child's production of 39 consonant sounds and blends. Its age range is 2-21 years, and age based standard scores have separate gender norms. In this revised edition, inappropriate stimulus words have been replaced based on multicultural review, and all new artwork is featured. Item number 190915116. *$229.99*

1113 HELP 1
LinguiSystems
3100 4th Avenue
East Moline, IL 61244
309-755-2300
800-776-4332
FAX 309-775-2375
TDY:800-933-8331
http://www.linguisystems.com
e-mail: service@linguisystems.com
Andrea Lazzari, Patricia Peters, Author
Linda Bowers, Co-Owner/Co-Founder
Rosemary Huisingh, Co-Owner/Co-Founder

Get the books clinicians have relied on for years as their number one therapy resource. Written by two speech-language pathologists who know language remediation, this series has set the industry standard for practical, pick-up-and-use-now language therapy activities. HELP 1 includes activities for auditory discrimination, question comprehension, auditory association, and auditory memory. *$39.95*
163 pages Ages 6-Adult

1114 HELP 2
LinguiSystems
3100 4th Avenue
East Moline, IL 61244
309-755-2300
800-776-4332
FAX 309-755-2377
TDY:800-933-8331
http://www.linguisystems.com
e-mail: service@linguisystems.com
Andrea Lazzari, Patricia Peters, Author
Linda Bowers, Co-Owner/Co-Founder
Rosemary Huisingh, Co-Owner/Co-Founder

Get the books clinicians have relied on for years as their number one therapy resource. Written by two speech-language pathologists who know language remediation, this series has set the industry standard for practical, pick-up-and-use-now language therapy activities. HELP 2 includes activities for word-finding, categorization, answering different question forms and grammar practice. *$39.95*

175 pages Ages 6-Adult

1115 HELP 3
LinguiSystems
3100 4th Avenue
East Moline, IL 61244
309-755-2300
800-776-4332
FAX 309-755-2377
TDY:800-933-8331
http://www.linguisystems.com
e-mail: service@linguisystems.com
Andrea Lazzari, Patricia Peters, Author
Linda Bowers, Co-Owner/Co-Founder
Rosemary Huisingh, Co-Owner/Co-Founder

Get the books clinicians have relied on for years as their number one therapy resource. Written by two speech-language pathologists who know language remediation, this series has set the industry standard for practical, pick-up-and-use-now language therapy activities. HELP 3 includes activities for basic concepts, paraphrasing, thinking and problem-solving, and social language skills. *$39.95*
194 pages Ages 6-Adult

1116 HELP 4
LinguiSystems
3100 4th Avenue
East Moline, IL 61244
309-755-2300
800-776-4332
FAX 309-755-2377
TDY:800-933-8331
http://www.linguisystems.com
e-mail: service@linguisystems.com
Andrea Lazzari, Patricia Peters, Author
Linda Bowers, Co-Owner/Co-Founder
Rosemary Huisingh, Co-Owner/Co-Founder

Get the books clinicians have relied on for years as their number one therapy resource. Written by two speech-language pathologists who know language remediation, this series has set the industry standard for practical, pick-up-and-use-now language therapy activities. HELP 4 includes activities for defining and describing activities, written language exercises, linguistic concepts, and the language of humor and riddles. *$39.95*
190 pages Ages 6-Adult

1117 HELP 5
LinguiSystems
3100 4th Avenue
East Moline, IL 61244
309-755-2300
800-776-4332
FAX 309-755-2377
TDY:800-933-8331
http://www.linguisystems.com
e-mail: service@linguisystems.com
Andrea Lazzari, Patricia Peters, Author
Linda Bowers, Co-Owner/Co-Founder
Rosemary Huisingh, Co-Owner/Co-Founder

Get the books clinicians have relied on for years as their number one therapy resource. Written by two speech-language pathologists who know language remediation, this series has set the industry standard for practical, pick-up-and-use-now lanuage therapy activities. HELP 5 includes activities for processing information and messages; comparing and contrasting words; understanding math language and concepts; and communicating needs, feelings, and opinions. *$39.95*
190 pages Ages 6-Adult

1118 HELP for Articulation
LinguiSystems
3100 4th Avenue
East Moline, IL 61244
309-755-2300
800-776-4332
FAX 309-755-2377
TDY:800-933-8331
http://www.linguisystems.com
e-mail: service@linguisystems.com
Andrea Lazzari, Author
Linda Bowers, Co-Owner/Co-Founder
Rosemary Huisingh, Co-Owner/Co-Founder

This pick-up-and-use resource gives you a great variety of target sounds and activities. The hierarchy of tasks ensures mastery along the way and keeps your articulation therapy organized. Best of all, it's designed to span ages 6 through adult so you'll have articulation practice for your entire caseload. *$39.95*

195 pages Ages 6-Adult

1119 HELP for Auditory Processing
LinguiSystems
3100 4th Avenue
East Moline, IL 61244
309-755-2300
800-776-4332
FAX 309-755-2377
TDY:800-933-8331
http://www.linguisystems.com
e-mail: service@linguisystems.com
Andrea Lazzari, Patricia Peters, Author
Linda Bowers, Co-Owner/Co-Founder
Rosemary Huisingh, Co-Owner/Co-Founder

Functional communication improves when auditory processing skills are strong. Work on skills necessary to receive, interpret, and internalize language. Work through a hierarchy of auditory processing strategies with exercises for processing information in word classes, following a variety of directions, listening for sounds in words, and more. *$39.95*
190 pages Ages 6-Adult

1120 HELP for Grammar
LinguiSystems
3100 4th Avenue
East Moline, IL 61244
309-755-2300
800-776-4332
FAX 309-755-2377
TDY:800-933-8331
http://www.linguisystems.com
e-mail: service@linguisystems.com
Andrea Lazzari, Author
Linda Bowers, Co-Owner/Co-Founder
Rosemary Huisingh, Co-Owner/Co-Founder

Get in-depth grammar practice arranged in developmental order so skill builds upon skill. Get grammar training and practice with oral and written language exercises including identifying and matching grammar types, categorizing grammar types, applying grammar skills in context, and more. *$39.95*
191 pages Ages 8-Adult

1121 HELP for Vocabulary
LinguiSystems
3100 4th Avenue
East Moline, IL 61244
309-755-2300
800-776-4332
FAX 309-755-2377
TDY:800-933-8331
http://www.linguisystems.com
e-mail: service@linguisystems.com
Andrea Lazzari, Author
Linda , Co-Owner/Co-Founder
Rosemary , Co-Owner/Co-Founder

Your students will expand word knowledge and learn to apply vocabulary skills in context with these great exercises. The hierarchy of tasks lets you see where breakdowns occur. Each page is a complete lesson with an IEP goal and ready-to-use exercise. *$39.95*
180 pages Ages 8-Adult

1122 HELP for Word Finding
LinguiSystems
3100 4th Avenue
East Moline, IL 61244
309-755-2300
800-776-4332
FAX 309-755-2377
TDY:800-933-8331
http://www.linguisystems.com
e-mail: service@linguisystems.com
Andera Lazzari, Patricia Peters, Author
Linda , Co-Owner/Co-Founder
Rosemary , Co-Owner/Co-Founder

Expand the speed, quality, and variety of word recall strategies within practical, everyday context. Stimulus items progress in difficulty within each task to cover a broad age range as well as range of ability. Clients practice word-finding strategies with exercises for automatic associations, words grouped in themes, and more. *$39.95*

179 pages Ages 6-Adult

1123 HearFones
Abilitations Speech Bin
PO Box 922668
Norcross, GA 30010
770-449-5700
800-850-8602
FAX 770-510-7290
http://www.speechbin.com
e-mail: info@speechbin.com
Tobi Isaacs, Catalog Director

This unique nonelectronic self-contained headset is made of composite and plastic materials, and it's easy to clean. It lets users hear themselves more directly and clearly so they can analyze their own speech sound production and voice quality. Item number N261. *$28.99*

1124 I Can Say R
Abilitations Speech Bin
PO Box 922668
Norcross, GA 30010
770-449-5700
800-850-8602
FAX 770-510-7290
http://www.speechbin.com
e-mail: info@speechbin.com
Tobi Isaacs, Catalog Director

Helping children overcome problems saying R sounds is one of the most perplexing dilemmas speech and language pathologists face in their caseloads. Here's a terrific book packed with innovative practice materials to make that task easier. Item number 190728116. *$26.99*

1125 Idiom's Delight
Academic Therapy Publications
20 Commercial Boulevard
Novato, CA 94949
415-883-3314
800-422-7249
FAX 888-287-9975
http://www.academictherapy.com
e-mail: sales@academictherapy.com
John Arena, Author
Jim Arena
Joanne Urban

Offers 75 idioms and accompanying reproducible activities. Delightful illustrations portraying humorous literal interpretations of idioms are sprinkled throughout the book to enhance enjoyment. *$14.00*
64 pages
ISBN 0-878798-89-7

1126 Island Reading Journey
Sunburst Technology
1550 Executive Drive
Elgin, IL 60123
800-321-7511
FAX 888-800-3028
http://http://store.sunburst.com/Home.aspx
e-mail: service@sunburst.com
Michael , Channel Sales/Marketing Manager

Enhance your reading program with meaningful summary and extension activities for 100 intermediate level books. Students read for meaning while they engage in activities that test for comprehension, build writing skills with reader response and essay questions, develop usage skills with cloze activities and improve vocabulary/word attack skills.

1127 Just for Kids: Apraxia
LinguiSystems
3100 4th Avenue
East Moline, IL 61244
309-755-2300
800-776-4332
FAX 309-755-2377
TDY:800-933-8331
http://www.linguisystems.com
e-mail: service@linguisystems.com
Martha Drake, Author
Linda Bowers, Co-Owner/Co-Founder
Rosemary Huisingh, Co-Owner/Co-Founder

Work through a sequence of skills to help your young students achieve intelligibility. Sessions are organized using the alphabet as a theme. Each phase gives you all the materials you need including goals, for moving to the nest phase, family letter for take-home practice, supplemental word lists, oral-mouth posture pictures, and ABC flash cards. *$39.95*
157 pages Ages 4-8

1128 Just for Kids: Articulation Stories
LinguiSystems
3100 4th Avenue
East Moline, IL 61244
309-755-2300
800-776-4332
FAX 309-755-2377
TDY:800-933-8331
http://www.linguisystems.com
e-mail: service@linguisystems.com
Jennifer Preschern, Author
Linda Bowers, Co-Owner/Co-Founder
Rosemary Huisingh, Co-Owner/Co-Founder

Work through target sounds at the word, carrier sentence, sentence, and conversation levels. For each target sound, you'll get a wonderful organized lesson with child-centered vocabulary, appealing pictures, fun stories and interactive activities. *$39.95*
175 pages Ages 4-9

1129 Just for Kids: Grammar
LinguiSystems
3100 4th Avenue
East Moline, IL 61244
309-755-2300
800-776-4332
FAX 309-755-2377
TDY:800-933-8331
http://www.linguisystems.com
e-mail: service@linguisystems.com
Janet Lanza, Lynn Flahive, Author
Linda Bowers, Co-Owner/Co-Founder
Rosemary Huisingh, Co-Owner/Co-Founder

This kid friendly approach to grammar teaches the parts of speech your students need to know. The practice centers around natural, meaningful activities. Each chapter includes a pre-and post-test, picture cards, sequence story, rebus story, and family letter. *$39.95*
186 pages Ages 4-9

1130 Just for Kids: Phonological Processing
LinguiSystems
3100 4th Avenue
East Moline, IL 61244
309-755-2300
800-776-4332
FAX 309-755-2377
TDY:800-933-8331
http://www.linguisystems.com
e-mail: service@linguisystems.com
Lynn Flahive, Janet Lanza, Author
Linda Bowers, Co-Owner/Co-Founder
Rosemary Huisingh, Co-Owner/Co-Founder

Teach phonological processing skills through fun, themed activities. You'll love each comprehensive, pick-up-and-use-now lesson! This terrific program gives you 22 theme-related lessons that target common phonological processes. *$39.95*
188 pages Ages 4-9

1131 Just for Me! Game
LinguiSystems
3100 4th Avenue
East Moline, IL 61244
309-755-2300
800-776-4332
FAX 309-755-2377
TDY:800-933-8331
http://www.linguisystems.com
e-mail: service@linguisystems.com
Margaret Warner, Author
Linda Bowers, Co-Owner/Co-Founder
Rosemary Huisingh, Co-Owner/Co-Founder

Follow-up on the early language skills from all five Just for Me! books with this fun new game. It's a hands-on approach as youngsters mix up specially designed puzzle pieces to make funny faces. Each piece gives you five questions. That's 360 questions in all! Each puzzle piece covers an early language skill and corresponds to one part of the face. *$37.95*

Ages 4-7

1132 Just for Me! Grammar
LinguiSystems
3100 4th Avenue
East Moline, IL 61244
309-755-2300
800-776-4332
FAX 309-755-2377
TDY:800-933-8331
http://www.linguisystems.com
e-mail: service@linguisystems.com
Margaret Warner, Author
Linda Bowers, Co-Owner/Co-Founder
Rosemary Huisingh, Co-Owner/Co-Founder

Teach oral grammar to your youngest students. Through a variety of engaging activities, your students will become familiar with basic parts of speech, correct word order, and simple grammar concepts. These activities provide a solid foundation for later formal grammar training in the classroom. *$24.95*
150 pages Ages 3-6

1133 Just for Me! Vocabulary
LinguiSystems
3100 4th Avenue
East Moline, IL 61244
309-755-2300
800-776-4332
FAX 309-755-2377
TDY:800-933-8331
http://www.linguisystems.com
e-mail: service@linguisystems.com
Margaret Warner, Author
Linda Bowers, Co-Owner/Co-Founder
Rosemary Huisingh, Co-Owner/Co-Founder

Your youngest students will love these fun cut-and-create activities for vocabulary. Each unit starts with poem introducing the key vocabulary words for the unit. *$24.95*
148 pages Ages 3-6

1134 Kaufman Speech Praxis Test
Abilitations Speech Bin
PO Box 922668
Norcross, GA 30010
770-449-5700
800-850-8602
FAX 770-510-7290
http://www.speechbin.com
e-mail: info@speechbin.com
Tobi Isaacs, Catalog Director

This standardized test utlilizes a hierarchy of simple to complex motor-speech movements, from oral movement and simple phonemic/syllable to complex phonemic/syllable level. The complete kit contains manual, guide, and 25 test booklets. Item number 192126116. *$161.99*

1135 LILAC
Abilitations Speech Bin
PO Box 922668
Norcross, GA 30010
770-449-5700
800-850-8602
FAX 770-510-7290
http://www.speechbin.com
e-mail: info@speechbin.com
Tobi Isaacs, Catalog Director

LILAC uses direct and naturalistic teaching in a creative approach that links spoken language learning to reading and writing. Activities to develop semantic, syntactic, expressive, and receptive language skills are presented sequentially from three-to five-year-old developmental levels. Item number 190825116. *$27.99*

1136 Language Activity Resource Kit: LARK
Abilitations Speech Bin
PO Box 922668
Norcross, GA 30010
770-449-5700
800-850-8602
FAX 770-510-7290
http://www.speechbin.com
e-mail: info@speechbin.com
Richard A Dressler, Author
Tobi Isaacs, Catalog Director

The LARK: Language Activity Resource Kit has been revised! This perennially popular language kit is now more portable and versatile for use with persons who have moderate to severe language disorders. Item number 190613116. *$ 217.99*

1137 Language Processing Kit
LinguiSystems
3100 4th Avenue
East Moline, IL 61244
309-755-2300
800-776-4332
FAX 309-755-2377
TDY:800-933-8331
http://www.linguisystems.com
e-mail: service@linguisystems.com
Gail Richard, Mary Anne Hanner, Author
Linda Bowers, Co-Owner/Co-Founder
Rosemary Huisingh, Co-Owner/Co-Founder

You'll get a variety of activities in developmental progression for improving processing skills. It's your comprehensive follow-up to the Language Processing Test-Revised. You'll also get an outline of compensatory cueing and prompting strategies with helpful tips on how to teach them. *$124.95*
143 pages Ages 5-11

1138 LanguageBURST: A Language and Vocabulary Game
LinguiSystems
3100 4th Avenue
East Moline, IL 61244
309-755-2300
800-776-4332
FAX 309-755-2377
TDY:800-933-8331
http://www.linguisystems.com
e-mail: service@linguisystems.com
Lauri Whiskeyman, Author
Linda Bowers, Co-Owner/Co-Founder
Rosemary Huisingh, Co-Owner/Co-Founder

Expand your student's language and vocabulary skills with this quick- thinking game. Many of the items are based on the curriculum for grades 3-8 so your therapy is classroom-relevant. Students think quickly as they practice skills in four key language areas: fill-in-the-blank; categories; comparing and contrasting; and attributes. *$37.95*
Ages 9-15

1139 Letter Sounds
Sunburst Technology
1550 Executive Drive
Elgin, IL 60123
800-321-7511
FAX 888-800-3028
http://http://store.sunburst.com/Home.aspx
e-mail: service@sunburst.com
Michael Guillory, Channel Sales/Marketing Manager

Students develop phonemic awareness skills as they make the connection between consonant letters and their sounds.

1140 Linamood Program (LIPS Clinical Version):Phoneme Sequencing Program
LinguiSystems
3100 4th Avenue
East Moline, IL 61244
309-755-2300
800-776-4332
FAX 309-755-2377
TDY:800-933-8331
http://www.linguisystems.com
e-mail: service@linguisystems.com
Patricia Lindamood, Phyllis Lindamood, Author
Linda Bowers, Co-Owner/Co-Founder
Rosemary Huisingh, Co-Owner/Co-Founder

Help your students develop phoneme awareness for competence in reading, spelling, and speech. This multisensory program meets the needs of the many children and adults who don't develop phonemic awareness through traditional methods. *$247.00*

Birth-Adult

1141 Listening Kit
LinguiSystems
3100 4th Avenue
East Moline, IL 61244
309-755-2300
800-776-4332
FAX 309-755-2377
TDY:800-933-8331
http://www.linguisystems.com
e-mail: service@linguisystems.com
Susan Simms, Mark Barrett, Rosemay Huisingh, Author
Linda Bowers, Co-Owner/Co-Founder
Rosemary Huisingh, Co-Owner/Co-Founder

This listening curriculum combines thinking, reasoning, and language skills for improved listening and attending. It's an unbeatable combination. The Listening Book organizes listening skills into the areas of paying attention, listening with an open mind and reasoning. *$119.95*
185 pages Ages 5-11

1142 Listening and Speaking for Job and Personal Use
AGS Globe
5910 Rice Creek Parkway
Shoreview, MN 55126
800-328-2560
http://www.agsglobe.com
e-mail: webmaster@agsglobe.com
L Ann Masters, Author
Karen Dahlen, Associate Director
Matt Keller, Marketing Manger

With an interest level of High School through Adult, and a reading level of Grade 5-6, this series has modules in Listening Skills and Speaking Skills. Self-paced texts have applications-oriented exercises.

1143 Listening for Articulation All Year 'Round
LinguiSystems
3100 4th Avenue
East Moline, IL 61244
309-755-2300
800-776-4332
FAX 309-755-2377
TDY:800-933-8331
http://www.linguisystems.com
e-mail: service@linguisystems.com
Brenda Brumbaugh, Nan Thompson-Trenta, Author
Linda Bowers, Co-Owner/Co-Founder
Rosemary Huisingh, Co-Owner/Co-Founder

Get your young students on their way to intelligible speech with this book devoted to early-developing sounds. Pictures and activities can be used for phonology or articulation therapy. The program includes practice with minimal pairs, tips for establishing production, a variety of stimulus pictures, and activity sheets organized by phoneme. *$39.95*
208 pages Ages 5-10

1144 Listening for Language All Year 'Round
LinguiSystems
3100 4th Avenue
East Moline, IL 61244
309-755-2300
800-776-4332
FAX 309-755-2377
TDY:800-933-8331
http://www.linguisystems.com
e-mail: service@linguisystems.com
Brenda Brumbaugh, Nan Thompson-Trenta, Author
Linda Bowers, Co-Owner/Co-Founder
Rosemary Huisingh, Co-Owner/Co-Founder

Reinforce word relationships while you teach these important language concepts: synonyms, antonyms, classification, comparisons, multiple meanings, and idioms. Special notebook activities give structured writing practice. *$39.95*
196 pages Ages 7-11

1145 Listening for Vocabulary All Year 'Round
LinguiSystems
3100 4th Avenue
East Moline, IL 61244
309-755-2300
800-776-4332
FAX 309-755-2377
TDY:800-933-8331
http://www.linguisystems.com
e-mail: service@linguisystems.com
Brenda Brumbaugh, Nan Thompson-Trenta, Author
Linda Bowers, Co-Owner/Co-Founder
Rosemary Huisingh, Co-Owner/Co-Founder

Save time and energy with these ready-to-use listening and vocabulary lessons that match the themes of your school year. This book includes language stories, hands-on listening activities, home lessons, and terrific artworks! *$ 39.95*
196 pages Ages 5-8

1146 Look! Listen! & Learn Language!: Software
Abilitations Speech Bin
PO Box 922668
Norcross, GA 30010
770-449-5700
800-850-8602
FAX 770-510-7290
http://www.speechbin.com
e-mail: info@speechbin.com
Tobi Isaacs, Catalog Director

Interactive activities for children with autism, PDD, Down syndrome, language delay, or apraxia include: hello; Match Same to Same; Quack; Let's talk About It; visual scanning/attention and match ups! Item number 190194116. *$98.99*

1147 M-SS-NG L-NKS
Sunburst Technology
1550 Executive Drive
Elgin, IL 60123
800-321-7511
FAX 888-800-3028
http://http://store.sunburst.com/Home.aspx
e-mail: service@sunburst.com
Michael Guillory, Channel Sales/Marketing Manager

This award-winning program is an engrossing language puzzle. A passage appears with letters or words missing. Students complete it based on their knowledge of word structure, spelling, grammar, meaning in context, and literary style.

1148 MCLA: Measure of Cognitive-Linguistic Abilities
Abilitations Speech Bin
PO Box 922668
Norcross, GA 30010
770-449-5700
800-850-8602
FAX 770-510-7290
http://www.speechbin.com
e-mail: info@speechbin.com
Wendy Ellmo, Jill Graser, Beth Krchnavek, Author
Tobi Isaacs, Catalog Director

MCLA evaluates your clients with cognitive-linguistic impairments caused by traumatic brain injuries (TBI). It determines their high level cognitive-linguistic deficits, reveals their strengths, and helps you plan treatment programs minimize effects of 'mild' deficits that may have a profound impact on their lives. Item number 192186116. *$109.99*

1149 Many Voices of Paws
Abilitations Speech Bin
PO Box 922668
Norcross, GA 30010
770-449-5700
800-850-8602
FAX 770-510-7290
http://www.speechbin.com
e-mail: info@speechbin.com
Julie Reville, Author
Tobi Isaacs, Catalog Director

The Many Voices of Paws shows young stuttering children how to modify their speaking rates and vocal behaviors in a way that's easy for them to understand. Beautifully illustrated, the story about Paws, the cat, combines pretending, talking, and playful interaction and helps children accept their disfluencies in a positive way. Item number 190868116. *$21.99*

64 pages
ISBN 0-937857-11-4

1150 **Max's Attic: Long & Short Vowels**
Sunburst Technology
1550 Executive Drive
Elgin, IL 60123
800-321-7511
FAX 888-800-3028
http://http://store.sunburst.com/Home.aspx
e-mail: service@sunburst.com
Michael Guillory, Channel Sales/Marketing Manager

Filled to the rafters with phonics fun, this animated program builds your students' vowel recognition skills.

1151 **Maxwell's Manor: A Social Language Game**
LinguiSystems
3100 4th Avenue
East Moline, IL 61244
309-755-2300
800-776-4332
FAX 309-755-2377
TDY:800-933-8331
http://www.linguisystems.com
e-mail: service@linguisystems.com
Carolyn LoGiudice, Nancy McConnell, Author
Linda Bowers, Co-Owner/Co-Founder
Rosemary Huisingh, Co-Owner/Co-Founder

This fun game will teach your students the social skills they need to get along with others, be more accepted by their peers, and be successful in the classroom. Maxwell, the loveable dog, leads the way as your students practice positive social language skills. *$44.95*

Ages 4-9

1152 **Middle School Language Arts**
Harcourt Achieve
Customer Service, 5th Floor
Orlando, FL 32887
800-284-7019
FAX 800-699-9459
http://www.harcourtachieve.com
e-mail: webmaster@harcourt.com
Steven , CEO
Randy , SVP National Sales

This skill-specific series reinforces and enhances the middle school language arts curriculum. It provides teachers and parents with a tool to focus on the skills that students need to review and reinforce. The lessons provide step-by-step instructions and follow-up activities to enable students to work independently.

1153 **Mike Mulligan & His Steam Shovel**
Sunburst Technology
1550 Executive Drive
Elgin, IL 60123
800-321-7511
FAX 888-800-3028
http://http://store.sunburst.com/Home.aspx
e-mail: service@sunburst.com
Michael Guillory, Channel Sales/Marketing Manager

This CD-ROM version of the Caldecott classic lets students experience interactive book reading and participate in four skills-based extension activities that promote memory, matching, sequencing, listening, pattern recognition and map reading skills.

1154 **Mouth Madness**
Abilitations Speech Bin
PO Box 922668
Norcross, GA 30010
770-449-5700
800-850-8602
FAX 770-510-7290
http://www.speechbin.com
e-mail: info@speechbin.com
Tobi Isaacs, Catalog Director

This unique manual uses oral imitation, motor planning, and breath control activities to improve the articulation and feeding skills of preschool and primary children. Games, manipulative tasks, silly sentences, rhymes, and funny faces target higher organizational levels of motor planning. Item number 192013116. *$54.99*

1155 **My First Phonics Book**
Speech Bin
PO Box 922668
Norcross, GA 30010
770-449-5700
800-850-8602
FAX 770-510-7290
http://www.speechbin.com
e-mail: info@speechbin.com
Shane Peters, Product Coordinator
Jen Binney, Owner

Shows that words are made of sounds, then helps to recognize the letter symbols for the sounds. It's organized in easy-to-locate alphabetical order of sounds, with one page for each of the 42 sounds of English. Item number H585. *$16.95*

1156 **Myrtle's Beach: A Phonological Awareness and Articulation Game**
LinguiSystems
3100 4th Avenue
East Moline, IL 61244
309-755-2300
800-776-4332
FAX 309-755-2377
TDY:800-933-8331
http://www.linguisystems.com
e-mail: service@linguisystems.com
LinguiSystems Staff, Author
Linda Bowers, Co-Owner/Co-Founder
Rosemary Huisingh, Co-Owner/Co-Founder

Myrtle's Beach is a fun place to practice phonological awareness, articulation, and language skills. The flexible format allows you to meet the varied needs of all the students in your speech and language groups. *$44.95*

Ages 4-9

1157 **No-Glamour Grammar**
LinguiSystems
3100 4th Avenue
East Moline, IL 61244
309-755-2300
800-776-4332
FAX 309-755-2377
TDY:800-933-8331
http://www.linguisystems.com
e-mail: service@linguisystems.com
Suzanna Mayer Watt, Author
Linda Bowers, Co-Owner/Co-Founder
Rosemary Huisingh, Co-Owner/Co-Founder

This best-selling grammar book teaches all the basic grammar skills your students need. The no-frills approach is great for students with language or learning disorders. You'll teach one skill at a time with tons of practice pages. The units progress in difficulty as students master each grammar skill. *$41.95*

415 pages Ages 8-12

1158 **No-Glamour Grammar 2**
LinguiSystems
3100 4th Avenue
East Moline, IL 61244
309-755-2300
800-776-4332
FAX 309-755-2377
TDY:800-933-8331
http://www.linguisystems.com
e-mail: service@linguisystems.com
Diane Hyde, Author
Linda Bowers, Co-Owner/Co-Founder
Rosemary Huisingh, Co-Owner/Co-Founder

Get more grammar skill practice with a variety of activity sheets. From nouns to verbs, adjectives to adverbs, your students will apply their knowledge to these challenging, fun activity pages. *$41.95*

320 pages Ages 8-12

1159 No-Glamour Vocabulary
LinguiSystems
3100 4th Avenue
East Moline, IL 61244
309-755-2300
800-776-4332
FAX 309-755-2377
TDY:800-933-8331
http://www.linguisystems.com
e-mail: service@linguisystems.com
Diane Hyde, Author
Linda Bowers, Co-Owner/Co-Founder
Rosemary Huisingh, Co-Owner/Co-Founder

With one vocabulary skill to a page, students can focus on the semantic areas that give them the most trouble. These vocabulary worksheets target absurdities, multiple meanings, associations, definitions, synonyms, antonyms, and more. *$41.95*
278 pages Ages 7-12

1160 Oral-Motor Activities for School-Aged Children
LinguiSystems
3100 4th Avenue
East Moline, IL 61244
309-755-2300
800-776-4332
FAX 309-755-2377
TDY:800-933-8331
http://www.linguisystems.com
e-mail: service@linguisystems.com
Elizabeth Mackie, Author
Linda Bowers, Co-Owner/Co-Founder
Rosemary Huisingh, Co-Owner/Co-Founder

Multisensory, oral-motor approach to treating articulation disorders. Great for older students with developmental delays or any student who needs to improve oral-motor function for better speech production. *$39.95*
171 pages Ages 7-12

1161 Oral-Motor Activities for Young Children
LinguiSystems
3100 4th Avenue
East Moline, IL 61244
309-755-2300
800-776-4332
FAX 309-755-2377
TDY:800-933-8331
http://www.linguisystems.com
e-mail: service@linguisystems.com
Elizabeth Mackie, Author
Linda Bowers, Co-Owner/Co-Founder
Rosemary Huisingh, Co-Owner/Co-Founder

Whether your are new to oral-motor skills training or an experienced oral-motor skills clinician, these activities get results. *$39.95*
119 pages Ages 3-8

1162 PLAID: Practical Lessons for Apraxia
Abilitations Speech Bin
PO Box 922668
Norcross, GA 30010
770-449-5700
800-850-8602
FAX 770-510-7290
http://www.speechbin.com
e-mail: info@speechbin.com
Tobi Isaacs, Catalog Director

PLAID is a top-notch clinical tool that gives you practical practice materials featuring twenty different phonemes — just what you need for your apraxic and aphasic adults — all in one resource. Item number 190746116. *$29.95*

1163 Pair-It Books: Early Emergent Stage 1
Harcourt Achieve
Customer Service, 5th Floor
Orlando, FL 32887
800-284-7019
FAX 800-699-9459
http://www.harcourtachieve.com
e-mail: webmaster@harcourt.com
Randy , SVP National Sales

Includes 30 eight-page books with simple concepts, predictable and repetitive text patterns, and a strong matching of art or photos to support the text.

1164 Pair-It Books: Early Emergent Stage 1 in Spanish
Harcourt Achieve
Customer Service, 5th Floor
Orlando, FL 32887
800-284-7019
FAX 800-699-9459
http://www.harcourtachieve.com
e-mail: webmaster@harcourt.com
Steven , CEO
Randy , SVP National Sales

Includes 30 eight-page books with simple concepts, predictable and repetitive text patterns, and a strong matching of art or photos to support the text. Six big books encourage shared reading and strategy instruction. Students can read these texts with ease and view themselves as successful readers.

1165 Pair-It Books: Early Emergent Stage 2
Customer Service, 5th Floor
Orlando, FL 32887
800-284-7019
FAX 800-699-9459
http://www.harcourtachieve.com
e-mail: webmaster@harcourt.com
Steven Korten, CEO
Randy Pennington, SVP National Sales

A series of 20 books, each containing 16 pages, that gradually become more difficult and reflect more complex text structures such as dialogue, content vocabulary and question and answer formats. All stories are available on audio cassette, and four are available in big book format.

1166 Pair-It Books: Early Emergent Stage 2 in S
Harcourt Achieve
Customer Service, 5th Floor
Orlando, FL 32887
800-284-7019
FAX 800-699-9459
http://www.harcourtachieve.com
e-mail: webmaster@harcourt.com
Steven Korten, CEO
Randy Pennington, SVP National Sales

A series of 20 books, each containing 16 pages, that encourage native Spanish speakers with early reading success in their first language. Simple concepts, predictable language, and well chosen art support students efforts.

1167 Pair-It Books: Early Fluency Stage 3
Harcourt Achieve
Customer Service, 5th Floor
Orlando, FL 32887
800-284-7019
FAX 800-699-9459
http://www.harcourtachieve.com
e-mail: webmaster@harcourt.com
Steven , CEO
Randy , SVP National Sales

A series of 30 books, each containing either 16 or 24 pages, and six big books that introduce tables, folktales, tall tales and plays that invite readers to respond in writing.

1168 Pair-It Books: Early Skills
Harcourt Achieve
Customer Service, 5th Floor
Orlando, FL 32887
800-284-7019
FAX 800-699-9459
http://www.harcourtachieve.com
e-mail: webmaster@harcourt.com
Steven Korten, CEO
Randy Pennington, SVP National Sales

Give students an early start on academic achievement with grade appropriate, cross-curricular excercises. Easy-to-understand lessons with helpful graphics are ideal for independent or small group learning.

1169 Pair-It Books: Fluency Stage 4
Harcourt Achieve
Customer Service, 5th Floor
Orlando, FL 32887
800-284-7019
FAX 800-699-9459
http://www.harcourtachieve.com
e-mail: webmaster@harcourt.com
Steven Korten, CEO
Randy Pennington, SVP National Sales

A series of 20 books, each containing 24 or 32 pages, and four big books. Readers encounter diaries, journals, biographies, and mysteries and explore written responses in a variety of formats. Students emerge as confident readers and writers of both narrative and informational texts.

1170 Pair-It Books: Proficiency Stage 5
Harcourt Achieve
Customer Service, 5th Floor
Orlando, FL 32887
800-284-7019
FAX 800-699-9459
http://www.harcourtachieve.com
e-mail: webmaster@harcourt.com
Steven Korten, CEO
Randy Pennington, SVP National Sales

A series of 30 books, each containing 32 or 40 pages, that take readers from fluency to proficiency, presenting a wide variety of genres and text structures. Offers helpful strategies and activities for improving phonics skills, vocabulary, and reading and language skills, as well as take-home letters in Spanish and English.

1171 Pair-It Books: Transition Stage 2-3
Harcourt Achieve
Customer Service, 5th Floor
Orlando, FL 32887
800-284-7019
FAX 800-699-9459
http://www.harcourtachieve.com
e-mail: webmaster@harcourt.com
Steven Korten, CEO
Randy Pennington, SVP National Sales

A series of 20 books, each containing 16 pages, that provide readers with a gradual transition into early fluency. All stories are available on audio cassette, and four are avaiable in big book format.

1172 Patterns Across the Curriculum
Harcourt Achieve
6277 Sea Harbor Drive
Orlando, FL 32887
252-480-3200
800-844-1464
FAX 800-269-5232
http://www.steckvaughn.com
e-mail: info@steckvaughn.com
Steck-Vaughn Staff, Author
Tim McEwen, President/CEO
Jeff Johnson, Dir Marketing Communications
Chris Lehmann, Team Coordinator
Develop students awareness and understanding of patterns in the real world. Exercises allow students to identify, complete, extend, and create patterns. Developed across math, language, social studies, and science. This flexible organization allows teachers to utilize content specific activities in coordination with other classroom assignments, providing additional richness in learning.

1173 Patty's Cake: A Describing Game
LinguiSystems
3100 4th Avenue
East Moline, IL 61244
309-755-2300
800-776-4332
FAX 309-755-2377
TDY:800-933-8331
http://www.linguisystems.com
e-mail: service@linguisystems.com
Julie Cole, Author
Linda Bowers, Co-Owner/Co-Founder
Rosemary Huisingh, Co-Owner/Co-Founder

Teach describing skills with Patty's Cake. Two levels of play in this fun game give you flexibility to meet individual students learning needs. Players describe age-appropriate picture vocabulary cards by naming attributes such as category, function, shape, color, or location. Your students will improve their skills in listening, memory, word retrieval, categorizing, naming attributes, formulating sentences, and giving descriptions. *$44.95*

Ages 4-9

1174 PhonicsMart CD-ROM
Harcourt Achieve
Customer Service, 5th Floor
Orlando, FL 32887
800-284-7019
FAX 800-699-9459
http://www.harcourtachieve.com
e-mail: webmaster@harcourt.com
Steven Korten, CEO
Randy Pennington, SVP National Sales

Five interactive games offer practice and reinforcement in 19 phonics skills at a variety of learning levels! Over 700 key words are vocalized, and each is accompanied by sound effects, colorful illustrations, animation, or video clips!

1175 Phonological Awareness Kit
LinguiSystems
3100 4th Avenue
East Moline, IL 61244
309-755-2300
800-776-4332
FAX 309-755-2377
TDY:800-933-8331
http://www.linguisystems.com
e-mail: service@linguisystems.com
Carolyn Robertson, Wanda Salter, Author
Linda Bowers, Co-Owner/Co-Founder
Rosemary Huisingh, Co-Owner/Co-Founder

Help your students learn to use phonological information to process oral and written language with this fantastic kit. Written by an SLP and special educator, this best-seller links sound awareness, oral language, and early reading and writing skills. The kit uses a multisensory approach to ensure success for all learning styles. *$69.95*
115 pages Ages 5-8

1176 Phonological Awareness Kit: Intermediate
LinguiSystems
3100 4th Avenue
East Moline, IL 61244
309-755-2300
800-776-4332
FAX 309-755-2377
TDY:800-933-8331
http://www.linguisystems.com
e-mail: service@linguisystems.com
Carolyn Robertson, Wanda Salter, Author
Linda Bowers, Co-Owner/Co-Founder
Rosemary Huisingh, Co-Owner/Co-Founder

Now there's hope for your older students who have struggled with reading through their early school years. Give them strategies to crack the reading code with this comprehensive program. Great for students with deficits in auditory processing, decoding, and written language. *$69.95*
116 pages Ages 9-14

1177 Phonological Awareness Test: Computerized Scoring
LinguiSystems
3100 4th Avenue
East Moline, IL 61244
309-755-2300
800-776-4332
FAX 800-577-4555
TDY:800-933-8331
http://www.linguisystems.com
e-mail: service@linguisystems.com
Carolyn Robertson, Wanda Salter, Author
Linda Bowers, Co-Owner/Co-Founder
Rosemary Huisingh, Co-Owner/Co-Founder

Designed to save time, this optional CD-ROM software allows you to accurately, conveniently, and quickly score The Phonological Awareness Test. Just plug in the raw scores and the program does everything else. You'll be able to print out all the scores you need to include in a student's assessment report. *$69.95*

Ages 5-9

1178 Phonology: Software

Abilitations Speech Bin
PO Box 922668
Norcross, GA 30010
770-449-5700
800-850-8602
FAX 770-510-7290
http://www.speechbin.com
e-mail: info@speechbin.com

Tobi Isaacs, Catalong Director

This unique software gives you six entertaining games to treat children's phonological disorders. The program uses target patterns in a pattern cycling approach to phonological processes. Item number 190215116. *$98.99*

1179 Plunk's Pond: A Riddles Game for Language

LinguiSystems
3100 4th Avenue
East Moline, IL 61244
309-755-2300
800-776-4332
FAX 309-755-2377
TDY:800-933-8331
http://www.linguisystems.com
e-mail: service@linguisystems.com

LinguiSystems Staff, Author
Linda Bowers, Co-Owner/Co-Founder
Rosemary Huisingh, Co-Owner/Co-Founder

Encourage divergent thinking, sharpen listening skills, and improve vocabulary with this fun riddle game. With a picture on one side and three clues on the other, these cards are great for all kinds of therapy games. Target attributes such as function, color, category, and more. *$44.95*

Ages 4-9

1180 Poetry in Three Dimensions: Reading, Writing and Critical Thinking Skills through Poetry

Educators Publishing Service
PO Box 9031
Cambridge, MA 02139
617-547-6706
800-225-5750
FAX 888-440-2665
http://www.epsbooks.com
e-mail: eps@epsbooks.com

Carol Clark, Alison Draper, Author
Gunnar Voltz, President
Jennifer Avery, Contact

Help your students improve their reading comprehension and writing through the study of poetry in this collection of multicultural poems. With poems and questions on facing pages, students are encouraged to annotate the text of the poem and to go back to the text to respond to the questions.

1181 Polar Express

Sunburst Technology
1550 Executive Drive
Elgin, IL 60123
800-321-7511
FAX 888-800-3028
http://http://store.sunburst.com/Home.aspx
e-mail: service@sunburst.com

Michael Guillory, Channel Sales/Marketing Manager

Share the magic and enchantment of the holiday season with this CD-ROM version of Chris Van Allsburg's Caldecott-winning picture book.

1182 Preschool Motor Speech Evaluation & Inter vention

Abilitations Speech Bin
PO Box 922668
Norcross, GA 30010
770-449-5700
800-850-8602
FAX 770-510-7290
http://www.speechbin.com
e-mail: info@speechbin.com

Margaret M Earnest, Author
Tobi Isaacs, Catalog Director

This comprehensive criterion-based assessment tool differentiates motor-based speech disorders from those of phonology and determines if speech difficulties of children 18 months to six years old are characteristic of: oral nonverbal apraxia; dysarthria; developmental verbal dyspraxia; hypersensitivity; differences in tone and hyposensitivity. Item number 190323116. *$65.99*

1183 Progress with Puppets: Speech and Language Activities for Children

Therapro
225 Arlington Street
Framingham, MA 01702
508-872-9494
800-257-5376
FAX 508-875-2062
http://www.theraproducts.com
e-mail: info@theraproducts.com

Joanne Hanson MS CCC-SLP, Author
Karen Conrad, Owner

A much needed book of activities to use during therapy with puppets. Great ideas for working on chewing and feeding, language stimulation, articulation training, fluency and more. Suggestions offered for use with the Puppets that Swallow. *$29.95*

1184 Promoting Communication in Infants 500 Ways

Abilitations Speech Bin
PO Box 922668
Norcross, GA 30010
770-449-5700
800-850-8602
FAX 770-510-7290
http://www.speechbin.com
e-mail: info@speechbin.com

Tobi Isaacs, Catalog Director

Gives you down-to-earth information, activities, and step-by-step suggestions for stimulating children's speech and language skills. Topics are conveniently organized, concisely presented, and written in easy-to-understand language. Item number 1512. *$17.95*

1185 Python Path Phonics Word Families

Sunburst Technology
1550 Executive Drive
Elgin, IL 60123
800-321-7511
FAX 888-800-3028
http://http://store.sunburst.com/Home.aspx
e-mail: service@sunburst.com

Michael Guillory, Channel Sales/Marketing Manager

Your students improve their word-building skills by playing three fun strategy games that involve linking one-or two-letter consonant beginnings to basic word endings.

1186 RULES

Speech Bin
PO Box 922668
Norcross, GA 30010
770-449-5700
800-850-8602
FAX 770-510-7290
http://www.speechbin.com
e-mail: info@speechbin.com

Shane Peters, Product Coordinator
Jen Binney, Owner

Faced with young children whose speech is unintelligible? RULES is the perfect program for these preschool and elementary children. It remediates the processes: cluster reduction;, final consonant deletion, stopping; and prevocalic voicing. Item number 1557. *$43.95*

1187 Receptive One-Word Picture Vocabulary Test (ROWPVT-2000)

Abilitations Speech Bin
PO Box 922668
Norcross, GA 30010
770-449-5700
800-850-8602
FAX 770-510-7290
http://www.speechbin.com
e-mail: info@speechbin.com

Rick Brownell, Author
Tobi Isaacs, Catalog Director

It is ideal for children unable or reluctant to speak because only a gestural response is required. ROWPVT-2000 requires only 15-20 minutes to give and score; it is co-normed with EOWPVT-2000 on 2,000 chilren. Item number 190076116. *$139.99*

1188 **Remediation of Articulation Disorders (RAD)**
Abilitations Speech Bin
PO Box 922668
Norcross, GA 30010
770-449-5700
800-850-8602
FAX 770-510-7290
http://www.speechbin.com
e-mail: info@speechbin.com
Tobi Isaacs, Catalog Director

RAD treats articulation and speech intelligibility as important parameters of language. It gives you thematic pictures and worksheets to facilitate the development of critical sounds. Each picture also has a problem-solving element that provides rich opportunities for discussion and narratives. Item number 1420. *$19.95*

1189 **Retell Stories**
Abilitations Speech Bin
PO Box 922668
Norcross, GA 30010
770-449-5700
800-850-8602
FAX 770-510-7290
http://www.speechbin.com
e-mail: info@speechbin.com
Tobi Isaacs, Catalog Director

You'll use them for pre-/post-testing, treatment sessions, and home practice. This approach emphasizes systematic training of error phonemes in a semantically potent core vocabulary of the child's own words. It enables children to use whole words intelligibly as powerful tools for real-life communication. Item number 1441. *$18.95*

1190 **Ridgewood Grammar**
Educators Publishing Service
PO Box 9031
Cambridge, MA 02139
617-547-6706
800-225-5750
FAX 888-440-2665
http://www.epsbooks.com
e-mail: eps@epsbooks.com
Terri Wiss, Nancy Bison, Author
Gunnar Voltz, President
Jennifer Avery, Contact

Grammar is an important part of any student's education. This new series, from the school district that developed the popular Ridgewood Analogies books, teaches 3rd, 4th, and 5th graders about the parts of speech and their use in sentences.

1191 **Rocky's Mountain: A Word-finding Game**
LinguiSystems
3100 4th Avenue
East Moline, IL 61244
309-755-2300
800-776-4332
FAX 309-755-2377
TDY:800-933-8331
http://www.linguisystems.com
e-mail: service@linguisystems.com
Gina Williamson, Susan Shields, Author
Linda Bowers, Co-Owner/Co-Founder
Rosemary Huisingh, Co-Owner/Co-Founder

Tackle stubborn word-finding problems with this fun game! Game cards are organized by four word-finding strategies so you can pick the strategy that best meets your students' needs. Teach these strategies for word-finding: visual imagery; word association; sound/letter cueing; and categories. *$44.95*

Ages 4-9

1192 **Room 14**
LinguiSystems
3100 4th Avenue
East Moline, IL 61244
309-755-2300
800-776-4332
FAX 309-755-2377
TDY:800-933-8331
http://www.linguisystems.com
e-mail: service@linguisystems.com
Carolyn Wilson, Author
Linda Bowers, Co-Owner/Co-Founder
Rosemary Huisingh, Co-Owner/Co-Founder

Build social skills by offering a variety of teaching approaches to meet the language and learning needs of your students. Through stories, comprehension activities, and organized lessons, students learn to: make and keep friends. fit in at school, handle feelings, and be responsible for their actions. *$59.95*
198 pages Ages 6-10

1193 **SLP's IDEA Companion**
LinguiSystems
3100 4th Avenue
East Moline, IL 61244
309-755-2300
800-776-4332
FAX 309-755-2375
TDY:800-933-8331
http://www.linguisystems.com
e-mail: service@linguisystems.com
Shaila Lucas, Author
Linda Bowers, Co-Owner/Co-Founder
Rosemary Huisingh, Co-Owner/Co-Founder

Set goals and objectives that match the guidelines outlined in the Individuals with Disabilities Education Act. You'll be able to link your therapy goals to the classroom curriculum, determine appropriate benchmarks for students, and determine levels of performance using the baseline measures provided in the book. *$39.95*
162 pages Ages 5-18

1194 **SPARC Artic Junior**
LinguiSystems
3100 4th Avenue
East Moline, IL 61244
309-755-2300
800-776-4332
FAX 309-755-2377
TDY:800-933-8331
http://www.linguisystems.com
e-mail: service@linguisystems.com
Beverly Plass, Author
Linda Bowers, Co-Owner/Co-Founder
Rosemary Huisingh, Co-Owner/Co-Founder

Reach intelligibility goals faster with these take-home exercises. The practice words have been carefully selected to control the phonetic context. It's a programmed, research-based approach that will get results. Activities are divided by primary and secondary phonological processes. *$39.95*
211 pages Ages 3-7

1195 **SPARC Artic Scenes**
LinguiSystems
3100 4th Avenue
East Moline, IL 61244
309-755-2300
800-776-4332
FAX 309-755-2377
TDY:800-933-8331
http://www.linguisystems.com
e-mail: service@linguisystems.com
Susan Rose Simms, Author
Linda Bowers, Co-Owner/Co-Founder
Rosemary Huisingh, Co-Owner/Co-Founder

Each picture scene is loaded with target sounds to get the most speech practice in your limited therapy time. You'll take care of your entire caseload with these articulation and language activities. Activities include vocabulary lists, story starts, thinking questions, categorizing and multiple meanings. *$39.95*

207 pages Ages 4-10

1196 **SPARC for Grammar**
LinguiSystems
3100 4th Avenue
East Moline, IL 61244
309-755-2300
800-776-4332
FAX 309-755-2377
TDY:800-933-8331
http://www.linguisystems.com
e-mail: service@linguisystems.com
Susan Thomsen, Kathy Donnelly, Author
Linda Bowers, Co-Owner/Co-Founder
Rosemary Huisingh, Co-Owner/Co-Founder

Teach grammar in meaningful contexts! The lessons provide a wealth of opportunities for your students to hear, repeat, answer questions and tell stories using targeted language structures. *$39.95*
165 pages Ages 4-10

1197 **SPARC for Phonology**
LinguiSystems
3100 4th Avenue
East Moline, IL 61244
309-755-2300
800-776-4332
FAX 309-755-2377
TDY:800-933-8331
http://www.linguisystems.com
e-mail: service@linguisystems.com
Susan Thomsen, Kathy Donnelly, Author
Linda Bowers, Co-Owner/Co-Founder
Rosemary Huisingh, Co-Owner/Co-Founder

This excellent resource includes 80 pages of 16 pictures each... that's 1280 pictures in all! Each picture page has corresponding 20-word auditory bombardment list. These great lessons cover syllable reduction, consonant deletion, cluster reduction, gliding, vowelization, fronting, backing, stopping, stridency deletion, affrication, deaffrication, voicing and devoicing. *$39.95*
165 pages Ages 4-10

1198 **SPARC for Vocabulary**
LinguiSystems
3100 4th Avenue
East Moline, IL 61244
309-755-2300
800-776-4332
FAX 309-755-2377
TDY:800-933-8331
http://www.linguisystems.com
e-mail: service@linguisystems.com
Susan Thomsen, Kathy Donnelly, Author
Linda Bowers, Co-Owner/Co-Founder
Rosemary Huisingh, Co-Owner/Co-Founder

Teach vocabulary skills through themes! Rapid-naming skills will improve as vocabulary knowledge increases. This invaluable picture resource gets your students learning and thinking about new words. *$39.95*
165 pages Ages 4-10

1199 **Scissors, Glue, and Artic, Too!**
LinguiSystems
3100 4th Avenue
East Moline, IL 61244
309-755-2300
800-776-4332
FAX 309-755-2377
TDY:800-933-8331
http://www.linguisystems.com
e-mail: service@linguisystems.com
Susan Rose Simms, Author
Linda Bowers, Co-Owner/Co-Founder
Rosemary Huisingh, Co-Owner/Co-Founder

Hands-on projects that beg to be talked about are perfect for young students in articulation therapy. This wonderfully illustrated manual is filled with puzzles, books, animals, and more that come to life in the hands of students. *$39.95*

189 pages Ages 4-9

1200 **Scissors, Glue, and Grammar, Too!**
LinguiSystems
3100 4th Avenue
East Moline, IL 61244
309-755-2300
800-776-4332
FAX 309-755-2377
TDY:800-933-8331
http://www.linguisystems.com
e-mail: service@linguisystems.com
Susan Boegler, Debbie Abruzzini, Author
Linda Bowers, Co-Owner/Co-Founder
Rosemary Huisingh, Co-Owner/Co-Founder

Even your youngest students can learn correct grammar and syntax skills. This interactive approach is the perfect resource. These cut-and-paste activities are so much fun, your students won't realize they're learning regular and irregular verbs, comparatives and superlatives, wh- questions, and more! *$39.95*
174 pages Ages 4-9

1201 **Scissors, Glue, and Phonological Processes, Too!**
LinguiSystems
3100 4th Avenue
East Moline, IL 61244
309-755-2300
800-776-4332
FAX 309-755-2377
TDY:800-933-8331
http://www.linguisystems.com
e-mail: service@linguisystems.com
Gayle H Daly, Author
Linda Bowers, Co-Owner/Co-Founder
Rosemary Huisingh, Co-Owner/Co-Founder

Eliminate error patterns with minimal pair contrasts at the word and phrase level. Watch your young students cut and paste their way to better speech with these engaging, interactive activities. *$39.95*
174 pages Ages 4-9

1202 **Scissors, Glue, and Vocabulary, Too!**
LinguiSystems
3100 4th Avenue
East Moline, IL 61244
309-755-2300
800-776-4332
FAX 309-755-2377
TDY:800-933-8331
http://www.linguisystems.com
e-mail: service@linguisystems.com
Barb Truman, Patti Halfman, Lauri Whiskeyman, Author
Linda Bowers, Co-Owner/Co-Founder
Rosemary Huisingh, Co-Owner/Co-Founder

These cut-and-paste activities keep young students motivated. The rich vocabulary content gets them using new words in new ways. You'll not only teach vocabulary skills but listening and following directions too. Each lesson gives you a list of key vocabulary, scripted directions, a family letter, and several enrichment activites. *$39.95*
187 pages Ages 4-9

1203 **Sequential Spelling 1-7 with Student Response Book**
AVKO Educational Research Foundation
3084 W Willard Road
Clio, MI 48420
810-686-1101
866-285-6612
FAX 810-686-1101
http://www.avko.org
e-mail: info@avko.org
Don McCabe, Author
Don Cabe, Research Director

Sequential Spelling uses immediate student self-correction. It builds from easier words of a word family such as all and then builds on them to teach; all, tall, stall, install, call, fall, ball, and their inflected forms such as: stalls, stalled, stalling, installing, installment. *$79.95*

72 pages
ISBN 1-664003-00-0

1204 **Silly Sentences**
Abilitations Speech Bin
PO Box 922668
Norcross, GA 30010
770-449-5700
800-850-8602
FAX 770-510-7290
http://www.speechbin.com
e-mail: info@speechbin.com
Tobi Isaacs, Catalog Director

Children love to have fun. Silly Sentences lets them have fun while they play these engaging card games to learn: subject verb agreement, speech sound articulation; S+ V+ O sentences, questioning and answering; humor and absurdities and present progressive verbs. Item number 190497116. *$47.99*

1205 **Soaring Scores CTB: TerraNova Reading and Language Arts**
Harcourt Achieve
Customer Service, 5th Floor
Orlando, FL 32887
800-284-7019
FAX 800-699-9459
http://www.harcourtachieve.com
e-mail: webmaster@harcourt.com
Steven Korten, CEO
Randy Pennington, SVP National Sales

Through a combination of targeted instructional practice and test-taking tips, these workbooks help students build better skills and improve CTB-TerraNova test scores. Initial lessons address reading comprehension and language arts. The authentic practice test mirrors the CTB's format and content.

1206 **Soaring Scores in Integrated Language Arts**
Harcourt Achieve
Customer Service, 5th Floor
Orlando, FL 32877
800-284-7019
FAX 800-699-9459
http://www.harcourtachieve.com
e-mail: webmaster@harcourt.com
Steven Korten, CEO
Randy Pennington, SVP National Sales

Help your students develop the right skills and strategies for success on integrated arts assessments. Soaring Scores presents three sets of two lengthy, thematically linked literature selections. Students develop higher-order thinking skills as they respond to open-ended questions about the selections.

1207 **Soaring Scores on the CMT in Language Arts& on the CAPT in Reading and Writing Across Disciplines**
Harcourt Achieve
Customer Service, 5th Floor
Orlando, FL 32887
800-284-7019
FAX 800-699-9459
http://www.harcourtachieve.com
e-mail: webmaster@harcourt.com
Steven Korten, CEO
Randy Pennington, SVP National Sales

Make every minute count when you are preparing for the CMT or CAPT. Fine tune your language arts test preparation with the program developed specifically for the Connecticut's assessments. Questions are correlated to Connecticut's content standards for reading and responding, producing text, applying English language conventions, and exploring and responding to texts.

1208 **Soaring Scores on the NYS English Language Arts Assessment**
Harcourt Achieve
Customer Service, 5th Floor
Orlando, FL 32887
800-284-7019
FAX 800-699-9459
http://www.harcourtachieve.com
e-mail: webmaster@harcourt.com
Steven Korten, CEO
Randy Pennington, SVP National Sales

With these workbooks, students receive instructional practice for approaching the assessment's reading, listening and writing questions.

1209 **Soaring on the MCAS in English Language Arts**
Harcourt Achieve
Customer Service, 5th Floor
Orlando, FL 32887
800-284-7019
FAX 800-699-9459
http://www.harcourtachieve.com
e-mail: webmaster@harcourt.com
Steven Korten, CEO
Randy Pennington, SVP National Sales

Instructional practice in the first section builds skills for the MCAS language, literacy, and composition questions. A practice test models the MCAS precisely in design and length.

1210 **Sound Connections**
Abilitations Speech Bin
PO Box 922668
Norcross, GA 30010
770-449-5700
800-850-8602
FAX 770-510-7290
http://www.speechbin.com
e-mail: info@speechbin.com
Tobi Isaacs, Catalog Director

This program teaches the critical connections between the sounds kids hear and speaking, reading, and writing. Dozens of activities and worksheets, 19 phoneme-based stories, and 100s of pictures. Item number 190805116. *$41.99*

1211 **Sounds Abound**
LinguiSystems
3100 4th Avenue
East Moline, IL 61244
309-755-2300
800-776-4332
FAX 309-755-2377
TDY:800-933-8331
http://www.linguisystems.com
e-mail: service@linguisystems.com
Hugh Catts, Tina Olsen, Author
Linda Bowers, Co-Owner/Co-Founder
Rosemary Huisingh, Co-Owner/Co-Founder

Delayed speech and language skills DO impact reading skills. Give your young students an edge with Sounds Abound. They'll connect letters with sounds as they meet their speech and language goals. This best-selling manual is loaded with activities for speech sound awareness, rhyming skills, beginning and ending sounds, segmenting and blending sounds, and putting sounds together with letters. *$37.95*
190 pages Ages 4-9

1212 **Sounds Abound Game**
LinguiSystems
3100 4th Avenue
East Moline, IL 61244
309-755-2300
800-776-4332
FAX 309-755-2377
TDY:800-933-8331
http://www.linguisystems.com
e-mail: service@linguisystems.com
Hugh Catts, Tina Olsen, Author
Linda Bowers, Co-Owner/Co-Founder
Rosemary Huisingh, Co-Owner/Co-Founder

Teach critical features about sounds in words for better language skills. Your students will love this fun game because it's easy to play. This game targets the sounds students use the most: f; s; p; t; and m. These essential sounds are critical for early literacy success. *$39.95*

Ages 4-9

1213 **Sounds Abound Multisensory Phonological Awareness**

LinguiSystems
3100 4th Avenue
East Moline, IL 61244
309-755-2300
800-776-4332
FAX 309-755-2377
TDY:800-933-8331
http://www.linguisystems.com
e-mail: service@linguisystems.com
Jill Teachworth, Author
Linda Bowers, Co-Owner/Co-Founder
Rosemary Huisingh, Co-Owner/Co-Founder

The multisensory approach in this phonological program reinforces knowledge and retention of sound-symbol correspondence. Students will learn through their best modality as they look, listen, feel, play, and even sing the sounds. *$37.95*

201 pages Ages 4-7

1214 **Source for Apraxia Therapy**

LinguiSystems
3100 4th Avenue
East Moline, IL 61244
309-755-2300
800-776-4332
FAX 309-755-2377
TDY:800-933-8331
http://www.linguisystems.com
e-mail: service@linguisystems.com
Kathryn J Tomlin, Author
Linda Bowers, Co-Owner/Co-Founder
Rosemary Huisingh, Co-Owner/Co-Founder

This resource combines a visual-auditory-kinesthetic approach to help your clients improve intelligibility. Three sections target phoneme production, articulation, fluency, and phrasing, and paralinguistic drills. You'll know just where to start therapy for clients with mild, moderate, or severe apraxia. *$41.95*

195 pages Adults

1215 **Source for Bilingual Students with Language Disorders**

LinguiSystems
3100 4th Avenue
East Moline, IL 61244
309-755-2300
800-776-4332
FAX 309-755-2377
TDY:800-933-8331
http://www.linguisystems.com
e-mail: service@linguisystems.com
Celeste Roseberry-McKibbin, Author
Linda Bowers, Co-Owner/Co-Founder
Rosemary Huisingh, Co-Owner/Co-Founder

Focus on teaching vocabulary and phonolgical awareness skills, the most important skills your bilingual students need for overall English proficiency and literacy. This resource gives you activities and materials based on a hierarchy of second language acquisition, *$41.95*

250 pages Ages 5-18

1216 **Source for Processing Disorders**

LinguiSystems
3100 4th Avenue
East Moline, IL 61244
309-755-2300
800-776-4332
FAX 309-755-2377
TDY:800-933-8331
http://www.linguisystems.com
e-mail: service@linguisystems.com
Gail J Richard, Author
Linda Bowers, Co-Owner/Co-Founder
Rosemary Huisingh, Co-Owner/Co-Founder

This great resource helps you differentiate between language processing disorders and auditory processing disorders. Chapters cover: the neurology of processing and learning; the central auditory processing model; the language processing model; and a lot more! *$41.95*

181 pages Ages 5-Adult

1217 **Source for Stuttering and Cluttering**

LinguiSystems
3100 4th Avenue
East Moline, IL 61244
309-755-2300
800-776-4332
FAX 309-755-2377
TDY:800-933-8331
http://www.linguisystems.com
e-mail: service@linguisystems.com
David A Daly, Author
Linda Bowers, Co-Owner/Co-Founder
Rosemary Huisingh, Co-Owner/Co-Founder

Author David Daly, a former stutterer and respected speech pathologist, puts his clinical expertise and personal passion into this comprehensive program. Your clients will become fluent, confident speakers with this excellent, field-tested resource. *$44.95*

210 pages Ages 13-Adult

1218 **Source for Syndromes**

LinguiSystems
3100 4th Avenue
East Moline, IL 61244
309-755-2300
800-776-4332
FAX 309-755-2377
TDY:800-933-8331
http://www.linguisystems.com
e-mail: service@linguisystems.com
Gail J Richard, Debra Reichert Hoge, Author
Linda Bowers, Co-Owner/Co-Founder
Rosemary Huisingh, Co-Owner/Co-Founder

Do you often wish someone would just tell you what to do with a specific youngster on your caseload? The Source for Syndromes can do just that. Learn about the speech-language characteristics for each sydrome with a focus on communication issues. This resource covers pertinent information for such sydromes such as Angelman, Asperger's, Autism, Rett's Tourette's, Williams, and more. *$41.95*

147 pages Ages Birth-18

1219 **Spectral Speech Analysis: Software**

Speech Bin
PO Box 922668
Norcross, GA 30010
770-449-5700
800-850-8602
FAX 770-510-7290
http://www.speechbin.com
e-mail: info@speechbin.com
Shane Peters, Product Coordinator
Jen Binney, Owner

This exciting new software uses visual feedback as an effective speech treatment tool. Speech-language pathologists can record speech and corresponding visual displays for clients who then try to match either auditory or visual targets. These built-in visual patterns can be displayed as either sophisticated spectrograms or real-time waveforms. Item number P227 — windows only. *$159.95*

1220 **Speech & Language & Voice & More**

Speech Bin
PO Box 922668
Norcross, GA 30010
770-449-5700
800-850-8602
FAX 770-510-7290
http://www.speechbin.com
e-mail: info@speechbin.com
Shane Peters, Product Coordinator
Jen Binney, Owner

Contains eighty-eight practically perfect reproducible games and activities ideal for your K-5 clients. It gives you: manipulable activities to keep active leaners learning; tasks to match a multitude of interests and abilities; and vocal hygiene worksheets targeted to reduce vocal abuse. Item number 1496. *$19.95*

1221 Speech Sports
Abilitations Speech Bin
PO Box 922668
Norcross, GA 30010
770-449-5700
800-850-8602
FAX 70-510-72906
http://www.speechbin.com
e-mail: info@speechbin.com
Janet M Shaw, Author
Tobi Isaacs, Catalog Director

Speech Sports makes every child in your caseload a shining sports star. Reproducible gameboards and language activities feature 19 different sports from boating to skating, bowling to running, basketball to soccer. Item number 190797116. *$29.95*

1222 Speech Viewer III
Speech Bin
PO Box 922668
Norcross, GA 30010
770-449-5700
800-850-8602
FAX 770-510-7290
http://www.speechbin.com
e-mail: info@speechbin.com
Shane Peters, Product Coordinator
Jen Binney, Owner

SpeechViewer III creates entertaining interactive displays that let them do just that! It has all the Visual Voice Tools and so much more! Begin with simple sound awareness and advance to complex speech tasks, increasing phoneme awareness and improving speech sound production. Users enjoy constant and objective real time visual feedback from graphical speech displayed. Item number E280 — windows only. *$899.00*

1223 Speech-Language Delights
Abilitations Speech Bin
PO Box 922668
Norcross, GA 30010
770-449-5700
800-850-8602
FAX 770-510-7290
http://www.speechbin.com
e-mail: info@speechbin.com
Janet M Shaw, Author
Tobi Isaacs, Catalog Director

Cook up lots of fun with Speech-Language Delights! Delectably delicious speech and language activities and games provide rich opportunities and hands-on activities with food-related themes to enrich K-8 kids. Item number 1541. *$ 29.95*

1224 SpeechCrafts
Abilitations Speech Bin
PO Box 922668
Norcross, GA 30010
770-449-5700
800-850-8602
FAX 770-510-7290
http://www.speechbin.com
e-mail: info@speechbin.com
Tobi Isaacs, Catalog Director

Children love to create decorative and useful objects. They also love the surprise of using common and ordinary objects in unexpected ways. Best of all, children learn best when engaged in tangible, concrete, hands-on projects that are designed to enhance learning. Activities develop skills in: sequencing; language; basic concepts; vocabulary; articulation and following directions. Item number 1490. *$23.99*

1225 Spelling: A Thematic Content-Area Approach
Harcourt Achieve
Customer Service, 5th Floor
Orlando, FL 32887
800-284-7019
FAX 800-699-9459
http://www.harcourtachieve.com
e-mail: webmaster@harcourt.com
Steven Korten, CEO
Randy Pennington, SVP National Sales

Help students master the words they will use most frequently in the classroom. Organized lessons incorporate word analysis of letter patterns, correlations to appropriate literature, writing exercises, and application and extension activities.

1226 Stepping Up to Fluency
Abilitations Speech Bin
PO Box 922668
Norcross, GA 30010
770-449-5700
800-850-8602
FAX 770-510-7290
http://www.speechbin.com
e-mail: info@speechbin.com
Tobi Isaacs, Catalog Director

Stepping Up to Fluency gives you a systematic program to help your clients from five years old to adults understand their disfluencies and gain control of their speech in 25-35 sessions. It presents high-interest strategies and materials in two levels, K-3 and grade 4 to adult. Item number 190862116. *$34.95*

1227 Stories and More: Time and Place
Riverdeep
100 Pine Street
San Francisco, CA 94111
415-659-2000
FAX 415-659-2020
http://www.riverdeep.net
e-mail: info@riverdeep.net
Barry O'Callaghan, Executive Chairman/CEO

Combines three well-loved stories - The House on Maple Street, Roxaboxen, and Galimoto with engaging activities that strengthen students' reading comprehension.

1228 Straight Speech
Abilitations Speech Bin
PO Box 922668
Norcross, GA 30010
770-449-5700
800-850-8602
FAX 770-510-7290
http://www.speechbin.com
e-mail: info@speechbin.com
Jane Folk, Author
Tobi Isaacs, Catalog Director

Straight Speech helps you with those pesky lateral lisps, one of the most perplexing articulation problems you encounter. It gives you an effective, easy-to-implement program for lateral lisps. Item number 190741116. *$19.99*

80 pages
ISBN 0-937857-32-7

1229 Stuttering: Helping the Disfluent Preschool Child
Abilitations Speech Bin
PO Box 922668
Norcross, GA 30010
770-449-5700
800-850-8602
FAX 770-510-7290
http://www.speechbin.com
e-mail: info@speechbin.com
Julie A Blonigen, Author
Tobi Isaacs, Catalog Director

Written in the warm encouraging style for which this author is known, Stuttering: Helping the Disfluent Preschool Child is the perfect tool for parents and teachers of young stuttering children. It uses a Speech Thermometer to show them ways to turn talking into an area of strength. Item number 190874116. *$13.99*

1230 Sunken Treasure Adventure: Beginning Blends
Sunburst Technology
1550 Executive Drive
Elgin, IL 60123
800-321-7511
FAX 888-800-3028
http://http://store.sunburst.com/Home.aspx
e-mail: service@sunburst.com
Michael Guillory, Channel Sales/Marketing Manager

Focus on beginning blends sounds and concepts with three high-spirited games that invite students to use two letter consonant blends as they build words.

1231 TARGET Technique for Aphasia Rehab
Abilitations Speech Bin
PO Box 922668
Norcross, GA 30010
770-449-5700
800-850-8602
FAX 770-510-7290
http://www.speechbin.com
e-mail: info@speechbin.com
Tobi Isaacs, Catalog Director

TARGET is the kind of resource aphasia clinicians beg for — a practical resource that answers not only the what and how questions of treatment but also the why. It describes dozens of treatment methods and gives you practical exercises and activities to implement each technique. Item number 1434. *$63.99*

1232 TOLD-P3: Test of Language Development Primary
Abilitations Speech Bin
PO Box 922668
Norcross, GA 30010
770-449-5700
800-850-8602
FAX 770-510-7290
http://www.speechbin.com
e-mail: info@speechbin.com
Tobi Isaacs, Catalog Director

This revised test of 4-8 year olds' language gives unbiased test items that reflect the most modern language theories, Two new subtests — Phonemic Analysis and Relational Vocabulary, full-color contemporary photos young children like and norms include minority and disability groups. Item number P501. *$255.99*

1233 TOPS Kit-Adolescent: Tasks of Problem Solving
LinguiSystems
3100 4th Avenue
East Moline, IL 61244
309-755-2300
800-776-4332
FAX 309-755-2377
TDY:800-933-8331
http://www.linguisystems.com
e-mail: service@linguisystems.com
Linda Bowers, Rosemary Huisingh, Mark Barrett, Author
Linda Bowers, Co-Owner/Co-Founder
Rosemary Huisingh, Co-Owner/Co-Founder

Teach your teens how to use their language skills to think, think, think. We combine literacy, thinking, writing, humor, and language arts practice to cover these thinking skills: using content to make references; analyzing information; taking another's point of view; and more. It's a literacy- based approach that gets dramatic results! *$59.95*
192 pages Ages 12-18

1234 TOPS Kit-Elementary: Tasks of Problem Solving
LinguiSystems
3100 4th Avenue
East Moline, IL 61244
309-755-2300
800-776-4332
FAX 309-755-2377
TDY:800-933-8331
http://www.linguisystems.com
e-mail: service@linguisystems.com
Linda Bowers, Rosemary Huisingh, Mark Barrett, Author
Linda Bowers, Co-Owner/Co-Founder
Rosemary Huisingh, Co-Owner/Co-Founder

Reveal thinking and language skills your students didn't know they had with this remarkable kit. TOPS Kit-Elementary combines thinking and expressive language skills to develop better communications. *$119.95*
209 pages Ages 6-12

1235 Take Home: Oral-Motor Exercises
LinguiSystems
3100 4th Avenue
East Moline, IL 61244
309-755-2300
800-776-4332
FAX 309-755-2377
TDY:800-933-8331
http://www.linguisystems.com
e-mail: service@linguisystems.com
Lisa Loncar-Belding, Author
Linda Bowers, Co-Owner/Co-Founder
Rosemary Huisingh, Co-Owner/Co-Founder

Stop writing your own take-home letters and exercises for carry-over! These homework pages work on the earliest developing vowel and consonant sounds. Created for use with deaf and hearing-impaired students, this resource is great for all of your oral-motor and articulation cases. *$31.95*
129 pages Ages 2-6

1236 Take Home: Phonological Awareness
LinguiSystems
3100 4th Avenue
East Moline, IL 61244
309-755-2300
800-776-4332
FAX 309-755-2377
TDY:800-933-8331
http://www.linguisystems.com
e-mail: service@linguisystems.com
Carolyn Robertson, Wanda Salter, Author
Linda Bowers, Co-Owner/Co-Founder
Rosemary Huisingh, Co-Owner/Co-Founder

These activities are easy for parents and caregivers to follow. Activities are organized at the word, syllable, phoneme, and grapheme level. You'll target these skills: rhyming; blending; isolation; segmentation; deletion; substitution; and phoneme-grapheme correspondence. *$31.95*
144 pages Ages 5-8

1237 Take Home: Preschool Language Development
LinguiSystems
3100 4th Avenue
East Moline, IL 61244
309-755-2300
800-776-4332
FAX 309-755-2377
TDY:800-933-8331
http://www.linguisystems.com
e-mail: service@linguisystems.com
Martha Drake, Author
Linda Bowers, Co-Owner/Co-Founder
Rosemary Huisingh, Co-Owner/Co-Founder

Home follow-up is essential for your little ones with speech and language delays. Get everything you need for a comprehensive take-home program with this time saver! Each take-home lesson is easy to follow. *$31.95*
191 pages Ages 1-5

1238 Talk About Fun
Abilitations Speech Bin
PO Box 922668
Norcross, GA 30010
770-449-5700
800-850-8602
FAX 770-510-7290
http://www.speechbin.com
e-mail: info@speechbin.com
Tobi Isaacs, Catalog Director

Talk About Fun takes advantage of children's natural love of play and making things to achieve your speech-language goals. Target phonemes featured include p-b-m, t-d-n, f, k-g, s, sh-ch-j, i, and consonant blends. Carryover projects, sequence stories, and letters to parents are an added bonus. Item number 190801116. *$29.99*

1239 Talkable Tales
Abilitations Speech Bin
PO Box 922668
Norcross, GA 30010
770-449-5700
800-850-8602
FAX 770-510-7290
http://www.speechbin.com
e-mail: info@speechbin.com
Tobi Isaacs, Catalog Director

Talkable Tales gives you a wealth of stories to build speech and language skills. Comprehension and challenge questions accompany each story. Stories are a uniform length so you may use them with groups working on multiple sounds. Each has ten key words containing the target sound. Item number 1540. *$25.95*

1240 Talking Time
Abilitations Speech Bin
PO Box 922668
Norcross, GA 30010
770-449-5700
800-850-8602
FAX 770-510-7290
http://www.speechbin.com
e-mail: info@speechbin.com
Jeanette Stickel, Author
Tobi Isaacs, Catalog Director

Talking times gives you sequenced activities to foster language and cognitive programs by parents, family members, and caregivers. Talking Time also includes guidelines for language development and directions and rationale for use. Item number 190837116. *$17.99*
64 pages

1241 Teaching Phonics: Staff Development Book
Harcourt Achieve
Customer Service, 5th Floor
Orlando, FL 32887
800-284-7019
FAX 800-699-9459
http://www.harcourtachieve.com
e-mail: webmaster@harcourt.com
Steven Korten, CEO
Randy Pennington, SVP National Sales

Fine-tune your instructional approach with fresh insights from phonics experts. This resource offers informative articles and timely tips for teaching phonics in the integrated language arts classroom.

1242 Test for Auditory Comprehension of Language: TACL-3
Abilitations Speech Bin
PO Box 922668
Norcross, GA 30010
770-449-5700
800-850-8602
FAX 770-510-7290
http://www.speechbin.com
e-mail: info@speechbin.com
Elizabeth Carrow-Woolfolk, Author
Tobi Isaacs, Catalog Director

The newly revised TACL-3 evaluates the 0-3 to 9-11 year-old's understanding of spoken language in three subtests: Vocabulary, Grammatical Morphemes and Elaborated Phrases and Sentences. Each test item is a word or sentence read aloud by the examiner; the child responds by pointing to one of three pictures. Item number 190237116. *$274.99*

1243 Test of Early Language Development 3rd Edition: TELD-3
Abilitations Speech Bin
PO Box 922668
Norcross, GA 30010
770-449-5700
800-850-8602
FAX 770-510-7290
http://www.speechbin.com
e-mail: info@speechbin.com
Wayne P Hresko, D Kim Reid, Donald D Hammill, Author
Tobi Isaacs, Catalog Director

Is a normed test appropriate for children 2-0 through 7-11. It quickly and easily measures Receptive and Expressive language and yields an overall Spoken Language Score. Item number 190129116. *$284.99*

1244 Test of Language Development: Intermediate (TOLD-I:3)
Abilitations Speech Bin
PO Box 922668
Norcross, GA 30010
770-449-5700
800-850-8602
FAX 770-510-7290
http://www.speechbin.com
e-mail: info@speechbin.com
Tobi Isaacs, Catalog Director

This well-normed test is one popular measure of language development; it's an ideal choice for speech-language pathologists' use in schools. The complete kit includes an examiner's manual, picture stimulus book, and 25 test forms. Item number 190178116. *$184.99*

1245 That's LIFE! Life Skills
LinguiSystems
3100 4th Avenue
East Moline, IL 61244
309-755-2300
800-776-4332
FAX 309-755-2377
TDY:800-933-8331
http://www.linguisystems.com
e-mail: service@linguisystems.com
Patricia Smith, Author
Linda Bowers, Co-Owner/Co-Founder
Rosemary Huisingh, Co-Owner/Co-Founder

Students get hands-on language experience in everyday events. Units are organized by consumer affairs, government, health concerns, money matters, going places, and homemaking. Tasks include identifying vocabulary, making inferences, predicting, and more. *$37.95*
192 pages Ages 12-18

1246 Therapy Guide for Language & Speech Disorders: Volume 1
Abilitations Speech Bin
PO Box 922668
Norcross, GA 30010
770-449-5700
800-850-8602
FAX 770-510-7290
http://www.speechbin.com
e-mail: info@speechbin.com
Kathryn M Kilpatrick, Author
Tobi Isaacs, Catalog Director

This structured language rehabilitation program contains 429 color-coded pages containing exercises for listening, reading comprehension, speech and language, gestures, writing, and number skills. A word communication notebook and worksheets suitable for carryover are included. Item number V368. *$49.95*

1247 Therapy Guide for Language and Speech Disorders: Volume 2
Abilitations Speech Bin
PO Box 922668
Norcross, GA 30010
770-449-5700
800-850-8602
FAX 770-510-7290
http://www.speechbin.com
e-mail: info@speechbin.com
Kathryn M Kilpatrick, Author
Tobi Isaacs, Catalog Director

Volume 2 answers your need for materials at a higher level. This large print workbook covers oral language comprehension, word retrieval, sentence formulation, general knowledge, thought organization, definitions, number skills, and daily needs. Item number 192220116. *$39.99*

1248 Thought Organization Workbook
Therapro
225 Arlington Street
Framingham, MA 01702
508-872-9494
800-257-5376
FAX 508-875-2062
http://www.theraproducts.com
e-mail: info@theraproducts.com
Therapro Staff, Author
Karen Conrad, Owner

Completing letter and word puzzles, composing sentences and organizing shapes, numbers, events and language. *$10.50*

1249 Tic-Tac-Artic and Match
LinguiSystems
3100 4th Avenue
East Moline, IL 61244
309-755-2300
800-776-4332
FAX 309-755-2377
TDY:800-933-8331
http://www.linguisystems.com
e-mail: service@linguisystems.com

Carol A Vaccariello, Author
Linda Bowers, Co-Owner/Co-Founder
Rosemary Huisingh, Co-Owner/Co-Founder

Tic-Tac-Artic and Match gives you five games on every page and tons of practice per session. Each page has 16 pictures for one target phoneme. To play Tic-Tac-Artic, use the special game template to create four different tic-tac-toe style games. *$34.95*
157 pages Ages 4-12

1250 **Visual Voice Tools**
Speech Bin
PO Box 922668
Norcross, GA 30010
770-449-5770
800-850-8602
FAX 770-510-7290
http://www.speechbin.com
e-mail: info@speechbin.com
Shane Peters, Product Coordinator
Jen Binney, Owner

Seven visual voice tools help your clients develop vocal control through engaging visual and auditory feedback. The tools include: Sound Presence; Loudness Range; Voice Presence; Voice Timing; Voice Onset; Pitch Range and Pitch Control. Item number E278. *$199.95*

1251 **Vocabulary Connections**
Harcourt Achieve
Customer Service, 5th Floor
Orlando, FL 32887
800-284-7019
FAX 800-699-9459
http://www.harcourtachieve.com
e-mail: webmaster@harcourt.com
Steven Korten, CEO
Randy Pennington, SVP National Sales

Keep students engaged in building vocabulary through crossword puzzles and cloze passages, and by using words in context and making analogies. Lessons build around thematically organized literature and nonfiction selections provide meaningful context for essential vocabulary words.

1252 **Vocabulary Play by Play**
LinguiSystems
3100 4th Avenue
East Moline, IL 61244
309-755-2300
800-776-4332
FAX 309-755-2377
TDY:800-933-8331
http://www.linguisystems.com
e-mail: service@linguisystems.com
Caolyn LoGiudice, Mike LoGiudice, Author
Linda Bowers, Co-Owner/Co-Founder
Rosemary Huisingh, Co-Owner/Co-Founder

Students with language-learning disabilities need ten times more encounters with new vocabulary words than their nondisabled peers. Vocabulary Play by Play gives students the built-in encounters with vocabulary they need for school success. *$44.95*
Ages 9-15

1253 **Vowel Patterns**
Sunburst Technology
1550 Executive Drive
Elgin, IL 60123
800-321-7511
FAX 888-800-3028
http://http://store.sunburst.com/Home.aspx
e-mail: service@sunburst.com
Michael Guillory, Channel Sales/Marketing Manager

Some vowels are neither long nor short. In this investigation, students explore and learn to use abstract vowels.

1254 **Vowel Scramble**
LinguiSystems
3100 4th Avenue
East Moline, IL 61244
309-755-2300
800-776-4332
FAX 309-755-2377
TDY:800-933-8331
http://www.linguisystems.com
e-mail: service@linguisystems.com
Carolyn LoGiudice, Author
Linda Bowers, Co-Owner/Co-Founder
Rosemary Huisingh, Co-Owner/Co-Founder

Your student will love this fun new way to practice spelling and phonological awareness skills. Players earn points by using letter tiles to complete words on the game board. *$44.95*
Ages 7-12

1255 **Warmups and Workouts**
Abilitations Speech Bin
PO Box 922668
Norcross, GA 30010
770-449-5700
800-850-8602
FAX 770-510-7290
http://www.speechbin.com
e-mail: info@speechbin.com
Jane Folk, Author
Tobi Isaacs, Catalog Director

Easy-to-follow step-by-step instructions demonstrate how to help children achieve reliable production of r sounds, practice them in words of increasing complexity, and improve their phonic skills simultaneously. Item number 190734116. *$26.99*

1256 **Weekly Language Practice**
Customer Service, 5th Floor
Orlando, FL 32887
800-281-7019
FAX 800-699-9459
http://www.harcourtachieve.com
e-mail: webmaster@harcourt.com
Steven Korten, CEO
Randy Pennington, SVP National Sales

Each activity page features five activity strips, one for each day of the week, and is backed up by a convenient answer key for the teacher that includes explanations and extensions.

1257 **Winning in Speech**
Abilitations Speech Bin
PO Box 922668
Norcross, GA 30010
770-449-5700
800-850-8602
FAX 770-510-7290
http://www.speechbin.com
e-mail: info@speechbin.com
Michelle Waugh, Author
Tobi Isaacs, Catalog Director

This delighful workbook gives your 7-14 year olds a wealth of information about stuttering and how to handle it. Winning in Speech shows them how they can modify their stuttering behaviors through everyday experiences. Item number 1594. *$22.99*
40 pages

1258 **Wizard of R'S**
Abilitations Speech Bin
PO Box 922668
Norcross, GA 30010
770-449-5700
800-850-8602
FAX 770-510-7290
http://www.speechbin.com
e-mail: info@speechbin.com
Tobi Isaacs, Catalog Director

This wizard makes those troublesome r problems diappear like magic! It gives you a practical approach with a wide range of scripted activities and helpful criterion-referenced testing, oral-motor exercises, remedial techniques and review of musculature. Item number 190377116. *$24.99*

1259 **Workbook for Aphasia**
Abilitations Speech Bin
PO Box 922668
Norcross, GA 30010
770-449-5700
800-850-8602
FAX 770-510-7290
http://www.speechbin.com
e-mail: info@speechbin.com
Susan Howell Brubaker, Author
Tobi Isaacs, Catalog Director

This book gives you materials for adults who have recovered a significant degree of speaking, reading, writing, and comprehension skills. It includes 106 excercises divided into eight target areas. Item number W331. *$69.99*

1260 **Workbook for Language Skills**
Abilitations Speech Bin
PO Box 922668
Norcross, GA 30010
770-449-5700
800-850-8602
FAX 770-510-7290
http://www.speechbin.com
e-mail: info@speechbin.com
Susan Howell Brubaker, Author
Tobi Isaacs, Catalog Director

This workbook features 68 real-world exercises designed for use with mildly to severely cognitive and language-impaired individuals. The workbook is divided in seven target areas: Sentence Completion; General Knowledge; Word Recall; Figurative Language; Sentence Comprehension; Sentence Construction and Spelling. Item number W333. *$53.99*

1261 **Workbook for Verbal Expression**
Abilitations Speech Bin
PO Box 922668
Norcross, GA 30010
770-449-5700
800-850-8602
FAX 770-510-7290
http://www.speechbin.com
e-mail: info@speechbin.com
Beth M Kennedy, Author
Tobi Isaacs, Catalog Director

Is a book of 100s of excerises from simple naming, automatic speech sequences, and repetition exercises to complex tasks in sentence formulation and abstract verbal reasoning. Item number 1435. *$49.99*

1262 **Writing Trek Grades 4-6**
Sunburst Technology
1550 Executive Drive
Elgin, IL 60123
800-321-7511
FAX 888-800-3028
http://http://store.sunburst.com/Home.aspx
e-mail: service@sunburst.com
Michael Guillory, Channel Sales/Marketing Manager

Enhance your students' experience in your English language arts classroom with twelve authentic writing projects that build students' competence while encouraging creativity.

1263 **Writing Trek Grades 6-8**
Sunburst Technology
1550 Executive Drive
Elgin, IL 60123
800-321-7511
FAX 888-800-3028
http://http://store.sunburst.com/Home.aspx
e-mail: service@sunburst.com
Michael Guillory, Channel Sales/Marketing Manager

Twelve authentic language arts projects, activities, and assignments develop your students' writing confidence and ability.

1264 **Writing Trek Grades 8-10**
Sunburst Technology
1550 Executive Drive
Elgin, IL 60123
800-321-7511
FAX 888-800-3028
http://http://store.sunburst.com/Home.aspx
e-mail: service@sunburst.com
Michael Guillory, Channel Sales/Marketing Manager

Help your students develop a concept of genre as they become familiar with the writing elements and characteristics of a variety of writing forms.

1265 **Your Child's Speech and Language**
Abilitations Speech Bin
PO Box 922668
Norcross, GA 30010
770-449-5700
800-850-8602
FAX 770-510-7290
http://www.speechbin.com
e-mail: info@speechbin.com
Tobi Isaacs, Catalog Director

This delightfully illustrated 52- page book provides helpful information about speech and language development from infancy through five years. It shows how to determine if speech is developing normally and ways to stimulate its growth. It's ideal for parent training and baby showers too! Item number P652. *$17.00*

Life Skills

1266 **Activities for the Elementary Classroom**
Curriculum Associates
PO Box 2001
North Billerica, MA 01862
800-225-0248
FAX 800-366-1158
http://www.curriculumassociates.com
e-mail: cainfo@curriculumassociates.com
Frank Ferguson, President

Challenge your students to make a hole in a 3" x 5" index card large enough to poke their heads through. Or offer to pour them a glass of air. You'll have their attenion — the first step toward learning — when you use the high-interest, hands-on activities in these exciting teacher resource books.

1267 **Activities of Daily Living: A Manual of Group Activities and Written Exercises**
Therapro
225 Arlington Street
Framingham, MA 01702
508-872-9494
800-257-5376
FAX 508-875-2062
http://www.theraproducts.com
e-mail: info@theraproducts.com
Karen McCarthy COTA/L, Author
Karen Conrad, Owner

Designed to provide group leaders easy access to structured plans for Activities of Daily Living (ADL) Groups. Organized into five modules: Personal Hygiene; Laundry Skills; Money Management; Leisure Skills and Nutrition. Each includes introduction, assessment guidelines, worksheets to copy, suggested board work, and wrap-up discussions. Appropriate for adult or adolescent programs, school systems and programs for the learning disabled. *$25.00*
136 pages

1268 **Aids and Appliances for Indepentent Living**
Maxi-Aids, Inc
42 Executive Boulevard
Farmingdale, NY 11735
631-752-0521
FAX 631-752-0689
http://www.maxiaids.com
Elliot Zaretsky, President
Barbara Collins, Contact

Thousands of products to make life easier. Eating, dressing, communications, bed, bath, kitchen, writing aids and more.

1269 Artic-Action
Abilitations Speech Bin
PO Box 922668
Norcross, GA 30010
770-449-5700
800-850-8602
FAX 770-510-7290
http://www.speechbin.com
e-mail: info@speechbin.com

Denise Grigas, Author
Tobi Isaacs, Catalog Director

Take the doldrums out of speech drills with this terrific collection of ideas! Clever tasks facilitate learning through hands-on experiences and provide a rich language learning environment for K-5 children. Activities encourage cooperative learning, turn taking, conversational discourse and social interaction. Item number 1524. *$18.99*
144 pages

1270 Barnaby's Burrow: An Auditory Processing Game
LinguiSystems
3100 4th Avenue
East Moline, IL 61244
309-755-2300
800-776-4332
FAX 309-755-2375
TDY:800-933-8331
http://www.linguisystems.com
e-mail: service@linguisystems.com

Barb Truman, Author
Linda Bowers, Co-Owner/Co-Founder
Rosemary Huisingh, Co-Owner/Co-Founder

Your students will practice good auditory processing skills as they help Barnaby the rabbit get to his burrow. This delightful game gives you tons of auditory processing tasks at increasing levels of difficulty. 300 game cards provide you stimulus items for phonological awareness, following directions, absurdities, and identifying main ideas and details. *$44.95*
Ages 4-9

1271 Boredom Rx
Abilitations Speech Bin
PO Box 922668
Norcross, GA 30010
770-449-5700
800-850-8602
FAX 770-510-7290
http://www.speechbin.com
e-mail: info@speechbin.com

Kristel Aderholdt, Author
Tobi Isaacs, Catalog Director

Fun-filled tasks help school-age kids improve their practical skills in listening, pragmatics, remembering, and following directions. Item number 1583. *$29.99*

1272 Brainopoly: A Thinking Game
LinguiSystems
3100 4th Avenue
East Moline, IL 61244
309-755-2300
800-776-4332
FAX 309-755-2377
TDY:800-933-8331
http://www.linguisystems.com
e-mail: service@linguisystems.com

LinguiSystems Staff, Author
Linda Bowers, Co-Owner/Co-Founder
Rosemary Huisingh, Co-Owner/Co-Founder

Target all the critical thinking, problem-solving, and decision-making skills your older students need to meet the demands of the classroom curriculum. Each game section has 50 questions divided into two levels of difficulty. That's 450 total questions! Students will practice using predicting, inferring, deduction skills, and more! *$44.95*
Ages 10-15

1273 Categorically Speaking
Abilitations Speech Bin
PO Box 922668
Norcross, GA 30010
770-449-5700
800-850-8602
FAX 770-510-7290
http://www.speechbin.com
e-mail: info@speechbin.com

Tobi Isaacs, Catalog Director

This game for two to four players or two teams gives 6-10 year-olds experience in asking questions, evaluating information they receive, and using it to solve problems. To play, they must use specified question formats to get clues about pictures, recognize similarities and differences, identify salient features of objects, and encode and decode messages. Item number Q849. *$56.99*

1274 Changes Around Us CD-ROM
Harcourt Achieve
Customer Service, 5th Floor
Orlando, FL 32887
800-284-7019
FAX 800-699-9459
http://www.harcourtachieve.com
e-mail: webmaster@harcourt.com

Steven Korten, CEO
Randy Pennington, SVP National Sales

Nature is the natural choice for observing change. By observing and researching dramatic visual sequences such as the stages of development of a butterfly, children develop a broad understanding of the concept of change. As they search this multimedia database for images and information about plant and animal life cycles and seasonal change, students strengthen their abilities in research, analysis, problem-solving, critical thinking and communication.

1275 Classroom Visual Activities
Therapro
225 Arlington Street
Framingham, MA 01702
508-872-9494
800-257-5376
FAX 508-875-2062
http://www.theraproducts.com
e-mail: info@theraproducts.com

Regina G Richards MA, Author
Karen Conrad, Owner

This work presents a wealth of activities for the development of visual skills in the areas of pursuit, scanning, aligning, and locating movements; eye hand coordination, and fixation activity. Each activity lists objectives and criteria for success and gives detailed instuctions. *$15.00*
80 pages

1276 Cognitive Strategy Instruction for Middle & High Schools
Brookline Books
PO Box 1209
Brookline, MA 02445
800-666-BOOK
http://www.brooklinebooks.com
e-mail: info@brooklinebooks.com

Eileen Wood, Vera Woloshyn, Teena Willoughby, Author
Milt Budoff, Founder/President

Presents cognitive strategies empirically validated for middle and high school students, with an emphasis for teachers on how to teach and support the strategies. *$26.95*
286 pages
ISBN 1-571290-07-9

1277 Complete Guide to Running, Walking and Fitness for Kids
Therapro
225 Arlington Street
Framingham, MA 01702
508-872-9494
800-257-5376
FAX 508-875-2062
http://www.theraproducts.com
e-mail: info@theraproducts.com

Tim Erson MS PT, Author
Karen Conrad, Owner

This should be every child's first book of fitness. Many tips on how to get started, such as stretching, dressing wisely, where to run, racing, aerobics and more. Includes a logbook and journal for 1 year, with weekly goals, encouraging messages, training notes, and so on. *$18.95*

263 pages

1278 Coping for Kids Who Stutter
Abilitations Speech Bin
PO Box 922668
Norcross, GA 30010
770-449-5700
800-850-8602
FAX 770-410-7290
http://www.speechbin.com
e-mail: info@speechbin.com
Tobi Isaacs, Catalog Director

Coping for Kids Who Stutter educates people of all ages about the confusing and frustrating communication disorder of stuttering. This matter-of-fact book presents a muiltitude of facts about stuttering and gives lots of good advice about what to do about it in a nonthreatening, convincing manner. Item number 1543. *$18.95*

1279 Definition Play by Play
LinguiSystems
3100 4th Avenue
East Moline, IL 61244
309-755-2300
800-776-4332
FAX 309-755-2377
TDY:800-933-8331
http://www.linguisystems.com
e-mail: service@linguisystems.com
Sharon Spencer, Author
Linda Bowers, Co-Owner/Co-Founder
Rosemary Huisingh, Co-Owner/Co-Founder

Teach your students to give accurate, cohesive definitions by identifying and organizing critical attributes of words. As players move along the board, they describe an object card by these attributes: function; what goes with it; size/shape; color; parts; what it's made of; and location. *$44.95*
Ages 8-14

1280 Effective Listening
Abilitations Speech Bin
PO Box 922668
Norcross, GA 30010
770-449-5700
800-850-8602
FAX 770-510-7290
http://www.speechbin.com
e-mail: info@speechbin.com
Tobi Isaacs, Catalog Director

Effective Listening gives you creative lessons in a stimulating format that takes the drudgery out of listening drills. Its LISTEN techniques provide structured strategies to improve auditory processing skills. Item number 1355. *$25.99*

1281 Fine Motor Activities Guide and Easel Activities Guide
Therapro
225 Arlington Street
Framingham, MA 01702
508-872-9494
800-257-5376
FAX 508-875-2062
http://www.theraproducts.com
e-mail: info@theraproducts.com
Jane Berry OTR/L, Author
Karen Conrad, Owner

These guides have always been included in the above kits and can now be purchased separately. Useful for activity plans or teacher-educator-parent consultations. Perfect hand-outs as part of your inservice packet (no need to write out ideas, photocopy materials, etc). Package of 10 booklets.

1282 Fine Motor Fun
Therapro
225 Arlington Street
Framingham, MA 01702
508-872-9494
800-257-5376
FAX 508-875-2062
http://www.theraproducts.com
e-mail: info@theraproducts.com
Maryanne Bruni BS OT, Author
Karen Conrad, Owner

Fine motor skills are the hand skills that allow us to do things like hold a pencil, cut with scissors, eat with a fork, and use a computer. This practical guide shows parents and professionals how to help children with Down Syndrome from infancy to 12 years improve fine motor functioning. *$16.95*
191 pages Ages Birth-12

1283 Finger Frolics: Fingerplays
Therapro
225 Arlington Street
Framingham, MA 01702
508-872-9494
800-257-5376
FAX 508-875-2062
http://www.theraproducts.com
e-mail: info@theraproducts.com
Liz Cromwell, Dixie Hibner, Author
Karen Conrad, Owner

Invaluable for occupational therapists, speech/language pathologists and teachers. Over 350 light and humorous fingerplays help children with rhyming and performing actions which develop fine motor and language skills. *$10.95*

1284 Follow Me!
LinguiSystems
3100 4th Avenue
East Moline, IL 61244
309-755-2300
800-776-4332
FAX 309-755-2377
TDY:800-933-8331
http://www.linguisystems.com
e-mail: service@linguisystems.com
Grace W Frank, Author
Linda Bowers, Co-Owner/Co-Founder
Rosemary Huisingh, Co-Owner/Co-Founder

Lessons are organized by grade level so you can control the lesson complexity as your students listen and follow oral directions. Get 91 listen-and-do lessons, each with a reproducible student worksheet to teach concepts such as location, association, exclusion, sequencing, and more. *$34.95*
187 pages Ages 5-9

1285 Follow Me! 2
LinguiSystems
3100 4th Avenue
East Moline, IL 61244
309-755-2300
800-776-4332
FAX 309-755-2377
TDY:800-933-8331
http://www.linguisystems.com
e-mail: service@linguisystems.com
Grace Frank, Author
Linda Bowers, Co-Owner/Co-Founder
Rosemary Huisingh, Co-Owner/Co-Founder

These activities are relevant to classroom listening demands. The directions relate specifically on an accompanying worksheet. It's a pick-up-and-use-now resource to teach the vocabulary of language arts, math, social studies and more. *$34.95*

201 pages Ages 7-11

1286 HELP Elementary
LinguiSystems
3100 4th Avenue
East Moline, IL 61244
309-755-2300
800-776-4332
FAX 309-755-2377
TDY:800-933-8331
http://www.linguisystems.com
e-mail: service@linguisystems.com
Andrea Lazzari, Patricia Peters, Author
Linda Bowers, Co-Owner/Co-Founder
Rosemary Huisingh, Co-Owner/Co-Founder

The look and content of these activities appeal specifically to your elementary-aged students. The no-frills, ready-to-use approach fits your precious time. These worksheets are perfect for oral or written practice. Help students improve question comprehension, association, specific word-finding, grammar, and more. *$39.95*

207 pages Ages 6-12

1287 HELP for Memory
LinguiSystems
3100 4th Avenue
East Moline, IL 61244
309-755-2300
800-776-4332
FAX 309-755-2377
TDY:800-933-8331
http://www.linguisystems.com
e-mail: service@linguisystems.com
Andrea Lazzari, Author
Linda Bowers, Co-Owner/Co-Founder
Rosemary Huisingh, Co-Owner/Co-Founder

Help clients and students acquire memory strategies they'll use in daily life. These exercises incorporate attention, discrimination, categorization, and association to cover the broad range of memory skills. These functional memory tasks are arranged in a hierarchy to build skill upon skill. Help clients organize and retrieve information through exercises for coding and grouping items for recall, applying memory techniques to daily life skills, and more. *$39.95*
178 pages Ages 8-Adult

1288 HELP for Middle School
LinguiSystems
3100 4th Avenue
East Moline, IL 61244
309-755-2300
800-776-4332
FAX 309-755-2377
TDY:800-933-8331
http://www.linguisystems.com
e-mail: service@linguisystems.com
Andrea Lazzari, Author
Linda Bowers, Co-Owner/Co-Founder
Rosemary Huisingh, Co-Owner/Co-Founder

Get ready-to-use activities relevant to middle school students. Your students will tune in and make progress! Middle school clinicians are singing the praises of this great resource. You'll get IEP goals and great language activities for vocabulary, grammer, question comprehension, following directions, test taking, and expression. *$39.95*
183 pages Ages 10-15

1289 Hands-On Activities for Exceptional Students
Peytral Publications
PO Box 1162
Minnetonka, MN 55345
952-949-8707
877-739-8725
FAX 952-906-9777
http://www.peytral.com
e-mail: help@peytral.com
Beverly Thorne, Author
Peggy Hammeken, President

This execptional new release is developed for educators of students who have cognitive delays who will eventually work in a sheltered employment environment. If you need new ideas at your fingertips, this practical book is for you. *$19.95*
112 pages Special Ed
ISBN 1-890455-31-8

1290 Health
Harcourt Achieve
Customer Service, 5th Floor
Orlando, FL 32887
800-284-7019
FAX 800-699-9459
http://www.harcourtachieve.com
e-mail: webmaster@harcourt.com
Steven Korten, CEO
Randy Pennington, SVP National Sales

Lessons and projects focus on nutrition, outdoor safety, smart choices, and exercise. Designed to make children more health conscious. Activity formats include fill in the blank, word puzzles, multiple choice, crosswords, and more.

1291 Hidden Senses: Your Balance Sense & Your Muscle Sense
Therapro
225 Arlington Street
Framingham, MA 01702
508-872-9494
800-257-5376
FAX 508-875-2062
http://www.theraproducts.com
e-mail: info@theraproducts.com
Jane Koomar PhD, Barbara Friedman MA, Author
Karen Conrad, Owner

These movement books are back in print! Help children discover the crucial, yet seldom mentioned body awareness senses that help them in movement, coordination, strength and perception. The authors, both practicing OTs, explain simply and clearly how the body senses work. Colorful and vibrant images bring the explanations to life.

1292 It's All in Your Head: A Guide to Understanding Your Brain and Boosting Your Brain Power
Therapro
225 Arlington Street
Framingham, MA 01702
508-872-9494
800-257-5376
FAX 508-875-2062
http://www.theraproducts.com
e-mail: info@theraproducts.com
Susan L Barrett, Author
Karen Conrad, Owner

By popular demand from therapists, we are carrying this popular book for children. An owners manual on the brain, written especially for kids, this upbeat, engaging book is great for ages 9-14. *$9.95*
151 pages

1293 Just for Me! Concepts
LinguiSystems
3100 4th Avenue
East Moline, IL 61244
309-755-2300
800-776-4332
FAX 309-755-2377
TDY:800-933-8331
http://www.linguisystems.com
e-mail: service@linguisystems.com
Margaret Warner, Author
Linda Bowers, Co-Owner/Co-Founder
Rosemary Huisingh, Co-Owner/Co-Founder

These fun color, cut, fold and play pages will keep youngsters busy learning basic concepts. Teach basic concepts in four areas: spatial, attributes, quantity, and temporal. *$24.95*
150 pages Ages 3-6

1294 Key Concepts in Personal Development
Marsh Media
8082 Ward Parkway Plaza
Kansas City, MO 64114
816-523-1059
800-821-3303
FAX 866-333-7421
http://www.marshmedia.com
e-mail: info@marshmedia.com
Joan Marsh, Owner
Liz Sweeney, Editorial Assistant

Puberty Education for Students with Special Needs. Comprehensive, gender-specific kits and supplemental paretn packets address human sexuality education for children with mild to moderate developmental disabilities.

1295 LD Teacher's IEP Companion Software
LinguiSystems
3100 4th Avenue
East Moline, IL 61244
309-755-2300
800-776-4332
FAX 309-755-2377
TDY:800-933-8331
http://www.linguisystems.com
e-mail: service@linguisystems.com

Molly Lyle, Author
Linda Bowers, Co-Owner/Co-Founder
Rosemary Huisingh, Co-Owner/Co-Founder

Create customized, professional reports with these terrific academic goals and objectives. You'll have individual objectives from nine skill areas at the click of your mouse! Save time with the software version of the best-selling book! For both PC and Macintosh. *$69.95*
Ages 5-18

1296 Life Management Skills I
Therapro
225 Arlington Street
Framingham, MA 01702
508-872-9494
800-257-5376
FAX 508-875-2062
http://www.theraproducts.com
e-mail: info@theraproducts.com
Therapro Staff, Author
Karen Conrad, Owner

Topics include: assertion; discharge planning; emotion identification; exercise; goal setting; leisure; motivation; nutrition; problem solving; risk taking; self awareness; self esteem; sleep; stress management; support systems; time management; and values clarification. *$39.95*

1297 Life Management Skills II
Therapro
225 Arlington Street
Framingham, MA 01702
508-872-9494
800-257-5376
FAX 508-875-2062
http://www.theraproducts.com
e-mail: info@theraproducts.com
Therapro Staff, Author
Karen Conrad, Owner

Topics include: activities of daily living; anger management; assertion; verbal and nonverbal communication; coping skills; grief/loss; humor; life balance; money management; parenting; reminiscence; safety issues; self esteem; image; steps to recovery; stress management; support systems and time management. *$41.95*

1298 Life Management Skills III
Therapro
225 Arlington Street
Framingham, MA 01702
508-872-9494
800-257-5376
FAX 508-875-2062
http://www.theraproducts.com
e-mail: info@theraproducts.com
Therapro Staff, Author
Karen Conrad, Owner

Using the same format as books I and II, this new book has 50 handouts including 5 forms on both men's and women's issues. Includes 9 pages of generic forms that everyone can use. Topics include: aging; body image; communication; conflict resolution; coping skills; creative expression; healthy living; job readiness; nurturance; relapse prevention; relationships and many more. *$41.95*

1299 Life Management Skills IV
Therapro
225 Arlington Street
Framingham, MA 01702
508-872-9494
800-257-5376
FAX 508-875-2062
http://www.theraproducts.com
e-mail: info@theraproducts.com
Therapro Staff, Author
Karen Conrad, Owner

Topics include: activities of daily living; combating stigma; communication; coping with serious mental illness; home management; humor; job readiness; journalizing; leisure; parenting; relationships; responsibility; self esteem; sexual health; social skills; stress mangagement; suicide isues and values. *$41.95*

1300 Life-Centered Career Education: Daily Living Skills
Council for Exceptional Children
1110 N Glebe Road
Arlington, VA 22201
703-245-0600
888-232-7733
FAX 703-264-9494
TDY:866-915-5000
http://www.cec.sped.org
e-mail: service@cec.sped.org
Donn Brolin, Author
Drew Albritten MD, Executive Director
Bruce Ramirez, Manager
Betty Bryant, LCCE Program Manager
LCCE teaches you to prepare students to function independently and productively as family members, citizens, and workers, and to enjoy fulfilling personal lives. LCCE is a motivating and effectiev classroom, home, and community-based curriculum.

1301 Listening for Basic Concepts All Year' Round
LinguiSystems
3100 4th Avenue
East Moline, IL 61244
309-755-2300
800-776-4332
FAX 309-755-2377
TDY:800-933-8331
http://www.linguisystems.com
e-mail: service@linguisystems.com
Brenda Brumbaugh, Nan Thompson-Trenta, Author
Linda Bowers, Co-Owner/Co-Founder
Rosemary Huisingh, Co-Owner/Co-Founder

Mastering concepts is guaranteed with this book because you teach them in fun, themed contexts. Teach 86 space, quanity, and attribute concepts. Concept tests give you built-in accountablility. *$39.95*
186 pages Ages 5-8

1302 Living Skills/Head Injured Child & Adolescents
Abilitations Speech Bin
PO Box 922668
Norcross, GA 30010
770-449-5700
800-850-8602
FAX 770-510-7290
http://www.speechbin.com
e-mail: info@speechbin.com
Tobi Isaacs, Catalog Director

Living Skills meets the challenges and special needs of children and adolescents with traumatic brain injury. A wealth of activities help restore cognitive, perceptual, and functional skills. Item number 1350. *$48.95*

1303 MORE: Integrating the Mouth with Sensory & Postural Functions
Therapro
225 Arlington Street
Framingham, MA 01702
508-872-9494
800-257-5376
FAX 508-875-2062
http://www.theraproducts.com
e-mail: info@theraproducts.com
Particia Oetter OTR/L, Eileen Richter OTR, Author
Karen Conrad, Owner

MORE is an acronym for Motor components, Oral organization, Respiratory demands and Eye contact and control; elements of toys and items that can be used to facilitate integration of the mouth with sensory and postural development, as well as self-regulation and attention. A theoretical framework for the treatment of both sensorimotor and speech/language problems is presented, methods for evaluating therapeutic potential of motor toys, and activities designed to improve functions. *$46.00*

1304 Memory Workbook
Therapro
225 Arlington Street
Framingham, MA 01702
508-872-9494
800-257-5376
FAX 508-875-2062
http://www.theraproducts.com
e-mail: info@theraproducts.com
Therapro Staff, Author
Karen Conrad, Owner

Recalling daily activities, seasons, months of the year, shapes, words and pictures. *$10.50*

1305 One-Handed in a Two-Handed World
Therapro
225 Arlington Street
Framingham, MA 01702
508-872-9494
800-257-5376
FAX 508-875-2062
http://www.theraproducts.com
e-mail: info@theraproducts.com
Tommye K Mayer, Author
Karen Conrad, Owner

A personal guide to managing single handed. Written by a woman who has lived one-handed for many years, this book shares a methodology and mindset necessary for managing. It details a wide array of topics including personal care, daily chores, office work, traveling, sports, relationships and many more. A must for patients and therapists. *$19.95*
250 pages

1306 Peabody Developmental Motor Scales-2
Speech Bin
PO Box 922668
Norcross, GA 30010
770-449-5700
800-850-8602
FAX 770-510-7290
http://www.speechbin.com
e-mail: info@speechbin.com
Rhonda Folio, Rebecca Fewell, Author
Shane Peters, Product Coordinator
Jen Binney, Owner

PDMS-2 gives you in-depth standardized assessment of motor skills in children birth to six years. Subtests include: fine motor object manipulation; grasping; gross motor; locomotion; reflexes; visual-motor integration and stationary. Item number P624. *$413.00*
Ages Birth-6

1307 People at Work
AGS Publishing
PO Box 99
Circle Pines, MN 55014
651-287-7220
800-328-2560
FAX 800-471-8457
http://www.agsnet.com
e-mail: agsmail@agsnet.com
Karen Dahlen, Associate Director
Matt Keller, Marketing Manager

With an interest level of High School through Adult, ABE and ESL and a reading level of Grades 3-4, this program is a simple, thorough teaching plan for every day of the school year. The program's 180 sessions are divided into eighteen study units that each survey an entire occupational cluster of eight jobs while focusing on one or two writing skills. *$26.95*

1308 Putting the Pieces Together: Volume 4
Abilitations Speech Bin
PO Box 922668
Norcross, GA 30010
770-449-5700
800-850-8602
FAX 770-510-7290
http://www.speechbin.com
e-mail: info@speechbin.com
Kathryn M Kilpatrick, Author
Tobi Isaacs, Catalog Director

This helpful volume gives you enjoyable materials and effective strategies for conceptualization, problem-solving, inductive and deductive reasoning, organization, judgement sequencing, attention/concentration, visual field neglect, and cognitve system reintegration. Item number V360. *$53.99*

1309 Reading and Writing Workbook
Therapro
225 Arlington Street
Framingham, MA 01702
508-872-9494
800-257-5376
FAX 508-875-2062
http://www.theraproducts.com
e-mail: info@theraproducts.com
Therapro Staff, Author
Karen Conrad, Owner

Writing checks and balancing a checkbook, copying words and sentences, and writing messages and notes. Helps with recognition and understanding of calendars, phone books and much more. *$10.50*

1310 Real World Situations
Harcourt Achieve
Customer Service, 5th Floor
Orlando, FL 32887
800-284-7019
FAX 800-69994597
http://www.harcourtachieve.com
e-mail: webmaster@harcourt.com
Steven Korten, CEO
Randy Pennington, SVP National Sales

Practice the practical problem-solving skills students need every day.

1311 Responding to Oral Directions
Abilitations Speech Bin
PO Box 922668
Norcross, GA 30010
770-449-5700
800-850-8602
FAX 770-510-7290
http://www.speechbin.com
e-mail: info@speechbin.com
Robert A Mancuso, Author
Tobi Isaacs, Catalog Director

Help children of all ages who function at first through sixth-grade levels learn to identify unclear directions and ask for clarification. Nine units teach them how to handle: recognizing directions, carryover and generalization; unreasonable, distorted, vague, unfamiliar, lenngthy, unknown, and mixed directions. Item number 190575116. *$56.99*

1312 SEALS II Self-Esteem and Life Skills II
Therapro
225 Arlington Street
Framingham, MA 01702
508-872-9494
800-257-5376
FAX 508-875-2062
http://www.theraproducts.com
e-mail: info@theraproducts.com
Therapro Staff, Author
Karen Conrad, Owner

Adapted from Life Management Skills III and IV, this book is for youth, ages 12-18 with age-appropriate language, graphics, and illustrations. Includes 80 activity-based handouts related to body image, communication, conflict resolution, coping skills, creative expression, humor, job readiness, leisure skills, nurturance and more. *$43.95*

1313 Scissors, Glue, and Concepts, Too!
LinguiSystems
3100 4th Avenue
East Moline, IL 61244
309-755-2300
800-776-4332
FAX 309-755-2377
TDY:800-933-8331
http://www.linguisystems.com
e-mail: service@linguisystems.com
Susan Boegler, Debbie Abruzzini, Author
Linda Bowers, Co-Owner/Co-Founder
Rosemary Huisingh, Co-Owner/Co-Founder

Your young students will learn to follow directions and understand basic concepts in context. Concepts for each activity are grouped as they naturally occur in our language. Teach over 50 concepts including right/left, above/below, empty/full, and more. *$39.95*

199 pages Ages 5-8

1314 **Sensory Motor Issues in Autism**
Speech Bin
PO Box 922668
Norcross, GA 30010
770-449-5700
800-850-8602
FAX 770-510-7290
http://www.speechbin.com
e-mail: info@speechbin.com
Shane Peters, Product Coordinator
Jen Binney, Owner

This resource for professionals and parents explains sensory processing disorders and their relationship to autism. It shows how to improve a child's responses to sensation, teach motor skills using daily living activities, and provide an effective learning environment. Item number C971. *$20.95*

1315 **So What Can I Do?**
Therapro
225 Arlington Street
Framingham, MA 01702
508-872-9494
800-257-5376
FAX 508-875-2062
http://www.theraproducts.com
e-mail: info@theraproducts.com
Gail Kushnir, Author
Karen Conrad, Owner

A book to help children develop their own solutions to everyday problems. Cartoon illustrations feature common situations for children to analyze. The adult asks the child, so what can you do? The child is then encouraged to think of creative solutions, developing their emotional intelligence and improving coping skills. 58 problems to solve. *$10.95*

1316 **Special Needs Program**
Dallas Metro Care
3330 S Lancaster Road
Dallas, TX 75216
214-941-6054
FAX 214-371-3933
Cecilia Castillo, Director
John Gorman, Supervisor
Cary Thomas, Manager
The special needs curriculum teaches students with disabilities the life skills they need to achieve self-sufficiency. The program focuses on and enhances coping skills.

1317 **Stepwise Cookbooks**
Therapro
225 Arlington Street
Framingham, MA 01702
508-872-9494
800-257-5376
FAX 508-875-2062
http://www.theraproducts.com
e-mail: info@theraproducts.com
Beth Jackson OTR, Author
Karen Conrad, Owner

A chance for children and adults at all developmental levels to participate in fun-filled hands-on cooking activities while developing independence. These cookbooks were developed by an OT working with children and teenagers with cognitive and physical challenges. Only one direction is presented on a page to reduce confusion. Recipes are represented by large Boardmaker symbols from Mayer Johnson. Large, easy-to-read text with dividing lines for visual clarity.

1318 **Strategies for Problem-Solving**
Harcourt Achieve
Customer Service, 5th Floor
Orlando, FL 32887
800-284-7019
FAX 800-699-9459
http://www.harcourtachieve.com
e-mail: webmaster@harcourt.com
Steven Korten, CEO
Randy Pennington, SVP National Sales

Show students more than one way to approach a problem, and you hand them the key to effective problem solving. These reproducible activities build math reasoning and critical thinking skills, reinforce core concepts, and reduce math anxiety too.

1319 **Survey of Teenage Readiness and Neurodevelopmental Status**
Educators Publishing Service
PO Box 9031
Cambridge, MA 02139
617-547-6706
800-225-5750
FAX 888-440-2665
http://www.epsbooks.com
e-mail: eps@epsbooks.com
Melvin D Levine MD FAAP, Author
Gunnar Voltz, President

Developed by Dr. Mel Livine and Dr.Stephen Hooper, The Survey of Teenage Readiness and Neurodevelopmental Status capitalizes on adolescents' evolving metacognitive abilities by directly asking them for their perceptions of how they are functioning in school and how they process information across a variety of neurocognitive and psychosocial domains.

1320 **Swallow Right**
Abilitations Speech Bin
PO Box 922668
Norcross, GA 30010
770-449-5700
800-850-8602
FAX 770-510-7290
http://www.speechbin.com
e-mail: info@speechbin.com
Tobi Isaacs, Catalog Director

This 12-session program evaluates and treats oral myofunctional disorders. 40 reproducible sequential exercises train individuals from five years to adult how to swallow correctly. Easy-to-use evaluation and tracking forms, checklist, and carryover strategies make this book a real time-saver! Item number Q858. *$52.99*

1321 **TARGET**
Abilitations Speech Bin
PO Box 922668
Norcross, GA 30010
770-449-5700
800-850-8602
FAX 770-510-7290
http://www.speechbin.com
e-mail: info@speechbin.com
Tobi Isaacs, Catalog Director

TARGET is the kind of resource aphasia clinicians beg for — a practical resource that answers not only the what and how questions of treatment but also the why. It describes dozens of treatment methods and gives you practical exercises and activities to implement each technique. Item number 1434. *$63.99*

1322 **TOPS Kit- Adolescent: Tasks of Problem Solving**
LinguiSystems
3100 4th Avenue
East Moline, IL 61244
309-755-2300
800-776-4332
FAX 309-755-2377
TDY:800-933-8331
http://www.linguisystems.com
e-mail: service@linguisystems.com
Linda Bowers, Rosemary Huisingh, Mark Barrett, Author
Linda Bowers, Co-Owner/Co-Founder
Rosemary Huisingh, Co-Owner/Co-Founder

Teach your teens how to use their language skills to think, think, think. We combine literacy, thinking, writing, humor, and language arts practice to cover these thinking skills: using content to make references; analyzing information; taking another's point of view; and more. It's a literacy-based approach that gets dramatic results! *$59.95*
192 pages Ages 12-18

1323 **TOPS Kit-Elementary: Tasks of Problem Solving**
LinguiSystems
3100 4th Avenue
East Moline, IL 61244
309-755-2300
800-776-4332
FAX 800-577-4555
TDY:800-933-8331
http://www.linguisystems.com
e-mail: service@linguisystems.com

Linda Bowers, Co-Owner/Co-Founder
Rosemary Huisingh, Co-Owner/Co-Founder

Reveal thinking and language skills your students didn't know they had with this remarkable kit. TOPS Kit-Elementary combines thinking and expressive language skills to develop better communications.
Ages 6-12

1324 Target Spelling
Harcourt Achieve
Customer Service, 5th Floor
Orlando, FL 32887
800-284-7019
FAX 800-699-9459
http://www.harcourtachieve.com
e-mail: webmaster@harcourt.com
Steven Korten, CEO
Randy Pennington, SVP National Sales

You can differentiate instructions to address a variety of learning styles and profiles and meet the needs of special education students.

1325 Teaching Dressing Skills: Buttons, Bows and More
Therapro
225 Arlington Street
Framingham, MA 01702
508-872-9494
800-257-5376
FAX 508-875-2062
http://www.theraproducts.com
e-mail: info@theraproducts.com
Marcy Coppelman Goldsmith OTR/L BCP, Author
Karen Conrad, Owner

Consists of 5 fold-out pamphlets for teaching children and adults of varying abilities the basic dressing skills: shoe tying, buttoning, zippering, dressing and undressing. Each task is broken down with every step clearly illustrated and specific verbal directions given to avoid confusion and to eliminate excess verbiage that can distract the learner. The author, an experienced OT, has included the needed prerequisites for each task, many great teaching tips and more. *$12.95*
5 Pamphlets

1326 That's Life Picture Stories
AGS Publishing
PO Box 99
Circle Pines, MN 55014
651-287-7220
800-328-2560
FAX 800-471-8457
http://www.agsnet.com
e-mail: agsmail@agsnet.com
Tana Reiff, Vince Clews, Author
Karen Dahlen, Associate Director
Matt Keller, Marketing Manager

With an interest level of high school through adult, ABE and ESL and a reading level of Grades 3-4, these eight picture stories describe how four families face daily challenges and solve practical problems. Features comic-book-style art and speech balloons. Families represent varied ethnic backgrounds. DramaTape cassettes featuring professional actors, music and sound effects available. *$105.99*

1327 That's Life! Social Language
LinguiSystems
3100 4th Avenue
East Moline, IL 61244
309-755-2300
800-776-4332
FAX 309-755-2377
TDY:800-933-8331
http://www.linguisystems.com
e-mail: service@linguisystems.com
Carolyn LoGiudice, Nancy McConnell, Author
Linda Bowers, Co-Owner/Co-Founder
Rosemary Huisingh, Co-Owner/Co-Founder

Teach your students to be effective and appropriate communicators in a wide variety of situations. Through direct instruction, role-playing activities, and discussion, your students will learn the how and why of social language interaction. *$37.95*
176 pages Ages 12-18

1328 That's Life: A Game of Life Skills
LinguiSystems
3100 4th Avenue
East Moline, IL 61244
309-755-2300
800-776-4332
FAX 309-755-2344
TDY:800-933-8331
http://www.linguisystems.com
e-mail: service@linguisystems.com
Patricia Smith, Author
Linda Bowers, Co-Owner/Co-Founder
Rosemary Huisingh, Co-Owner/Co-Founder

Help your older students refine their language skills to negotiate the real-world with this fun game. Get 100 thinking and language questions for each of these life areas: consumer affairs; government; health concerns; money matters; going places; and homemaking. *$44.95*
Ages 12-18

1329 ThemeWeavers: Animals Activity Kit
Riverdeep
100 Pine Street
San Francisco, CA 94111
415-659-2000
FAX 415-659-2020
http://www.riverdeep.net
e-mail: info@riverdeep.net
Barry O'Callaghan, Executive Chairman/CEO

ThemeWeavers: Animals is the essential companion for theme-based teaching. Dozens of animal-themed, interactive activities immediately engage your students to practice fundamental skills in math, language arts, science, social studies and more. Easy-to-use tools allow you to modify these activities or create your own to meet specific classroom needs.

1330 ThemeWeavers: Nature Activity Kit
Riverdeep
100 Pine Street
San Francisco, CA 94111
415-659-2000
FAX 415-659-2020
http://www.riverdeep.net
e-mail: info@riverdeep.net
Barry O'Callaghan, Executive Chairman/CEO

ThemeWeavers: Nature Activity Kit is an all-in-one solution for theme-based teaching. In just a few minutes, you can select from dozens of ready-to-use activities centering on the seasons and weather and be ready for the next day's lesson! Interactive and engaging activities cover multiple subject areas such as language arts, math, science, social studies and art.

1331 Thinkin' Science ZAP
Riverdeep
100 Pine Street
San Francisco, CA 94111
415-659-2000
FAX 415-659-2020
http://www.riverdeep.net
e-mail: info@riverdeep.net
Barry O'Callaghan, Executive Chairman/CEO

It is a dark and stormy night as you step backstage to be guest director at the Wonder Dome, the world-famous auditorium of light, sound, and electricity. But great zotz! The Theater has been zapped by lightning, and the Laser Control System is on the fritz! Can you learn all about light, sound and electricity to rescue the show? *$69.95*

1332 Time: Concepts & Problem-Solving
Harcourt Achieve
Customer Service, 5th Floor
Orlando, FL 32887
800-284-7019
FAX 800-699-9459
http://www.harcourtachieve.com
e-mail: webmaster@harcourt.com
Steven Korten, CEO
Randy Pennington, SVP National Sales

Develop concepts of telling time, identifying intervals, calculating elapsed time, and solving problems that deal with time changes, lapses, and changes over the AM/PM cusp.

1333 Tips for Teaching Infants & Toddlers
Abilitations Speech Bin
PO Box 922668
Norcorss, GA 30010
770-449-5700
800-850-8602
FAX 770-510-7290
http://www.speechbin.com
e-mail: info@speechbin.com
Tobi Isaacs, Catalog Director

This multisensory approach to Early Intervention is a whole year's worth of weekly thematic lessons which let children see, hear, feel, manipulate, smell, and taste. Item number 1235. *$47.99*

1334 Travel the World with Timmy Deluxe
Riverdeep
100 Pine Street
San Francisco, CA 94111
415-659-2000
FAX 415-659-2020
http://www.riverdeep.net
e-mail: info@riverdeep.net
Barry O'Callaghan, Executive Chairman/CEO

France and Russia are the newest destinations for Edmark's favorite world traveler, Timmy! In this delightful and improved program, students will enjoy expanding their understanding of the world around them. With wonderful stories, songs, games, and printable crafts, early learners discover how their international neighbors live, dress, sing, eat and play.

1335 Visual Perception and Attention Workbook
Therapro
225 Arlington Street
Framingham, MA 01702
508-872-9494
800-257-5376
FAX 508-875-2062
http://www.theraproducts.com
e-mail: info@theraproducts.com
Therapro Staff, Author
Karen Conrad, Owner

Simple mazes, visual discrimination and visual form constancy task, telling time and much more! *$10.50*

1336 Workbook for Cognitive Skills
Abilitations Speech Bin
PO Box 922668
Norcross, GA 30010
770-449-5700
800-850-8602
FAX 770-510-7290
http://www.speechbin.com
e-mail: info@speechbin.com
Susan Howell Brubaker, Author
Tobi Isaacs, Catalog Director

This workbook of perceptual and problem-solving exercises provides challenging material that's easy to read. Designed for adults and adolescents who have cognitive disorders. Item number W336. *$57.99*

1337 Workbook for Memory Skills
Abilitations Speech Bin
PO Box 922668
Norcorss, GA 30010
770-449-5700
800-850-8602
FAX 770-510-7290
http://www.speechbin.com
e-mail: info@speechbin.com
Beth M Kennedy, Author
Tobi Isaacs, Catalog Director

Helpful in treating individuals with deficits in attention and memory skills secondary to: traumatic brain injury; cognitive disorganization; early stage dementia; brain damage; learning disability; and progressive disease. Item number 1488. *$47.99*

1338 Workbook for Reasoning Skills
Abilitations Speech Bin
PO Box 922668
Norcorss, GA 30010
770-449-5700
800-850-8602
FAX 770-510-7290
http://www.speechbin.com
e-mail: info@speechbin.com
Susan Howell Brubaker, Author
Tobi Isaacs, Catalog Director

This workbook is designed for adults and children who need practice in reasoning, thinking, and organizing. Includes 67 exercises created for individuals with closed head injuries and mild to moderate cognitive deficits. Item number W332. *$57.99*

1339 Workbook for Word Retrieval
Abilitations Speech Bin
PO Box 922668
Norcross, GA 30010
770-449-5700
800-850-8602
FAX 770-510-7290
http://www.speechbin.com
e-mail: info@speechbin.com
Beth M Kennedy, Author
Tobi Isaacs, Catalog Director

Helpful materials treat individuals with deficits in attention and memory skills secondary to: Traumatic brain injury, Congnitive disorganization, Early stage dementia, Brain damage, Learning disability and Progressive disease. Item number 1523. *$42.99*
248 pages

1340 Working With Words-Volume 3
Abilitations Speech Bin
PO Box 922668
Norcross, GA 30010
770-449-5700
800-850-8602
FAX 770-510-7290
http://www.speechbin.com
e-mail: info@speechbin.com
Kathryn M Kilpatrick, Author
Tobi Isaacs, Catalog Director

Stimulate the reasoning skills of your brain-injured patients with this large print workbook of puzzles and word games. Activities include word builders, word hunters, word puzzlers, and word games challenging exercises for older children and adults. Item number V371. *$42.99*

1341 Working for Myself
AGS Publishing
PO Box 99
Circle Pines, MN 55014
651-287-7220
800-328-2560
FAX 800-471-8457
http://www.agsnet.com
e-mail: agsmail@agsnet.com
Tana Reiff, Author
Karen Dahlen, Associate Director
Matt Keller, Marketing Manager

With an interest level of High School through Adult, ABE and ESL and a reading level of Grades 3-4, this series of ten easy-to-read books tells the stories of ordinary people who successfully build small businesses. Students will learn that energy, problem-solving skills and thorough preparation can make the difference between success and failure.

Math

1342 Algebra Stars
Sunburst Technology
1550 Executive Drive
Elgin, IL 60123
800-321-7511
FAX 888-800-3028
http://http://store.sunburst.com/Home.aspx
e-mail: service@sunburst.com
Michael Guillory, Channel Sales/Marketing Manager

Students build their understanding of algebra by constructing, categorizing, and solving equations and classifying polynomial expressions using algebra tiles.

1343 **American Guidance Service Learning Disabilities Resources**
Instruction & Assessment AGS Special Needs Catalog
PO Box 716
Bryn Mawr, PA 19010
610-525-8336
800-869-8336
FAX 610-525-8337
http://www.ldonline.org
Dr. Richard Cooper, Author

A collection of alternative techniques which Dr. Cooper has found useful in teaching arithmetic to individuals with learning problems. *$9.95*

1344 **Attack Math**
Educators Publishing Service
PO Box 9031
Cambridge, MA 02139
617-547-6706
800-225-5750
FAX 888-440-2665
http://www.epsbooks.com
e-mail: eps@epsbooks.com
Carol Greenes, George Immerzeel, Linda Shulman, Author
Gunnar Voltz, President

This series, for grades 1-6, teaches the four arithmetic operations: addition, subtraction, multiplication and division. Each operation is covered in three books, with book one teaching the basic facts and books two and three teaching multi-digit computation with whole numbers. A checkpoint and testpoint monitor progress at the middle and end of each book.

1345 **Awesome Animated Monster Maker Math**
Sunburst Technology
1550 Executive Drive
Elgin, IL 60123
800-321-7511
FAX 888-800-3028
http://http://store.sunburst.com/Home.aspx
e-mail: service@sunburst.com
Michael Guillory, Channel Sales/Marketing Manager

With an emphasis on building core math skills, this humorous program incorporates the monstrous and the ridiculous into a structured learning environment. Students choose from six skill levels tailored to the 3rd to 8th grade.

1346 **Awesome Animated Monster Maker Math & Monster Workshop**
Sunburst Technology
1550 Executive Drive
Elgin, IL 60123
800-321-7511
FAX 888-800-3028
http://http://store.sunburst.com/Home.aspx
e-mail: service@sunburst.com
Michael Guillory, Channel Sales/Marketing Manager

Students develop money and strategic thinking skills with this irresistable game that has them tinker about making monsters.

1347 **Awesome Animated Monster Maker Number Drop**
Sunburst Technology
1550 Executive Drive
Elgin, IL 60123
800-321-7511
FAX 888-800-3028
http://http://store.sunburst.com/Home.aspx
e-mail: service@sunburst.com
Michael Guillory, Channel Sales/Marketing Manager

Your students will think on their mathematical feet estimating and solving thousands of number problems in an arcade-style game designed to improve their performance in numeration, money, fractions, and decimals.

1348 **Basic Essentials of Mathematics**
Harcourt Achieve
Customer Service, 5th Floor
Orlando, FL 32887
800-284-7019
FAX 800-699-9459
http://www.harcourtachieve.com
e-mail: webmaster@harcourt.com
Steven Korten, CEO
Randy Pennington, SVP National Sales

Ideal for basic math skill instruction, test practice, or any situation requiring a thorough, confidence-building review. It provides a complete lesson - instruction, examples, and computation exercises.

1349 **Basic Math for Job and Personal Use**
AGS Publishing
PO Box 99
Circle Pines, MN 55014
651-287-7220
800-328-2560
FAX 800-471-8457
http://www.agsnet.com
e-mail: agsmail@agsnet.com
Merle Wood, Jeanette Powell, Author
Karen Dahlen, Associate Director
Matt Keller, Marketing Manager

With an interest level of high school through adult, and a reading level of Grade 3-4, this series has modules in addition, subtraction, multiplication and division.

1350 **Building Mathematical Thinking**
Educators Publishing Service
PO Box 9031
Cambridge, MA 02139
617-547-6706
800-225-5750
FAX 888-440-2665
http://www.epsbooks.com
e-mail: eps@epsbooks.com
Marsha Stanton, Author
Gunnar Voltz, President

In this new math program, the units covered are presented as a series of Skinny Concepts that serve as manageable building blocks that eventually become entire topics. The Students Journal provides exercises for each Skinny Concept, encourages students to seek their own conclusions for problem solving, and provides space for the students ideas.

1351 **Building Perspective**
Sunburst Technology
1550 Executive Drive
Elgin, IL 60123
800-321-7511
FAX 888-800-3028
http://http://store.sunburst.com/Home.aspx
e-mail: service@sunburst.com
Michael Guillory, Channel Sales/Marketing Manager

Develop spatial perception and reasoning skills with this award-winning program that will sharpen your students' problem-solving abilities.

1352 **Building Perspective Deluxe**
Sunburst Technology
1550 Executive Drive
Elgin, IL 60123
800-321-7511
FAX 888-800-3028
http://http://store.sunburst.com/Home.aspx
e-mail: service@sunburst.com
Michael Guillory, Channel Sales/Marketing Manager

New visual thinking challenges await your students as they engage in three spacial reasoning activities that develop their 3D thinking, deductive reasoning and problem solving skills

1353 Calculator Math for Job and Personal Use

PO Box 99
Circle Pines, MN 55014
651-287-7220
800-328-2560
FAX 800-471-8457
http://www.agsnet.com
e-mail: agsmail@agsnet.com

With an interest level of high school through adult, and a reading level of Grade 3-4, this series has modules in basic math with a calculator and fractions, decimals, and percentages using a calculator.

1354 Combining Shapes

Sunburst Technology
1550 Executive Drive
Elgin, IL 60123
800-321-7511
FAX 888-800-3028
http://http://store.sunburst.com/Home.aspx
e-mail: service@sunburst.com
Michael Guillory, Channel Sales/Marketing Manager

Students discover the properties of simple geometric figures through concrete experience combining shapes. Measurements, estimating and operation skills are part of this fun program.

1355 Combining and Breaking Apart Numbers

Sunburst Technology
1550 Executive Drive
Elgin, IL 60123
800-321-7511
FAX 888-800-3028
http://http://store.sunburst.com/Home.aspx
e-mail: service@sunburst.com
Michael Guillory, Channel Sales/Marketing Manager

Students develop their number sense as they engage in "real life" dilemmas, which demonstrates the basic concepts of operations.

1356 Comparing with Ratios

Sunburst Technology
1550 Executive Drive
Elgin, IL 60123
800-321-7511
FAX 888-800-3028
http://http://store.sunburst.com/Home.aspx
e-mail: service@sunburst.com
Michael Guillory, Channel Sales/Marketing Manager

Students learn that ratio is a way to compare amounts by using multiplication and division. Through five engaging activities, students recognize and describe ratios, develop proportional thinking skills, estimate ratios, determine equivalent ratios, and use ratios to analyze data.

1357 Concert Tour Entrepreneur

Sunburst Technology
1550 Executive Drive
Elgin, IL 60123
800-321-7511
FAX 888-800-3028
http://http://store.sunburst.com/Home.aspx
e-mail: service@sunburst.com
Michael Guillory, Channel Sales/Marketing Manager

Your students improve math, planning and problem solving skills as they manage a band in this music management business simulation.

1358 Creating Patterns from Shapes

Sunburst Technology
1550 Executive Drive
Elgin, IL 60123
800-321-7511
FAX 888-800-3028
http://http://store.sunburst.com/Home.aspx
e-mail: service@sunburst.com
Michael Guillory, Channel Sales/Marketing Manager

Students discover patterns by exploring the properties of radiating and tiling patterns through Native American basket weaving and Japanese fish print themes.

1359 Data Explorer

Sunburst Technology
1550 Executive Drive
Elgin, IL 60123
800-321-7511
FAX 888-800-3028
http://http://store.sunburst.com/Home.aspx
e-mail: service@sunburst.com
Michael Guillory, Channel Sales/Marketing Manager

This easy-to-use CD-ROM provides the flexibility needed for eleven different graph types including tools for long-term data analysis projects.

1360 Decimals and Percentages for Job and Personal Use

AGS Publishing
PO Box 99
Circle Pines, MN 55014
651-287-7220
800-328-2560
FAX 800-471-8457
http://www.agsnet.com
e-mail: agsmail@agsnet.com
Merle Wood, Jeanette Powell, Author
Karen Dahlen, Associate Director
Matt Keller, Marketing Manager

With an interest level of high school through adult, and a reading level of Grade 3-4, this series has modules in decimals, fractions and percentages.

1361 Decimals: Concepts & Problem-Solving

Harcourt Achieve
Customer Service, 5th Floor
Orlando, FL 32887
800-284-7019
FAX 800-699-9459
http://www.harcourtachieve.com
e-mail: webmaster@harcourt.com
Steven Korten, CEO
Randy Pennington, SVP National Sales

This easy to implement, flexible companion to the classroom mathematics curriculum emcompasses decimal concepts such as values and names, equivalent decimals, mixed decimals, patterns, comparing, ordering, estimating and more.

1362 ESPA Math Practice Tests D

Harcourt Achieve
Customer Service, 5th Floor
Orlando, FL 32887
800-284-7019
FAX 800-699-9459
http://www.harcourtachieve.com
e-mail: webmaster@harcourt.com
Steven Korten, CEO
Randy Pennington, SVP National Sales

If you are concerned about your students' performance on the math portion of the ESPA, these workbooks can give them the boost they need. Each follows the New Jersey State standards in mathematics, giving students additional practice with the same kinds of questions they will face on the test day. Workbooks include three practice tests, with 50 multiple choice and open-ended questions each.

1363 ESPA Success in Mathematics

Harcourt Achieve
Customer Service, 5th Floor
Orlando, FL 32887
800-284-7019
FAX 800-699-9459
http://www.harcourtachieve.com
e-mail: webmaster@harcourt.com
Steven Korten, CEO
Randy Pennington, SVP National Sales

Ensure a positive experience on the ESPA with the preparatory program that follows the New Jersey State standards in mathematics, including instruction and practice in all five content clusters. Modeled instruction provides strategies to help students get the right answer on both multiple choice and open-ended questions.

1364 **Elementary Math Bundle**
Sunburst Technology
1550 Executive Drive
Elgin, IL 60123
800-321-7511
FAX 888-800-3028
http://http://store.sunburst.com/Home.aspx
e-mail: service@sunburst.com
Michael Guillory, Channel Sales/Marketing Manager

Number sense and operations are the focus of the Elementary Math Bundle. Students engage in activities that reinforce basic addition and subtraction skills. This product comes with Splish Splash Math, Ten Tricky Tiles and Numbers Undercover.

1365 **Equation Tile Teaser**
Sunburst Technology
1550 Executive Drive
Elgin, IL 60123
800-321-7511
FAX 888-800-3028
http://http://store.sunburst.com/Home.aspx
e-mail: service@sunburst.com
Michael Guillory, Channel Sales/Marketing Manager

Students develop logic thinking and pre-algebra skills solving sets of numbers equations in three challenging problem-solving activities.

1366 **Equivalent Fractions**
Sunburst Technology
1550 Executive Drive
Elgin, IL 60123
800-321-7511
FAX 888-800-3028
http://http://store.sunburst.com/Home.aspx
e-mail: service@sunburst.com
Michael Guillory, Channel Sales/Marketing Manager

This exciting investigation develops students' conceptual understanding that every fraction can be named in many different but equivalent ways.

1367 **Estimation**
Harcourt Achieve
Customer Service, 5th Floor
Orlando, FL 32887
800-284-7019
FAX 800-699-9459
http://www.harcourtachieve.com
e-mail: webmaster@harcourt.com
Steven Korten, CEO
Randy Pennington, SVP National Sales

Students learn to make sensible estimates, educated guesses, and logical choices, then use tools to check their estimates for accuracy. Practice includes estimation in measurement of length, weight, capacity, temperature, time and money.

1368 **Factory Deluxe**
Sunburst Technology
1550 Executive Drive
Elgin, IL 60123
800-321-7511
FAX 888-800-3028
http://http://store.sunburst.com/Home.aspx
e-mail: service@sunburst.com
Michael Guillory, Channel Sales/Marketing Manager

Five activities explore shapes, rotation, angles, geometric attributes, area formulas, and computation. Includes journal, record keeping, and on-screen help. This program helps sharpen geometry, visual thinking and problem solving skills.

1369 **Focus on Math**
Harcourt Achieve
Customer Service, 5th Floor
Orlando, FL 32887
800-284-7019
FAX 800-699-9459
http://www.harcourtachieve.com
e-mail: webmaster@harcourt.com
Steven Korten, CEO
Randy Pennington, SVP National Sales

Consists of four sections and in each you will learn more about addition and subtraction, multiplication and division, fractions, decimals, measurements, geometry and problem solving.

1370 **Follow Me! 2**
LinguiSystems
3100 4th Avenue
East Moline, IL 61244
309-755-2300
800-776-4332
FAX 309-755-2377
TDY:800-933-8331
http://www.linguisystems.com
e-mail: service@linguisystems.com
Grace Frank, Author
Linda Bowers, Co-Owner/Co-Founder
Rosemary Huisingh, Co-Owner/Co-Founder

These activities are relevant to classroom listening demands. The directions relate specifically on an accompanying worksheet. It's a pick-up-and-use-now resource to teach the vocabulary of language arts, math, social studies, and more.
$34.95
201 pages Ages 7-11

1371 **Fraction Attraction**
Sunburst Technology
1550 Executive Drive
Elgin, IL 60123
800-321-7511
FAX 888-800-3028
http://http://store.sunburst.com/Home.aspx
e-mail: service@sunburst.com
Michael Guillory, Channel Sales/Marketing Manager

Build the fraction skills of ordering, equivalence, relative sizes and multiple representations with four, multi-level, carnival style games.

1372 **Fraction Operations**
Sunburst Technology
1550 Executive Drive
Elgin, IL 60123
800-321-7511
FAX 888-800-3028
http://http://store.sunburst.com/Home.aspx
e-mail: service@sunburst.com
Michael Guillory, Channel Sales/Marketing Manager

Students build on their concepts of fraction meaning and equivalence as they learn how to perform operations with fractions.

1373 **Fractions: Concepts & Problem-Solving**
Harcourt Achieve
Customer Service, 5th Floor
Orlando, FL 32887
800-284-7019
FAX 800-699-9459
http://www.harcourtachieve.com
e-mail: webmaster@harcourt.com
Steven Korten, CEO
Randy Pennington, SVP National Sales

This companion to the classroom mathematics curriculum emcompasses many of the standards established at each grade level. Each activity page targets a specific skill to help bolster students who need additional work in a particular area of fractions.

1374 **Funny Monster for Tea**
Sunburst Technology
1550 Executive Drive
Elgin, IL 60123
800-321-7511
FAX 888-800-3028
http://http://store.sunburst.com/Home.aspx
e-mail: service@sunburst.com
Michael Guillory, Channel Sales/Marketing Manager

This interactive, read-along rhyme features six activities for young students to learn about time, practice spelling, investigate math and explore poetry, music and art.

1375 **GEPA Success in Language Arts Literacy and Mathematics**
Harcourt Achieve
Customer Service, 5th Floor
Orlando, FL 32887
800-284-7019
FAX 800-699-9459
http://www.harcourtachieve.vom
e-mail: webmaster@harcourtacheive.com
Steck-Vaughn Staff, Author
Tim McEwen, President/CEO
Susan Canizares, SVP Publisher
Lee Wilson, VP Marketing
Build skills as you improve scores on the GEPA. Better test scores don't always mean better skills. With these workbooks, you can ensure that your students are becoming more proficient users of language and math as well as more skilled test-takers. Your students will gain valuable practice answering the types of questions found on the GEPA, such as open-ended and enhanced multiple-choice items. *$15.60*

1376 **Geometry for Primary Grades**
Harcourt Achieve
Customer Service, 5th Floor
Orlando, FL 32887
800-284-7019
FAX 800-699-9459
http://www.harcourtachieve.com
e-mail: webmaster@harcourt.com
Steven Korten, CEO
Randy Pennington, SVP National Sales

Self-explanatory lessons ideal for independent work or as homework. Transitions from concrete to pictorial to abstract.

1377 **Get Up and Go!**
Sunburst Technology
1550 Executive Drive
Elgin, IL 60123
800-321-7511
FAX 888-800-3028
http://http://store.sunburst.com/Home.aspx
e-mail: service@sunburst.com
Michael Guillory, Channel Sales/Marketing Manager

Students interpret and construct timelines through three descriptive activities in the animated program. Students are introduced to timelines as they participate in an interactive story.

1378 **Grade Level Math**
Harcourt Achieve
Customer Service, 5th Floor
Orlando, FL 32887
800-284-7019
FAX 800-699-9459
http://www.harcourtachieve.com
e-mail: webmaster@harcourt.com
Steven Korten, CEO
Randy Pennington, SVP National Sales

Easy to understand practice exercises help students build conceptual knowledge and computation skills together. Each book addresses essential grade appropriate math areas.

1379 **Graphers**
Sunburst Technology
1550 Executive Drive
Elgin, IL 60123
800-321-7511
FAX 888-800-3028
http://http://store.sunburst.com/Home.aspx
e-mail: service@sunburst.com
Michael Guillory, Channel Sales/Marketing Manager

Students develop data analysis skills with this easy to use graphing tool. With over 30 pictorial data sets and 16 lessons, students learn to construct and interpret six different graph types.

1380 **Green Globs & Graphing Equations**
Sunburst Technology
1550 Executive Drive
Elgin, IL 60123
800-321-7511
FAX 888-800-3028
http://http://store.sunburst.com/Home.aspx
e-mail: service@sunburst.com
Michael Guillory, Channel Sales/Marketing Manager

As students explore parabolas, hyperbolas, and other graphs, they discover how altering an equation changes a graph's shape or position.

1381 **Grouping and Place Value**
Sunburst Technology
1550 Executive Drive
Elgin, IL 60123
800-321-7511
FAX 888-800-3028
http://http://store.sunburst.com/Home.aspx
e-mail: service@sunburst.com
Michael Guillory, Channel Sales/Marketing Manager

Students develop their understanding of our number system, learning to think about numbers in groups of ones, tens, and hundreds, and discovering the meaning of place value.

1382 **Hidden Treasures of Al-Jabr**
Sunburst Technology
1550 Executive Drive
Elgin, IL 60123
800-321-7511
FAX 888-800-3028
http://http://store.sunburst.com/Home.aspx
e-mail: service@sunburst.com
Michael Guillory, Channel Sales/Marketing Manager

Beginning algebra students undertake three challenges that develop skills in the areas of solving linear equations, substituting variables, grouping like variables, using systems of equations and translating algebra word problems into equations.

1383 **High School Math Bundle**
Sunburst Technology
1550 Executive Drive
Elgin, IL 60123
800-321-7511
FAX 888-800-3028
http://http://store.sunburst.com/Home.aspx
e-mail: service@sunburst.com
Michael Guillory, Channel Sales/Marketing Manager

Each program in this bundle focuses on a specific area to ensure that your students master the math skills they need. This bundle allows students to master basics of Algebra, explore equations and graphs, practice learning with algebra graphs, use trigonometric functions, apply math concepts to practical situations and improve problem solving and data analysis skills.

1384 Higher Scores on Math Standardized Tests
Harcourt Achieve
Customer Service, 5th Floor
Orlando, FL 32887
800-284-7019
FAX 800-699-9459
http://www.harcourtachieve.com
e-mail: webmaster@harcourt.com
Steven Korten, CEO
Randy Pennington, SVP National Sales

These grade level math test preparation series provide focused practice in areas where students have shown a weakness in previous standardized tests. Improves test scores by zeroing in on the skills requiring remediation.

1385 Hot Dog Stand: The Works
Sunburst Technology
1550 Executive Drive
Elgin, IL 60123
800-321-7511
FAX 888-800-3028
http://http://store.sunburst.com/Home.aspx
e-mail: service@sunburst.com
Michael Guillory, Channel Sales/Marketing Manager

Students practice math, problem-solving, and communication skills in a multimedia business simulation that challenges students with unexpected events.

1386 How the West Was 1+3x4
Sunburst Technology
1550 Executive Drive
Elgin, IL 60123
800-321-7511
FAX 888-800-3028
http://http://store.sunburst.com/Home.aspx
e-mail: service@sunburst.com
Michael Guillory, Channel Sales/Marketing Manager

Students use order of operations to construct equations and race along number line trails.

1387 Ice Cream Truck
Sunburst Technology
1550 Executive Drive
Elgin, IL 60123
800-321-7511
FAX 888-800-3028
http://http://store.sunburst.com/Home.aspx
e-mail: service@sunburst.com
Michael Guillory, Channel Sales/Marketing Manager

Elementary students learn important problem solving, strategic planning and math operation skills, as they become owners of a busy ice cream truck.

1388 Intermediate Geometry
Harcourt Achieve
Customer Service, 5th Floor
Orlando, FL 32887
800-284-7019
FAX 800-699-9459
http://www.harcourtachieve.com
e-mail: webmaster@harcourt.com
Steven Korten, CEO
Randy Pennington, SVP National Sales

Prepares intermediate and middle school students for a successful experience in high school geometry. Intermediate geometry provides a study of the concepts, computation, problem-solving, and enrichment of topics identified by NCTM standards. This three-book series links the informal explorations of geometry in primary grades to more formalized processes taught in high school.

1389 Introduction to Patterns
Sunburst Technology
1550 Executive Drive
Elgin, IL 60123
800-321-7511
FAX 888-800-3028
http://http://store.sunburst.com/Home.aspx
e-mail: service@sunburst.com
Michael Guillory, Channel Sales/Marketing Manager

Students discover patterns found in art and nature, exploring linear and geometric designs, predicting outcomes and creating patterns of their own.

1390 It's Elementary!
Educators Publishing Service
PO Box 9031
Cambridge, MA 02139
617-547-6706
800-225-5750
FAX 888-440-2665
http://www.epsbooks.com
e-mail: eps@epsbooks.com
M J Owen, Author
Gunnar Voltz, President

These new books helps make math word problems less intimidating for students in grades 2 through 5 by teaching them how to identify key words, draw pictures, and disregard unnecessary information. Captivating illustrations provide visual reinforcement of addition, subtraction, multiplication and division problems.

1391 Maps & Navigation
Sunburst Technology
1550 Executive Drive
Elgin, IL 60123
800-321-7511
FAX 888-800-3028
http://http://store.sunburst.com/Home.aspx
e-mail: service@sunburst.com
Michael Guillory, Channel Sales/Marketing Manager

This exciting nautical simulation provides students with opportunities use their math and science skills.

1392 Mastering Math
Harcourt Achieve
Customer Service, 5th Floor
Orlando, FL 32887
800-284-7019
FAX 800-699-9459
http://www.harcourtachieve.com
e-mail: webmaster@harcourt.com
Steven Korten, CEO
Randy Pennington, SVP National Sales

Now low level readers can succeed at math with this easy to read presentation. Makes basic math concepts accessible to all students.

1393 Math Assessment System
Harcourt Achieve
Customer Service, 5th Floor
Orlando, FL 32887
800-284-7019
FAX 800-699-9459
http://www.harcourtachieve.com
e-mail: webmaster@harcourt.com
Steven Korten, CEO
Randy Pennington, SVP National Sales

This easy-to-administer program generates individual scores, class scores, and an item analysis two times per year, providing a benchmark and two clear indicators of student progress.

1394 Math Detectives
Harcourt Achieve
Customer Service, 5th Floor
Orlando, FL 32887
800-284-7019
FAX 800-699-9459
http://www.harcourtachieve.com
e-mail: webmaster@harcourt.com
Steven Korten, CEO
Randy Pennington, SVP National Sales

Put student sleuths on the trail of mathematical problem solving and critical thinking with short mysteries even limited readers can manage. Use these motivating, grade-level mysteries as individual assignments, math center materials, group projects, or whole-class activities.

1395 Math Enrichment
Harcourt Achieve
Customer Service, 5th Floor
Orlando, FL 32887
800-284-7019
FAX 800-699-9459
http://www.harcourtachieve.com
e-mail: webmaster@harcourt.com
Steven Korten, CEO
Randy Pennington, SVP National Sales

Features alternate ways to help children become mathematical thinkers and master the basic rules and concepts. It has relevance to the reader, promoting and expanding critical thinking skills through puzzles, mazes, games, charts, tables, symbols and codes, and more.

1396 Math Scramble
LinguiSystems
3100 4th Avenue
East Moline, IL 61244
309-755-2300
800-776-4332
FAX 309-755-2377
TDY:800-933-8331
http://www.linguisystems.com
e-mail: service@linguisystems.com
Paul F Johnson, Author
Linda Bowers, Co-Owner/Co-Founder
Rosemary Huisingh, Co-Owner/Co-Founder

It's great for students with learning disabilities who need a different approach to learning and memorizing basic math facts. Students can play with your guidance or as independent practice.
$44.95
Ages 5-12

1397 Mathematics Skills Books
Harcourt Achieve
Customer Service, 5th Floor
Orlando, FL 32887
800-284-7019
FAX 800-699-9459
http://www.harcourtachieve.com
e-mail: webmaster@harcourt.com
Steven Korten, CEO
Randy Pennington, SVP National Sales

Affordable, focused reviews of fundamental math principles. Six 48 page books. Complete series of focused books offers practice in all basic mathematics skill areas with a consistent approach.

1398 Maximize Math Success for the Special Populations You Serve
Saxon Publishers
Harcourt 6277 C. Harvard Drive Seah
Norman, FL
405-329-7071
800-284-7019
FAX 866-378-2249
http://www.saxonpublishers.com
e-mail: info@saxonpublishers.com
Tim Mcquine, President/CEO

An adaptation that helps special populations with math where other teaching methods have failed.

1399 Maya Math
Sunburst Technology
1550 Executive Drive
Elgin, IL 60123
800-321-7511
FAX 888-800-3028
http://http://store.sunburst.com/Home.aspx
e-mail: service@sunburst.com
Michael Guillory, Channel Sales/Marketing Manager

Students discover the importance of place value and the number zero as they learn a different number and calendar system.

1400 Measurement: Practical Applications
Harcourt Achieve
Customer Service, 5th Floor
Orlando, FL 32887
800-284-7019
FAX 800-699-9459
http://www.harcourtachieve.com
e-mail: webmaster@harcourt.com
Steven Korten, CEO
Randy Pennington, SVP National Sales

Concentrated practice on the measurement skills we use on a daily basis. This practical presentation of both customary and metric units helps the student to understand the importance of measurement skills in everyday life. Hands on activities and real life situations create logical applications so measurements make sense.

1401 Memory Fun!
Sunburst Technology
1550 Executive Drive
Elgin, IL 60123
800-321-7511
FAX 888-800-3028
http://http://store.sunburst.com/Home.aspx
e-mail: service@sunburst.com
Michael Guillory, Channel Sales/Marketing Manager

Welcome to Tiny's attic where students build memory, matching, counting and money sense through a variety of fun matching activities.

1402 Middle School Geometry: Basic Concepts
Harcourt Achieve
Customer Service, 5th Floor
Orlando, FL 32887
800-284-7019
FAX 800-699-9459
http://www.harcourtachieve.com
e-mail: webmaster@harcourt.com
Steven Korten, CEO
Randy Pennington, SVP National Sales

Provides students with enough comprehensive, skill specific practice in the key areas of geometry to ensure mastery. Ideal for junior high or high school students in need of remediation.

1403 Middle School Math
Harcourt Achieve
Customer Service, 5th Floor
Orlando, FL 32887
800-284-7019
FAX 800-699-9459
http://www.harcourtachieve.com
e-mail: webmaster@harcourt.com
Steven Korten, CEO
Randy Pennington, SVP National Sales

This skill-specific series reinforces and enhances the middle school math curriculum. It provides teachers and parents with a tool to focus on the skills that students need to review and reinforce. The lessons provide step-by-step instructions, sample problems, and practices that enable students to work independently.

1404 Middle School Math Bundle
Sunburst Technology
1550 Executive Drive
Elgin, IL 60123
800-321-7511
FAX 888-800-3028
http://http://store.sunburst.com/Home.aspx
e-mail: service@sunburst.com
Michael Guillory, Channel Sales/Marketing Manager

This bundle helps improve student's logical thinking, number sense and operation skills. This product comes with Math Arena, Building Perspective Deluxe, Equation Tile Teasers and Easy Sheet.

1405 MindTwister Math
Riverdeep
100 Pine Street
San Francisco, CA 94111
415-659-2000
FAX 415-659-2020
http://www.riverdeep.net
e-mail: info@riverdeep.net
Barry O'Callaghan, Executive Chairman/CEO

MindTwister Math provides a challenging review of third grade math and problem-solving skills in a fast-paced, multi-player game show format. Thousands of action-packed challenges encourage students to practice essential math facts including addition, subtraction, mutiplication and division and develop more advanced mathematical problem-solving skills such as visualization, deduction, sequencing, estimating and pattern recognition.

1406 Mirror Symmetry
Sunburst Technology
1550 Executive Drive
Elgin, IL 60123
800-321-7511
FAX 888-800-3028
http://http://store.sunburst.com/Home.aspx
e-mail: service@sunburst.com
Michael Guillory, Channel Sales/Marketing Manager

Students advance their understanding of geometric properties and spatial relationships by exploring lines of symmetry within a single geometric shape.

1407 Multiplication & Division
Harcourt Achieve
Customer Service, 5th Floor
Orlando, FL 32887
800-284-7019
FAX 800-699-9459
http://www.harcourtachieve.com
e-mail: webmaster@harcourt.com
Steven Korten, CEO
Randy Pennington, SVP National Sales

Skill specific activities focus on the concepts and inverse relationships of multiplication and division. Explains in simplified terms how the process of multiplication undoes the process of division, and vice versa.

1408 My Mathematical Life
Sunburst Technology
1550 Executive Drive
Elgin, IL 60123
800-321-7511
FAX 888-800-3028
http://http://store.sunburst.com/Home.aspx
e-mail: service@sunburst.com
Michael Guillory, Channel Sales/Marketing Manager

Students discover the math involved in everyday living as they take a character from high school graduation to retirement, advising on important health, education, career, and financial decisions.

1409 Number Meanings and Counting
Sunburst Technology
1550 Executive Drive
Elgin, IL 60123
800-321-7511
FAX 888-800-3028
http://http://store.sunburst.com/Home.aspx
e-mail: service@sunburst.com
Michael Guillory, Channel Sales/Marketing Manager

Students develop their understanding of number meaning and uses with experiences practicing estimating, using number meanings, and making more-and-less comparisons.

1410 Number Sense & Problem Solving CD-ROM
Sunburst Technology
1550 Executive Drive
Elgin, IL 60123
800-321-7511
FAX 888-800-3028
http://http://store.sunburst.com/Home.aspx
e-mail: service@sunburst.com
Michael Guillory, Channel Sales/Marketing Manager

Build number and operation skills with these three programs: How the West Was One + Three x Four, Divide and Conquer and Puzzle Tanks.

1411 Numbers Undercover
Sunburst Technology
1550 Executive Drive
Elgin, IL 60123
800-321-7511
FAX 888-800-3028
http://http://store.sunburst.com/Home.aspx
e-mail: service@sunburst.com
Michael Guillory, Channel Sales/Marketing Manager

As children try to solve the case of missing numbers, they practice telling time, measuring and estimating, counting, and working with money.

1412 Patterns Across the Curriculum
Harcourt Achieve
6277 Sea Harbor Drive
Orlando, FL 32887
252-480-3200
800-844-1464
FAX 800-269-5232
http://www.steckvaughn.com
e-mail: info@steckvaughn.com
Steck-Vaughn Staff, Author
Tim McEwen, President/CEO
Jeff Johnson, Dir Marketing Communications
Chris Lehmann, Team Coordinator
Develop students awareness and understanding of patterns in the real world. Exercises allow students to identify, complete, extend, and create patterns. Developed across four curriculum areas: math, language, social studies, and science. Flexible organization allows teachers to utilize content specific activities in coordination with other classroom assignments, providing additional richness in learning.

1413 Penny Pot
Sunburst Technology
1550 Executive Drive
Elgin, IL 60123
800-321-7511
FAX 888-800-3028
http://http://store.sunburst.com/Home.aspx
e-mail: service@sunburst.com
Michael Guillory, Channel Sales/Marketing Manager

Students learn about money as they count combinations of coins in this engaging program.

1414 Problemas y mas
Harcourt Achieve
Customer Service, 5th Floor
Orlando, FL 32887
800-284-7019
FAX 800-699-9459
http://www.harcourtachieve.com
e-mail: webmaster@harcourt.com
Tim McEwen, President/CEO
Susan Canizares, SVP Publisher
Lee Wilson, VP Marketing
This ESL math practice and strategy tool is in three levels the same as Problems Plus, but expressly for your Spanish fluent ESL learners. *$13.40*
1995Grade Range: Grades 2-4
ISBN 0-811495-91-4

1415 Problems Plus Levels B-H
Harcourt Achieve
Customer Service, 5th Floor
Orlando, FL 32887
800-284-7019
FAX 800-699-9459
http://www.harcourtachieve.com
e-mail: webmaster@harcourt.com
Steck-Vaughn Staff, Author
Tim McEwen, President/CEO
Susan Canizares, SVP Publisher
Lee Wilson, VP Marketing
A one-of-a-kind guide to solving open-ended math problems. Doesn't just give answers to test questions. With its innovative problem-solving plan, this series teaches math thinking and problem attack strategies, plus offers practice in higher order thinking skills students need to solve open-ended math problems successfully. *$3.30*

1416 Puzzle Tanks
Sunburst Technology
1550 Executive Drive
Elgin, IL 60123
800-321-7511
FAX 888-800-3028
http://http://store.sunburst.com/Home.aspx
e-mail: service@sunburst.com
Michael Guillory, Channel Sales/Marketing Manager

A problem-solving program that uses logic puzzles involving liquid measurements.

1417 Representing Fractions
Sunburst Technology
1550 Executive Drive
Elgin, IL 60123
800-321-7511
FAX 888-800-3028
http://http://store.sunburst.com/Home.aspx
e-mail: service@sunburst.com
Michael Guillory, Channel Sales/Marketing Manager

In this investigation students work with one interpretation of a fraction and the relationship between parts and wholes by working with symbolic and visual representations.

1418 Sequencing Fun!
Sunburst Technology
1550 Executive Drive
Elgin, IL 60123
800-321-7511
FAX 888-800-3028
http://http://store.sunburst.com/Home.aspx
e-mail: service@sunburst.com
Michael Guillory, Channel Sales/Marketing Manager
Katie Birmingham, Office Manager
Text, pictures, animation, and video clips provide a fun-filled program that encourages critical thinking skills.

1419 Shape Up!
Sunburst Technology
1550 Executive Drive
Elgin, IL 60123
800-321-7511
FAX 888-800-3028
http://http://store.sunburst.com/Home.aspx
e-mail: service@sunburst.com
Michael Guillory, Channel Sales/Marketing Manager
Katie Birmingham, Office Manager
Students actively create and manipulate shapes to discover important ideas about mathematics in an electronic playground of two and three dimensional shapes.

1420 Shapes Within Shapes
Sunburst Technology
1550 Executive Drive
Elgin, IL 60123
800-321-7511
FAX 888-800-3028
http://http://store.sunburst.com/Home.aspx
e-mail: service@sunburst.com
Michael Guillory, Channel Sales/Marketing Manager
Katie Birmingham, Office Manager
Students identify shapes within shapes, then rearrange them to develop spatial sense and deepen their understanding of the properties of shapes.

1421 Soaring Scores AIMS Mathematics
Harcourt Achieve
Customer Service, 5th Floor
Orlando, FL 32887
800-284-7019
FAX 800-699-9459
http://www.harcourtachieve.com
e-mail: webmaster@harcourtachieve.com
Steck-Vaughn Staff, Author
Tim McEwen, President/CEO
Susan Canizares, SVP Publisher
Lee Wilson, VP Marketing
Emphasize problem-solving and conceptual understanding to succeed with Arizona mathematics standards such as number sense, data analysis and probability, patterns, algebra and functions, measurement and discrete mathematics, and mathematics structure. *$61.90*

ISBN 0-739834-86-X

1422 Soaring Scores in Math Assessment
Harcourt Achieve
Customer Service, 5th Floor
Orlando, FL 32887
800-284-7019
FAX 800-699-9459
http://www.harcourtachieve.com
e-mail: webmaster@harcourt.com
Steck-Vaughn Staff, Author
Tim McEwen, President/CEO
Susan Canizares, SVP Publisher
Lee Wilson, VP Marketing
Students get 48 pages of modeled instruction and practice tests covering exactly the types of questions they'll face on assessments, which include open-ended, multiple choice, and free response problems with fill in grids. A review test helps assess, diagnose, and prescribe additional work quickly. *$54.50*

1423 Soaring Scores on the CMT in Mathematics & Soaring Scores on the CAPT in Mathematics
Harcourt Achieve
Customer Service, 5th Floor
Orlando, FL 32887
800-284-7019
FAX 800-699-9459
http://www.harcourtachieve.com
e-mail: webmaster@harcourt.com
Steck-Vaughn Staff, Author
Tim McEwen, President/CEO
Susan Canizares, SVP Publisher
Lee Wilson, VP Marketing

Build the skills, strategies, and confidence your students need to do their best on the mathematics portion of the CMT and CAPT with this focused test preparation program. The instructional portion offers hints and strategies for each type of question students will face. Content standards and strands accompany each modeled problem. *$56.90*

1424 Soaring Scores on the CSAP Mathematics Assessment
Harcourt Achieve
Customer Service, 5th Floor
Orlando, FL 32887
800-284-7019
FAX 800-699-9459
http://www.harcourtachieve.com
e-mail: webmaster@harcourt.com
Steck-Vaughn Staff, Author
Tim McEwen, President/CEO
Susan Canizares, SVP Publisher
Lee Wilson, VP Marketing
Make the most of your CSAP test preparation. The best way to prepare your students for Colorado's unique achievement assessment is to use the program designed specifically for that purpose. *$56.90*

1425 Soaring Scores on the ISAT Mathematics
Harcourt Achieve
Customer Service, 5th Floor
Orlando, FL 32887
800-284-7019
FAX 800-699-9459
http://www.harcourtachieve.com
e-mail: webmaster@harcourt.com
Steck-Vaughn Staff, Author
Tim McEwen, President/CEO
Susan Canizares, SVP Publisher
Lee Wilson, VP Marketing
Developed to ensure peak performance on Illinois new math assessment. This test preparation product offers grade specific materials and authentic practice designed to help students approach the ISAT in mathematics strategically and confidently. *$56.90*

1426 Soaring Scores on the MEAP Math Test
Harcourt Achieve
Customer Service, 5th Floor
Orlando, FL 32887
800-284-7019
FAX 800-699-9459
http://www.harcourtachieve.com
e-mail: webmaster@harcourt.com
Steck-Vaughn Staff, Author
Tim McEwen, President/CEO
Susan Canizares, SVP Publisher
Lee Wilson, VP Marketing
Focus your MEAP math preparation where it will do the most good. This targeted test preparation program delivers the instruction, strategies, and practice your students need to be accomplished test takers. *$50.20*

1427 Spatial Relationships
Sunburst Technology
1550 Executive Drive
Elgin, IL 60123
800-321-7511
FAX 888-800-3028
http://http://store.sunburst.com/Home.aspx
e-mail: service@sunburst.com
Michael Guillory, Channel Sales/Marketing Manager

Students explore location by identifying the positions of objects and creating paths between places. Children develop spatial abilities and language needed to communicate about our world.

1428 Spatial Sense CD-ROM
Sunburst Technology
1550 Executive Drive
Elgin, IL 60123
800-321-7511
FAX 888-800-3028
http://http://store.sunburst.com/Home.aspx
e-mail: service@sunburst.com
Michael Guillory, Channel Sales/Marketing Manager

Your students will strenghten their spatial perception, spatial reasoning and problem-solving skills with three great programs now on one CD-ROM.

1429 Splish Splash Math
Sunburst Technology
1550 Executive Drive
Elgin, IL 60123
800-321-7511
FAX 888-800-3028
http://http://store.sunburst.com/Home.aspx
e-mail: service@sunburst.com
Michael Guillory, Channel Sales/Marketing Manager

Students learn and practice basic operation skills as they engage in this high interest program that keeps them motivated. Great visual rewards and three levels of difficulty keep students challanged.

1430 Statistics & Probability
Harcourt Achieve
Customer Service, 5th Floor
Orlando, FL 32887
800-284-7019
FAX 800-699-9459
http://www.harcourtachieve.com
e-mail: webmaster@harcourt.com
Steck-Vaughn Staff, Author
Tim McEwen, President/CEO
Susan Canizares, SVP Publisher
Lee Wilson, VP Marketing
A working knowledge of statistics and probability increases problem solving skills, and provides students with the skills to be able to more effectively gather, describe, organize, and interpret information in their world.

1431 Strategic Math Series
Edge Enterprises
708 W 9th Street
Lawrence, KS 66044
785-749-1473
877-767-1487
FAX 785-749-0207
e-mail: info@edgenterprise.inc.com
Cecil D Mercer and Susan Peterson Miller, Author
Jacqueline Schafer, Managing Editor
Sue Vernon, Manager
Carolyn Mitchell, Accounting
The Strategic Math Series are a group of seven manuals designed for any aged student who needs to learn basic math facts and operations. Each manual is built upon the concrete-representational-abstract method of instruction. Within this approach, understanding of mathematics is developed through the use of concrete objects, representational drawings and an easy-to-learn strategy that turns all students into active problem-solvers. Available as a series or individually.

1432 Strategies for Problem-Solving
Harcourt Achieve
Customer Service, 5th Floor
Orlando, FL 32887
800-284-7019
FAX 800-699-9459
http://www.harcourtachieve.com
e-mail: webmaster@harcourt.com
Steck-Vaughn Staff, Author
Tim McEwen, President/CEO
Susan Canizares, SVP Publisher
Lee Wilson, VP Marketing
Show students more than one way to approach a problem, and you hand them the key to effective problem solving. These reproducible activities build math reasoning and critical thinking skills, reinforce core concepts, and reduce math anxiety, too. *$11.99*

ISBN 0-817267-62-X

1433 Strategies for Success in Mathematics

Harcourt Achieve
Customer Service, 5th Floor
Orlando, FL 32887
800-284-7019
FAX 800-699-9459
http://www.harcourtachieve.com
e-mail: webmaster@harcourt.com

Steck-Vaughn Staff, Author
Tim McEwen, President/CEO
Susan Canizares, SVP Publisher
Lee Wilson, VP Marketing

Teach your students specific problem-solving skills and test taking strategies for success with math and math assessments. Practice thoroughly covers five math clusters: numerical operations, patterns and functions, algebraic concepts, measurement and geometry, and data analysis. *$3.30*

1434 Sunbuddy Math Playhouse

Sunburst Technology
1550 Executive Drive
Elgin, IL 60123
800-321-7511
FAX 888-800-3028
http://http://store.sunburst.com/Home.aspx
e-mail: service@sunburst.com

Michael Guillory, Channel Sales/Marketing Manager

An entertaining play, hidden math-related animations, and four multi-level interactive activities encourage children to explore math and reading.

1435 Take Off With...

Harcourt Achieve
6277 Sea Harbor Drive
Orlando, FL 32887
252-480-3200
800-531-5015
FAX 800-699-9459
http://www.steckvaughn.com
e-mail: info@steckvaughn.com

Steck-Vaughn Staff, Author
Tim McEwen, President/CEO
Jeff Johnson, Dir Marketing Communications
Chris Lehmann, Team Coordinator

Youngsters build number sense with concepts such as counting, sequencing and dividing, sorting, sets, and graphing, memory games, board games, and guessing games.

1436 Teddy Bear Press

Teddy Bear Press
3639 Midway Drive
San Diego, CA 92110
858-560-8718
FAX 858-674-0423
http://www.teddybearpress.net
e-mail: fparker@teddybearpress.net

Fran Parker, Author
Fran Parker, President

Introduces number concepts 1-10 using the pre-primer words found in the I Can Read series. *$20.00*

1437 Ten Tricky Tiles

Sunburst Technology
1550 Executive Drive
Elgin, IL 60123
800-321-7511
FAX 888-800-3028
http://http://store.sunburst.com/Home.aspx
e-mail: service@sunburst.com

Michael Guillory, Channel Sales/Marketing Manager

Students develop their arithmetic and logic skills with three levels of activities that involve solving sets of numbers sentences.

1438 Weekly Math Practice

Harcourt Achieve
6277 Sea Harbor Drive
Orlando, FL 32887
252-480-3200
800-531-5015
FAX 800-699-9459
http://www.steckvaughn.com
e-mail: info@steckvaughn.com

Steck-Vaughn Staff, Author
Tim McEwen, President/CEO
Jeff Johnson, Dir Marketing Communications
Chris Lehmann, Team Coordinator

Keep students sharp throughout the year with 36 weeks of brief, daily activities in math. Each activity page features five activity strips, one for each day of the week, and is backed up by a convenient answer key for the teacher that includes explanations and extensions.

1439 Zap! Around Town

Sunburst Technology
1550 Executive Drive
Elgin, IL 60123
800-321-7511
FAX 888-800-3028
http://http://store.sunburst.com/Home.aspx
e-mail: service@sunburst.com

Michael Guillory, Channel Sales/Marketing Manager

Students develop mapping and direction skills in this easy-to-use, animated program featuring Shelby, your friendly Sunbuddy guide.

Preschool

1440 2's Experience Fingerplays

Therapro
225 Arlington Street
Framingham, MA 01702
508-872-9494
800-257-5376
FAX 508-875-2062
http://www.theraproducts.com
e-mail: info@theraproducts.com

Liz Wilmes, Dick Wilmes, Author
Karen Conrad, Owner

A wonderful collection of fingerplays, songs and rhymes for the very young child. Fingerplays are short, easy to learn, and full of simple movement. Chant or sing the fingerplays and then enjoy the accompanying games and activities. *$12.95*
159 pages

1441 28 Instant Song Games

Therapro
225 Arlington Street
Framingham, MA 01702
508-872-9494
800-257-5376
FAX 508-875-2062
http://www.theraproducts.com
e-mail: info@theraproducts.com

MaBoAubLo, Barbara Sher, Author
Karen Conrad, Owner

Gets kids up and moving in no time! Includes numerous games of body awareness, movement play, self expression, imagination and language play. Booklet and 75 minute audio tape. *$21.00*
Audio Tape

1442 Artic Shuffle

LinguiSystems Incorporated.
3100 4th Avenue
East Moline, IL 61244
309-755-2300
800-776-4332
FAX 309-755-2377
TDY:800-933-8331
http://www.linguisystems.com
e-mail: service@linguisystems.com

Tobie Nan Kaufman, Author
Linda Bowers, Co-Owner/Co-Founder
Rosemary Huisingh, Co-Owner/Co-Founder

Why are these card decks best-sellers? Because they're real playing cards! Your students can play Go Fish, Crazy Eights, or Concentration while they practice their target sounds. Use them for vocabulary drills or naming practice. *$89.95*
Ages 5-Adult

1443 Curious George Preschool Learning Games
Sunburst Technology
1550 Executive Drive
Elgin, IL 60123
800-321-7511
FAX 888-800-3028
http://http://store.sunburst.com/Home.aspx
e-mail: service@sunburst.com
Michael Guillory, Channel Sales/Marketing Manager

Join Curious George in Fun Town and play five arcade-style games that promote the visual and auditory discrimination skills all students need before they begin to read. Mac/Win CD-ROM

1444 Devereux Early Childhood Assessment (DECA)
Kaplan Early Learning Company
1310 Lewisville-Clemmons Road
Lewisville, NC 27023
800-334-2014
FAX 800-452-7526
http://www.kaplanco.com
e-mail: info@kaplanco.com
David Kulick

Strength-based standardized, norm-referenced behavior rating scale designed to promote resilience and measure protective factors in children ages 2-5. Through the program, early childhood professionals and families learn specific strategies to support young children's social and emotional development and to enhance the ovall quality of early childhood programs.

1445 Devereux Early Childhood Assessment: Clinical Version (DECA-C)
Kaplan Early Learning Company
1310 Lewisville-Clemmons Road
Lewisville, NC 27023
800-334-2014
FAX 800-452-7526
http://www.kaplanco.com
e-mail: info@kaplanco.com
Paul LeBuffe, Author
David Kulick

DECA-C is designed to support early intervention efforts to reduce or eliminate significant emotional and behavioral concerns in preschool children. This can be used for guide interventions, identify children needing special services, assess outcomes and help programs meet Head Start, IDEA, and similar requirements. Kit includes: 1 Manual, 30 Record Forms, and 1 Norms Reference Card. *$125.95*

1446 Early Movement Skills
Therapro
225 Arlington Street
Framingham, MA 01702
508-872-9494
800-257-5376
FAX 508-875-2062
http://www.theraproducts.com
e-mail: info@theraproducts.com
Naomi Benari, Author
Karen Conrad, Owner

Easy to follow, reproducible gross motor activities are graded from very simple (even for the passive child) to more demanding (folk dancing). Each of the 150 pages offers an activity with its objective, a clear instruction of the activity, rationale, and alternative movements and games. Many activities involve music and rythm. A great source for early intervention and early childhood programs. *$58.00*

1447 Early Screening Inventory: Revised
Harcourt
6277 Sea Harbor Drive
Orlando, FL 32887
407-345-2000
http://www.harcourt.com
Patrick Tierrey, CEO
Gail Ribalta, Marketing VP

A developmental screening instrument for 3-to-6-year olds. Provides a norm-referenced overview of visual-motor/adaptive, language and cognition, and gross motor development. Meets IDEA and Head Start requirements for early identification and parental involvement. Test in English or Spanish in 15-20 minutes. Training video and materials available.

1448 Early Sensory Skills
Therapro
225 Arlington Street
Framingham, MA 01702
508-872-9494
800-257-5376
FAX 508-875-2062
http://www.theraproducts.com
e-mail: info@theraproducts.com
Jackie Cooke, Author
Karen Conrad, Owner

A wonderful book filled with practical and fun activities for stimulating vision, touch, taste and smell. Invaluable for anyone working with children 6 months to 5 years, this manual outlines basic principals followed by six sections containing activities, games and topics to excite the senses. Introductions are easy to follow, and materials for the sensory work are readily accessible in the everyday environment. *$52.50*

1449 Early Visual Skills
Therapro
225 Arlington Street
Framingham, MA 01702
508-872-9494
800-257-5376
FAX 508-875-2062
http://www.theraproducts.com
e-mail: info@theraproducts.com
Diana Williams, Author
Karen Conrad, Owner

A beautifully designed, easy to follow reproducible book for working with young children on visual perceptual skills. Most of the activities are nonverbal and can be used with children who have limited language. Each section has both easy and challenging activities for school and for parents working with children at home. Activities include sorting, color and shape matching, a looking walk, games to develop visual memory and concentration and many more. *$52.50*
208 pages

1450 Family Literacy Package
Harcourt Achieve
Customer Service, 5th Floor
Orlando, FL 32887
800-284-7019
FAX 800-699-9459
http://www.harcourtachieve.com
e-mail: webmaster@harcourt.com
Steck-Vaughn Staff, Author
Tim McEwen, President/CEO
Susan Canizares, SVP Publisher
Lee Wilson, VP Marketing
Parent Package: includes materials that provide valuable academic and life coping resources for parents. Manual and companion video tapes prepare staff members for effective implementation. Child Package: includes materials that develop reading readiness and encourage positive parent-child interaction. Manual and companion video tapes prepare staff members to direct preschool learning and to facilitate supportive new relationships. *$231.10*

1451 Fluharty Preschool Speech & Language Screening Test-2
Abilitations Speech Bin
PO Box 922668
Norcross, GA 30010
770-449-5700
800-850-8602
FAX 770-510-7290
http://www.speechbin.com
e-mail: info@speechbin.com

Tobi Isaacs, Catalog Director

Carefully normed on 705 children, the Fluharty yields standard scores, percentiles, and age equivalents. The form features space for speech-language pathologist to note phonological processes, voice quality, and fluency; a Teacher Questionnaire is also provided. Item number P882 *$167.99*

1452 For Parents and Professionals: Preschool

LinguiSystems
3100 4th Avenue
East Moline, IL 61244
309-755-2300
800-776-4332
FAX 309-755-2377
TDY:800-933-8331
http://www.linguisystems.com
e-mail: service@linguisystems.com
Marilyn A Ianni, Karin A Mullin, Author
Linda Bowers, Co-Owner/Co-Founder
Rosemary Huisingh, Co-Owner/Co-Founder

Get tips and activities to facilitate developing communication skills in young children. You'll target social development, fine and gross motor development, cognitive growth, and receptive and expressive language skills. Each activity gives you three levels of increasing complexity for children functioning at different developmental levels. *$37.95*

181 pages Ages 2-5

1453 Funology Fables

Abilitations Speech Bin
PO Box 922668
Norcross, GA 30010
770-449-5700
800-850-8602
FAX 770-510-7290
http://www.speechbin.com
e-mail: info@speechbin.com
Tobi Isaacs, Catalog Director

Funology Fables targets specific phonemes and critical early concepts, such as matching, sequencing, opposites, comparisons, quantity, size, and space. Reproducible Talking Tales and activities include 32 six-part sequence stories. Item number 1484. *$47.95*

1454 Goal Oriented Gross & Fine Motor Lesson Plans for Early Childhood Classes

Therapro
225 Arlington Street
Framingham, MA 01702
508-872-9494
800-257-5376
FAX 508-875-2062
http://www.theraproducts.com
e-mail: info@theraproducts.com
Donna Weiss MA OTR, Author
Karen Conrad, Owner

Practical and convinient format covers 224 activities grouped into 12 monthly units, making it easy to incorporate gross and fine motor activities into a daily class schedule. Provides challenges for groups whose abilities span early childhood, from 2.5 to 5.5 years of age. *$32.00*

77 pages

1455 HELP for Preschoolers at Home

Therapro
225 Arlington Street
Framingham, MA 01702
508-872-9494
800-257-5376
FAX 508-875-2062
http://www.theraproducts.com
e-mail: info@theraproducts.com
Therapro Staff, Author
Karen Conrad, Owner

Three hundred pages of practical, home-based activities that can be easily administered by the parents or the child's home-care provider. Upon completion of their assessments, teachers and therapists provide parents with these handouts to help them work on skills at home in conjunction with the program. *$72.50*

Ages 3-6

1456 IEP Companion Software

LinguiSystems
3100 4th Avenue
East Moline, IL 61244
309-755-2300
800-776-4332
FAX 309-755-2377
TDY:800-933-8331
http://www.linguisystems.com
e-mail: service@linguisystems.com
Carolyn Wilson, Janet Lanza, Jeannie Evans, Author
Linda Bowers, Co-Owner/Co-Founder
Rosemary Huisingh, Co-Owner/Co-Founder

Get IEP goals from the best-selling book with the click of your mouse. Writing complete reports is easy! You'll get to choose from hundreds of individual and classroom goals and objectives for all the important speech and language areas. Just click on the specific goals you want to create your individualized report. *$69.95*

Birth-Adult

1457 Just for Me! Grammar

LinguiSystems
3100 4th Avenue
East Moline, IL 61244
309-755-2300
800-776-4332
FAX 309-755-2377
TDY:800-933-8331
http://www.linguisystems.com
e-mail: service@linguisystems.com
Margaret Warner, Author
Linda Bowers, Co-Owner/Co-Founder
Rosemary Huisingh, Co-Owner/Co-Founder

Teach oral grammar to your youngest students! Through a variety of engaging activities, your students will become familiar with basic parts of speech, correct word order, and simple grammar concepts. These activities provide a solid foundation for later formal grammar training in the classroom. *$24.95*

150 pages Ages 3-6

1458 LAP-D Kindergarten Screen Kit

Kaplan Early Learning Company
1310 Lewisville-Clemmons Road
Lewisville, NC 27023
800-334-2014
FAX 800-452-7526
http://www.kaplanco.com
e-mail: info@kaplanco.com
David Kulick

Concise, standardized screening deice normed on 5 year old children. Tasks are in four domains: fine, motor, gross motor, cognititve, and language. The Kindergarten Kit includes the technical manual, examiners, manual, and materials to assist in determining pure outcomes. *$124.95*

1459 LILAC

Abilitations Speech Bin
PO Box 922668
Norcross, GA 30010
770-449-5700
800-850-8602
FAX 770-510-7290
http://www.speechbin.com
e-mail: info@speechbin.com
Tobi Isaacs, Catalog Director

LILAC uses direct and naturalistic teaching in a creative approach that links spoken language learning to reading and writing. Activities to develop semantic, syntactic, expressive, and receptive language skills are presented sequentially from three-to-five-year old developmental levels. Item number 1428. *$27.99*

1460 Learning Accomplishment Profile Diagnostic Normed Screens for Age 3-5

Kaplan Early Learning Company
1310 Lewisville-Clemmons Road
Lewisville, NC 27023
800-334-2014
FAX 800-452-7526
http://www.kaplanco.com
e-mail: info@kaplanco.com

David Kulick

For 3-5 years. Create reliable developmental snapshots in fine motor, gross motor, cognitive, language, personal/social, and self-help skill domains. *$349.95*

1461 Learning Accomplishment Profile (LAP-R) KIT

Kaplan Early Learning Company
1310 Lewisville-Clemmons Road
Lewisville, NC 27023
800-334-2014
FAX 800-452-7526
http://www.kaplanco.com
e-mail: info@kaplanco.com
David Kulick

A criterion-referenced assessment instrument measuring development in six domains: gross motor, fine motor, cognitive, language, self-help and social/emotional. Kit includes all materials necessary for assessing 20 children. *$ 299.95*

1462 Learning Accomplishment Profile Diagnostic Normed Assessment (LAP-D)

Kaplan Early Learning Company
1310 Lewisville-Clemmons Road
Lewisville, NC 27023
800-334-2014
FAX 800-452-7526
http://www.kaplanco.com
e-mail: info@kaplanco.com
David Kulick

A comprehensive developemtal assessment tool for children between the ages of 30 and 72 months. LAP-D consists of a hierarchy of developmental skills arranged in four developmental domains: fine motor, gross motor, cognitive and language. *$624.95*

1463 Linamood Program (LIPS Clinical Version)-Phoneme Sequencing Program for Reading, Spelling,Speech

LinguiSystems
3100 4th Avenue
East Moline, IL 61244
309-755-2300
800-776-4332
FAX 309-755-2377
TDY:800-933-8331
http://www.linguisystems.com
e-mail: service@linguisystems.com
Patricia Linamood, Phyllis Linamood, Author
Linda Bowers, Co-Owner/Co-Founder
Rosemary Huisingh, Co-Owner/Co-Founder

Help your students develop phoneme awareness for competence in reading, spelling, and speech. This multisensory program meets the needs of the many children and adults who don't develop phonemic awareness through traditional methods. *$247.00*

Birth-Adult

1464 Make Every Step Count: Birth to 1 Year

Therapro
225 Arlington Street
Framingham, MA 01702
508-872-9494
800-257-5376
FAX 508-875-2062
http://www.theraproducts.com
e-mail: info@theraproducts.com
Stephanie Parks MA, Author
Karen Conrad, Owner

A great book with many ideas for parents to use at home to foster child development. *$16.50*

94 pages

1465 Make It Today for Pre-K Play

Therapro
225 Arlington Street
Framingham, MA 01702
508-872-9494
800-257-5376
FAX 508-875-2062
http://www.theraproducts.com
e-mail: info@theraproducts.com
Joyce Hamman, Author
Karen Conrad, Owner

Many ideas for making and using toys for motor development. Includes a nice checklist for balance, directional terms, body awareness, and gross and fine motor skills. For each piece of equipment, specific directions are given on how to make it; teaching tips, many ideas for using in curriculum integration. *$7.95*

1466 Mouth Madness

Abilitations Speech Bin
PO Box 922668
Norcross, GA 30010
770-449-5700
800-850-8602
FAX 770-510-7290
http://www.speechbin.com
e-mail: info@speechbin.com
Tobi Isaacs, Catalog Director

This unique manual uses oral imitation, motor planning, and breath control activities to improve the articulation and feeding skills of preschool and primary children. Games, manipulative tasks, silly sentences, rhymes, and funny faces target higher organizational levels of motor planning. Item number C758. *$54.99*

1467 Partners for Learning (PFL)

Kaplan Early Learning Company
1310 Lewisville-Clemmons Road
Lewisville, NC 27023
336-766-7374
800-334-2014
FAX 800-452-7526
http://www.kaplanco.com
e-mail: info@kaplanco.com
David Kulick

This resource uses cards, books, posters, and support materials to supply teaching ideas and to support child development. PARTNERS for Learning encourages cognitive, social, motor, and language development. The kit provides materials for curriculum planning and self-assessment. *$199.95*

1468 Preschool

Harcourt Achieve
Customer Service, 5th Floor
Orlando, FL 32887
800-284-7019
FAX 800-699-9459
http://www.harcourtachieve.com
e-mail: webmaster@harcourt.com
Tim McEwen, President/CEO
Susan Canizares, SVP Publisher
Lee Wilson, VP Marketing

This series provides age appropriate activities to foster childrens' desire to read and create a print rich classroom to enhance their emergent literacy. Multiple lesson plans save teachers time by providing suggested lessons that cover the purpose, materials, direct teaching, and application of new skills. This is a great resource for center ideas that provide opportunities for children to think creatively, explore new ideas, and use problem-solving skills.

320 pages
ISBN 0-739885-58-8

1469 Preschool Motor Speech Evaluation & Intervention

Abilitations Speech Bin
PO Box 922668
Norcross, GA 30010
770-449-5700
800-850-8602
FAX 770-510-7290
http://www.speechbin.com
e-mail: info@speechbin.com
Margaret M Earnest, Author
Tobi Isaacs, Catalog Director

This comprehensive criterion-based assessment tool differentiates motor-based speech disorders from those of phonology and determines if speech difficulties of children 18 months to six years old are characteristic of: oral nonverbal apraxia; dysarthria; developmental verbal dyspraxia; hypersensitivity; differences in tone and hyposensitivity. Item number J322. *$65.99*

1470 Promoting Communication in Infants & Children
Abilitations Speech Bin
PO Box 922668
Norcross, GA 30010
770-449-5700
800-850-8602
FAX 770-510-7290
http://www.speechbin.com
e-mail: info@speechbin.com
Tobi Isaacs, Catalog Director

Promoting Communication in Infants and Young Children gives you down-to-earth information, activities, and step-by-step suggestions for stimulating children's speech and language skills. Topics are conveniently organized, concisely presented, and written in easy-to-understand language. Item number 1512. *$17.95*

1471 RULES
Abilitations Speech Bin
PO Box 922668
Norcross, GA 30010
770-449-5700
800-850-8602
FAX 770-510-7290
http://www.speechbin.com
e-mail: info@speechbin.com
Jane C Webb, Barbara Duckett, Author
Tobi Isaacs, Catalog Director

Faced with young children whose speech is unintelligible? RULES is the perfect program for these preschool and elementary children. It remediates the processes: cluster reduction; final consonant deletion; stopping and prevocalic voicing. Item number 1557. *$58.99*

1472 Receptive One-Word Picture Vocabulary Test (ROWPVT-2000)
Abilitations Speech Bin
PO Box 922668
Norcross, GA 30010
770-449-5700
800-850-8602
FAX 770-510-7290
http://www.speechbin.com
e-mail: info@speechbin.com
Rick Brownell, Author
Tobi Isaacs, Catalog Director

This administered, untimed measure assessess the vocabulary comprehension of 0-2 through 11-18 years. New full-color test pictures are easy to recognize; many new test items have been added. It is ideal for children unable or reluctant to speak because only a gestural response is required. Item number A305. *$139.99*

1473 Right from the Start: Behavioral Intervention for Young Children with Autism: A Guide
Therapro
225 Arlington Street
Framingham, MA 01702
508-872-9494
800-257-5376
FAX 508-875-2062
http://www.theraproducts.com
e-mail: info@theraproducts.com
Mary Jane Weiss PhD, Sandra Harris PhD, Author
Karen Conrad, Owner

This informative and user-friendly guide helps parents and service providers explore programs that use early intensive behavioral intervention for young children with autism and related disorders. Within these programs, many children improve in intellectual, social and adaptive functioning, enabling them to move on to regular elementary and preschools. Benefits all children, but primarily useful for children age five and younger. *$14.95*
138 pages

1474 SPARC Artic Junior
LinguiSystems
3100 4th Avenue
East Moline, IL 61244
309-755-2300
800-776-4332
FAX 309-755-2377
TDY:800-933-8331
http://www.linguisystems.com
e-mail: service@linguisystems.com
Beverly Plass, Author
Linda Bowers, Co-Owner/Co-Founder
Rosemary Huisingh, Co-Owner/Co-Founder

Reach intelligibility goals faster with these take-home exercises. The practice words have been carefully selected to control the phonetic context. It's a programmed, research-based approach that will get results. Activities are divided by primary and secondary phonological processes. *$39.95*
211 pages Ages 3-7

1475 Sensory Motor Activities for Early Development
Therapro
225 Arlington Street
Framingham, MA 01702
508-872-9494
800-257-5376
FAX 508-875-2062
http://www.theraproducts.com
e-mail: info@theraproducts.com
Chia Swee Hong, Helen Gabriel, Cathy St John, Author
Karen Conrad, Owner

A complete package of tried and tested gross and fine motor activities. Many activities to stimulate sensory and body awareness, encourage basic movement, promote hand skills, and enhance spatial/early perceptual skills. Master handouts throughout to give to parents for home practice activities for working in small groups. *$44.50*

1476 Silly Sentences
Abilitations Speech Bin
PO Box 922668
Norcross, GA 30010
770-449-5700
800-850-8602
FAX 770-510-7290
http://www.speechbin.com
e-mail: info@speechbin.com
Tobi Isaacs, Catalog Director

Children love to have fun. Silly Sentences lets them have fun while they play these engaging card games to learn: subject verb agreement; speech sound articulation; S+ V+ O sentences; questioning and answering; humor and absurdities; and present progressive verbs. Item number P506. *$47.99*

1477 Sound Connections
Abilitations Speech Bin
PO Box 922668
Norcross, GA 30010
770-449-5700
800-850-8602
FAX 770-510-7290
http://www.speechbin.com
e-mail: info@speechbin.com
Tobi Isaacs, Catalog Director

This program teaches the critical connections between the sounds kids hear and speaking, reading, and writing. Dozens of activities and worksheets, 19 phoneme-based stories, and 100s of pictures. Item number 1487. *$41.99*

1478 Source for Early Literacy Development
LinguiSystems
3100 4th Avenue
East Moline, IL 61244
309-755-2300
800-776-4332
FAX 309-755-2377
TDY:800-933-8331
http://www.linguisystems.com
e-mail: service@linguisystems.com
Linda K Crowe, Sara S Reichmuth, Author
Linda Bowers, Co-Owner/Co-Founder
Rosemary Huisingh, Co-Owner/Co-Founder

This great resource gives you the latest information on children's emergent reading and writing from birth through age eight. You'll also get helpful strategies to facilitate literacy development for future academic success! *$ 41.95*

151 pages Birth-8

1479 Stuttering: Helping the Disfluent Preschool Child
Abilitations Speech Bin
PO Box 922668
Norcross, GA 30010
770-449-5700
800-850-8602
FAX 770-510-7290
http://www.speechbin.com
e-mail: info@speechbin.com
Julie A Blonigen, Author
Tobi Isaacs, Catalog Director

Written in the warm encouraging style for which this author is known, Stuttering: Helping the Disfluent Preschool Child is the perfect tool for parents and teachers of young stuttering children. It uses a Speech Thermometer to show them ways to turn talking into an area of strength. Item number 1489. *$13.95*

1480 Take Home: Preschool Language Development
LinguiSystems
3100 4th Avenue
East Moline, IL 61244
309-755-2300
800-776-4332
FAX 309-755-2377
TDY:800-933-8331
http://www.linguisystems.com
e-mail: service@linguisystems.com
Martha Drake, Author
Linda Bowers, Co-Owner/Co-Founder
Rosemary Huisingh, Co-Owner/Co-Founder

Home follow-up is essential for your little ones with speech and language delays. Get everything you need for a comprehensive take-home program with this time saver! Each take-home lesson is easy to follow. *$31.95*
191 pages Ages 1-5

1481 Test for Auditory Comprehension of Language: TACL-3
Abilitations Speech Bin
PO Box 922668
Norcross, GA 30010
770-449-5700
800-850-8602
FAX 770-510-7290
http://www.speechbin.com
e-mail: info@speechbin.com
Tobi Isaacs, Catalog Director

The newly revised TACL-3 evaluates the 0-3 to 9-11-year old's understanding of spoken language in three subtests: Vocabulary, Grammatical Morphemes and Elaborated Phrases and Sentences. Each test item is a word or sentence read aloud by the examiner; the child responds by pointing to one of three pictures. Item number P792. *$274.99*

1482 Tips for Teaching Infants & Toddlers
Abilitations Speech Bin
PO Box 922668
Norcross, GA 30010
770-449-5700
800-850-8602
FAX 770-510-7290
http://www.speechbin.com
e-mail: info@speechbin.com
Tobi Isaacs, Catalog Director

This multisensory approach to Early Intervention is a whole year's worth of weekly thematic lessons which let children see, hear, feel, manipulate, smell, and taste. Item number 1235. *$47.99*

1483 What Am I? Game
Harcourt Achieve
6277 Sea Harbor Drive
Orlando, FL 32887
252-480-3200
800-531-5015
FAX 800-699-9459
http://www.steckvaughn.com
e-mail: info@steckvaughn.com
Steck-Vaughn Staff, Author
Tim McEwen, President/CEO
Jeff Johnson, Dir Marketing Communications
Chris Lehmann, Team Coordinator

Turn animal identity into a guessing game. Children guess the identities of amazing animals from a series of clues and up close views. A world map pinpoints each animal's habitat, and a quick quiz reinforces fun facts.

1484 When Pre-Schoolers are Not on Target: Guide for Parents & Early Childhood Educators
Learning Disabilities Association of America
4156 Library Road
Pittsburgh, PA 15234
412-341-1515
FAX 412-344-0224
http://www.ldaamerica.org
e-mail: info@ldaamerica.org
Sheila Buckley, Executive Director

Booklet provides information on early identification of learning disabilities and appropriate intervention strategies to professionals who work with preschool children. Available in Spanish. Discounts for multiples. *$4.00*

1485 Your Child's Speech and Language
Abilitations Speech Bin
PO Box 922668
Norcross, GA 30010
770-449-5700
800-850-8602
FAX 770-510-7290
http://www.speechbin.com
e-mail: info@speechbin.com
Tobi Isaacs, Catalog Director

This delightfully illustrated 52- page book provides helpful information about speech and language development from infancy through five years. It shows how to determine if speech is developing normally and ways to stimulate its growth. It's ideal for parent training and baby showers too! Item number P652. *$17.00*

Reading

1486 100% Reading: 2-Book Intermediate Set
LinguiSystems
3100 4th Avenue
East Moline, IL 61244
309-755-2300
800-776-4332
FAX 309-755-2377
TDY:800-933-8331
http://www.linguisystems.com
e-mail: service@linguisystems.com
LinguiSystems Staff, Author
Linda Bowers, Co-Owner/Co-Founder
Rosemary Huisingh, Co-Owner/Co-Founder

Our reading series uses a developmental approach based on the latest research in phonological awareness and early reading skills. Intermediate books are for ages 8-10. Great as a reading curriculum or to supplement your current reading program. *$69.90*
200 pages Ages 8-10

1487 100% Reading: 3-Book Primary Set
LinguiSystems
3100 4th Avenue
East Moline, IL 61244
309-755-2300
800-776-4332
FAX 309-755-2377
TDY:800-933-8331
http://www.linguisystems.com
e-mail: service@linguisystems.com
LinguiSystems Staff, Author
Linda Bowers, Co-Owner/Co-Founder
Rosemary Huisingh, Co-Owner/Co-Founder

Our reading series uses a developmental approach based on the latest research in phonological awareness and early reading skills. Primary books are for ages 5-7. Great as a reading curriculum or to supplement your current reading program. *$104.85*

200 pages Ages 5-7

1488 100% Reading: Decoding and Word Recognition: 5-book set
LinguiSystems
3100 4th Avenue
East Moline, IL 61244
309-755-2300
800-776-4332
FAX 309-755-2377
TDY:800-933-8331
http://www.linguisystems.com
e-mail: service@linguisystems.com
LinguiSystems Staff, Author
Linda Bowers, Co-Owner/Co-Founder
Rosemary Huisingh, Co-Owner/Co-Founder

Our reading series uses a developmental approach based on the latest research in phonological awareness and early reading skills. Primary books are for ages 5-7. Intermediate books are for ages 8-10. Great as a reading curriculum or to supplement your current reading program. *$174.75*
200 pages Ages 5-10

1489 100% Reading: Intermediate Book 1
LinguiSystems
3100 4th Avenue
East Moline, IL 61244
309-755-2300
800-776-4332
FAX 309-755-2377
TDY:800-933-8331
http://www.linguisystems.com
e-mail: service@linguisystems.com
LinguiSystems Staff, Author
Linda Bowers, Co-Owner/Co-Founder
Rosemary Huisingh, Co-Owner/Co-Founder

Our reading series uses a developmental approach based on the latest research in phonological awareness and early reading skills. Great as a reading curriculum or to supplement your current reading program. Intermediate Book 1 covers: schwa, vowel sounds, consonant sounds, hard and soft c and g sound, and silent letters. *$34.95*
211 pages Ages 8-10

1490 100% Reading: Intermediate Book 2
LinguiSystems
3100 4th Avenue
East Moline, IL 61244
309-755-2300
800-776-4332
FAX 309-755-2377
TDY:800-933-8331
http://www.linguisystems.com
e-mail: service@linguisystems.com
LinguiSystems Staff, Author
Linda Bowers, Co-Owner/Co-Founder
Rosemary Huisingh, Co-Owner/Co-Founder

Our reading series uses a developmental approach based on the latest research in phonological awareness and early reading skills. Great as a reading curriculum or to supplement your current reading program. Intermediate Book 2 covers: syllables, root words and affixes, plurals and possessive, contractions, homonyms, and word endings. *$34.95*
221 pages Ages 8-10

1491 100% Reading: Primary Book 1
LinguiSystems
3100 4th Avenue
East Moline, IL 61244
309-755-2300
800-776-4332
FAX 309-755-2377
TDY:800-933-8331
http://www.linguisystems.com
e-mail: service@linguisystems.com
LinguiSystems Staff, Author
Linda Bowers, Co-Owner/Co-Founder
Rosemary Huisingh, Co-Owner/Co-Founder

Our reading series uses a developmental approach based on the latest research in phonological awareness and early reading skills. Primary books are ages 5-7. Great as a reading curriculum or to supplement your current reading program. Primary Book 1 covers: sight words, short vowels, long vowels, and sorry vowels oo, ow, oi, aw, er. *$34.95*
194 pages Ages 5-7

1492 100% Reading: Primary Book 2
LinguiSystems
3100 4th Avenue
East Moline, IL 61244
309-755-2300
800-776-4332
FAX 309-755-2377
TDY:800-933-8331
http://www.linguisystems.com
e-mail: service@linguisystems.com
LinguiSystems Staff, Author
Linda Bowers, Co-Owner/Co-Founder
Rosemary Huisingh, Co-Owner/Co-Founder

Our reading series uses a developmental approach based on the latest research in phonological awareness and early reading skills. Primary books are ages 5-7. Great as a reading curriculum or to supplement your current reading program. Primary Book 2 covers: sight words, beginning consonants, and ending constants. *$34.95*
200 pages Ages 5-7

1493 100% Reading: Primary Book 3
LinguiSystems
3100 4th Avenue
East Moline, IL 61244
309-755-2300
800-776-4332
FAX 309-755-2377
TDY:800-933-8331
http://www.linguisystems.com
e-mail: service@linguisystems.com
LinguiSystems Staff, Author
Linda Bowers, Co-Owner/Co-Founder
Rosemary Huisingh, Co-Owner/Co-Founder

Our reading series uses a developmental approach based on the latest research in phonological awareness and early reading skills. Primary books are ages 5-7. Great as a reading curriculum or to supplement your current reading program. Primary Book 3 covers: intial blends, final blends, consonant digraphs, vowel digraphs, vowel dipthongs, sounds of y. *$34.95*
233 pages Ages 5-7

1494 125 Ways to Be a Better Reader
LinguiSystems
3100 4th Avenue
East Moline, IL 61244
309-755-2300
800-776-4332
FAX 309-755-2377
TDY:800-933-8331
http://www.linguisystems.com
e-mail: service@linguisystems.com
Elizabeth M Wadlington, Paula S Currie, Author
Linda Bowers, Co-Owner/Co-Founder
Rosemary Huisingh, Co-Owner/Co-Founder

Get 125 strategies to improve decoding and conprehension skills. You'll improve reading abilities and attitudes in seven major areas including: getting ready to read, decoding, comprehension, content area reading, reading for test, reading reference materials, and the reading-writing connection. *$35.95*
180 pages Ages 10-16

1495 Animals of the Rain Forest: Steadwell
Harcourt Achieve
Customer Service, 5th Floor
Orlando, FL 32887
800-284-7019
FAX 800-699-9459
http://www.harcourtachieve.com
e-mail: webmaster@harcourt.com
Steck-Vaughn Staff, Author
Tim McEwen, President/CEO
Susan Canizares, SVP Publisher
Lee Wilson, VP Marketing
When reading is a struggle, academic success is even harder to achieve. Now you can put social studies and science curriculum content within reach of every student with this series. Designed specifically for limited readers. *$ 44.40*

ISBN 0-739849-32-8

1496 Ants in His Pants: Absurdities and Realities of Special Education

Peytral Publications
PO Box 1162
Minnetonka, MN 55345
952-949-8707
877-739-8725
FAX 952-906-9777
http://www.peytral.com
e-mail: help@peytral.com

Michael F Giangreco, Author
Kevin Ruelle, Illustrator
Peggy Hammeken, President

With wit, humor and profound one liners, Michael Giagreco will transform your thinking as you take a lighter look at the sometimes comical and occasionally harsh truths in the ever changing field of special education. *$19.95*

128 pages
ISBN 1-890455-42-3

1497 AppleSeeds

Cobblestone Publishing - Division of Cane Pub. Co.
30 Grove Street
Peterborough, NH 03458
603-924-7209
800-821-0115
FAX 603-924-7380
http://www.cricketmag.com
e-mail: swbuc@aol.com

Susan Buckley, Editor
Annabel Wildrick, Associate Editor

An award winning magazine of adventure and exploration for children ages 7 to 9. Provides kids with themed issues that explore a different topic with insightful articles, cool photographs, and a unique you-are-there perspective on culture and history. *$29.95*

36 pages 9 times a year

1498 Basic Level Workbook for Aphasia

Abilitations Speech Bin
PO Box 922668
Norcross, GA 30010
770-449-5700
800-850-8602
FAX 770-510-7290
http://www.speechbin.com
e-mail: info@speechbin.com

Susan Howell Brubaker, Author
Tobi Isaacs, Catalog Director

If you work with adolescents and adults with mild to moderate language deficits or limited, impaired, or emerging reading skills, this workbook is what you've been waiting for! The mMaterial is relevant to their lives, interests, experiences, and vocabulary. Item number W324. *$54.29*

1499 Beyond the Code

Educators Publishing Service
PO Box 9031
Cambridge, MA 02139
617-547-6706
800-225-5750
FAX 888-440-2665
http://www.epsbooks.com
e-mail: eps@epsbooks.com

Nancy M Hall, Author
Gunnar Voltz, President

Beyond the Code gives beginning readers experience reading original stories as well as thinking about what they have read. This companion series follows the same phonetic progression as the frist 4 books of the popular Explode the Code program.

1500 Book Reports Plus

Harcourt Achieve
6277 Sea Harbor Drive
Orlando, FL 32887
252-480-3200
800-531-5015
FAX 800-699-9459
http://www.steckvaughn.com
e-mail: info@steckvaughn.com

Steck-Vaughn Staff, Author
Tim McEwen, President/CEO
Jeff Johnson, Dir Marketing Communications
Chris Lehmann, Team Coordinator

Readers of all levels and abilities will be able to participate in activities that allow them to respond to literature in nontraditional ways. Six units include written and oral reports, dramatizations, and other expressive media. Multiple graphic organizers reinforce the habits of planning and preparing for reading, writing, and presenting.

96 pages

1501 Bridges to Reading Comprehension

Harcourt Achieve
6277 Sea Harbor Drive
Orlando, FL 32887
252-480-3200
800-531-5015
FAX 800-699-9459
http://www.steckvaughn.com
e-mail: info@steckvaughn.com

Steck-Vaughn Staff, Author
Tim McEwen, President/CEO
Jeff Johnson, Dir Marketing Communications
Chris Lehmann, Team Coordinator

Lets your readers build skills in the context of high quality fiction and nonfiction selections.

1502 Careers

Harcourt Achieve
6277 Sea Harbor Drive
Orlando, FL 32887
252-480-3200
800-531-5015
FAX 800-699-9459
http://www.steckvaughn.com
e-mail: info@steckvaughn.com

Heyworth, Author
Tim McEwen, President/CEO
Jeff Johnson, Dir Marketing Communications
Chris Lehmann, Team Coordinator

Develop reading skills while expanding students frames of reference in employment. A highly accessible preview of vocational, technical, and professional career opportunities on both today's and tomorrow's job market. Eight thematic units per title present overviews of careers in health, science, community service, agriculture and forestry circuitry, communications, entertainment and the creative industries.

1503 Claims to Fame

Educators Publishing Service
PO Box 9031
Cambridge, MA 02139
617-547-6706
800 225-5750
FAX 888-440-2665
http://www.epsbooks.com
e-mail: eps@epsbooks.com

Carol Einstein, Author
Gunnar Voltz, President

The three exercises after each reading are tailored to the content of each story. In Thinking About What You Have Read, students check and extend their understanding of the story. Working with Words asks students to think about and experiment with vaious word meanings.

1504 Clues to Meaning

Educators Publishing Service
PO Box 9031
Cambridge, MA 02139
617-547-6706
800-225-5750
FAX 888-440-2665
http://www.epsbooks.com
e-mail: eps@epsbooks.com

Ann L Staman, Author
Gunnar Voltz, President

A versatile series which teaches beginning readers to use the sounds of letters as one strategy among many in learning to read.

Ages 6-10

1505 Connect-A-Card
Abilitations Speech Bin
PO Box 922668
Norcross, GA 30010
770-449-5700
800-850-8602
FAX 770-510-7290
http://www.speechbin.com
e-mail: info@speechbin.com
Tobi Isaacs, Catalog Director

How to teach your 6-12 year olds how to build tons of sentences, each using two illustrated phrase cards plus a common conjunction. Word cards feature four coordinating and, but, or, yet and eleven subordinating after, although, because, before, if, since, so that, unless, until, when, while conjunctions; clear black and white picture cards foster creative sentence construction. Item number Q974. *$40.99*

1506 Cosmic Reading Journey
Sunburst Technology
1550 Executive Drive
Elgin, IL 60123
800-321-7511
FAX 888-800-3028
http://http://store.sunburst.com/Home.aspx
e-mail: service@sunburst.com
Michael Guillory, Channel Sales/Marketing Manager

This reading comprehension program provides meaningful summary and writing activities for the 100 books that early readers and their teachers love most.

1507 Creepy Cave Initial Consonants
Sunburst Technology
1550 Executive Drive
Elgin, IL 60123
800-321-7511
FAX 888-800-3028
http://http://store.sunburst.com/Home.aspx
e-mail: service@sunburst.com
Michael Guillory, Channel Sales/Marketing Manager

Help your students develop letter recognition and phonemic awareness skills matching words with the same initial consonant letter in a Creepy Cave.

1508 Curious Creatures Program: Owls-Spiders-Wolves-Snakes-Bats
Curriculum Associates
PO Box 2001
North Billerica, MA 01862
800-225-0248
FAX 800-366-1158
http://www.curriculumassociates.com
e-mail: cainfo@curriculumassociates.com
Louis Jame Taris, James Robert Taris, Author
Frank Ferguson, President

Users of this award-winning multimedia program say awesome! They learn little known facts about animals that make most of us cringe. Designed to encourage reluctant readers in grades 4 and above, the program is also appropriate for on-level students in grades 2-3. Students learn the language of life science as they strengthen their reading and comprehension skills.

1509 Decoding Games
LinguiSystems
3100 4th Ave
East Moline, IL 61244
309-755-2300
800-776-4332
FAX 309-755-2377
TDY:800-933-8331
http://www.linguisystems.com
e-mail: service@linguisystems.com
Tina Sanford, Author
Linda Bowers, Co-Owner/Co-Founder
Rosemary Huisingh, Co-Owner/Co-Founder

Get three fun games in one handy case. These colorful games target tricky decoding skills your students need for strong reading skills. *$39.95*

1510 Dyslexia Training Program
Educators Publishing Service
PO Box 9031
Cambridge, MA 02139
617-547-6706
800-225-5750
FAX 888-440-2665
http://www.epsbooks.com
e-mail: eps@epsbooks.com
Texas Scottish Rite Hospital For Children, Author
Gunnar Voltz, President

Introduces reading and writing skills to dyslexic children through a two-year, cumulative series of daily one-hour videotaped lessons and accompanying student's books and teacher's guides.

1511 Earobics® Clinic Version 1 for Adolescents & Adults
Abilitations Speech Bin
PO Box 922668
Norcross, GA 30010
770-449-5700
800-850-8602
FAX 770-510-7290
http://www.speechbin.com
e-mail: info@speechbin.com
Tobi Isaacs, Catalog Director

The Clinician/Specialist Version has twelve name slots per workstation and goal writing and charting capability to save professional time. This level is also available in a Home Version limited to two users. Both versions offer hundreds of levels of play, appealing graphics, and entertaining music. Item number C486. *$298.99*

1512 Earobics® Clinic Version Step 1
Abilitations Speech Bin
PO Box 922668
Norcross, GA 30010
770-449-5700
800-850-8602
FAX 770-510-7290
http://www.speechbin.com
e-mail: info@speechbin.com
Tobi Isaacs, Catalog Director

Earobics is a dazzling software that teaches phonological awareness and auditory processing. It systematically — anf enjoyably — trains these critical skills for development ages four to seven years. Item number C482. *$298.99*

1513 Earobics® for Adolescents & Adults Home Version
Abilitations Speech Bin
PO Box 922668
Norcross, GA 30010
770-449-5700
800-850-8602
FAX 770-510-7290
http://www.speechbin.com
e-mail: info@speechbin.com
Tobi Isaacs, Catalog Director

Two users may use the Home Version which offers hundreds of levels of play, age-appropriate graphics, and entertaining music. This level is also available in a professional version for specialists and clinicians. Item number C485. *$58.99*

1514 EarobicsM® Step 1 Home Version
Abilitations Speech Bin
PO Box 922668
Norcross, GA 30010
770-449-5700
800-850-8602
FAX 770-510-7290
http://www.speechbin.com
e-mail: info@speechbin.com
Tobi Isaacs, Catalog Director

Step 1 offers hundreds of levels of play, appealing graphics, and entertaining music to train the critical auditory skills young children need for success in learning. Item number C481. *$58.99*

1515 **Emergent Reader**
Sunburst Technology
1550 Executive Drive
Elgin, IL 60123
800-321-7511
FAX 888-800-3028
http://http://store.sunburst.com/Home.aspx
e-mail: service@sunburst.com
Michael Guillory, Channel Sales/Marketing Manager

This story-reading program supports the efforts of beginning readers by developing their sight word vocabularies.

1516 **Every Child a Reader**
Sunburst Technology
1550 Executive Drive
Elgin, IL 60123
800-321-7511
FAX 888-800-3028
http://http://store.sunburst.com/Home.aspx
e-mail: service@sunburst.com
Michael Guillory, Channel Sales/Marketing Manager

Traditional reading strategies in a rich literary context. Designed to promote independent reading and develop oral and written language expression.

1517 **Explode the Code**
Educators Publishing Service
PO Box 9031
Cambridge, MA 02139
617-547-6706
800-225-5750
FAX 888-440-2665
http://www.epsbooks.com
e-mail: eps@epsbooks.com
Nancy M Hall, Rena Price, Author
Gunnar Voltz, President

Explode the Code provides a sequential, systematic approach to phonics in which students blend sounds to build vocabulary and read words, phrases, sentences, and stories.

1518 **Expressway to Reading**
Harcourt Achieve
Customer Service, 5th Floor
Orlando, FL 32887
800-284-7019
FAX 800-699-9459
http://www.harcourtachieve.com
e-mail: webmaster@harcourt.com
Davis, Author
Tim McEwen, President/CEO
Susan Canizares, SVP Publisher
Lee Wilson, VP Marketing
Now parents can make everyday activities fun exercises in reading. These skill building and practice activities turn ordinary errands into opportunities for progress. *$518.40*

ISBN 0-739829-95-5

1519 **Funology Fables**
Abilitations Speech Bin
PO Box 922668
Norcross, GA 30010
770-449-5700
800-850-8602
FAX 770-510-7290
http://www.speechbin.com
e-mail: info@speechbin.com
Tobi Isaacs, Catalog Director

Funology Fables targets specific phonemes and critical early concepts, such as matching, sequencing, opposites, comparisons, quantity, size, and space. Reproducible Talking Tales and activities include 32 six-part sequence stories. Item number 1484. *$47.95*

1520 **Great Series Great Rescues**
Harcourt Achieve
Customer Service, 5th Floor
Orlando, FL 32887
800-284-7019
FAX 800-699-9459
http://www.harcourtachieve.com
e-mail: webmaster@harcourt.com
Tim McEwen, President/CEO
Susan Canizares, SVP Publisher
Lee Wilson, VP Marketing
Human drama makes beginning reading worth the effort. Eight exciting titles build confidence as they build skills. Short, easy-to-read selections enable limited readers to succeed with material that matters. *$15.00*

ISBN 0-811441-76-8

1521 **Handprints**
Educators Publishing Service
PO Box 9031
Cambridge, MA 02139
617-547-6706
800-225-5750
FAX 888-440-2665
http://www.epsbooks.com
e-mail: eps@epsbooks.com
Ann L Staman, Author
Gunnar Voltz, President

Handprints is a set of 50 storybooks and 4 workbooks for beginning readers in kindergarten and first grade. The storybooks increase in difficulty very gradually and encourage the new readers to use meaning, language, and print cues as they read.

1522 **High Interest Nonfiction**
Harcourt Achieve
Customer Service, 5th Floor
Orlando, FL 32887
800-284-7019
FAX 800-699-9459
http://www.harcourtachieve.com
e-mail: webmaster@harcourt.com
Steck-Vaughn Staff, Author
Tim McEwen, President/CEO
Susan Canizares, SVP Publisher
Lee Wilson, VP Marketing
Whether you want to promote the joy of reading or the thrill of reading riveting nonfiction, this series does the job. Amazing stories of adventure, mystery, escape, disaster, rescue, challenge, firsts, and heroes capture and hold student interest. *$11.99*

1523 **High Interest Nonfiction for Primary Grades**
Harcourt Achieve
Customer Service, 5th Floor
Orlando, FL 32887
800-284-7019
FAX 800-699-9459
http://www.harcourtachieve.com
e-mail: webmaster@harcourt.com
Steck-Vaughn Staff, Author
Tim McEwen, President/CEO
Susan Canizares, SVP Publisher
Lee Wilson, VP Marketing
Introduce students to a new type of reading in which the reader gains information! As students read nonfiction, they continue to develop and build reading comprehension skills and reading strategies. Fun and exciting stories are organized into four units that support the curriculum, such as people, animals, Earth and space , and more. *$11.99*

1524 **High Noon Books**
Academic Therapy Publications
20 Commercial Boulevard
Novato, CA 94949
415-883-3314
800-422-7249
FAX 888-287-9975
http://www.academictherapy.com
e-mail: sales@academictherapy.com
Jim Arena
Joanne Urban

Serving the field of learning disabilities for 35 years. High-interest books for reluctant readers, phonic remedial reading lessons, streamlined Shakespeare, etc.

1525 I Can Read
Teddy Bear Press
3639 Midway Drive
San Diego, CA 92110
858-560-8718
FAX 858-874-0423
http://www.teddybearpress.net
e-mail: fparker@teddybearpress.net
Fran Parker, Author
Fran Parker, President

A series of 7 reading books and 7 workbooks, a set of 52 flashcards and teacher manual which uses a sight word approach to teach beginning readers. These teacher created books and workbooks present an easy to use beginning reading program which provides repetition, visual motor, visual discrimination and word comprehension activities. It was created to teach young, learning disabled children and has been successfully employed to teach beginning readers of varying ages and abilities. *$80.00*

1526 I Can See the ABC's
Teddy Bear Press
3639 Midway Drive
San Diego, CA 92110
858-560-8718
FAX 858-874-0423
http://www.teddybearpress.net
e-mail: fparker@teddybearpress.net
Fran Parker, Author
Fran Parker, President

A big 11x17 which contains the pre-primer words found in the I Can Read program while introducing the alphabet. *$20.00*

1527 Inclusion: Strategies for Working with Young Children
Peytral Publications
PO Box 1162
Minnetonka, MN 55345
952-949-8707
877-739-8725
FAX 952-906-9777
http://www.peytral.com
e-mail: help@peytral.com
Lorraine O Moore PhD, Author
Peggy Hammeken, President

This exceptional resource is a gold mine of developmentally based ideas to help children between the ages of 3-7 or older students who may be developmentally delayed. This is a very practical and easy-to-use publication which is appropriate for early childhood teachers, K-2 general and special education teachers. *$21.95*

185 pages Educators
ISBN 1-890455-33-4

1528 Island Reading Journey
Sunburst Technology
1550 Executive Drive
Elgin, IL 60123
800-321-7511
FAX 888-800-3028
http://http://store.sunburst.com/Home.aspx
e-mail: service@sunburst.com
Michael Guillory, Channel Sales/Marketing Manager

Enhance your reading program with meaningful summary and extension activities for 100 intermediate level books. Students read for meaning while they engage in activities that test for comprehension, build writing skills with reader response and essay questions, develop usage skills with cloze activities and improve vocabulary/word attack skills.

1529 It's a...Safari: Software
Abilitations Speech Bin
PO Box 922668
Norcross, GA 30010
770-449-5700
800-850-8602
FAX 770-510-7290
http://www.speechbin.com
e-mail: info@speechbin.com
Tobi Isaacs, Catalog Director

It's a Safari improves these critical skills: auditory processing; reading; spelling and comprehension. This unique Locu Tour language software presents a total of 100 short stories which describe the animals and people of Africa. Item number L190. *$28.99*

1530 Just for Me! Phonological Awareness
LinguiSystems
3100 4th Avenue
East Moline, IL 61244
309-755-2300
800-776-4332
FAX 309-755-2377
TDY:800-933-8331
http://www.linguisystems.com
e-mail: service@linguisystems.com
Margaret Warner, Author
Linda Bowers, Co-Owner/Co-Founder
Rosemary Huisingh, Co-Owner/Co-Founder

Youngsters will love this cut, color, and create approach to sound awareness. You'll love how they begin to learn strong reading and literacy skills. The hands-on activities help students learn rhyming, syllables, compound words, beginning and ending sounds, short and long vowels, and beginning blends. *$24.95*

154 pages Ages 3-6

1531 Kids Media Magic 2.0
Sunburst Technology
1550 Executive Drive
Elgin, IL 60123
800-321-7511
FAX 888-800-3028
http://http://store.sunburst.com/Home.aspx
e-mail: service@sunburst.com
Michael Guillory, Channel Sales/Marketing Manager

The first multimedia word processor designed for young children. Help your child become a fluent reader and writer. The Rebus Bar automatically scrolls over 45 vocabulary words as students type.

1532 LD Teacher's IEP Companion
LinguiSystems
3100 4th Avenue
East Moline, IL 61244
309-755-2300
800-776-4332
FAX 309-755-2377
TDY:800-933-8331
http://www.linguisystems.com
e-mail: service@linguisystems.com
Molly Lyle, Author
Linda Bowers, Co-Owner/Co-Founder
Rosemary Huisingh, Co-Owner/Co-Founder

These IEP goals are organized developmentally by skill area with individual objectives and classroom activity suggestions. Goals and objectives cover these academic areas: math; reading; writing; literacy concepts; attention skills; study skills; classroom behavior; social interaction; and transition skills. *$39.95*
169 pages Ages 5-18

1533 Learning 100 Computerized Reading Skills
Harcourt Achieve
Customer Service, 5th Floor
Orlando, FL 32887
800-284-7019
FAX 800-699-9459
http://www.harcourtachieve.com
e-mail: webmaster@harcourt.com
Steck-Vaughn Staff, Author
Tim McEwen, President/CEO
Susan Canizares, SVP Publisher
Lee Wilson, VP Marketing
Now you can determine each individual's precise reading level and mastery of individual comprehension skills automatically with this extraordinary accurate, easy-to-use program. Computer-administered cloze and criterion referenced tests yield the results you need as well as personalized prescriptions. *$410.80*

1534 **Learning 100 Computerized Reading Skills: Inventory**
Harcourt Achieve
6277 Sea Harbor Drive
Orlando, FL 32887
252-480-3200
800-531-5015
FAX 800-699-9459
http://www.steckvaughn.com
e-mail: info@steckvaughn.com
Steck-Vaughn Staff, Author
Tim McEwen, President/CEO
Jeff Johnson, Dir Marketing Communications
Chris Lehmann, Team Coordinator
Planning and placement without the guesswork. Now you can determine each individual's precise reading level and mastery of individual comprehension skills automatically with this extraordinary accurate, easy-to-use program.

1535 **Learning 100 Go Books**
Harcourt Achieve
6277 Sea Harbor Drive
Orlando, FL 32887
252-480-3200
800-531-5015
FAX 800-699-9459
http://www.steckvaughn.com
e-mail: info@steckvaughn.com
Steck-Vaughn Staff, Author
Tim McEwen, President/CEO
Jeff Johnson, Dir Marketing Communications
Chris Lehmann, Team Coordinator
Go Books offer readers at all levels the opportunity to experience reading success with real-life content in an enjoyable environment. Softcover anthologies offer variety. Each book contains stories dealing with real-life situations in both fiction and nonfiction presentations.

1536 **Learning 100 Language Clues Software**
Harcourt Achieve
6277 Sea Harbor Drive
Orlando, FL 32887
252-480-3200
800-531-5015
FAX 800-699-9459
http://www.steckvaughn.com
e-mail: info@steckvaughn.com
Steck-Vaughn Staff, Author
Tim McEwen, President/CEO
Jeff Johnson, Dir Marketing Communications
Chris Lehmann, Team Coordinator
When learners have control over their instruction, they are motivated to succeed. This program lets users customize instruction to their individual needs. They can control the speed of presentation, the number of times a word is used, and the length of time each word appears.

1537 **Learning 100 System**
Harcourt Achieve
6277 Sea Harbor Drive
Orlando, FL 32887
252-480-3200
800-531-5015
FAX 800-699-9459
http://www.steckvaughn.com
e-mail: info@steckvaughn.com
Steck-Vaughn Staff, Author
Tim McEwen, President/CEO
Jeff Johnson, Dir Marketing Communications
Chris Lehmann, Team Coordinator
Deliver research-based reading strategies in the context of real-life stories. If your readers need extra motivation, this program is a must. Compelling, relevant stories coupled with audio instruction build vocabulary, comprehension, and confidence. Built on findings from 40 years of reading research, Learning 100 Reading Strategies is a proven performer for low-level readers.

1538 **Learning 100 Write and Read**
Harcourt Achieve
6277 Sea Harbor Drive
Orlando, FL 32887
252-480-3200
800-531-5015
FAX 800-699-9459
http://www.steckvaughn.com
e-mail: info@steckvaughn.com
Steck-Vaughn Staff, Author
Tim McEwen, President/CEO
Jeff Johnson, Dir Marketing Communications
Chris Lehmann, Team Coordinator
Helps learners succeed with reading and writing opportunities they encounter every day. Learners improve grammar, mechanics, usage, style, and paragraphing skills through a proven program based on more than 40 years of research.

1539 **Let's Go Read 1: An Island Adventure**
Riverdeep
100 Pine Street
San Francisco, CA 94111
415-659-2000
FAX 415-659-2020
http://www.riverdeep.net
e-mail: info@riverdeep.net
Barry O'Callaghan, Executive Chairman/CEO

Take off with Robby the Raccoon, Emily the Squirrel and the Reading Rover on an exciting adventure to an island inhabited by the alphabet. Motivated by the delight of mastering new challenges, your child will play through more than 35 fun activties that install and reinforce the essential skills for successful reading.

1540 **Let's Go Read 2: An Ocean Adventure**
Riverdeep
100 Pine Street
San Francisco, CA 94111
415-659-2000
FAX 415-659-2020
http://www.riverdeep.net
e-mail: info@riverdeep.net
Barry O'Callaghan, Executive Chairman

Building upon your child's mastery of letters, Let's Go Read: 2 explores how letters combine to form words, and how words combine to express meaning. Dozens of captivating, skill-building activities teach your child the skills to sound out, recognize, build and comprehend hundreds of new words. It's an endlessly fun voyage toward reading fluency!

1541 **Let's Read**
Educators Publishing Service
PO Box 9031
Cambridge, MA 02139
617-547-6706
800-225-5750
FAX 888-440-2665
http://www.epsbooks.com
e-mail: eps@epsbooks.com
Leonard Bloomfield, Clarence and Robert Barnhart, Author
Gunnar Voltz, President

Using a linguistic approach to teaching reading skills, this series emphasizes relationship of spelling to sound, presenting the concepts together, and providing nine reading books and accompanying workbooks for practice. Provides classroom directions and suggestions for supplementary exercises.

1542 **Lighthouse Low Vision Products**
Lighthouse International
Sol & Lillian Goldman Building
New York, NY 10022
212-821-9200
800-829-0500
FAX 212-821-9707
http://www.lighthouse.org
e-mail: info@lighthouse.com
Jeffrey Eaton, Stewardship Manager

Helping people who are blind or partially sighted to lead independent and productive lives.

1543 **Linamood Program (LIPS Clinical Version):Phoneme Sequencing Program for Reading, Spelling,Speech**

LinguiSystems
3100 4th Avenue
East Moline, IL 61244
309-755-2300
800-776-4332
FAX 309-755-2377
TDY:800-933-8331
http://www.linguisystems.com
e-mail: service@linguisystems.com
Patricia Linamood, Phyllis Linamood, Author
Linda Bowers, Co-Owner/Co-Founder
Rosemary Huisingh, Co-Owner/Co-Founder

Help your students develop phoneme awareness for competence in reading, spelling, and speech. This multisensory program meets the needs of the many children and adults who don't develop phonemic awareness through traditional methods. *$247.00*

Birth-Adult

1544 **Mastering Reading Series**

AGS Publishing
PO Box 99
Circle Pines, MN 55014
651-287-7220
800-328-2560
FAX 800-471-8457
http://www.agsnet.com
e-mail: agsmail@agsnet.com
Kevin Brueggeman, President
Matt Keller, Marketing Manager

With an interest level of High School through Adult, and a reading level of Grade 3-7, this series will help your students build reading and life skills while learning about specific occupations. Each series features four books of increasing complexity in reading level, allowing learners to work at their own pace to master essential reading skills. The five series titles are: Office Work; Health Care; Commercial Trucking; Food Service and Manufacturing.

1545 **Megawords**

Educators Publishing Service
PO Box 9031
Cambridge, MA 02139
617-547-6706
800-225-5750
FAX 888-440-2665
http://www.epsbooks.com
e-mail: eps@epsbooks.com
Kristin Johnson, Polly Baird, Author
Gunnar Voltz, President

A series with a systematic, multisensory approach to learning the longer words encountered from fourth grade on. Students first work with syllables, then combine the syllables into words, use them in context, and work to increase their reading and spelling proficiency. Teacher's Guide and Answer Key available.

1546 **Mike Mulligan & His Steam Shovel**

Sunburst Technology
1550 Executive Drive
Elgin, IL 60123
800-321-7511
FAX 888-800-3028
http://http://store.sunburst.com/Home.aspx
e-mail: service@sunburst.com
Michael Guillory, Channel Sales/Marketing Manager

This CD-ROM version of the Caldecott classic lets students experience interactive book reading and participate in four skills-based extension activities that promote memory, matching, sequencing, listening, pattern recognition and map reading skills.

1547 **More Primary Phonics**

Educators Publishing Service
PO Box 9031
Cambridge, MA 02139
617-547-6706
800-225-5750
FAX 888-440-2665
http://www.epsbooks.com
e-mail: eps@epsbooks.com
Barbara Makar, Author
Gunnar Voltz, President

Reinforces and expands skills developed in Primary Phonics. Workbooks and storybooks contain the same phonetic elements, sight words and phonetic sequences as workbooks 1 and 2.

1548 **Mythopoly**

LinguiSystems
3100 4th Avenue
East Moline, IL 61244
309-755-2300
800-776-4332
FAX 309-755-2377
TDY:800-933-8331
http://www.linguisystems.com
e-mail: service@linguisystems.com
Mike LoGiudice, Carolyn LoGiudice, Author
Linda Bowers, Co-Owner/Co-Founder
Rosemary Huisingh, Co-Owner/Co-Founder

Boost your student's reading and listening comprehension skills with this wonderful game. Engaging stories from classical mythology help students understand references to mythological concepts in literature and everyday life. The reading level of the 25 stories ranges from grades 3.5 to 5.2. *$44.95*

Ages 10-18

1549 **New Way: Learning with Literature**

Harcourt Achieve
6277 Sea Harbor Drive
Orlando, FL 32887
252-480-3200
800-531-5015
FAX 800-699-9459
http://www.steckvaughn.com
e-mail: info@steckvaughn.com
Steck-Vaughn Staff, Author
Tim McEwen, President/CEO
Jeff Johnson, Dir Marketing Communications
Chris Lehmann, Team Coordinator

Do you need additional literature your primary readers can read independently? Steck-Vaughn offers a large collection of developmentally appropriate titles at attractive prices.

1550 **Next Stop**

Educators Publishing Service
PO Box 9031
Cambridge, MA 02139
617-547-6706
800-225-5750
FAX 888-440-2665
http://www.epsbooks.com
e-mail: eps@epsbooks.com
Tanya Auger, Author
Gunnar Voltz, President

Increase reading and language skills while exploring different literacy genres. This series is intended for students who are ready to move beyond phonetically controlled readers to the nest stop-real chapter books that will help prepare them for the more challenging literature they will encounter in later grades.

1551 **PATHS**

Abilitations Speech Bin
PO Box 922668
Norcross, GA 30010
770-449-5700
800-850-8602
FAX 770-510-7290
http://www.speechbin.com
e-mail: info@speechbin.com
Tobi Isaacs, Catalog Director

PATHS gives you a step-by-step comprehensive program for students who have experienced difficulty in academic learning. It targets skills critical for academic achievements: phonological awareness; phonemic relationships; phonemic processing; and listening and memory. Item number 1491. *$22.95*

1552 Patterns of English Spelling
AVKO Educational Research Foundation
3084 W Willard Road
Clio, MI 48420
810-686-1101
866-285-6612
FAX 810-686-1101
http:// www.spelling.org
e-mail: info@avko.org

Don McCabe, Author
Don Cabe, Research Director

Use the index to locate the page upon which you can find all the words that share the same patterns. If you look up the word cat, you will find all the pages where all the at words are located. If you look up the word precious you will find all the words ending in cious. There are ten volumes which can be purchased all together or separately. *$119.95*

Whole set

1553 Phonemic Awareness: The Sounds of Reading
Peytral Publication
PO Box 1162
Minnetonka, MN 55345
952-949-8707
877-739-8725
FAX 952-906-9777
http://www.peytral.com
e-mail: help@peytral.com

Victoria Groves Scott, Author
Peggy Hammeken, President
Peggy Peytral, Publisher
Victoria Scott, Author

In this dynamic new video, Dr. Scott demonstrates the principal components of phonemic awareness: identification; comparison; segmentation; blending and rhyming. This video will help you to better understand phonemic awareness training and will show you how to apply these components not only to the reading curriculum but to all subjects through the school day. Filmed in actual classroom settings. *$59.95*

25 minute video
ISBN 1-890455-29-6

1554 Phonological Awareness Kit
LinguiSystems
3100 4th Avenue
East Moline, IL 61244
309-755-2300
800-776-4332
FAX 309-755-2377
TDY:800-933-8331
http://www.linguisystems.com
e-mail: service@linguisystems.com

Carolyn Robertson, Wanda Salter, Author
Linda Bowers, Co-Owner/Co-Founder
Rosemary Huisingh, Co-Owner/Co-Founder

Help your students learn to use phonological information to process oral and written language with this fantastic kit. Written by an SLP and special educator, this best-seller links sound awareness, oral language, and early reading and writing skills. The kit uses a multisensory approach to ensure success for all learning styles. *$69.95*

115 pages Ages 5-8

1555 Poetry in Three Dimensions: Reading, Writing and Critical Thinking Skills through Poetry
Educators Publishing Service
PO Box 9031
Cambridge, MA 02139
617-547-6706
800-225-5750
FAX 888-440-2665
http://www.epsbooks.com
e-mail: eps@epsbooks.com

Carol Clark, Alison Draper, Author
Gunnar Voltz, President

Help your students improve their reading comprehension and writing through the study of poetry in this collection of multicultural poems. With poems and questions on facing pages, students are encouraged to annotate the text of the poem and to go back to the text to respond to the questions.

1556 Polar Express
Sunburst Technology
1550 Executive Drive
Elgin, IL 60123
800-321-7511
FAX 888-800-3028
http://http://store.sunburst.com/Home.aspx
e-mail: service@sunburst.com

Michael Guillory, Channel Sales/Marketing Manager

Share the magic and enchantment of the holiday season with this CD-ROM version of Chris Van Allsburg's Caldecott-winning picture book.

1557 Prehistoric Creaures Then & Now: Steadwell
Harcourt Achieve
Customer Service, 5th Floor
Orlando, FL 32887
800-284-7019
FAX 800-699-9459
http://www.harcourtachieve.com
e-mail: webmaster@harcourt.com

Steck-Vaughn Staff, Author
Tim McEwen, President/CEO
Susan Canizares, SVP Publisher
Lee Wilson, VP Marketing

When reading is a struggle, academic success is even harder to achieve. Now you can put social studies and science curriculum content within reach of every students with Steadwell Books — the series designed specifically for limited readers. Attention-getting photos and informative illustrations, maps, and time lines communicate the social studies and science concepts found in the text. *$44.40*

ISBN 0-739822-07-1

1558 Primary Phonics
Educators Publishing Service
PO Box 9031
Cambridge, MA 02139
617-547-6706
800-225-5750
FAX 888-440-2665
http://www.epsbooks.com
e-mail: eps@epsbooks.com

Barbara Makar, Author
Gunnar Voltz, President

This revised program of storybooks and coordinated workbooks teaches reading for grades K-2. There is a set of ten storybooks to go with each of the first five workbooks. A Primary Phonics Picture Dictionary contains 2,500 commonly used words, including most of the words in the series. This series' individualized nature permits students to progress at their own speed. Teacher's manual available.

1559 Racing Through Time on a Flying Machine
Harcourt Achieve
6277 Sea Harbor Drive
Orlando, FL 32887
252-480-3200
800-531-5015
FAX 800-699-9459
http://www.steckvaughn.com
e-mail: info@steckvaughn.com

Elizabeth Werley-Prieto, Mike Lester, Author
Tim McEwen, President/CEO
Jeff Johnson, Dir Marketing Communications
Chris Lehmann, Team Coordinator

Traveling through time to visit Thomas Edison and Leonardo da Vinci inspires young Keene to become an inventor himself.

1560 Read On! Plus
Sunburst Technology
1550 Executive Drive
Elgin, IL 60123
800-321-7511
FAX 888-800-3028
http://http://store.sunburst.com/Home.aspx
e-mail: service@sunburst.com

Michael Guillory, Channel Sales/Marketing Manager

Promote skills and strategies that improve reading comprehension, and build appreciation for literature and the written word.

1561 **Read-A-Bit**
LinguiSystems
3100 4th Avenue
East Moline, IL 61244
309-755-2300
800-776-4332
FAX 309-755-2377
TDY:800-933-8331
http://www.linguisystems.com
e-mail: service@linguisystems.com
Dagmar Kafka, Author
Linda Bowers, Co-Owner/Co-Founder
Rosemary Huisingh, Co-Owner/Co-Founder

Get 15 games in one box! Six decks of cards with different levels of reading difficulty work with and without the colorful game board to give you plenty of flexibility. You'll work through a hierarchy of reading skills from primer to grade 3. Students practice consonants, vowels, controlled R sounds, sight words, and more. *$41.95*
Ages 5-9

1562 **Reader's Quest I**
Sunburst Technology
1550 Executive Drive
Elgin, IL 60123
800-321-7511
FAX 888-800-3028
http://http://store.sunburst.com/Home.aspx
e-mail: service@sunburst.com
Michael Guillory, Channel Sales/Marketing Manager

These reading workshops provide students with direct reading instruction, interactive practice activities, and practical strategies to ensure reading success.

1563 **Reader's Quest II**
Sunburst Technology
1550 Executive Drive
Elgin, IL 60123
800-321-7511
FAX 888-800-3028
http://http://store.sunburst.com/Home.aspx
e-mail: service@sunburst.com
Michael Guillory, Channel Sales/Marketing Manager

These reading workshops provide students with direct reading instruction, interactive practice activities, and practical strategies to ensure reading success.

1564 **Reading Comprehension Bundle**
Sunburst Technology
1550 Executive Drive
Elgin, IL 60123
800-321-7511
FAX 888-800-3028
http://http://store.sunburst.com/Home.aspx
e-mail: service@sunburst.com
Michael Guillory, Channel Sales/Marketing Manager

This collection for the intermediate-level classroom develops the skills students need to read for meaning and understanding.

1565 **Reading Comprehension Game Intermediate**
LinguiSystems
3100 4th Avenue
East Moline, IL 61244
309-755-2300
800-776-4332
FAX 309-755-2377
TDY:800-933-8331
http://www.linguisystems.com
e-mail: service@linguisystems.com
Linda Bowers, Rosemary Huisingh, Carolyn LoGiudice, Author
Linda Bowers, Co-Owner/Co-Founder
Rosemary Huisingh, Co-Owner/Co-Founder

This game gives you fun, repetitive practice in three essential reading comprehension skills. The first is Reading for Details including cloze, referents, sequencing, describing, and more! The second is Reading for Understanding including main idea, paraphrasing, context clues, defining, and more. The thrid area is Going Beyond including making references, predicting, and making associations. *$44.95*
Ages 12-18

1566 **Reading Comprehension Materials (Volume 5)**
Abilitations Speech Bin
PO Box 922668
Norcross, GA 30010
770-449-5700
800-850-8602
FAX 770-510-7290
http://www.speechbin.com
e-mail: info@speechbin.com
Kathryn M Kilpatrick, Author
Tobi Isaacs, Catalog Director

Three hundred and fifty-one pages of practical large-print materials give older children and adults practice thinking about words, following directions, and telling what/who stories, stories in part, short stories, and more. Stories are either high-interest factual stories or relate to everyday experiences. Tasks are versatile and a variety of difficulties for maximum use. Item number V372. *$56.29*

1567 **Reading Comprehension Series**
Harcourt Achieve
Customer Service, 5th Floor
Orlando, FL 32887
800-284-7019
FAX 800-699-9459
http://www.harcourtachieve.com
e-mail: webmaster@harcourt.com
Tim McEwen, President/CEO
Susan Canizares, SVP Publisher
Lee Wilson, VP Marketing
Develop basic reading skills! Short stories sustain interest! Brief, captivating selections feature children and animals in contemporary situations. Exercises build comprehension skills! Exercises cover all aspects of reading comprehension, including main idea, sequencing, facts, and inferences. *$95.40*

1568 **Reading Comprehension in Varied Subject Matter**
Educators Publishing Service
PO Box 9031
Cambridge, MA 02139
617-547-6706
800-225-5750
FAX 888-440-2665
http://www.epsbooks.com
e-mail: eps@epsbooks.com
Jane Ervin, Author
Gunnar Voltz, President

Ten workbooks that present a wide range of people and situations with new reading selections, new vocabulary, and a new writing exercise. Each book contains 31 selections in the subject areas of social studies, science, literature, mathematics, philosophy, logic, language, and the arts.

1569 **Reading Pen**
Wizcom Technologies
234 Littleton Road
Westford, MA 01886
978-727-0026
FAX 978-727-0032
http://www.wizcomtech.com
e-mail: usa.info@wizcomtech.com
Michael Kenan, CEO

Portable assitive reading device that reads words aloud and can be used anywhere. Scans a word from printed text, displays the word in large characters, reads the word aloud from built-in speaker or ear phones and defines the word with the press of a button. Displays syllables, keeps a history of scanned words, adjustable for left or right-handed use. Includes a tutorial video and audio cassette. Not recommended for persons with low vision or impaired fine motor control. *$279.00*

Teach beginning reading skills effectively with phonics instruction built into engaging games and puzzles that have children asking for more.

1570 Reading Power Modules Books
Harcourt Achieve
Customer Service, 5th Floor
Orlando, FL 32887
800-284-7019
FAX 800-699-9459
http://www.harcourtachieve.com
e-mail: webmaster@harcourt.com
Steven Korten, CEO
Randy Pennington, SVP National Sales

Supplementary reading based on 4 decades of reading research. Companion books give students and teachers a choice of formats. High interest stories reinforce reading comprehension skills while building vocabulary, spelling skills, reading fluency, and speed.

1571 Reading Power Modules Software
Harcourt Achieve
6277 Sea Harbor Drive
Orlando, FL 32887
252-480-3200
800-531-5015
FAX 800-699-9459
http://www.steckvaughn.com
e-mail: info@steckvaughn.com
Steck-Vaughn Staff, Author
Tim McEwen, President/CEO
Jeff Johnson, Dir Marketing Communications
Chris Lehmann, Team Coordinator
This program provides practice and reinforcement of reading comprehension skills while building spelling and reading skills and vocabulary. Exercises include requiring learners to type the new vocabulary word after it flashes on the screen, fill-in-the-blank exercises, timed reading exercises, comprehension checks, vocabulary review in multiple-choice format, and vocabulary games.

1572 Reading Readiness
Harcourt Achieve
6277 Sea Harbor Drive
Orlando, FL 32887
252-480-3200
800-531-5015
FAX 800-699-9459
http://www.steckvaughn.com
e-mail: info@steckvaughn.com
Steck Vaughn Staff, Author
Tim McEwen, President/CEO
Jeff Johnson, Dir Marketing Communications
Chris Lehmann, Team Coordinator
Build a firm foundation for reading success with thematic workbooks that introduce readiness skills through literature. Fun-filled nursery rhymes, riddles, and tongue twisters focus on the key words and sound/letter patterns that precede decoding skills.

1573 Reading Skills Bundle
Sunburst Technology
1550 Executive Drive
Elgin, IL 60123
800-321-7511
FAX 888-800-3028
http://http://store.sunburst.com/Home.aspx
e-mail: service@sunburst.com
Michael Guillory, Channel Sales/Marketing Manager

Teach beginning reading with teacher-developed programs that sequentially present phonics, phonemic awareness, word recognition, and reading comprehension concepts.

1574 Reading Who? Reading You!
Sunburst Technology
1550 Executive Drive
Elgin, IL 60123
800-321-7511
FAX 888-800-3028
http://http://store.sunburst.com/Home.aspx
e-mail: service@sunburst.com
Michael Guillory, Channel Sales/Marketing Manager

1575 Reading and Writing Workbook
Therapro
225 Arlington Street
Framingham, MA 01702
508-872-9494
800-257-5376
FAX 508-875-2062
http://www.theraproducts.com
e-mail: info@theraproducts.com
Therapro Staff, Author
Karen Conrad, Owner

Writing checks and balancing a checkbook, copying words and sentences, and writing messages and notes. Helps with recognition and understanding of calendars, phone books and much more. *$10.50*

1576 Reading for Content
Educators Publishing Service
PO Box 9031
Cambridge, MA 02139
617-547-6706
800-225-5750
FAX 888-440-2665
http://www.epsbooks.com
e-mail: eps@epsbooks.com
Carol Einstein, Author
Gunnar Voltz, President

Reading for Content is a series of 4 books designed to help students improve their reading comprehension skills. Each book contains 43 pasages followed by 4 questions. Two questions ask for a recall of main ideas, and two ask the student to draw conclusions from what they have just read.

1577 Reading for Job and Personal Use
AGS Publishing
PO Box 99
Circle Pines, MN 55014
651-287-7220
800-328-2560
FAX 800-471-8457
http://www.agsnet.com
e-mail: agsmail@agsnet.com
Joyce Hing-McGowan, Author
Kevin Brueggeman, President
Matt Keller, Marketing Manager

The practical, real-life exercises in these texts teach students how to read and comprehend catalogs, training manuals, letters and memos, signs, reports, charts, and more. *$14.95*

1578 Ready to Read
Educators Publishing Service
PO Box 9031
Cambridge, MA 02139
617-547-6706
800-225-5750
FAX 888-440-2665
http://www.epsbooks.com
e-mail: eps@epsbooks.com
Phyllis Bertin, Eileen Perlman, Author
Gunnar Voltz, President

Ready to Read contains activities for teaching sound/symbol association, blending, word recognition, reading, spelling and handwriting, including individual words, phrases, sentences, and connected text.

1579 Reasoning & Reading Series
Educators Publishing Service
PO Box 9031
Cambridge, MA 02139
617-547-6706
800-225-5750
FAX 888-440-2665
http://www.epsbooks.com
e-mail: eps@epsbooks.com
Joanne Carlisle, Author
Gunnar Voltz, President

These workbooks develop basic language and thinking skills that build the foundation for reading comprehension. Exercises reinforce reading as a critical reasoning activity. Many exercises encourage students to come up with their own response in instances where there is no single correct answer. In other cases, exercises lend themselves to students working collaboratively to see how many different answers satisfy a question.

1580 Right into Reading: A Phonics-Based Reading and Comprehension Program

Educators Publishing Service
PO Box 9031
Cambridge, MA 02139
617-547-6706
800-225-5750
FAX 888-440-2665
http://www.epsbooks.com
e-mail: eps@epsbooks.com
Jane Ervin, Author
Gunnar Voltz, President

Right into Reading introduces phonics skills in a carefully ordered sequence of bite-size lessons so that students can progress easily and successfully from one reading level to the next. The stories and selections are unusually diverse and interactive.

1581 Roots, Prefixes & Suffixes

Sunburst Technology
1550 Executive Drive
Elgin, IL 60123
800-321-7511
FAX 888-800-3028
http://http://store.sunburst.com/Home.aspx
e-mail: service@sunburst.com
Michael Guillory, Channel Sales/Marketing Manager

Students learn to decode difficult and more complex words as they engage in six activities where they construct and dissect words with roots, prefixes and suffixes.

1582 See Me Add

Teddy Bear Press
3639 Midway Drive
San Diego, CA 92110
858-560-8718
FAX 858-874-0423
http://www.teddybearpress.net
e-mail: fparker@teddybearpress.net
Fran Parker, Author
Fran Parker, President

Introduces the concept of addition using simple story problems and the basic sight word vocabulary found in the I Can Read and Reading Is Fun programs. *$20.00*

1583 See Me Subtract

Teddy Bear Press
3639 Midway Drive
San Diego, CA 92110
858-560-8718
FAX 858-874-0423
http://www.teddybearpress.net
e-mail: fparker@teddybearpress.net
Fran Parker, Author
Fran Parker, President

Introduces the concept of subtraction using simple story problems. *$20.00*

1584 Short Classics

Harcourt Achieve
Customer Service, 5th Floor
Orlando, FL 32887
800-284-7019
FAX 800-699-9459
http://www.harcourtachieve.com
e-mail: webmaster@harcourt.com
Steck-Vaughn Staff, Author
Tim McEwen, President/CEO
Susan Canizares, SVP Publisher
Lee Wilson, VP Marketing

These shortened easy-to-read presentations use carefully controlled vocabulary while maintaining the style of the original authors. Your students can broaden their horizons and build self-esteem as they succeed with literary classics. *$168.60*

1585 Soaring Scores CTB: Reading and LanguageArts

Harcourt Achieve
Customer Service, 5th Floor
Orlando, FL 32887
800-284-7019
FAX 800-699-9459
http://www.harcourtachieve.com
e-mail: webmaster@harcourt.com
Steck-Vaughn Staff, Author
Tim McEwen, President/CEO
Susan Canizares, SVP Publisher
Lee Wilson, VP Marketing

Through a combination of targeted instructional practice and testing-taking tips, these workbooks help students build better skills and improve CTB-TerraNova tests scores. Initial lessons address reading comprehension and language arts. The authentic practice test mirrors the CTB's format and content. *$56.30*

1586 Soaring Scores on the ISAT Reading and Writing

Harcourt Achieve
Customer Service, 5th Floor
Orlando, FL 32887
800-284-7019
FAX 800-699-9459
http://www.harcourtachieve.com
e-mail: webmaster@harcourt.com
Steck-Vaughn Staff, Author
Tim McEwen, President/CEO
Susan Canizares, SVP Publisher
Lee Wilson, VP Marketing

Highly targeted instruction and practice tests help students approach the ISAT strategically and confidently. Writing prompts ask students to write a persuasive, expository, or narrative essay. Modeled questions practice both multiple-choice and open-ended queries. *$61.90*

1587 Sounds Abound Program

LinguiSystems
3100 4th Avenue
East Moline, IL 61244
309-755-2300
800-776-4332
FAX 309-755-2377
TDY:800-933-8331
http://www.linguisystems.com
e-mail: service@linguisystems.com
Orna Lenchner PhD, Blanche Podhajski PhD, Author
Linda Bowers, Co-Owner/Co-Founder
Rosemary Huisingh, Co-Owner/Co-Founder

This program boosts emergent reading and beginning literacy through a hierarchy of skills. Activities target rhyming, syllables, sound recognition, sound production, sound blending, phoneme-grapheme correspondence, and more phonological skills. *$109.95*

112 pages Ages 4-8

1588 Source for Aphasia Therapy

LinguiSystems
3100 4th Avenue
East Moline, IL 61244
309-755-2300
800-776-4332
FAX 309-755-2377
TDY:800-933-8331
http://www.linguisystems.com
e-mail: service@linguisystems.com
Lisa A Arnold, Author
Linda Bowers, Co-Owner/Co-Founder
Rosemary Huisingh, Co-Owner/Co-Founder

Therapy exercises are organized into three groups: receptive language, reading comprehension, and expressive language. Each section is organized in a hierarchy to meet each client's individual needs. You'll cover imitating gestures, following commands, understanding symbols and signs, naming and describing objects, and much more! *$41.95*

183 pages Adults

1589 Source for Dyslexia and Dysgraphia
LinguiSystems
3100 4th Avenue
East Moline, IL 61244
309-755-2300
800-776-4332
FAX 309-755-2377
TDY:800-933-8331
http://www.linguisystems.com
e-mail: service@linguisystems.com
Regina G Richards, Author
Linda Bowers, Co-Owner/Co-Founder
Rosemary Huisingh, Co-Owner/Co-Founder

From diagnosis to developmental strategies to how-to techniques, this is the definitivie SOURCE on students who have difficulty with the reading and writing process. *$41.95*
308 pages Ages 6-18

1590 Source for Early Literacy Development
LinguiSystems
3100 4th Avenue
East Moline, IL 61244
309-755-2300
800-776-4332
FAX 309-755-2377
TDY:800-933-8331
http://www.linguisystems.com
e-mail: service@linguisystems.com
Linda K Crowe, Sara S Reichmuth, Author
Linda Bowers, Co-Owner/Co-Founder
Rosemary Huisingh, Co-Owner/Co-Founder

This great resource gives you the latest information on children's emergent reading and writing from birth through age eight. You'll also get helpful strategies to facilitate literacy development for future academic success! *$ 41.95*
151 pages Birth-8

1591 Specialized Program Individualizing Reading Excellence (SPIRE)
Educators Publishing Service
PO Box 9031
Cambridge, MA 02139
617-547-6706
800-225-5750
FAX 207-985-3878
http://www.espbooks.com
e-mail: spire@espbooks.com
Gunnar Voltz, President

SPIRE is a comprehensive multisensory reading and language arts program for students with learning differences.

1592 Starting Comprehension
Educators Publishing Service
PO Box 9031
Cambridge, MA 02139
617-547-6706
800-225-5750
FAX 888-440-2665
http://www.epsbooks.com
e-mail: eps@epsbooks.com
Ann L Staman, Author
Gunnar Voltz, President

A reading series of 12 workbooks that develops essential comprehension skills at the earliest reading level. It is divided into two different strands, one for students who have a strong visual sense, the other for those who learn sounds easily. Vocabulary introduced within context of exercises, using most of the words in the books. Student relates the details of the passage to the main idea.

1593 Stories and More: Animal Friends
Riverdeep
100 Pine Street
San Francisco, CA 94111
415-659-2000
FAX 415-659-2020
http://www.riverdeep.net
e-mail: info@riverdeep.net
Barry O'Callaghan, Executive Chairman

Stories and More: Animal Friends features three well-known stories — The Gunnywolf, The Trek, and Owl and the Moon — with engaging activities that strengthen students reading comprehension. A scaffolding of pre-reading, reading, and post-reading activities for each story helps kindergarten and 1st grade students practice prediction and sequencing skills; appreciate the importance of character and setting; and respond to literature through writing, drawing, and speaking. *$ 69.95*

1594 Stories and More: Time and Place
Riverdeep
100 Pine Street
San Francisco, CA 94111
415-659-2000
FAX 415-659-2020
http://www.riverdeep.net
e-mail: info@riverdeep.net
Barry O'Callaghan, Executive Chairman

Stories and More: Time and Place combines three well-loved stories — The House on Maple Street, Roxaboxen, and Galimoto — with — angaging activities that strengthen students' reading comprehension. In these books, the setting plays a primary role. Second and third grade students learn the importance of time, culture, and place in our lives.

1595 Success Stories 1, 2
Educators Publishing Service
PO Box 9031
Cambridge, MA 02139
617-547-6706
800-225-5750
FAX 888-440-2665
http://www.epsbooks.com
e-mail: eps@epsbooks.com
Elizabeth H Butcher, Nancy A Simonetti, Author
Gunnar Voltz, President

These workbooks contain high-interest phonetically structured stories. Each book contains 60 stories, each story focusing on an individual grapheme or syllable pattern.

1596 Take Me Home Pair-It Books
Harcourt Achieve
Customer Service, 5th Floor
Orlando, FL 32887
800-284-7019
FAX 800-699-9459
http://www.harcourtachieve.com
e-mail: webmaster@harcourt.com
Park, Author
Tim McEwen, President/CEO
Susan Canizares, SVP Publisher
Lee Wilson, VP Marketing
Make reading time a family favorite. Our most popular Pair-It Book titles in convenient take-home packages make it easy to get parents involved in reinforcing reading. *$346.10*

1597 Taking Your Camera To...Steadwell
Harcourt Achieve
Customer Service, 5th Floor
Orlando, FL 32887
800-284-7019
FAX 800-699-9459
http://www.harcourtachieve.com
e-mail: webmaster@harcourt.com
Park, Author
Tim McEwen, President/CEO
Susan Canizares, SVP Publisher
Lee Wilson, VP Marketing
Give limited readers unlimited access to major countries! Each title devotes a spread to the land, the people, major cities, lifestyles, places to visit, government and religion, earning a living, sports and school, food and holidays, quick facts, statistics and maps, and the future. *$7.80*

1598 That's LIFE! Reading Comprehension
LinguiSystems
3100 4th Avenue
East Moline, IL 61244
309-755-2300
800-776-4332
FAX 309-755-2377
TDY:800-933-8331
http://www.linguisystems.com
e-mail: service@linguisystems.com
LinguiSystems Staff, Author
Linda Bowers, Co-Owner/Co-Founder
Rosemary Huisingh, Co-Owner/Co-Founder

Get two programs in one. Each high-interest reading passage is written at an upper and lower reading level to meet your students' needs. These lessons are great for individuals or classroom istruction. Each story is followed by thought-provoking comprehension questions, including multiple choice, fill-in-the-blank, true/false, and critical thinking questions. *$37.95*
191 pages Ages 11-18

1599 Tic-Tac-Read and Match: Fun Phonics Games
LinguiSystems
3100 4th Avenue
East Moline, IL 61244
309-755-2300
800-776-4332
FAX 309-755-2377
TDY:800-933-8331
http://www.linguisystems.com
e-mail: service@linguisystems.com
Carol A Vaccariello, Author
Linda Bowers, Co-Owner/Co-Founder
Rosemary Huisingh, Co-Owner/Co-Founder

Two-books set offers fun activities to reinforce reading. Use the whole page to play Read and Match. Use the nine shaded areas to play Tic-Tac-Read. Students move progressively through a hierarchy of phonics skills as they read the words aloud while playing. *$38.90*
160 pages Ages 7-14

1600 Transition Stage 2-3
Harcourt Achieve
Customer Service, 5th Floor
Orlando, FL 32887
800-284-7019
FAX 800-699-9459
http://www.harcourtachieve.com
e-mail: webmaster@harcourt.com
Steck-Vaughn Staff, Author
Tim McEwen, President/CEO
Susan Canizares, SVP Publisher
Lee Wilson, VP Marketing
A series of 20 books, each containing 16 pages, that provide readers with a gradual transition into early fluency. All stories are available on audio cassette, and four are available in big book format. *$951.80*

1601 Understanding Me
Churchill Center and School
1035 Price School Lane
Saint Louis, MO 63124
314-997-4343
FAX 314-997-2760
http://www.churchillschool.org
e-mail: info@churchstl.org
Michele Berg, PhD, Director

A student workbook of activities that have been developed to reinforce the language and vocabulary found in 'Keeping Ahead in School' by Dr. Melvin Levine. The workbook is comprised of blackline masters which can be reproduced. *$ 20.00*

1602 Vocabulary
Harcourt Achieve
Customer Service, 5th Floor
Orlando, FL 32887
800-284-7019
FAX 800-699-9459
http://www.harcourtachieve.com
e-mail: webmaster@harcourt.com
Steck-Vaughn Staff, Author
Tim McEwen, President/CEO
Susan Canizares, SVP Publisher
Lee Wilson, VP Marketing
Improve reading comprehension where it matters most by introducing new words in the context of content area articles. Twenty-five highly visual lessons include a high-interest story with vocabulary words highlighted, a full-page graphic application activity, and reinforcement and extension activities presented as computer pull-down menus.

1603 Vowels: Short & Long
Sunburst Technology
1550 Executive Drive
Elgin, IL 60123
800-321-7511
FAX 888-800-3028
http://http://store.sunburst.com/Home.aspx
e-mail: service@sunburst.com
Michael Guillory, Channel Sales/Marketing Manager

Introduce students to vowels and the role they play in the structure of words. By engaging in word building activities, students learn to identify short and long vowels and regular spelling patterns.

1604 Warmups and Workouts
Abilitations Speech Bin
PO Box 922668
Norcross, GA 30010
770-449-5700
800-850-8602
FAX 770-510-7290
http://www.speechbin.com
e-mail: info@speechbin.com
Jane Folk, Author
Tobi Isaacs, Catalog Director

Easy-to-follow step-by-step instructions demonstrate how to help children achieve reliable production of r sounds, practice them in words of increasing complexity, and improve their phonic skills simultaneously. Item number 1486. *$26.99*

1605 Wilson Language Training
Wilson Reading System
47 Old Webster Road
Oxford, MA 01540
508-368-2399
FAX 508-368-2300
http://www.wilsonlanguage.com
e-mail: info@wilsonlanguage.com
Barbara Wilson, Owner
Judith Nicholas, Administrator Training

Our mission is to instruct teachers, or other professionals in a related field, how to succeed with students who have not learned to read, write and spell despite great effort. Established in order to provide training in the Wilson Reading System, the Wilson staff provides Two-Day Overview Workshops as well as certified Level I and II training.

1606 Word Parts
Sunburst Technology
1550 Executive Drive
Elgin, IL 60123
800-321-7511
FAX 888-800-3028
http://http://store.sunburst.com/Home.aspx
e-mail: service@sunburst.com
Michael Guillory, Channel Sales/Marketing Manager

Students build skills with compound and polysyllabic words by learning to chunk big words into manageable parts.

1607 Word Scramble 2
LinguiSystems
3100 4th Avenue
East Moline, IL 61244
309-755-2300
800-776-4332
FAX 309-755-2377
TDY:800-933-8331
http://www.linguisystems.com
e-mail: service@linguisystems.com

Paul F Johnson, Author
Linda Bowers, Co-Owner/Co-Founder
Rosemary Huisingh, Co-Owner/Co-Founder

Customers loved the best-selling Word Scramble game and kept asking for more. Take your students to a new level of decoding practice with Word Scramble 2. This game is perfect for your students who've mastered CVC words and are ready for more challenging decoding practice. *$44.95*
Ages 7-14

1608 **Wordly Wise 3000 ABC 1-9**
Educators Publishing Service
PO Box 9031
Cambridge, MA 02139
617-547-6706
800-225-5750
FAX 888-440-2665
http://www.epsbooks.com
e-mail: eps@epsbooks.com
Kenneth Hodkinson, Sandra Adams, Author
Gunnar Voltz, President

Three thousand new and carefully selected words taken from literature, textbooks and SAT-prep books, are the basis of this new series that teaches vocabulary through reading, writing, and a variety of exercises for grades 4-12.

1609 **Wordly Wise ABC 1-9**
Educators Publishing Service
PO Box 9031
Cambridge, MA 02139
617-547-6706
800-225-5750
FAX 888-440-2665
http://www.epsbooks.com
e-mail: eps@epsbooks.com
Kenneth Hodkinson, Author
Gunnar Voltz, President

Vocabulary workbook series employs crossword puzzles, riddles, word games and a sense of humor to make the learning of new words an interesting experience.

1610 **Workbook for Aphasia**
Abilitations Speech Bin
PO Box 922668
Norcross, GA 30010
770-449-5700
800-850-8602
FAX 770-510-7290
http://www.speechbin.com
e-mail: info@speechbin.com
Susan Howell Brubaker, Author
Tobi Isaacs, Catalog Director

This book gives you materials for adults who have recovered a significant degree of speaking, reading, writing, and comprehension skills. It includes 106 excercises divide into eight target areas. Item number W331. *$69.99*

Science

1611 **Animals and Their Homes CD-ROM**
Harcourt Achieve
6277 Sea Harbor Drive
Orlando, FL 32887
252-480-3200
800-531-5015
FAX 800-699-9459
http://www.steckvaughn.com
e-mail: info@steckvaughn.com
Steck-Vaughn Staff, Author
Tim McEwen, President/CEO
Jeff Johnson, Dir Marketing Communications
Chris Lehmann, Team Coordinator
This interactive simulation encourages students to explore animals habitats and environmental needs and create appropriate environments for a variety of animals. Students use the Animal Book to create a customized habitat display and write or record their own observations and ideas.

1612 **Animals in Their World CD-ROM**
Harcourt Achieve
6277 Sea Harbor Drive
Orlando, FL 32887
252-480-3200
800-531-5015
FAX 800-699-9459
http://www.steckvaughn.com
e-mail: info@steckvaughn.com
Steck-Vaughn Staff, Author
Tim McEwen, President/CEO
Jeff Johnson, Dir Marketing Communications
Chris Lehmann, Team Coordinator
This multimedia database motivates children to explore, compare, and contrast habitats, behaviors, and physicl characteristics of 58 animals in nine categories, such as carnivore or herbivore, hatched or born, and with or without backbone.

1613 **Curious Creatures Program: Owls-Spiders-Wolves-Snakes-Bats**
Curriculum Associates
PO Box 2001
North Billerica, MA 01862
800-225-0248
FAX 800-366-1158
http://www.curriculumassociates.com
e-mail: cainfo@curriculumassociates.com
Louis James Taris, James Robert Taris, Author
Frank Ferguson, President

Users of this award-winning multimedia program say awesome! They learn little known facts about animals that make most of us cringe. Designed to encourage reluctant readers in grades 4 and above, the program is also appropriate for on-level students in grades 2-3. Students learn the language of life science as they strengthen their reading and comprehension skills.

1614 **Deep in the Rain Forest**
Harcourt Achieve
6277 Sea Harbor Drive
Orlando, FL 32887
252-480-3200
800-531-5015
FAX 800-699-9459
http://www.steckvaughn.com
e-mail: info@steckvaughn.com
Pirotta, Author
Tim McEwen, President/CEO
Jeff Johnson, Dir Marketing Communications
Chris Lehmann, Team Coordinator
Now even young readers can investigate the wonder and importance of the rain forest. Hands-on activities, large photos, and meaningful tests in each of these titles relate rain forest facts to a child's world and introduce conservation and environmental protection issues.

1615 **Dive to the Ocean Deep: Voyages of Exploration and Discovery**
Harcourt Achieve
6277 Sea Harbor Drive
Orlando, FL 32819
252-480-3200
800-531-5015
FAX 800-699-9459
http://www.steckvaughn.com
e-mail: info@steckvaughn.com
Steck-Vaughn Staff, Author
Tim McEwen, President/CEO
Jeff Johnson, Dir Marketing Communications
Chris Lehmann, Team Coordinator
These exciting titles draw readers in with true tales of discovery using a documentary approach. Renowned scientists show real world science at work in the depths of the ocean. *$27.11*
64 pages

1616 **Harcourt Brace: The Science Book of....**
Harcourt Achieve
6277 Sea Harbor Drive
Orlando, FL 32887
252-480-3200
800-531-5015
FAX 800-699-9459
http://www.steckvaughn.com
e-mail: info@steckvaughn.com

Ardley, Author
Tim McEwen, President/CEO
Jeff Johnson, Dir Marketing Communications
Chris Lehmann, Team Coordinator
Encourage independent scientific inquiry. Set up a classroom library of 16 hardcover titles that offer dozens of exploration opportunities with basic science principles. Ordinary classroom or household materials are all you need. Full-color photos of preparations and experiments are ideal for independent work. Practical examples relate each experiment to real world.

1617 Learn About Life Science: Animals

Sunburst Technology
1550 Executive Drive
Elgin, IL 60123
800-321-7511
FAX 888-800-3028
http://http://store.sunburst.com/Home.aspx
e-mail: service@sunburst.com
Michael Guillory, Channel Sales/Marketing Manager

Learn about animal classification, adaptation to climate, domestication and special relationships between humans and animals.

1618 Learn About Life Science: Plants

Sunburst Technology
1550 Executive Drive
Elgin, IL 60123
800-321-7511
FAX 888-800-3028
http://http://store.sunburst.com/Home.aspx
e-mail: service@sunburst.com
Michael Guillory, Channel Sales/Marketing Manager

Students explore the world of plants. From small seeds to tall trees students learn what plants are and what they need to grow.

1619 Learn About Physical Science: Simple Machines

Sunburst Technology
1550 Executive Drive
Elgin, IL 60123
800-321-7511
FAX 888-800-3028
http://http://store.sunburst.com/Home.aspx
e-mail: service@sunburst.com
Michael Guillory, Channel Sales/Marketing Manager

Students delve into the mechanical world learning about the ways simple machines make our work easier.

1620 Life Cycles

Harcourt Achieve
Customer Service, 5th Floor
Orlando, FL 32887
800-284-7019
FAX 800-699-9459
http://www.harcourtachieve.com
e-mail: webmaster@harcourt.com
Hogan, Author
Tim McEwen, President/CEO
Susan Canizares, SVP Publisher
Lee Wilson, VP Marketing

Dramatic photos tell the story of animal growth and development. This softcover series enriches any classroom science curriculum. Animal development is a complex subject but this series makes it understandable for young readers with simple text and informative images that follow each animal from birth to maturity. *$7.80*

1621 Maps & Navigation

Sunburst Technology
1550 Executive Drive
Elgin, IL 60123
800-321-7511
FAX 888-800-3028
http://http://store.sunburst.com/Home.aspx
e-mail: service@sunburst.com
Michael Guillory, Channel Sales/Marketing Manager

This exciting nautical simulation provides students with opportunities to use their math and science skills.

1622 Our Universe: Steadwell

Harcourt Achieve
Customer Service, 5th Floor
Orlando, FL 32887
800-284-7019
FAX 800-699-9459
http://www.harcourtachieve.com
e-mail: webmaster@harcourt.com
Vogt, Author
Tim McEwen, President/CEO
Susan Canizares, SVP Publisher
Lee Wilson, VP Marketing

Unravel the mysteries of space! A complex universe becomes amazingly clear in these easy-to-read titles. *$88.90*

ISBN 0-739833-55-3

1623 Prehistoric Creaures Then & Now: Steadwell

Harcourt Achieve
Customer Service, 5th Floor
Orlando, FL 32887
800-284-7019
FAX 800-699-9459
http://www.harcourtachieve.com
e-mail: webmaster@harcourt.com
Steck-Vaughn Staff, Author
Tim McEwen, President/CEO
Susan Canizares, SVP Publisher
Lee Wilson, VP Marketing

Now limited readers can dig into the details of dinosaurs! Each information-packed title includes a special spread with a project, a profile of a dinosaur expert, or a description of a recent dinosaur discovery. *$44.90*

ISBN 0-739849-32-8

1624 Space Academy GX-1

Riverdeep
100 Pine Street
San Francisco, CA 94111
415-659-2000
FAX 415-659-2020
http://www.riverdeep.net
e-mail: info@riverdeep.net
Barry O'Callaghan, Executive Chairman/CEO

Explore the solar system with Space Academy GX-1! Fully aligned with national science standards and state curricula, Space Academy GX-1, students investigate the astronomical basis for seasons, phases of the moon, gravity, orbits, and more. As students succeed, Grow Slides adjust to offer more advanced topics and problems.

1625 Steck-Vaughn Science Centers

Harcourt Achieve
6277 Sea Harbor Drive
Orlando, FL 32887
252-480-3200
800-531-5015
FAX 800-699-9459
http://www.harcourtachieve.com
e-mail: info@harcourtachieve.com
Steck-Vaughn Staff, Author
Tim McEwen, President/CEO
Jeff Johnson, Dir Marketing Communications
Chris Lehmann, Team Coordinator

Organized by theme, these books will supplement the study of weather, prehistoric life, plants, animals of the ocean, animals of the rain forest, earth and space, and energy.

1626 Talking Walls

Riverdeep
100 Pine Street
San Francisco, CA 94111
415-659-2000
FAX 415-659-2020
http://www.riverdeep.net
e-mail: info@riverdeep.net
Barry O'Callaghan, Executive Chairman/CEO

The Talking Walls Software Series is a wonderful springboard for a student's journey of exploration and discovery. This comprehensive collection of researched resources and materials enables students to focus on learning while conducting a guided search for information.

1627 Talking Walls: The Stories Continue

Riverdeep
100 Pine Street
San Francisco, CA 94111
415-659-2000
FAX 415-659-2020
http://www.riverseep.net
e-mail: info@riverdeep.net
Barry O'Callaghan, Executive Chairman/CEO

Using the Talking Walls Software Series, students discover the stories behind some of the world's most fascinating walls. The award-winning books, interactive software, carefully chosen Web sites, and suggested classroom activities build upon each other, providing a rich learning experience that includes text, video, and hands-on projects.

1628 ThemeWeavers: Nature Activity Kit

Riverdeep
100 Pine Street
San Francisco, CA 94111
415-659-2000
FAX 415-659-2020
http://www.riverdeep.net
e-mail: info@riverdeep.net
Barry O'Callaghan, Executive Chairman/CEO

ThemeWeavers: Nature Activity Kit is an all-in-one solution for theme-based teaching. In just a few minutes, you can select from dozens of ready-to-use activities centering on the seasons and weather and be ready for the next day's lesson! Interactive and engaging activities cover multiple subject areas such as language arts, math, science, social studies and art.

1629 Thinkin' Science

Sunburst Technology
1550 Executive Drive
Elgin, IL 60123
800-321-7511
FAX 888-800-3028
http://http://store.sunburst.com/Home.aspx
e-mail: service@sunburst.com
Michael Guillory, Channel Sales/Marketing Manager

Five environments introduce students to the scientific methods and concepts needed to understand basic earth, life and physical sciences. Students learn to think like scientists as they solve problems using hypothesis, experimentation, observation and deduction.

1630 Thinkin' Science ZAP!

Sunburst Technology
1550 Executive Drive
Elgin, IL 60123
800-321-7511
FAX 888-800-3028
http://http://store.sunburst.com/Home.aspx
e-mail: service@sunburst.com
Michael Guillory, Channel Sales/Marketing Manager

Working with laser beams, electrical circuits, and "visible" sound waves, students practice valuable thinking skills, observation, prediction, dedutive reasoning, conceptual modeling, theory building and hypothesis testing while experimenting within scientifically accurate learning environment.

1631 True Tales

Harcourt Achieve
Customer Service, 5th Floor
Orlando, FL 32887
800-284-7019
FAX 800-699-9459
http://www.harcourtachieve.com
e-mail: webmaster@harcourt.com
Billings, Author
Tim McEwen, President/CEO
Susan Canizares, SVP Publisher
Lee Wilson, VP Marketing

If you have been looking for reading comprehension materials for limited readers, your search is over. True Tales presents powerful real-lfe events with direct connections to geography and science at reading level 3. Gripping accounts of personal triumph and tragedy put geography and science in a very real context. Accompanying activities develop reading and language arts, science, and geography skills students need to boost test scores. *$185.80*

ISBN 0-739834-49-5

1632 Turnstone Explorer Kits

Harcourt Achieve
6277 Sea Harbor Drive
Orlando, FL 32887
252-480-3200
800-531-5015
FAX 800-699-9459
http://www.steckvaughn.com
e-mail: info@steckvaughn.com
Steck-Vaughn Staff, Author
Tim McEwen, President/CEO
Jeff Johnson, Dir Marketing Communications
Chris Lehmann, Team Coordinator

Encourage inquiry with an insider's look at science exploration! Energize discovery-based learning through nonfiction literature, hands-on exploration, and challenging application projects. Put budding scientists in touch with real thing. Action-packed kits bring the experience of scientific exploration to life.

1633 Untamed World

Harcourt Achieve
6277 Sea Harbor Drive
Orlando, FL 32887
252-480-3200
800-531-5015
FAX 800-699-9459
http://www.steckvaughn.com
e-mail: info@steckvaughn.com
Karen Dudley, Marie Levine, Patricia Schroeder, Author
Tim McEwen, President/CEO
Jeff Johnson, Dir Marketing Communications
Chris Lehmann, Team Coordinator

A vivid view of wild animals through science and literature! Awe-inspiring creatures of the land and sea are as fascinating in fact as in folklore. These titles offer both views, combining a thorough nonfiction resource with riveting reading. Topics include life span, classification, the food chain, social organization, communication, and seasonal activities.

1634 Virtual Labs: Electricity

Riverdeep
100 Pine Street
San Francisco, CA 94111
415-659-2000
FAX 415-659-2020
http://www.riverdeep.net
e-mail: info@riverdeep.net
Barry O'Callaghan, Executive Chairman/CEO

Five environments introduce students to the scientific methods and conepts needed to understand basic Earth, life, and physical sciences. Students will learn to think like scientists as they solve problems using hypothesis, experimentation, observation, and deduction. *$69.95*

1635 Virtual Labs: Light

Riverdeep
100 Pine Street
San Francisco, CA 94111
415-659-2000
FAX 415-659-2020
http://www.riverdeep.net
e-mail: info@riverdeep.com
Barry O'Callaghan, Executive Chairman/CEO

Designed to integrate directly into the physcial science curricula, Virtual Labs: Light combines easy-to-use experiments and highly accurate simulations with over 40 reproducible lab worksheets. Carefully sequenced levels of virtual experiments — basic, extension, and challenge — provide a safe means for students to perform hands-on activities with lasers and an assortment of optical tools.

Social Skills

1636 2's Experience Fingerplays
Therapro
225 Arlington Street
Framingham, MA 01702
508-872-9494
800-257-5376
FAX 508-875-2062
http://www.theraproducts.com
e-mail: info@theraproducts.com
Liz Wilmes, Dick Wilmes, Author
Karen Conrad, Owner

A wonderful collection of fingerplays, songs and rhymes for the very young child. Fingerplays are short, easy to learn, and full of simple movement. Chant or sing the fingerplays and then enjoy the accompanying games and activities. *$12.95*
159 pages

1637 28 Instant Song Games
Therapro
225 Arlington Street
Framingham, MA 01702
508-872-9494
800-257-5376
FAX 508-875-2062
http://www.theraproducts.com
e-mail: info@theraproducts.com
MaBoAubLo, Barbara Sher, Author
Karen Conrad, Owner

Gets kids up and moving in no time! Includes numerous games of body awareness, movement play, self expression, imagination and language play. Booklet and 75 minute audio tape. *$21.00*
Audio Tape

1638 Active Learning Series
Therapro
225 Arlington Street
Framingham, MA 01702
508-872-9494
800-257-5376
FAX 508-875-2062
http://www.theraproducts.com
e-mail: info@theraproducts.com
Therapro Staff, Author
Karen Conrad, Owner

A favorite of parents and caregivers. Over 300 innovative and easy-to-do activities in each book. The activities are easy to read and can be done with one child in a group. Helps caregivers to choose the right activities for each child. Ideas on setting up environments, and an easy system for writing plans, helps caregivers set the stage for a good activity program. Each book contains a complete planning guide. Activities for listening, talking, physical development and more.

1639 Activities Unlimited
Therapro
225 Arlington Street
Framingham, MA 01702
508-872-9494
800-257-5376
FAX 508-875-2062
http://www.theraproducts.com
e-mail: info@theraproducts.com
A Cleveland, B Caton, L Adler, Author
Karen Conrad, Owner

Helps young children develop fine and gross motor skills, increase their language, become self-reliant and play cooperatively. An innovative resource that immediately attracts and engages children. Short of time? Need a good idea? Count on Activites Unlimited. *$19.95*

1640 Activity Schedules for Children with Autism: Teaching Independent Behavior
Therapro
225 Arlington Street
Framingham, MA 01702
508-872-9494
800-257-5376
FAX 508-875-2062
http://www.theraproducts.com
e-mail: info@theraproducts.com
Lynn McClannahan PhD, Patricia Krantz PhD, Author
Karen Conrad, Owner

An activity schedule is a set of pictures or words that cue a child to follow a sequence of activities. When mastered, the children are more self-directed and purposeful at home, school and leisure activites. In this book, parents and professionals can find detailed instructions and examples, assess a child's readiness to use activity schedules, and understand graduated guidance and progress monitoring. Great for promoting independence in children with autism. *$14.95*
117 pages

1641 Alert Program With Songs for Self-Regulation
Therapro
225 Arlington Street
Framingham, MA 01702
508-872-9494
800-257-5376
FAX 508-875-2062
http://www.theraproducts.com
e-mail: info@theraproducts.com
Mary Sue Williams OTR, Sherry Shellenberger OTR, Author
Karen Conrad, Owner

This program compares the body to an engine, running either high, low, or just right. Side A is an overview, Side B has 15 songs for self-regulation. Extremely successful in helping kids recognize and change their own engine speeds.
Audio Tape

1642 An Introduction to How Does Your Engine Run?
Therapro
225 Arlington Street
Framingham, MA 01702
508-872-9494
800-257-5376
FAX 508-875-2062
http://www.theraproducts.com
e-mail: info@theraproducts.com
Mary Sue Williams OTR, Sherry Shellenberger OTR, Author
Karen Conrad, Owner

Introduces the entire Alert Program, which explains how we regulate our arousal states. Describes the use of sensorimotor strategies to manage levels of alertness. This program is fun for students and the adults working with them, and translates easily into real life. *$40.00*

1643 Andy and His Yellow Frisbee
Therapro
225 Arlington Street
Framingham, MA 01702
508-872-9494
800-257-5376
FAX 508-875-2062
http://www.theraproducts.com
e-mail: info@theraproducts.com
Mary Thompson, Author
Karen Conrad, Owner

A heartwarming story about Andy, a boy with autism. Like many children with autism, Andy has a fascination with objects in motion. His talent for spinning his Frisbee and a new classmate's curiosity set this story in motion. Rosie, the watchful and protective sister, supplies backround on Andy and autism, as well as a sibling's perspective. *$14.95*
19 pages

1644 Artic-Riddles
Abilitations Speech Bin
PO Box 922668
Norcross, GA 30010
770-449-5700
800-850-8602
FAX 770-510-7290
http://www.speechbin.com
e-mail: info@speechbin.com
Tobi Isaacs, Catalog Director

Tired of the same old games? Artic-Riddles is a collection of speech materials with a tantalizing new twist! Each deck of twenty cards has an eye-catching picture on the front and five riddle clues on the back. Games provide speech sound practice; at the same time, they develop and reinforce skills in listening, turn taking, recalling, reasoning, vocabulary, naming, inferring, answering questions, and drawing conclusions. Item numbers 1408, 1409, 1412, 1415.

1645 Autism & PDD: Primary Social Skills Lessons

LinguiSystems
3100 4th Avenue
East Moline, IL 61244
309-755-2300
800-776-4332
FAX 309-755-2377
TDY:800-933-8331
http://www.linguisystems.com
e-mail: service@linguisystems.com
Pam Britton Reese, Nena C Challenner, Author
Linda Bowers, Co-Owner/Co-Founder
Rosemary Huisingh, Co-Owner/Co-Founder

These structured lessons teach social skills through rebus stories. The pictures help students read the lesson with you. Here are just some of the social skill areas you'll address: using a quiet voice, self-care skills, school behavior, hurting self or others, table social skills, getting a check-up. *$109.75*
60 pages Ages 3-8

1646 Autism & PPD: Adolescent Social Skills Lessons

LinguiSystems
3100 4th Avenue
East Moline, IL 61244
309-755-2300
800-776-4332
FAX 309-755-2377
TDY:800-933-8331
http://www.linguisystems.com
e-mail: service@linguisystems.com
Pam Britton Reese, Nena C Challenner, Author
Linda Bowers, Co-Owner/Co-Founder
Rosemary Huisingh, Co-Owner/Co-Founder

These lessons target the social skills your students with autism need to succeed in school and in life. From school schedule changes to staying healthy to job skills, you'll cover all the important skills your students need. Each book includes instructional and behavioral lessons. *$109.75*
65 pages Ages 12-18

1647 Autism & PPD: Adolescent Social Skills Lessons-Health & Hygiene

LinguiSystems
3100 4th Avenue
East Moline, IL 61244
309-755-2300
800-776-4332
FAX 309-755-2377
TDY:800-933-8331
http://www.linguisystems.com
e-mail: service@linguisystems.com
Pam Britton Reese, Nena C Challenner, Author
Linda Bowers, Co-Owner/Co-Founder
Rosemary Huisingh, Co-Owner/Co-Founder

Use these rebus story lessons to teach your students important social skills related to health and hygiene. The instructional lessons teach what to say or do in social situations that are sometimes overwhelming to the student with autism and PPD. The behavioral lessons target specific social problems that need to be stopped. *$21.95*
63 pages Ages 12-18

1648 Breakthroughs Manual: How to Reach Students with Autism

Therapro
225 Arlington Street
Framingham, MA 01702
508-872-9494
800-257-5376
FAX 508-875-2062
http://www.theraproducts.com
e-mail: info@theraproducts.com
Karen Sewell, Author
Karen Conrad, Owner

This manual features practical suggestions for everyday use with preschool through high school students. Covers communication, behavior, academics, self-help, life and social skills. Includes reproducible lesson plans and up to date listing of classroom materials and catalog supply companies. *$59.00*
243 pages

1649 Broccoli-Flavored Bubble Gum

Harcourt Achieve
6277 Sea Harbor Drive
Orlando, FL 32887
252-480-3200
800-531-5015
FAX 800-699-9459
http://www.steckvaughn.com
e-mail: info@steckvaughn.com
Justin McGivern, Patrick Girouard, Author
Tim McEwen, President/CEO
Jeff Johnson, Dir Marketing Communications
Chris Lehmann, Team Coordinator

A young boy gains fame and fortune encouraging kids to eat their vegetables.
32 pages

1650 Busy Kids Movement

Therapro
225 Arlington Street
Framingham, MA 01702
508-872-9494
800-257-5376
FAX 508-875-2062
http://www.theraproducts.com
e-mail: info@theraproducts.com
Therapro Staff, Author
Karen Conrad, Owner

Full of ideas for developing youngsters' gross motor skills. Games, dramatics, action songs, music and rythm activities. *$9.95*
64 pages

1651 Calm Down and Play

Childswork
2 Skyline Drive
Hawthorne, NY 10532
888-367-6368
FAX 914-347-1805
http://www.sunburstvm.com
e-mail: zstarr@sunburstvm.com
Zena Starr

Filled with fun and effective activities to help children: calm down and control their impulses; focus, concentrate, and organize their thoughts; identify and verbalize feelings; channel and release excess energy appropriately; and build self-esteem and confidence. *$17.95*
Ages 5-12

1652 Case of the Crooked Candles

Harcourt Achieve
6277 Sea Harbor Drive
Orlando, FL 32887
252-480-3200
800-531-5015
FAX 800-699-9459
http://www.steckvaughn.com
e-mail: info@steckvaughn.com
Jonathan Conn, Author
Tim McEwen, President/CEO
Jeff Johnson, Dir Marketing Communications
Chris Lehmann, Team Coordinator

A pair of felonious fruit bats is no match for Detective Dog and his alert animal assistants.
32 pages

1653 Cooperative Thinking Strategies

Edge Enterprises
708 W 9th Street
Lawrence, KS 66044
785-749-1473
FAX 785-749-0207
e-mail: edge@midusa.net
D Sue Vernon, Donald Deshler, Jean Schumaker, Author
Jacqueline Schafer, Managing Editor
Sue Vernon, Manager

Cooperative Thinking Strategies are a group of strategies students can use to think, learn and work together productively. The strategies are designed to improve the students' ability to interact and work with others as they restructure and manipulate information in group tasks. Instruction in these strategies has been designed to be delivered in general education classes in which a diversity of students are enrolled, including students with disabilities. Available as a series or individually.

1654 Courageous Pacers Classroom Chart
Therapro
225 Arlington Street
Framingham, MA 01702
508-872-9494
800-257-5376
FAX 508-875-2062
http://www.theraproducts.com
e-mail: info@theraproducts.com
Therapro Staff, Author
Karen Conrad, Owner

Highly recommended to accompany the Courageous Pacers Program. Assists in keeping record of 12 students' progress in walking and lifting. A great visual tool to view progress.

1655 Courageous Pacers Program
Therapro
225 Arlington Street
Framingham, MA 01702
508-872-9494
800-257-5376
FAX 508-875-2062
http://www.theraproducts.com
e-mail: info@theraproducts.com
Tim Erson MS PT, Author
Karen Conrad, Owner

This fun and easy program was developed to help students become more active. Research shows that students who are more active, do better in school. The goal of the program is simple: get students to walk 100 miles and lift 10,000 pounds in a year.
92 pages

1656 Dance Land
Therapro
225 Arlington Street
Framingham, MA 01702
508-872-9494
800-257-5376
FAX 508-875-2062
http://www.theraproducts.com
e-mail: info@theraproducts.com
Fitz-Taylor, McDonald, Hicman, Lande, Wiz, Author
Karen Conrad, Owner

Safe fun for kids of all abilities. Engages listeners in rythmic expression, which is fundamental to physical, cognitive and emotional development. Dance activities designed by physical and occupational therapists. 33 page book included. Many sensory motor activites included. 50 minute audio tape. *$21.00*
Audio Tape

1657 Eden Family of Services
One Eden Way
Princeton, NJ 08540
609-987-0099
FAX 609-987-0243
http://www.edenservices.org
e-mail: info@edenservices.org
David Holmes EdD, Executive Director
Tom Cool, President
Joani Truch, Administration/Communications
Provides year round educational services, early intervention, parent training, respite care, outreach services, community based residential services and employment opportunities for individuals with autism.

1658 Emotions Activity Manuals
Therapro
225 Arlington Street
Framingham, MA 01702
508-872-9494
800-257-5376
FAX 508-875-2062
http://www.theraproducts.com
e-mail: info@theraproducts.com
Therapro Staff, Author
Karen Conrad, Owner

Great new manuals to use with the EMOTIONS products (poster, cards and flashcards). 63 different tried and true activities from therapists, educators and counselors form the US and Canada. Simply produced, includes an EMOTIONS page.

1659 Expression Connection
Abilitations Speech Bin
PO Box 922668
Norcross, GA 30010
770-449-5700
800-850-8602
FAX 770-510-7290
http://www.speechbin.com
e-mail: info@speechbin.com
Tobi Isaacs, Catalog Director

This criterion-referenced assessment protocol and structured instructional program moves elementary school children from simple narratives to complex stories and establishes the critical concepts that underline coherent oral expression. Item number 1586. *$46.99*

1660 Expressive Language Kit
LinguiSystems
3100 4th Avenue
East Moline, IL 61244
309-755-2300
800-776-4332
FAX 309-755-2377
TDY:800-933-8331
http://www.linguisystems.com
e-mail: service@linguisystems.com
Linda Bowers, Rosemary Huisingh, Carolyn LoGiudice, Author
Linda Bowers, Co-Owner/Co-Founder
Rosemary Huisingh, Co-Owner/Co-Founder

It's our biggest language therapy kit ever. The focus is on strengthening expressive language skills so your students will become effective communicators. A combination of colorful photographs, picture cards, and activity sheets work together to create an outstanding expressive language program. A comprehension therapy manual is included to help you direct this incredibly wide variety of language activities. *$149.95*
250 pages Ages 5-11

1661 Face to Face: Resolving Conflict Without Giving in or Giving Up
National Association for Community Mediation
1527 New Hampshire Avenue NW
Washington, DC 20036
202-667-9700
FAX 202-667-8629
http://www.nafcm.org
e-mail: nafcm@nafcm.org
Jan Bellard,Hilda Gutierrez Baldoquin,Andrew Sachs, Author
Mary Ellen Bowen

Modular curriculum for training program for AmeriCorps members. Addresses conflict at the personal level, interpersonal level, and group collaboration. Includes workbook. *$69.95*
266 pages

1662 Forms for Helping the ADHD Child
Childswork
45 Executive Drive
Plainview, NY 11803
516-349-6274
800-962-1141
FAX 877-434-6553
http://www.childswork.com
Sally Germain, Editorial

Forms, charts, and checklists for treating children with Attention Deficit Hyperactivity Disorder cover a wide range of approaches. Includes effective aids in assessing, treating, and monitoring the progress of the ADHD child. *$ 31.95*
100 pages

1663 Friendzee: A Social Skills Game
LinguiSystems
3100 4th Avenue
East Moline, IL 61244
309-755-2300
800-776-4332
FAX 309-755-2377
TDY:800-933-8331
http://www.linguisystems.com
e-mail: service@linguisystems.com

Diane A Figula, Author
Linda Bowers, Co-Owner/Co-Founder
Rosemary Huisingh, Co-Owner/Co-Founder

This game uses a communication-based approach to teaching social skills. Skills are taught through the themes of home, school, and community. Stimulus items teach these social skills: body language; tone of voice; polite forms; giving information; listening; asking questions; and problem solving. *$39.95*
Ages 7-11

1664 Funsical Fitness With Silly-cise CD: Motor Development Activities
Therapro
225 Arlington Street
Framingham, MA 01702
508-872-9494
800-257-5376
FAX 508-875-2062
http://www.theraproducts.com
e-mail: info@theraproducts.com
Karen Conrad, Owner

This unique blending of developmentally appropriate gross motor, sensory integration, and aerobic activities is guaranteed to build children's strength, balance endurance, coordination, and self confidence. Leads children through four 15-minute classes of Wacky Walking, Grinnastics, Brain Gym, Warm Ups, Adventurobics, and Chill Out activities. *$15.00*
Ages 3-9

1665 Games We Should Play in School
Therapro
225 Arlington Street
Framingham, MA 01702
508-872-9494
800-257-5376
FAX 508-875-2062
http://www.theraproducts.com
e-mail: info@theraproducts.com
Frank Aycox, Author
Karen Conrad, Owner

Includes over 75 interactive, fun, social games; describes how to effectively lead Social Play sessions in the classroom. Students become more cooperative, less antagonistic and more capable of increased attentiveness. Contains the secrets to enriching the entire school environment. *$16.50*
154 pages

1666 Goal Oriented Gross & Fine Motor Lesson Plans for Early Childhood Classes
Therapro
225 Arlington Street
Framingham, MA 01702
508-872-9494
800-257-5376
FAX 508-875-2062
http://www.theraproducts.com
e-mail: info@theraproducts.com
Donna Weiss MA OTR, Author
Karen Conrad, Owner

Practical and convinient format covers 224 activities grouped into 12 monthly units, making it easy to incorporate gross and fine motor activities into a daily class schedule. Provides challenges for groups whose abilities span early childhood, from 2.5 to 5.5 years of age. *$32.00*
77 pages

1667 Hidden Child: Linwood Method for Reaching the Autistic Child
Therapro
225 Arlington Street
Framingham, MA 01702
508-872-9494
800-257-5376
FAX 508-875-2062
http://www.theraproducts.com
e-mail: info@theraproducts.com
Jeanne Simmons, Sabine Oiski PhD, Author
Karen Conrad, Owner

This book provides an explanation of autism, then a step-by-step analysis of the Linwood method of establishing relationships, patterning good behavior, overcoming compulsions, developing skills, and fostering social and emotional development. This guidebook for teachers and therapists also has a message for parents.

1668 High Interest Sports
Harcourt Achieve
6277 Sea Harbor Drive
Orlando, FL 32887
252-480-3200
800-531-5015
FAX 800-699-9459
http://www.steckvaughn.com
e-mail: info@steckvaughn.com
Fetty, Author
Tim McEwen, President/CEO
Jeff Johnson, Dir Marketing Communications
Chris Lehmann, Team Coordinator
Exercise is an important part of a healthy lifestyle. By providing a variety of activities, games, and sports, we give students as opportunity to choose the exercise that fits their personal needs. These books provide the basic framework of a variety of sports and schoolyard games, making it an excellent resource for the classroom teacher.

1669 Inclusive Early Childhood Classroom: Easy Ways to Adapt Learning Centers for All Children
Therapro
225 Arlington Street
Framingham, MA 01702
508-872-9494
800-257-5376
FAX 508-875-2062
http://www.theraproducts.com
e-mail: info@theraproducts.com
Patti Gould, Joyce Sullivan, Author
Karen Conrad, Owner

A great inclusion resource! This long awaited book by two experienced occupational therapists offers many concrete suggestions that are easy to implement. Gives teachers tools to make classrooms more effective environments for ALL students. *$24.95*
203 pages

1670 Jarvis Clutch: Social Spy
Educators Publishing Service
PO Box 9031
Cambridge, MA 02139
617-547-6706
800-225-5750
FAX 888-440-2665
http://www.epsbooks.com
e-mail: eps@epsbooks.com
Melvin D Levine MD FAAP, Author
Gunnar Voltz, President

In Jarvis Clutch social spy, Dr. Mel Levine teams up with eight grader Jarvis Clutch for an insider's look at life on the middle school social scene. Jarvis's wry and insightful observations of student interactions at Eastern Middle School bring to light the myriad social challenges that adolescents face every day, including peer pressure, the need to seem cool, the perils of dating., Include the commentary in Jarivs' Spy Notes!

1671 Kids with Special Needs: Information & Activities to Promote Awareness & Understanding
Therapro
225 Arlington Street
Framingham, MA 01702
508-872-9494
800-257-5376
FAX 508-875-2062
http://www.theraproducts.com
e-mail: info@theraproducts.com
Dee Konczal, Veronica Getskow, Author
Karen Conrad, Owner

Children with disabilities have a need to be accepted and understood by other children. This book provides simulation activities to better understand what it's like to have a disability. Background information about communicative developmental, physical and learning disabilities is also offered. Includes a comprehensive resource list. *$16.95*

200 pages

1672 Learning in Motion
Therapro
225 Arlington Street
Framingham, MA 01702
508-872-9494
800-257-5376
FAX 508-875-2062
http://www.theraproducts.com
e-mail: info@theraproducts.com
Angermeir, Krzyzanowski, Keller-Moir, Author
Karen Conrad, Owner

Written by 3 OTs, this book is for the busy therapist or teacher of preschoolers to second graders. Provides group activities using gross, fine andsensory motor skills in theme based curricula. Every lesson plan contains goals, objectives, materials and adaptations to facilitate inclusion and multilevel instructions. Includes 130 lesson plans with corresponding parent letters that explain the lesson and provide home follow-up activities. *$50.00*
379 pages

1673 Look At It This Way
Therapro
225 Arlington Street
Framingham, MA 01702
508-872-9494
800-257-5376
FAX 508-875-2062
http://www.theraproducts.com
e-mail: info@theraproducts.com
Roma Lee, Author
Karen Conrad, Owner

Although the play and toy activities in this book are designed for children with visual impairment, they can be used with other children as well. Chapters include Learning to Look, Learning to Listen, Learning to Feel, and Using the Sense of Smell. *$32.00*
129 pages

1674 Maxwell's Manor: A Social Language Game
LinguiSystems
3100 4th Avenue
East Moline, IL 61244
309-755-2300
800-776-4332
FAX 309-755-2377
TDY:800-933-8331
http://www.linguisystems.com
e-mail: service@linguisystems.com
Carolyn LoGiudice, Nancy McConnell, Author
Linda Bowers, Co-Owner/Co-Founder
Rosemary Huisingh, Co-Owner/Co-Founder

This fun game will teach your students the social skills they need to get along with others, be more accepted by their peers, and be successful in the classroom. Maxwell, the loveable dog, leads the way as your students practice positive social language skills. *$44.95*
Ages 4-9

1675 Moving Right Along
Therapro
225 Arlington Street
Framingham, MA 01702
508-872-9494
800-257-5376
FAX 508-875-2062
http://www.theraproducts.com
e-mail: info@theraproducts.com
Barbara Sher MA OTR, Author
Karen Conrad, Owner

A collection of 264 easy, spur of the moment, movement games for young children to increase coordination, balance, rythm and enhance their sense of mastery. Great resource for parents, teachers, PT's and OT's. *$14.50*

1676 Moving and Learning Across the Curriculum: 315 Games to Make Learning Fun
Therapro
225 Arlington Street
Framingham, MA 01702
508-872-9494
800-257-5376
FAX 508-875-2062
http://www.theraproducts.com
e-mail: info@theraproducts.com
Rae Pica, Author
Karen Conrad, Owner

Gives children the chance to be physically involved in the experience of learning concepts. A great way to include gross motor skills across 6 major content areas: art; language arts; mathematics; music; science and social studies. *$4.00*

1677 New Language of Toys: Teaching Communication Skills to Children with Special Needs
Therapro
225 Arlington Street
Framingham, MA 01702
508-872-9494
800-257-5376
FAX 508-875-2062
http://www.theraproducts.com
e-mail: info@theraproducts.com
Sue Schwarz PhD, Joan Heller Miller EdM, Author
Karen Conrad, Owner

Play time becomes a fun and educational experience with this revised hands-on approach for developing communication skills using everyday toys. Includes a fresh assortment of toys, books and new chapters on computer technology, language learning, videotapes and television. *$16.95*
289 pages Ages Birth-6

1678 Patterns Across the Curriculum
Harcourt Achieve
Customer Service, 5th Floor
Orlando, FL 32887
800-284-7019
FAX 800-699-9459
http://www.harcourtachieve.com
e-mail: webmaster@harcourt.com
Steven Korten, CEO
Randy Pennington, SVP National Sales

Develop students' awareness and understanding of patterns in the real world! Exercises allow students to identify, complete, extend, and create patterns. Developed across four curriculum areas: Math; Language; Social Studies; and Science. Flexible organization allows teachers to utilize content-specific activities in coordination with other classroom assignments, providing additional richness in learning.

1679 Peer Pals
AGS Publishing
4201 Woodland Road
Circle Pines, MN 55014
763-786-4343
800-328-2560
FAX 800-471-8457
http://www.agsnet.com
e-mail: agsmail@agsnet.com
Robert P Bowman, John N Chanaca, Author
Kevin Brueggeman, Manager
Matt Keller, Marketing Manager

A peer helping program designed to improve study skills, self-esteem, and decision making. The program uses a big sister/big brother approach, as grade 3-6 students are paired with grade K-2 students. *$33.99*

ISBN 0-886711-62-2

1680 Play Helps: Toys and Activities for Children with Special Needs
Therapro
225 Arlington Street
Framingham, MA 01702
508-872-9494
800-257-5376
FAX 508-875-2062
http://www.theraproducts.com
e-mail: info@theraproducts.com
Roma Lear, Author
Karen Conrad, Owner

This unique book features many homemade ideas for all ages, including the very young child. All the toys can be adapted to meet individual needs. The text is divided into sections on each of the five senses: sight, hearing, touch, taste and smell. Anyone working with children will find this book indispensable. *$42.00*

200 pages 3rd Edition

1681 **Reaching Out, Joining In: Teaching Social Skills to Young Children with Autism**
Therapro
225 Arlington Street
Framingham, MA 01702
508-872-9494
800-257-5376
FAX 508-875-2062
http://www.theraproducts.com
e-mail: info@theraproducts.com
Mary Jane Weiss PhD BCBA, Sandra Harris PhD, Author
Karen Conrad, Owner

Describes how to help young children diagnosed within the autism spectrum with one of their most challenging areas of development, social behavior. Focuses on four broad topics: play skills; the language of social skills; undestanding another person's perspective; and using these skills in an inclusive classroon. The authors present concrete strategies to teach basic play skills, how to play with others, to recognize social cues and engage in social conversation. Practical and accessible. *$16.95*
215 pages

1682 **Right from the Start: Behavioral Intervention for Young Children with Autism: A Guide**
Therapro
225 Arlington Street
Framingham, MA 01702
508-872-9494
800-257-5376
FAX 508-875-2062
http://www.theraproducts.com
e-mail: info@theraproducts.com
Mary Jane Weiss PhD BCBA, Sandra Harris PhD, Author
Karen Conrad, Owner

This informative and user-friendly guide helps parents and service providers explore programs that use early intensive behavioral intervention for young children with autism and related disorders. Within these programs, many children improve in intellectual, social and adaptive functioning, enabling them to move on to regular elementary and preschools. Benefits all children, but primarily useful for children age five and younger. *$14.95*
138 pages

1683 **Room 14**
LinguiSystems
3100 4th Avenue
East Moline, IL 61244
309-755-2300
800-776-4332
FAX 309-755-2377
TDY:800-933-8331
http://www.linguisystems.com
e-mail: service@linguisystems.com
Carolyn Wilson, Author
Linda Bowers, Co-Owner/Co-Founder
Rosemary Huisingh, Co-Owner/Co-Founder

Build social skills by offering a variety of teaching approaches to meet the language and learning needs of your students. Through stories, comprehension activities, and organized lessons, students learn to: make and keep friends: fit in at school; handle feelings; and be responsible for their actions. *$59.95*
198 pages Ages 6-10

1684 **S'Cool Moves for Learning: A Program Designed to Enhance Learning Through Body-Mind**
Therapro
225 Arlington Street
Framingham, MA 01702
508-872-9494
800-257-5376
FAX 508-875-2062
http://www.theraproducts.com
e-mail: info@theraproducts.com
Debra Heiberger MA, Margot Heiniger-White MA, Author
Karen Conrad, Owner

The movement activities described in this book are organized in a way that is easy to integrate into the class routine throughout the day. The Minute Moves for the Classroom included in several chapters is a handy reference of movement activities which help make the transition from one activity to another fun and smooth. *$35.00*

1685 **Self-Perception: Organizing Functional Information Workbook**
Therapro
225 Arlington Street
Framingham, MA 01702
508-872-9494
800-257-5376
FAX 508-875-2062
http://www.theraproducts.com
e-mail: info@theraproducts.com
Therapro Staff, Author
Karen Conrad, Owner

Recognizing human and animal body parts, discriminating between right and left, and exploring attitudes, emotions, humor and personal problem-solving. *$10.50*

1686 **Simple Steps: Developmental Activities for Infants, Toddlers & Two Year-Olds**
Therapro
225 Arlington Street
Framingham, MA 01702
508-872-9494
800-257-5376
FAX 508-875-2062
http://www.theraproducts.com
e-mail: info@theraproducts.com
Karen Miller, Author
Karen Conrad, Owner

Three hundred activities linked to the latest research in brain development. Outlines a typical developmental sequence in 10 domains: social/emotional, fine motor; gross motor; language; cognition; sensory; nature; music and movement; creativity and dramatic play. Chapters on curriculum development and learning environment also included. *$24.95*
293 pages

1687 **Solutions Kit for ADHD**
Childswork
45 Executive Drive
Plainview, NY 11803
516-349-6274
800-962-1141
FAX 877-434-6553
http://www.childswork.com
Sally Germain, Editorial

This comprehensive kit is packed with hands-on materials for a multi-modal approach to working with ADHD kids aged 5 through 12. *$105.00*
Ages 5-12

1688 **Song Games for Sensory Integration**
Therapro
225 Arlington Street
Framingham, MA 01702
508-872-9494
800-257-5376
FAX 508-875-2062
http://www.theraproducts.com
e-mail: info@theraproducts.com
Aubrey Carton, Lois Hickman, Author
Karen Conrad, Owner

For young children with sensory processing challenges, 15 play-along routines help remediate everything from bilateral skills to vestibular dysfunction. Narrative is helpful for parents. Includes a 51 page book filled with ideas for extending therapeutic value of these activites. 87 minute audio tape. *$21.00*
Audio Tape

1689 **Source for Syndromes**
LinguiSystems
3100 4th Avenue
East Moline, IL 61244
309-755-2300
800-776-4332
FAX 309-755-2377
TDY:800-933-8331
http://www.linguisystems.com
e-mail: service@linguisystems.com
Gail J Richard, Debra Reichert Hoge, Author
Linda Bowers, Co-Owner/Co-Founder
Rosemary Huisingh, Co-Owner/Co-Founder

Do you often wish someone would just tell you what to do with a specific youngster on your caseload? The Source for Syndromes can do just that. Learn about the speech-language characteristics for each sydrome with a focus on communication issues. This resource covers pertinent information for such sydromes such as Angelman, Asperger's, Autism, Rett's Tourette's, Williams, and more. *$41.95*

117 pages Ages Birth-18

1690 Start to Finish: Developmentally Sequenced Fine Motor Activities for Preschool Children

Therapro
225 Arlington Street
Framingham, MA 01702
508-872-9494
800-257-5376
FAX 508-875-2062
http://www.theraproducts.com
e-mail: info@theraproducts.com

Nory Marsh, Author
Karen Conrad, Owner

Seventy stimulating activities target 4 areas of fine motor development normally acquired between 3 and 5: hand manipulation, pencil grasp, scissors skill and grasp, and visual motor skills. Each 30 minute activity has skills, projected goal, supplies needed, instructions and modifications provided and needs limited preparation time. *$57.50*

1691 Stop, Relax and Think

Childswork
45 Executive Drive
Plainview, NY 11803
516-349-6274
800-962-1141
FAX 877-434-6553
http://www.childswork.com

Sally Germain, Editorial

In this board game, active impulsive children learn motor control, relaxation skills, how to express their feelings, and how to problem-solve. Can be used both as a diagnostic and a treatment tool, and behaviors learned in the game can be generalized into the home or classroom. *$52.00*

Ages 6-12

1692 Stop, Relax and Think Ball

Childswork
45 Executive Drive
Plainview, NY 11803
516-349-6274
800-962-1141
FAX 877-434-6553
http://www.childswork.com

Sally Germain, Editorial

This ball teaches children to control their impulsivity by helping them understand and control their actions. *$22.00*

1693 Stop, Relax and Think Card Game

Childswork
45 Executive Drive
Plainview, NY 11803
516-349-6274
800-962-1141
FAX 877-434-6553
http://www.childswork.com

Sally Germain, Editorial

Players are dealt Stop, Relax and Think cards and also Stressed Out, Confused, and Discouraged cards. As they acquire more cards, they must choose different self-control skills, and they learn the value of patience and cooperating with others to achieve a goal. *$21.95*

Ages 6-12

1694 Stop, Relax and Think Scriptbook

Childswork
45 Executive Drive
Plainview, NY 11803
516-349-6274
800-962-1141
FAX 877-434-6553
http://www.childswork.com

Sally Germain, Editorial

In this uniquely designed book, children can practice what to say and how to act in eight different scenarios common to children with behavioral problems. The counselor and the child sit across from each other and read the scripts. *$24.95*

Ages 8-12

1695 Stop, Relax and Think Workbook

Childswork
45 Executive Drive
Plainview, NY 11803
516-349-6274
800-257-5376
FAX 877-434-6553
http://www.childswork.com

Sally Germain, Editorial

This new workbook contains more than 60 paper and pencil activities that teach children such important skills as: thinking about consequences, staying focused and completing a task, engaging in quiet activities without disturbing others, and more. *$19.95*

Ages 6-12

1696 Successful Movement Challenges

Therapro
225 Arlington Street
Framingham, MA 01702
508-872-9494
800-257-5376
FAX 508-875-2062
http://www.theraproducts.com
e-mail: info@theraproducts.com

Jack Capon, Author
Karen Conrad, Owner

Extensive and exciting movement activities for children in preschool, elementary and special education. Includes movement exploration challenges using parachutes, balls, hoops, ropes, bean bags, rythm sticks, scarves and much more. This popular publication also includes body conditioning, mat activities and playground apparatus activities. Everyone enjoys the creative and carefully designed movement experiences. *$14.25*

127 pages

1697 Surface Counseling

Edge Enterprises
708 W 9th Street
Lawrence, KS 66044
785-749-1473
FAX 785-749-0207
e-mail: nfo@edgenterprise.inc.com

Joe N Crank, Donald D Deshler, Jean B Schumaker, Author
Sue Vernon, Manager
Jacqueline Schafer, Managing Editor
Carolyn Mitchell, Accounting

Details a set of relationship-building skills necessary for establishing a trusting, cooperative relationship between adults and youths and a problem-solving strategy that youths can learn to use by themselves. Includes study guide questions, model dialogues and role-play activities. Useful for any adult who has daily contact with children and adolescents.

60 pages Paperback

1698 Survival Guide for Kids with LD

Therapro
225 Arlington Street
Framingham, MA 01702
508-872-9494
800-257-5376
FAX 508-875-2062
http://www.theraproducts.com
e-mail: info@theraproducts.com

Gary Fisher PhD, Rhonda Cummings EdD, Author
Karen Conrad, Owner

Popular book that is highly reccommended. Contains vital information, practical advice, step-by-step strategies, and encouragement for children labeled Learning Disabled. *$9.95*

1699 Taking Part

AGS Publishing
PO Box 99
Circle Pines, MN 55014
651-287-7220
800-328-2560
FAX 800-471-8457
http://www.agsnet.com
e-mail: agsmail@agsnet.com

Gwendolyn Cartledge, James Kleefield, Author
Kevin Brueggeman, President
Matt Keller, Marketing Manager

A social skills program for students in preschool to grade 3 that teaches skills identified by research to be essential to social development: expressing oneself; playing with peers; responding to aggression; cooperating with peers; communicating nonverbally and making conversation. The program focuses on cooperative or group play skills and conflict resolution. Materials include a manual, puppets, stickers and posters. *$90.99*

ISBN 0-886714-21-4

1700 That's Life! Social Language

LinguiSystems
3100 4th Avenue
East Moline, IL 61244
309-755-2300
800-776-4332
FAX 309-755-2377
TDY:800-933-8331
http://www.linguisystems.com
e-mail: service@linguisystems.com
Linda Bowers, Co-Owner/Co-Founder
Rosemary Huisingh, Co-Owner/Co-Founder

Teach your students to be effective and appropriate communicators in a wide variety of situations. Through direct instruction, role-playing activities, and discussion, your students will learn the how and why of social language interaction.

Ages 12-18

1701 Tools for Students Video

Therapro
225 Arlington Street
Framingham, MA 01702
508-872-9494
800-257-5376
FAX 508-875-2062
http://www.theraproducts.com
e-mail: info@theraproducts.com
Therapro Staff, Author
Karen Conrad, Owner

This 30 minute video is a fun and participatory how-to video which provides solutions to the problems indentified in the Tools for Teachers Video. It can be used by teachers in the classroom and by parents at home. There are 25 sensory tools for movement, proprioception, mouth and hand fidgets, calming and recess. Pencil-holding and hand games to develop hand manipulation skills are also demonstrated. *$25.95*

Video

1702 Tools for Teachers Video

Therapro
225 Arlington Street
Framingham, MA 01702
508-872-9494
800-257-5376
FAX 508-875-2062
http://www.theraproducts.com
e-mail: info@theraproducts.com
Therapro Staff, Author
Karen Conrad, Owner

This video, designed by an OT to provide a logical approach to sensory integration and hand skill strategies for anyone to use, is ideal for in-services. Within 20 minutes, you'll learn how to help students calm down, focus, and increase their self-awareness. This is a great tool for teachers and therapists (shows how to inplement sensory diet into classroom), administrators and parents. *$25.95*

Video

1703 Understanding Argumentative Communication: How Many Ways Can You Ask for a Cookie?

Therapro
225 Arlington Street
Framingham, MA 01702
508-872-9494
800-257-5376
FAX 508-875-2062
http://www.theraproducts.com
e-mail: info@theraproducts.com
Christine Derse MEd, Janice Lopes MSEd, Author
Karen Conrad, Owner

Ten uncomplicated lesson plans for classroom use. Teach a complete overview of all that Argumentative Communication encompasses or give students a brief awareness lesson about just one type of communication. Lessons can be used either consecutively or singly. Includes defining communication, gestures, sign language, object boards, picture boards, headsticks, eye pointing, scanning with picture boards, picture boards in sentence format and computers for argumentative communication. *$17.95*

142 pages

1704 Updown Chair

R.E.A.L. Design
187 S Main Street
Dolgeville, NY 13329
315-429-3071
800-696-7041
FAX 315-429-3071
http://www.realdesigninc.com
e-mail: rdesign@twcny.rr.com
Kris Wohnsen, Co-Owner
Sam Camarello, Co-Owner

The updown chair is designed for children from 43"-63" in height. It combines optimal positioning and sitting comfort with ease of adjustment. Changing the seat height can be done quickly and safely with our exclusive foot lever activation which uses a pneumatic cylinder assist. Children can be elevated to just the right position for floor or table top activities.

5-15 years

1705 What's Up? A That's LIFE! Game of Social Language

LinguiSystems
3100 4th Avenue
East Moline, IL 61244
309-755-2300
800-776-4332
FAX 309-755-2377
TDY:800-933-8331
http://www.linguisystems.com
e-mail: service@linguisystems.com
Carolyn LoGiudice, Nancy McConnell, Author
Linda Bowers, Co-Owner/Co-Founder
Rosemary Huisingh, Co-Owner/Co-Founder

Here's a game with strategy, fast action, and competition. Your older students will love it! Teach appropriate social communication with this game. Peer evaluation is built-in so students can track progress. *$44.95*

Ages 12-16

1706 Who Cares?

Therapro
225 Arlington Street
Framingham, MA 01702
508-872-9494
800-257-5376
FAX 508-875-2062
http://www.theraproducts.com
e-mail: info@theraproducts.com
Therapro Staff, Author
Karen Conrad, Owner

This series of small handbooks for children teaches them about diversity. *$7.99*

32 pages Hardcover

1707 Wikki Stix Hands On-Learning Activity Book

Therapro
225 Arlington Street
Framingham, MA 01702
508-872-9494
800-257-5376
FAX 508-875-2062
http://www.theraproducts.com
e-mail: info@theraproducts.com
Therapro Staff, Author
Karen Conrad, Owner

Loaded with great ideas for using Wikki Stix. For all ages and curriculums. *$3.50*

1708 Workbook for Verbal Expression

Abilitations Speech Bin
PO Box 922668
Norcross, GA 30010
770-449-5700
800-850-8602
FAX 770-510-7290
http://www.speechbin.com
e-mail: info@speechbin.com

Beth M Kennedy, Author
Tobi Isaacs, Catalog Director

A book of 100s of excercises from simple naming, automatic speech sequences, and repetition exercises to complex tasks in sentence formulation and abstract verbal reasoning. Item number 1435. *$49.99*

Social Studies

1709 A Knock at the Door
Harcourt Achieve
6277 Sea Harbor Drive
Orlando, FL 32887
252-480-3200
800-531-5015
FAX 800-699-9459
http://www.steckvaughn.com
e-mail: info@steckvaughn.com
Eric Sonderling, Wendy Wassink Ackison, Author
Tim McEwen, President/CEO
Jeff Johnson, Dir Marketing Communications
Chris Lehmann, Team Coordinator
The frightened stranger's identity remains a secret until the day a Nazi soldier knocks on the door.

1710 A World So Different
Harcourt Achieve
6277 Sea Harbor Drive
Orlando, FL 32887
252-480-3200
800-531-5015
FAX 800-699-9459
http://www.steckvaughn.com
e-mail: info@steckvaughn.com
Steck-Vaughn Staff, Author
Tim McEwen, President/CEO
Jeff Johnson, Dir Marketing Communications
Chris Lehmann, Team Coordinator
As generations of family members recall how dramatically technology has changed everyday life, Sarah wonders what changes are in store for her generation.

1711 American Government Today: Steadwell
Harcourt Achieve
Customer Service, 5th Floor
Orlando, FL 32887
800-284-7019
FAX 800-699-9459
http://www.harcourtachieve.com
e-mail: webmaster@harcourt.com
Sanders, Author
Tim McEwen, President/CEO
Susan Canizares, SVP Publisher
Lee Wilson, VP Marketing
Give limited readers unlimited access to social studies and citizenship topics! Whether applying for citizenship or studying for GED Test, learners need to know about our nation's capital and the democracy it hosts. In this series, even limited readers can get a clear picture of a complex system. *$44.40*

1712 Calliope
Cobblestone Publishing
30 Grove Street
Peterborough, NH 03458
603-924-7209
800-821-0115
FAX 603-924-7380
http://www.cricketmag.com
e-mail: custsvc@cobblestone.mv.com
Rosalie Baker, Editor

Kid's world history magazine written for kids ages 9 to 14, goes beyond the facts to explore provocative issues. *$29.95*
49 pages 9x/year 1981

1713 Discoveries: Explore the Desert Ecosystem
Sunburst Technology
1550 Executive Drive
Elgin, IL 60123
800-321-7511
FAX 888-800-3028
http://http://store.sunburst.com/Home.aspx
e-mail: service@sunburst.com
Michael Guillory, Channel Sales/Marketing Manager

This program invites students to explore the plants, animals, culture and georgraphy of the Sonoran Desert by day and by night.

1714 Discoveries: Explore the Everglades Ecosystem
Sunburst Technology
1550 Executive Drive
Elgin, IL 60123
800-321-7511
FAX 888-800-3028
http://http://store.sunburst.com/Home.aspx
e-mail: service@sunburst.com
Michael Guillory, Channel Sales/Marketing Manager

This multi curricular research program takes students to the Everglades where they anchor their exploration photo realistic panaramas of the habitiat.

1715 Discoveries: Explore the Forest Ecosystem
Sunburst Technology
1550 Executive Drive
Elgin, IL 60123
800-321-7511
FAX 888-800-3028
http://http://store.sunburst.com/Home.aspx
e-mail: service@sunburst.com
Michael Guillory, Channel Sales/Marketing Manager

This theme based CD-ROM enables students of all abilities to actively research a multitude of different forest ecosystems in the Appalachian National Park.

1716 Easybook Deluxe Writing Workshop: Colonial Times
Sunburst Technology
1550 Executive Drive
Elgin, IL 60123
800-321-7511
FAX 888-800-3028
http://http://store.sunburst.com/Home.aspx
e-mail: service@sunburst.com
Michael Guillory, Channel Sales/Marketing Manager

Writing workshops combine theme-based activities with the award-winning EasyBook Deluxe.

1717 Easybook Deluxe Writing Workshop: Immigration
Sunburst Technology
1550 Executive Drive
Elgin, IL 60123
800-321-7511
FAX 888-800-3028
http://http://store.sunburst.com/Home.aspx
e-mail: service@sunburst.com
Michael Guillory, Channel Sales/Marketing Manager

Writing workshops combine theme-based activities with the award-winning EasyBook Deluxe.

1718 Easybook Deluxe Writing Workshop: Rainforest & Astronomy
Sunburst Technology
1550 Executive Drive
Elgin, IL 60123
800-321-7511
FAX 888-800-3028
http://http://store.sunburst.com/Home.aspx
e-mail: service@sunburst.com
Michael Guillory, Channel Sales/Marketing Manager

Writing workshops combine theme-based activities with the award-winning EasyBook Deluxe.

1719 **Explorers & Exploration: Steadwell**
Harcourt Achieve
Customer Service, 5th Floor
Orlando, FL 32887
800-284-7019
FAX 800-699-9459
http://www.harcourtachieve.com
e-mail: webmaster@harcourt.com
Steck-Vaughn Staff, Author
Tim McEwen, President/CEO
Susan Canizares, SVP Publisher
Lee Wilson, VP Marketing
Long ago adventures are still a thrill in these vividly illustrated titles. Maps, diagrams, and contemporary prints lend an authenic air. A time line and list of events in the appropriate century put history in perspective. *$44.40*

ISBN 0-739822-05-5

1720 **First Biographies**
Harcourt Achieve
Customer Service, 5th Floor
Orlando, FL 32887
800-284-7019
FAX 800-699-9459
http://www.harcourtachieve.com
e-mail: webmaster@harcourt.com
Steck-Vaughn Staff, Author
Tim McEwen, President/CEO
Susan Canizares, SVP Publisher
Lee Wilson, VP Marketing
True stories of true legends! Legendary figures triumph over tough challenges in these brief biographies. Beginning readers learn about favorite heroes and heroines in books they can read for themselves. *$98.80*

ISBN 0-817268-91-X

1721 **Imagination Express Destination Time Trip USA**
Sunburst Technology
1550 Executive Drive
Elgin, IL 60123
800-321-7511
FAX 888-800-3028
http://http://store.sunburst.com/Home.aspx
e-mail: service@sunburst.com
Michael Guillory, Channel Sales/Marketing Manager

Student's travel through time to explore the history and development of a fictional New England town. An online scrapbook lets them learn about architecture, fashion, entertainment and events of the six major periods in U.S. history.

1722 **Make-a-Map 3D**
Sunburst Technology
1550 Executive Drive
Elgin, IL 60123
800-321-7511
FAX 888-800-3028
http://http://store.sunburst.com/Home.aspx
e-mail: service@sunburst.com
Michael Guillory, Channel Sales/Marketing Manager

Students learn basic mapping, geography and navigation skills. Students design maps of their immediate surroundings by dragging and dropping roads and buildings and adding landmarks, land forms and traffic signs.

1723 **Maps & Navigation**
Sunburst Technology
1550 Executive Drive
Elgin, IL 60123
800-321-7511
FAX 888-800-3028
http://http://store.sunburst.com/Home.aspx
e-mail: service@sunburst.com
Michael Guillory, Channel Sales/Marketing Manager

This exciting nautical simulation provides students with opportunities to use their math and science skills.

1724 **Patterns Across the Curriculum**
Harcourt Achieve
6277 Sea Harbor Drive
Orlando, FL 32887
252-480-3200
800-531-5015
FAX 800-699-9459
http://www.steckvaughn.com
e-mail: info@steckvaughn.com
Steck-Vaughn Staff, Author
Tim McEwen, President/CEO
Jeff Johnson, Dir Marketing Communications
Chris Lehmann, Team Coordinator
Develop students' awareness and understanding of patterns in the real world. Exercises allow students to identify, complete, extend, and create patterns. Developed across math, language, social studies, and science. This flexible organization allows teachers to utilize content specific activities in coordination with other classroom assignments, providing additional richness in learning.

1725 **Prehistoric Creaures Then & Now: Steadwell**
Harcourt Achieve
Customer Service, 5th Floor
Orlando, FL 32887
800-284-7019
FAX 800-699-9459
http://www.harcourtachieve.com
e-mail: webmaster@harcourt.com
Steck-Vaughn Staff, Author
Tim McEwen, President/CEO
Susan Canizares, SVP Publisher
Lee Wilson, VP Marketing
Now limited readers can dig into the details of dinosaurs! Each information-packed title includes a special spread with a project, a profile of a dinosaur expert, or a description of a recent dinosaur discovery. *$44.40*

ISBN 0-739822-07-1

1726 **Story of the USA**
Educators Publishing Service
PO Box 9031
Cambridge, MA 02139
617-547-6706
800-225-5750
FAX 888-440-2665
http://www.epsbooks.com
e-mail: eps@epsbooks.com
Franklin Escher Jr, Author
Gunnar Voltz, President

A series of four workbooks for grades 4-8 which presents basic topics in American History: Book 1, Explorers and Settlers - Book 2, A Young Nation Solves Its Problems - Book 3, America Becomes A Giant - and Book 4, Modern America. A list of vocabulary words introduces each chapter and study questions test students' knowledge.

1727 **Talking Walls Bundle**
Sunburst Technology
1550 Executive Drive
Elgin, IL 60123
800-321-7511
FAX 888-800-3028
http://http://store.sunburst.com/Home.aspx
e-mail: service@sunburst.com
Michael Guillory, Channel Sales/Marketing Manager

Broaden students' perspective of cultures around the world with this two program CD-ROM bundle. From the Great Wall of China to the Berlin Wall to the Vietnam Memorial, students explore 28 "walls" that represent examples of the greatest human achievements to the most intimate expressions of individuality.

1728 **Test Practice Success: American History**
Harcourt Achieve
Customer Service, 5th Floor
Orlando, FL 32887
800-284-7019
FAX 800-699-9459
http://www.harcourtachieve.com
e-mail: webmaster@harcourt.com

Steck-Vaughn Staff, Author
Tim McEwen, President/CEO
Susan Canizares, SVP Publisher
Lee Wilson, VP Marketing
When you are trying to meet history standards, standardized test preparation is hard to schedule. Now you can do both at the same time. Steck-Vaughn/Berrent Test Practice Success: American History refreshes basic skills, familiarizes students with test formats and directions, and teaches test-taking strategies, while drawing on the material students are studying in class. *$16.30*

ISBN 0-739831-31-3

1729 **True Tales**
Harcourt Achieve
Customer Service, 5th Floor
Orlando, FL 32877
800-284-7019
FAX 800-699-9459
http://www.harcourtachieve.com
e-mail: webmaster@harcourt.com
Billings, Author
Tim McEwen, President/CEO
Susan Canizares, SVP Publisher
Lee Wilson, VP Marketing
If you have been looking for reading comprehension materials for limiteed readers, your search is over. True Tales presents powerful real-lfe events with direct connections to geography and science at reading level 3. Gripping accounts of personal triumph and tragedy put geography and science in a very real context. Accompanying activities develop reading and language arts, science, and geography skills students need to boost test scores. *$185.80*

ISBN 0-739834-49-5

Study Skills

1730 **125 Ways to Be a Better Student**
LinguiSystems
3100 4th Avenue
East Moline, IL 61244
309-755-2300
800-776-4332
FAX 309-755-2377
TDY:800-933-8331
http://www.linguisystems.com
e-mail: service@linguisystems.com
Paula Currie, Mary deBrueys, Jill Exnicios, Author
Linda Bowers, Co-Owner/Co-Founder
Rosemary Huisingh, Co-Owner/Co-Founder

Eliminate poor study habits! Help your students develop positive attitudes toward school with these study strategies. Students will get organized and take responsibility for their classroom attitude with these terrific lessons. Lessons are complete with key vocabulary, informative handouts, and practice activities. *$35.95*
136 pages Ages 10-18

1731 **125 Ways to Be a Better Test-Taker**
LinguiSystems
3100 4th Avenue
East Moline, IL 61244
309-755-2300
800-776-4332
FAX 309-755-2377
TDY:800-933-8331
http://www.linguisystems.com
e-mail: service@linguisystems.com
Andrea M Lazzari, Judy W Wood, Author
Linda Bowers, Co-Owner/Co-Founder
Rosemary Huisingh, Co-Owner/Co-Founder

Help your students with test-taking strategies they can use right away. Through activities and practice tests, students learn test-taking strategies including: looking for key words in true/false questions;, answering the multiple-choice questions you know first;, drawing lines through answers you've used in matching questions, re-reading passages for comprehension tasks;, and adding details to a main idea in an essay test. *$35.95*
150 pages Ages 12-18

1732 **Crash Course for Study Skills**
LinguiSystems
3100 4th Avenue
East Moline, IL 61244
309-755-2300
800-776-4332
FAX 309-755-2377
TDY:800-933-8331
http://www.linguisystems.com
e-mail: service@linguisystems.com
Marty Soper, Author
Linda Bowers, Co-Owner/Co-Founder
Rosemary Huisingh, Co-Owner/Co-Founder

These helpful study strategies teach your students to take responsibility for their own learning. It's a practical, motivating approach that works! Students will learn to set goals, manage time, take notes, improve study habits, and understand their personal learning styles. *$35.95*
172 pages Ages 12-18

1733 **Experiences with Writing Styles**
Harcourt Achieve
Customer Service, 5th Floor
Orlando, FL 32887
800-284-7019
FAX 800-699-9459
http://www.harcourtachieve.com
e-mail: webmaster@harcourt.com
Steck-Vaughn Staff, Author
Tim McEwen, President/CEO
Susan Canizares, SVP Publisher
Lee Wilson, VP Marketing
Give your students experience applying the writing process in nine relevant situations, from personal narratives to persuasive paragraphs to research reports. Units provide a clear definition of each genre and plenty of practice with prewriting, writing, revising, proofreading, and publishing. *$11.99*

1734 **INSPECT: A Strategy for Finding and Correcting Spelling Errors**
Edge Enterprises
708 W 9th Street
Lawrence, KS 66044
785-749-1473
FAX 785-749-0207
e-mail: nfo@edgenterprise.inc.com
David B McNaughton and Charles A Hughes, Author
Jacqueline Schafer, Managing Editor
Sue Schafer, Manager
Carolyn Mitchell, Accounting
A strategy for detecting and correcting spelling errors in work generated with a word processing-based spellchecker. Can also be adapted for use with hand-held spellcheckers. The manual comes with IBM and Macintosh computer disks containing practice passages appropriate for upper elementary-aged students, junior-high students and high-school students. The passages can be used with such word processing programs as MS Word, Claris Works and MS Works.
36 pages Paperback

1735 **Keyboarding Skills**
Educators Publishing Service
PO Box 9031
Cambridge, MA 02139
617-547-6706
800-225-5750
FAX 888-440-2665
http://www.epsbooks.com
e-mail: eps@epsbooks.com
Diana Hanbury King, Author
Gunnar Voltz, President

This innovative touch typing method enables students of all ages to learn to type quickly and easily. After learning the alphabet, students can practice words, phrases, numbers, symbols and punctuation.

1736 **LD Teacher's IEP Companion**
LinguiSystems
3100 4th Avenue
East Moline, IL 61244
309-755-2300
800-776-4332
FAX 309-755-2377
TDY:800-933-8331
http://www.linguisystems.com
e-mail: service@linguisystems.com
Molly Lyle, Author
Linda Bowers, Co-Owner/Co-Founder
Rosemary Huisingh, Co-Owner/Co-Founder

These IEP goals are organized developmentally by skill area with individual objectives and classroom activity suggestions. Goals and objectives cover these academic areas: math, reading, writing, literacy concepts, attention skills, study skills, classroom behavior, social interaction, and transition skills. *$39.95*
169 pages Ages 5-18

1737 **Learning Strategies Curriculum**
Edge Enterprises
708 W 9th Street
Lawrence, KS 66044
785-749-1473
FAX 785-749-0207
e-mail: nfo@edgenterprise.inc.com
Jacqueline Schafer, Managing Editor
Sue Vernon, Manager
Carolyn Mitchell, Accounting
A learning strategy is an individual's approach to a learning task. It includes how a person thinks and acts when planning, executing and evaluating performance on the task and its outcomes. In short, learning strategy instruction focuses on how to learn and how to effectively use what has been learned. Manuals range from sentence writing to test taking. All require training. For information, contact the Kansas Center for Research on Learning, 3061 Dole Center, Lawrence 66045 (785-864-4780)

1738 **Peer Pals**
AGS Publishing
4201 Woodland Road
Circle Pines, MN 55014
763-786-4343
800-328-2560
FAX 800-471-8457
http://www.agsnet.com
e-mail: agsmail@agsnet.com
Robert P Bowman,John N Chanaca, Author
Kevin Brueggeman, Manager
Matt Keller, Marketing Manager

A peer helping program designed to improve study skills, self-esteem, and decision-making. The program uses a big sister/big brother approach, as grade 3-6 students are paired with grade K-2 students. *$33.99*

ISBN 0-886711-62-2

1739 **Resource Room**
608 S Race Street
Urbana, IL 61801
217-367-6218
http://www.resourceroom.net
e-mail: info@resourceroom.net
Susan Jones, President/Founder

Tools, strategies, and structured explorations for interesting learners. Resources for people who learn differently, or have learning difficulties or learning disabilities such as dyslexia, dysgraphia, or dyscalculia.

1740 **SLANT: A Starter Strategy for Class Participation**
Edge Enterprises
708 W 9th Street
Lawrence, KS 66044
785-749-1473
FAX 785-749-0207
e-mail: nfo@edgenterprise.inc.com
Edwin S Ellis, Author
Jacqueline Schafer, Managing Editor
Sue Vernon, Manager
Carolyn Mitchell, Accounting

An easy-to-learn strategy that students of all ages can use to combine nonverbal, cognitive and verbal behaviors to increase their class participation. Specifically, students learn how to use appropriate posture, track the speaker, activate their thinking and contribute information. Once exposed to this strategy, students not only increase their amount of class participation, but understand how their use of positive participation behaviors can influence the reactions of others.
8 pages Pamphlet

1741 **School Power: Strategies for Succeeding in School**
Therapro
225 Arlington Street
Framingham, MA 01702
508-872-9494
800-257-5376
FAX 508-875-2062
http://www.theraproducts.com
e-mail: info@theraproducts.com
Jeanne Schumm PhD, Marguite Radencich PhD, Author
Karen Conrad, Owner

A great book for students, parents and teachers. Helps students get organized, take notes, study smarter, write better, handle homework and more. Includes 17 reproducible handout masters. *$16.95*
136 pages

1742 **Study Skills and Learning Strategies for Transition**
HEATH Resource Center
2121 K Street NW
Washington, DC 20037
202-337-7600
800-544-3284
FAX 202-973-0908
http://www.heath.gwu.gov
e-mail: askheath@gwu.edu
Pamela Ekpone MD, Director
Janine Heath, Manager

The curriculum guide provides students with learning disabilities the skills and strategies they will need to increase their level of success within the high school curriculum. *$15.00*

1743 **Super Study Wheel: Homework Helper**
Therapro
225 Arlington Street
Framingham, MA 01702
508-872-9494
800-257-5376
FAX 508-875-2062
http://www.theraproducts.com
e-mail: info@theraproducts.com
Therapro Staff, Author
Karen Conrad, Owner

The fun and simple way to find study tips. Developed by learning specialists and an occupational therapist, the Super Study Wheel is an idea-packed resource (with 101 tips) to improve study skills in 13 areas. As a visual, motor and kinesthetic tool, it is very helpful to students with unique learning styles. *$6.95*

Toys & Games, Catalogs

1744 **Enabling Devices/Toys for Special Children**
Enabling Devices
385 Warburton Avenue
Hastings on Hudson, NY 10706
914-478-0960
800-832-8697
FAX 914-478-7030
http://www.enablingdevices.com
e-mail: info@enablingdevices.com
Steven Kanor PhD, Owner

A designer, manufacturer and distributor of unique and affordable assitive and adaptive technologies for the physically and mentally challenged, ED/TFSC's products are sought by parents, teachers, and professionals alike.

1745 **Maxi Aids**
Maxi-Aids, Inc
42 Executive Boulevard
Farmingdale, NY 11735
631-752-0521
FAX 631-752-0689
http://www.maxiaids.com

Aids and appliances for independent living with products designed especially for the visually impaired, blind, hard of hearing, deaf, deaf-blind, arthritic and the physically challenged. New educational games and toys section.

1746 PCI Educational Publishing

4560 Lockhill Road
San Antonio, TX 78249
800-594-4263
FAX 888-259-8284
http://www.pcieducation.com
e-mail: returns@pcieducation.com

Robert Pici, President
Janie Haugen-McLane, Senior VP/Founder
Resnik VP Sales/Marketing, Sales VP/Marketing

Offers 14 programs in a gameboard format to improve life and social skills including Cooking Class, Community Skills, Looking Good, Eating Skills, Workplace Skills, Behavior Skills, Time Skills, Money Skills, Safety Skills, Household Skills, Social Skills, Health Skills, Survival Skills and Recreation Skills. Also offers a Life Skills catalog with over 140 additional products.

1747 School Specialties

Guidance Channel
PO Box 9120
Plainview, NY 11803
516-349-5520
800-962-9020
FAX 800-262-1886
http://www.childswork.com
e-mail: info@childswork.com

Carmine Russo, Manager

The most complete source for toys, books and games to help children with their mental health needs, including hundreds of items that deal with ADD, behavior problems, learning disabilities, physical disabilities, sleep disorders, stress and more.

1748 Therapro

225 Arlington Street
Framingham, MA 01702
508-872-9494
800-257-5376
FAX 508-875-2062
http://www.theraproducts.com
e-mail: info@theraproducts.com

Karen Conrad, Owner

Therapro offers for families and professionals a 100+ page catalog with the following: handwriting and fine motor products; perceptual, cognitive and language activities; publications and assessments.
116 pages

Toys & Games, Products

1749 Animal Match-Ups

Therapro
225 Arlington Street
Framingham, MA 01702
508-872-9494
800-257-5376
FAX 508-875-2062
http://www.theraproducts.com
e-mail: info@theraproducts.com

Therapro Staff, Author
Karen Conrad, Owner

A wonderful visual memory game designed to appeal to young children. Learn to recognize 28 animals by collecting matching pairs from remembered positions. Develops attention and memory. *$8.95*
Ages 3+

1750 Artic Shuffle

LinguiSystems
3100 4th Avenue
East Moline, IL 61244
309-755-2300
800-776-4332
FAX 309-755-2377
TDY:800-933-8331
http://www.linguisystems.com
e-mail: service@linguisystems.com

Tobie Nan Kaufman, Author
Linda Bowers, Co-Owner/Co-Founder
Rosemary Huisingh, Co-Owner/Co-Founder

Why are these card decks best-sellers? Because they're real playing cards! Your students can play Go Fish, Crazy Eights, or Concentration while they practice their target sounds. Use them for vocabulary drills or naming practice. *$89.95*
Ages 5-Adult

1751 ArticBURST Articulation Practice for S, R, Ch, and Sh

LinguiSystems
3100 4th Avenue
East Moline, IL 61244
309-755-2300
800-776-4332
FAX 309-755-2377
TDY:800-933-8331
http://www.linguisystems.com
e-mail: service@linguisystems.com

LinguiSystems Staff, Author
Linda Bowers, Co-Owner/Co-Founder
Rosemary Huisingh, Co-Owner/Co-Founder

Here's a fun quick-thinking game for your older students and clients who continue to need articulation therapy. You'll get a set of cards for each of the toughest sounds. Players have to think of a word with their target sound in these four areas: rhyming, compounds, antonyms, and synonyms. *$37.95*
Ages 10-Adult

1752 BUSY BOX Activity Centers

Enabling Devices
385 Warburton Avenue
Hastings on Hudson, NY 10706
914-478-0960
800-832-8697
FAX 914-478-7030
http://www.enablingdevices.com
e-mail: info@enablingdevices.com

Steven Kanor PhD, Owner
Karen O'Connor, Operations VP

With their bright colors and exciting variety of textures and shapes that are designed to invite exploration that results in rewards including buzzers, music box melodies, radio, vibrations, puffs of air, flashing lights, and even a model that talks. Encourages hand-eye coordination, fine motor skills, gross arm movement. A full line of activity centers are available to meet the needs of the learning disabled, hearing impaired, visually impaired and multisensory impaired.

1753 Barnaby's Burrow: An Auditory Processing Game

LinguiSystems
3100 4th Avenue
East Moline, IL 61244
309-755-2300
800-776-4332
FAX 309-755-2377
TDY:800-933-8331
http://www.linguisystems.com
e-mail: service@linguisystems.com

Barb Truman, Author
Linda Bowers, Co-Owner/Co-Founder
Rosemary Huisingh, Co-Owner/Co-Founder

Your students will practice good auditory processing skills as they help Barnaby the rabbit get to his burrow. This delightful game gives you tons of auditory processing tasks at increasing levels of difficulty. 300 game cards provide stimulus items for: phonological awareness; following directions; absurdities; and identifying main idea and details. *$44.95*
Ages 4-9

1754 Beads and Baubles

Therapro
225 Arlington Street
Framingham, MA 01702
508-872-9494
800-257-5376
FAX 508-875-2062
http://www.theraproducts.com
e-mail: info@theraproducts.com

Therapro Staff, Author
Karen Conrad, Owner

A basic stringing activity great for developing fine motor skills. Over 100 pieces in various shapes, colors, and sizes to string on a lace. Three laces included. *$7.50*

1755 **Beads and Pattern Cards: Complete Set**
Therapro
225 Arlington Street
Framingham, MA 01702
508-872-9494
800-257-5376
FAX 508-875-2062
http://www.theraproducts.com
e-mail: info@theraproducts.com
Therapro Staff, Author
Karen Conrad, Owner

Colorful wooden sphers, cubes, cylinders and laces provide pre-reading/early math practice and help develop shape/color sorting and recognition skills. *$26.50*

1756 **Big-Little Pegboard Set**
Therapro
225 Arlington Street
Framingham, MA 01702
508-872-9494
800-257-5376
FAX 508-875-2062
http://www.theraproducts.com
e-mail: info@theraproducts.com
Therapro Staff, Author
Karen Conrad, Owner

Kids love to play with this set of 25 safe, brightly colored hardwood pegs and a durable foam rubber board. *$16.99*

1757 **Blend It! End It!**
LinguiSystems
3100 4th Avenue
East Moline, IL 61244
309-755-2300
800-776-4332
FAX 309-755-2377
TDY:800-933-8331
http://www.linguisystems.com
e-mail: service@linguisystems.com
Heather Koepke, Author
Linda Bowers, Co-Owner/Co-Founder
Rosemary Huisingh, Co-Owner/Co-Founder

Get this fun, quick-thinking game to work on phonics and spelling skills. Players write as many words as they can that include a specific initial blend or word ending. You get 36 initial word blends including: bl-, cr-, spl-. sk-, th-, tw-. *$42.95*
Ages 7-14

1758 **Brainopoly: A Thinking Game**
LinguiSystems
3100 4th Avenue
East Moline, IL 61244
309-755-2300
800-776-4332
FAX 309-755-2377
TDY:800-933-8331
http://www.linguisystems.com
e-mail: service@linguisystems.com
LinguiSystems Staff, Author
Linda Bowers, CEO
Rosemary Huisingh, Co-Owner/Co-Founder

Target all the critical thinking, problem-solving, and decision-making skills your older students need to meet the demands of the classroom curriculum. Each game section has 50 questions divided into two levels of difficulty. That's 450 total questions! Students will practice using predicting, inferring, deduction skills, and more! *$44.95*
Ages 10-15

1759 **Categorically Speaking**
Abilitations Speech Bin
PO Box 922668
Norcross, GA 30010
770-449-5700
800-850-8602
FAX 770-510-7290
http://www.speechbin.com
e-mail: info@speechbin.com
Tobi Isaacs, Catalog Director

This game for two to four players or two teams gives 6-10 years-olds experience in asking questions, evaluating information they receive, and using it to solve problems. To play, they must use specified question formats to get clues about pictures, recognize similarities and differences, identify salient features of objects, and encode and decode messages. Item number Q849. *$56.99*

1760 **Children's Cabinet**
1090 S Rock Boulevard
Reno, NV 89502
775-856-6200
FAX 775-856-6208
http://www.childrenscabinet.org
e-mail: mail@childrenscabinet.org
Laura Marineau, Community Educator

The Children's Cabinet is our community's stand to ensure every child and family has the services and resources to meet fundamental development, care, and learning needs.

1761 **Clip Art Collections: The Environment & Space**
1550 Executive Drive
Elgin, IL 60123
800-321-7511
FAX 888-800-3028
Mark Sotir, CEO
Morton Cohen, VP/CFO
Daniel Figurski, VP Sales
This thematic clip art collection is a perfect creativity tool for the classroom.

1762 **Clip Art Collections: The US & The World**
Sunburst Technology
1550 Executive Drive
Elgin, IL 60123
FAX 888-800-3028
http://http://store.sunburst.com/Home.aspx
e-mail: service
Michael Guillory, Channel Sales/Marketing Manager

This thematic clip art collection is a perfect tool for the classroom.

1763 **Colored Wooden Counting Cubes**
Therapro
225 Arlington Street
Framingham, MA 01702
508-872-9494
800-257-5376
FAX 508 875 2062
http://www.theraproducts.com
e-mail: info@theraproducts.com
Therapro Staff, Author
Karen Conrad, Owner

100 cubes in 6 colors are perfect for counting, patterning, and building activities. Activity Guide included. *$19.95*

1764 **Come Play with Me**
Therapro
225 Arlington Street
Framingham, MA 01702
508-872-9494
800-257-5376
FAX 508-875-2062
http://www.theraproducts.com
e-mail: info@theraproducts.com
Therapro Staff, Author
Karen Conrad, Owner

This three-dimensional game is so much fun while working on language, matching and visual observation skills. Toys are everywhere! Balls in the livingroom, trains in the kitchen, bears in the bedroom. Look, I found the blocks! Can you be the first to collect all of the toys you need for your toybox? *$19.95*
Ages 3-6

1765 **Communication Aids**
Enabling Devices
385 Warburton Avenue
Hastings on Hudson, NY 10706
914-478-0960
800-832-8697
FAX 914-478-7030
http://www.enabling devices. com
e-mail: info@enablingdevices.com
Steven Kanor PhD, Owner
Karen O'Connor, Operations VP

Designed to encourage independence by allowing the user to speak your pre-recorded messages.

1766 Create-A-Story
Speech Bin
PO Box 922668
Norcross, GA 30010
770-449-5700
800-850-8602
FAX 770-510-7290
http://www.speechbin.com
e-mail: info@speechbin.com
Shane Peters, Product Coordinator
Jen Binney, Owner

Here's a powerful language learning game that simplifies the creative process of story-telling and writing for 5-99 years-olds. It fosters their imaginations, organizes their thoughts, and boosts their confidence as they build a narrative. The game can be played by 1-6 players as groups or individuals. Item number C151. *$44.95*

1767 Decoding Games
LinguiSystems
3100 4th Avenue
East Moline, IL 61244
309-755-2300
800-776-4332
FAX 309-755-2377
TDY:800-933-8331
http://www.linguisystems.com
e-mail: service@linguisystems.com
Tina Sanford, Author
Linda Bowers, Co-Owner/Co-Founder
Rosemary Huisingh, Co-Owner/Co-Founder

Get three fun games in one handy case. These colorful games target tricky decoding skills your students need for strong reading skills. *$39.95*
Ages 6-10

1768 Definition Play by Play
LinguiSystems
3100 4th Avenue
East Moline, IL 61244
309-755-2300
800-776-4332
FAX 309-755-2377
TDY:800-933-8331
http://www.linguisystems.com
e-mail: service@linguisystems.com
Sharon Spencer, Author
Linda Bowers, Co-Owner/Co-Founder
Rosemary Huisingh, Co-Owner/Co-Founder

Teach your students to give accurate, cohesive definitions by identifying and organizing critical attributes of words. As players move along the board, they describe an object card by these attributes: function; what goes with it; size/shape; color; parts; what it's made of; and location. *$44.95*
Ages 8-14

1769 Disc-O-Bocce
Therapro
225 Arlington Street
Framingham, MA 01702
508-872-9494
800-257-5376
FAX 508-875-2062
http://www.theraproducts.com
e-mail: info@theraproducts.com
Therapro Staff, Author
Karen Conrad, Owner

Requested by therapists working with adults, this item is also great for children. Hundreds of uses include tossing the discs onto the ground and stepping on them to follow their path, tossing and trying to hit the same color disc on the floor, or using the discs to toss in a game of tic-tac-toe on the floor. Includes 12 colorful bocce discs in a storage box with handle. *$17.95*

1770 Earobics® Clinic Version Step 2
Abilitations Speech Bin
PO Box 922668
Norcross, GA 30010
770-449-5700
800-850-8602
FAX 770-510-7290
http://www.speechbin.com
e-mail: info@speechbin.com
Tobi Isaacs, Catalog Director

Earobics features: Tasks and Level Counter with real time display, adaptive training technology for individualized programs and reporting to track and evaluate each individual's progress. Step 2 teaches critical language comprehension skills and trains the critical auditory skills children need for success in learning. Item number C484. *$298.99*

1771 Earobics® Home Version Step 2
Abilitations Speech Bin
PO Box 922668
Norcross, GA 30010
770-449-5700
800-850-8602
FAX 770-510-7290
http://www.speechbin.com
e-mail: info@speechbin.com
Tobi Isaacs, Catalog Director

Step 2 teaches critical language comprehension skills and trains the critical auditory skills children need for success in learning. It offers hundreds of levels of play, appealing graphics, and entertaining music to train the critical auditory skills young children need for success in learning. Item number C483. *$58.99*

1772 Earobics® Step 1 Home Version
Abilitations Speech Bin
PO Box 922668
Norcross, GA 30010
770-449-5700
800-850-8602
FAX 770-510-7290
http://www.speechbin.com
e-mail: info@speechbin.com
Tobi Isaacs, Catalog Director

Step 1 offers hundreds of levels of play, appealing graphics, and entertaining music to train the critical auditory skills young children need for success in learning. Item number C481. *$58.99*

1773 Eye-Hand Coordination Boosters
Therapro
225 Arlington Street
Framingham, MA 01702
508-872-9494
800-257-5376
FAX 508-875-2062
http://www.theraproducts.com
e-mail: info@theraproducts.com
Therapro Staff, Author
Karen Conrad, Owner

A book of 92 masters that can be used over and over again with work sheets that are appropriate for all ages. These are perceptual motor activities that involve copying and tracing in the areas of visual tracking, discrimination and spatial relationships. *$14.00*
92 pages

1774 Familiar Things
Therapro
225 Arlington Street
Framingham, MA 01702
508-872-9494
800-257-5376
FAX 508-875-2062
http://www.theraproducts.com
e-mail: info@theraproducts.com
Therapro Staff, Author
Karen Conrad, Owner

Identify and match shapes of common objects with these large square, rubber pieces. *$19.99*

1775 Fishing!
Therapro
225 Arlington Street
Framingham, MA 01702
508-872-9494
800-257-5376
FAX 508-875-2062
http://www.theraproducts.com
e-mail: info@theraproducts.com
Therapro Staff, Author
Karen Conrad, Owner

Encourages eye-hand coordination. Rubber hook safely catches velcro on chipboard fish. *$6.95*

1776 **Flagship Carpets**
Blue Ridge Industries
PO Box 507
Ellijay, GA 30540
706-695-4055
800-848-4055
FAX 706-276-1980
http://www.flagshipcarpets.com
e-mail: info@flagshipcarpets.com
Jeremy Barton, Manager
Vicki Winkler, Sales Director

Offers a variety of carpet games like hopscotch, the alphabet, geography maps, custom logo mats and more.

1777 **Geoboard Colored Plastic**
Therapro
225 Arlington Street
Framingham, MA 01702
508-872-9494
800-257-5376
FAX 508-875-2062
http://www.theraproducts.com
e-mail: info@theraproducts.com
Therapro Staff, Author
Karen Conrad, Owner

Teach eye/hand coordination skills while strengthening pincher grasp with rubber bands. *$3.25*

1778 **Geometrical Design Coloring Book**
Therapro
225 Arlington Street
Framingham, MA 01702
508-872-9494
800-257-5376
FAX 508-875-2062
http://www.theraproducts.com
e-mail: info@theraproducts.com
Spyros Horemis, Author
Karen Conrad, Owner

Color these 46 original designs of pure patterns and abstract shapes for a striking and beautiful result, regardless of skill level. Most designs are made of a combination of small and large areas. *$3.95*
48 pages

1779 **Geosafari**
Lakeshore Learning Materials
2695 E Dominguez Street
Carson, CA 90895
800-421-5354
FAX 800-537-5403
http://www.lakeshorelearning.com
e-mail: lakeshore@lakeshorelearning.com
Ethelyn Kaplan

A fast-paced electronic game teaching geography in an exciting new way. *$99.50*
Item #ED8700

1780 **Get in Shape to Write**
Therapro
225 Arlington Street
Framingham, MA 01702
508-872-9494
800-257-5376
FAX 508-875-2062
http://www.theraproducts.com
e-mail: info@theraproducts.com
Phillip Bongiorno MA OTR, Author
Karen Conrad, Owner

Practice the visula perceptual motor skills needed for writing with these colorful, fun, and engaging activities. The 23 reusuable activities will keep a student's interest while they learn to process auditory, visual, and motoor movement patterns. In addition, learn concepts of matching and sorting colors, shapes and familiar objects. *$12.95*
Ages 3+

1781 **Gram's Cracker: A Grammar Game**
LinguiSystems
3100 4th Avenue
East Moline, IL 61244
309-755-2300
800-776-4332
FAX 309-755-2377
TDY:800-933-8331
http://www.linguisystems.com
e-mail: service@linguisystems.com
Julie Cole, Author
Linda Bowers, Co-Owner/Co-Founder
Rosemary Huisingh, Co-Owner/Co-Founder

Gram the mouse is in the house! Students will love helping Gram get to his mouse hole as they practice these grammar skills: pronouns; plurals; possessives; past tense verbs; comparatives and superlatives; copulas; present progressives; has and have; and negatives. *$44.95*
Ages 4-9

1782 **Grammar Scramble: A Grammar and Sentence-Building Game**
LinguiSystems
3100 4th Avenue
East Moline, IL 61244
309-755-2300
800-776-4332
FAX 309-755-2377
TDY:800-933-8331
http://www.linguisystems.com
e-mail: service@linguisystems.com
Rick Bowers, Linda Bowers, Author
Linda Bowers, Co-Owner/Co-Founder
Rosemary Huisingh, Co-Owner/Co-Founder

Students will improve their grammar and thinking skills as they form intersecting sentences in crossword style. Students receive word tiles divide into these parts of speech: nouns; verbs; pronouns; adjectives; adverbs; articles; interrogatives; prepositions; and conjunctions. *$44.95*
Ages 8-Adult

1783 **Gramopoly: A Parts of Speech Game**
LinguiSystems
3100 4th Avenue
East Moline, IL 61244
309-755-2300
800-776-4332
FAX 309-755-2377
TDY:800-933-8331
http://www.linguisystems.com
e-mail: service@linguisystems.com
Raelene Hudson, Author
Linda Bowers, Co-Owner/Co-Founder
Rosemary Huisingh, Co-Owner/Co-Founder

This best-selling game turns on the grammar lights for your older students. Assign each player a sentence from three levels of difficulty. Players must purchase parts of speech to complete their sentence. *$44.95*
Ages 10-15

1784 **Half and Half Design and Color Book**
Therapro
225 Arlington Street
Framingham, MA 01702
508-872-9494
800-257-5376
FAX 508-875-2062
http://www.theraproducts.com
e-mail: info@theraproducts.com
Therapro Staff, Author
Karen Conrad, Owner

Geometric designs appropriate for all ages. The client draws over dotted lines to finish the other half of the printed design. *$15.00*
72 pages

1785 **Hands, Feet and Arrows**
Therapro
225 Arlington Street
Framingham, MA 01702
508-872-9494
800-257-5376
FAX 508-875-2062
http://www.theraproducts.com
e-mail: info@theraproducts.com

Therapro Staff, Author
Karen Conrad, Owner

This kit has many possibilities for working on gross motor, sensory integration and academic skills. Its variety and ability to easily change to new tasks challenges all levels of abilities. Includes: 12 round sturdy plastic pieces (3 red, 3 yellow, 3 blue and 3 green) and stickers to go on the plastic pieces (3 right & 3 left feet, 3 right & 3 left hands, and 3 arrows). Guaranteed to provide many hours of fun. *$52.95*

1786 Hooray I Can Read!
Therapro
225 Arlington Street
Framingham, MA 01702
508-872-9494
800-257-5376
FAX 508-875-2062
http://www.theraproducts.com
e-mail: info@theraproducts.com
Ravensburger, Author
Karen Conrad, Owner

Have fun learning letters, sounds and more with 200 age appropriate questions and answers. Turn the dial until a question appears in the window, choose an answer and flip up the question mark to check it. 1-2 Players. *$18.95*
Ages 6-8

1787 Huffy Woofers
Therapro
225 Arlington Street
Framingham, MA 01702
508-872-9494
800-257-5376
FAX 508-875-2062
http://www.theraproducts.com
e-mail: info@theraproducts.com
Therapro Staff, Author
Karen Conrad, Owner

Safe giant ring toss game. Great for either indoor or outdoor activity. Includes a foam base and 6 rings, 3 red and 3 blue. *$18.95*

1788 Idiom Game
LinguiSystems
3100 4th Avenue
East Moline, IL 61244
309-755-2300
800-776-4332
FAX 309-755-2377
TDY:800-933-8331
http://www.linguisystems.com
e-mail: service@linguisystems.com
Dave Wisniewski, Author
Linda Bowers, Co-Owner/Co-Founder
Rosemary Huisingh, Co-Owner/Co-Founder

Idioms give our language richness but confuse our students! Give your students practice with 800 of the most commonly used idiomatic expressions in our language. Each card provides multiple-choice questions at a lower and upper level. *$44.95*
Ages 10-16

1789 Just for Me! Game
LinguiSystems
3100 4th Avenue
East Moline, IL 61244
309-755-2300
800-776-4332
FAX 309-755-2377
TDY:800-933-8331
http://www.linguisystems.com
e-mail: service@linguisystems.com
Margaret Warner, Author
Linda Bowers, Co-Owner/Co-Founder
Rosemary Huisingh, Co-Owner/Co-Founder

Follow-up on the early language skills from all five Just for Me! books with this fun new game. It's a hands-on approach as youngsters mix up specially-designed puzzle pieces to make funny faces. Each piece gives you five questions. That's 360 questions in all! Each puzzle piece covers an early language skill and corresponds to one part of the face. *$37.95*
Ages 4-7

1790 LanguageBURST: A Language and Vocabulary Game
LinguiSystems
3100 4th Avenue
East Moline, IL 61244
309-755-2300
800-776-4332
FAX 309-755-2377
TDY:800-933-8331
http://www.linguisystems.com
e-mail: service@linguisystems.com
Lauri Whiskeyman, Author
Linda Bowers, Co-Owner/Co-Founder
Rosemary Huisingh, Co-Owner/Co-Founder

Expand your students' language and vocabulary skills with this quick- thinking game. Many of the items are based on the curriculum for grades 3-8 so your therapy is classroom-relevent. Students think quickly as they practice skills in four key language areas: fill-in-the-blank; categories; comparing and contrasting; and attributes. *$37.95*
Ages 9-15

1791 Link N' Learn Activity Book
Therapro
225 Arlington Street
Framingham, MA 01702
508-872-9494
800-257-5376
FAX 508-875-2062
http://www.theraproducts.com
e-mail: info@theraproducts.com
Therapro Staff, Author
Karen Conrad, Owner

A nice accompaniment to the color rings. There are great cognitive activities included. *$8.95*
80 pages

1792 Link N' Learn Activity Cards
Therapro
225 Arlington Street
Framingham, MA 01702
508-872-9494
800-257-5376
FAX 508-875-2062
http://www.theraproducts.com
e-mail: info@theraproducts.com
Therapro Staff, Author
Karen Conrad, Owner

Learn patterning, sequencing and color discrimination and logic skills with this set of 20 cards that show life-sized links. An instructor's guide is included. *$6.95*

1793 Link N' Learn Color Rings
Therapro
225 Arlington Street
Framingham, MA 01702
508-872-9494
800-257-5376
FAX 508-875-2062
http://www.theraproducts.com
e-mail: info@theraproducts.com
Therapro Staff, Author
Karen Conrad, Owner

These easy to hook and separate colorful 1-1/2" plastic rings can be used in color sorting, counting, sequencing, and other perceptual/cognitive activities. *$6.95*

1794 Magicatch Set
Therapro
225 Arlington Street
Framingham, MA 01702
508-872-9494
800-257-5376
FAX 508-875-2062
http://www.theraproducts.com
e-mail: info@theraproducts.com
Therapro Staff, Author
Karen Conrad, Owner

This Velcro catch game offers a much higher degree of success and feeling of security than traditional ball tossing games. 7 1/2 inch neon catching paddles and 2 1/2 inch ball, in a mesh bag. No latex. *$7.50*

1795 **Magnetic Fun**

Therapro
225 Arlington Street
Framingham, MA 01702
508-872-9494
800-257-5376
FAX 508-875-2062
http://www.theraproducts.com
e-mail: info@theraproducts.com
Therapro Staff, Author
Karen Conrad, Owner

One swipe of the magic wand can pick up small objects without the need for a refined pincher grasp. *$13.95*

1796 **Maxwell's Manor: A Social Language Game**

LinguiSystems
3100 4th Avenue
East Moline, IL 61244
309-755-2300
800-776-4332
FAX 309-755-2377
TDY:800-933-8331
http://www.linguisystems.com
e-mail: service@linguisystems.com
Carolyn LoGiudice, Nancy McConnell, Author
Linda Bowers, Co-Owner/Co-Founder
Rosemary Huisingh, Co-Owner/Co-Founder

This fun game will teach your students the social skills they need to get along with others, be more accepted by their peers, and be successful in the classroom. Maxwell, the loveable dog, leads the way as your students practice positive social language skills. *$44.95*

Ages 4-9

1797 **Maze Book**

Therapro
225 Arlington Street
Framingham, MA 01702
508-872-9494
800-257-5376
FAX 508-875-2062
http://www.theraproducts.com
e-mail: info@theraproducts.com
Therapro Staff, Author
Karen Conrad, Owner

Significantly more challenging than the ABC Mazes; rich in perceptual activities. *$10.00*

32 pages

1798 **Myrtle's Beach: A Phonological Awareness and Articulation Game**

LinguiSystems
3100 4th Avenue
East Moline, IL 61244
309-755-2300
800-776-4332
FAX 309-755-2377
TDY:800-933-8331
http://www.linguisystems.com
e-mail: service@linguisystems.com
LinguiSystems Staff, Author
Linda Bowers, Co-Owner/Co-Founder
Rosemary Huisingh, Co-Owner/Co-Founder

Myrtle's Beach is a fun place to practice phonologial awareness, articulation, and language skills. The flexible format allows you to meet the varied needs of all the students in your speech and language groups. *$44.95*

Ages 4-9

1799 **Opposites Game**

Therapro
225 Arlington Street
Framingham, MA 01702
508-872-9494
800-257-5376
FAX 508-875-2062
http://www.theraproducts.com
e-mail: info@theraproducts.com
Therapro Staff, Author
Karen Conrad, Owner

Children can explore the concept of opposites by matching and then joining these tiles. Self correcting feature allows for both independent and supervised play. Helps build observation and recognition skills. *$8.50*

1800 **PLAID Practical Lessons for Apraxia**

Abilitations Speech Bin
PO Box 922668
Norcross, GA 30010
770-449-5700
800-850-8602
FAX 770-510-7290
http://www.speechbin.com
e-mail: info@speechbin.com
Tobi Isaacs, Catalog Director

PLAID is a top-notch clinical tool that gives you practical practice materials featuring twenty different phonemes — just what you need for your apraxic and aphasic adults — all in one resource. Item number 1424. *$29.99*

1801 **Parquetry Blocks & Pattern Cards**

Therapro
225 Arlington Street
Framingham, MA 01702
508-872-9494
800-257-5376
FAX 508-875-2062
http://www.theraproducts.com
e-mail: info@theraproducts.com
Therapro Staff, Author
Karen Conrad, Owner

Encourages visual perceptual skills and challenges a person's sense of design and color with squares, triangles, and rhombuses in six colors.

1802 **Patty's Cake: A Describing Game**

LinguiSystems
3100 4th Avenue
East Moline, IL 61244
309-755-2300
800-776-4332
FAX 309-755-2377
TDY:800-933-8331
http://www.linguisystems.com
e-mail: service@linguisystems.com
Julie Cole, Author
Linda Bowers, Co-Owner/Co-Founder
Rosemary Huisingh, Co-Owner/Co-Founder

Teach describing skills with Patty's Cake. Two levels of play in this fun game give you flexibility to meet individual students' learning needs. Players describe age-appropriate picture vocabulary cards by naming attributes such as category, function, shape, color, or location. Your students will improve their skills in: listening; memory; word retrieval; categorizing; naming attributes; formulating sentences; and giving descriptions. *$44.95*

Ages 4-9

1803 **Peabody Artic Decks**

Abilitations Speech Bin
PO Box 922668
Norcross, GA 30010
770-449-5700
800-850-8602
FAX 770-510-7290
http://www.speechbin.com
e-mail: info@speechbin.com
Tobi Isaacs, Catalog Director

You'll use these colorful stimulus cards in dozens of games and activities. Ten PAD decks — 480 cards — feature 18 frequently misarticulated consonants and blends. Each deck includes 40 picture cards, word list, two response cards, and five blank cards. Item number A180. *$164.99*

1804 **Pegboard Set**

Therapro
225 Arlington Street
Framingham, MA 01702
508-872-9494
800-257-5376
FAX 508-875-2062
http://www.theraproducts.com
e-mail: info@theraproducts.com
Therapro Staff, Author
Karen Conrad, Owner

Pegboard has 100 holes and measures 5-3/4 inch square. The pegs come in six bright colors. The 20 double-sided pattern cards or 40 different patterns present 5 levels of difficulty. *$14.99*

1805 Phonology 1: Software
Abilitations Speech Bin
PO Box 922668
Norcross, GA 30010
770-449-5700
800-850-8602
FAX 770-510-7290
http://www.speechbin.com
e-mail: info@speechbin.com
Tobi Isaacs, Catalog Director

This unique software gives you six entertaining games to treat children's phonological disorders. The program uses target patterns in a pattern cycling approach to phonological processes. Item number L183. *$98.99*

1806 Plastic Cones
Therapro
225 Arlington Street
Framingham, MA 01702
508-872-9494
800-257-5376
FAX 508-875-2062
http://www.theraproducts.com
e-mail: info@theraproducts.com
Therapro Staff, Author
Karen Conrad, Owner

The 12-inch versions of the construction project cones are bright orange and made of lightweigth vinyl. Hole in top. *$5.95*

1807 Plunk's Pond: A Riddles Game for Language
LinguiSystems
3100 4th Avenue
East Moline, IL 61244
309-755-2300
800-776-4332
FAX 309-755-2377
TDY:800-933-8331
http://www.linguisystems.com
e-mail: service@linguisystems.com
LinguiSystems Staff, Author
Linda Bowers, Co-Owner/Co-Founder
Rosemary Huisingh, Co-Owner/Co-Founder

Encourage divergent thinking, sharpen listening skills, and improve vocabulary with this fun riddle game. With a picture on one side and three clues on the other, these cards are great for all kinds of therapy games. Target attributes such as function, color, category, and more! *$44.95*
Ages 4-9

1808 Primer Pak
Therapro
225 Arlington Street
Framingham, MA 01702
508-872-9494
800-257-5376
FAX 508-875-2062
http://www.theraproducts.com
e-mail: info@theraproducts.com
Therapro Staff, Author
Karen Conrad, Owner

A challenging sampler of manipulatives. Four Fit-A-Space disk puzzles with basic shapes, an 8x8 Alphabet Puzzle, three Lacing Shapes for primary lacing, and 24 Locktagons to form structures. *$14.99*

1809 Punctuation Play-by-Play
LinguiSystems
3100 4th Avenue
East Moline, IL 61244
309-755-2300
800-776-4332
FAX 309-755-2377
TDY:800-933-8331
http://www.linguisystems.com
e-mail: service@linguisystems.com
Carolyn LoGiudice, Mike LoGiudice, Author
Linda Bowers, Co-Owner/Co-Founder
Rosemary Huisingh, Co-Owner/Co-Founder

Punctuation Play-by-Play engages students in a lively game as they practice essential punctuation skills including: capitalization; end marks; apostrophes; commas; quotation marks; colons; semicolons. Question cards are divided into two levels of difficulty. *$44.95*
Ages 10-18

1810 Read-A-Bit
LinguiSystems
3100 4th Avenue
East Moline, IL 61244
309-755-2300
800-776-4332
FAX 309-755-2377
TDY:800-933-8331
http://www.linguisystems.com
e-mail: service@linguisystems.com
Dagmar Kafka, Author
Linda Bowers, Co-Owner/Co-Founder
Rosemary Huisingh, Co-Owner/Co-Founder

Get 15 games in one box! Six decks of cards with different levels of reading difficulty work with and without the colorful game board to give you plenty of flexibility. You'll work through a hierarchy of reading skills from primer to grade 3. Students practice consonants, vowels, controlled R sounds, sight words, and more. *$41.95*
Ages 5-9

1811 Reading Comprehension Game Intermediate
LinguiSystems
3100 4th Avenue
East Moline, IL 61244
309-755-2300
800-776-4332
FAX 309-755-2377
TDY:800-933-8331
http://www.linguisystems.com
e-mail: service@linguisystems.com
Linda Bowers, Rosemary Huisingh, Carolyn LoGiudice, Author
Linda Bowers, Co-Owner/Co-Founder
Rosemary Huisingh, Co-Owner/Co-Founder

This game gives you fun, repetitive practice in three essential reading comprehension skills. The first is Reading for Details including cloze, referents, sequencing, describing, and more! The second is Reading for Understanding including main idea, paraphrasing, context clues, defining, and more. The third area is Going Beyond including making references, predicting, and making associations. *$44.95*
Ages 12-18

1812 Rhyming Sounds Game
Therapro
225 Arlington Street
Framingham, MA 01702
508-872-9494
800-257-5376
FAX 508-875-2062
http://www.theraproducts.com
e-mail: info@theraproducts.com
Therapro Staff, Author
Karen Conrad, Owner

Introduces 32 different rhyming sounds as players match the ending sound of the picture tile to the corresponding object on the category boards. Includes sorting/storage tray, 56 picture tiles, and 4 category cards with self-checking feature. No reading required. *$9.95*

1813 Rocky's Mountain: A Word-finding Game
LinguiSystems
3100 4th Avenue
East Moline, IL 61244
309-755-2300
800-776-4332
FAX 309-755-2377
TDY:800-933-8331
http://www.linguisystems.com
e-mail: service@linguisystems.com
Gina Williamson, Susan Shields, Author
Linda Bowers, Co-Owner/Co-Founder
Rosemary Huisingh, Co-Owner/Co-Founder

Tackle stubborn word-finding problems with this fun game! Game cards are organized by four word-finding strategies so you can pick the strategy that best meets your students' needs. Teach these strategies for word-finding: visual imagery; word association; sound/letter cueing; and categories. *$44.95*

Ages 4-9

1814 **SPARC for Grammar**
LinguiSystems
3100 4th Avenue
East Moline, IL 61244
309-755-2300
800-776-4332
FAX 309-755-2377
TDY:800-933-8331
http://www.linguisystems.com
e-mail: service@linguisystems.com
Susan Thomsen, Kathy Donnelly, Author
Linda Bowers, Co-Owner/Co-Founder
Rosemary Huisingh, Co-Owner/Co-Founder

Teach grammar in meaningful contexts! The lessons provide a wealth of opportunities for your students to hear, repeat, answer questions and tell stories using targeted language structures. *$39.95*

165 pages Ages 4-10

1815 **Self-Control Games & Workbook**
Western Psychological Services
12031 Wilshire Boulevard
Los Angeles, CA 90025
800-648-8857
FAX 310-478-7838
http://portal.wpspublish.com
e-mail: research@wpspublish.com
Berthold Berg, PhD, Author
Greg Gilmore, Vice President

This game is designed to teach self-control in academic and social situations. Addresses a total of 24 impulsive, inattentive and hyperactive behaviors. The companion workbook reinforces the use of positive self-statements, and problem-solving techniques, instead of expressing anger. *$62.50*

1816 **Sequenced Inventory of Communication Development Revised(SICD)**
Abilitations Speech Bin
PO Box 922668
Norcross, GA 30010
770-449-5700
800-850-8602
FAX 770-510-7290
http://www.speechbin.com
e-mail: info@speechbin.com
Dona Hedrick, Elizabeth Prather, Annette Tobin, Author
Tobi Isaacs, Catalog Director

SICD uses appealing toys to assess communication skills of children at all levels of ability including those with impaired hearing or vision. SICD looks at child and environment, measuring receptive and expressive language. Item number W710. *$438.99*

1817 **Shape and Color Sorter**
Therapro
225 Arlington Street
Framingham, MA 01702
508-872-9494
800-257-5376
FAX 508-875-2062
http://www.theraproducts.com
e-mail: info@theraproducts.com
Therapro Staff, Author
Karen Conrad, Owner

This simple and safe task of perception includes 25 crepe foam rubber pieces to sort by shape or color. Comes in five bright colors, each color representing a shape. Shapes fit nicely onto five large pegs. *$14.99*

1818 **Shapes**
Therapro
225 Arlington Street
Framingham, MA 01702
508-872-9494
800-257-5376
FAX 508-875-2062
http://www.theraproducts.com
e-mail: info@theraproducts.com
Therapro Staff, Author
Karen Conrad, Owner

This 8 1/2 x 11 inch high quality coloring book will help children learn to recognize shapes while improving their fine motor and perceptual skills. *$1.50*

30 pages

1819 **Silly Sentences**
Abilitations Speech Bin
PO Box 922668
Norcross, GA 30010
770-449-5700
800-850-8602
FAX 770-510-7290
http://www.speechbin.com
e-mail: info@speechbin.com
Tobi Isaacs, Catalog Director

Children love to have fun. Silly Sentences lets them have fun while they play these engaging card games to learn: subject + verb agreement; speech sound articulation; S+ V+ O sentences; questioning and answering; humor and absurdities and present progressive verbs. Item number P506. *$47.99*

1820 **Snail's Pace Race Game**
Therapro
225 Arlington Street
Framingham, MA 01702
508-872-9494
800-257-5376
FAX 508-875-2062
http://www.theraproducts.com
e-mail: info@theraproducts.com
Therapro Staff, Author
Karen Conrad, Owner

This classic, easy color game is back and is fun for all to play. Roll the colored dice to see which wooden snail will move closer to the finish line. Promotes color recognition, understanding of taking turns, and sharing. *$ 19.95*

1821 **Sounds Abound Game**
LinguiSystems
3100 4th Avenue
East Moline, IL 61244
309-755-2300
800-776-4332
FAX 309-755-2377
TDY:800-933-8331
http://www.linguisystems.com
e-mail: service@linguisystems.com
Orna Lenchner PhD, Blanche Podhajski PhD, Author
Linda Bowers, Co-Owner/Co-Founder
Rosemary Huisingh, Co-Owner/Co-Founder

Teach critical features about sounds in words for better language skills. Your students will love this fun game because it's easy to play. This game targets the sounds students use the most — f, s, p, t, and m. These essential sounds are critical for early literacy success. *$109.95*

112 pages Ages 4-8

1822 **Speech & Language & Voice & More...**
Abilitations Speech Bin
PO Box 922668
Norcross, GA 30010
770-449-5700
800-850-8602
FAX 770510072906
http://www.speechbin.com
e-mail: info@speechbin.com
Tobi Isaacs, Catalog Director

Contains 88 practically perfect reproducible games and activities ideal for your K-5 clients. It gives you: manipulable activities to keep active leaners learning; tasks to match a multitude of interests and abilities and vocal hygiene worksheets targeted to reduce vocal abuse. Item number 1496. *$21.95*

1823 **Speech Sports**
Abilitations Speech Bin
PO Box 922668
Norcross, GA 30010
770-449-5700
800-850-8602
FAX 770-510-7290
http://www.speechbin.com
e-mail: info@speechbin.com
Janet M Shaw, Author
Tobi Isaacs, Catalog Director

Speech Sports makes every child in your caseload a shining sports star. Reproducible gamesboards and language activities feature 19 different sports from boating to skating, bowling to running, basketball to soccer. Item number 1590. *$24.99*

1824 **Speech-Language Delights**
Abilitations Speech Bin
PO Box 922668
Norcross, GA 30010
770-449-5700
800-850-8602
FAX 770-510-7290
http://www.speechbin.com
e-mail: info@speechbin.com
Janet M Shaw, Author
Tobi Isaacs, Catalog Director

Cook up lots of fun with Speech-Language Delights! Delectably delicious speech and language activities and games provide rich opportunities and hands-on activities with food-related themes to enrich K-8 kids. Item number 1541. *$ 29.95*

1825 **Spider Ball**
Therapro
225 Arlington Street
Framingham, MA 01702
508-872-9494
800-257-5376
FAX 508-875-2062
http://www.theraproducts.com
e-mail: info@theraproducts.com
Therapro Staff, Author
Karen Conrad, Owner

Easy to catch, won't roll away! This foam rubber ball has rubber legs that make it incredibly easy to catch. Invented by a PE teacher to help children improve their ball playing skills. The Spiderball's legs act as brakes bringing it to a stop when rolled and minimizing the time needed to chase a missed ball. 2 1/4 inch diameter. *$4.50*

1826 **Squidgie Flying Disc**
Therapro
225 Arlington Street
Framingham, MA 01702
508-872-9494
800-257-5376
FAX 508-875-2062
http://www.theraproducts.com
e-mail: info@theraproducts.com
Therapro Staff, Author
Karen Conrad, Owner

This is a great flexible flying disc that is amazingly easy to throw and travels over long distances. It is soft and easy to catch. It will even float in the pool! *$4.95*

1827 **String-A-Long Lacing Activity**
Therapro
225 Arlington Street
Framingham, MA 01702
508-872-9494
800-257-5376
FAX 508-875-2062
http://www.theraproducts.com
e-mail: info@theraproducts.com
Therapro Staff, Author
Karen Conrad, Owner

A lacing activity that develops hand eye coordination and concentration as children create 2 colorful bead buddies. Each buddy has 4 laces attached to its painted heal now build the body with 23 beads! *$18.00*
Ages 4+

1828 **That's Life: A Game of Life Skills**
LinguiSystems
3100 4th Avenue
East Moline, IL 61244
309-755-2300
800-776-4332
FAX 309-755-2377
TDY:800-933-8331
http://www.linguisystems.com
e-mail: service@linguisystems.com
Patricia Smith, Author
Linda Bowers, Co-Owner/Co-Founder
Rosemary Huisingh, Co-Owner/Co-Founder

Help your older students refine their language skills to negotiate the real world with this fun game. Get 100 thinking and language questions for each of these life area: consumer affairs, government, health concerns, money matters, going places, and homemaking. *$44.95*
Ages 12-18

1829 **Things in My House: Picture Matching Game**
Therapro
225 Arlington Street
Framingham, MA 01702
508-872-9494
800-257-5376
FAX 508-875-2062
http://www.theraproducts.com
e-mail: info@theraproducts.com
Therapro Staff, Author
Karen Conrad, Owner

Strengthen visual discrimination, sorting, and organizing skills. Young children enjoy finding correct matches in this fun first game. The colorful graphics depicting familiar household objects and activities encourage verbalization and imaginative play. *$10.95*

1830 **Tic-Tac-Artic and Match**
LinguiSystems
3100 4th Avenue
East Moline, IL 61244
309-755-2300
800-776-4332
FAX 309-755-2377
TDY:800-933-8331
http://www.linguisystems.com
e-mail: service@linguisystems.com
Carol A Vaccariello, Author
Linda Bowers, Co-Owner/Co-Founder
Rosemary Huisingh, Co-Owner/Co-Founder

Tic-Tac-Artic and Match gives you five games on every page and tons of practice per session. Each page has 16 pictures for one target phoneme. To play Tic-Tac-Artic, use the special game template to create four different tic-tac-toe style games. *$34.95*
Ages 4-12

1831 **Toddler Tote**
Therapro
225 Arlington Street
Framingham, MA 01702
508-872-9494
800-257-5376
FAX 508-875-2062
http://www.theraproducts.com
e-mail: info@theraproducts.com
Therapro Staff, Author
Karen Conrad, Owner

Offers one Junior Fit-A-Space panel that has large geometric shapes; 4 Shape Squares providing basic shapes in a more challenging size; 2 Peg Play Vehicles and Pegs introducing early peg board skills; 3 Familiar Things and 2 piece puzzles and a handy take-along bag. *$14.99*

1832 **Tools of the Trade Game**
Therapro
225 Arlington Street
Framingham, MA 01702
508-872-9494
800-257-5376
FAX 508-875-2062
http://www.theraproducts.com
e-mail: info@theraproducts.com
Therapro Staff, Author
Karen Conrad, Owner

Introduces 32 different occupations and the tools they use. Tool picture tiles are sorted into compartments which correspond to the category card, showing people dressed for their jobs. Includes sorting tray, 56 tool tiles and 4 category cards with self-checking feature. No reading required. *$9.95*

1833 **Vowel Scramble**
LinguiSystems
3100 4th Avenue
East Moline, IL 61244
309-755-2300
800-776-4332
FAX 309-755-2377
TDY:800-933-8331
http://www.linguisystems.com
e-mail: service@linguisystems.com
Carolyn LoGiudice, Author
Linda Bowers, Co-Owner/Co-Founder
Rosemary Huisingh, Co-Owner/Co-Founder

Your student will love this fun new way to practice spelling and phonological awareness skills. Players earn points by using letter tiles to complete words on the game board. *$44.95*
Ages 7-12

1834 Whistle Set
Therapro
225 Arlington Street
Framingham, MA 01702
508-872-9494
800-257-5376
FAX 508-875-2062
http://www.theraproducts.com
e-mail: info@theraproducts.com
Therapro Staff, Author
Karen Conrad, Owner

The whistles in this collection are colorful and sturdy. Most feature moving parts as well as noise-makers to stimulate both ocular and oral motor skills. Includes nine whistles. Respiratory demand ranges from easy to difficult. *$17.50*

1835 Wikki Stix-Neon & Primary
Therapro
225 Arlington Street
Framingham, MA 01702
508-872-9494
800-257-5376
FAX 508-875-2062
http://www.theraproducts.com
e-mail: info@theraproducts.com
Therapro Staff, Author
Karen Conrad, Owner

Colorful, nontoxic waxed strings which are easily molded to create various forms, shapes and letters. Combine motor planning skill with fine motor skill by following simple shapes with Wikki Stix and then coloring in the shape. *$4.95*
Each

1836 Wonder Ball
Therapro
225 Arlington Street
Framingham, MA 01702
508-872-9494
800-257-5376
FAX 508-875-2062
http://www.theraproducts.com
e-mail: info@theraproducts.com
Therapro Staff, Author
Karen Conrad, Owner

This 3 inch ball made of many small suction cups feels good in the palm of the hand and, when thrown against a smooth surface, will firmly stick. Pulling it from the surface requires strength, resulting in proprioceptive stimulation. *$1.95*

1837 Wooden Pegboard
Therapro
225 Arlington Street
Framingham, MA 01702
508-872-9494
800-257-5376
FAX 508-875-2062
http://www.theraproducts.com
e-mail: info@theraproducts.com
Therapro Staff, Author
Karen Conrad, Owner

This 10 inch square, laquer-finished wooden board has 100 drilled holes. *$10.95*

1838 Wooden Pegs
Therapro
225 Arlington Street
Framingham, MA 01702
508-872-9494
800-257-5376
FAX 508-875-2062
http://www.theraproducts.com
e-mail: info@theraproducts.com
Therapro Staff, Author
Karen Conrad, Owner

Smooth 2 inch pegs in 6 colors for use in design and pattern making with the wooden pegboard above. Set of 100 pegs. *$4.95*

1839 WriteOPOLY
LinguiSystems
3100 4th Avenue
East Moline, IL 61244
309-755-2300
800-776-4332
FAX 309-755-2377
TDY:800-933-8331
http://www.linguisystems.com
e-mail: service@linguisystems.com
Paul F Johnson, Author
Linda Bowers, Co-Owner/Co-Founder
Rosemary Huisingh, Co-Owner/Co-Founder

End writer's block for even your most reluctant writers with this fun game. Improve written language skills with WriteOPOLY. Students travel around a colorful game board buying properties and filling out Writing Plan sheets. *$ 44.95*
Ages 9-14

Writing

1840 100% Grammar
LinguiSystems
3100 4th Avenue
East Moline, IL 61244
309-755-2300
800-776-4332
FAX 309-755-2377
TDY:800-933-8331
http://www.linguisystems.com
e-mail: service@linguisystems.com
Mike LoGiudice, Carolyn LoGiudice, Author
Linda Bowers, Co-Owner/Co-Founder
Rosemary Huisingh, Co-Owner/Co-Founder

Make the link between grammar and communication skills with this incredible resource. You'll get relevant, fun activities to develop clear, accurate, excellent communication skills. 100% Grammar thoroughly covers all the essential grammar areas including: nouns; pronouns; complements; verbals; clauses; and fine points. *$37.95*
174 pages Ages 9-14

1841 100% Grammar LITE
LinguiSystems
3100 4th Avenue
East Moline, IL 61244
309-755-2300
800-776-4332
FAX 309-755-2377
TDY:800-933-8331
http://www.linguisystems.com
e-mail: service@linguisystems.com
Mike LoGiudice, Carolyn LoGiudice, Author
Linda Bowers, Co-Owner/Co-Founder
Rosemary Huisingh, Co-Owner/Co-Founder

Teach one grammar concept at a time. Compared to 100% Grammar, this resource is lighter in the amount of content per page and contextual demands of the practice items. The fun art and light approach will appeal to your hardest-to-teach students. The book is divided into two sections covering parts of speech and sentence structures. *$37.95*
178 pages Ages 4-19

1842 100% Punctuation
LinguiSystems
3100 4th Avenue
East Moline, IL 61244
309-755-2300
800-776-4332
FAX 309-755-2377
TDY:800-933-8331
http://www.linguisystems.com
e-mail: service@linguisystems.com
Mike LoGiudice, Carolyn LoGiudice, Author
Linda Bowers, Co-Owner/Co-Founder
Rosemary Huisingh, Co-Owner/Co-Founder

Good written language requires the appropriate touches. On-target punctuation is essential for clear writing. This resource puts fun, zip, and humor into teaching this necessary skill. Each unit gives you a teacher guide, a skill overview, light-hearted activity sheets, and a handy quiz for accountability. *$37.95*

179 pages Ages 9-14

1843 100% Punctuation LITE
LinguiSystems
3100 4th Avenue
East Moline, IL 61244
309-755-2300
800-776-4332
FAX 309-755-2377
TDY:800-933-8331
http://www.linguisystems.com
e-mail: service@linguisystems.com
LinguiSystems Staff, Author
Linda Bowers, Co-Owner/Co-Founder
Rosemary Huisingh, Co-Owner/Co-Founder

Good punctuation is essential for clear written communication. This light approach makes it fun to teach and fun to learn. Get practice pages for: capitals; end marks; apostrophes; commas; quotation marks; letters; abbreviations; colons; and semicolons. *$37.95*
183 pages Ages 9-14

1844 100% Spelling
LinguiSystems
3100 4th Avenue
East Moline, IL 61244
309-755-2300
800-776-4332
FAX 309-755-2377
TDY:800-933-8331
http://www.linguisystems.com
e-mail: service@linguisystems.com
LinguiSystems Staff, Author
Linda Bowers, Co-Owner/Co-Founder
Rosemary Huisingh, Co-Owner/Co-Founder

Demystify spelling by helping students tackle one pattern at a time. Your students will discover and retain spelling rules by searching for spelling patterns. Each set of three lessons targets a specific spelling pattern. These activity sheets are great for independent work, group work, and take-home practice. *$37.95*
187 pages Ages 8-14

1845 100% Story Writing
LinguiSystems
3100 4th Avenue
East Moline, IL 61244
309-755-2300
800-776-4332
FAX 309-755-2377
TDY:800-933-8331
http://www.linguisystems.com
e-mail: service@linguisystems.com
Dave Wisniewski, Katarina Hempstead, Author
Linda Bowers, Co-Owner/Co-Founder
Rosemary Huisingh, Co-Owner/Co-Founder

Your students experience success with writing because you give them strategies to sequence, plan, and write a great story! You'll get 50 well-developed topics for your students to choose from. Work on organizing thoughts before writing, sequencing story events, writing paragraphs, and using storyboards to visualize a story. *$37.95*
149 pages Ages 9-14

1846 100% Writing 4-book Set
LinguiSystems
3100 4th Avenue
East Moline, IL 61244
309-755-2300
800-776-4332
FAX 309-755-2377
TDY:800-933-8331
http://www.linguisystems.com
e-mail: service@linguisystems.com
Dave Wisniewski, Author
Linda Bowers, Co-Owner/Co-Founder
Rosemary Huisingh, Co-Owner/Co-Founder

Awaken the slumbering interest in writing that your students unknowingly possess. This set of books shows students how to organize thoughts into cohesive, interesting writing. Even students who hate to write will produce solidly-crafted products. *$131.80*

150 pages Ages 12-15

1847 100% Writing: Comparison and Contrast
LinguiSystems
3100 4th Avenue
East Moline, IL 61244
309-755-2300
800-776-4332
FAX 309-755-2377
TDY:800-933-8331
http://www.linguisystems.com
e-mail: service@linguisystems.com
Dave Wisniewski, Author
Linda Bowers, Co-Owner/Co-Founder
Rosemary Huisingh, Co-Owner/Co-Founder

Help your students to learn to write comparison and contrast with this helpful resource. Chapters walk students through introductory, body, and concluding paragraphs. Along the way they'll practice helpful strategies of identifying workable comparisons and meaningful contrasts. *$37.95*
183 pages Ages 12-15

1848 100% Writing: Exposition
LinguiSystems
3100 4th Avenue
East Moline, IL 61244
309-755-2300
800-776-4332
FAX 309-755-2377
TDY:800-933-8331
http://www.linguisystems.com
e-mail: service@linguisystems.com
Dave Wisniewski, Author
Linda Bowers, Co-Owner/Co-Founder
Rosemary Huisingh, Co-Owner/Co-Founder

Get helpful handouts, instructions, and practice sheets to help students learn all about expository writing. Chapters cover introductory paragraph, building body paragraphs, concluding paragraph, using quotations in definition, and much more! *$37.95*
143 pages Ages 12-15

1849 100% Writing: Narration
LinguiSystems
3100 4th Avenue
East Moline, IL 61244
309-755-2300
800-776-4332
FAX 309-755-2377
TDY:800-933-8331
http://www.linguisystems.com
e-mail: service@linguisystems.com
Dave Wisniewski, Author
Linda Bowers, Co-Owner/Co-Founder
Rosemary Huisingh, Co-Owner/Co-Founder

Your students will learn all they need to know about narrative writing with this incredible resource. Chapters cover introducing narration, consistency of tense, use of dialogue sequencing an incident, using specific vocabulary, variety in sentence structure, character and setting development, and much more! *$37.95*

187 pages Ages 12-15

1850 100% Writing: Persuasion
LinguiSystems
3100 4th Avenue
East Moline, IL 61244
309-755-2300
800-776-4332
FAX 309-755-2377
TDY:800-933-8331
http://www.linguisystems.com
e-mail: service@linguisystems.com
Dave Wisniewski, Author
Linda Bowers, Co-Owner/Co-Founder
Rosemary Huisingh, Co-Owner/Co-Founder

Teach all the basics of writing persuasion. Students will learn how to write a simple five-paragraph persuasion, understand fact vs. opinion, circling in persuasion, appealing to logic and emotion, and much more. *$37.95*

143 pages Ages 12-15

1851 125 Ways to Be a Better Writer

LinguiSystems
3100 4th Avenue
East Moline, IL 61244
309-755-2300
800-776-4332
FAX 309-755-2377
TDY:800-933-8331
http://www.linguisystems.com
e-mail: service@linguisystems.com
Paul F Johnson, Author
Linda Bowers, Co-Owner/Co-Founder
Rosemary Huisingh, Co-Owner/Co-Founder

Your students will be eager to write in these fun, relevant contexts. Train functional, confident writers with 125 strategies for better writing skills. Easy-to-grasp strategies and practice pages help your students learn the writing process, express their thoughts clearly, write better sentences and paragraphs, and more. *$35.95*
166 pages Ages 12-18

1852 125 Writing Projects

LinguiSystems
3100 4th Avenue
East Moline, IL 61244
309-755-2300
800-776-4332
FAX 309-755-2377
TDY:800-933-8331
http://www.linguisystems.com
e-mail: service@linguisystems.com
Paul F Johnson, Author
Linda Bowers, Co-Owner/Co-Founder
Rosemary Huisingh, Co-Owner/Co-Founder

Help your students discover themselves as successful writers. This handy resource gives you activities arranged in a hierarchy to meet the needs of all the levels you teach. *$35.95*
171 pages Ages 10-17

1853 Author's Toolkit

Sunburst Technology
1550 Executive Drive
Elgin, IL 60123
800-321-7511
FAX 888-800-3028
http://http://store.sunburst.com/Home.aspx
e-mail: service@sunburst.com
Michael Guillory, Channel Sales/Marketing Manager

Students can use this comprehensive tool to organize ideas, make outlines, rough drafts, edit and print all their written work.

1854 Blend It! End It!

LinguiSystems
3100 4th Avenue
East Moline, IL 61244
309-755-2300
800-776-4332
FAX 309-755-2377
TDY:800-933-8331
http://www.linguisystems.com
e-mail: service@linguisystems.com
Heather Koepke, Author
Linda Bowers, Co-Owner/Co-Founder
Rosemary Huisingh, Co-Owner/Co-Founder

Get this fun quick-thinking game to work on phonics and spelling skills. Players write as many words as they can including a specific initial blend or word ending. You get 36 initial word blends including: bl-, cr-, spl-. sk-, th-, tw-. *$42.95*
Ages 7-14

1855 Callirobics: Advanced Exercises

Therapro
225 Arlington Street
Framingham, MA 01702
508-872-9494
800-257-5376
FAX 508-875-2062
http://www.theraproducts.com
e-mail: info@theraproducts.com
Therapro Staff, Author
Karen Conrad, Owner

Allows those who have finished earlier Callirobics programs to continue improving their handwriting in a fun and creative way. Callirobics Advanced lets one create shapes to popular music from around the world. *$27.95*
Book and CD

1856 Callirobics: Exercises for Adults

Therapro
225 Arlington Street
Framingham, MA 01702
508-872-9494
800-257-5376
FAX 508-875-2062
http://www.theraproducts.com
e-mail: info@theraproducts.com
Therapro Staff, Author
Karen Conrad, Owner

Callirobics-for-Adults is a program designed to help adults regain handwriting skills to music. The music assists as an auditory cue in initiating writing movements, and will help develop a sense of rhythm in writing. The program consists of two sections: exercises of simple graphical shapes that help adults gain fluency in the writing movement, and exercises of various combinations of cursive letters. *$30.95*

1857 Callirobics: Handwriting Exercises to Music

Therapro
225 Arlington Street
Framingham, MA 01702
508-872-9494
800-257-5376
FAX 508-875-2062
http://www.theraproducts.com
e-mail: info@theraproducts.com
Therapro Staff, Author
Karen Conrad, Owner

Ten structured sessions, each with 2 exercises and 2 pieces of music. Includes stickers and a certificate book. *$27.95*
Book and CD

1858 Callirobics: Prewriting Skills with Music

Therapro
225 Arlington Street
Framingham, MA 01702
508-872-9494
800-257-5376
FAX 508-875-2062
http://www.theraproducts.com
e-mail: info@theraproducts.com
Therapro Staff, Author
Karen Conrad, Owner

These 11 handwriting exercises are a series of simple and enjoyable graphical patterns to be traced by the child while listening to popular melodies. *$27.95*
Book and CD

1859 Caps, Commas and Other Things

Academic Therapy Publications
20 Commercial Boulevard
Novato, CA 94949
415-883-3314
800-422-7249
FAX 888-287-9975
http://www.academictherapy.com
e-mail: sales@academictherapy.com
Sheryl Pastorek, Author
Jim Arena
Joanne Urban

A writing program for regular, remedial and EST students in grades 3 through 12 and adults in basic education classes remedial ESL. Six levels on capitalization and punctuation, four levels on written expression. Specific lesson plans with reproducible worksheets. *$20.00*
264 pages
ISBN 0-878793-25-9

1860 Create-A-Story

Speech Bin
PO Box 922668
Norcross, GA 30010
770-449-5700
800-850-8602
FAX 770-510-7290
http://www.speechbin.com
e-mail: info@speechbin.com

Shane Peters, Product Coordinator
Jen Binney, Owner

Here's a powerful language learning game that simplifies the creative process of storytelling and writing for 5-99 year olds. It fosters their imaginations, organizes their thoughts, and boosts their confidence as they build a narrative. The game can be played by 1-6 players as groups or individuals. Item number C151. *$44.95*

1861 D'Nealian Handwriting from A to Z
Therapro
225 Arlington Street
Framingham, MA 01702
508-872-9494
800-257-5376
FAX 508-875-2062
http://www.theraproducts.com
e-mail: info@theraproducts.com
Donald Thurber, Author
Karen Conrad, Owner

Up to date books for D'Nealian manuscript and cursive handwriting. In the manuscript children master each lowercase and uppercase letter in natural progressive stages first by tracing with their fingers, then by writing the letters, and finally by writing words that begin with the letter. *$9.95*

1862 Daily Starters: Quote of the Day
LinguiSystems
3100 4th Avenue
East Moline, IL 61244
309-755-2300
800-776-4332
FAX 309-755-2377
TDY:800-933-8331
http://www.linguisystems.com
e-mail: service@linguisystems.com
Dave Wisniewski, Author
Linda Bowers, Co-Owner/Co-Founder
Rosemary Huisingh, Co-Owner/Co-Founder

Get your students off to a focused start in therapy or in the classroom. These quick activities help older students integrate several language arts skills at once including writing, thinking, grammar, punctuation, vocabulary, and more. *$21.95*
142 pages Ages 12-18

1863 Do-A-Dot Activity Books
Therapro
225 Arlington Street
Framingham, MA 01702
508-872-9494
800-257-5376
FAX 508-875-2062
http://www.theraproducts.com
e-mail: info@theraproducts.com
Therapro Staff, Author
Karen Conrad, Owner

Do-A-Dot Activity Books are great for pre-writing skill books, printed on heavy paper stock, with each page perforated for easy removal. They promote eye-hand coordination and visual recognition. *$4.95*

1864 Draw-Write-Now, A Drawing and Handwriting Course for Kids
Therapro
225 Arlington Street
Framingham, MA 01702
508-872-9494
800-257-5376
FAX 508-875-2062
http://www.theraproducts.com
e-mail: info@theraproducts.com
Therapro Staff, Author
Karen Conrad, Owner

A great way to incorporate visual motor skills and handwriting with curriculum studies. Based on a teacher's idea that handwriting utilizes many of the same skills as drawing, these books feature easy to follow drawing lessons that are broken down into a series of steps. Students can use the practice text provided to write about their drawings. The books cover a variety of themes and subjects. *$10.95*

1865 Dysgraphia: Why Johnny Can't Write: 3rd Edition
Therapro
225 Arlington Street
Framingham, MA 01702
508-872-9494
800-257-5376
FAX 508-875-2062
http://www.theraproducts.com
e-mail: info@theraproducts.com
D Cavey, Author
Karen Conrad, Owner

Dysgraphia is a serious writing difficulty. This book provides guidelines for recognizing dysgraphic children and explains their special writing needs. Offers valuable tips, ideas and methods to promote success and self regard. *$15.95*
61 pages

1866 Easybook Deluxe
Sunburst Technology
1550 Executive Drive
Elgin, IL 60123
800-321-7511
FAX 888-800-3028
http://http://store.sunburst.com/Home.aspx
e-mail: service@sunburst.com
Michael Guillory, Channel Sales/Marketing Manager

Designed to support the needs of a wide range of writers, this book publishing tool provides students with a creative environment to write, design and illustrate stories and reports, and to print their work in book formats.

1867 Easybook Deluxe Writing Workshop: Colonial Times
Sunburst Technology
1550 Executive Drive
Elgin, IL 60123
800-321-7511
FAX 888-800-3028
http://http://store.sunburst.com/Home.aspx
e-mail: service@sunburst.com
Michael Guillory, Channel Sales/Marketing Manager

Writing workshops combine theme-based activities with the award-winning EasyBook Deluxe.

1868 Easybook Deluxe Writing Workshop: Immigration
Sunburst Technology
1550 Executive Drive
Elgin, IL 60123
800-321-7511
FAX 888-800-3028
http://http://store.sunburst.com/Home.aspx
e-mail: service@sunburst.com
Michael Guillory, Channel Sales/Marketing Manager

Writing workshops combine theme-based activities with the award-winning EasyBook Deluxe.

1869 Easybook Deluxe Writing Workshop: Rainforest & Astronomy
Sunburst Technology
1550 Executive Drive
Elgin, IL 60123
800-321-7511
FAX 888-800-3028
http://http://store.sunburst.com/Home.aspx
e-mail: service@sunburst.com
Michael Guillory, Channel Sales/Marketing Manager

Writing workshops combine theme-based activities with the award-winning EasyBook Deluxe.

1870 Easybook Deluxe Writing Workshop: Whales & Oceans

Sunburst Technology
1550 Executive Drive
Elgin, IL 60123
800-321-7511
FAX 888-800-3028
http://http://store.sunburst.com/Home.aspx
e-mail: service@sunburst.com
Michael Guillory, Channel Sales/Marketing Manager

Writing workshops combine theme-based activities with the award-winning EasyBook Deluxe.

1871 Experiences with Writing Styles
Harcourt Achieve
Customer Service, 5th Floor
Orlando, FL 32887
800-284-7019
FAX 800-699-9459
http://www.harcourtachieve.com
e-mail: webmaster@harcourt.com
Steck-Vaughn Staff, Author
Tim McEwen, President/CEO
Susan Canizares, SVP Publisher
Lee Wilson, VP Marketing
Give your students experience applying the writing process in nine relevant situations, from personal narratives to persuasive paragraphs to research reports. Units provide a clear definition of each genre and plenty of practice with prewriting, writing, revising, proofreading, and publishing. *$11.99*

1872 Fonts 4 Teachers
Therapro
225 Arlington Street
Framingham, MA 01702
508-872-9494
800-257-5376
FAX 508-875-2062
http://www.theraproducts.com
e-mail: info@theraproducts.com
Therapro Staff, Author
Karen Conrad, Owner

A software collection of 31 True Type fonts for teachers, parents and students. Fonts include Tracing, lined and unlined Traditional Manuscript and Cursive (similar to Zaner Blouser and D'Nealian), math, clip art, decorative, time, American Sign Language symbols and more. The included manual is very informative, with great examples of lesson plans and educational goals. *$39.95*
Windows/Mac

1873 From Scribbling to Writing
Therapro
225 Arlington Street
Framingham, MA 01702
508-872-9494
800-257-5376
FAX 508-875-2062
http://www.theraproducts.com
e-mail: info@theraproducts.com
Suzanne Naville, Pia Marbacher, Author
Karen Conrad, Owner

Ideas, exercises and practice pages for all children preparing to write. Contains line drawing exercises, forms to complete, and forms for encouraging good flow of movement during writing. *$29.95*
99 pages

1874 Fun with Handwriting
Therapro
225 Arlington Street
Framingham, MA 01702
508-872-9494
800-257-5376
FAX 508-875-2062
http://www.theraproducts.com
e-mail: info@theraproducts.com
Therapro Staff, Author
Karen Conrad, Owner

One hundred and one ways to improve handwriting. Includes key to writing legibly, chalkboard activities, evaluation tips, and real world handwriting projects. *$16.00*
160 pages Spiral-bound

1875 Getting It Write
Therapro
225 Arlington Street
Framingham, MA 01702
508-872-9494
800-257-5376
FAX 508-875-2062
http://www.theraproducts.com
e-mail: info@theraproducts.com
LouAnne Audette OTR, Anne Karson OTR, Author
Karen Conrad, Owner

A 6-week course for individuals or groups of 4-10 children, 6-12 years. Weekly, 1/2 hour classes begin with a short orientation followed by 25 minutes of games and sensory motor activities, from prewriting to writing practice, from basic strokes to letter formation. Reproducible manuscript and cursive worksheets are included along with homework assignments. *$58.95*
215 pages

1876 Getting Ready to Write: Preschool-K
Therapro
225 Arlington Street
Framingham, MA 01702
508-872-9494
800-257-5376
FAX 508-875-2062
http://www.theraproducts.com
e-mail: info@theraproducts.com
Therapro Staff, Author
Karen Conrad, Owner

A wonderful little book for any handwriting program. Includes many basic skills needed for beginning writing such as matching like objects, finding differences, writing basic strokes, left to right sequence, etc. *$6.50*
97 pages

1877 Getty-Dubay Italic Handwriting Series: The Natural Way to Write
Therapro
225 Arlington Street
Framingham, MA 01702
508-872-9494
800-257-5376
FAX 508-875-2062
http://www.theraproducts.com
e-mail: info@theraproducts.com
Barbara Getty, Inga Dubay, Author
Karen Conrad, Owner

This method produces fast and legible handwriting by consistently using an elliptical shape and letter slope (5 degrees) which conforms to natural hand movements and requires very few pencil lifts. A great handwriting program for all children and for adults. Also, use this method with student's handwriting problems. You will see an immediate difference. Has long term effects, when the practice stops, the good handwriting continues!
Video available

1878 Grammar Scramble: A Grammar and Sentence-Building Game
LinguiSystems
3100 4th Avenue
East Moline, IL 61244
309-755-2300
800-776-4332
FAX 309-755-2377
TDY:800-933-8331
http://www.linguisystems.com
e-mail: service@linguisystems.com
Rick Bowers, Linda Bowers, Author
Linda Bowers, Co-Owner/Co-Founder
Rosemary Huisingh, Co-Owner/Co-Founder

Students will improve their grammar and thinking skills as they form intersecting sentences in crossword style. Students receive word tiles divided into these parts of speech: nouns; verbs; pronouns; adjectives; adverbs; articles; interrogatives; prepostions; and conjunctions. *$44.95*

Ages 8-Adult

1879 Grammar and Writing for Job and Personal Use
AGS Publishing
PO Box 99
Circle Pines, MN 55014
651-287-7220
800-328-2560
FAX 800-471-8457
http://www.agsnet.com
e-mail: agsmail@agsnet.com
Joyce Hing-McGowan, Author
Kevin Brueggeman, President
Matt Keller, Marketing Manager

With an interest level of high school through adult, and a reading level of Grade 5-6, this series has modules in Improving Basic Grammar and Writing Skills and Writing for Employment. Self-paced texts are filled with exercises that teach students the basic rules of English grammar and how to apply them to actual writing situations.

1880 Gramopoly: A Parts of Speech Game
LinguiSystems
3100 4th Avenue
East Moline, IL 61244
309-755-2300
800-776-4332
FAX 309-755-2377
TDY:800-933-8331
http://www.linguisystems.com
e-mail: service@linguisystems.com
Raelene Hudson, Author
Linda Bowers, Co-Owner/Co-Founder
Rosemary Huisingh, Co-Owner/Co-Founder

This best-selling game turns on the grammar lights for your older students. Assign each player a sentence from three levels of difficulty. Players must purchase parts of speech to complete their sentence. *$44.95*
Ages 10-15

1881 HELP for Grammar
LinguiSystems
3100 4th Avenue
East Moline, IL 61244
309-755-2300
800-776-4332
FAX 309-755-2377
TDY:800-933-8331
http://www.linguisystems.com
e-mail: service@linguisystems.com
Andrea Larazzi, Author
Linda Bowers, Co-Owner/Co-Founder
Rosemary Huisingh, Co-Owner/Co-Founder

Get in-depth grammar practice arranged in developmental order so skill builds upon skill. Get grammar training and practice with oral and written language exercises including identifying and matching grammar types, categorizing grammar types, applying grammar skills in context, and more. *$39.95*
191 pages Ages 8-Adult

1882 Handwriting Readiness for Preschoolers
Therapro
225 Arlington Street
Framingham, MA 01702
508-872-9494
800-257-5376
FAX 508-875-2062
http://www.theraproducts.com
e-mail: info@theraproducts.com
Donald Thurber, Author
Karen Conrad, Owner

As teacher recites directions, children trace lower case manuscript letters with finger (Book 1) or crayon (Book 2), developing letter recognition skills and writing readiness. *$9.95*
32 pages

1883 Handwriting Without Tears
8801 Macarthur Boulevard
Cabin John, MD 20818
301-263-2700
FAX 301-263-2707
http://www.hwtears.com
Jan Olsen, President

An easy and fun method for children of all abilities to learn printing and cursive.

1884 Handwriting without Tears Workbooks
Therapro
225 Arlington Street
Framingham, MA 01702
508-872-9494
800-257-5376
FAX 508-875-2062
http://www.theraproducts.com
e-mail: info@theraproducts.com
Therapro Staff, Author
Karen Conrad, Owner

These workbooks are excellent for both classroom and individual instruction. Minimal preparation time is needed to use the clear and easy-to-follow lesson guides. *$5.95*

1885 Handwriting: Cursive ABC Book
Therapro
225 Arlington Street
Framingham, MA 01702
508-872-9494
800-257-5376
FAX 508-875-2062
http://www.theraproducts.com
e-mail: info@theraproducts.com
Therapro Staff, Author
Karen Conrad, Owner

The perfect at-home reinforcement with fully illustrated excerpts from children's literature, model letters, practice space and tear-out alphabet cards. *$9.95*
56 pages

1886 Handwriting: Manuscript ABC Book
Therapro
225 Arlington Street
Framingham, MA 01702
508-872-9494
800-257-5376
FAX 508-875-2062
http://www.theraproducts.com
e-mail: info@theraproducts.com
Therapro Staff, Author
Karen Conrad, Owner

Illustrated rhymes, practice letters and words, coloring and tear out alphabet cards teach letter formation. *$9.95*
56 pages

1887 Home/School Activities Manuscript Practice
Therapro
225 Arlington Street
Framingham, MA 01702
508-872-9494
800-257-5376
FAX 508-875-2062
http://www.theraproducts.com
e-mail: info@theraproducts.com
Therapro Staff, Author
Karen Conrad, Owner

Directions for forming lower and upper case letters, and numbers, with space for practice. Activities use letters in words and sentences. *$9.95*
64 pages

1888 Introduction to Journal Writing
Harcourt Achieve
Customer Service, 5th Floor
Orlando, FL 32887
800-284-7019
FAX 800-699-9459
http://www.harcourtachieve.com
e-mail: webmaster@harcourt.com
Steck-Vaughn Staff, Author
Tim McEwen, President/CEO
Susan Canizares, SVP Publisher
Lee Wilson, VP Marketing
The more students write as young children, the higher quality their writing will be, now and as they go on through life. Journal Writing is not about spelling and grammar. It's a highly personal outpouring of thoughts and experiences. *$11.99*

1889 Just for Kids: Grammar
LinguiSystems
3100 4th Avenue
East Moline, IL 61244
309-755-2300
800-776-4332
FAX 309-755-2377
TDY:800-933-8331
http://www.linguisystems.com
e-mail: service@linguisystems.com
Janet Lanza, Lynn Flahive, Author
Linda Bowers, Co-Owner/Co-Founder
Rosemary Huisingh, Co-Owner/Co-Founder

This kid-friendly approach to grammar teaches the parts of speech your students need to know. The practice centers around natural, meaningful activities. Each chapter includes: a pre-and post-test, picture cards, sequence story, rebus story, and family letter. *$39.95*
186 pages Ages 4-9

1890 LD Teacher's IEP Companion
LinguiSystems
3100 4th Avenue
East Moline, IL 61244
309-755-2300
800-776-4332
FAX 309-755-2377
TDY:800-933-8331
http://www.linguisystems.com
e-mail: service@linguisystems.com
Molly Lyle, Author
Linda Bowers, Co-Owner/Co-Founder
Rosemary Huisingh, Co-Owner/Co-Founder

These IEP goals are organized developmentally by skill area with individual objectives and classroom activity suggestions. Goals and objectives cover these academic areas: math; reading; writing; literacy concepts; attention skills; study skills; classroom behavior; social interaction; and transition skills. *$39.95*
169 pages Ages 5-18

1891 Learning 100 Writing Strategies
Harcourt Achieve
6277 Sea Harbor Drive
Orlando, FL 32887
252-480-3200
800-531-5015
FAX 800-699-9459
http://www.steckvaughn.com
e-mail: info@steckvaughn.com
Steck-Vaughn Staff, Author
Tim McEwen, President/CEO
Jeff Johnson, Director Marketing Communication
Chris Lehmann, Team Coordinator
Use the writing process as a tool to build reading comprehension, writing proficiency, and learner confidence. Help learners make a successful connection between reading and writing. Writing Strategies gives learners thorough instruction in the writing process and challenges them to apply their new skills in an everyday writing task that provides ongoing success and encouragement.

1892 Learning Grammar Through Writing
Educators Publishing Service
PO Box 9031
Cambridge, MA 02139
617-547-6706
800-225-5750
FAX 888-440-2665
http://www.epsbooks.com
e-mail: eps@epsbooks.com
Sandra M Bell, James I Wheeler, Author
Gunnar Voltz, President

Learning Grammar through Writing contains grammar and composition rules explained and reference-numbered. Basic grammatical rules, common stylistic and grammatical writing errors, and commonly confused words and expressions are a few of the topics.

1893 Let's Write Right: Teacher's Edition
AVKO'S Educational Research Foundation
3084 W Willard Road
Clio, MI 48420
810-686-1101
866-285-6612
FAX 810-686-1101
http://www.spelling.org
e-mail: info@avko.org
Don McCabe, Author
Don Cabe, Research Director

This is a teacher's lesson plan book which uses an approach designed specifically for dyslexics to teach reading and spelling skills through the side door of penmanship exercises with an empasis on legibility. Student books are handy but are not required. *$19.95*

1894 Let's-Do-It-Write: Writing Readiness Workbook
Therapro
225 Arlington Street
Framingham, MA 01702
508-872-9494
800-257-5376
FAX 508-875-2062
http://www.theraproducts.com
e-mail: info@theraproducts.com
Gail Kushnir, Author
Karen Conrad, Owner

A great variety of prewriting activities and exercises focusing on development of eye-hand coordination and motor, sensory and cognitive skills. Also, helps improve sitting posture, cutting skills, pencil grasp, spatial orientation and problem-solving. Written by an occupational therapist who is a special educator. *$19.95*
112 pages

1895 Linamood Program (LIPS Clinical Version):Phoneme Sequencing Program for Reading, Spelling,Speech
LinguiSystems
3100 4th Avenue
East Moline, IL 61244
309-755-2300
800-776-4332
FAX 309-755-2377
TDY:800-933-8331
http://www.linguisystems.com
e-mail: service@linguisystems.com
Patricia Linamood, Phyllis Linamood, Author
Linda Bowers, Co-Owner/Co-Founder
Rosemary Huisingh, Co-Owner/Co-Founder

Help your students develop phoneme awareness for competence in reading, spelling, and speech. This multisensory program meets the needs of the many children and adults who don't develop phonemic awareness through traditional methods. *$247.00*
Birth-Adult

1896 MAXI
Aids and Appliances for Independent Living
42 Executive Boulevard
Farmingdale, NY 11735
631-752-0521
FAX 516-752-0689
http://www.maxiaids.com
Elliot Zaretsky, President

Thousands of products to make life easier. Eating, dressing, communications, bed, bath, kitchen, writing aids and more.

1897 Manual for Learning to Use Manuscript and Cursive Handwriting
Educators Publishing Service
PO Box 9031
Cambridge, MA 02139
617-547-6706
800-225-5750
FAX 888-440-2665
http://www.epsbooks.com
e-mail: eps@epsbooks.com
Beth Slingerland, Author
Gunnar Voltz, President

This multisensory handwriting program is divided into two parts, manuscript and cursive, which can be used either consecutively or independently.

1898 Media Weaver 3.5
Sunburst Technology
1550 Executive Drive
Elgin, IL 60123
800-321-7511
FAX 888-800-3028
http://http://store.sunburst.com/Home.aspx
e-mail: service@sunburst.com
Michael Guillory, Channel Sales/Marketing Manager

Publishing becomes a multimedia event with this dynamic word processor that contains hundreds of media elements and effective process writing resources.

1899 Middle School Writing: Expository Writing
Harcourt Achieve
Customer Service, 5th Floor
Orlando, FL 32887
800-284-7019
FAX 800-699-9459
http://www.harcourtachieve.com
e-mail: webmaster@harcourt.com
Steck-Vaughn Staff, Author
Tim McEwen, President/CEO
Susan Canizares, SVP Publisher
Lee Wilson, VP Marketing
An effective comprehensive review and reinforcement of the writing and research skills students will need. Effectively used in both school and home setting. Ideal for junior high or high school students in need of remediation. *$ 7.99*

ISBN 0-739829-28-9

1900 My Handwriting Word Book
Therapro
225 Arlington Street
Framingham, MA 01702
508-872-9494
800-257-5376
FAX 508-875-2062
http://www.theraproducts.com
e-mail: info@theraproducts.com
Therapro Staff, Author
Karen Conrad, Owner

Children practice writing everyday words — two letter words, words for days, months, numbers, family names and more. *$9.95*

64 pages

1901 PAF Handwriting Programs for Print, Cursive (Right or Left-Handed)
Educators Publishing Service
PO Box 9031
Cambridge, MA 02139
617-547-6706
800-225-5750
FAX 888-440-2665
http://www.epsbooks.com
e-mail: eps@epsbooks.com
Phyllis Bertin, Eileen Perlman, Author
Gunnar Voltz, President

These workbooks can be used in conjunction with the PAF curriculum or independently as a classroom penmanship program. They were specifically designed to accommodate all students including those with fine-motor, visual-motor and graphomotor weaknesses. The workbooks contain both large models for introducing motor patterns and smaller models to facilitate the transition to primary and loose-leaf papers. A detailed instruction booklet accompanies each workbook.

1902 PATHS
Abilitations Speech Bin
3155 Northwoods Parkway
Norcross, GA 30071
770-449-5700
800-477-3324
FAX 770-510-7290
http://www.speechbin.com
e-mail: info@speechbin.com
Suzanne Wilkerson, Catalog Director

PATHS gives you a step-by-step comprehensive program for students who have experienced difficulty in academic learning. It targets skills critical for academic achievements: phonological awareness, phonemic relationships, phonemic processing and listening and memory. Item number 1491. *$22.95*

1903 Phonological Awareness Kit
LinguiSystems
3100 4th Avenue
East Moline, IL 61244
309-755-2300
800-776-4332
FAX 309-755-2377
TDY:800-933-8331
http://www.linguisystems.com
e-mail: service@linguisystems.com
Carolyn Robertson, Wanda Salter, Author
Linda Bowers, Co-Owner/Co-Founder
Rosemary Huisingh, Co-Owner/Co-Founder

Help your students learn to use phonological information to process oral and written language with this fantastic kit. Written by an SLP and special educator, this best-seller links sound awareness, oral language, and early reading and writing skills. The kit uses a multisensory approach to ensure success for all learning styles. *$69.95*
115 pages Ages 5-8

1904 Phonological Awareness Kit: Intermediate
LinguiSystems
3100 4th Avenue
East Moline, IL 61244
309-755-2300
800-776-4332
FAX 309-755-2377
TDY:800-933-8331
http://www.linguisystems.com
e-mail: service@linguisystems.com
Carolyn Robertson, Wanda Salter, Author
Linda Bowers, Co-Owner/Co-Founder
Rosemary Huisingh, Co-Owner/Co-Founder

Now there's hope for your older students who have struggled with reading through their early school years. Give them strategies to crack the reading code with this comprehensive program. Great for students with deficits in auditory processing, decoding, and written language. *$69.95*
116 pages Ages 9-14

1905 Prewriting Curriculum Enrichment Series
Therapro
225 Arlington Street
Framingham, MA 01702
508-872-9494
800-257-5376
FAX 508-875-2062
http://www.theraproducts.com
e-mail: info@theraproducts.com
Peggy Hundley Spitz OTR, Author
Karen Conrad, Owner

This series offers a wide variety of thematically related developmental activities: Trace & Draw; Crafts and Costumes; Cooking; Stories to Color & Read; and Games. Enough activities for several years. Many reproducable worksheets are included. Ideal for preschool programs. Helps all levels of development with hand skills, eye-hand coordination, perception and sensory motor awareness. *$22.50*
180 pages

1906 Punctuation Play-by-Play
LinguiSystems
3100 4th Avenue
East Moline, IL 61244
309-755-2300
800-776-4332
FAX 309-755-2377
TDY:800-933-8331
http://www.linguisystems.com
e-mail: service@linguisystems.com
Carolyn LoGiudice, Mike LoGiudice, Author
Linda Bowers, Co-Owner/Co-Founder
Rosemary Huisingh, Co-Owner/Co-Founder

Punctuation Play-by-Play engages students in a lively game as they practice essential punctuation skills including: capitalization; end marks; apostrophes; commas; quotation marks; colons; semicolons. Question cards are divides into two levels of difficulty. *$44.95*

Ages 10-18

1907 Punctuation, Capitalization, and Handwriting for Job and Personal Use
AGS Publishing
PO Box 99
Circle Pines, MN 55014
651-287-7220
800-328-2560
FAX 800-471-8457
http://www.agsnet.com
e-mail: agsmail@agsnet.com
Renae B Humberg, Author
Kevin Brueggeman, President
Matt Keller, Marketing Manager

With an interest level of high school through adult, and a reading level of Grade 5-6, this series has modules in Punctuation, Capitalization and Handwriting. *$299.00*

1908 Reading and Writing Workbook
Therapro
225 Arlington Street
Framingham, MA 01702
508-872-9494
800-257-5376
FAX 508-875-2062
http://www.theraproducts.com
e-mail: info@theraproducts.com
Therapro Staff, Author
Karen Conrad, Owner

Writing checks and balancing a checkbook, copying words and sentences, and writing messages and notes. Helps with recognition and understanding of calendars, phone books and much more. *$10.50*

1909 Report Writing
Harcourt Achieve
6277 Sea Harbor Drive
Orlando, FL 32887
252-480-3200
800-531-5015
FAX 800-699-9459
http://www.steckvaughn.com
e-mail: info@steckvaughn.com
Steck-Vaughn Staff, Author
Tim McEwen, President/CEO
Jeff Johnson, Director Marketing Communication
Chriss Lehmann, Team Coordinator
Here is the complete, step-by-step guide to learning the tools, skills, and time management techniques necessary for researching, organizing, outlining, and writing reports.

1910 SLP's IDEA Companion
LinguiSystems
3100 4th Avenue
East Moline, IL 61244
309-755-2300
800-776-4332
FAX 309-755-2377
TDY:800-933-8331
http://www.linguisystems.com
e-mail: service@linguisystems.com
Shaila Lucas, Author
Linda Bowers, Co-Owner/Co-Founder
Rosemary Huisingh, Co-Owner/Co-Founder

Get goals and objectives that match the guidelines outlined in the individuals with Disabilities Education Act. You'll be able to link your therapy goals to the classroom curriculum, determine appropriate benchmarks for students, and determine levels of performance using the baseline measures provided in the book. *$39.95*

162 pages Ages 5-18

1911 Soaring Scores on the ISAT Reading and Writing
Harcourt Achieve
Customer Service, 5th Floor
Orlando, FL 32887
800-284-7019
FAX 800-699-9459
http://www.harcourtachieve.com
e-mail: webmaster@harcourt.com
Steck-Vaughn Staff, Author
Tim McEwen, President/CEO
Susan Canizares, SVP Publisher
Lee Wilson, VP Marketing

Highly targeted instruction and practice tests help students approach the ISAT strategically and confidently. Writing prompts ask students to write a persuasive, expository, or narrative essay. Modeled questions practice both multiple-choice and open-ended queries. *$61.90*

1912 Spelling Charts: Intermediate
LinguiSystems
3100 4th Avenue
East Moline, IL 61244
309-755-2300
800-776-4332
FAX 800-577-4555
TDY:800-933-8331
http://www.linguisystems.com
e-mail: service@linguisystems.com
Linda Bowers, Co-Owner/Co-Founder
Rosemary Huisingh, Co-Owner/Co-Founder

Good spelling doesn't stop in the primary grades. Help your older students understand word families with this great resource. It's a valuable tool for spelling, writing, and vocabulary skills. You get 45 full-color cards to use as charts, overheads, or take-home practice.

1913 Spelling Charts: Primary
LinguiSystems
3100 4th Avenue
East Moline, IL 61244
309-755-2300
800-776-4332
FAX 800-577-4555
TDY:800-933-8331
http://www.linguisystems.com
e-mail: service@linguisystems.com
Linda Bowers, Co-Owner/Co-Founder
Rosemary Huisingh, Co-Owner/Co-Founder

Tap into phonological awareness skills with these full-color charts. Use them as classroom charts, overheads, or take-home practice. They're great for large group, small group, or individual teaching. Each chart features words grouped by rhyming families or similar word endings.

1914 Spelling for Job and Personal Use
AGS Publishing
PO Box 99
Circle Pines, MN 55014
651-287-7220
800-328-2560
FAX 800-471-8457
http://www.agsnet.com
e-mail: agsmail@agsnet.com
Merle Wood, Author
Kevin Brueggeman, President
Matt Keller, Marketing Manager

With an interest level of high school through adult, and a reading level of Grade 5-6, this series has modules in Using the Dictionary, Guides to Spelling and Spelling the 100 Most Used Words.

1915 StartWrite
Therapro
225 Arlington Street
Framingham, MA 01702
508-872-9494
800-257-5376
FAX 508-875-2062
http://www.theraproducts.com
e-mail: info@theraproducts.com
Therapro Staff, Author
Karen Conrad, Owner

With this easy-to-use software package, you can make papers and handwriting worksheets to meet individual student's needs. Type letters, words, or numbers and they appear in a dot format on the triple line guide. Change letter size, add shading, turn on or off guide lines and arrow strokes and place provided clipart. Fonts include Manuscript and Cursive, Modern Manuscript and Cursive and Italic Manuscript and Cursive. Useful manual included. *$39.95*

Windows/Mac

1916 Strategies for Success in Writing
Harcourt Achieve
Customer Service, 5th Floor
Orlando, FL 32887
800-284-7019
FAX 800-699-9459
http://www.harcourtachieve.com
e-mail: webmaster@harcourt.com
Steck-Vaughn Staff, Author
Tim McEwen, President/CEO
Susan Canizares, SVP Publisher
Lee Wilson, VP Marketing
Help your students gain success and master all the steps in writing through essay-writing strategies and exercises in proofreading, editing, and revising written work. This program also helps students approach tests strategically. *$3.30*

1917 Sunbuddy Writer
Sunburst Technology
1550 Executive Drive
Elgin, IL 60123
800-321-7511
FAX 888-800-3028
http://http://store.sunburst.com/Home.aspx
e-mail: service@sunburst.com
Michael Guillory, Channel Sales/Marketing Manager

An easy-to-use picture and word processor designed especially for young writers.

1918 TOPS Kit: Adolescent-Tasks of Problem Solving
LinguiSystems
3100 4th Avenue
East Moline, IL 61244
309-755-2300
800-776-4332
FAX 309-755-2377
TDY:800-933-8331
http://www.linguisystems.com
e-mail: service@linguisystems.com
Linda Bowers, Rosemary Huisingh, Mark Barrett, Author
Linda Bowers, Co-Owner/Co-Founder
Rosemary Huisingh, Co-Owner/Co-Founder

Teach your teens how to use their language skills to think, think, think. We combine literacy, thinking, writing, humor, and language arts practice to cover these thinking skills: using content to make references; analyzing information; taking another's point of view; and more. It's a literacy- based approach that gets dramatic results! *$59.95*
192 pages Ages 12-18

1919 Tool Chest: For Teachers, Parents and Students
Therapro
225 Arlington Street
Framingham, MA 01702
508-872-9494
800-257-5376
FAX 508-875-2062
http://www.theraproducts.com
e-mail: info@theraproducts.com
Henry OT Services, Author
Karen Conrad, Owner

Ideas for self-regulation and handwriting skills. 26+ activities, each on its own page, with rationale, supplies needed, instructions and related projects. Provides a fast way to prepare for OT activities. Supports the videotapes Tools for Teachers and Tools for Students. *$19.95*

1920 Type-It
Educators Publishing Service
PO Box 9031
Cambridge, MA 02139
617-547-6706
800-225-5750
FAX 888-440-2666
http://www.epsbooks.com
e-mail: eps@epsbooks.com

Joan Duffy, Author
Gunnar Voltz, President

A linguistically oriented beginning 'touch-system' typing manual. A progress chart allows students to pace their progress in short, easily attainable units, often enabling them to proceed with little or no supervision.

1921 Vowel Scramble
LinguiSystems
3100 4th Avenue
East Moline, IL 61244
309-755-2300
800-776-4332
FAX 309-755-2377
TDY:800-933-8331
http://www.linguisystems.com
e-mail: service@linguisystems.com
Carolyn LoGiudice, Author
Linda Bowers, Co-Owner/Co-Founder
Rosemary Huisingh, Co-Owner/Co-Founder

Your student will love this fun new way to practice spelling and phonological awareness skills. Players earn points by using letter tiles to complete words on the game board. *$44.95*
Ages 7-12

1922 Workbook for Aphasia
Abilitations Speech Bin
PO Box 922668
Norcross, GA 30010
770-499-5700
800-850-8602
FAX 770-510-7290
http://www.speechbin.com
e-mail: info@speechbin.com
Susan Howell Brubaker, Author
Tobi Isaacs, Catalog Director

This book gives you materials for adults who have recovered a significant degree of speaking, reading, writing, and comprehension skills. It includes 106 exercises divided into eight target areas. Item number W331. *$69.99*

1923 Write On! Plus: Beginning Writing Skills
Sunburst Technology
1550 Executive Drive
Elgin, IL 60123
800-321-7511
FAX 888-800-3028
http://http://store.sunburst.com/Home.aspx
e-mail: service@sunburst.com
Michael Guillory, Channel Sales/Marketing Manager

This classic process writing series teaches a wide range of core writing and literature skills through hundreds of motivating and challenging activities.

1924 Write On! Plus: Elementary Writing Skills
Sunburst Technology
1550 Executive Drive
Elgin, IL 60123
800-321-7511
FAX 888-800-3028
http://http://store.sunburst.com/Home.aspx
e-mail: service@sunburst.com
Michael Guillory, Channel Sales/Marketing Manager

This classic process writing series teaches a wide range of core writing and literature skills through hundreds of motivating and challenging activities.

1925 Write On! Plus: Essential Writing
Sunburst Technology
1550 Executive Drive
Elgin, IL 60123
800-321-7511
FAX 888-800-3028
http://http://store.sunburst.com/Home.aspx
e-mail: service@sunburst.com
Michael Guillory, Channel Sales/Marketing Manager

This classic process writing series teaches a wide range of core writing and literature skills through hundreds of motivating and challenging activities.

1926 Write On! Plus: Growing as a Writer
Sunburst Technology
1550 Executive Drive
Elgin, IL 60123
800-321-7511
FAX 888-800-3028
http://http://store.sunburst.com/Home.aspx
e-mail: service@sunburst.com
Michael Guillory, Channel Sales/Marketing Manager

This classic process writing series teaches a wide range of core writing and literature skills through hundreds of motivating and challenging activities.

1927 Write On! Plus: High School Writing Skills
Sunburst Technology
1550 Executive Drive
Elgin, IL 60123
800-321-7511
FAX 888-800-3028
http://http://store.sunburst.com/Home.aspx
e-mail: service@sunburst.com
Michael Guillory, Channel Sales/Marketing Manager

This classic process writing series teaches a wide range of core writing and literature skills through hundreds of motivating and challenging activities.

1928 Write On! Plus: Literature Studies
Sunburst Technology
1550 Executive Drive
Elgin, IL 60123
800-321-7511
FAX 888-800-3028
http://http://store.sunburst.com/Home.aspx
e-mail: service@sunburst.com
Michael Guillory, Channel Sales/Marketing Manager

This classic process writing series teaches a wide range of core writing and literature skills through hundreds of motivating and challenging activities.

1929 Write On! Plus: Middle School Writing Skills
Sunburst Technology
1550 Executive Drive
Elgin, IL 60123
800-321-7511
FAX 888-800-3028
http://http://store.sunburst.com/Home.aspx
e-mail: service@sunburst.com
Michael Guillory, Channel Sales/Marketing Manager

This classic process writing series teaches a wide range of core writing and literature skills through hundreds of motivating and challenging activities.

1930 Write On! Plus: Responding to Great Literature
Sunburst Technology
1550 Executive Drive
Elgin, IL 60123
800-321-7511
FAX 888-800-3028
http://http://store.sunburst.com/Home.aspx
e-mail: service@sunburst.com
Michael Guillory, Channel Sales/Marketing Manager

This classic process writing series teaches a wide range of core writing and literature skills through hundreds of motivating and challenging activities.

1931 Write On! Plus: Spanish/ English Literacy Series
Sunburst Technology
1550 Executive Drive
Elgin, IL 60123
800-321-7511
FAX 888-800-3028
http://http://store.sunburst.com/Home.aspx
e-mail: service@sunburst.com
Michael Guillory, Channel Sales/Marketing Manager

This classic process writing series teaches a wide range of core writing and literature skills through hundreds of motivating and challenging activities.

1932 Write On! Plus: Steps to Better Writing
Sunburst Technology
1550 Executive Drive
Elgin, IL 60123
800-321-7511
FAX 888-800-3028
http://http://store.sunburst.com/Home.aspx
e-mail: service@sunburst.com
Michael Guillory, Channel Sales/Marketing Manager

This classic process writing series teaches a wide range of core writing and literature skills through hundreds of motivating and challenging activities.

1933 Write On! Plus: Writing with Picture Books
Sunburst Technology
1550 Executive Drive
Elgin, IL 60123
800-321-7511
FAX 888-800-3028
http://http://store.sunburst.com/Home.aspx
e-mail: service@sunburst.com
Michael Guillory, Channel Sales/Marketing Manager

This classic process writing series teaches a wide range of core writing and literature skills through hundreds of motivating and challenging activities.

1934 Write from the Start
Therapro
225 Arlington Street
Framingham, MA 01702
508-872-9494
800-257-5376
FAX 508 875 2062
http://www.theraproducts.com
e-mail: info@theraproducts.com
Ion Teodorescu, Lois M Addy, Author
Karen Conrad, Owner

This program addresses the handwriting process in two ways. First, it assists in developing the intrinsic muscles of the hand to gain the control required to form letter shapes and to create appropriate spaces between words. Secondly, it helps to develop perceptual skills that are required to orient letters and organize the page. Each book has sections to be copied. Two books consisting of eye hand, spatial organization, graphic and perceptual challenges.
128 pages

1935 WriteOPOLY
LinguiSystems
3100 4th Avenue
East Moline, IL 61244
309-755-2300
800-776-4332
FAX 309-755-2377
TDY:800-933-8331
http://www.linguisystems.com
e-mail: service@linguisystems.com
Paul F Johnson, Author
Linda Bowers, Co-Owner/Co-Founder
Rosemary Huisingh, Co-Owner/Co-Founder

End writer's block for even your most reluctant writers with this fun game. Improve written language skills with WriteOPOLY. Students travel around a colorful game board buying properties and filling out Writing Plan sheets. *$ 44.95*
Ages 9-14

1936 Writer's Resources Library 2.0
Sunburst Technology
1550 Executive Drive
Elgin, IL 60123
800-321-7511
FAX 888-800-3028
http://http://store.sunburst.com/Home.aspx
e-mail: service@sunburst.com

Michael Guillory, Channel Sales/Marketing Manager

Students quickly access seven reference resources with this indispensable writing tool.

1937 Writestart
Therapro
225 Arlington Street
Framingham, MA 01702
508-872-9494
800-257-5376
FAX 508-875-2062
http://www.theraproducts.com
e-mail: info@theraproducts.com
Therapro Staff, Author
Karen Conrad, Owner

A great prewriting kit with 30 beautifully illustrated 8x8 reusable cards. The activities progress from simple pre-writing activities such as mazes and tracking, up to formation of upper and lower case letters, all hosted by a green dinosaur. Includes a special pencil and triangular grip. *$16.95*

1938 Writing Trek Grades 4-6
Sunburst Technology
1550 Executive Drive
Elgin, IL 60123
800-321-7511
FAX 888-800-3028
http://http://store.sunburst.com/Home.aspx
e-mail: service@sunburst.com
Michael Guillory, Channel Sales/Marketing Manager

Enhance your students' experience in your English language arts classroom with twelve authentic writing projects that build students' competence while encouraging creativity.

1939 Writing Trek Grades 6-8
Sunburst Technology
1550 Executive Drive
Elgin, IL 60123
800-321-7511
FAX 888-800-3028
http://http://store.sunburst.com/Home.aspx
e-mail: service@sunburst.com
Michael Guillory, Channel Sales/Marketing Manager

Twelve authentic language arts projects, activities, and assignments develop your students' writing confidence and ability.

1940 Writing Trek Grades 8-10
Sunburst Technology
1550 Executive Drive
Elgin, IL 60123
800-321-7511
FAX 888-800-3028
http://http://store.sunburst.com/Home.aspx
e-mail: service@sunburst.com
Michael Guillory, Channel Sales/Marketing Manager

Help your students develop a concept of genre as they become familiar with the writing elements and characteristics of a variety of writing forms.

Learning Disabilities

1941 Active Parenting Workshops
Active Parenting Publishers
1955 Vaughn Road NW
Kennesaw, GA 30144
770-429-0565
800-825-0060
FAX 770-429-0334
http://www.activeparenting.com
e-mail: cservice@activeparenting.com
Michael Popkin PhD, Founder/President

Conducts nationwide parenting workshops recognized by the National Board of Certified Counselors. Offers parenting education curriculum for parents of ADD/ADHD children.

1942 American Council on Rural Special Education Conference
Utah State University
2865 Old Main Hl
Logan, UT 84322
435-797-3243
FAX 801-626-7427
http://extension.usu.edu
e-mail: jmayhew@weber.edu
Ben Lignugaris-Kra, Manager

Conference of special educators, teachers and professors working with exceptional needs students. Keynote speakers, silent auction.
March

1943 American Counseling Association Convention
ACA Membership Division
5999 Stevenson Avenue
Alexandria, VA 22304
800-347-6647
FAX 800-473-2329
http://www.counseling.org
e-mail: webmaster@counseling.org
Brian Canfield, President

Keynote speakers and workshops as well as exhibits are offered.

March

1944 American Speech-Language-Hearing Association Annual Convention
American Speech Language-Hearing Association
10801 Rockville Pike
Bethesda, MD 20852
800-638-8255
FAX 240-333-4705
http://www.asha.org
e-mail: convention@asha.org
Arlene Pietranton, Executive Director
Cheyrl Russel, Convention/Meetings

Topics addressed include hearing impairments, special education and speech communication. 10,000 attendees.
November

1945 Annual International Technology & PersonsDisabilities Conference
Center on Disabilities/CSU - Northbridge
18111 Nordhoff Street
Northridge, CA 91330
818-677-2578
FAX 818-677-4929
TDY:818-677-2579
http://www.csun.edu/cod
e-mail: conference@csun.edu
Sandy Plotin, Managing Director

Comprehensive, international conference, where all technologies across all ages, disabilities, levels of education and training, employment and independent living are addressed. It is the largest conference of its kind with exhibit halls open free to public.

1946 Annual Postsecondary Disability Training Institute
University of Connecticut
249 Glenbrook Road
Storrs Mansfield, CT 06269
860-486-3321
FAX 860-486-5799
http://www.cped.uconn.edu
e-mail: carrol.waite@uconn.edu
Stan Shaw, Institute Coordinator
Carrol Waite, Program Assistant

Focus of the Institute is to assist concerned professionals to meet the unique needs of college students with disabilities.
June

1947 Assessing Learning Problems Workshop
Learning Disabilities Resources
PO Box 716
Bryn Mawr, PA 19010
610-525-8336
800-869-8336
FAX 610-525-8337
http://www.ldonline.org
This workshop includes behavioral manifestations of information processing problems and how to relate these to learning processes.

1948 Association Book Exhibit: Brain Research
Association Book Exhibit
8727a Cooper Road
Alexandria, VA 22309
703-619-5030
FAX 703-619-5035
http://www.bookexhibit.com
e-mail: info@bookexhibit.com
Mark Trocchi, Vice President

Attendence is 800-1,000. Every serious publisher of Neuroscience material represented.

1949 CACLD Spring & Fall Conferences
Connecticut Assoc. for Children & Adults with LD
25 Van Zant Street
Norwalk, CT 06855
203-838-5010
FAX 203-866-6108
http://www.CACLD.org
e-mail: cacld@optonline.net
Beryl Kaufman, Conference Coordinator

Offers speakers, workshops, presentations and more for professionals and parents dealing with learning disability and attention disorder in their daily life. Also offers a strand on college for students with LD and ADD, exhibitors and a giant bookstore.

1950 CEC Federation Conference: Arkansas
Council for Exceptional Children
PO Box 928
Russellville, AR 72801
479-967-6025
FAX 479-967-6056
http://www.cec.sped.org
e-mail: chris.foley@rsdmail.k12.ar.us
Jill Simpson, President, Arkansas CEC
Chris Foley, Conference Chair

Annual conference held at Hot Springs Convention Centerin Hot Springs, AR.
November

1951 CEC Federation Conference: Kansas
Council for Exceptional Children
1011 Price Boulevard
Atchison, KS 66002
785-462-2940
http://www.kansascec.org
e-mail: aoelke@nkesc.org
Anita Oelke, President Elect/Conference Chair

Exhibits and workshop sessions for educators building a brighter tomorrow.
October

1952 CEC Federation Conference: Pennsylvania
Council of Exceptional Children
309 B Recitation Hall
West Chester, PA 19383
610-436-1060
FAX 610-436-3102
http://www.pacec.sped.org
e-mail: vmcginley@wcupa.edu

Laura Receveur, President-Elect
Cathy McCarthy, Vice President
Darlene Perner, Conference Chair
The convention offers opportunities to learn about new research, new technology and best practice in the profession plus a chance to meet and share with exceptional individuals who are dedicated to children and education.
November

1953 **CEC Federation Conference: Virginia**
Council for Exceptional Children
1110 N Glebe Road
Arlington, VA 22201
703-245-0600
FAX 703-264-1637
http://www.cec.sped.org
e-mail: victore@cec.sped.org
Victor Erickson, Exhibits Manager
Liz Martinez, Publications Director
Bruce Ramirez, Manager
Find a wealth of information targeted just for educators. Choose from more than 600 workshops, lectures, demonstrations, mini workshops, panels and poster sessions.
April

1954 **Center on Disabilities Conference**
California State University Northridge
18111 Nordhoff Street
Northridge, CA 91330
818-677-2578
FAX 818-677-4929
http://www.csun.edu
e-mail: conference@csun.edu
Sandy Plotin, Managing Director

Focuses on issues pertaining to the disabled learner and gifted education. 2,000 attendees.

1955 **Closing the Gap Conference**
526 Main Street
Henderson, MN 56044
507-248-3294
FAX 507-248-3810
http://www.closingthegap.com
e-mail: ckneip@closingthegap.com
Connie Kneip, VP/General Manager

Annual international conference with over 100 exhibitors concerned with the use of assistive technology in special education and rehabilitation.
October

1956 **College Students with Learning Disabilities Workshop**
Learning Disabilities Resources
PO Box 716
Bryn Mawr, PA 19010
610-525-8336
800-869-8336
FAX 610-525-8337
http://www.ldonline.org
This workshop is designed to provide both information and motivation to both students and college personnel.

1957 **Communication Aid Manufacturers Association (CAMA) Workshops**
205 W Randolf Street
Evanston, IL 60204
847-869-2122
800-441-2262
FAX 847-869-2161
TDY:800-441-2262
http://www.aacproducts.org
e-mail: cama@northshore.net
James Neils, Association Administrator
Chris Murin, Workshop Coordinator

CAMA sponsors workshops throughout the US and Canada that demonstrates a variety of communication products from leading manufacturers. The Association strives to keep up with the latest in augmentative and alternative communication (ACC) technology, and promotes understanding of software and hardware, appropriate for clients with learning disabilities. Members teach functional use in a variety of speaking situations.

1958 **ConnSENSE Conference**
University of Connecticut
233 Glenbrook Road, Unit 4171
Storrs Mansfield, CT 06269
860-486-2020
FAX 860-486-4412
TDY:860-486-2077
http://www.csd.uconn.edu
e-mail: csd@uconn.edu
Donna Korbel, Director

Annual conference on technology for people with special needs.

1959 **Council for Exceptional Children: Teacher Education Division Conference**
Peabody College/Vanderbilt University
2201 W End Avenue
Nashville, TN 37235
615-322-7311
FAX 615-343-5555
Harry Jacobson, Plant Manager
Patricia Gegelka, Contact Person

Topics addressed include personnel, productivity and teacher education.

1960 **Council for Learning Disabilities International Conference**
Council for Learning Disabilities
1184 Antioch Road
Overland, KS 66210
913-491-1011
FAX 913-491-1012
http://www.cldinternational.org
e-mail: lnease@cldinternational.org
Linda Nease, Executive Director
Mary Provost, Conference Director

Focuses on all aspects pertaining to learning disabled individuals from a teaching and research perspective.
October

1961 **Council of Administrators of Special Education Conference**
Fort Valley State University
1005 State University Drive
Fort Valley, GA 31030
478-825-7667
FAX 478-825-7811
http://www.casecec.org
e-mail: lpurcell@bellsouth.net
Christy Chambers, President
Luann Purcell, Executive Director

To provide leadership and support to members by shaping policies and practices impact the quality of education
January

1962 **Counseling Individuals with Learning Disabilities Workshop**
Learning Disabilities Resources
PO Box 716
Bryn Mawr, PA 19010
610-525-8336
800-869-8336
FAX 610-525-8337
http://www.ldonline.org
Richard Cooper, Author

In this workshop, Dr. Cooper discusses reasons why some individuals with learning disabilities often do respond well to traditional therapies.

1963 **Creative Mind Workshop: Making Magic with Children and Art**
P Buckley Moss Foundation for Children's Education
152 P Buckley Moss Drive
Waynesboro, VA 22980
540-932-1728
FAX 540-941-8865
http://www.mossfoundation.org
e-mail: foundation@mossfoundation.org
Pat Moss

Instructional and collaborative strategies for including the visual and performing arts in the education of students with special needs.

1964 Eden Family of Services
Eden Services
1 Eden Way
Princeton, NJ 08540
609-987-0099
FAX 609-987-0243
http://www.edenservices.org
e-mail: info@edenservices.org
Tom Cool, President
Anne Holmes, Director Outreach Support
Joani Truch, Administration/Communications
Provides year-round educational services, early intervention, parent training and workshops, respite care, outreach services, community based residential services and employment opportunities for individuals with autism.

1965 Educating Children Summer Training Institute (ECSTI)
Muskingum College - Graduate & Continuing Studies
163 Stormont Street
New Concord, OH 43762
740-826-8211
http://www.muskingum.edu
e-mail: ecsti@muskingum.edu
Sheila Ellenberger, Executive Director

ECSIT offers graduate teacher education and continuing professional development through a series of week long courses. An innovative immersion program, ECSTI offers over 40 course options.

1966 Educational Computer Conference
Annual International Conference
19 Calvert Court
Piedmont, CA 94611
510-594-1249
888-594-1249
FAX 510-594-1838
http://www.trld.com
e-mail: registration@trld.com
Diane Frost, CEO

Focusing on actual classroom and administrative applications for technology, reading and learning difficulties. Hands on workshops are featured.
January

1967 Educational Options for Students with Learning Disabilities and LD/HD
Connecticut Assoc. for Children & Adults with LD
25 Van Zant Street
Norwalk, CT 06855
203-838-5010
FAX 203-866-6108
http://www.CACLD.org
e-mail: cacld@optonline.net
Beryl Kaufman, Conference Coordinator

Conference held for parents, students and professionals. Features workshops, panels, exhibitors and a bookstore.
Spring

1968 Inclusion of Learning Disabled Students in Regular Classrooms Workshop
Learning Disabilities Resources
PO Box 716
Bryn Mawr, PA 19010
610-525-8336
800-869-8336
FAX 610-525-8337
http://www.ldonline.org
This workshop provides teachers with practical suggestions and techniques for including students with learning problems.

1969 Innovative Instructional Techniques Workshop
Learning Disabilities Resources
PO Box 716
Bryn Mawr, PA 19010
610-525-8336
800-869-8336
FAX 610-525-8337
http://www.ldonline.org
Richard Cooper, Author

In this workshop, Dr. Cooper provides an overview of the various techniques he has developed for helping students with learning problems in reading, writing, spelling and math.

1970 Interest-Driven Learning Master Class/Workshop
199 NE Burr Oak Court
Lees Summit, MO 64064
816-478-4824
800-245-5733
FAX 816-478-4824
http://www.drpeet.com
e-mail: drpeet@drpeet.com
Bill Peet MD, CEO

Provides master classes or workshops on how to use talking word processors and interactive fiction to create highly effective supplemental reading and writing activities for learners of varying abilities aged three to eight. Assistive technology access channels provided for all disabilities. All strategies taught reference the results of 25 years or research.

1971 International Adolescent Conference: Programs for Adolescents
Behavioral Institute for Children and Adolescents
3585 Lexington Avenue N
Arden Hills, MN 55126
651-484-5510
FAX 651-483-3879
http://www.behavioralinstitute.org
e-mail: info@behavioralinstitute.org
Sheldon Braaten, Executive Director
Melissa Knoll, Managing Director
Jackie Borock, Director
Information on programs for the developmental needs of children and adolescents with behavioral disorders. Transdisciplinary knowledge and skill, training related, to serve children and youth who have emotional/behavioral disorders.

1972 International Dyslexia Association Conference: Maryland
International Dyslexia Association
40 York Road
Baltimore, MD 21206
410-296-0232
800-ABC-D123
FAX 410-321-5069
http://www.interdys.org
e-mail: info@interdys.org
Megan Cohen, Executive Director
Mike Hayes, Director Marketing
Elaine Niefeld, Director of Publications
Each year IDA sponsors an international conference. Sessions meet the needs and interests of a wide range of consumers.
November

1973 International Dyslexia Association Conference: Illinois
Illinois Branch of the International Dyslexia Asso
751 Roosevelt Road
Glen Ellyn, IL 60137
630-469-6900
FAX 630-469-6810
http://www.readibida.org
e-mail: info@readibida.org
Jo Ann Paldo, President
Kathleen L Wgner, Executive Director

This conference will have approximately 500 attendees and 20 exhibitors.
November

1974 LDR Workshop: What Are Learning Disabilities, Problems and Differences?
Learning Disabilities Resources
PO Box 716
Bryn Mawr, PA 19010
610-525-8336
800-869-8336
FAX 610-525-8337
http://www.ldonline.org
Richard Cooper, Author

In this workshop, Dr. Cooper draws on personal experiences with a learning disability and on his clinical work with thousands of individuals with a wide variety of learning problems to provide the participants with an understanding of the positive and negative aspects of being, living and learning differently.

1975 Landmark School Outreach Program
Landmark School
429 Hale Street
Prides Crossing, MA 01965
978-236-3216
FAX 978-927-7268
http://www.landmarkoutreach.org
e-mail: outreach@landmarkschool.org

Dan Ahearn, Director

Provides consultation and professional development to schools, professional organizations, parent groups, and businesses on topics related to individuals with learning disabilities. Services are individually designed to meet the client's specific needs and can range from a two-hour workshop to a year-long collaboration. Options include: annual Professional Development Institute at Landmark School; on-site professional development programs at schools; online professional development program.

1976 Learning Disabilities Association Conference: International

4156 Library Road
Pittsburgh, PA 15234
412-341-1515
FAX 412-344-0224
http://www.ldaamerica.org
e-mail: info@ldaamerica.org
Shiela Buckley, Executive Director
Sharon Tanner, Membership Coordinator

Topics addressed at the conference include advocacy, adult literacy and learning disabled education.
March

1977 Learning Disabilities Association of Texas Conference

1011 W 31st Street
Austin, TX 78705
512-458-8234
800-604-7500
FAX 512-458-3826
http://www.ldat.org
e-mail: contact@ldat.org
Jean Kueker, President
Ann Robinson, State Coordinator

Promotes the educational and general welfare of individuals with learning disabilities.

1978 Learning Disabilities and the World of Work Workshop

Learning Disabilities Resources
PO Box 716
Bryn Mawr, PA 19010
610-525-8336
800-869-8336
FAX 610-525-8337
http://www.ldonline.org

This workshop is designed for employers, parents or professionals working with individuals with learning disabilities.

1979 Learning Problems and Adult Basic Education Workshop

Learning Disabilities Resources
PO Box 716
Bryn Mawr, PA 19010
610-525-8336
800-869-8336
FAX 610-525-8337
http://www.ldonline.org

This workshop for adult educators discusses the manifestations of learning problems in adults.

1980 Life Lines in the Classroom: LR Consulting & Workshops

925 S Mason Road
Katy, TX 77450
281-395-4978
FAX 281-392-8379
http://www.lrconsulting.com
Marlene Johnson, Curriculum and Instruction
Mary Fitzgerald, Special Education

Offers a variety of staff development training options regarding inclusive and special educational issues.

1981 Lindamood-Bell Learning Processes Professional Development

Lindamood-Bell Learning Processes
416 Higuera Street
San Luis Obispo, CA 93401
805-541-3836
800-233-1819
FAX 805-541-9332
http://www.lblp.com
e-mail: rbell@lblp.com
Rodney Bell, Conferences/Prof Workshops Dir

Offers workshops nationwide for educators in the internationally acclaimed Lindamood-Bell teaching methods. Approximately 40 workshops hosted annually across the United State and Internationally. Inservices also available.

1982 Melvin-Smith Learning Center Annual Conference

EDU-Therapeutics
1900 Garden Road
Monterey, CA 93940
831-484-0994
800-505-3276
FAX 831-484-0998
http://www.edu-therapeutics.com
e-mail: joan_smith@comcast.net
Joan Smith, Director

National conference entitled Strategies for Success in Overcoming Learning Handicaps. Special Sessions: 1) Strategic Planning for Learning Centers; 2) Administration and Interpretation of Receptive Expressive Observation of Memory Skills. Workshops: 1) Reading for Nonreaders; 2) Setting Structure for Homework Success; 3) Developing Attention Focus Skills and many more. Call for conference program. Exhibitors welcome.

1983 National Center for Family Literacy Conference

325 W Main Street
Louisville, KY 40202
502-584-1133
FAX 502-584-0172
http://www.famlit.org
e-mail: ncfl@famlit.org
Sharon Darling, President

National Center for Family Literacy will be holding a conference with approximately 40-50 exhibitors and 2,000-2,400 attendees.
March

1984 National Head Start Association Academy Workshop

1651 Prince Street
Alexandria, VA 22314
703-739-0875
FAX 703-739-0878
http://www.nhsa.org
e-mail: ojarvis@nhsa.org
Oletha Jarvis

Both Adminstrator and Mid-Manager credentials are offered in a six day, institute style setting, workshop. Family Services and Health credentials are offered through a self study format.
September

1985 National Head Start Association Parent Conference

1651 Prince Street
Alexandria, VA 22314
703-739-0875
FAX 703-739-0878
http://www.nhsa.org
e-mail: rlewisriar@nhsa.org
Sarah Greene, CEO
Diane Whitehead, Program Development
Cheyrl Thompson, Conferences

Newest information on enhancing parent involvement, child development, and sharpening parenting skills. More than 100 workshops.

1986 New England Joint Conference on Specific Learning Disabilities

58 Prince Street
Needham, MA 02492
781-455-9895
FAX 781-449-1332
http://www.addinfonetwork.org
e-mail: adin@gis.net
Linda Downer, Conference Coordinator

Dynamic, informative conference with the goal being to improve services for language/learning-disabled individuals by encouraging dialogue among the many disciplines, organizations and professions involved in the field of learning disabilities.

1987 North American Montessori Teachers' Association Conference

13693 Butternut Road
Burton, OH 44021
440-834-4011
FAX 440-834-4016
http://www.montessori-namta.org
e-mail: staff@montessori-namta.org

Maria Montessori, Founder

Montessori method of teaching is discussed as well as topics pertaining to all levels of special education. This and other conferences are held in different locations and months throughout the year. Please contact us for more information.
Quarterly

1988 Pacific Rim Conference on Disabilities
University of Hawaii Center on Disability Studies
1776 University Avenue
Honolulu, HI 96822
808-956-5739
FAX 808-956-7878
http://www.pacrim.hawaii.edu
e-mail: prinfo@hawaii.edu

Steve Potts, Organizer
Valerie Shearer, Organizer

Participants from the US and other Pacific Rim nations study such topics in disabilities as lifelong inclusion in education and community, new technology, family support, employment and adult services.
March

1989 Pennsylvania Training and Technical Assistance Network Workshops
6340 Flank Drive
Harrisburg, PA 17112
717-541-4960
800-360-7282
FAX 717-541-4968
http://www.pattan.net
e-mail: askpattan@pattan.net

Fran Warkomski, Director

Supports the Department of Education's efforts to lead and serve the educational community by offering professional development that builds the capacity of loacl educational agencies to meet students' needs. PaTTAN's primary focus is special education. However, services are also provided to support Early Intervention, student assessment, tutoring and other partnership efforts, all designed to help students succeed.

1990 Social Skills Workshop
Learning Disabilities Resources
PO Box 716
Bryn Mawr, PA 19010
610-525-8336
800-869-8336
FAX 610-525-8337
http://www.ldonline.org

This workshop is relevant for individuals with learning disabilities, parents or professionals.

1991 Son-Rise Program®
Autism Treatment Center of America™
2080 S Undermountain Road
Sheffield, MA 01257
413-229-2100
800-714-2779
FAX 413-229-8931
http://www.autismtreatment.com
e-mail: autism@option.org

Tracy Baisden, Marketing Associate
Barry Neil Kaufman, Co-Founder

Since 1983, the Autism Treatment Center of America has provided innovative training programs for parents and professionals caring for children challenged by Autism, Autism Spectrum Disorders, Pervasive Developmental Disorder (PDD) and other developmental difficulties. The Son-Rise Program teaches a specific yet comprehensive system of treatment and education designed to help families and caregivers enable their children to dramatically improve in all areas of learning.

1992 Symposium Series on Assistive Technology
Center on Disabilities/California State University
18111 Nordhoff Street
Northridge, CA 91330
818-677-2684
FAX 818-677-4929
http://www.csun.edu/cod
e-mail: codss@csun.edu

Sonya Hernandez, Conference Coordinator

Series of workshops that will address specific areas of assistive technology through in depth one and two day training workshops.

1993 TASH Annual Conference
1025 Vermont Avenue
Washington, DC 20005
202-263-5600
FAX 202-637-0138
http://www.tash.org
e-mail: info@tash.org

Nancy Weiss, Executive Director

Progressive international conference that focuses on strategies for achieving full inclusion for people with disabilities. This invigorating conference, which brings together the best hearts and minds in the disability movement, features over 450 breakout sessions, exhibits, roundtable discussions, poster sessions and much more.
December

1994 Teaching Math Workshop
Learning Disabilities Resources
PO Box 716
Bryn Mawr, PA 19010
610-525-8336
800-869-8336
FAX 610-525-8337
http://www.ldonline.org

A workshop for teachers on how to teach math to individuals with learning problems.

1995 Teaching Reading Workshop
Learning Disabilities Resources
PO Box 716
Bryn Mawr, PA 19010
610-525-8336
800-869-8336
FAX 610-525-8337
http://www.ldonline.org

This workshop explains how to teach individuals with reading problems, dyslexia, ADD, and specific learning disabilities.

1996 Teaching Spelling Workshop
Learning Disabilities Resources
PO Box 716
Bryn Mawr, PA 19010
610-525-8336
800-869-8336
FAX 610-525-8337
http://www.ldonline.org

Spelling is a problem which directly affects an individual's ability to write.

1997 Technology & Persons with Disabilities Conference
California State University, Northridge
18111 Nordhoff Street
Northridge, CA 91330
818-349-4357
FAX 818-677-4929
http://www.csun.edu/cod
e-mail: conference@csun.edu

Jolene Koester, President
Kyndra Till-Gonzalez, Exhibits Coordinator
Jessie Baker, Registration Coordinator

Comprehensive, international conference where technologies across all ages, disabilities, levels of education and training, employment and independent living are addressed.
March

1998 Tic Tac Toe: Math Training Workshop
Learning Disabilities Resources
PO Box 716
Bryn Mawr, PA 19010
610-525-8336
800-869-8336
FAX 610-525-8337
http://www.ldonline.org

This two hour workshop provides teachers with instruction in Tic Tac Toe Math and how to teach it.

1999 Wilson Language Training
Wilson Reading System
175 W Main Street
Millbury, MA 01527
508-865-3656
800-599-8454
FAX 508-865-9644
http://www.wilsonlanguage.com
e-mail: info@wilsonlanguage.com

Barbara Wilson, Owner
Judith Nicholas, Administrator Training

Our workshops instruct teachers, or other professionals in a related field, how to succeed with students who have not learned to read, write and spell despite great effort. Established in order to provide training in the Wilson Reading System, the Wilson staff provides Two-Day Overview Workshops as well as certified Level I and II training.

2000 Wilson Reading System

Wilson Language Training
47 Old Webster Road
Oxford, MA 01540
508-751-8546
800-899-8454
FAX 508-865-9644
http://www.wilsonlanguage.com
Judith Nicholas, Administrator Training
Duane Armstrong

Wilson Reading System workshops are research-based programs designed for individuals who have difficulty with written language in the areas of decoding and spelling. Wilson Language Training was established in order to provide training in the Wilson Reading System. The Wilson staff provides two-day Overview Workshops as well as certified Level I and Level II training. A noncertified Level I training is now offered on line.

2001 Young Adult Institute Conference on Developmental Disabilities

460 W 34th Street
New York, NY 10001
212-273-6100
FAX 212-629-4113
http://www.yai.org
e-mail: ahorowitz@yai.org
Philip Levy, Manager

Annual conference of developmental disabilities. In-depth sessions on the keys to success in developmental and learning disabilities.

May

Assistive Devices

2002 **ABLEDATA**
USDE National Institution on Disability and Rehabi
8630 Fenton Street
Silver Spring, MD 20910
800-227-0216
800-227-0216
FAX 301-608-8958
http://www.abledata.com
e-mail: abledata@verizon.net
Katherine Belknap, Project Director
Janice Benton, Information Services Manager
David Johnson, Publications Director
Database contains descriptions of more than 38,000 commercially available, one-of-a-kind, and do-it-yourself products for rehabilitation and independent living. A wealth of information on assistive technology.

2003 **ARTIC Technologies**
1000 John R. Road
Troy, MI 48083
248-588-7370
FAX 248-588-2650
http://www.artictech.com
e-mail: info@artictech.com
Dale McDaniels, President

Manufacturers of speed boards for the blind and visually impaired. Accessibility appliances for low vision and blindness.

2004 **Ablenet**
2808 Fairview Avenue N
Roseville, MN 55113
651-294-2200
800-322-0956
FAX 651-294-2259
http://www.ablenetinc.com
e-mail: customerservice@ablenetinc.com
Cheryl Volkman, CEO
Richard J. Osterhaus, Chief Executive Officer/Presiden

2005 **Adaptive Device Locator System (ADLS)**
Academic Software
3504 Tates Creek Road
Lexington, KY 40517
859-552-1020
FAX 859-273-1943
http://www.acsw.com
e-mail: asistaff@acsw.com
Warren E Lacefield, President
Penelope D Ellis, COO/Dir Sales/Marketing

System describes thousands of devices, cross references over 600 vendors and illustrates devices graphically. The ADLS databases include a full spectrum of living aids, products ranging from specialized eating utensils to dressing aids, electronic switches, computer hardware and software, adapted physical education devices and much more. Now accessible on the internet through Adaptworld.com and Acsw.com *$195.00*

2006 **Braille' n Speak Classic**
American Printing House for the Blind
1839 Frankfort Avenue
Louisville, KY 40206
502-895-2405
800-223-1839
FAX 502-899-2274
http://www.aph.org
e-mail: info@aph.org
Tuck Tinsley, President
Fred Gissoni, Technical Support Specialist
Allan Lovell, Customer Relations Manager
This computerized, talking device has many features useful to student and adult braille users (word processors, print-to-braille translator, talking clocks/calculators and much more). *$929.95*

2007 **CCT Telephone Interface**
Consultants for Communication Technology
508 Bellevue Terrace
Pittsburgh, PA 15202
412-761-6062
FAX 412-761-7336
http://www.concommtech.com
e-mail: kathy@concommtech.com
Kathleen Miller, Owner
Sharon Money, Office Manager

Device allows output from your communication software to be transmitted directly through the telephone. Requires CCT software. *$300.00*

2008 **Communication Aids: Manufacturers Association**
205 W Randolph Street
Chicago, IL 60606
312-229-5444
800-441-2262
FAX 312-229-5445
TDY:800-441-2262
http://www.aacproducts.org
e-mail: cama@northshore.net
James Neils, President

A nonprofit organization of the world's leading manufacturers of augmentative and alternative communication software and hardware.

2009 **Connect Outloud**
Freedon Scientific
11800 31st Court North
St Petersburg, FL 33716
727-803-8000
800-444-4443
FAX 727-803-8001
http://www.freedomscientific.com
e-mail: info@freedomscientific.com
Lee Hamilton, CEO/President

Designed to allow beginners through experienced blind or low vision computer users to access the Internet through speech and Braille output. Based on our JAWS for Windows technology, and offers additional access to Windows XP. *$ 249.00*

2010 **Consultants for Communication Technology**
Consultants for Communication Technology
508 Bellevue Terrace
Pittsburgh, PA 15202
412-761-6062
FAX 412-761-7336
http://www.concommtech.com
e-mail: cct@concommtech.com
Kathleen Miller, Owner
Sharon Money, Office Manager

Manufactures and distributes a line of augmentative communication products for persons with speech impairments. In addition we have software products for environmental control, word processing and phone management. All products can be used with only one muscle movement or from the full keyboard.

2011 **Controlpad 24**
Genovation
17741 Mitchell N
Irvine, CA 92614
949-833-3355
800-822-4333
FAX 949-833-0322
http://www.genovation.com
e-mail: sales@genovation.com
Leonard Genest, Owner
Edward Lopez, Assistant Project Manager
Chris Fructus, Marketing Director
Fully programmable 24 key pad. Its principal purpose is to provide single keystroke macros.

2012 **Creature Games Series**
Dunamis
3545 Cruse Road
Lawrenceville, GA 30044
770-279-1144
800-828-2443
FAX 770-279-0809
http://www.dunamisinc.com
e-mail: info@dunamisinc.com
Pat Satterfield, Owner
Ben Satterfield, President
Matt Satterfield, College/LD Sales
Everybody loves computer games, but these games are unique. They can be enjoyed by children with severe/profound disabilities, including those functioning as low as 4 months of age. *$80.00*

2013 **Dunamis**
Dunamis
3545 Cruse Road
Lawrenceville, GA 30044
770-279-1144
800-828-2443
FAX 770-279-0809
http://www.dunamisinc.com
e-mail: info@dunamisinc.com
Pat Satterfield, Owner
Ben Satterfield, President
Matt Satterfield, College/LD Sales
Since 1984 we have been committed to helping you find the technology you need to accomplish your goals and realize your dreams. We offer assistive technology that is the most appropriate available, at the highest quality and the most competitive price possible.

2014 **Dyna Vox Technologies**
2100 Wharton Street
Pittsburgh, PA 15203
412-381-4883
866-396-2869
FAX 412-381-5241
http://www.dynavoxtech.com
e-mail: sale@dynavoxtech.com
Joe Swenson, President & CEO
Joanne Kaufmann, Public Relations Supervisor

DynaVox Technologies develops, manufactures, distributes and supports a variety of speech-output devices that allow individuals challenged by speech, lanugage and learning disabilities to make meaningful connections with their world. The company's products allow individuals of all ages and abilities to initiate and participate in conversations at home, work, in school and throughout the community. *$4500.00*

2015 **EZ Keys**
Words+
42505 10th Street W
Lancaster, CA 93534
661-723-6523
800-869-8521
FAX 661-723-2114
http://www.words-plus.com
e-mail: info@word-plus.com
Jeff Dahlen, President
Walt Wolosz, Manager
Janet Aviles, Sales Supervisor
Assistance program that provides keyboard control, dual word prediction, abbreviation-expansion and speech output while running standard software. *$695.00*

2016 **Franklin Language Master**
Freedon Scientific
11800 31st Court North
St Petersburg, FL 33716
727-803-8000
800-444-4443
FAX 727-803-8001
http://www.freedomscientific.com
e-mail: info@freedomscientific.com
Lee Hamilton, CEO

Versatile hand-held dictionary full speech controls to read screens or speak individual words at the speed you choose. At less than 6 inches square, this lightweight tool is designed for maximum efficiency. Large-type display, high contrast screen and black on white QWERTY keyboard. For blind users, orientation features include active screen announcing and raised dots on location keys. *$450.00*

2017 **Genie Color TV**
TeleSensory
650 Vaqueros Avenue
Sunnyvale, CA 94085
408-616-8700
800-227-8418
FAX 408-616-8720
http://www.telesensory.com
e-mail: info@insiphil.com
Soon Seng Ng, President
Anita Thibeaux, Operation Manager
Jennifer Street, Marketing Director
Brings clarity and comfort to reading and writing. Since many people with low vision find that specific color combinations enhance legibility, VersiColor offers 24 customized foreground and background color combinations to choose from in addition to a full color mode. Genie can also connect to a computer for use with Telesensory's Vista screen magnification system. *$2995.00*

2018 **Genovation**
17741 Mitchell N
Irvine, CA 92614
949-833-3355
800-822-4333
FAX 949-822-4333
http://www.genovation.com
e-mail: sales@genovation.com
Leonard Genest, Owner
Edward Lopez, Assistant Project Manager
Chris Fructus, Marketing Director
Produces a wide variety of computer input devices for data-entry, and custom applications. Produces the Function Keypad 682 for people with limited dexterity. It is programmable, allowing the user to store macros (selected patterns of key strokes) into memory, and relegendable keys allow easy labeling of user-programmed functions. Additional options such as larger keys (1x2), allow reconfiguration to meet the user's needs. Call toll-free for pricing and availability.

2019 **Home Row Indicators**
Hooleon Corporation
304 West Denby Ave.
Melrose, NM 88124
505-253-4503
800-937-1337
FAX 505-253-4299
http://www.hooleon.com
e-mail: sales@hooleon.com
Joan Crozier, President

Plastic adhesive labels with a raised bump in the center allowing the user to designate home row keys, or any other key, for quick recognition.

2020 **Hub**
Alliance for Technology Access
1304 Southpoint Boulevard
Petaluma, CA 94954
707-778-3011
707-778-3015
FAX 707-765-2080
TDY:707-778-3015
http://www.ataccess.org
e-mail: ATAinfo@ataccess.org
Mary Lester, Executive Director

Interactive information service provides quick and efficient access to information on assistive technology tools and services to consumers, families and service providers.

2021 **IBM Independence Series**
IBM
11400 Burnet Road
Austin, TX 78758
512-823-4400
800-IBM-4YOU
FAX 512-838-9367
http://www.IBM.com/able
Dennis O'Brien, Product Manager

A group of products designed to help individuals with disabilities to achieve greater personal and professional independence through the use of technology. Products include Keyguard, AccessDOS, THINKable/2, Screen Reader/2, Screen Magnifier/2, SpeechViewer II, THINKable/DOS and Screen Reader/DOS.

2022 **IntelliKeys**
IntelliTools
1720 Corporate Circle
Petaluma, CA 94954
707-773-2000
800-899-6687
FAX 707-773-2001
http://www.intellitools.com
e-mail: info@intellitools.com
Beth Davis, Director
Arjan Khalsa, CEO

Alternative, touch-sensitive keyboard. Plugs into any MAC, APPLE, or IBM compatible computer, no interface needed. *$395.00*

2023 JAWS for Windows
Freedon Scientific
11800 31st Court N
St Petersburg, FL 33716
727-803-8000
800-444-4443
FAX 727-803-8001
http://www.freedomscientific.com
e-mail: info@freedomscientific.com
Lee Hamilton, CEO/President

Works with your PC to provide access to today's software applications and the internet. With its internal software speech synthesizer and the computer's sound card, information from the screen is read aloud, providing technology to access a wide variety of information, education and job related applications.

2024 Large Print Keyboard
Hooleon Corporation
304 W Denby Avenue
Melrose, NM 88124
505-253-4503
800-937-1337
FAX 505-253-4299
http://www.hooleon.com
e-mail: sales@hooleon.com
Joan Crozier, President

Keyboard with 104 keys features large print on all the keys.

2025 Large Print Lower Case Labels
Hooleon Corporation
304 W Denby Avenue
Melrose, NM 88124
505-253-4503
800-937-1337
FAX 505-253-4299
http://www.hooleon.com
e-mail: sales@hooleon.com
Joan Crozier, President

For children learning the keyboard.

2026 Lekotek of Georgia Shareware
Lekotek of Georgia
1955 Cliff Valley Way NE
Atlanta, GA 30329
404-633-3430
FAX 404-633-1242
http://www.lekotekga.org
e-mail: lekotekga@mindspring.com
Helene Prokesch, Executive Director
Peggy McWilliams, Tech Specialist

Software created by our staff using Intellipics, Intellipics Studio or Hyperstudio. Players are included to run this shareware. Color overlays for intellomusic are included. Input methods are mouse, switch, touch window, head mouse and intellikeys if applicable. Subjects are colors and emotions, early childhood music in English and Spanish, shapes and sounds, pictures and letters.

2027 Micro IntroVoice
Voice Connexion
2324 N Batavia Street
Orange, CA 92865
714-685-1066
FAX 714-685-1070
http://www.voicecnx.com
e-mail: voicecnx_@aol.com
Shirley Dworak, Vice President Marketing

A complete voice input/output system which provides voice recognition of 1,000 words with accuracy of 98 percent and unlimited text-to-speech and recorded speech for voice prompting and varification. Micro IntroVoice works with DOS and Windows applications for entering commands or data. *$1095.00*

2028 Open Book
Freedon Scientific
11800 31st Court N
St Petersburg, FL 33716
727-803-8000
800-444-4443
FAX 727-803-8001
http://www.freedomscientific.com
e-mail: info@freedomscientific.com
Lee Hamilton, CEO

Allows you to convert printed documents or graphic based text into an electronic text format using accurate optical character recognition and quality speech. The many powerful low vision tools allow you to customize how the document appears on your screen, while other features provide portability. *$995.00*

2029 OutSPOKEN
Alva Access Group
436 14th Street
Oakland, CA 94612
510-451-2582
888-318-2582
FAX 510-451-0878
http://www.aagi.com
e-mail: info@aagi.com
Larry Lake, Owner

Gives blind and learning disabled persons access to mainstream Macintosh software via speech output. *$395.00*

2030 PCD Communication Device
ABOVO
96 Rhinebeck Avenue
Springfield, MA 1129
860-623-7364
FAX 860-623-2941
http://www.dcdinc.com
e-mail: info@dcdinc.com
A portable, handheld electronic device designed for single finger communication by people who wish to communicate through typing.

2031 Phonic Ear Auditory Trainers
Phonic Ear
3880 Cypress Drive
Petaluma, CA 94954
707-769-1110
800-227-0735
FAX 707-769-9624
TDY: 707-769-126
http://www.phonicear.com
e-mail: customerservice@phonicear.com
Rick Pimentel, President
Paul Hickey, Sales VP
Cindy Pedersen, Customer Service Manager
A line of learning disabled communication equipment.

2032 QuicKeys
Startly Technologies
PO Box 65580
West Des Moines, IA 50265
515-221-1801
800-523-7638
FAX 515-221-1806
http://www.startly.com
e-mail: sales@cesoft.com
Jim Kirk, Manager
Joe Gray, Human Resources Director
John Kirk, Controller
Assigns Macintosh functions to one keystroke.

2033 Reading Pen
Wizcom Technologies
234 Littleton Road
Westford, MA 1886
978-727-0026
888-777-0552
FAX 978-727-0032
http://www.wizcomtech.com
e-mail: usa.info@wizcomtech.com
Randy Green, President
Raz Itzhaki, President
Peter Lovitz, Office Manager
Portable assistive reading device that reads words aloud and can be used anywhere. Scans a word from printed text, displays the word in large characters, reads the word aloud from built-in speaker or ear phones and defines the word with the press of a button. Displays syllables, keeps a history of scanned words, adjustable for left or right-handed use. Includes a tutorial video and audio cassette. Not recommended for persons with low vision or impaired fine motor control.

2034 Scan It-Switch It
UCLA Intervention Program for Handicapped Children
1000 Veteran Avenue
Los Angeles, CA 90095
310-825-4821
800-899-6687
FAX 310-206-7744
http://www.bol.ucla.edu
e-mail: consult@ucla.edu

Kit Kehr, Executive Director

Helps teach horizontal and vertical scanning using a single switch or TouchWindow. Instruction progresses through five levels of difficulty from capturing a single object with a moving box to using scanning to select matching items. *$45.00*

2035 Self-Adhesive Braille Keytop Labels
Hooleon Corporation
304 W Denby Avenue
Melrose, NM 88124
505-253-4503
800-937-1337
FAX 505-253-4299
http://www.hooleon.com
e-mail: sales@hooleon.com

Joan Crozier, President

Transparent with raised braille allows both sighted and nonsighted users to use same keyboard.

2036 Switch Accessible Trackball
Lekotek of Georgia
1955 Cliff Valley Way NE
Atlanta, GA 30329
404-633-3430
FAX 404-633-1242
http://www.lekotekga.org
e-mail: email@lekotekga.com

Helene Prokesch, Executive Director
Peggy McWilliams, Tech Specialist

Universal to Mac or Windows, this device aids computer navigation where traditional devices are not used. Trackball guards available. *$125.00*

2037 Switch It Software Bundle
Dunamis
3423 Fowler Boulevard
Lawrenceville, GA 30044
770-279-1144
800-828-2443
FAX 770-279-0809
http://www.dunamisinc.com
e-mail: info@dunamisinc.com

Pat Satterfield, Owner
Ben Satterfield, President
Matt Satterfield, College/LD Sales
Collection of 4 software programs that follow a developmental learning sequence.

2038 SwitchIt! Arcade Adventure
Dunamis
3545 Cruse Road
Lawrenceville, GA 30044
770-279-1144
800-828-2443
FAX 770-279-0809
http://www.dunamisinc.com
e-mail: info@Dunamisinc.com

Pat Satterfield, Owner
Ben Satterfield, President/CEO
Matt Satterfield, College/LD Sales
Game-style program helps more advanced switch users build hand-eye coordination and problem solving skills. *$50.00*

2039 Talking Typer for Windows
American Printing House for the Blind
1839 Frankfort Avenue
Louisville, KY 40206
502-895-2405
800-223-1839
FAX 502-899-2274
http://www.aph.org
e-mail: info@aph.org

Tuck Tinsley, President
Allan Lovell, Customer Relations Manager
Fred Gissoni, Customer Support

Designed to reinforce keyboarding skills for visually impaired PC users and their teachers.

2040 Talking Utilities for DOS 3.3
American Printing House for the Blind
1839 Frankfort Avenue
Louisville, KY 40206
502-895-2405
800-223-1839
FAX 502-899-2274
http://www.aph.org
e-mail: info@aph.org

Tuck Tinsley, President
Allan Lovell, Customer Relations Manager
Fred Gissoni, Customer Support
A talking version of System Master with features added for speech synthesis users. *$15.00*

2041 Talking Utilities for ProDOS
American Printing House for the Blind
1839 Frankfort Avenue
Louisville, KY 40206
502-895-2405
800-223-1839
FAX 502-899-2274
http://www.aph.org
e-mail: info@aph.org

Tuck Tinsley, President
Allan Lovell, Customer Relations Manager
Fred Gissoni, Customer Support
A speech-accessible version of Apple's ProDOS User's Disk. *$10.00*

2042 Text 2000
American Printing House for the Blind
1839 Frankfort Avenue
Louisville, KY 40206
502-895-2405
800-223-1839
FAX 502-899-2274
http://www.aph.org
e-mail: info@aph.org

Tuck Tinsley, President
Fred Gissoni, Customer Support
Allows students to read textbooks in a number of ways, including synthetic speech, large type sized to the screen and refreshable braille. *$112.00*

2043 Ufonic Voice System
Compass Learning
7878 N 16th Street203 Colorado St.
PhoenixAustin, AZ 850207870
512-478-9600
800-422-4339
FAX 602-230-7034
http://www.compasslearning.com
e-mail: mholt@compasslearning.com

Eric Leoffel, President
Curt Hedges, Vice President and Corporate Con
Mark Holt, Office Manager
Consists of the interface card, amplifier/speaker with dual headphones and volume control, and provides human sounding speech in instructional software developed for this use. *$245.00*

2044 Unicorn Expanded Keyboard
IntelliTools
1720 Corporate Circle
Petaluma, CA 94954
707-773-2000
800-899-6687
FAX 707-773-2001
http://www.intellitools.com
e-mail: info@intellitools.com

Beth Davis, Director
Arjan Khalsa, CEO

Alternative keyboard with large, user-defined keys, requires interface. Smaller version is also available. *$315.00*

2045 Unicorn Smart Keyboard
IntelliTools
55 Leveroni Court
Novato, CA 94949
415-382-5959
800-899-6687
FAX 415-382-5950
http://www.intellitools.com
e-mail: info@intellitools.com

Beth Davis, Director
Arjan Khlasa, CEO

Works with any standard keyboard and offers seven overlays and a cable for one type of computer.

2046 Universal Numeric Keypad
Genovation
17741 Mitchell North
Irvine, CA 92614
949-833-3355
800-822-4333
FAX 949-833-0322
http://www.genovation.com
e-mail: sales@genovation.com
Max Rahim Zadeh, President
Chris Fructus, Marketing Director
Edward Lopez, Product Manager
A 21 key numeric keypad that works with any laptop or portable computer.

2047 Up and Running
IntelliTools
1720 Corporate Circle
Petaluma, CA 94954
707-773-2000
800-899-6687
FAX 707-773-2001
http://www.intellitools.com
e-mail: info@intellitools.com
Beth Davis, Director
Arjan Khlasa, CEO

A custom overlay kit for the Unicorn Keyboard that provides instant access to a wide range of software including over 60 popular educational programs. *$69.95*

2048 VISTA
TeleSensory
650 Vaqueros Avenue
Sunnyvale, CA 94085
408-616-8700
800-804 8004
FAX 408-616-8720
http://www.telesensory.com
e-mail: info@insiphil.com
Soon Seng Ng, President
Anita Thibeaux, Operation Manager
Jennifer Street, Marketing
Image enlarging system that magnifies the print and graphics on the screen from three to 16 times. *$2495.00*

2049 Visagraph II Eye-Movement Recording System
Taylor Associated Communications
200 East Second Street
Huntington Station, NY 11746
631-549-3000
800-732-3758
FAX 631-549-3156
http://www.readingplus.com
e-mail: info@readingplus.com
Stanford Taylor, Owner
D.J. Ware, Sales Representative

Measures reading performance efficiency, visual and functional proficiency, perceptual development, and information processing competence.

2050 VoiceNote
Pulse Date Human Ware
175 Mason Circle
Concord, CA 94520
925-680-7100
800-722-3393
FAX 925-681-4630
http://www.pulsedata.com
e-mail: us.info@humanware.com
Peter Standish, President
Phil Rance, President and CEO

Speech synthesizer without a braille display. Most of the great features that are on BrailleNote are here, but on a smaller and lighter unit. Choose from either a braille key or a QWERTY input, depending on your preference.

2051 Window-Eyes
GW Micro
725 Airport North Office Park
Fort Wayne, IN 46825
260-489-3671
FAX 260-489-2608
http://www.gwmicro.com
e-mail: support@gwmicro.com
Dan Weirich, Vice President Sales and Marketi
Mike Lawler, Development Liaison and Technica

Screen reader that is adaptable to your specific needs and preferances. Works automatically so you can focus on your application program, not so much on operating the screen reader.

Books & Periodicals

2052 AppleWorks Education
AACE
PO Box 1545
Chesapeake, VA 23327
757-366-5606
FAX 703-997-8760
http://www.aace.org
e-mail: info@aace.org
Gary Marks, Publisher
Tracy Jacobs, Office Manager

Covers educational uses of AppleWorks software. *$25.00*

2053 AppleWorks Manuals: Special Editions
American Printing House for the Blind
1839 Frankfort Avenue
Louisville, KY 40206
502-895-2405
800-223-1839
FAX 502-899-2274
http://www.aph.org
e-mail: info@aph.org
Tuck Tinsley, President
Allan Lovell, Customer Relations Manager
Fred Gissoni, Customer Support
Designed for visually impaired users. Includes AppleWorks tutorials on cassette and AppleWorks Reference Manual on computer diskette. *$23.90*

2054 Art Express and the Literacy Curriculum
Center for Best Practices in Early Childhood
Western Illinois University
Macomb, IL 61455
309-298-1634
FAX 309-298-2305
http://www.wiu.edu/thecenter
e-mail: PL-Hutinger@wiu.edu
Patricia Hutinger EdD, Director
Joyce Johanson, Coordinator

Make your classroom come alive with art, music, movement, and dramatic play. Innovative, yet practical guide for helping teachers implement a comprehensive expressive arts curriculum in their classrooms include tips for arranging the environment. *$20.00*
16-20 pages

2055 Bibliography of Journal Articles on Microcomputers & Special Education
Special Education Resource Center
25 Industrial Park Road
Middletown, CT 6457
860-632-1485
800-842-8678
FAX 860-632-8870
http://www.ctserc.org
e-mail: info@ctserc.org
Marianne Kirner Ph.D., Executive Director

This pamphlet offers information on a wide variety of professional journals in the fields of microcomputers and special education.

2056 Closing the Gap Newsletter
526 Main Street
Henderson, MN 56044
507-248-3294
FAX 507-248-3810
http://www.closingthegap.com
e-mail: info@closingthegap.com
Dolores Hagen, President
Jan Latzke, Communications

Bimonthly newsletter on the use of computer technology in special education and rehabilitation. CTG also sponsors an annual international conference. *$34.00*

40 pages
ISSN 0886-1935

2057 Computer Access-Computer Learning
Special Needs Project
324 State Street
Santa Barbara, CA 93101
800-333-6867
FAX 805-962-5087
http://www.specialneeds.com
e-mail: books@specialneeds.com
Ginny LaVine, Author
Hod Gray, Director
Laraine Gray, Conference Coordinator

A resource manual in adaptive technology. *$22.50*
226 pages

2058 MACcessories: Guide to Peripherals
Western Illinois University: Macomb Projects
Western Illinois University
Macomb, IL 61455
309-298-1955
FAX 309-298-2305
http://www.wiu.edu/thecenter
e-mail: PL-Hutinger@wiu.edu
Amanda Silberer, Manager
Joyce Johanson, Coordinator

Designed to help the Macintosh user understand peripheral devices. Includes descriptions of each device, advantages and disadvantages of each, procedures for installation, troubleshooting tips, suggested software and company resources. *$15.00*
41 pages

2059 Opening Windows: A Talking and Tactile Tutorial for Microsoft Windows
American Printing House for the Blind
PO Box 6085
Louisville, KY 40206
502-895-2405
800-223-1839
FAX 502-895-1509
http://www.aph.org
e-mail: info@aph.org
Tuck Tinsley, President
Allan Lovell, Customer Relations Manager
Fred Gissoni, Customer Support
Includes raised line graphics, cassette and computer diskette designed to acquaint visually impaired computer users with Windows 3.1 operating environment. *$50.00*

2060 Switch to Turn Kids On
Western Illinois University: Macomb Projects
Horrabin Hall 71B, 1 University Cir
Macomb, IL 61455
800-322-3905
FAX 309-298-2288
http://www.wiu.edu/users/micpc
e-mail: www.wiu.edu/cpc
Raemarie Oatman, Director
Susan Schoonover, Chief Clerk

Guide to homemade switches gives information on conducting a switch workshop and constructing a battery interrupter as well as various kinds of switches (tread switches, ribbon switches, mercury switches, pillow switches). Contains illustrations and step-by-step instructions. *$12.00*
47 pages

Centers & Organizations

2061 Activating Children Through Technology (ACCT)
Western Illinois University: Macomb Projects
27 Horrabin Hall
Macomb, IL 61455
309-298-1634
FAX 309-298-2305
http://www.wiu.edu/thecenter/littech/
e-mail: PL-Hutinger@wiu.edu
Patricia Hutinger, Principal Investigator
Joyce Johanson, Project Co-Director

ACTT integrates assistive technology into early childhood services for children with disabilities from birth to 8 years old. It helps them gain control over their environment, develop autonomy, communicate, develop problem-solving skills and participate in an inclusive environment. ACTT provides training to families and educators and has written materials and software available. *$16.00*

2062 Adaptive Technology Laboratory
Center for Adaptive Technology Department
1 Oxford Street
Cambridge, MA 2138
617-496-8800
FAX 203-392-5796
http://www.southernct.edu
e-mail: atl@fas.harvard.edu
Louise Russell, Director

Helps individuals with visual, orthopedic and learning disabilities to gain computer access through the use of the latest technology.

2063 American Foundation for the Blind
American Foundation for the Blind
11 Penn Plaza
New York, NY 10001
212-502-7600
800-232-5463
FAX 212-502-7777
http://www.afb.org
e-mail: afbinfo@afb.net
Carl R. Augusto, President & CEO

Is a national nonprofit that expands possibilities for people with vision loss. AFB's priorities include broadening access to technology; elevating the quality of information and tools for the professionals who serve people with vision loss; and promoting independent and healthy living for people with vision loss by providing them and their families with relevant and timely resources.

2064 Artificial Language Laboratory
Michigan State University
405 Computer Center
East Lansing, MI 48824
517-353-0870
FAX 517-353-4766
http://www.msu.edu/unit/artlang/
e-mail: artlang@pilot.msu.edu
John Eulenberg PhD, Director
Stephen Blosser, Rehab Engineer

Multidisciplinary teaching and research center involved in basic and applied research concerning the computer processing of formal linguistic structures.

2065 Association for Educational Communications and Technology
Association for Educational Communications and Tec
1800 N Stonelake Drive
Bloomington, IN 47404
812-335-7675
877-677-AECT
FAX 812-335-7678
http://www.aect.org
e-mail: aect@aect.org
Phillip Harris MD, Executive Director
Larry Vernon, Director Electronic Services
Ned Shaw, Dir Marketing/Communications
Provides leadership in educational communications and technology by linking professionals holding a common interest in the use of educational technology and its application to the learning process.

2066 Birmingham Alliance for Technology Access Center
Birmingham Independent Living Center
206 13th Street S
Birmingham, AL 35233
205-251-2223
FAX 205-251-0605
e-mail: minorris@bellsouth.net
Mike Norris, Information Specialist
Daniel Kessler, Executive Director

Information dissemination, network, referral service, support services, and training. Disabilities served are cognitive, hearing, learning, physical, speech and vision.

2067 **Bluegrass Technology Center**
961 Beasley Street
Lexington, KY 40509
859-294-4343
800-209-7769
FAX 859-294-0704
TDY:800-209-7767
http://www.bluegrass-tech.org
e-mail: office@bluegrass-tech.org
Jean Isaacs Bramlette, Technology Specialist
Penny Ellis, Special Education Consultant
Penny Ellis, Assistive Technology Consultant
Provides support to all persons with disabilities in their efforts to access technology and to increase awareness and understanding of how that technology can enhance their abilities to participate more fully in their community, assisting individuals directly or indirectly by working with their caregivers, therapists, vocational counselors, case managers, educators, employers, and community members.

2068 **CAST**
40 Harvard Mill Square
Wakefield, MA 1880
781-245-2212
(781) 245-93
FAX 781-245-5212
TDY:781-245-9320
http://www.cast.org
e-mail: cast@cast.org
Anne Meyer, Founder,Chief of Education Desig
David Rose, Founder,Chief Education Officer
Linda Encarnacao, Executive Assistant
A nonprofit organization that works to expand learning opportunities for all individuals, especially those with disabilities, through the research and development of innovative, technology-based educational resources and strategies.

2069 **CITE Technology Access Center**
215 E New Hampshire Street
Orlando, FL 32804
407-898-2483
FAX 407-895-5255
http://www.centralfloridalighthouse.org
e-mail: jgideons@cite-fl.com
Lee Nasehi, Executive Director
Karen Morehouse, Director of Children's Services

Community based technology resource center seeks to redefine human potential by making technology a regular part of the lives of people with disabilities. Dedicated to increasing the use of technology by children and adults with disabilities, their families, educators and employers. CITE exists to solve the problem of where people can find out about the power of technology and get the expertise and assistance they need to make computers work for them.

2070 **CMECSU Technology Project for Learners with Low Incidence Disabilities**
3335 W Saint Germain Street
Saint Cloud, MN 56301
763-255-4913
Dixie Anderson

A regional educational organization that works within a nine county region. Maintains a demonstration center with about 500 public domain software programs. Offers specialized equipment for loan to students.

2071 **Carolina Computer Access Center**
PO Box 247
Cramerton, NC 28032
704-342-3004
888-342-3004
FAX 704-342-1513
http://http.ccac.ataccess.org
e-mail: ccacnc@carolina.rr.com
Linda Schilling, Executive Director
Allison Schilling, Communications Specialist
Lynn Koch, Herzog Keyboarding Trainer
Demonstrations, assessments, workshops, and information on assistive technologies. Training available for: WYNN, TextHELP, INTELLITOOLS, JAWS, ZoomText.

2072 **Center for Accessible Technology**
Center for Accessible Technology
2547 8th Street
Berkeley, CA 94710
510-841-3224
FAX 510-841-7956
http://www.cforat.org
e-mail: info@cforat.org
Eric Smith, Associate Director
Dmitri Belser, Executive Director

Resource center for parents, professionals, developers and individuals with disabilities, filled with computers, software, adapted toys and adaptive technology.

2073 **Center for Enabling Technology**
College of New Jersey
2000 Pennington Rd.
Ewing, NJ 8628
609-771-3016
FAX 609-637-5172
http://www.tcnj.edu
e-mail: educat@tcnj.edu
William Behre, Dean
Christine Schindler, Assistive Technology Specialist
Amy Dell, Executive Director
Ongoing projects that match assistive devices to the children who need them. Training and educational workshops.

2074 **Comprehensive Services for the Disabled**
Comprehensive Services for the Disabled
1605 Belmar & Woodfield Avenue
Wall, NJ 7719
732-681-5632
800-784-2919
FAX 732-681-5632
Donald DeSanto, Executive Director

Helps special students realize their potential and bring college admission a step closer. Program designed to meet the needs and maximize the unique talents of each individual. The staff consists of highly qualified teachers who see beyond labels and reach the person inside. By pacing scholastics to each student's ability, the college increases understanding and makes learning a positive experience. Instruction is tailored to each individual.

2075 **Computer Access Center**
Computer Access Center
6234 West 87th St.
Los Angeles, CA 90045
310-338-1597
FAX 310-338-9318
http://www.cac.org
e-mail: info@cac.org
Marcy Kaplan, Executive Director

Computer resource center serving primarily as a place where people with all types of disabilities can preview equipment. Workshops, seminars, after school clubs for children and individual consultations are provided.

2076 **Computer Accommodation Lab**
Woodrow Wilson Rehab Center
PO Box 1500
Fishersville, VA 22939
540-332-7000
800-345-9972
FAX 540-332-7132
http://www.wwrc.net
e-mail: colemawl@wwrc.state.va.us
Richard L. Sizemore, Director

Provides assessments for adolescents and adults in appropriate access to computers, including alternative input strategies, mouse applications, and software solutions.

2077 **Computer Learning Foundation**
P.O. Box 60007
Palo Alto, CA 94306
408-720-8898
FAX 408- 730-119
http://www.computerlearning.org
e-mail: clf@computerlearning.org
Sally Alden, Executive Director

An international nonprofit educational foundation, dedicated to improving the quality of education and preparation of youth for the workplace through the use of technology. To accomplish its mission, the foundation provides numerous projects and materials to help parents and educators use technology effectively with children.

2078 Council for Exceptional Children (ECER)
Council for Exceptional Children
1110 N Glebe Road
Arlington, VA 22201
703-620-3660
888-232-7733
FAX 703-264-9494
http://www.cec.sped.org
e-mail: service@cec.sped.org
Bruce Ramirez, Interim Executive Director
Victor Erickson, Director
Liz Martinez, Publications Director
This database contains citations and abstracts of print and nonprint materials dealing with exceptional children, those who have disabilities and those who are gifted. Resources in all areas of special education and related services (including services provided by audiologists, speech therapists, occupational therapists, physical therapists, and educational psychologists) are covered in ECER.

2079 Dialog Information Services
Dialog Information Services
11000 Regency Parkway
Cary, NC 27518
919-462-8600
800-334-2564
FAX 919-468-9890
http://www.dialog.com
e-mail: customer@dialog.com
Roy Martin, President, CEO

Offers access to over 390 data bases containing information on various aspects of disabling conditions and services to disabled individuals.

2080 Eastern Tennessee Technology Access Center
4918 N Broadway Street
Knoxville, TN 37918
865-219-0130
FAX 865-219-0137
http://www.korrnet.org/ettac
e-mail: etstactn@aol.com
Lois Symington, Executive Director

Assistive technology resource and information center for individuals with disabilities, their families and professionals who work with them. Workshops, consultations, tutoring, information and product reviews available.

2081 High Tech Center Training Unit
Foothill-DeAnza Community College District
21050 McClellan Road
Cupertino, CA 95014
408-996-4636
800-411-8954
FAX 408-996-6042
http://www.htctu.fhda.edu
Carl Brown, Director
Bong Deiparine, Staff

Provides training for faculty and staff of the California community colleges in access technologies.

2082 Iowa Program for Assistive Technology
IA University Assistive Technology
100 Hawkins Drive
Iowa City, IA 52242
319-353-8502
800-331-3027
FAX 319-353-5139
http://www.uiowa.edu/infotech
e-mail: jane-gay@uiowa.edu
Jane Gay, Director

Computer accesssed solutions for physically challenged students.

2083 Learning Independence Through Computers
LINC
1001 Eastern Avenue
Baltimore, MD 21202
410-659-5462
FAX 410-659-5472
http://www.linc.org
e-mail: info@linc.org
Christine L. Oughton, President
Hugh M. Evans III, Vice-President

Resource center that offers specially adapted computer technology to children and adults with a variety of disabilities. State-of-the-art systems allow consumers to achieve their potential for productivity and independence at home, school, work and in the community. Also offers a quarterly newsletter called Connections.

2084 New Breakthroughs
89911 Greenwood Drive
Leaburg, OR 97489
541-741-5070
FAX 541-896-0123
e-mail: breakthrus@aol.com
Carol Berger, Contact

Facilitated communication and information in all areas of assistive, alternative communication. Technological education materials, workshops and training in new special education advancements are available.

2085 Northern Illinois Center for Adaptive Technology
3615 Louisiana Road
Rockford, IL 61108
815-229-2163
FAX 815-229-2135
http://www.nicat.ataccess.org
e-mail: davegrass@earthlink.net
Dave Grass, Director

Nonprofit computer and adaptive devices resource center operated by parents, consumers, volunteers and professionals dedicated to providing information, seminars and individual needs technology. It is the goal of the center to help people with disabilities reach their full potential by providing them with information on the latest technology and by matching adaptive devices to their disabilities allowing them to more effectively interface with their environment.

2086 Project TECH
Massachusetts Easter Seal Society
484 Main Street
Worcester, MA 1608
508-757-2756
800-922-8290
FAX 508-831-9768
http://www.eastersealsma.org
e-mail: info@eastersealsma.org
Kirk Joslin, President
Mary D'Antonio, Information Specialist

Assistive technology services, suited to an individual's needs. Transition from school to work, employment planning, occupational skills and more are coached here.

2087 RESNA Technical Assistance Project
Rehabilitation Engineering & Asst Technology: NA
1700 N Moore Street
Arlington, VA 22209
703-524-6686
FAX 703-524-6630
http://www.resna.org
e-mail: info@resna.org
Glenn Hedman, President
Thomas A. Gorski, Executive Director
Nell Bailey, Director Projects
Provides technical assistance to states in the development and implementation of consumer responsive statewide programs of technology-related assistance under the Technology Related Assistance for Individuals with Disabilities Act of 1988.

2088 Special Education Preview Center
Ruth Eason School
648 Old Mill Road
Millersville, MD 21108
410-222-3815
FAX 410-222-3817
http://www.aacps.org
e-mail: schoolsite@aacps.org
Carol Mohsberg, Principal
Linda Abe, Secretary

2089 Star Center
1119 Old Humboldt Road
Jackson, TN 38305
731-668-3888
800-464-5619
FAX 731-668-1666
http://www.starcenter.tn.org
e-mail: information@starcenter.tn.org

Margaret Doumitt, Executive Director
Judy Duke, Information/Outreach Manager
Joan Page, Administrative Assistant
Technology center for people with disabilities. Some of the services are: music therapy, art therapy, augmentative communication evaluation and training, vocational evaluation, job placement, vision department, environmental controls.

2090 Tech-Able
Tech-Able
1114 Brett Drive
Conyers, GA 30094
770-922-6768
FAX 770-992-6769
http://www.techable.org
e-mail: techweb@techable.org
Joe Tedesco, Executive Director
Pat Hanus, Program Manager
Joe Tedesco, Assistive Tech. Practitioner
Assistive technology demonstration and information center. Provides demonstrations of computer hardware and software specially designed to assist people with disabilities. Serves a wide range of disabilities and virtually all age groups. Also custom fabrication of key guards and switches.

2091 Technology Access Center
2222 Metrocenter Boulevard
Nashville, TN 37228
615-248-6733
800-368-4651
FAX 615-259-2536
TDY:615-248-6733
http://www.tac.ataccess.org
e-mail: techaccess@tacnashville.com
Bob Kibler, Director
Lynn Magner, Service Coordinator

Serves the community as a resource center and carries out specific projects related to assistive technology.

2092 Technology Access Foundation
Technology Access Foundation
3803 S. Edmunds Street
Seattle, WA 98118
206-725-9095
FAX 206-725-9097
http://www.techaccess.org
e-mail: taf@techaccess.org
Trish Millines-Dziko, Co-founder, Executive Director
Sherry Williams, Director of External Relations

Provides information, consultation and technical assistance on assistive technology for people with disabilities, including computer hardware and software technology, and adaptive and assistive equipment.

2093 Technology Assistance for Special Consumers
United Cerebral Palsy
2075 Max Luther Drive
Huntsville, AL 35810
256-852-5600
FAX 256-852-6722
http://www.tasc.ataccess.org
e-mail: tasc@hiwaay.net
Cherly Smith, Executive Director
Lisa Snyder, Resource Center Coordinator
Sandra Schmidt, Office Manager
Offers a computer resource center which has both computers and software for use at the center or for short-term.

2094 Technology Utilization Program
National Aeronautics and Space Administration
300 E Street NE
Washington, DC 20002
202-358-0000
FAX 202-358-4338
http://www.hq.nasa.gov
e-mail: hqhompag@hq.nasa.gov
Sean O'Keith, President
Michael Griffin, CEO

Adapts aerospace technology to the development of equipment for the disabled, sick and elderly persons.

2095 Technology for Language and Learning
PO Box 327
East Rockaway, NY 11518
516-625-4550
FAX 516-621-3321
e-mail: ForTLL@aol.com
Joan Tanenhaus, Executive Director

An organization dedicated to advancing the use of computers and technology for children and adults with special language and learning needs. Public domain computer software for special education.

2096 Tidewater Center for Technology Access
Laskin Road Annex
1413 Laskin Road
Virginia Beach, VA 23451
757-263-2829
FAX 757-263-2801
http://www.tcta.ataccess.org
e-mail: myra.flint@vbschools.com
Myra Jessie Flint, Assistive Technology Specialist

Offers resources and information, equipment loans, hands-on exploration of assistive technologies, equipment and software awareness, consultations and interagency collaborations.

Games

2097 A Day at Play
Don Johnston
26799 W Commerce Drive
Volo, IL 60073
847-740-0749
800-999-4660
FAX 847-740-7326
http://www.donjohnston.com
e-mail: info@donjohnston.com
Ruth Ziolkowski, President
Angie Leboida, Marketing/Channel Development

A Day at Play and Out and About, programs in the UKanDu Little Books Series, are early literacy programs that consist of several create-your-own four-page animated stories that help build language experience for early readers. Students fill in the blanks to complete a sentence on each page and then watch the page come alive with animation and sound. After completing the story, students can print it out to make a book which can be read over and over again.

2098 Academic Drill Builders: Wiz Works
SRA Order Services
220 E Danieldale Road
Desoto, TX 75115
1-888-772-45
800-843-8855
FAX 1-972-228-19
http://www.sraonline.com
e-mail: SRA_CustomerService@mcgraw-hill.com
Jerry Chaffin, Author
Peter Sayeski, President

A program using an arcade game format for the creation, editing, pacing and monitoring of 36 drill and practice games. *$49.00*

2099 Adaptive Physical Education Program
One Eden Way
Princeton, NJ 8540
609-987-0099
FAX 609-987-0243
http://www.edenservices.org
e-mail: info@edenservices.org
Dr. Thomas McCool, Executive Director
Diane Van Driesen, EI Program Director
Anne Holmes, Outreach/Support Director
This volume contains teaching programs in the area of sensory integration and adaptive physical education for students with autism. *$50.00*

2100 Alpine Tram Ride
Merit Software
132 W 21st Street
New York, NY 10001
212-675-8567
800-753-6488
FAX 212-675-8607
http://www.meritsoftware.com
e-mail: sales@meritsoftware.com
Ben Weintrap, President

Teaches cognitive redevelopment skills. *$12.95*

2101 Blocks in Motion
Don Johnston
26799 W Commerce Drive
Volo, IL 60073
847-740-0749
800-999-4660
FAX 847-740-7326
http://www.donjohnston.com
e-mail: info@donjohnston.com
Ruth Ziolkowski, President
Angie Leboida, Marketing/Channel Development

An art and motion program that makes drawing, creating and animating fun and educational for all users. Based on the Piagetian theory for motor-sensory development, this program promotes the concept that the process is as educational and as much fun as the end result. Good fine motor skills are not required for students to be successful and practice critical thinking. *$99.00*

2102 CONCENTRATE! On Words and Concepts
Laureate Learning Systems
110 East Spring Street
Winooski, VT 5404
802-655-4755
800-562-6801
FAX 802-655-4757
http://www.laureatelearning.com
e-mail: info@lauretelearning.com
Mary Sweig Wilson, Owner
Bernard J. Fox, Founder

A series of educational games that reinforces the lessons of the Words and Concepts Series while developing short term memory skills. *$105.00*

2103 Camp Frog Hollow
Don Johnston
26799 West Commerce Drive
Volo, IL 60073
847-740-0749
800-999-4660
FAX 847-740-7326
http://www.donjohnston.com
e-mail: info@donjohnston.com
Ruth Ziolkowski, President
Angie Leboida, Marketing Director/Channel Devel

Camp Frog Hollow chronicles the further adventures of K.C. and Clyde as they head off to summer camp. This entertaining approach to reading, literacy and learning can be beneficial for individual reading lessons or large group activities. The journaling feature provides students the opportunity to record their thoughts and feelings while the tracking feature provides a record of progress for the teacher/parent.

2104 Create with Garfield
SRA Order Services
220 East Danieldale Road
Desoto, TX 75115
888-772-4543
800-843-8855
FAX 972-228-1982
http://www.sraonline.com
e-mail: mhls_ecommerce_custserv@mcgraw-hill.com
Peter Sayeski, President

For students to create cartoons, posters and labels by choosing a variety of backgrounds, props and Garfield characters.

2105 Create with Garfield: Deluxe Edition
SRA Order Services
220 East Danieldale Road
Desoto, TX 75115
888-772-4543
800-843-8855
FAX 972-228-1982
http://www.sraonline.com
e-mail: mhls_ecommerce_custserv@mcgraw-hill.com
Ahead Designes, Author
Peter Sayeski, President

A program to be used by children to create and print cartoons, posters or labels featuring Garfield and his friends.

2106 Dino-Games
Academic Software
3504 Tates Creek Road
Lexington, KY 40517
859-552-1020
859-552-1040
FAX 253-799-4012
http://www.acsw.com
e-mail: asistaff@acsw.com
Dr. Warren E Lacefield, President & Senior Research Edit
Penelope D. Ellis, COO/Dir Sales/Marketing

Single switch software programs designed for early switch practice. CD-ROM for Mac or PC. Visit web site for demonstrations. *$39.00*

2107 Dinosaur Days
Queue
1 Controls Drive
Shelton, CT 6484
203-446-8100
800-232-2224
FAX 800-775-2729
http://www.queueinc.com
e-mail: jdk@queueinc.com
Monica Kantrowitz, Owner
Jonathan Kantrowitz, Owner

Students can create their own unique dinosaurs choosing from hundreds of prehistoric parts. *$49.95*

2108 ECS Music Education Software
Electronic Courseware Systems
1713 S State St.
Champaign, IL 61820
800-832-4965
217-359-7099
FAX 217-359-6578
http://www.ecsmedia.com
e-mail: sales@ecsmedia.com
G. David Peters, President
Jodie Varner, Marketing/Sales Director

A fun program designed to help students practice in matching pitches. Two pitches are played with the second one sounding out of tune with the first. The student adjusts the second pitch until it matches the first. Records are kept for students' scores. Tune It II is one of 80 programs in music education published by Electronic Courseware Systems.

2109 Early Games for Young Children
Software to Go-Gallaudet University
800 Florida Avenue NE
Washington, DC 20002
202-651-5220
FAX 202-651-5109
http://www.clerccenter.gallaudet.edu
e-mail: afbinfo@afb.net
Ken Kurlychek, Electronic Information Specialis
Karen Kautz, Administrative Secretary

2110 Eency-Weency Spider Game
UCLA Intervention Program for Handicapped Children
1000 Veteran Avenue
Los Angeles, CA 90095
562-825-4821
FAX 310-206-7744
http://www.bol.ucla.edu
e-mail: consult@ucla.edu
Kit Kehr, Executive Director
Scott Waugh, Executive Vice Chancellor

Board game with spiders moving up the drain spout to win. The scanner randomly selects the sun (move up one space) or rain (move down one space). Scan speed can be modified to allow children with various abilities to compete more equally. *$35.00*

2111 Every Day Is a Holiday: Seasons
UCLA Intervention Program for Handicapped Children
1000 Veteran Avenue
Los Angeles, CA 90095
562-825-4821
FAX 310-206-7744
http://www.bol.ucla.edu
e-mail: consult@ucla.edu

Kit Kehr, Executive Director
Scott Waugh, Executive Vice Chancellor

Explore the major holidays of the year. Summer/Fall includes July 4th, Birthday, Halloween and Thanksgiving. *$45.00*

2112 Fast Food Game
UCLA Intervention Program for Handicapped Children
1000 Veteran Avenue
Los Angeles, CA 90095 562-825-4821
FAX 310-206-7744
http://www.bol.ucla.edu
e-mail: consult@ucla.edu
Kit Kehr, Executive Director
Scott Waugh, Executive Vice Chancellor

Board game activity where players advance by selecting Fast Food items. The children press their switches to spin a spinner which randomly points to a fast food item or sick face. Press the switch to move to the next square with the selected item on it. If you get a sick face you lose your turn. *$35.00*

2113 Frisian Phonology
UCLA Intervention Program for Handicapped Children
1000 Veteran Avenue
Los Angeles, CA 90024 562-825-4821
FAX 310-206-7744
http://www.bol.ucla.edu
e-mail: consult@ucla.edu
Kit Kehr, Executive Director

Five familiar zoo animals: kangaroo, elephant, monkey, giraffe and bird are depicted on an overlay. Level I, the child selects any animal. Level II, the child selects an animal by name. Level III, the child selects an animal by its actions. *$35.00*

2114 Garfield Trivia Game
SRA Order Services
220 East Danieldale Road
Desoto, TX 75115 888-772-4543
800-843-8855
FAX 972-228-1982
http://www.sraonline.com
e-mail: mhls_ecommerce_custserv@mcgraw-hill.com
Jerry Chaffin, Author
Peter Sayeski, President

Designed for the student's creative side. Students can apply their knowledge to 300 intriguing questions about Garfield and his friends.

2115 Incredible Adventures of Quentin
Queue
1 Controls Drive
Shelton, CT 6484 203-446-8100
800-232-2224
FAX 800-775-2729
http://www.queueinc.com
e-mail: jdk@queueinc.com
Monica Kantrowitz, President
Jonathan Kantrowitz, CEO

Students can interact with the story on a screen, with wonderful visual and sound effects, animation and music, for a multisensory learning experience. *$225.00*

2116 KC & Clyde in Fly Ball
Don Johnston
26799 West Commerce Drive
Volo, IL 60073 847-740-0749
800-999-4660
FAX 847-740-7326
http://www.donjohnston.com
e-mail: info@donjohnston.com
Ruth Ziolkowski, President
Angie Leboida, Director of Marketing

In the UKanDu Series of interactive software which is designed to promote learning, independence, and accommodate special needs. Word interaction and context are stressed as students progress through the story and make decisions on how the storyline will advance. Active interaction at the word level is encouraged by UKanDu the wordbird, the tour guide to language in this story. *$95.00*

2117 Listen with Your Ears
UCLA Intervention Program for Handicapped Children
1000 Veteran Avenue
Los Angeles, CA 90095 562-825-4821
FAX 310-206-7744
http://www.bol.ucla.edu
e-mail: consult@ucla.edu
Norman Abrams, Chancellor
Scott Waugh, Executive Vice Chancellor

Auditory discrimination game in which the user identifies an object or action by the sound it makes. Twenty-four choices include: snoring, laughing, cat, doorbell, fire truck, dog, cow, and many more. *$45.00*

2118 Maze-O
Software to Go by Gallaudet University
800 Florida Avenue NE
Washington, DC 20002 202-651-5220
FAX 202-651-5109
http://www.clerccenter.gallaudet.edu
e-mail: afbinfo@afb.net
Ken Kurlychek, Electronic Information Specialis
Karen Kautz, Administrative Secretary

2119 Mind Over Matter
Learning Well
111 Kane Street
Baltimore, MD 21224 516-326-2101
800-645-6564
FAX 800-413-7442
Michael Heins, Author
Joyce Dash

A game program that challenges students to solve 185 visual word puzzles or create their own puzzles, using symbols and graphics.

2120 Monkey Business
Merit Software
121 West 27th Street
New York, NY 10011 212-675-8567
800-753-6488
FAX 212-675-8607
http://www.meritsoftware.com
e-mail: sales@meritsoftware.comfeedback@meritsoftwar
Ben Weintrap, President

Choose one of the three levels of difficulty and play until a minimum score is reached. *$10.95*

2121 Monsters & Make-Believe
Queue
1 Controls Drive
Shelton, CT 6484 203-446-8100
800-232-2224
FAX 800-775-2729
http://www.queueinc.com
e-mail: jdk@queueinc.com
Monica Kantrowitz, President
Jonathan Kantrowitz, Owner, CEO

Children of all ages will love making monsters from over 100 body parts. Use the text processor to write about characters and add speech bubbles and type to the dialogue. *$49.95*

2122 Monty Plays Scrabble
Software to Go-Gallaudet University
800 Florida Avenue NE
Washington, DC 20002
202-651-5220
FAX 202-651-5109
http://www.clerccenter.gallaudet.edu
e-mail: afbinfo@afb.net
Ken Kurlychek, Project Coordinator
Karen Kauutz, Admin. Secretary I

2123 Multi-Scan
Academic Software
3504 Tates Creek Road
Lexington, KY 40517
859-552-1020
FAX 859-273-1943
http://www.acsw.com
e-mail: asistaff@acsw.com
Warren E Lacefield, President
Penelope D Ellis, COO/Sales & Marketing Director

Single switch activity center containing educational games such as numerical dot to dot, concentration, mazes, and matching, for PCs and Macintosh CD-ROM. Handbook for adaptive switches available. *$149.00*

2124 Note Speller
Electronic Courseware Systems
1713 S State St.
Champaign, IL 61820
800-832-4965
217-359-7099
FAX 217-359-6578
http://www.ecsmedia.com
e-mail: Sales@ecsmedia.com
G. David Peters, President
Jodie Varner, Marketing/Sales Director

A drill-and-practice game designed to teach notes presented on the alto, treble, or bass staff. Note Speller has four levels of difficulty. This is one of eighty music education titles published by Electronic Courseware Systems. May be used in Spanish or English. *$39.95*

2125 On a Green Bus
Don Johnston
26799 West Commerce Drive
Volo, IL 60073
847-740-0749
800-999-4660
FAX 847-740-7326
http://www.donjohnston.com
e-mail: info@donjohnston.com
Ruth Ziolkowski, President
Angie Leboida, Marketing/Channel Development

An early literacy program in the UKandDu Little Books Series consisting of several create-your-own four-page animated stories that help build language experience for early readers. Students fill in the blanks, completing sentences on each page. After completing the story, students can print it out to make a book which can be read over and over again.

2126 Path Tactics
Software to Go-Gallaudet University
800 Florida Avenue NE
Washington, DC 20002
202-651-5220
FAX 202-651-5109
http://www.clerccenter.gallaudet.edu
e-mail: afbinfo@afb.net
Charles Kelly, Coordinator, Professional Develo
Karen Kautz, Admin. Secretary I

2127 Pitch Challenger: Music Education Software
Electronic Courseware Systems
1713 S State St.
Champaign, IL 61820
800-832-4965
217-359-7099
FAX 217-359-6578
http://www.ecsmedia.com
e-mail: sales@ecsmedia.com
G. David Peters, President
Jodie Varner, Marketing/Sales Director

Enables a computer to detect pitches produced by voice or instruments. Comes with microphone and is geared towards elementary and junior high students. Available for Mac or IBM. *$295.00*

2128 Seek and Find
UCLA Intervention Program for Handicapped Children
1000 Veteran Avenue
Los Angeles, CA 90024
562-825-4821
FAX 310-206-7744
http://www.bol.ucla.edu
e-mail: consult@ucla.edu
Kit Kehr, Executive Director

Game promoting matching, figure/ground, and auditory discrimination utilizing four scenes: park; campground; city; play room. *$55.00*

2129 Ships Ahoy
Software to Go-Gallaudet University
800 Florida Avenue NE
Washington, DC 20002
202-651-5220
FAX 202-651-5109
http://www.clerccenter.gallaudet.edu
e-mail: afbinfo@afb.net
Charles Kelly, Coordinator, Professional Develo
Karen Kautz, Admin. Secretary I

2130 Son of Seek and Find
UCLA Intervention Program for Handicapped Children
1000 Veteran Avenue
Los Angeles, CA 90024
562-825-4821
FAX 310-206-7744
http://www.bol.ucla.edu
e-mail: consult@ucla.edu
Kit Kehr, Executive Director

Game promoting matching, figure/ground, and auditory discrimination utilizing three scenes: farm; classroom; house. *$55.00*

2131 Switch It-See It
UCLA Intervention Program for Handicapped Children
1000 Veteran Avenue
Los Angeles, CA 90024
562-825-4821
FAX 310-206-7744
http://www.bol.ucla.edu
e-mail: consult@ucla.edu
Kit Kehr, Executive Director

Colorful animated graphics and sound effects encourage visual tracking from left to right, up and down, and on the diagonal. Graphics include: bear; fish; mouse; rocket; and others. *$35.00*
Mac

2132 Teddy Barrels of Fun
SRA Order Services
220 E Danieldale Road
Desoto, TX 75115
877-833-5524
1-888-772-45
FAX 972-228-1982
http://www.sraonline.com
e-mail: mhls_ecommerce_custserv@mcgraw-hill.com
A graphic design program that includes over 200 pieces of art for creating pictures, posters and labels, and word processing capabilities to develop writing skills and creative thinking. *$42.00*

2133 Tennis Anyone?
Software to Go-Gallaudet University
800 Florida Avenue NE
Washington, DC 20002
202-651-5220
FAX 202-651-5109
http://www.clerccenter.gallaudet.edu
e-mail: afbinfo@afb.net
Charles Kelly, Coordinator, Professional Develo
Karen Kautz, Admin. Secretary I

448 pages Video

2134 Worm Squirm
UCLA Intervention Program for Handicapped Children
1000 Veteran Avenue
Los Angeles, CA 90095
562-825-4821
FAX 310-206-7744
http://www.kloo.bol.ucla.edu
Kit Kehr, Executive Director

Maze game designed to teach directionality. A worm is directed through the maze by pushing the appropriate arrows on the overlay. *$35.00*

Language Arts

2135 Alphabet Circus
SRA Order Services
220 East Danieldale Road
Desoto, TX 75115
877-833-5524
1-888-772-45
FAX 972-228-1982
http://www.sraonline.com
e-mail: mhls_ecommerce_custserv@mcgraw-hill.com
Software to teach letter recognition. *$35.00*

2136 Alphabetizing
Aquarius Instructional
13064 Indian Rocks Road
Largo, FL 33774
800-255-9085
FAX 877-595-2685
http://www.phillIproy.com
e-mail: info@philliproy.com
Ruth Farmand, Owner
Ruth Bragman, President
Ashley Sutton, Office Manager
Teaches language arts skills to early childhood students. *$45.00*

2137 American Sign Language Dictionary: Software
Speech Bin
P.O. Box 922668
Norcross, GA 30010
770-449-5700
800-850-8602
FAX 888-329-2246
http://www.speechbin.com
e-mail: info@speechbin.com
Shane Peters, Product Coordinator
Jen Binney, Owner

The CD includes captivating video clips that show 2,500+ words, phrases, and idioms in sign language. The videos may be played at normal speed, slow motion, and stop action. Animations explain origins of selected signs; drills and games are provided to reinforce learning. Item number M545 for Windows $24.95 Item number M540 for MAC. *$29.95*

2138 American Sign Language Video Dictionary &Inflection Guide
Harris Communications
15155 Technology Drive
Eden Prairie, MN 55344
952-906-1180
800-825-6758
FAX 952-906-1099
TDY:952-906-1180
http://www.harriscomm.com
e-mail: info@harriscomm.com
Robert Harris, Owner
Lori Foss, Marketing Director

Combines text, video, and animation to create a leading interactive reference tool that makes learning ASL easy and fun. Contains 2700 signs, searching capabilities in 5 languages, new learning games, and expanded sections in fingerspelling. *$49.95*

2139 AtoZap!
Sunburst Technology
1550 Executive Drive
Elgin, IL 60123
888-492-8817
FAX 888-800-3028
http://www.sunburst.com
e-mail: Service@sunburst.com
Mark Sotir, President
Tara Green, Marketing Executive
Katie Birmingham, Office Manager
When users select an A, little airplanes that fly madly about appear. Users select T and students have their own telephone to talk to any one of nine animated friends. This program for prereaders has an activity for every letter.

2140 Auditory Skills
Psychological Software Services
6555 Carrollton Avenue
Indianapolis, IN 46220
317-257-9672
FAX 317-257-9674
http://www.neuroscience.cnter.com
e-mail: nsc@neuroscience.cnter.com
Odie Bracy MD, Director
Nancy Bracy, Office Manager

Four computer programs designed to aid in the remediation of auditory discrimination problems. *$50.00*

2141 Basic Language Units: Grammar
Continental Press
520 E Bainbridge Street
Elizabethtown, PA 17022
717-367-1836
800-233-0759
FAX 888-834-1303
http://www.continentalpress.com
Daniel Raffensperger, President

Sentence disks include sentence types, subjects and predicates and phrases and clauses (Apple).

2142 Basic Skills Products
EDCON Publishing Group
30 Montauk Boulevard
Oakdale, NY 11769
631-567-7227
888-553-3266
FAX 631-567-8745
TDY:631-567-7227
http://www.edconpublishing.com
e-mail: info@edconpublishing.com
Deals with basic math and language arts. Free catalog available.

2143 Blackout! A Capitalization Game
Software to Go-Gallaudet University
800 Florida Avenue NE
Washington, DC 20002
202-651-5031
FAX 202-651-5109
http://www.clerccenter.gallaudet.edu
e-mail: afbinfo@afb.net
Ken Kurlychek, Electronic Information Specialis
Karen Kautz, Administrative Secretary

2144 Boppie's Great Word Chase
SRA Order Services
220 E Danieldale Road
DeSoto, TX 75115
888-772-4543
800-843-8855
FAX 972-228-1982
http://www.sraonline.com
e-mail: SRA_CustomerService@mcgraw-hill.com
Stephen Schlapp, Author

A program that helps refine spelling and word recognition skills.

2145 **Bubblegum Machine**
Kid Smart, LLC.
8252 S Harvard Avenue
Tulsa, OK 74137
918-494-7878
800-285-3475
FAX 800-285-4018
http://www.heartsoft.com
e-mail: sales@heartsoft.com
A vocabulary enrichment program that challenges students to rhyme, build words out of provided vocabulary or a user-created one. *$39.95*

2146 **Capitalization Plus**
Software to Go-Gallaudet University
800 Florida Avenue NE
Washington, DC 20002
202-651-5031
FAX 202-651-5109
http://www.clerccenter.gallaudet.edu
e-mail: afbinfo@afb.net
Ken Kurlychek, Electronic Information Specialis
Karen Kauutz, Administrative Secretary

2147 **Challenging Our Minds**
Psychological Software Services
6555 Carrollton Avenue
Indianapolis, IN 46220
317-257-9672
FAX 317-257-9674
http://www.challenging-our-minds.com
e-mail: info@challenging-our-minds.com
Odie Bracy, Director
Nancy Bracy, Office Manager

Challenging our Minds (COM) is a cognitive enhancement system designed by a neuropsychologist to develop and enhance cognitive functions across the domains of attention, executive skills, memory, visuospatial skills, problem solving skills, communication and psychosocial skills. COM is a subscription website providign online cognitive enhancement applications for all children.

2148 **Character Education/Life Skills Online Education**
Phillip Roy
13064 Indian Rocks Road
Largo, FL 33774
727-593-2700
800-255-9085
FAX 877-595-2685
http://www.philliproy.com
e-mail: info@philliproy.com
Ruth Bragman PhD, President
Phillip Roy, Owner
Ashley Nipper, Office Manager
Includes 77 CDs, 77 books and unlimited interactive online access, per purchasing site. All print materials are also available to be Brailled and all CDs come with complete audio components along with interactive graphics. Pre/post tests included along with teacher's guide and lesson plans. All materials can be duplicated at purchasing site. No yearly fees. *$3950.00*

2149 **Circletime Tales Deluxe**
Don Johnston
26799 W Commerce Drive
Volo, IL 60073
847-740-0749
800-999-4660
FAX 847-740-7326
http://www.donjohnston.com
e-mail: info@donjohnston.com
Ruth Ziolkowski, President
Angie Leboida, Marketing/Channel Development

An interactive CD-ROM that introduces and reinforces pre-literacy concepts using nursery rhymes and songs familiar to many children. This English/Spanish program emphasizes listening to and learning basic concepts such as opposites, directionality, colors and counting.

2150 **Cognitive Rehabilitation**
Technology for Language and Learning
PO Box 327
East Rockaway, NY 11518
516-625-4550
FAX 516-621-3321
A series of public domain programs that strengthen cognitive skills, memory, language and visual motor skills. *$20.00*

2151 **Construct-A-Word I & II**
SRA Order Services
220 E Danieldale Road
Desoto, TX 75115
1-888-772-45
800-843-8855
FAX 1-972-228-19
http://www.sraonline.com
e-mail: SRA_CustomerService@mcgraw-hill.com
Students blend beginnings and endings to create words. *$99.00*

2152 **Crypto Cube**
Software to Go-Gallaudet University
800 Florida Avenue NE
Washington, DC 20002
202-651-5031
FAX 202-651-5109
http://www.clerccenter.gallaudet.edu
e-mail: afbinfo@afb.net
Ken Kurlychek, Electronic Information Specialis
Karen Kautz, Admin. Secretary I

2153 **Curious George Pre-K ABCs**
Sunburst Technology
1550 Executive Drive
Elgin, IL 60123
914-747-3310
800-321-7511
FAX 888-800-3028
http://www.sunburst.com
e-mail: Support@sunburst.com
Mark Sotir, President
Katie Birmingham, Office Manager
Children go on a lively adventure with Curious George visiting six multi level activities that provide an animated introduction to letters and their sounds. Students discover letter names and shapes, initial letter sounds, letter pronunciations, the order of the alphabet and new vocabulary words during the fun exursions with Curious George. Mac/Win CD-ROM

2154 **Double-Up**
Research Design Associates
5 Main Street
Freeville, NY 13068
607-844-4601
FAX 607-844-3310
e-mail: adra@twcny.rr.com
Brian Buttner, CEO

Takes one or two sentences and puts words in alphabetical order. *$139.95*

2155 **Easy as ABC**
Software to Go-Gallaudet University
800 Florida Avenue NE
Washington, DC 20002
202-651-5031
FAX 202-651-5109
http://www.clerccenter.gallaudet.edu
e-mail: afbinfo@afb.net
Ken Kurlychek, Electronic Information Specialis
Karen Kautz, Admin. Secretary I

2156 **Eden Institute Curriculum: Classroom**
1 Eden Way
Princeton, NJ 8540
609-987-0099
FAX 609-987-0243
http://www.edenservices.org
e-mail: info@edenservices.org
Tom McCool, President
David Holmes, Executive Director
Anne Holmes, Outreach/Support Director
This volume is geered toward students with autism who have mastered some basic academic skills and are able to learn in a small group setting. Teaching programs include academics, domestic and social skills. *$100.00*

2157 Elephant Ears: English with Speech
Ballard & Tighe
PO Box 219
Brea, CA 92821
714- 990-433
800-321-4332
FAX 714-255-9828
http://www.ballard-tighe.com
e-mail: info@ballard-tighe.com
Dorothy Roberts, CEO
Dr. Roberta Stathis, President

Features instruction and assessment of prepositions in a 3-part diskette. *$49.00*

2158 Emerging Literacy
Technology for Language and Learning
PO Box 327
East Rockaway, NY 11518
516-625-4550
FAX 516-621-3321
A five-volume set of stories. *$25.00*

2159 English 4-Pack
Dataflo Computer Services
531 Us Route 4
Lebanon, NH 3766
603-448-2223
These programs provide various spelling problems through word scrambling, letter substitution and spelling bee simulation. *$39.95*

2160 Essential Learning Systems (ELS)
Creative Education Institute
1105 Wooded Acres
Waco, TX 76710
254-751-1188
800-234-7319
FAX 888-475-2402
http://www.ceilearning.com
e-mail: info@ceilearning.com
Terry Irwin, CEO
Ric Klein, Marketing Director

Enables special education, learning disabled and dyslexic students to develop the skills they need to learn. Using computer exercises to appropriately stimulate the brain's language areas, the lagging learning skills can be developed and patterns of correct language taught.

2161 First Phonics
Sunburst Technology
1550 Executive Drive
Elgin, IL 60123
914-747-3310
800-321-7511
FAX 888-800-3028
http://www.sunburst.com
e-mail: Service@sunburst.com
Mark Sotir, CEO
Tara Green, Marketing Executive
Katie Birmingham, Office Manager
Targets the phonics skills that all children need to develop, sounding out the first letter of a word. This program offers four different engaging activities that you can customize to match each child's specific need.

2162 Grammar Examiner
Software to Go-Gallaudet University
800 Florida Avenue NE
Washington, DC 20002
202-651-5220
FAX 202-651-5109
http://http://clerccenter.gallaudet.edu
e-mail: Karen.Kautz@gallaudet.edu
Ken Kurlychek, Electronic Information Specialis
Karen Kautz, Administrative Assistant

2163 Grammar Toy Shop
Software to Go-Gallaudet University
800 Florida Avenue NE
Washington, DC 20002
202-651-5220
FAX 202-651-5109
http://http://clerccenter.gallaudet.edu
e-mail: Karen.Kautz@gallaudet.edu
Ken Kurlychek, Electronic Information Specialis
Karen Kautz, Administrative Assistant

2164 Gremlin Hunt
Merit Software
121 West 27th Street
New York, NY 10001
212-675-8567
800-753-6488
FAX 212-675-8607
http://www.meritsoftware.com
e-mail: sales@meritsoftware.com
Ben Weintraub, CEO

Gremlins test visual discrimination and memory skills at three levels. *$9.95*

2165 High Frequency Vocabulary
Technology for Language and Learning
PO Box 327
East Rockaway, NY 11518
516-625-4550
FAX 516-621-3321
Each volume of the series has 10 stories that teach specific vocabulary. *$35.00*

2166 Hint and Hunt I & II
SRA Order Services
220 E Danieldale Road
Desoto, TX 75115
888-772-4543
800-843-8855
FAX 972-228-1982
http://www.sraonline.com
e-mail: mhls_ecommerce_custserv@mcgraw-hill.com
With these programs, students can actually see and hear how changing vowels can make a new word. *$99.00*

2167 Homonyms
Software to Go-Gallaudet University
800 Florida Avenue NE
Washington, DC 20002
202-651-5220
FAX 202-651-5109
http://http://clerccenter.gallaudet.edu
e-mail: Karen.Kautz@gallaudet.edu
Ken Kurlychek, Electronic Information Specialis
Karen Kautz, Administrative Assistant

2168 HyperStudio Stacks
Technology for Language and Learning
PO Box 327
East Rockaway, NY 11518
516-625-4550
FAX 516-621-3321
Offers various volumes in language arts, social studies and reading. *$10.00*

2169 Hyperlingua
Research Design Associates
5 Main Street
Freeville, NY 13068
607-844-4601
FAX 607-844-3310
e-mail: adra@twcny.rr.com
Brian Buttner, President

Allows teachers to create on-screen printing language drills. *$69.95*

2170 IDEA Cat I, II and III
Ballard & Tighe
PO Box 219
Brea, CA 92821
714-990-4332
800-321-4332
FAX 714-255-9828
http://www.ballard-tighe.com
e-mail: info@ballard-tighe.com
Richard Bullard, Manager
Robert Batson, Finance/Operations VP

Computer-assisted teaching of English language lessons reinforces skills of Level I, II, and III of the IDEA Oral Program. *$142.00*

2171 **Improving Reading/Spelling Skills via Keyboarding**

AVKO Educational Research Foundation
3084 W Willard Road
Clio, MI 48420
810-686-9283
866-2856-612
FAX 810-686-1101
http://www.spelling.org
e-mail: avkoemail@aol.com

Don McCabe, Author
Don McCabe, Research Director
Devorah Wolf, President

Students learn spelling patterns and acquire important word recognition skills as they slowly and methodically learn proper fingering and keystrokes on a typewriter or computer keyboard.
$12.95

ISBN 1-564004-01-5

2172 **Katie's Farm**

Lawrence Productions
1800 S 35th Street
Galesburg, MI 49053
269-665-7075
800-421-4157
FAX 269-665-7060
http://www.lpi.com
e-mail: sales@lpi.com

John Lawrence, Owner
Edwin Wright, President
Karen Morehouse, Operations Manager

Designed to encourage exploration and language development.
$29.95

2173 **Key Words**

Humanities Software
408 Columbia Street, Suite 222
Hood River, OR 97031
541-386-6737
800-245-6737
FAX 541-386-1410
http://www.humanitiessoftware.com
e-mail: info@humanitiessoftware.com

Peggy Menasco, Development Support Supervisor
Charlotte Arnold, Marketing Director

Learning to keyboard goes hand-in-hand with language play, learning word families, and phonics rules. Six original passages at each of sixteen levels provide reading pleasure and finger dances that pop. You'll tell your students to stop. Key Words is available in versions for all your needs — elementary, high school, emergent literacy and remedial education. One computer, lab pack and school community site and network license.
$49.00

2174 **Keys to Success: Computer Keyboard Skills for Blind Children**

Life Science Associates
1 Fennimore Road
Bayport, NY 11705
631-472-2111
FAX 631-472-8146
http://www.lifesciassoc.home.pipeline.com
e-mail: lifesciassoc@pipeline.com

A voice output program to help blind and partially sighted children learn the computer keyboard layout. Program includes keyboard tutorial, keyboard practice, timed keyboard practice, and a timed game for two players.

2175 **Kid Pix**

Riverdeep
222 3rd Avenue SE
Cedar Rapids, IA 52401
319-395-9626
800-362-2890
FAX 319-395-0217
http://www.riverdeep.net
e-mail: info@riverdeep.net

Barry O'Callaghan, Executive Chairman & Chief Execu

A painting program that combines special effect art tools, sounds and magic screen transformations. *$59.95*

2176 **Kids Media Magic 2.0**

Sunburst Technology
1550 Executive Drive
Elgin, IL 60123
914-747-3310
800-321-7511
FAX 888-800-3028
http://www.sunburst.com
e-mail: Service@sunburst.com

Mark Sotir, CEO
Tara Green, Marketing Executive
Katie Birmingham, Office Manager

The first multimedia word processor designed for young children. Help your child become a fluent reader and writer. The Rebus Bar automatically scrolls over 45 vocabulary words as students type.

2177 **Language Carnival I**

SRA Order Services
220 E Danieldale Road
Desoto, TX 75115
888-772-4543
800-843-8855
FAX 972-228-1982
http://www.sraonline.com
e-mail: mhls_ecommerce_custserv@mcgraw-hill.com

David Ertmer, Author

A diskette of four games using humor to help students develop language and thinking skills.

2178 **Language Carnival II**

SRA Order Services
220 E Danieldale Road
Desoto, TX 75115
888-772-4543
800-843-8855
FAX 972-228-1982
http://www.sraonline.com
e-mail: mhls_ecommerce_custserv@mcgraw-hill.com

David Ertmer, Author

A diskette of four games using humor to help students develop language and thinking skills.

2179 **Language Master: MWD-640**

Franklin Learning Resources
1 Franklin Plaza
Burlington, NJ 8016
800-525-9673
800-266-5626
FAX 609-239-5948
http://www.franklin.com
e-mail: service@franklin.com

Barry Lipsky, CEO and President
John Applegate, Director

A language master without speech defining over 83,000 words, spelling correction capability, pick/edit feature, vocabulary enrichment activities and advanced word list. *$79.95*

2180 **Learn to Match**

Technology for Language and Learning
PO Box 327
East Rockaway, NY 11518
516-625-4550
FAX 516-621-3321

Joan Tanenhaus, Founder

Ten volume set of picture-matching disks. *$50.00*

2181 **Letter Sounds**

Sunburst Technology
400 Columbus Avenue
Valhalla Pleasantville, NY 10595
914-747-3310
800-321-7511
FAX 914-747-4109
http://www.sunburst.com
e-mail: support@nysunburst.com

Mark Sotir, CEO
Tara Green, Marketing Executive
Katie Birmingham, Office Manager

Students develop phonemic awareness skills as they make the connection between consonant letters and their sounds.

2182 Letters and First Words
C&C Software
5713 Kentford Circle
Wichita, KS 67220
316-683-6056
800-752-2086
Carol Clark, President

Helps children learn to identify letters and recognize their associated sounds. *$30.00*

2183 Lexia Phonics Based Reading
Lexia Learning Systems
200 Baker Ave. Extension
Concord, MA 1742
800-435-3942
800-435-3942
FAX 978-287-0062
http://www.lexialearning.com
e-mail: info@lexialearning.com
Nicholas C. Gaehde, President and C.E.O.

Five activity areas with 64 branching units and practice with 535 one-syllable words and 90 two-syllable words, sentences and stories. *$250.00*

2184 Look! Listen! & Learn Language!: Software
Abilitations Speech Bin
3155 Northwoods Parkway
Norcross, GA 30071
800-477-3324
800-477-3324
FAX 888-329-2246
http://www.speechbin.com
e-mail: info@speechbin.com
Tobi Isaacs, Catalog Director

Interactive activities for children with autism, PDD, Down syndrome, language delay, or apraxia include: hello; Match Same to Same; Quack; Let's talk About It; visual scanning/attention and match ups! Item number L177. *$98.99*

2185 M-ss-ng L-Nks Single Educational Software
Sunburst Technology
400 Columbus Avenue
Valhalla Pleasantville, NY 10595
914-747-3310
800-321-7511
FAX 914-747-4109
http://www.sunburst.com
e-mail: support@nysunburst.com
Mark Sotir, CEO
Tara Green, Marketing Executive
Katie Birmingham, Office Manager
This award-winning program is an engrossing language puzzle. A passage appears with letters or words missing. Students complete it based on their knowledge of word structure, spelling, grammar, meaning in context, and literary style.

2186 Make It Go
KidTECH
4181 Pinewood Lake Drive
Bakersfield, CA 93309
661-396-8676
FAX 661-396-8760
Joyce Meyer, President

A collection of seven original cause and effect programs. *$20.00*

2187 Make-A-Flash
Teacher Support Software
325 North Kirkwood Road
St. Louis, MO 63122
888-726-8100
888-351-4199
FAX 314-984-8063
http://www.siboneylearninggroup.com
e-mail: info@siboneylearninggroup.com
Alan Stern, Regional Manager

A flash card program displaying and printing large, easy-to-read letters or numbers. *$69.95*

2188 Mark Up
Research Design Associates
5 Main Street
Freeville, NY 13068
607-844-4601
FAX 607-844-3310
e-mail: adra@twcny.rr.com
Brian Buttner, CEO

A sentence reconstruction program which presents learners with four options for the study of grammar. *$49.95*

2189 Max's Attic: Long & Short Vowels
Sunburst Technology
400 Columbus Avenue
Valhalla Pleasantville, NY 10595
914-747-3310
800-321-7511
FAX 914-747-4109
http://www.sunburst.com
e-mail: support@nysunburst.com
Mark Sotir, CEO
Tara Green, Marketing Executive
Katie Birmingham, Office Manager
Filled to the rafters with phonics fun, this animated program builds your students' vowel recognition skills.

2190 McGee
Lawrence Productions
1800 South 35th Street
Galesburg, MI 49053
269-665-7075
800-421-4157
FAX 269-665-7060
http://www.lpi.com
e-mail: sales@lpi.com
Edwin Wright, President and C.E.O.
John Lawrence, Owner

An independent exploration with no words. Available in IBM, Mac and IIGS formats. *$34.95*

2191 Memory I
Psychological Software Services
6555 Carrollton Avenue
Indianapolis, IN 46220
317-257-9672
FAX 317-257-9674
http://www.neuroscience.cnter.com
e-mail: nsc@netdirect.net
Odie L. Bracy MD, Director
Nancy Bracy, Office Manager

Consists of four computer programs designed to provide verbal and nonverbal memory exercises. *$110.00*

2192 Memory II
Psychological Software Services
6555 Carrollton Avenue
Indianapolis, IN 46220
317-257-9672
FAX 317-257-9674
http://www.neuroscience.cnter.com
e-mail: nsc@netdirect.net
Odie L. Bracy MD, Director
Nancy Bracy, Office Manager

These programs allow for work with encoding, categorizing and organizing skills. *$150.00*

2193 Microcomputer Language Assessment and Development System
Laureate Learning Systems
110 East Spring Street
Winooski, VT 5404
802-655-4755
800-562-6801
FAX 802-655-4757
http://www.laureatelearning.com
e-mail: info@laureatelearning.com
Mary Sweig Wilson, President and C.E.O.
Bernard J. Fox, Vice President

A series of seven diskettes designed to teach over 45 fundamental syntactic rules. Students are presented two or three pictures, depending on the grammatical construction being trained with optional speech and/or text and asked to select the picture which represents the correct construction. *$775.00*

2194 Mike Mulligan & His Steam Shovel

Sunburst Technology
400 Columbus Avenue
Valhalla Pleasantville, NY 10595
914-747-3310
800-321-7511
FAX 914-747-4109
http://www.sunburst.com
e-mail: support@nysunburst.com

Mark Sotir, CEO
Tara Green, Marketing Executive
Katie Birmingham, Office Manager

This CD-ROM version of the Caldecott classic lets students experience interactive book reading and participate in four skills-based extension activities that promote memory, matching, sequencing, listening, pattern recognition and map reading skills.

2195 My Action Book

KidTECH
4300 Stine Road
Bakersfield, CA 93313
661-396-8676
FAX 661-396-8760
http://www.softtouch.com
e-mail: sales@softtouch.com

Joyce Meyer, President

Designed to teach familiar action vocabulary through live voice, song and animation. *$30.00*

2196 Old MacDonald II

UCLA Intervention Program for Handicapped Children
1000 Veteran Avenue
Los Angeles, CA 90095
562-825-4821
FAX 310-206-7744
http://www.bol.ucla.edu
e-mail: consult@ucla.edu

Kit Kehr, Executive Director
Scott Waugh, Acting Executive Vice Chancellor

An early preposition program involving in, on top, behind, in front of, next to and between depicted in a farm scene. *$35.00*

2197 Optimum Resource

18 Hunter Road
Hilton Head Island, SC 29926
843-689-8000
888-784-2592
FAX 843-689-8008
http://www.stickybear.com
e-mail: stickyb@stickybear.com

Chris Gintz, CEO
Christopher Hefter, Product VP

An educational software publishing company for grades K-12. Our software titles are available in Consumer, School, Labpack or Site License versions. Please call for further details. Prices range from $59.95 for Consumer to $699.95 for Site Licenses.

2198 Padded Food

UCLA Intervention Program for Handicapped Children
1000 Veteran Avenue
Los Angeles, CA 90095
562-825-4821
FAX 310-206-7744
http://www.bol.ucla.edu
e-mail: consult@ucla.edu

Kit Kehr, Executive Director
Scott Waugh, Acting Executive Vice Chancellor

Program overlay depicts familiar foods and can be used as a matching or categorizing program. *$35.00*
Mac

2199 Phonology: Software

Abilitations Speech Bin
3155 Northwoods Parkway
Norcross, GA 30071
800-477-3324
800-477-3324
FAX 888-329-2246
http://www.speechbin.com
e-mail: info@speechbin.com

Tobi Isaacs, M.Ed., Catalog Director

This unique software gives you six entertaining games to treat children's phonological disorders. The program uses target patterns in a pattern cycling approach to phonological processess. Item number L183. *$98.99*

2200 Prefixes

American Printing House for the Blind
1839 Frankfort Avenue
Louisville, KY 40206
502-895-2405
800-223-1839
FAX 502-899-2274
http://www.aph.org
e-mail: info@aph.org

Tuck Tinsley, President
Bob Brasher, Vice President Advisory Services
Fred Gissoni, Customer Support

An interactive software program that teaches about five common prefixes — un, re, dis, pre, and in — for Apple II computers. *$34.95*

2201 Python Path Phonics Word Families

Sunburst Technology
1550 Executive Drive
Elgin, IL 60123
914-747-3310
800-321-7511
FAX 888-800-3028
http://www.sunburst.com
e-mail: Service@sunburst.com

Mark Sotir, CEO
Tara Green, Marketing Executive
Katie Birmingham, Office Manager

Your child improves their word-building skills by playing three fun strategy games that involve linking one-or two-letter consonant beginnings to basic word endings.

2202 Read, Write and Type! Learning System

Talking Fingers
830 Rincon Way
San Rafael, CA 94901
415-472-3103
800-674-9126
FAX 415-472-7812
http://www.readwritetype.com
e-mail: contact@talkingfingers.com

Jeannine Herron, President

This 40-lesson adventure is a powerful tool for 6-8 year-olds just learning to read, for children of other cultures learning to read and write in English, and for students of any age who are struggling to become successful readers and writers.

2203 Reading Riddles with the Boars

Queue
1 Controls Drive
Shelton, CT 6484
203-446-8100
800-232-2224
FAX 800-775-2729
http://www.queueinc.com
e-mail: jdk@queueinc.com

Monica Kantrowitz, President
Jonathan Kantrowitz, CEO
Peter Uhrynowski, Controller

Children are naturally curious about pictures. This program uses pictures to teach over 1,000 vocabulary words. *$39.95*

2204 Reading Rodeo

Heartsoft
8252 S Harvard Avenue
Tulsa, OK 74137
800-285-3475
800-285-4018
FAX 800-285-4018
http://www.heartsoft.com
e-mail: sales@heartsoft.com

Utilizes over 100 artist drawn pictures to show students how to distinguish between words beginning with different initial consonant sounds. *$39.95*

2205 Rhubarb

Research Design Associates
5 Main Street
Freeville, NY 13068
607-844-4601
FAX 607-844-3310
e-mail: adra@twcny.rr.com

Brian Buttner, CEO

Allows teachers to quickly and easily enter reading passages tailored to needs of their classes. *$69.95*

2206 Same or Different
Merit Software
121 West 27th Street
New York, NY 10001
212-675-8567
800-753-6488
FAX 212-675-8607
http://www.meritsoftware.com
e-mail: sales@meritsoftware.com
Ben Weintrap, President

Requires students to make important visual discriminations which involve shape, color and whole/part relationships. *$9.95*

2207 Sensible Speller: Talking APH Edition
American Printing House for the Blind
1839 Frankfort Avenue
Louisville, KY 40206
502-895-2405
800-223-1839
FAX 502-899-2274
http://www.aph.org
e-mail: info@aph.org
Tuck Tinsley, President
Bob Brasher, Vice President Advisory Services
Fred Gissoni, Customer Support
A speech output version of the spelling checker program from Sensible Software, for Apple IIs using the ProDOS Operating System. *$65.00*

2208 Sequencing Fun!
Sunburst Technology
1550 Executive Drive
Elgin, IL 60123
914-747-3310
800-321-7511
FAX 888-800-3028
http://www.sunburst.com
e-mail: Service@sunburst.com
Mark Sotir, CEO
Tara Groon, Marketing Executive
Katie Birmingham, Office Manager
Text, pictures, animation and video clips provide a fun filled program that encourages critical thinking skills.

2209 Show Time
Software to Go - Gallaudet University
800 Florida Avenue NE
Washington, DC 20002
202-651-5220
FAX 202-651-5109
http://http://clerccenter.gallaudet.edu
e-mail: afbinfo@afb.net
Ken Kurlychek, Electronic Information Specialis
Karen Kautz, Administrative Secretary

2210 Sight Words
UCLA Intervention Program for Handicapped Children
1000 Veteran Avenue
Los Angeles, CA 90095
562-825-4821
FAX 310-206-7744
http://www.bol.ucla.edu
e-mail: consult@ucla.edu
Norman Abrams, Chancellor
Scott Waugh, Executive Vice Chancellor

Early sight vocabulary program with six categories to choose from: school; outside; home; toys; food; clothing. Teacher options include: scan speed selection; switch or spacebar selection. *$35.00*
Mac

2211 Soft Tools
Psychological Software Services
6555 Carrollton Avenue
Indianapolis, IN 46220
317-257-9672
FAX 317-257-9674
http://www.neuroscience.cnter.com
e-mail: nsc@neuroscience.cnter.com
Odie L. Bracy MD, Director
Nancy Bracy, Office Manager

Menu-driven disk versions of the computer programs published in the Cognitive Rehabilitation Journal. *$50.00*

2212 Sound Match
Enable/Schneier Communication Unit
1603 Court Street
Syracuse, NY 13208
315-455-7591
315-455-1794
FAX 315-455-7591
http://www.enablecny.org
e-mail: info@enablecny.orgÿÿ
Clement Nadeau, President
Leola Rodgers, Executive Vice President

Presents a variety of sounds/noises requiring gross levels of auditory discrimination and matching. *$25.00*

2213 Speaking Language Master Special Edition Model Number: LM-60
Franklin Learning Resources
1 Franklin Plaza
Burlington, NJ 8016
609-386-8997
800-525-9673
FAX 609-387-1787
http://www.franklin.com
e-mail: service@franklin.com
Barry Lipsky, CEO
John Applegate, Customer Relations Sr. Manager

A language master with speech defining over 110,000 words, spelling correction capability, pick/edit feature, vocabulary enrichment activities and advanced word list. *$79.95*

2214 Speaking Speller
American Printing House for the Blind
1839 Frankfort Avenue
Louisville, KY 40206
502-895-2405
800-223-1839
FAX 502-899-2274
http://www.aph.org
e-mail: info@aph.org
Tuck Tinsley, President
Bob Brasher, Vice President Advisory Services
Fred Gissoni, Customer Support
A spelling program with speech output for students and teachers. For Apple II computers using either ProDOS or DOS 3.3. *$28.95*

2215 Spell-a-Word
RJ Cooper & Associates
27601 Forbes Road
Laguna Niguel, CA 92677
949-582-2572
800-752-6673
FAX 949-582-3169
http://www.rjcooper.com
e-mail: info@rjcooper.com
RJ Cooper, Owner

A large print, talking, spelling program. It uses an errorless learning method. It has both a drill and test mode, which a supervisor can set. Letters, words or phrases are entered by a supervisor and recorded by supervisor, peer, or sibling. Available for Mac, Windows. *$99.00*

2216 Spellagraph
Software to Go-Gallaudet University
800 Florida Avenue NE
Washington, DC 20002
202-651-5220
FAX 202-651-5109
http://http://clerccenter.gallaudet.edu
e-mail: afbinfo@afb.net
Ken Kurlychek, Electronic Information Specialis
Karen Kautz, Administrative Secretary

2217 **Spelling Ace**
Franklin Learning Resources
One Franklin Plaza
Burlington, NJ 8016
609-386-2500
800-266-5626
FAX 609-239-5948
http://www.franklin.com
e-mail: service@franklin.com
Barry Lipsky, CEO and President

The basic spelling corrector with 80,000 words. Sound-Alikes feature identifies commonly confused words. *$25.00*

2218 **Spelling Mastery**
SRA/McGraw-Hill
220 East Danieldale Road
Desoto, TX 75115
888-SRA-4543
800-843-8855
FAX 972-228-1892
http://www.sraonline.com
e-mail: SRA_CustomerService@mcgraw-hill.com
Peter Sayeski, President

Spelling Mastery teaches students dependable spelling skills by blending the phonemic, morphemic, and whole word approaches.

2219 **Stanley Sticker Stories**
Riverdeep
222 3rd Avenue SE
Cedar Rapids, IA 52401
319-395-9626
800-362-2890
FAX 800-567-2714
http://www.riverdeep.net
Barry O'Callaghan, Executive Chairman & CEO
Jim Ruddy, Chief Revenue Officer

Kids love Mille, Bailey, Sammy and Trudy, the characters from Edmark's award-winning Early Learning Series. Now they can feature these and other Edmark characters in their very own animated storybooks building spelling and writing skills and expanding creativity along the way. The fun-filled program from the educational software experts at Edmark gives kids the power to build stories that come to life right on screen. *$59.95*

2220 **Stickybear Software**
Optimum Resource
18 Hunter Road
Hilton Head Island, SC 29926
843-689-8000
888-784-2592
FAX 843-689-8008
http://www.stickybear.com
e-mail: stickyb@stickybear.com
Chris Gintz, CEO
Christopher Hefter, Vice President of Product Develo

An educational software publishing company for grades K-12. Our software titles are available in Consumer, School, Labpack, Site License and Network versions. Please call for further details. Prices range from $59.95 for Consumer to $699.95 for Site Licenses.

2221 **Sunken Treasure Adventure: Beginning Blends**
Sunburst Technology
1550 Executive Drive
Elgin, IL 60123
914-747-3310
800-321-7511
FAX 888-800-3028
http://www.sunburst.com
e-mail: Service@sunburst.com
Mark Sotir, CEO
Tara Green, Marketing Executive
Katie Birmingham, Office Manager
Focus on beginning blends sounds and concepts with three high-spirited games that invite students to use two letter consonant blends as they build words.

2222 **Syllasearch I, II, III, IV**
SRA Order Services
220 East Danieldale Road
Desoto, TX 75115
888-SRA-4543
800-843-8855
FAX 972-228-1982
http://www.sraonline.com
e-mail: SRA_CustomerService@mcgraw-hill.com
Students learn how to read multi-syllable words accurately and automatically with this new game that uses actual human speech for instruction and correction. *$99.00*

2223 **Talking Nouns**
Laureate Learning Systems
110 E Spring Street
Winooski, VT 5404
802-655-4755
800-562-6801
FAX 802-655-4757
http://www.laureatelearning.com
e-mail: info@laureatelearning.com
Mary Wilson, CEO
Bernard Fox, Vice President

An interactive communication product that helps build expressive language and augmentative communication skills. *$130.00*

2224 **Talking Nouns II**
Laureate Learning Systems
110 E Spring Street
Winooski, VT 5404
802-655-4755
800-562-6801
FAX 802-655-4757
http://www.laureatelearning.com
e-mail: info@laureatelearning.com
Mary Wilson, CEO
Bernard Fox, Vice President

Designed to build expressive language and augmentative communication skills. *$130.00*

2225 **Talking Verbs**
Laureate Learning Systems
110 E Spring Street
Winooski, VT 5404
802-655-4755
800-562-6801
FAX 802-655-4757
http://www.laureatelearning.com
e-mail: info@laureatelearning.com
Mary Wilson, CEO
Bernard Fox, Vice President

Builds expressive language and augmentative communication skills. *$130.00*

2226 **Texas School for the Deaf Sign Language**
Harris Communications
15155 Technology Drive
Eden Prairie, MN 55344
952-906-1180
800-825-6758
FAX 952-906-1099
TDY:952-906-1198
http://www.harriscomm.com
e-mail: info@harriscomm.com
Texas School for the Deaf, Author
Robert Harris, Owner
Patty Johnson, President

Colorful picture book of four popular fables with fun animation on CD-ROM. Has the option to have the story voiced, with computer highlighting words as they are spoken. *$79.95*
CD-ROM

2227 **Twenty Categories**
Laureate Learning Systems
110 E Spring Street
Winooski, VT 5404
802-655-4755
800-562-6801
FAX 802-655-4757
http://www.laureatelearning.com
e-mail: info@laureatelearning.com

Mary S Wilson, Author
Mary Wilson, CEO
Bernard Fox, Vice President

Designed to use with children and adults, these two diskettes provide instruction in both abstracting the correct category for a noun and placing a noun in the appropriate category. *$100.00*

2228 Type to Learn 3
Sunburst Technology
1550 Executive Drive
Elgin, IL 60123
914-747-3310
800-321-7511
FAX 888-800-3028
http://www.sunburst.com
e-mail: Service@sunburst.com
Mark Sotir, CEO
Tara Green, Marketing Executive
Katie Birmingham, Office Manager
With the 25 lessons in this animated update of Type to Learn, students embark on time travel missions to learn keyboarding skills.

2229 Type to Learn Jr.
Sunburst Technology
1550 Executive Drive
Elgin, IL 60123
914-747-3310
800-321-7511
FAX 888-800-3028
http://www.sunburst.com
e-mail: Service@sunburst.com
Mark Sotir, CEO
Tara Green, Marketing Executive
Katie Birmingham, Office Manager
One of the first steps to literacy is learning how to use the keyboard. Age appropriate instruction and three practice activities help students use the computer with greater ease.

2230 Type to Learn Jr. New Keys for Kids
Sunburst Technology
1550 Executive Drive
Elgin, IL 60123
914-747-3310
800-321-7511
FAX 888-800-3028
http://www.sunburst.com
e-mail: Service@sunburst.com
Mark Sotir, CEO
Tara Green, Marketing Executive
Katie Birmingham, Office Manager
With new keys to learn, your early keyboarders focus on using the letter and number keys, the shift key, home row and are introduced to selected internet symbols.

2231 Vowel Patterns
Sunburst Technology
1550 Executive Drive
Elgin, IL 60123
914-747-3310
800-321-7511
FAX 888-800-3028
http://www.sunburst.com
e-mail: Service@sunburst.com
Mark Sotir, CEO
Tara Green, Marketing Executive
Katie Birmingham, Office Manager
Some vowels are neither long nor short. In this investigation, students explore and learn to use abstract vowels.

2232 Word Invasion: Academic Skill Builders in Language Arts
SRA Order Services
220 East Danieldale Road
Desoto, TX 75115
888-SRA-4543
800-843-8855
FAX 972-228-1982
http://www.sraonline.com
e-mail: SRA_CustomerService@mcgraw-hill.com
Jerry Chaffin, Author

A program using an arcade game format to provide practice in identifying words representing six parts of speech: nouns; pronouns; verbs; adjectives; adverbs and prepositions. *$49.00*

2233 Word Master: Academic Skill Builders in Language Arts
SRA Order Services
220 East Danieldale Road
Desoto, TX 75115
888-SRA-4543
800-843-8855
FAX 972-228-1982
http://www.sraonline.com
e-mail: SRA_CustomerService@mcgraw-hill.com
Jerry Chaffin, Author

A program using arcade game format to provide practice in identifying parts of antonyms, synonyms or homonyms at three difficulty levels. *$49.00*

2234 Word Wise I and II: Better Comprehension Through Vocabulary
SRA Order Services
220 East Danieldale Road
Desoto, TX 75115
888-SRA-4543
800-843-8855
FAX 972-228-1982
http://www.sraonline.com
e-mail: SRA_CustomerService@mcgraw-hill.com
Isabel Beck, Author

A series of two software programs for developing and improving reading comprehension by building vocabulary knowledge.

Life Skills

2235 Big/Little I
UCLA Intervention Program for Handicapped Children
1000 Veteran Avenue
Los Angeles, CA 90024
562-825-4821
FAX 310-206-7744
http://www.bol.ucla.edu
e-mail: consult@ucla.edu
Kit Kehr, Executive Director

Program for one to four players in which a little bear scans big and little objects commonly seen by young children. *$35.00*
Mac

2236 Big/Little II
UCLA Intervention Program for Handicapped Children
1000 Veteran Avenue
Los Angeles, CA 90024
562-825-4821
FAX 310-206-7744
http://www.bol.ucla.edu
e-mail: consult@ucla.edu
Kit Kehr, Executive Director

Children construct a big or little bear by choosing the appropriate size body parts and articles of clothing.

2237 Boars Tell Time
Queue
1 Controls Drive
Shelton, CT 6484
203-446-8100
800-232-2224
FAX 800-775-2729
http://www.queueinc.com
e-mail: jdk@queueinc.com
Monica Kantrowitz, President
Jonathan Kantrowitz, CEO
Peter Uhrynowski, Controller
The Boars help youngsters to learn both analog and digital time.
$39.95

2238 Bozons' Quest
Laureate Learning Systems
110 E Spring Street
Winooski, VT 5404
802-655-4755
800-562-6801
FAX 802-655-4757
http://www.laureatelearning.com
e-mail: info@laureatelearning.com
Mary Wilson, CEO
Bernard Fox, Vice President

A computer game designed to teach cognitive skills and strategies and left/right discrimination skills. *$32.50*

2239 Braille 'n Speak Scholar
American Printing House for the Blind
1839 Frankfort Avenue
Louisville, KY 40206
502-895-2405
800-223-1839
FAX 502-899-2274
http://www.aph.org
e-mail: info@aph.org
Tuck Tinsley, President
Allan Lovell, Customer Relations Manager
Frank Gissone, Customer Support
This portable, computerized, talking device has many features useful to student and adult braille users (word processors, print-to-braille translator, talking clocks/calculators and much more). *$929.95*

2240 Buddy's Body
UCLA Intervention Program for Handicapped Children
1000 Veteran Avenue
Los Angeles, CA 90095
310-825-4821
FAX 310-206-7744
http://www.bol.ucla.edu
e-mail: consult@ucla.edu
Kit Kehr, Executive Director

Body parts program containing two levels with animation. Level I contains facial features. Level II contains larger body parts. In each level, children are asked to identify body parts by pressing the part on the overlay. Each level has its own overlay. *$35.00*

2241 Calendar Fun with Lollipop Dragon
SVE & Churchill Media
6465 North Avondale Avenue
Chicago, IL 60631
773-775-9433
800-829-1900
FAX 773-775-9855
http://www.clearvue.com
e-mail: clearvue_service@discovery.com
Mark Ventling, President

Young students learn the calendar basics. *$84.00*

2242 Coin Changer
Kid Smart, LLC.
8252 S Harvard Avenue
Tulsa, OK 74137
918-494-7878
800-285-3475
FAX 800-285-4018
e-mail: sales@hearsoft.com
Uses large coin graphics which help teach money skills. *$39.95*

2243 Comparison Kitchen
SRA Order Services
220 E Danieldale Road
Desoto, TX 75115
888-772-4543
800-843-8855
FAX 1-972-228-19
http://www.sraonline.com
e-mail: SRA_CustomerService@mcgraw-hill.com
Strengthens students' visual perception of sizes and amounts as well as their visual discrimination of objects by color, shape and size. *$35.00*

2244 Early Learning: Preparing Children for School
Phillip Roy
13064 Indian Rocks Road
Largo, FL 33774
727-593-2700
800-255-9085
FAX 877-595-2685
http://www.philliproy.com
e-mail: info@philliproy.com
Ruth Bragman, President
Phillip Roy, Manager
Ashley Nipper, Office Manager
This program includes unlimited online access to 42 interactive lessons per individual. This pre-kindergarten curriculum has over 250 activities which include: Math, Problem-Solving, Reading, Language Development, Physical Skills, Self-Esteem, Your Community, and Healthy Habits. Includes audio and interactive graphics. Allows parents to work with their children at home or any place. Can be duplicated at the purcashing school. No yearly fees. *$995.00*

2245 Eden Institute Curriculum: Volume I
Eden Services
One Eden Way
Princeton, NJ 8540
609-987-0099
FAX 609-987-0243
http://www.members.aol.com/edensvcs
e-mail: info@edenservices.org
Tom McCool, Executive Director
David Holmes, President, CEO
Anne Holmes, Outreach/Support Director
Learning readiness, preacademic, academic, prevocational, self-care, domestic, social and play skills programs for young students with autism. *$200.00*

2246 Electric Crayon
Merit Software
121 West 27th Street
New York, NY 10011
212-675-8567
800-753-6488
FAX 212-675-8607
http://www.meritsoftware.com
e-mail: sales@meritsoftware.com
Ben Weintrap, President

A tool to help preschool and primary aged children learn about and enjoy the computer. *$14.95*

2247 Family Fun
UCLA Intervention Program for Handicapped Children
1000 Veteran Avenue
Los Angeles, CA 90095
310-825-4821
FAX 310-206-7744
http://www.bol.ucla.edu
e-mail: consult@ucla.edu
Kit Kehr, Executive Director

FamilyFun is a pre-reading tutorial *$35.00*

2248 Feelings
UCLA Intervention Program for Handicapped Children
1000 Veteran Avenue
Los Angeles, CA 90095
310-825-4821
FAX 310-206-7744
http://www.bol.ucla.edu
e-mail: consult@ucla.edu
Kit Kehr, Executive Director

Five feelings: happy, sad, scared, love and tired, are depicted on an overlay. Level I describes each emotion. Level II, the child associates an emotion with an action. Level III, the child chooses a picture to describe his or her feelings. *$35.00*

2249 First Categories
Laureate Learning Systems
110 E Spring Street
Winooski, VT 5404
802-655-4755
800-562-6801
FAX 802-655-4757
http://www.laureatelearning.com
e-mail: info@laureatelearning.com
Mary Wilson, Owner
Bernard Fox, Vice President

A program that trains categorization skills with a natural sounding voice and pictures of 60 nouns in six categories. *$100.00*

2250 **First R**
Milliken Publishing
3190 Rider Trail South
Earth City, MO 63045
314-991-4220
800-325-4136
FAX 314-991-4807
http://www.millikenpub.com
e-mail: webmaster@millikenpub.com
Thomas Moore, President

A phonetically-based word recognition program with emphasis on comprehension. *$325.00*

2251 **First Verbs**
Laureate Learning Systems
110 E Spring Street
Winooski, VT 5404
802-655-4755
800-562-6801
FAX 802-655-4757
http://www.laureatelearning.com
e-mail: info@laureatelearning.com
Mary Wilson, Owner
Bernard Fox, Vice President

A program that trains and tests 40 early developing verbs using animated pictures and a natural sounding female voice. *$225.00*

2252 **First Words**
Laureate Learning Systems
110 E Spring Street
Winooski, VT 5404
802-655-4755
800-562-6801
FAX 802-655-4757
http://www.laureatelearning.com
e-mail: info@laureatelearning.com
Mary Wilson, Owner
Bernard Fox, Vice President

A talking program that trains and tests 50 early developing nouns presented within 10 categories. *$225.00*

2253 **First Words II**
Laureate Learning Systems
110 E Spring Street
Winooski, VT 5404
802-655-4755
800-562-6801
FAX 802-655-4757
http://www.laureatelearning.com
e-mail: info@laureatelearning.com
Mary Wilson, Owner
Bernard Fox, Vice President

Continues the training of First Words with training and testing of an additional 50 early developing nouns presented within the same 10 categories as used in First Words. *$225.00*

2254 **Fish Scales**
SRA Order Services
220 E Danieldale Road
Desoto, TX 75115
888-772-4543
800-843-8855
FAX 1-972-228-19
http://www.sraonline.com
e-mail: SRA_CustomerService@mcgraw-hill.com

Graphics, animation and sound will capture players' attention as they learn how things are measured for height, length and distance. *$35.00*

2255 **Following Directions: Left and Right**
Laureate Learning Systems
110 E Spring Street
Winooski, VT 5404
802-655-4755
800-562-6801
FAX 802-655-4757
http://www.laureatelearning.com
e-mail: info@laureatelearning.com
Mary Wilson, Owner
Bernard Fox, Vice President

Provides practice in following directions and exercises short-term memory while reinforcing left/right discrimination concepts. *$165.00*

2256 **Following Directions: One and Two-Level Commands**
Laureate Learning Systems
110 E Spring Street
Winooski, VT 5404
802-655-4755
800-562-6801
FAX 802-655-4757
http://www.laureatelearning.com
e-mail: info@laureatelearning.com
Eleanor Semel, Author
Mary Wilson, Owner
Bernard Fox, Vice President

Designed for a broad range of students experiencing difficulty in processing, remembering and following oral commands, a program of exercises on short and long-term memory highlighting specific spatial, directional and ordinary vocabulary.

2257 **Food Facts**
American Printing House for the Blind
1839 Frankfort Avenue
Louisville, KY 40206
502-895-2405
800-223-1839
FAX 502-899-2274
http://www.aph.org
e-mail: info@aph.org
Tuck Tinsley, President
Allan Lovell, Customer Relations Manager
Fred Gissoni, Customer Support

An interactive software program for Apple II computer that teaches about nutrition of common foods. *$39.70*

2258 **Functional Skills System and MECA**
Conover Company, Division of Oakwood Solution
1789 North Oakwood Road
Oshkosh, WI 54904
920-231-4667
800-933-1933
FAX 920-231-4809
http://www.conovercompany.com
e-mail: sales@conovercompany.com
Terry Schmitz, President
Becky Schmitz, Member

Functional Skills System software assists in the transition from school to the community and workplace. Functional literary, functional life skills, functional social skills, functional work skills. MECA - The system for creating post-secondary transition outcomes and the instructional services to support them. *$2535.00*

2259 **Getting Clean with Herkimer I**
UCLA Intervention Program for Handicapped Children
1000 Veteran Avenue
Los Angeles, CA 90095
310-825-4821
FAX 310-206-7744
http://www.bol.ucla.edu
e-mail: consult@ucla.edu
Kit Kehr, Executive Director

Help Herkimer, the visitor from outer space, find the things he can use to get clean and look good in the bath, at the sink, or in the shower. Grooming items such as brush, comb, soap, towel, washcloth, toothbrush, tooth paste, sponge and bubble bath are illustrated. *$75.00*

2260 **Getting Clean with Herkimer II**
UCLA Intervention Program for Handicapped Children
1000 Veteran Avenue
Los Angeles, CA 90095
310-825-4821
FAX 310-206-7744
http://www.bol.ucla.edu
e-mail: consult@ucla.edu
Kit Kehr, Executive Director

Find the things that Herkimer cannot use to get clean or look good. *$45.00*

2261 **Getting Clean with Herkimer III**
UCLA Intervention Program for Handicapped Children
1000 Veteran Avenue
Los Angeles, CA 90095
310-825-4821
FAX 310-206-7744
http://www.bol.ucla.edu
e-mail: consult@ucla.edu
Kit Kehr, Executive Director

Emphasis is on grooming items, with cooking and health care items also shown. Teaches children to categorize objects according to their functions. *$45.00*

2262 **Information Station**
SVE & Churchill Media
6465 North Avondale Avenue
Chicago, IL 60631
773-775-9433
800-253-2788
FAX 773-775-9855
http://www.clearvue.com
e-mail: clearvue service@discovery.com
Mark Ventling, President

Students who boot up this software will find themselves floating miles above the earth orbiting the planet in an information station satellite. *$144.00*

2263 **Job Readiness Software**
Lawrence Productions
1800 S 35th Street
Galesburg, MI 49053
269-665-7075
800-421-4157
FAX 269-665-7060
http://www.lpi.com
e-mail: sales@lpi.com
John Lawrence, Chairman
Jerry Brown, President
Karen Morehouse, Operations Manager
Four programs: Job Attitudes: Assessment and Improvement; Filling Out Job Applications; Successful Job Interviewing; and Resumes Made Easy. *$99.00*
CD

2264 **Knowledgeworks Company**
Milliken Publishing
11643 Lilburn Park Drive
Saint Louis, MO 63146
314-991-4220
800-325-4136
FAX 314-991-4807
http://www.knowledgeworksnc.com
e-mail: customercare@knowledgeworksnc.com
Thomas Moore, President
Victoria Scott, Sales Manager
Lourie Avery, Accountant
Math and reading software for on track and remediation.
Price varies

2265 **Let's Go Shopping I: Toys and Groceries**
UCLA Intervention Program for Handicapped Children
1000 Veteran Avenue
Los Angeles, CA 90095
310-825-4821
FAX 310-206-7744
http://www.bol.ucla.edu
e-mail: consult@ucla.edu
Kit Kehr, Executive Director

Classification game in which children select the appropriate items that belong in the corresponding store (toy or grocery). *$35.00*

2266 **Let's Go Shopping II: Clothes & Pets**
UCLA Intervention Program for Handicapped Children
1000 Veteran Avenue
Los Angeles, CA 90095
310-825-4821
FAX 310-206-7744
http://www.bol.ucla.edu
e-mail: consult@ucla.edu
Kit Kehr, Executive Director

Classification game in which children select the appropriate items that belong in the corresponding store (clothes or pet).

2267 **Lion's Workshop**
Merit Software
121 West 27th Street
New York, NY 10001
212-675-8567
800-753-6488
FAX 212-675-8607
http://www.meritsoftware.com
e-mail: sales@meritsoftware.com
Ben Weintrap, President

Presents various objects with parts missing or with like objects to be matched. *$9.95*

2268 **Marsh Media**
Marshware
PO Box 8082
Shawnee Mission, KS 66208
816-523-1059
800-821-3303
FAX 866-333-7421
http://www.marshmedia.com
e-mail: info@marshmedia.com
Joan K. Marsh, President

Marsh Media publishes closed captioned health and guidance videos for the classroom and school library. Catalog available.

2269 **Math Spending and Saving**
World Class Learning
406 Main Street
Reisterstown, MD 21136
800-638-6470
FAX 800-638-6499
http://www.wclm.com
e-mail: jdash@wclm.com
Paul Edwards, Author
Bruce Brown, President

Designed for secondary students and adults, this program focuses on personal financial management, comparison shopping and calculation of essential banking transactions.

2270 **Money Skills**
MarbleSoft
12301 Central Avenue NE
Blaine, MN 55434
763-755-1402
FAX 763-862-2920
http://www.marblesoft.com
e-mail: mail@marblesoft.com
Money Skills 2.0 includes five activities that teach counting money and making change: Coins and Bills; Counting Money; Making Change; how much change? and the Marblesoft Store. Teaches American, Canadian and European money using clear, realistic pictures of the money. Single and dual-switch scanning options on all difficulty levels. Runs on Macintosh and Windows computers. *$60.00*

2271 **My House: Language Activities of Daily Living**
Laureate Learning Systems
110 East Spring Street
Winooski, VT 5404
802-655-4755
800-562-6801
FAX 802-655-4757
http://www.laureatelearning.com
e-mail: info@laureatelearning.com
Mary Wilson, President
Bernard Fox, Vice President

A language-simulation program designed for communicatively low-functioning clients. *$1200.00*

2272 **NOMAD Talking Touch Pad**
American Printing House for the Blind
1839 Frankfort Avenue
Louisville, KY 40206
502-895-2405
800-223-1839
FAX 502-895-1509
http://www.aph.org
e-mail: info@aph.org
Tuck Tinsley, President
Rosanne Broome, Customer Relations Manager
Fred Gissoni, Customer Support

Connects to a computer to make tactile pictures talk. Uses include teaching about tactile graphics, training in orientation and mobility, and a talking directory for buildings and campuses. *$750.00*

2273 Occupations
UCLA Intervention Program for Handicapped Children
1000 Veteran Avenue
Los Angeles, CA 90024
562-825-4821
FAX 310-206-7744
http://www.bol.ucla.edu
Kit Kehr, Executive Director

Companion game to Community Vehicles. Game identifying 6 community helpers: Fireman, teacher, police officer, gas station attendant, dentist, and doctor. Level I, the child selects any community helper. Level II, the child chooses the community helper associated with the scene. *$36.00*

2274 Optimum Resource
18 Hunter Road
Hilton Head Island, SC 29926
843-689-8000
888-784-2592
FAX 843-689-8008
http://www.stickybear.com
e-mail: stickyb@stickybear.com
Christopher Gintz, CEO
Robert Stangroom, Product Manager

An educational software publishing company for grades K-12. Our software titles are available in Consumer, School, Labpack or Site License versions. Please call for further details. Prices range from $59.95 for Consumer to $699.95 for Site Licenses.

2275 PAVE: Perceptual Accuracy/Visual Efficiency
Software to Go-Gallaudet University
800 Florida Avenue NE
Washington, DC 20002
202-651-5220
FAX 202-651-5109
http://www.clerccenter.gallaudet.edu
e-mail: afbinfo@afb.net
Ken Kurlychek, Elelctronic Information Speciali
Karen Kautz, Admin. Secretary

2276 Padded Vehicles
UCLA Intervention Program for Handicapped Children
1000 Veteran Avenue
Los Angeles, CA 90024
562-825-4821
FAX 310-206-7744
http://www.bol.ucla.edu
Kit Kehr, Executive Director

Children Identify 10 Vehicles — airplane, helicopter, motorcycle, police car, truck, ambulance, garbage truck, school bus, fire engine and tractor, which are illustrated on the overlay. Level I, the child selects any vehicle, Level II, the child selects the vehicle by name. *$36.00*

2277 Paper Dolls I: Dress Me First
UCLA Intervention Program for Handicapped Children
1000 Veteran Avenue
Los Angeles, CA 90024
562-825-4821
FAX 310-206-7744
http://www.bol.ucla.edu
Kit Kehr, Executive Director

Five articles of clothing (shoes, socks, jacket, pants, and T-shirt for boy, overall and dress for girl) are depicted on an overlay to dress the paper doll. *$36.00*

2278 Paper Dolls II: Dress Me Too
UCLA Intervention Program for Handicapped Children
1000 Veteran Avenue
Los Angeles, CA 90024
562-825-4821
FAX 310-206-7744
http://www.bol.ucla.edu
Kit Kehr, Executive Director

Twelve articles of clothing are depicted on an overlay to dress the paper doll (boy or girl). Options include dressing for: school day; sunny day; rainy day; or silly day. *$36.00*

2279 Personal Life Skills Curriculum
Aquarius Instructional
13064 Indian Rocks Road
Largo, FL 33774
1-800-255-90
800-338-2644
FAX 877-595-2685
http://www.philliproy.com
e-mail: info@philliproy.com
Phillip Roy, Owner
Ruth Bragman, President
Ashley Sutton, Office Manger
Through the use of high-interest, low-reading levels, these programs promote self-concept. *$115.00*

2280 Pick a Meal
UCLA Intervention Program for Handicapped Children
1000 Veteran Avenue
Los Angeles, CA 90095
310-825-4821
FAX 310-206-7744
http://www.bol.ucla.edu
e-mail: consult@ucla.edu
Kit Kehr, Executive Director

This game is designed to promote good nutrition for children and/or individuals who are low functioning. Level I teaches the 4 basic food groups. Level II helps the individual learn how to select balanced meals for each meal of the day. There is no print-out data collection, but scan speed selection is available. *$35.00*

2281 Pictalk
UCLA Intervention Program for Handicapped Children
1000 Veteran Avenue
Los Angeles, CA 90024
562-825-4821
FAX 310-206-7744
http://www.bol.ucla.edu
Kit Kehr, Executive Director

Developed as a pre-primer for an alternative communication device for nonreaders who are severely physically disabled. Program includes 6 categories— places, things, action, foods, and feelings — with 54 picture vocabulary. *$ 35.00*

2282 Print Shop Deluxe 15, EEV
Riverdeep
222 3rd Avenue SE
Cedar Rapids, IA 52401
319-395-9626
800-362-2890
FAX 319-395-0217
http://www.riverdeep.net
David Valsam, Author
Barry O'Callaghan, Executive Chairman & CEO
Jim Ruddy, Chief Revenue Officer

A program allowing the user to automatically design and print greeting cards, letterhead stationery, banners, signs and other graphic designs on regular computer paper.

2283 Puzzle Works Readiness
Continental Press
520 E Bainbridge Street
Elizabethtown, PA 17022
717-367-1836
800-233-0759
FAX 888-834-1303
http://www.continentalpress.com
Daniel Raffensperger, President

This series of five disks uses colorful graphics and reward techniques that are especially suited to the interests and needs of special learners. *$25.95*

2284 Quiz Castle
Software to Go-Gallaudet University
800 Florida Avenue NE
Washington, DC 20002
202-651-5220
FAX 202-651-5109
http://www.clerccenter.gallaudet.edu
e-mail: afbinfo@afb.net
Ken Kurlychek, Project Coordinator
Karen Kauutz, Administrative Assistant

2285 Remembering Numbers and Letters
Relevant Publications
13200 106th Ave. N.
Largo, FL 33774
727-595-7890
800-338-2644
FAX 727-595-2685
http://www.relevantpublications.com
e-mail: info@relevantpublications.com
Ruth Farmand, Owner
Phil Padol, Director

Students work at their own pace and select their own numbers and letters with which to work. *$29.95*

2286 Resumes Made Easy
Lawrence Productions
1800 South 35th Street
Galesburg, MI 49053
616-454-4380
800-421-4157
FAX 616-454-4711
http://www.lpi.com
e-mail: sales@lpi.com
George Spengler, Author
John Lawrence, Chairman
Jerry Brown, President
Karen Morehouse, Operations Manager
An interactive program covering what a resume is, how a resume is prepared and what is to be included in a resume. *$29.95*

2287 Seasons
UCLA Intervention Program for Handicapped Children
1000 Veteran Avenue
Los Angeles, CA 90095
310-825-4821
FAX 310-206-7744
http://www.bol.ucla.edu
e-mail: consult@ucla.edu
Kit Kehr, Executive Director

Game is designed to help teach children and/or low functioning individuals to identify attributes of the four seasons. Students select a season from the menu, then objects from each season scan the bottom of the screen. The child selects items matching the season using the mouse, switch, space bar, or TouchWindows. When a season is completed, there is an option to type a brief statement about the scene. *$45.00*

2288 Secondary Print Pack
Failure Free
140 Cabarrus Avenue W
Concord, NC 28025
704-786-7838
800-542-2170
FAX 704-785-8940
http://www.failurefree.com
e-mail: info@failurefree.com
Vince Vezza, Vice President of Sales and Mark

Thousands of independent activities teaching over 750 words. *$1929.00*

2289 Stickybear Software
Optimum Resource
18 Hunter Road
Hilton Head Island, SC 29926
843-689-8000
FAX 843-689-8008
http://www.stickybear.com
e-mail: stickyb@stickybear.com
Christopher Gintz, CEO

An educational software publishing company for grades K-12. Our software titles are available in Consumer, School, Labpack or Site License versions. Please call for further details. Prices range from $59.95 for Consumer to $699.95 for Site Licenses.

2290 Switch It-Change It
UCLA Intervention Program for Handicapped Children
1000 Veteran Avenue
Los Angeles, CA 90095
310-825-4821
FAX 310-206-7744
http://www.bol.ucla.edu
e-mail: consult@ucla.edu
Kit Kehr, Executive Director

Switch-activated cause and effect program presents colorful, common objects. Designed to be paired with three-dimensional objects for matching, identification and selection. Geared toward the young and/or low functioning. *$35.00*
Mac

2291 Tea Party
UCLA Intervention Program for Handicapped Children
1000 Veteran Avenue
Los Angeles, CA 90095
310-825-4821
FAX 310-206-7744
http://www.bol.ucla.edu
e-mail: consult@ucla.edu
Kit Kehr, Executive Director

Follow-up classification game to Let's Go Shopping. Children shop at four different stores to select items for a tea party. *$36.00*

2292 Teenage Switch Progressions
RJ Cooper & Associates
27601 Forbes Road
Laguna Niguel, CA 92677
949-582-2572
800-752-6673
FAX 949-582-3169
http://www.rjcooper.com
e-mail: info@rjcooper.com
RJ Cooper, Owner

Five activities for teenage persons working on switch training, attention training, life skills simulation and following directions. *$75.00*

2293 TeleSensory
Telesensory
650 Vaqueros Avenue
Sunnyvale, CA 94085
408-616-8700
FAX 408-616-8720
http://www.telesensory.com
e-mail: info@insiphil.com
Soon Seng Ng, President
Anita Thibeaux, Operation Manager
Jennifer Street, Marketing Director
Helps visually impaired people become more independent with the most comprehensive products available anywhere for reading, writing, taking notes and using computers.

2294 This Is the Way We Wash Our Face
UCLA Intervention Program for Handicapped Children
1000 Veteran Avenue
Los Angeles, CA 90095
310-825-4821
FAX 310-206-7744
http://www.bol.ucla.edu
e-mail: consult@ucla.edu
Kit Kehr, Executive Director

Familiar Nursery song with singing and animation depicted in picture form on an overlay. Five verses are: washing your face; brushing your teeth; combing your hair; getting dressed; and eating. *$36.00*

Math

2295 2+2
RJ Cooper & Associates
27601 Forbes Road
Laguna Niguel, CA 92677
949-582-2572
800-752-6673
FAX 949-582-3169
http://www.rjcooper.com
e-mail: info@rjcooper.com

RJ Cooper, Owner

This large print, talking, early academic program is for drilling math facts, including addition, subtraction, multiplication and division. It uses an errorless learning method. Available for Mac, Windows. *$89.00*

2296 Access to Math
Don Johnston
26799 West Commerce Drive
Volo, IL 60073
847-740-0749
800-999-4660
FAX 847-740-7326
http://www.donjohnston.com
e-mail: info@donjohnston.com
Ruth Ziolkowski, President
Mindy Brown, Marketing

The Macintosh talking math worksheet program that's two products in one. For teachers, it makes customized worksheets in a snap. For students who struggle, it provides individualized on-screen lessons.

2297 Algebra Stars
Sunburst Technology
1550 Executive Drive
Elgin, IL 60123
888-492-8817
FAX 888-800-3028
http://www.sunburst.com
e-mail: service@sunburst.com
Mark Sotir, CEO
Mike Gavelek, Senior Vice President of Marketi
Katie Birmingham, Office Manager
Students build their understanding of algebra by constructing, categorizing, and solving equations and classifying polynomial expressions using algebra tiles.

2298 Alien Addition: Academic Skill Builders in Math
SRA Order Services
220 East Danieldale Road
Desoto, TX 75115
877-833-5524
FAX 972-228-1982
http://www.sraonline.com
Jerry Chaffin, Author

A program using an arcade game format to provide practice in addition of numbers 0 through 9. *$49.00*

2299 Awesome Animated Monster Maker Math
Sunburst Technology
1550 Executive Drive
Elgin, IL 60123
888-492-8817
FAX 888-800-3028
http://www.sunburst.com
e-mail: service@sunburst.com
Mark Sotir, CEO
Mike Gavelek, Senior Vice President of Marketi
Katie Birmingham, Office Manager
With an emphasis on building core math skills, this humorous program incorporates the monstrous and the ridiculous into a structured learning environment. Students choose from six skill levels tailored to the 3rd to 8th grade.

2300 Awesome Animated Monster Maker Math and Monster
Sunburst Technology
1550 Executive Drive
Elgin, IL 60123
888-492-8817
FAX 888-800-3028
http://www.sunburst.com
e-mail: service@sunburst.com
Mark Sotir, CEO
Mike Gavelek, Senior Vice President of Marketi
Katie Birmingham, Office Manager
Students develop money and strategic thinking skills with this irresistable game that has them tinker about making monsters.

2301 Awesome Animated Monster Maker Number Drop
Sunburst Technology
1550 Executive Drive
Elgin, IL 60123
888-492-8817
FAX 888-800-3028
http://www.sunburst.com
e-mail: service@sunburst.com
Mark Sotir, CEO
Mike Gavelek, Senior Vice President of Marketi
Katie Birmingham, Office Manager
Your students will think on their mathematical feet estimating and solving thousands of number problems in an arcade-style game designed to improve their performance in numeration, money, fractions, and decimals.

2302 Basic Math Competency Skill Building
Educational Activities Software
PO Box 220790
St. Louis, MO 63122
866-243-8464
FAX 239-225-9299
http://www.ea-software.com
e-mail: jwest@siboneylg.com
Michael Conlon, Author
Alan Stern, Manager

An interactive, tutorial and practice program to teach competency with arithmetic operations, decimals, fractions, graphs, measurement and geometric concepts. *$369.00*

2303 Basic Skills Products
EDCON Publishing Group
30 Montauk Boulevard
Oakdale, NY 11769
631-567-7227
888-553-3266
FAX 631-567-8745
TDY:631-567-7227
http://www.edconpublishing.com
e-mail: info@edconpublishing.com
Dale Solimene, Publisher
Roberto Fuentes, Office Manager

Deals with basic math and language arts. Free catalog available.

2304 Big: Calc
Don Johnston
26799 West Commerce Drive
Volo, IL 60073
847-740-0749
800-999-4660
FAX 847-740-7326
http://www.donjohnston.com
e-mail: info@donjohnston.com
Ruth Ziolkowski, President
Mindy Brown, Marketing

A Macintosh calculator program for people with special needs but also beneficial for users who need the auditory reinforcement of a talking calculator. Features include big numbers, high-quality speech and versatile layouts. Encourages math motivation.

2305 Boars 1, 2, 3! Counting with the Boars
Queue
1 Controls Drive
Shelton, CT 6484
203-446-8100
800-232-2224
FAX 800-775-2729
http://www.qworkbooks.com
e-mail: jdk@queueine.com
Monica Kantrowitz, President
Jonathan Kantrowitz, CEO
Peter Uhrynowski, Controller
The Boars teach young learners basic keyboard skills while they identify numbers from 1-10 and count familiar objects in a variety of colorful scenes. *$39.95*

2306 Boars Store
Queue
1 Controls Drive
Shelton, CT 6484
203-446-8100
800-232-2224
FAX 800-775-2729
http://www.qworkbooks.com
e-mail: jdk@queueine.com
Monica Kantrowitz, President
Jonathan Kantrowitz, CEO
Peter Uhrynowski, Controller
Shopping at the Boars Store offers students an exciting way to learn to count money and make change. *$39.95*

2307 Building Perspective
Sunburst Technology
1550 Executive Drive
Elgin, IL 60123
888-492-8817
FAX 888-800-3028
http://www.sunburst.com
e-mail: service@sunburst.com
Mark Sotir, CEO
Mike Gavelek, Senior Vice President of Marketi
Katie Birmingham, Office Manager
Develop spatial perception and reasoning skills with this award-winning program that will sharpen your students' problem-solving abilities.

2308 Building Perspective Deluxe
Sunburst Technology
1550 Executive Drive
Elgin, IL 60123
888-492-8817
FAX 888-800-3028
http://www.sunburst.com
e-mail: service@sunburst.com
Mark Sotir, CEO
Mike Gavelek, Senior Vice President of Marketi
Katie Birmingham, Office Manager
New visual thinking challenges await your students as they engage in three spacial reasoning activities that develop their 3D thinking, deductive reasoning and problem solving skills

2309 Combining Shapes (Tenth Planet)
Sunburst Technology
1550 Executive Drive
Elgin, IL 60123
888-492-8817
FAX 888-800-3028
http://www.sunburst.com
e-mail: service@sunburst.com
Mark Sotir, CEO
Mike Gavelek, Senior Vice President of Marketi
Katie Birmingham, Office Manager
Students discover the properties of simple geometric figures through concrete experience combining shapes. Measurements, estimating and operation skills are part of this fun program.

2310 Combining and Breaking Apart Numbers
Sunburst Technology
1550 Executive Drive
Elgin, IL 60123
888-492-8817
FAX 888-800-3028
http://www.sunburst.com
e-mail: service@sunburst.com
Mark Sotir, CEO
Mike Gavelek, Senior Vice President of Marketi
Katie Birmingham, Office Manager
Students explore part-whole relationships and develop number sense by combining and breaking apart numbers in a variety of problem-solving situations.

2311 Comparing with Ratios
Sunburst Technology
1550 Executive Drive
Elgin, IL 60123
888-492-8817
FAX 888-800-3028
http://www.sunburst.com
e-mail: service@sunburst.com
Mark Sotir, CEO
Mike Gavelek, Senior Vice President of Marketi
Katie Birmingham, Office Manager
Students learn that ratio is a way to compare amounts by using multiplication and division. Through five engaging activities, students recognize and describe ratios, develop proportional thinking skills, estimate ratios, determine equivalent ratios, and use ratios to analyze data.

2312 Conceptual Skills
Psychological Software Services
6555 Carrollton Avenue
Indianapolis, IN 46220
317-257-9672
FAX 317-257-9674
http://www.neuroscience.cnter.com
e-mail: nsc@neuroscience.cnter.com
Odie Bracy PhD HSPP, Director, Clinical Neuropsycholo
Nancy Bracy, Office Manager

Twelve programs designed to enhance skills involved in relationships, comparisons and number concepts. *$50.00*

2313 Concert Tour Entrepreneur
Sunburst Technology
1550 Executive Drive
Elgin, IL 60123
888-492-8817
FAX 888-800-3028
http://www.sunburst.com
e-mail: service@sunburst.com
Mark Sotir, CEO
Mike Gavelek, Senior Vice President of Marketi
Katie Birmingham, Office Manager
Your students improve math, planning and problem solving skills as they manage a band in this music management business simulation.

2314 Counters
Software to Go-Gallaudet University
800 Florida Avenue NE
Washington, DC 20002
202-651-5231
FAX 202-651-5109
http://http://clerccenter.gallaudet.edu
e-mail: products.clerccenter@gallaudet.edu
Ken Kurlychek, Electronic Information Specialis
Karen Kautz, Admin. Secretary I

2315 Counting Critters
Software to Go-Gallaudet University
800 Florida Avenue NE
Washington, DC 20002
202-651-5231
FAX 202-651-5109
http://http://clerccenter.gallaudet.edu
e-mail: products.clerccenter@gallaudet.edu
Ken Kurlychek, Electronic Information Specialis
Karen Kautz, Admin. Secretary I

2316 DLM Math Fluency Program: Addition Facts
SRA Order Services
220 East Danieldale Road
Desoto, TX 75115
888-772-4543
888-772-4543
FAX 972-228-1982
http://www.sraonline.com
e-mail: SRA_CustomerService@mcgraw-hill.com
Ted Hasselbring, Author
Peter Sayeski, President

A program using drill and practice, arcade games, student record keeping, worksheet production and testing to develop the ability to recall basic addition math facts. *$32.00*

2317 DLM Math Fluency Program: Division Facts

SRA Order Services
220 East Danieldale Road
Desoto, TX 75115
888-772-4543
888-772-4543
FAX 972-228-1982
http://www.sraonline.com
e-mail: SRA_CustomerService@mcgraw-hill.com
Ted Hasselbring, Author
Peter Sayeski, President

A series of 10-minute sessions in this diskette program easily retrieves answers to basic division facts up to 144 divided by 12.

2318 DLM Math Fluency Program: Multiplication Facts

SRA Order Services
220 East Danieldale Road
Desoto, TX 75115
888-772-4543
888-772-4543
FAX 972-228-1982
http://www.sraonline.com
e-mail: SRA_CustomerService@mcgraw-hill.com
Ted Hasselbring, Author
Peter Sayeski, President

A series of 10-minute sessions easily retrieves answers to basic multiplication facts up to 12x12. *$32.00*

2319 DLM Math Fluency Program: Subtraction Facts

SRA Order Services
220 East Danieldale Road
Desoto, TX 75115
888-772-4543
888-772-4543
FAX 972-228-1982
http://www.sraonline.com
e-mail: SRA_CustomerService@mcgraw-hill.com
Ted Hasselbring, Author
Peter Sayeski, President

A series of sessions that easily retrieve answers to basic subtraction facts up to 24x12. *$32.00*

2320 Data Explorer

Sunburst Technology
1550 Executive Drive
Elgin, IL 60123
888-492-8817
FAX 888-800-3028
http://www.sunburst.com
e-mail: Service@sunburst.com
Mark Sotir, CEO
Katie Birmingham, Office Manager

This easy-to-use CD-ROM provides the flexibility needed for eleven different graph types including tools for long-term data analysis projects.

2321 Dragon Mix: Academic Skill Builders in Math

SRA Order Services
220 East Danieldale Road
Desoto, TX 75115
888-772-4543
888-772-4543
FAX 1-972-228-19
http://www.sraonline.com
e-mail: SRA_CustomerService@mcgraw-hill.com
Jerry Chaffin, Author
Peter Sayeski, President

A program providing practice in multiplication of numbers 0 through 9 and division of problems with answers 0 through 9. *$49.00*

2322 Elementary Math Bundle

Sunburst Technology
1550 Executive Drive
Elgin, IL 60123
888-492-8817
FAX 888-800-3028
http://www.sunburst.com
e-mail: Service@sunburst.com
Mark Sotir, CEO
Katie Birmingham, Office Manager

Number sense and operations are the focus of the Elementary Math Bundle. Students engage in activities that reinforce basic addition and subtraction skills. This product comes with Splish Splash Math, Ten Tricky Tiles and Numbers Undercover.

2323 Elements of Mathematics

Electronic Courseware Systems
1713 S State Street
Champaign, IL 61820
217-359-7099
800-832-4965
FAX 217-359-6578
http://www.ecsmedia.com
e-mail: sales@ecsmedia.com
G. David Peters, President
Jodie Varner, Education/Marketing Director

This program includes two lessons and a test in the addition of simple and complex fractions. Test results are stored for both student and instructor accessibility. Includes such graphics as pie slices. Elements of Mathematics is one of several programs published by Electronic Courseware Systems.

2324 Equation Tile Teaser

Sunburst Technology
1550 Executive Drive
Elgin, IL 60123
888-492-8817
FAX 888-800-3028
http://www.sunburst.com
e-mail: Service@sunburst.com
Mark Sotir, CEO
Katie Birmingham, Office Manager

Students develop logic thinking and pre-algebra skills solving sets of numbers equations in three challenging problem-solving activities.

2325 Equations

Software to Go-Gallaudet University
800 Florida Avenue NE
Washington, DC 20002
202-651-5877
FAX 202-651-5109
http://www.clerccenter.gallaudet.edu
Ken Kurlychek, Electronic Information Specialis
Karen Kautz, Administrative Secretary I / ISC

2326 Equivalent Fractions

Sunburst Technology
1550 Executive Drive
Elgin, IL 60123
888-492-8817
FAX 888-800-3028
http://www.sunburst.com
e-mail: Service@sunburst.com
Mark Sotir, CEO
Katie Birmingham, Office Manager

This exciting investigation develops students' conceptual understanding that every fraction can be named in many different but equivalent ways.

2327 Factory Deluxe

Sunburst Technology
1550 Executive Drive
Elgin, IL 60123
888-492-8817
FAX 888-800-3028
http://www.sunburst.com
e-mail: Service@sunburst.com

Mark Sotir, CEO
Katie Birmingham, Office Manager
Five activities explore shapes, rotation, angles, geometric attributes, area formulas, and computation. Includes journal, record keeping, and on-screen help. This program helps sharpen geometry, visual thinking and problem solving skills.

2328 Fast-Track Fractions
SRA Order Services
220 East Danieldale Road
Desoto, TX 75115
888-772-4543
888-772-4543
FAX 972-228-1982
http://www.sraonline.com
e-mail: SRA_CustomerService@mcgraw-hill.com
Peter Sayeski, President

Students solve problems that compare, add, subtract, multiply and divide fractions. *$46.00*

2329 Fifth Through Seventh Grade Math Competencies
Aquarius Instructional
13064 Indian Rocks Road
Largo, FL 33774
727-593-2700
800-255-9085
FAX 877-595-2685
http://www.philliproy.com
e-mail: info@philliproy.com
Phillip Roy, Owner
Ruth Bragman, President
Ashley Sutton, Office Manager
Offers 32 disks on reading money values, ordering numbers, multiplying whole numbers, dividing whole numbers, adding and subtracting decimals and more. *$995.00*

2330 Fraction Attraction
Sunburst Technology
1550 Executive Drive
Elgin, IL 60123
203-446-8100
888-492-8817
FAX 888-800-3028
http://www.sunburst.com
e-mail: Service@sunburst.com
Mark Sotir, CEO
Katie Birmingham, Office Manager
Build the fraction skills of ordering, equivalence, relative sizes and multiple representations with four, multi-level, carnival style games.

2331 Fraction Fairy Tales with the Boars
Queue
1 Controls Drive
Shelton, CT 6484
800-232-2224
FAX 800-775-2729
http://www.queueinc.com
e-mail: jdk@queueinc.com
Monica Kantrowitz, President
Jonathan Kantrowitz, CEO
Peter Uhrynowski, Controller
The Boars teach students about fractions in their favorite fairy tale surroundings. *$39.95*

2332 Fraction Fuel-Up
SRA Order Services
220 East Danieldale Road
Desoto, TX 75115
888-772-4543
888-772-4543
FAX 972-228-1982
http://www.sraonline.com
e-mail: SRA_CustomerService@mcgraw-hill.com
Peter Sayeski, President

Players practice reducing, renaming, finding equivalent fractions and adding/subtracting fractions. *$46.00*

2333 Fraction Operations
Sunburst Technology
1550 Executive Drive
Elgin, IL 60123
888-492-8817
FAX 888-800-3028
http://www.sunburst.com
e-mail: Service@sunburst.com
Mark Sotir, CEO
Katie Birmingham, Office Manager
Students build on their concepts of fraction meaning and equivalence as they learn how to perform operations with fractions.

2334 Get Up and Go!
Sunburst Technology
1550 Executive Drive
Elgin, IL 60123
888-492-8817
FAX 888-800-3028
http://www.sunburst.com
e-mail: Service@sunburst.com
Mark Sotir, CEO
Katie Birmingham, Office Manager
Students interpret and construct timelines through three descriptive activities in the animated program. Students are introduced to timelines as they participate in an interactive story.

2335 Handling Money
Aquarius Instructional
13064 Indian Rocks Road
Largo, FL 33774
727-593-2700
800-255-9085
FAX 877-595-2685
http://www.philliproy.com
e-mail: info@philliproy.com
Phillip Roy, Owner
Ruth Bragman, President
Ashley Sutton, Office Manager
This program teaches students how to count money and make change in paper and coin. *$75.00*

2336 Hey, Taxi!
Queue
1 Controls Drive
Shelton, CT 6484
203-446-8100
800-232-2224
FAX 800-775-2729
http://www.qworkbooks.com
e-mail: jdk@queueinc.com
Monica Kantrowitz, President
Jonathan Kantrowitz, CEO
Peter Uhrynowski, Controller
Children maneuver their cab through the city streets to pick up passengers that solve basic math facts problems to collect their fares. *$39.95*

2337 Learning About Numbers
C&C Software
5713 Kentford Circle
Wichita, KS 67220
316-683-6056
800-752-2086
Carol Clark, President

Three segments use computer graphics to provide students with an experience in working with numbers. *$25.00*

2338 Math Machine
Software to Go-Gallaudet University
800 Florida Avenue, NE
Washington, DC 20002
202-651-5220
FAX 202-651-5109
http://http://clerccenter.gallaudet.edu
e-mail: Karen.Kautz@gallaudet.edu
Ken Kurlychek, Electron Information Specialists
Karen Kautz, Administrative Assistant

2339 Math Masters: Addition and Subtraction

SRA Order Services
220 E Danieldale Road
Desoto, TX 75115
888-SRA-4543
800-843-8855
FAX 972-228-1982
http://www.sraonline.com
e-mail: SRA_CustomerService@mcgraw-hill.com
Jerry Chaffin, Author

Designed to supplement math curriculum, this program covers addition and subtraction for all numbers from 0 through 25.

2340 Math Masters: Multiplication and Division

SRA Order Services
220 E Danieldale Road
Desoto, TX 75115
888-SRA-4543
800-843-8855
FAX 972-228-1982
http://www.sraonline.com
e-mail: SRA_CustomerService@mcgraw-hill.com
Jerry Chaffin, Author

Designed to supplement math curriculum, this program covers multiplication and division for all numbers from 0 through 25.

2341 Math Shop

Software to Go-Gallaudet University
800 Florida Avenue NE
Washington, DC 20002
202-651-5220
FAX 202-651-5109
http://http://clerccenter.gallaudet.edu
e-mail: products.clerccenter@gallaudet.edu
Ken Kurlychek, Electron Information Specialists
Karen Kautz, Administrative Assistant

2342 Math Skill Games

Software to Go-Gallaudet University
800 Florida Avenue NE
Washington, DC 20002
202-651-5220
FAX 202-651-5109
http://http://clerccenter.gallaudet.edu
e-mail: products.clerccenter@gallaudet.edu
Ken Kurlychek, Electron Information Specialists
Karen Kautz, Administrative Assistant

2343 Math for Everyday Living

Educational Activities Software
PO Box 87
Baldwin, NY 11510
516-867-7878
1-800-797-32
FAX 1-516-623-92
http://www.edact.com
e-mail: learn@edact.com

Ann Edson, Author
Alan Stern, Manager

Designed for secondary students, a tutorial and practice program with simulated activities for applying math skills in making change, working with sales slips, unit pricing, computing gas mileage and sales tax. *$129.00*

2344 Mighty Math Astro Algebra

Riverdeep
222 3rd Avenue SE
Cedar Rapids, IA 52401
319-395-9626
800-362-2890
FAX 319-395-0217
http://www.riverdeep.net
e-mail: info@riverdeep.net
Barry O'Callaghan, Executive Chairman & Chief Execu
Jim Ruddy, Chief Revenue Officer

In Astro Algebra, you're the captain of the Algebra Centauri spaceship! Traveling through the galaxy, you meet fascinating alien species and use algebra to help them out of predicaments. Four expert crew members Skler, Max, Mialee and Tyric are standing by to help you understand, strategize, calculate and check your work. *$59.95*

2345 Mighty Math Calculating Crew

Riverdeep
222 3rd Avenue SE
Cedar Rapids, IA 52401
319-395-9626
800-362-2890
FAX 319-395-0217
http://www.riverdeep.net
e-mail: info@riverdeep.net
Barry O'Callaghan, Executive Chairman & Chief Execu
Jim Ruddy, Chief Revenue Officer

Calculating Crew teaches your 3rd, 4th, 5th, or 6th grader the concepts, facts and thinking skills necessary to build math confidence and develop a strong, lasting understanding of math! Wanda Wavelet, Captain Nick Knack and Dr. Gee guide your child through thousands of skill-building problems! *$59.95*

2346 Mighty Math Carnival Countdown

Riverdeep
222 3rd Avenue SE
Cedar Rapids, IA 52401
319-395-9626
800-362-2890
FAX 319-395-0217
http://www.riverdeep.net
e-mail: info@riverdeep.net
Barry O'Callaghan, Executive Chairman & Chief Execu
Jim Ruddy, Chief Revenue Officer

Kids love to visit Carnival Countdown, where addition, subtraction, early multiplication, division and logic are always center ring! This breakthrough math progam offers your child three years of math learning and ensures math success by teaching kindergarten through 2nd grade math concepts and problem-solving. With Carnival Countdown, learning math is as much fun as a trip to the circus! *$59.95*

2347 Mighty Math Cosmic Geometry

Riverdeep
222 3rd Avenue SE
Cedar Rapids, IA 52401
319-395-9626
800-362-2890
FAX 319-395-0217
http://www.riverdeep.net
e-mail: info@riverdeep.net
Barry O'Callaghan, Executive Chairman & Chief Execu
Jim Ruddy, Chief Revenue Officer

Cosmic Gemetry teaches you the concepts and problem-solving skills you need to master geometry and build math confidence! Polyhedral characters such as Dodeca, Hexa and Lcosa are your guides on this fun-filled exploration of Planet Geometry. *$59.95*

2348 Mighty Math Number Heroes

Riverdeep
222 3rd Avenue SE
Cedar Rapids, IA 52401
319-395-9626
800-362-2890
FAX 319-395-0217
http://www.riverdeep.net
e-mail: info@riverdeep.net
Barry O'Callaghan, Executive Chairman & Chief Execu
Jim Ruddy, Chief Revenue Officer

Number Heroes teaches kids the basics and problem-solving skills they need to succeed in math. With the help of Fraction Man, Star Brilliant and other math superheroes, kids understand dozens of math concepts and solve thousands of problems while learning multiplication and division, fractions, 2D geometry and probability. Help your children master 3rd through 6th-grade math with the Number Heroes! *$59.95*

2349 Mighty Math Zoo Zillions
Riverdeep
222 3rd Avenue SE
Cedar Rapids, IA 52401
319-395-9626
800-362-2890
FAX 319-395-0217
http://www.riverdeep.net
e-mail: info@riverdeep.net
Barry O'Callaghan, Executive Chairman & Chief Execu
Jim Ruddy, Chief Revenue Officer

Mighty Math Zoo Zillions teaches your kindergartener, 1st grader or 2nd grader the concepts, facts and thinking skills necessary to build math confidence and develop a strong, lasting understanding of math! Armadillo Annie, the Otter Twins and other animal friends guide your child on this exciting mathematical adventure! *$59.95*

2350 Millie's Math House
Riverdeep
222 3rd Avenue SE
Cedar Rapids, IA 52401
319-395-9626
800-362-2890
FAX 319-395-0217
http://www.riverdeep.net
e-mail: info@riverdeep.net
Tina Martin, Education Marketing

Now featuring addition, subtraction and counting to 30, the award-winning Millie's Math House has been enhanced to offer even more learning! In seven activities, children explore numbers, shapes, sizes, patterns, addition and subtraction as they build mouse houses, create wacky bugs, count animated critters, make jellybean cookies and answer math challenges posed by Dorothy the Duck! *$59.95*

2351 Number Farm
Software to Go-Gallaudet University
800 Florida Avenue NE
Washington, DC 20002
202-651-5220
FAX 202-651-5109
http://http://clerccenter.gallaudet.edu
e-mail: products.clerccenter@gallaudet.edu
Ken Kurlychek, Electron Information Specialists
Karen Kautz, Administrative Assistant

2352 Number Please
Merit Software
121 West 27th Street
New York, NY 10001
212-675-8567
800-753-6488
FAX 212-675-8607
http://www.meritsoftware.com
e-mail: sales@meritsoftware.com
Ben Weintraub, Chief Executive Officer

Students are challenged to remember combinations of 4, 7 and 10 digit numbers. *$9.95*

2353 Number Sense and Problem Solving
Sunburst Technology
1550 Executive Drive
Elgin, IL 60123
888-492-8817
FAX 888-800-3028
http://www.sunburst.com
e-mail: Service@sunburst.com
Mark Sotir, President
Tara Green, Marketing Executive
Katie Birmingham, Office Manager
Build number and operation skills with these three programs: How the West Was One + Three x Four, Divide and Conquer and Puzzle Tank.

2354 Number Stumper
Software to Go-Gallaudet University
800 Florida Avenue NE
Washington, DC 20002
202-651-5220
FAX 202-651-5109
http://www.clerccenter.gallaudet.edu
e-mail: afbinfo@afb.net
Ken Kurlychek, Project Coordinator
Karen Kauutz, Administrative Assistant

2355 Optimum Resource
18 Hunter Road
Hilton Head Island, SC 29926
843-689-8000
888-784-2592
FAX 843-689-8008
http://www.stickybear.com
e-mail: stickyb@stickybear.com
Christopher Gintz, CEO
Robert Stangroom, Product Manager

An educational software publishing company for grades K-12. Our software titles are available in Consumer, School, Labpack or Site License versions. Please call for further details. Prices range from $59.95 for Consumer to $699.95 for Site Licenses.

2356 Race Car 'rithmetic
Software to Go-Gallaudet University
800 Florida Avenue NE
Washington, DC 20002
202-651-5220
FAX 202-651-5109
http://www.clerccenter.gallaudet.edu
e-mail: afbinfo@afb.net
Ken Kurlychek, Project Coordinator
Karen Kauutz, Administrative Assistant

2357 Read and Solve Math Problems #1
Educational Activities
P.O. Box 87
Baldwin, NY 11510
516-223-4666
800-797-3223
FAX 516-623-9282
http://www.edact.com
e-mail: learn@edact.com
Ann Edson, Author
Alfred Harris, President
Rose Falco, Sales/Marketing Director

A tutorial and practice program for students which focuses on recognition of key words in solving arithmetic word problems, writing equations and solving word problems. *$109.00*

2358 Read and Solve Math Problems #2
Educational Activities
P.O. Box 87
Baldwin, NY 11510
516-223-4666
800-797-3223
FAX 516-623-9282
http://www.edact.com
e-mail: learn@edact.com
Ann Edson, Author
Alfred Harris, President
Rose Falco, Sales/Marketing Director

A tutorial and practice program for students which focuses on recognition of key words in solving two-step arithmetic problems, writing equations and solving two-step word problems. *$109.00*

2359 Read and Solve Math Problems #3 Fractions, Two-Step Problems
Educational Activities
P.O. Box 87
Baldwin, NY 11510
516-223-4666
800-797-3223
FAX 516-623-9282
http://www.edact.com
e-mail: learn@edact.com
Ann Edson, Author
Alfred Harris, President
Rose Falco, Sales/Marketing Director

Designed for students, this tutorial and practice program provides initial instruction and experience in critical thinking and problem-solving using fractions and mixed numbers. *$109.00*

2360 Shape Up!
Sunburst Technology
1550 Executive Drive
Elgin, IL 60123
914-747-3310
888-492-8817
FAX 888-800-3028
http://www.sunburst.com
e-mail: Service@sunburst.com
Mark Sotir, President
Tara Green, Marketing Executive
Katie Birmingham, Office Manager
Students actively create and manipulate shapes to discover important ideas about mathematics in an electronic playground of two and three dimensional shapes.

2361 Spatial Sense CD-ROM
Sunburst Technology
1550 Executive Drive
Elgin, IL 60123
914-747-3310
888-492-8817
FAX 888-800-3028
http://www.sunburst.com
e-mail: Service@sunburst.com
Mark Sotir, President
Tara Green, Marketing Executive
Katie Birmingham, Office Manager
Your students will strenghten their spatial perception, spatial reasoning and problem-solving skills with three great programs now on one CD-ROM.

2362 Splish Splash Math
Sunburst Technology
1550 Executive Drive
Elgin, IL 60123
914-747-3310
888-492-8817
FAX 888-800-3028
http://www.sunburst.com
e-mail: Service@sunburst.com
Mark Sotir, President
Tara Green, Marketing Executive
Katie Birmingham, Office Manager
Students learn and practice basic operation skills as they engage in this high interest program that keeps them motivated. Great visual rewards and three levels of difficulty keep students challanged.

2363 This Old Man
UCLA Intervention Program for Handicapped Children
1000 Veteran Avenue
Los Angeles, CA 90024
562-825-4821
FAX 310-206-7744
http://www.bol.ucla.edu
Kit Kehr, Executive Director

Uses the song This Old Man in singing and signing to teach numbers and counting 1-10. *$35.00*

2364 WORLD*CLASS Learning Materials
World Class Learning
406 Main Street
Reisterstown, MD 21136
800-638-6470
FAX 800-638-6499
http://www.wclm.com
e-mail: dealers@wclm.comjdash@wclm.com
Paul Edwards, Author
Bruce Brown, President

Designed for secondary students and adults, this program focuses on personal financial management, comparison shopping and calculation of essential banking transactions.

2365 Zap! Around Town
Sunburst Technology
1550 Executive Drive
Elgin, IL 60123
914-747-3310
888-492-8817
FAX 888-800-3028
http://www.sunburst.com
e-mail: Service@sunburst.com
Mark Sotir, President
Tara Green, Marketing Executive
Katie Birmingham, Office Manager
Students develop mapping and direction skills in this easy-to-use, animated program featuring Shelby, your friendly Sunbuddy guide.

Preschool

2366 Creature Series
Laureate Learning Systems
110 East Spring Street
Winooski, VT 5404
802-655-4755
800-562-6801
FAX 802-655-4757
http://www.laureatelearning.com
e-mail: info@laureatelearning.com
Mary Wilson, Owner
Bernard Fox, Vice President

Programs designed to improve visual and auditory attention and teach cause and effect, turn taking, and switch use. *$95.00*

2367 Curious George Visits the Library
Software to Go-Gallaudet University
800 Florida Avenue NE
Washington, DC 20002
202-651-5220
FAX 202-651-5109
http://www.clerccenter.gallaudet.edu
e-mail: afbinfo@afb.net
Ken Kurlychek, Project Coordinator
Karen Kauutz, Administrative Assistant

2368 Dinosaur Game
UCLA Intervention Program for Handicapped Children
1000 Veteran Avenue
Los Angeles, CA 90024
562-825-4821
FAX 310-206-7744
http://www.bol.ucla.edu
Kit Kehr, Executive Director

Game board format where dinosaurs race each other home. Children press their switches to spin a spinner which randomly selects the color of the square. Children then move their dinosaurs by pressing their switches. Accommodates 1-4 players. *$35.00*

2369 Early Discoveries: Size and Logic
Software to Go-Gallaudet University
800 Florida Avenue NE
Washington, DC 20002
202-651-5220
FAX 202-651-5109
http://www.clerccenter.gallaudet.edu
e-mail: afbinfo@afb.net
Ken Kurlychek, Project Coordinator
Karen Kauutz, Administrative Assistant

2370 Early Emerging Rules Series
Laureate Learning Systems
110 East Spring Street
Winooski, VT 5404
802-655-4755
800-562-6801
FAX 802-655-4757
http://www.laureatelearning.com
e-mail: info@laureatelearning.com

Mary Wilson, Owner
Bernard Fox, Vice President

Three programs that introduce early developing grammatical constructions and facilitate the transition from single words to word combinations. *$175.00*

2371 Early Learning I
MarbleSoft
12301 Central Avenue NE
Blaine, MN 55434
763-755-1402
FAX 763-862-2920
http://www.marblesoft.com
e-mail: mail@marblesoft.com
Valerie Reit, Sales

Early Learning 2.0 includes four activities that teach prereading skills. Single and dual-switch scanning are built in and special prompts allow blind students to use all levels of difficulty. Includes Matching Colors, Learning Shapes, Counting Numbers and Letter Match. Runs on Macintosh and Windows computers. *$70.00*

2372 Early Music Skills
Electronic Courseware Systems
1713 S State Street
Champaign, IL 61820
217-359-7099
800-832-4965
FAX 217-359-6578
http://www.ecsmedia.com
e-mail: sales@ecsmedia.com
G Peters, President

Covers four basic music reading skills. *$39.95*

2373 Early and Advanced Switch Games
RJ Cooper & Associates
27601 Forbes Road
Laguna Niguel, CA 92677
949-582-2571
800-752-6673
FAX 949-582-3169
http://www.rjcooper.com
e-mail: info@rjcooper.com
RJ Cooper, Owner

Thirteen single switch games that start at cause/effect, work through timing and selection and graduate with matching and manipulation tasks. *$75.00*

2374 Edustar's Early Childhood Special Education Programs

Edustar America
6220 S Orange Blossom Trail
Orlando, FL 32809
561-638-8733
800-952-3041
FAX 561-330-0849
David Zeldin, Marketing Manager
Stewart Holtz, Curriculum Director

Integrated software program that incorporates manipulatives and special tables for learning early childhood subjects. Features include an illuminated six key keyboard. A special U-shaped touch table for the physically challenged and changeable mats and keys for different subject areas.

2375 Electric Coloring Book
Heartsoft
8252 S Harvard Avenue
Tulsa, OK 74137
918-494-7878
800-285-3475
FAX 800-285-4018
http://www.heartsoft.com
e-mail: sales@heartsoft.com
Benjamin P. Shell Jr., President and Chief Executive Of
Juanita L. Seng, Vice President of Sales and Mark

Teaches young students the alphabet, numbers and basic keyboarding skills by using a graphic coloring concept. *$39.95*

2376 If You're Happy and You Know It
UCLA Intervention Program for Handicapped Children
1000 Veteran Avenue
Los Angeles, CA 90095
562-825-4821
800-899-6687
FAX 310-206-7744
http://www.bol.ucla.edu
e-mail: consult@ucla.edu
Norman Abrams, Chancellor
Scott Waugh, Executive Vice Chancellor

A nursery school song with five verses depicted in picture form. *$35.00*

2377 Joystick Games
Technology for Language and Learning
PO Box 327
East Rockaway, NY 11518
516-625-4550
FAX 516-621-3321
Joan Tanenhaus, Founder

Five volumes of public domain joystick programs. *$28.50*

2378 Kindercomp Gold
Software to Go-Gallaudet University
800 Florida Avenue NE
Washington, DC 20002
202-651-5220
FAX 202-651-5109
http://www.clerccenter.gallaudet.edu
Ken Kurlychek, Electronic Information Specialis
Karen Kautz, Administrative Secretary

2379 Old MacDonald's Farm Deluxe
KidTECH
4300 Stine Road
Bakersfield, CA 93313
661-396-8676
FAX 661-396-8760
http://www.softtouch.com
e-mail: sales@softtouch.com
Joyce Meyer, President

Utilizes the all-time favorite children's song to teach vocabulary and animal sounds to young children. *$30.00*

2380 Old MacDonald's Farm I
UCLA Intervention Program for Handicapped Children
1000 Veteran Avenue
Los Angeles, CA 90095
562-825-4821
800-899-6687
FAX 310-206-7744
http://www.bol.ucla.edu
e-mail: consult@ucla.edu
Norman Abrams, Chancellor
Scott Waugh, Executive Vice Chancellor

Nursery School song depicting a farmer, his wife, and 6 farm animals — cow, sheep, rooster, pig, and duck — displayed on as overlay. Level I, the child selects any animal. Level II, the child selects an animal by name. Level III, the child selects an animal by its sound. *$35.00*

2381 Optimum Resource
18 Hunter Road
Hilton Head Island, SC 29926
843-689-8000
888-784-2592
FAX 843-689-8008
http://www.stickybear.com
e-mail: stickyb@stickybear.com
Christopher Gintz, CEO
Robert Stangroom, Publisher

An educational software publishing company for grades K-12. Our software titles are available in Consumer, School, Labpack or Site License versions. Please call for further details. Prices range from $59.95 for Consumer to $699.95 for Site Licenses.

2382 Padded Vehicles
UCLA Intervention Program for Handicapped Children
1000 Veteran Avenue
Los Angeles, CA 90024
562-825-4821
800-899-6687
FAX 310-206-7744
http://www.bol.ucla.edu
e-mail: consult@ucla.edu
Norman Abrams, Chancellor
Scott Waugh, Executive Vice Chancellor

Children identify 10 vehicles — airplane, helicopter, motorcycle, police car, truck, ambulance, garbage truck, school bus, fire engine, and tractor — which are depicted on an overlay. Level I, the child selects any vehicle. Level II, the child selects the vehicle by name. *$35.00*

2383 Shape and Color Rodeo
SRA Order Services
220 East Danieldale Road
Desoto, TX 75115
888-772-4543
800-843-8855
FAX 972-228-1892
http://www.sraonline.com
e-mail: SRA_CustomerService@mcgraw-hill.com
Peter Sayeski, President

Children learn recognition and identification of common shapes and color discriminations. *$35.00*

2384 Silly Sandwich
UCLA Intervention Program for Handicapped Children
1000 Veteran Avenue
Los Angeles, CA 90095
562-825-4821
800-899-6687
FAX 310-206-7744
http://www.bol.ucla.edu
e-mail: consult@ucla.edu
Norman Abrams, Chancellor
Scott Waugh, Executive Vice Chancellor

Build a silly sandwich selecting from six to twelve different items depicted on a PowerPad overlay. *$35.00*

2385 Switch It - Change It
UCLA Intervention Program for Handicapped Children
1000 Veteran Avenue
Los Angeles, CA 90095
562-825-4821
800-899-6687
FAX 310-206-7744
http://www.bol.ucla.edu
e-mail: consult@ucla.edu
Norman Abrams, Chancellor
Scott Waugh, Executive Vice Chancellor

Cause and effect program presents color-animated common objects. *$35.00*
Mac

2386 Trudy's Time and Place House
Riverdeep
222 3rd Avenue SE
Cedar Rapids, IA 52401
319-395-9626
800-362-2890
FAX 800-567-2714
http://www.riverdeep.net
Barry O'Callaghan, Executive Chairman & CEO
Jim Ruddy, Chief Revenue Officer

In Trudy's Time and Place House, children enjoy exploring geography and time with Trudy's whimsical friends! Ann and Dan, Joe Crow and Nellie the Elephant invite kids to: build time-telling skills; develop mapping and direction skills; and travel the world learning about continents, oceans and landmarks. *$59.95*

2387 Wheels on the Bus I: Intellipics Activity
UCLA Intervention Program for Handicapped Children
1000 Veteran Avenue
Los Angeles, CA 90095
562-825-4821
800-899-6687
FAX 310-206-7744
http://www.bol.ucla.edu
e-mail: consult@ucla.edu
Norman Abrams, Chancellor
Scott Waugh, Executive Vice Chancellor

This native Macintosh activity requires Intellipics to run. It includes 6 verses (Baby, Bus, Doors, Horn, Kids, Mommy) with digitalized sound and color animations. It can be used with intellipics options such as color and a number selection, and includes both free choice and quiz options. *$25.00*

2388 Wheels on the Bus II
UCLA Intervention Program for Handicapped Children
1000 Veteran Avenue
Los Angeles, CA 90095
562-825-4821
800-899-6687
FAX 310-206-7744
http://www.bol.ucla.edu
e-mail: consult@ucla.edu
Norman Abrams, Chancellor
Scott Waugh, Executive Vice Chancellor

Popular nursery school song that is activated to sing 5 verses by pressing the corresponding picture on an overlay. Verses are driver, wheel, wiper, windows, daddy. *$36.00*

2389 Wheels on the Bus III
UCLA Intervention Program for Handicapped Children
1000 Veteran Avenue
Los Angeles, CA 90095
562-825-4821
800-899-6687
FAX 310-206-7744
http://www.bol.ucla.edu
e-mail: consult@ucla.edu
Norman Abrams, Chancellor
Scott Waugh, Executive Vice Chancellor

Popular nursery school song that is activated to sing 5 verses of the song by pressing the corresponding picture on an overlay. Verses are: People, money, brakes, seatbelt, wheelchair lift. *$36.00*

2390 Where is Puff?
UCLA Intervention Program for Handicapped Children
1000 Veteran Avenue
Los Angeles, CA 90095
562-825-4821
800-899-6687
FAX 310-206-7744
http://www.bol.ucla.edu
e-mail: consult@ucla.edu
Norman Abrams, Chancellor
Scott Waugh, Executive Vice Chancellor

Early preposition program that includes six prepositions illustrated by Puff the cat: in, on, next to, under, in front of, in back of. Features include: scan speed selection and data collection. *$35.00*

2391 Word Pieces
Software to Go-Gallaudet University
800 Florida Avenue NE
Washington, DC 20002
202-651-5220
FAX 202-651-5109
http://www.clerccenter.gallaudet.edu
Ken Kurlychek, Electronic Information Specialis
Karen Kautz, Administrative Secretary

Problem Solving

2392 Captain's Log
BrainTrain
727 Twinridge Lane
Richmond, VA 23235
804-320-0120
800-822-0538
FAX 804-320-0242
http://www.braintrain.com
e-mail: info@braintrain.com

Joseph Sandford, Director
Virginia Sandford, Sales/Marketing VP

A comprehensive, multilevel computerized mental gym to help people with brain injuries, learning disabilities, developmental disabilities, ADD, ADHD and psychiatric disorders improve their cognitive skills. *$2695.00*

ISBN 3-490019-95-0

2393 Changes Around Us CD-ROM
Steck-Vaughn Company
6277 Sea Harbor Dr.
Orlando, FL 32887 407-345-3800
800-531-5015
FAX 800-699-9459
http://www.steck-vaughn.com
e-mail: info@steck-vaughn.com
Connie Alden, Vice President of Human Resource

Nature is the natural choice for observing change. By observing and researching dramatic visual sequences such as the stages of development of a butterfly, children develop a broad understanding of the concept of change. As they search this multimedia database for images and information about plant and animal life cycles and seasonal change, students strengthen their abilities in research, analysis, problem-solving, critical thinking and communication.

2394 Factory Deluxe: Grades 4 to 8
Sunburst Technology
1550 Executive Drive
Elgin, IL 60123
888-492-8817
FAX 888-800-3028
http://www.sunburst.com
e-mail: Service@sunburst.com
Mark Sotir, CEO
Katie Birmingham, Office Manager
Five activities explore shapes, rotation, angles, geometric attributes, area formulas, and computation. Includes journal, record keeping, and on-screen help. This program helps sharpen geometry, visual thinking and problem solving skills.

2395 Freddy's Puzzling Adventures
SRA Order Services
220 East Danieldale Road
Desoto, TX 75115 888-SRA-4543
800-843-8855
FAX 972-228-1892
http://www.sraonline.com
e-mail: SRA_CustomerService@mcgraw-hill.com
Peter Sayeski, President

Helps students acquire problem solving and logical thinking skills with three activities. *$34.00*

2396 Guessing and Thinking
Software to Go-Gallaudet University
800 Florida Avenue NE
Washington, DC 20002 202-651-5231
FAX 202-651-5109
http://http://clerccenter.gallaudet.edu
e-mail: products.clerccenter@gallaudet.edu
Ken Kurlychek, Electronic Information Specialis
Karen Kautz, Admin. Secretary I

2397 High School Math Bundle
Sunburst Technology
1550 Executive Drive
Elgin, IL 60123
888-492-8817
FAX 888-800-3028
http://www.sunburst.com
e-mail: Service@sunburst.com
Mark Sotir, CEO
Mike Gavelek, Vice President of Marketing
Katie Birmingham, Office Manager

Each program in this bundle focuses on a specific area to ensure that your students master the math skills they need. This bundle allows students to master basics of Algebra, explore equations and graphs, practice learning with algebra graphs, use trigonometric functions, apply math concepts to practical situations and improve problem solving and data analysis skills.

2398 Ice Cream Truck
Sunburst Technology
1550 Executive Drive
Elgin, IL 60123
888-492-8817
FAX 888-800-3028
http://www.sunburst.com
e-mail: Service@sunburst.com
Mark Sotir, CEO
Mike Gavelek, Vice President of Marketing
Katie Birmingham, Office Manager
Elementary students learn important problem solving, strategic planning and math operation skills, as they become owners of a busy ice cream truck.

2399 Lesson Maker: Do-It-Yourself Computer Program
Harris Communications
15155 Technology Drive
Eden Prairie, MN 55344 952-906-1180
800-825-6758
FAX 952-906-1099
TDY:952-906-1198
http://www.harriscomm.com
e-mail: info@harriscomm.com
Robert Harris, Owner
Bill Williams, National Sales Manager

For teachers, parents and students who want to create their own computer lessons. Choose any topic from Vocabulary to Volcanoes. For each lesson enter eight of your own questions or prompts with eight answers or desired responses. Lesson Maker automatically inputs information into 4 separate fun games for each lesson: Spinmeister; Matching; Paired Squares; and Pop Quiz. Up to 15 individual lessons can be made for one Unit. *$24.95*
Diskettes

2400 Memory Match
Software to Go-Gallaudet University
800 Florida Avenue NE
Washington, DC 20002 202-651-5231
FAX 202-651-5109
http://http://clerccenter.gallaudet.edu
e-mail: products.clerccenter@gallaudet.edu
Ken Kurlychek, Electronic Information Specialis
Karen Kautz, Admin. Secretary I

2401 Memory: A First Step in Problem Solving
Software to Go-Gallaudet University
800 Florida Avenue NE
Washington, DC 20002 202-651-5220
FAX 202-651-5109
http://www.clerccenter.gallaudet.edu
Ken Kurlychek, Electronic Information Specialis
Karen Kautz, Admin. Secretary I

2402 Merit Software
Merit Software
121 West 27th Street
New York, NY 10001 212-675-8567
800-753-6488
FAX 212-675-8607
http://www.meritsoftware.com
Ben Weintraub, Marketing Manager

Deductive logic and problem solving are the primary skills developed in the variation of the game MASTERMIND. *$9.95*

2403 Middle School Math Bundle
Sunburst Technology
1550 Executive Drive
Elgin, IL 60123
888-492-8817
FAX 888-800-3028
http://www.sunburst.com
e-mail: Service@sunburst.com
Mark Sotir, CEO
Mike Gavelek, Vice President of Marketing
Katie Birmingham, Office Manager
This bundle helps improve student's logical thinking, number sense and operation skills. This product comes with Math Arena, Building Perspective Deluxe, Equation Tile Teasers and Easy Sheet.

2404 Nordic Software
PO Box 5403
Lincoln, NE 68505
402-489-1557
800-306-6502
FAX 402-489-1560
http://www.nordicsoftware.com
e-mail: webmaster@nordicsoftware.com
James Wrenholt, Owner/President

Develops and publishes entertaining, educational software. Children ages three and up can build math skills, expand their vocabulary and increase proficiency in spelling, among other subjects. *$59.95*

2405 Number Sense & Problem Solving CD-ROM
Sunburst Technology
1550 Executive Drive
Elgin, IL 60123
888-492-8817
FAX 888-800-3028
http://www.sunburst.com
e-mail: Service@sunburst.com
Mark Sotir, CEO
Mike Gavelek, Vice President of Marketing
Katie Birmingham, Office Manager
Build number and operation skills with these three programs: How the West Was One + Three x Four, Divide and Conquer and Puzzle Tank.

2406 Problem Solving
Psychological Software Services
6555 Carrollton Avenue
Indianapolis, IN 46220
317-257-9672
FAX 317-257-9674
http://www.neuroscience.cnter.com
e-mail: nsc@neuroscience.cnter.com
Odie Bracy PhD HSPP, Director, Clinical Neuropsycholo
Nancy Bracy, Office Manager

Nine computer programs designed to challenge high functioning patients/students with tasks requiring logic. *$150.00*

2407 Single Switch Games
MarbleSoft
12301 Central Avenue NE
Blaine, MN 55434
763-755-1402
FAX 763-862-2920
http://www.marblesoft.com
e-mail: mail@marblesoft.com
Valerie Reit, Sales

There's a lot of educational software for single switch users, but how about something that's just for fun? We've taken some games similar to the ones you enjoyed as a kid and made them work just right for single switch users. Includes Single Switch Maze, A Frog's Life, Switching Lanes, Switch Invaders, Slingshot Gallery and Scurry. Runs on Macintosh and Windows computers. *$30.00*

2408 Sliding Block
Merit Software
121 West 27th Street
New York, NY 10001
212-675-8567
800-753-6488
FAX 212-675-8607
http://www.meritsoftware.com
Ben Weintraub, Marketing Manager

Learners rearrange one of the four pictures which can be scrambled at five separate levels to test visual discrimination and problem solving skills. *$9.95*

2409 SmartDriver
BrainTrain
727 Twinridge Lane
Richmond, VA 23235
804-320-0120
800-822-0538
FAX 804-320-0242
http://www.braintrain.com
e-mail: info@braintrain.com
Joseph Sandford, Owner/President
Virginia Sandford, Sales/Marketing VP

Visual attention building software where you 'win' by driving defensively and following the rules of the road. Children love this driving game that teaches visual attention, visual tracking, patience, following the rules, planning, and hand-eye coordination.

2410 SoundSmart
BrainTrain
727 Twinridge Lane
Richmond, VA 23235
804-320-0120
800-822-0538
FAX 804-320-0242
http://www.braintrain.com
e-mail: info@braintrain.com
Joseph Sandford, Owner/President
Virginia Sandford, Sales/Marketing VP

Auditory Attention Building software to help improve phonenic awareness, listening skills, working memory, mental processing speech and self-control. *$549.00*

2411 Strategy Challenges Collection: 1
Riverdeep
222 3rd Avenue SE
Cedar Rapids, IA 52401
319-395-9626
800-362-2890
FAX 319 395 0217
http://www.riverdeep.net
e-mail: info@riverdeep.net
Barry O'Callaghn, CEO

Play Mancala, Go-Muku and Nine Men's Morris- the three games in Strategy Challenges Collection 1 against Game Masters from around the world! Why? Because you'll learn important problem-solving and strategies thinking skills you can use throughout life in games, in school and in jobs. *$39.95*

2412 Strategy Challenges Collection: 2
Riverdeep
222 3rd Avenue SE
Cedar Rapids, IA 52401
319-395-9626
800-362-2890
FAX 319-395-0217
http://www.riverdeep.net
e-mail: info@riverdeep.net
Barry O'Callaghn, CEO

Strategy Challenges Collection: 2 — featuring Jungle Chess, Surakarta and Tablut — boosts your thinking power! How does it work? Six diverse Opponents challenge you to build a repertoire of powerful problem-solving strategies and skills. You'll also meet Strategy Coaches who offer offensive and defensive tips that can improve your game and be applied throughout life. *$39.95*

2413 Switch Arcade
UCLA Intervention Program for Handicapped Children
1000 Veteran Avenue
Los Angeles, CA 90024
310-825-4821
FAX 310-206-7744
http://www.bol.ucla.edu
e-mail: consult@ucla.edu
Kit Kehr, Coordinator

Three switch games are presented: Tug of War; Racing; Fishing. The racing game allows children to choose from several racers including cars, wheelchairs, and animals using a single switch. The game is designed for two players using two switches to play competitive, cooperative games together. Can be used to promote social interaction and eye-hand coordination. *$45.00*

Mac

2414 **Thinkin' Things C1 Toony the Loons Lagoon**
Riverdeep
222 3rd Avenue SE
Cedar Rapids, IA 52401
319-395-9626
800-362-2890
FAX 319-395-0217
http://www.riverdeep.net
e-mail: info@riverdeep.net
Barry O'Callaghan, Executive Chairman & Chief Execu
Jim Ruddy, Chief Revenue Officer

Toony the Loon's Lagoon sparkles with dozens of fun loving characters and activities that help kids learn how to be better thinkers. Toony, Oranga and other jungle friends guide your child toward success in six unique locations — plus there's a fun, new online puzzle each week.

2415 **Thinkin' Things Collection 3: Galactic**
Riverdeep
222 3rd Avenue SE
Cedar Rapids, IA 52401
319-395-9626
800-362-2890
FAX 319-395-0217
http://www.riverdeep.net
e-mail: info@riverdeep.net
Barry O'Callaghan, Executive Chairman & Chief Execu
Jim Ruddy, Chief Revenue Officer

Become a strong thinker with Thinkin' Things Collection 3 and build thinking skills you can use wherever you are in anything you do! Make trades with brokers from around the world, program a half-time show and solve the Case of the Empty Fripple House. You'll improve deductive and inductive reasoning, synthesis and analysis, while building problem-solving skills essential for success!

2416 **Thinkin' Things: All Around Frippletown**
Riverdeep
222 3rd Avenue SE
Cedar Rapids, IA 52401
319-395-9626
800-825-4420
FAX 319-395-0217
http://www.riverdeep.net
e-mail: info@riverdeep.net
Barry O'Callaghn, CEO

Welcome to FrippleTown, where dozens of fun-loving Fripples will tickle your funny bone and challenge your brain. Discover and use the best of your creative thinking skills! Think through problems and explore solutions to furnish the Fripples with artful flags, crazy cookies, door-to-door surprises and more. Every visit to FrippleTown is a chance to discover something new.

2417 **Thinkin' Things: Collection 1**
Riverdeep
222 3rd Avenue SE
Cedar Rapids, IA 52401
319-395-9626
800-825-4420
FAX 319-395-0217
http://www.riverdeep.net
e-mail: info@riverdeep.net
Barry O'Callaghn, CEO

Good thinkers learn quickly, adapt to change easily and accomplish remarkable things. That's why we created Thinkin' Things Collection 1, a powerful set of tools and toys to help children strengthen observation and memory, improve problem solving and encourage creativity. Thinkin' Things Collection 1 will help your child build a solid foundation for successful learning!

2418 **Thinkin' Things: Collection 2**
Riverdeep
222 3rd Avenue SE
Cedar Rapids, IA 52401
319-395-9626
800-362-2890
FAX 319-395-0217
http://www.riverdeep.net
e-mail: info@riverdeep.net
Barry O'Callaghan, Executive Chairman & Chief Execu
Jim Ruddy, Chief Revenue Officer

In this rapidly changing world, kids with strong thinking skills will thrive and excel. That's why the educators at Edmark developed Thinkin' Things Collection 2, a powerful set of tools and toys that strengthen observation and analysis, develop spatial awareness, improve memory and foster creativity. With a strong grasp of these skills, your child is ready to succeed!

2419 **Thinkin' Things: Sky Island Mysteries**
Riverdeep
222 3rd Avenue SE
Cedar Rapids, IA 52401
319-395-9626
800-362-2890
FAX 319-395-0217
http://www.riverdeep.net
e-mail: info@riverdeep.net
Barry O'Callaghan, Executive Chairman & Chief Execu
Jim Ruddy, Chief Revenue Officer

Inspector Cluestoe needs help cracking 14 zany mysteries to nab a slew of crafty culprits. Visit each island and put your best thinking skills to work to collect the clues! Prioritize tasks, apply your powers of observation and logic, and draw valid conclusions to solve the mysteries of the Sky Islands.

Professional Resources

2420 **Accurate Assessments**
1016 Leavenworth Street
Omaha, NE 68102
1-402-341-88
800-324-7966
FAX 402-341-8911
http://www.myaccucare.com
e-mail: info@orionhealthcare.com
Bill Allen, Owner

Accurate Assessments offers a full range of superior innovative technological services and expertise to the behavioral health industry. Our premier product, AccuCare Behavioral Healthcare System, was developed by teams of experts in their respective fields, insuring our products are truly useful to clinicians and are easy to use. This innovative software program is a comprehensive and adaptable approach to the behavioral health practice environment.

2421 **Analytic Learning Disability Assessment Computer Report**
Southern Micro Systems
4265 Brownsboro Road
Winston-Salem, NC 27106
336-759-7477
FAX 336-759-7212
http://www.smsi.net
Sandra Miller Jones, Chairman and Founder
Lafayette Jones, President and CEO

This software provides an interpretation of the ALDA assessment results. The report describes to the professional the most efficient method for this child to learn the basic subjects of Reading, Spelling, Math and Handwriting. The report can be given to the professional or parent and may be used to design remedial approaches and improve academic functioning. *$195.00*

2422 **Beyond Drill and Practice: Expanding the Computer Mainstream**
Council for Exceptional Children
655 Tyee Road
Victoria, BC V9A 6X5
250-412-3258
888-232-7733
FAX 703-264-9494
http://www.abebooks.com/sell
e-mail: sellbooks@abebooks.com
Richard Davies, PR & Publicity Manager
Bruce Ramirez, Manager

Provides informative guidelines and examples for teachers who want to expand the use of the computer as a learning tool. *$10.00*

120 pages

2423 CE Software
PO Box 65580
West Des Moines, IA 50265
515-221-1801
FAX 515-221-1806
http://www.cesoft.com
e-mail: sales@cesoft.com
Eric Conrad, Director
Jim Kirk, Manager

International software developer. Many products for adaptive technology.

2424 CRISP (Computer Retrieval of Information on Scientific Project)
National Institute of Health
9000 Rockville Pike
Bethesda, MD 20892
301-402-2900
FAX 301-480-2845
http://www.crisp.cit.nih.gov/
e-mail: commons@od.nih.gov
Nancy Morris, Manager
Dorrette Finch, Research Documentation Div. Dir.

A major scientific information system containing data on the research programs supported by the US Public Health Service.

2425 Classification Series
Aquarius Instructional
13064 Indian Rocks Road
Largo, FL 33774
1-800-255-90
800-338-2644
FAX 877-595-2685
http://www.phillipoy.com
e-mail: Info@PhillipRoy.com
Ruth Farmand, Owner
Ruth Bragman, President
Philip Padole, Vice President
Curriculum-based programs are learning units containing matching, sorting, form and object, and familiar settings. *$75.00*

2426 Compass Learning
203 Colorado Street
Austin, TX 78701
512-478-9600
800-422-4339
FAX 858-587-1629
http://www.compasslearning.com
e-mail: lkrauss@compasslearning.com
Eric Loeffel, President
Bill Willis, Chief Operating Officer

Educational software for teachers of K-12.

2427 Conover Company
1789 North Oakwood Road
Oshkosh, WI 54904
920-231-4667
FAX 920-231-4809
http://www.conovercompany.com
e-mail: sales@conovercompany.com
Terry Schmitz, Owner
Kris Volkman, Software Developer

2428 DC Health and Company
222 Berckly Street
Boston, MA 02116
617-351-5000
FAX 617-351-1110
http://www.hmco.com
Anthony Lucki, Chairman, President and CEO
Gerald Hughes, Executive Vice President, Chief

Helping people with learning disabilities.

2429 Developmental Profile
Western Psychological Services
12031 Wilshire Boulevard
Los Angeles, CA 90025
310-478-2061
800-648-8857
FAX 310-478-7838
http://www.wpspublish.com
e-mail: customerservice@wpspublish.com
Greg Gillmar, Vice President

This computer program substantially reduces the time educators spend on preparing Individualized Educational Plans (IEPs). The system allows the user to use any IEP format. Simply type the format into the computer, and the program will customize the system to your district's specifications. *$115.00*

2430 FileMaker Inc.
5201 Patrick Henry Drive
Santa Clara, CA 95054
408-987-7000
800 -725-274
FAX 408-987-3932
http://www.claris.com
e-mail: filemakerstore_licensing@filemaker.com
Dominique Ph Goupil, President
Bill Epling, Senior Vice President Finance an

Company that produces a variety of Macintosh Documentation.

2431 Filling Out Job Applications
Lawrence Productions
1800 S. 35Th Street
Galesburg, MI 49053
800 421 4157
616 450 4380
FAX 616 454 4711
http://www.lpi.com
e-mail: sales@lpi.com
Holly Argue, Author
Edwin Wright, President
John Lawrence, Owner

Designed for adolescents and adults in basic education classes providing one step analysis and completion of typical job applications. *$29.95*

2432 HEATH Resource Center People with Handicaps
HEATH Resource Center
2134 G Street, N.W.
Washington, DC 20052
202-337-7600
202 - 973 -
FAX 202 - 994 -
http://www.heath.gwu.edu
e-mail: askheath@gwu.edu
Dr. Lynda West, Principal Investigator
Dr. Joel Gomez, Co-Principal Investigator

$1.00

2433 IEP Companion Software
LinguiSystems
3100 4th Avenue
East Moline, IL 61244
309-755-2300
800-776-4332
FAX 309-755-2377
TDY:800-933-8331
http://www.linguisystems.com
e-mail: service@linguisystems.com
Carolyn Wilson, Janet Lanza, Jeannie Evans, Author
Linda Bowers, Co-owners/Founders
Rosemary Huisingh, Co-owners/Founders

Get IEP goals from the best-selling book with the click of your mouse. Writing complete reports is easy! You'll get to choose from hundreds of individual and classroom goals and objectives for all the important speech and language areas. Just click on the specific goals you want to create your individualized report. *$69.95*

Birth-Adult

2434 Interest Driven Learning
199 NE Burr Oak Court
Lees Summit, MO 64064
1-800-245-57
800-245-5733
FAX 1-816-478-48
http://www.drpeet.com
e-mail: drpeet@drpeet.com
Bill Peet MD, CEO

Our mission is to provide affordable low and high-tech tools that will help people of all ages and abilities learn to read, write and communicate with support from assistive technology as needed.

2435 International Society for Technology in Education (ISTE)
University of Oregon
480 Charnelton St
Eugene, OR 97401
541-302-3777
800-366-5191
FAX 541-3023781
http://www.iste.org
e-mail: iste@iste.org

Don Knezek, CEO
Deborah Carver, Manager
Lorraine Davis, Vice President
A nonprofit professional organization dedicated to promoting appropriate uses of information technology to support and improve learning, teaching, and administration in K-12 education and teacher education.

2436 KidDesk
Riverdeep
222 3rd Avenue SE
Cedar Rapids, IA 52401
319-395-9626
800-362-2890
FAX 319-395-0217
http://www.riverdeep.net
e-mail: info@riverdeep.net
Barry O'Callaghan, Executive Chairman & CEO
Jim Ruddy, Chief Revenue Officer

A hard disk security program, KidDesk makes it easy for kids to launch their programs, but impossible for them to access adult programs. Includes interactive desktop accessories including desktop-to-desktop electronic mail, and voice mail. *$24.95*

2437 KidDesk: Family Edition
Riverdeep
222 3rd Avenue SE
Cedar Rapids, IA 52401
319-395-9626
800-362-2890
FAX 319-395-0217
http://www.riverdeep.net
e-mail: info@riverdeep.net
Barry O'Callaghan, Executive Chairman & CEO
Jim Ruddy, Chief Revenue Officer

Now kids can launch their programs, but can't access yours! With KidDesk Family Edition, you can give your children the keys to the computer without putting your programs and files at risk! The auto-start option provides constant hard drive security — any time your computer is turned on, KidDesk will appear. *$24.95*

2438 LD Teacher's IEP Companion Software
LinguiSystems
3100 4th Avenue
East Moline, IL 61244
309-755-2300
800-776-4332
FAX 309-755-2377
TDY:800-933-8331
http://www.linguisystems.com
e-mail: service@linguisystems.com

Molly Lyle, Author
Linda Bowers, CEO
Rosemary Huisingh, Owner

Create customized, professional reports with these terrific academic goals and objectives. You'll have individual objectives from nine skill areas at the click of your mouse! Save time with the software version of the best-selling book! For both PC and Macintosh. *$69.95*

Ages 5-18

2439 Laureate Learning Systems
110 E Spring Street
Winooski, VT 05404
802-655-4755
800-652-6801
FAX 802-655-4757
http://www.laureatelearning.com
e-mail: laureate-customer-service@laureatelearning.co
Mary S. Wilson, President and CEO
Bernard J. Fox, Vice President

Provides resources for people with learning disabilities.

2440 Learning Company
Riverdeep
100 Pine Street
San Francisco, CA 94111
415-659-2000
800-852-2255
FAX 319-395-0217
http://www.riverdeep.net
e-mail: info@riverdeep.net
Barry O'Callaghan, Executive Chairman & CEO
Jim Ruddy, Chief Revenue Officer

2441 Microsoft Corporation
One Microsoft Way
Redmond, WA 98052
800-642-7676
FAX 425-936-7329
http://www.microsoft.com
Steve Ballmer, Chief Executive Officer

Our mission is to enable people and businesses throughout the world to realize their full potential.

2442 Print Module
Failure Free
140 West Cabarrus Ave.
Concord, NC 28025
704-786-7838
800-542-2170
FAX 704-785-8940
http://www.failurefree.com
e-mail: info@failurefree.com
Vincent Vezza, VP Sales and Marketing

Includes teacher's manual, instructional readers, flashcards, independent activities and illustrated independent reading booklets. *$499.00*

2443 PsycINFO Database
American Psychological Association
750 First Street, NE
Washington, DC 20002
202-336-5500
800-374-2721
FAX 202-336-5997
TDY:202-336-6123
http://www.apa.org
e-mail: mis@apa.org

Sharon S. Brehm, PhD, President
Marion Harrell, Assistant Director

An online abstract database that provides access to citations to the international serial literature in psychology and related disciplines from 1887 to present. Available via PsycINFO Direct at www.psycinfo.com.

2444 Public Domain Software
Kentucky Special Ed TechTraining Center
229 Taylor Education Building
Lexington, KY 40506
859-257-4713
FAX 859-257-1325
TDY:859-257-4714
http://www.serc.gws.uky.edu
Debra A. Harley, Professor and Department Chair
Marcia Bowling, Administrative Assistant

Entire collections of Macintosh, MS-DOS or Apple II software.

2445 **Pugliese, Davey and Associates**
Adaptive Technology Institutes
5 Bessom Street
Marblehead, MA 01945
781-639-1930
FAX 781-631-9928
TDY:617-224-2521
Madalaine Pugliese, President

Offers computer lab courses for Apple IIGS and Macintosh LC.

2446 **Riverdeep**
100 Pine Street
San Francisco, CA 94111
415-659-2000
FAX 415-659-2020
http://www.riverdeep.net
e-mail: info@riverdeep.net
Barry O'Callaghan, Executive Chairman & CEO
Jim Ruddy, Chief Revenue Officer
Fiona O'Carroll, EVP Marketing/Development
Developer of educational software, including software for mathematics instruction.

2447 **Scholastic**
2931 East McCarty Street
Jefferson City, MO 65101
573-636-5271
800-541-5513
FAX 573-632-5271
http://www.scholastic.com
e-mail: custserv@scholastic.com
Maureen O'Connell, Executive VP/CAO/CEO
Larry Holland, Human Resources Director

2448 **Speech Bin Abilitations**
3155 Northwoods Parkway
Norcross, GA 30071
770-449-5700
800-477-3324
FAX 888-329-2246
http://www.speechbin.com
e-mail: info@speechbin.com
Tobi Isaacs, M.Ed., Catalog Director

The Speech Bin offers materials to help persons of all ages who have special needs. We specialize in products for children and adults who have communication disorders.

2449 **Sunburst Communications**
400 Columbus Avenue
Valhalla Pleasantville, NY 10595
800-321-7511
914-747-4109
FAX 888-800-3028
http://www.sunburst.com
e-mail: support@nysunburst.com
Mark Sotir, CEO
Katie Birmingham, Office Manager

2450 **Testmaster**
Research Design Associates
5 Main Street
Freeville, NY 13068
607-844-4601
FAX 607-844-3310
Brian Buttner, CEO

A new concept in question and answer testing with an Exploratory Mode which allows students to explore a range of answers. *$199.95*

Reading

2451 **Adaptive Technology Tools**
Freedom Scientific
11800 31st Court North
St. Petersburg, FL 33716
727-803-8000
800-444-4443
FAX 727-803-8001
http://www.freedomscientific.com
e-mail: info@FreedomScientific.com
Lee Hamilton, President & CEO

A wide variety of adaptive technology tools for the visually or reading impaired person.

2452 **An Open Book**
Freedom Scientific
11800 31st Court North
St Petersburg, FL 33716
727-803-8000
800-444-4443
FAX 727-803-8001
http://www.freedomscientific.com
e-mail: info@FreedomScientific.com
Lee Hamilton, President & CEO

The stand-alone reading machine, An Open Book, is an easy-to-use appliance for noncomputer users that comes equipped with a Hewlett Packard ScanJet IIP scanner, DECtalk PC speech synthesizer and a 17 key keypad. An Open Book uses Calera WordScan optical character recognition (OCR) to convert pages into text, then reads it aloud with a speech synthesizer.

2453 **An Open Book Unbound**
Freedom Scientific
11800 31st Court North
St. Petersburg, FL 33716
727-803-8000
800-444-4443
FAX 727-803-8001
http://www.freedomscientific.com
e-mail: info@FreedomScientific.com
Lee Hamilton, President & CEO

PC-based OCR and reading software. Together with a scanner and a speech synthesizer, this software provides everything needed to make an IBM-compatible PC into a talking reading machine. The system includes automatic page orientation, automatic contrast control, decolumnization of multicolumn documents and recognition of a wide variety of type fonts and sizes. *$995.00*

2454 **Bailey's Book House**
Riverdeep
222 3rd Avenue SE
Cedar Rapids, IA 52401
319-395-9626
FAX 319-395-0217
http://www.riverdeep.net
e-mail: info@riverdeep.net
Barry O'Callaghan, Executive Chairman & CEO
Jim Ruddy, Chief Revenue Officer

The award-winning Bailey's Book House now features 2 new activities! Bailey and his friends encourage young children to build important literacy skills while developing a love for reading. In seven activities, kids explore the sounds and meanings of letters, words, sentences, rhymes and stories. No reading skills are required: all directions and written words are spoken. *$59.95*

2455 **Banner Books**
Queue
1 Control Drive
Shelton, CT 06484
203-446-8100
800-232-2224
FAX 800-775-2729
http://www.qworkbooks.com
e-mail: jdk@queueinc.com
Monica Kantrowitz, President
Jonathan Kantrowitz, CEO
Peter Uhrynowski, Controller
This is a format students and teachers will love. Students select a variety of backgrounds and watch as they move by on the screen. Students then add clip art and text to create their own Banner Book pages. Offers various programs. *$49.95*

2456 **Boars in Camelot**
Queue
1 Control Drive
Shelton, CT 06484
203-446-8100
800-232-2224
FAX 800-775-2729
http://www.qworkbooks.com
e-mail: jdk@queueinc.com
Monica Kantrowitz, President
Jonathan Kantrowitz, CEO
Peter Uhrynowski, Controller

Written in an upbeat and amusing style to capture students' interest as they interact with the story by answering questions about what they have read. *$45.00*

2457 Comprehension Connection
Milliken Publishing
PO Box 21579
Saint Louis, MO 63132
314-991-4220
800-325-4136
FAX 314-991-4807
http://www.millikenpub.com
Thomas Moore, President

Comprehension Connection improves reading comprehension by stressing basic skills that combine the reading process with relevant activities and interesting, thought-provoking stories. This award-winning software package spans six reading levels that increase in difficulty. Passages range from 150-300 words. *$150.00*

2458 Compu-Teach
Compu-Teach
16541 Redmond Way
Redmond, WA 98052
425-885-0517
800-448-3224
FAX 425-883-9169
http://www.compu-teach.com
e-mail: info@compu-teach.com
David Urban, President

Higher resolution graphics, digitized voice, MIDI music, animation and sound effects make this program one of America's favorites. Children have never had so much fun learning the basics of reading, language and math! Includes letter recognition, counting, adding and sentence structure. This wonderful series will provide an exciting learning experience for any child between the ages of 2 and 7. The bonus pack contains six separate learning activities which have won many software awards. *$59.95*
Ages 4-7

2459 Cosmic Reading Journey
Sunburst Technology
1550 Executive Drive
Elgin, IL 60123
914-747-3310
888-492-8817
FAX 888-800-3028
http://www.sunburst.com
e-mail: service@sunburst.com
Mark Sotir, President
Tara Green, Marketing Executive
Katie Birmingham, Office Manager
This reading comprehension program provides meaningful summary and writing activities for the 100 books that early readers and their teachers love most.

2460 Don Johnston Reading
Don Johnston
26799 W Commerce Drive
Volo, IL 60073
847-740-0749
800-999-4660
FAX 847-740-7326
http://www.donjohnston.com
e-mail: info@donjohnston.com
Ruth Ziolkowski, President
Mindy Brown, Marketing Director

Don Johnston Inc. is a provider of quality products and services that enable people with special needs to discover their potential and experience success. Products are developed for the areas of computer access and for those who struggle with reading and writing.

2461 Failure Free Reading
140 West Cabarrus Avenue
Concord, NC 28025
704-786-7838
800-542-2170
FAX 704-785-8940
http://www.failurefree.com
e-mail: info@failurefree.com
Vincent Vezza, VP Sales/Marketing and Professio

Curriculum areas covered: reading for those with learning disabilities and moderate mentally disabled/emotionally disabled.

2462 Judy Lynn Software
PO Box 373
East Brunswick, NJ 08816
732-390-8845
FAX 732-390-8845
http://www.judylynn.com
e-mail: techsupt@judylynn.com
Elliot Pludwinski, Founder/President

Offers switch computer programs for windows.The programs are geared towards children with a cognitive age level from 9 months to 4 years. Programs use bright colorful animation with captivating sounds to maintain attention span. Programs are reasonably priced from $20-$39. Recipient of a Parents' Choice Honor.
1991

2463 Kurzweil 3000
Kurzweil Educational Systems
100 Crosby Drive
Bedford, MA 01730
781-276-0600
FAX 781-276-0650
http://www.kurzweiledu.com
e-mail: info@kurzweiledu.cc
Christina Newman, Marketing Communications Manager

Kurzweil Educational's flagship product for struggling readers and writers. It is widely recognized as the most comprehensive and integrated solution for addressing language and literacy difficulties. The software uses a multisensory approach — presenting printed or electronic text on the computer screen with added visual and audible accessibility. The product incorporates a host of dynamic features including powerful decoding, study skills tools and test taking tools.

2464 Lexia Cross-Trainer
Lexia Learning Systems
200 Baker Avenue Extension
Concord, MA 01742
781-259-8752
800-435-3942
FAX 978-287-0062
http://www.lexialearning.com
e-mail: info@lexialearning.com
Nicholas C. Gaehde, President and C.E.O.
Robert A. Lemire, Founder, Treasurer and Chairman

Interactive software with an engaging video-gme interface that is designed to strengthen cognitive skills. Activities that advance visual-spatial and logical reasoning skills are designed to improve the memory, critical thinking, and problem solving abilities necessary for academic success in all subjects. *$250.00*

2465 Lexia Early Reading
Lexia Learning Systems
200 Baker Avenue Extension
Concord, MA 01742
781-259-8752
800-435-3942
FAX 978-287-0062
http://www.lexialearning.com
e-mail: info@lexialearning.com
Nicholas C. Gaehde, President and C.E.O.
Robert A. Lemire, Founder, Treasurer and Chairman

Engaging, interactive software fochildren aged four to six that introduces and develops proficiency with phonological principles and the alphabet - both proven indicators of later reading success.

2466 Lexia Primary Reading
Lexia Learning Systems
200 Baker Avenue Extension
Concord, MA 01742
781-259-8752
800-435-3942
FAX 978-287-0062
http://www.lexialearning.com
e-mail: info@lexialearning.com
Nicholas C. Gaehde, President and C.E.O.
Robert A. Lemire, Founder, Treasurer and Chairman

Interactive software designed to ensure mastery of basic phonological skills and introduce more advanced phonics priciples. five levels of engaging activities deliver practice in phonemic awareness, sight-word recognition, word attack strategies, sound-symbol correspondence, listening and reading comprehension. *$50.00*

2467 Lexia Strategies for Older Students

Lexia Learning Systems
200 Baker Avenue Extension
Concord, MA 01742
781-259-8752
800-435-3942
FAX 978-287-0062
http://www.lexialearning.com
e-mail: info@lexialearning.com
Nicholas C. Gaehde, President and C.E.O.
Robert A. Lemire, Founder, Treasurer and Chairman

Reading skills software program specifically designed for ages 9-adult. Five levels of activities provide extensive practice in everything from basic phonological awareness to advanced word attack strategy and vocabulary development based on Greek and Laitn word roots. *$250.00*

2468 Mike Mulligan & His Steam Shovel

Sunburst Technology
1550 Executive Drive
Elgin, IL 60123
914-747-3310
888-492-8817
FAX 888-800-3028
http://www.sunburst.com
e-mail: service@sunburst.com
Mark Sotir, President
Tara Green, Marketing Executive
Katie Birmingham, Office Manager

This CD-ROM version of the Caldecott classic lets students experience interactive book reading and participate in four skills-based extension activities that promote memory, matching, sequencing, listening, pattern recognition and map reading skills.

2469 Optimum Resource

18 Hunter Road
Hilton Head Island, SC 29926
843-689-8000
888-784-2592
FAX 843-689-8008
http://www.stickybear.com
e-mail: stickyb@stickybear.com
Christopher Gintz, CEO
Robert Stangroom, Product Manager

An educational software publishing company for grades K-12. Our software titles are available in Consumer, School, Labpack or Site License versions. Please call for further details. Prices range from $59.95 for Consumer to $699.95 for Site Licenses.

2470 Polar Express

Sunburst Technology
1550 Executive Drive
Elgin, IL 60123
914-747-3310
888-492-8817
FAX 888-800-3028
http://www.sunburst.com
e-mail: service@sunburst.com
Mark Sotir, President
Tara Green, Marketing Executive
Katie Birmingham, Office Manager

Share the magic and enchantment of the holiday season with this CD-ROM version of Chris Van Allsburg's Caldecott-winning picture book.

2471 Prolexia

4726 13th Avenue NW
Rochester, MN 55901
507-780-1859
888-776-5394
FAX 507-252-0131
http://www.prolexia.com
e-mail: info@prolexia.com
John Rylander, President

UltraPhonics Tutor software teaches reading, spelling, handwriting, & pronunication to beginners and those with dyslexia via multisensory structured phonics.

2472 Read On! Plus

Sunburst Technology
1550 Executive Drive
Elgin, IL 60123
914-747-3310
888-492-8817
FAX 888-800-3028
http://www.sunburst.com
e-mail: service@sunburst.com
Mark Sotir, President
Tara Green, Marketing Executive
Katie Birmingham, Office Manager

Promote skills and strategies that improve reading comprehension, and build appreciation for literature and the written word.

2473 Read, Write and Type! Learning Systems

Talking Fingers
830 Rincon Way
San Rafael, CA 94901
415-472-3103
800-674-9126
FAX 415-472-7812
TDY:415-472-3106
http://www.readwritetype.com
e-mail: contact@talkingfingers.com
Jeannine Herron, Director
Kris Kuebler

A 40-level software adventure providing highly motivating instruction and practice in phonics, reading, writing, spelling and typing. This multisensory program includes 9 levels of assessment and reports. Classroom packs available.

2474 Reading Power Modules Books

Steck-Vaughn Company
6277 Sea Harbor Dr.
Orlando, FL 32887
800-531-5015
800-225-5425
FAX 800-699-9459
http://www.steck-vaughn.com
e-mail: info@steck-vaughn.com
Connie Alden, Vice President of Human Resource
Michael Ruecker, Vice President of Human Resource

Supplementary reading based on 4 decades of reading research. Companion books give students and teachers a choice of formats. High interest stories reinforce reading comprehension skills while building vocabulary, spelling skills, reading fluency, and speed.

2475 Reading Realities Elementary Series

Teacher Support Software
3542 NW 97th Boulevard
Gainesville, FL 32606
877-833-5524
800-228-2871
FAX 972-228-1982
http://www.tssoftware.com
Ruth Smith, Manager

Students will read about topics that focus on issues they face in their everyday lives. Over 1000 students contributed stories that make up the program. Students will benefit from prereading, reading and follow-up activities in a directed reading-thinking format. The manager tracks reading ability and class and student progress. Vocabulary support and speech make this a nonthreatening atmosphere for sharing and learning.

2476 Reading Skills Bundle

Sunburst Technology
1550 Executive Drive
Elgin, IL 60123
888-492-8817
FAX 888-800-3028
http://www.sunburst.com
e-mail: service@sunburst.com
Mark Sotir, CEO
Mike Gavelek, Senior VP/Marketing
Katie Birmingham, Office Manager

Teach beginning reading with teacher-developed programs that sequentially present phonics, phonemic awareness, word recognition, and reading comprehension concepts.

2477 Reading Who? Reading You!
Sunburst Technology
1550 Executive Drive
Elgin, IL 60123
888-492-8817
FAX 888-800-3028
http://www.sunburst.com
e-mail: service@sunburst.com
Mark Sotir, CEO
Mike Gavelek, Senior VP/Marketing
Katie Birmingham, Office Manager
Teach beginning reading skills effectively with phonics instruction built into engaging games and puzzles that have children asking for more.

2478 Roots, Prefixes & Suffixes
Sunburst Technology
1550 Executive Drive
Elgin, IL 60123
888-492-8817
FAX 888-800-3028
http://www.sunburst.com
e-mail: service@sunburst.com
Mark Sotir, CEO
Mike Gavelek, Senior VP/Marketing
Katie Birmingham, Office Manager
Students learn to decode difficult and more complex words as they engage in six activities where they construct and dissect words with roots, prefixes and suffixes.

2479 Sentence Master: Level 1, 2, 3, 4
Laureate Learning Systems
110 E Spring Street
Winooski, VT 05404
802-655-4755
800-562-6801
FAX 802-655-4757
http://www.laureatelearning.net
e-mail: info@laureatelearning.com
Mary Wilson, Owner
Bernard Fox, VP

A revolutionary way to teach beginning reading. Avoiding the confusing rules of phonics and the complexity of whole language, The Sentence Master focuses on the most frequently-used words of our language; i.e. the, is, but, and, etc., by truly teaching these little words, The Sentence Master gives students control over the majority of text they will ever encounter. *$475.00*

2480 Simon Sounds It Out
Don Johnston
26799 West Commerce Drive
Volo, IL 60073
847-740-0749
800-999-4660
FAX 847-740-7326
http://www.donjohnston.com
e-mail: info@donjohnston.com
Ruth Ziolkowski, President
Mindy Brown, Marketing Director

Struggling students who can recite the alphabet and recognize letters on a page may still have trouble making connections between letters and sounds. This creates a barrier to recognizing and learning words which prevents your students from reading and writing successfully. Simon Sounds It Out provides the vital practice and repetition they need to overcome the letter-to-sound barrier. *$59.00*

2481 Stickybear Software
Optimum Resource
18 Hunter Road
Hilton Head Island, SC 29926
843-689-8000
888-784-2592
FAX 843-689-8008
http://www.stickybear.com
e-mail: stickyb@stickybear.com
Christopher Gintz, CEO
Robert Stangroom, Product Manager

An educational software publishing company for grades K-12. Our software titles are available in Consumer, School, Labpack or Site License versions. Please call for further details. Prices range from $59.95 for Consumer to $699.95 for Site Licenses.

2482 Time for Teachers Online
Stern Center for Language and Learning
135 Allen Brook Lane
Williston, VT 05495
802-878-2332
800-544-4863
FAX 802-878-0230
http://www.sterncenter.org
e-mail: learning@sterncenter.org
Blanche Podhajsk MD, President
Mary Stifler, Vice President

A 45 hour course completed entirely on the internet, designed to help teachers implement research-based best practices in reading instruction. *$525.00*

Science

2483 Changes Around Us CD-ROM
Steck-Vaughn Company
6277 Sea Harbor Dr.
Orlando, FL 32887
800-531-5015
800-531-5015
FAX 800-699-9459
http://www.steck-vaughn.com
e-mail: info@steck-vaughn.com
Connie Alden, Vice President of Human Resource
Michael Ruecker, Vice President of Human Resource

Nature is the natural choice for observing change. By observing and researching dramatic visual sequences such as the stages of development of a butterfly, children develop a broad understanding of the concept of change. As they search this multimedia database for images and information about plant and animal life cycles and seasonal change, students strengthen their abilities in research, analysis, problem-solving, critical thinking and communication.

2484 Exploring Heat
TERC
2067 Massachusetts Avenue
Cambridge, MA 02140
617-547-0430
FAX 617-349-3535
http://www.terc.edu
e-mail: communications@terc.edu
Dennis Bartels, President
Sarah Glatt, Administrative Assistant

A combination of lessons, software, temperature probes and activity sheets, specifically designed for the learning disabled child. *$160.00*

2485 Field Trip Into the Sea
Sunburst Technology
1550 Executive Drive
Elgin, IL 60123
888-492-8817
FAX 888-800-3028
http://www.sunburst.com
e-mail: service@sunburst.com
Mark Sotir, CEO
Mike Gavelek, Senior VP/Marketing
Katie Birmingham, Office Manager
Visit a kelp forest and the rocky shore with this information packed guide that lets your students learn about the plants, animals and habitats of coastal environments.

2486 Field Trip to the Rain Forest
Sunburst Technology
1550 Executive Drive
Elgin, IL 60123
888-492-8817
FAX 888-800-3028
http://www.sunburst.com
e-mail: service@sunburst.com
Mark Sotir, CEO
Mike Gavelek, Senior VP/Marketing
Katie Birmingham, Office Manager

Visit a Central American rainforest to learn more about its plants and animals with this dynamic research program that includes a useful information management tool.

2487 Learn About Life Science: Animals
Sunburst Technology
1550 Executive Drive
Elgin, IL 60123
888-492-8817
FAX 888-800-3028
http://www.sunburst.com
e-mail: service@sunburst.com
Mark Sotir, CEO
Mike Gavelek, Senior VP/Marketing
Katie Birmingham, Office Manager
Learn about animal classification, adaptation to climate, domestication and special relationships between humans and animals.

2488 Learn About Life Science: Plants
Sunburst Technology
1550 Executive Drive
Elgin, IL 60123
888-492-8817
FAX 888-800-3028
http://www.sunburst.com
e-mail: service@sunburst.com
Mark Sotir, CEO
Mike Gavelek, Senior VP/Marketing
Katie Birmingham, Office Manager
Students explore the world of plants. From small seeds to tall trees students learn what plants are and what they need to grow.

2489 Milliken Science Series: Circulation and Digestion
Milliken Publishing
11643 Liburn Park Road
Saint Louis, MO 63146
314-991-4220
800-325-4136
FAX 314-991-4807
http://www.milikenpub.com
Delores Boufard, Author
Thomas Moore, President

A program designed to introduce students to two subsystems of the human body. Provides practice using the correct terms for the various organs that make up each system, illustrating how the parts of each subsystem work together, and ensuring that students can explain the functions of the subsystems and their parts.

2490 NOMAD Graphics Packages
American Printing House for the Blind
1839 Frankfort Avenue
Louisville, KY 40206
502-895-2405
800-223-1839
FAX 502-899-2274
http://www.aph.org
e-mail: info@aph.org
Tuck Tinsley, President
Fred Gissoni, Customer Support

Offers a variety of ready-made graphics as well as preprogrammed computer files, for use with NOMAD Talking Touch Pad. Topics include geography, orientation and mobility, and Star Trek.

2491 Sammy's Science House
Riverdeep
222 3rd Avenue SE
Cedar Rapids, IA 52401
319-395-9626
319-395-0217
FAX 800-567-2714
http://www.riverdeep.net
e-mail: info@riverdeep.net
Tina Martin, Education Marketing

Developed by early learning experts, the award-winning Sammy's Science House builds important early science skills, encourages wonder and joy as children discover the world of science around them. Five engaging activities help children practice sorting, sequencing, observing, predicting and constructing. They'll learn about plants, animals, minerals, fun seasons and weather, too! *$59.95*

2492 Talking Walls
Riverdeep
500 Redmond Boulevard
Novato, CA 94947
415-763-4940
800-362-2890
FAX 415-763-4385
http://www.elmark.com
e-mail: info@riverdeep.net
Barry O'Callaghan, Chairman
Simon Calver, CEO
John Rim, CFO
The Talking Walls Software Series is a wonderful springboard for a student's journey of exploration and discovery. This comprehensive collection of researched resources and materials enables students to focus on learning while conducting a guided search for information.

2493 Talking Walls: The Stories Continue
Riverdeep
500 Redmond Boulevard
Novato, CA 94947
415-763-4940
800-362-2890
FAX 415-763-4385
http://www.elmark.com
e-mail: info@riverdeep.net
Barry O'Callaghan, Chairman
Simon Calver, CEO
John Rim, CFO
Using the Talking Walls Software Series, students discover the stories behind some of the world's most fascinating walls. The award-winning books, interactive software, carefully chosen Web sites, and suggested classroom activities build upon each other, providing a rich learning experience that includes text, video, and hands-on projects.

Social Studies

2494 Discoveries: Explore the Desert Ecosystem
Sunburst Technology
1550 Executive Drive
Elgin, IL 60123
888-492-8817
FAX 888-800-3028
http://www.sunburst.com
e-mail: service@sunburst.com
Mark Sotir, CEO
Mike Gavelek, Senior VP/Marketing
Katie Birmingham, Office Manager
This program invites students to explore the plants, animals, culture and georgraphy of the Sonoran Desert by day and by night.

2495 Discoveries: Explore the Everglades Ecosystem
Sunburst Technology
1550 Executive Drive
Elgin, IL 60123
800-321-7511
888-492-8817
FAX 888-800-3028
http://www.sunburst.com
e-mail: Service@sunburst.com
Mark Sotir, President
Tara Green, Marketing Executive
Katie Birmingham, Office Manager
This multi curricular research program takes students to the Everglades where they anchor their exploration photo realistic panaramas of the habitiat.

2496 Discoveries: Explore the Forest Ecosystem
Sunburst Technology
1550 Executive Drive
Elgin, IL 60123
800-321-7511
888-492-8817
FAX 888-800-3028
http://www.sunburst.com
e-mail: Service@sunburst.com
Mark Sotir, President
Tara Green, Marketing Executive
Katie Birmingham, Office Manager

This theme based CD-ROM enables students of all abilities to actively research a multitude of different forest ecosystems in the Appalachian National Park.

2497 Imagination Express Destination: Castle
Riverdeep
222 3rd Avenue SE
Cedar Rapids, IA 52401
319-395-9626
888-242-6747
FAX 319-395-0217
http://www.riverdeep.net
e-mail: info@riverdeep.net
Barry O'Callaghan, Executive Chairman & Chief Execu
Jim Ruddy, Chief Revenue Officer

Kids enter a medieval kingdom where knights, jesters, wild boars and falconers become actors in their own interactive stories. As kids cast characters, develop plots, narrate and write and record dialogue, they become enthusiastic writers, editors, producers and publishers! *$59.95*

2498 Imagination Express Destination: Neighborhood
Riverdeep
222 3rd Avenue SE
Cedar Rapids, IA 52401
319-395-9626
888-242-6747
FAX 319-395-0217
http://www.riverdeep.net
e-mail: info@riverdeep.net
Barry O'Callaghan, Executive Chairman & Chief Execu
Jim Ruddy, Chief Revenue Officer

In Destination: Neighborhood, familiar settings and characters encourage kids to write about actual or imagined adventures. Kids enjoy developing creativity, writing and communication skills as they explore the neighborhood and all the people who live there. As kids select scenes, choose and animate stickers, write, narrate, add music and record dialogue, their stories, journals, letters and poems come alive! *$59.95*

2499 Imagination Express Destination: Ocean
Riverdeep
222 3rd Avenue SE
Cedar Rapids, IA 52401
319-395-9626
888-242-6747
FAX 319-395-0217
http://www.riverdeep.net
e-mail: info@riverdeep.net
Barry O'Callaghan, Executive Chairman & Chief Execu
Jim Ruddy, Chief Revenue Officer

The fascinating shores and depths of Destination: Ocean inspire kids to create interactive stories and movies. Using exciting new technology, kids make stickers move across each scene: sharks swim through the sea kelp while dolphins leap above waves! With Destination: Ocean, your child's writing and creativity will soar! *$59.95*

2500 Imagination Express Destination: Pyramids
Riverdeep
222 3rd Avenue SE
Cedar Rapids, IA 52401
319-395-9626
888-242-6747
FAX 319-395-0217
http://www.riverdeep.net
e-mail: info@riverdeep.net
Barry O'Callaghan, Executive Chairman & Chief Execu
Jim Ruddy, Chief Revenue Officer

Kids can create interactive electronic books and movies featuring pharaohs, mummies and life on the Nile. Builds writing, creativity and communication skills as they learn about and explore this captivating destination. Kids select scenes, choose and animate characters, plan plots, write stories, narrate pages and add music, dialogue and sound effects to make their own adventures. *$59.95*

2501 Imagination Express Destination: Rain Forest
Riverdeep
222 3rd Avenue SE
Cedar Rapids, IA 52401
319-395-9626
888-242-6747
FAX 319-395-0217
http://www.riverdeep.net
e-mail: info@riverdeep.net
Barry O'Callaghan, Executive Chairman & Chief Execu
Jim Ruddy, Chief Revenue Officer

Rain Forest invities kids to step into a Panamanian rain forest, where they craft exciting, interactive adventures filled with exotic plants, insects, waterfalls and Kuna Indians. Kids build essential communication skills as they select scenes and characters, plan plots, write, narrate, animate and record dialogue to create remarkable adventures! *$59.95*

2502 Imagination Express Destination: Time Trip USA
Riverdeep
222 3rd Avenue SE
Cedar Rapids, IA 52401
319-395-9626
888-242-6747
FAX 319-395-0217
http://www.riverdeep.net
e-mail: info@riverdeep.net
Barry O'Callaghan, Executive Chairman & Chief Execu
Jim Ruddy, Chief Revenue Officer

Children will love traveling through time to create interactive electronic books and movies set in a fictional New England town. As students select scenes, cast charcters, develop plots, narrate, write and record dialogue, they'll bring the town's history to life through their own exciting adventures. *$59.95*

2503 NOMAD Graphics Packages
American Printing House for the Blind
1839 Frankfort Avenue
Louisville, KY 40206
502-895-2405
800-223-1839
FAX 502-899-2274
http://www.aph.org
e-mail: info@aph.org
Tuck Tinsley, President
Kathy Smiddy, Executive Secretary
Fred Gissoni, Customer Support
Offers a variety of ready-made graphics as well as preprogrammed computer files, for use with NOMAD Talking Touch Pad. Topics include geography, orientation and mobility, and Star Trek.

Speech

2504 Eden Institute Curriculum: Speech and Language, Volume IV
1 Eden Way
Princeton, NJ 08540
609-987-0099
FAX 609-987-0243
http://www.edenservices.org
e-mail: info@edenservices.org
Tom Cool, President/CEO
David Holmes, Founder/Director
Anne Holmes, Outreach/Support Director
Peceptive, expressive and pragmatic language skills programs for students with autism. *$170.00*

2505 Spectral Speech Analysis: Software
Speech Bin
PO Box 922668
Norcross, GA 30010
770-449-5700
1-800-850-86
FAX 1-888-329-22
http://www.speechbin.com
e-mail: info@speechbin.com
Tobi Isaacs, Catalog Director

This exciting new software uses visual feedback as an effective speech treatment tool. Speech-language pathologists can record speech and corresponding visual displays for clients who then try to match either auditory or visual targets. These built-in visual patterns can be displayed as either sophisticated spectrograms or real-time waveforms. Item number P227. *$159.95*

Word Processors

2506 Braille' n Speak Classic
American Printing House for the Blind
1839 Frankfort Avenue
Louisville, KY 40206
502-895-2405
800-223-1839
FAX 502-899-2274
http://www.aph.org
e-mail: info@aph.org
Fred Gissoni, Technical Support Specialist
Kathy Smiddy, Executive Secretary
Fred Gissoni, Customer Support
This computerized, talking device has many features useful to student and adult braille users (word processors, print-to-braille translators, talking clocks/calculators and much more). *$929.95*

2507 Dr. Peet's TalkWriter
Interest Driven Learning
446 Bouchelle Drive #303
New Smyrna Beach, FL 32169
386-427-4473
800-245-5733
FAX 816-478-4824
http://www.drpeet.com
e-mail: drpeet@drpeet.com
William Peet PhD, CEO/Owner
Libby Peet EdD, Adaptive Access Specialist, and

A talking, singing word processor designed to meet the needs of young learners from three to eight. Runs on Windows.

2508 Kids Media Magic 2.0
Sunburst Technology
1550 Executive Drive
Elgin, IL 60123
800-321-7511
888-492-8817
FAX 888-800-3028
http://www.sunburst.com
e-mail: Service@sunburst.com
Mark Sotir, President
Tara Green, Marketing Executive
Katie Birmingham, Office Manager
The first multimedia word processor designed for young children. Help your child become a fluent reader and writer. The Rebus Bar automatically scrolls over 45 vocabulary words as students type.

2509 Media Weaver 3.5
Sunburst Technology
1550 Executive Drive
Elgin, IL 60123
800-321-7511
888-492-8817
FAX 888-800-3028
http://www.sunburst.com
e-mail: Service@sunburst.com
Mark Sotir, President
Tara Green, Marketing Executive
Katie Birmingham, Office Manager
Publishing becomes a multimedia event with this dynamic word processor that contains hundreds of media elements and effective process writing resources.

2510 Sunbuddy Writer
Sunburst Technology
1550 Executive Drive
Elgin, IL 60123
800-321-7511
888-492-8817
FAX 888-800-3028
http://www.sunburst.com
e-mail: Service@sunburst.com
Mark Sotir, President
Tara Green, Marketing Executive
Katie Birmingham, Office Manager
An easy-to-use picture and word processor designed especially for young writers.

2511 Write: Outloud to Go
Don Johnston
26799 W Commerce Drive
Volo, IL 60073
847-740-0749
800-999-4660
FAX 847-740-7326
http://www.donjohnston.com
e-mail: info@donjohnston.com
Ruth Ziolkowski, President
Mindy Brown, Marketing Director

A flexible and user-friendly talking word processor that offers multisensory learning and positive reinforcement for writers of all ages and ability levels. Powerful features include a talking spell checker, on-screen speech and file management and color capabilities that allow for customization to meet individual needs or preferences. Requires Macintosh computer. Voted Best Special Needs Product by the Software Publishers Association. *$99.00*

Writing

2512 Abbreviation/Expansion
Zygo Industries
PO Box 1008
Portland, OR 97207
503-684-6006
800-234-6006
FAX 503-684-6011
http://www.zygo-usa.com
e-mail: zygo@zygo-usa.com
Lawrence Weiss, President

Allows the individual to define and store word/phrase abbreviations to achieve efficiency and accelerated entry rate of text. *$95.00*

2513 Author's Toolkit
Sunburst Technology
1550 Executive Drive
Elgin, IL 60123
800-321-7511
888-492-8817
FAX 888-800-3028
http://www.sunburst.com
e-mail: Service@sunburst.com
Mark Sotir, President
Tara Green, Marketing Executive
Katie Birmingham, Office Manager
Students can use this comprehensive tool to organize ideas, make outlines, rough drafts, edit and print all their written work.

2514 Dr. Peet's Picture Writer
Interest Driven-Learning
446 Bouchelle Drive #303
New Smyrna Beach, FL 32169
386-427-4473
800-245-5733
FAX 816-478-4824
http://www.drpeet.com
e-mail: drpeet@drpeet.com
William Peet PhD, Owner/Chief Executive Officer
Libby Peet EdD, Adaptive Access Specialist, and

A talking picture-writer. It guides novice writers, regardless of age, motivation or ability, in creating simple talking picture sentences about things that are interesting and important to them. *$500.00*

2515 Easybook Deluxe
Sunburst Technology
1550 Executive Drive
Elgin, IL 60123
888-492-8817
FAX 888-800-3028
http://www.sunburst.com
e-mail: Service@sunburst.com
Mark Sotir, CEO
Mike Gavelek, Senior Vice President of Marketi
Katie Birmingham, Office Manager

Designed to support the needs of a wide range of writers, this book publishing tool provides students with a creative environment to write, design and illustrate stories and reports, and to print their work in book formats.

2516 Fonts4Teachers

Therapro
225 Arlington Street
Framingham, MA 01702
508-872-9494
800-257-5376
FAX 508-875-2062
http://www.theraproducts.com
e-mail: info@theraproducts.com
Karen Conrad, President

A software collection of 31 True Type fonts for teachers, parents and students. Fonts include Tracing, lined and unlined Traditional Manuscript and Cursive (similar to Zaner Blouser and D'Nealian), math, clip art, decorative, time, American Sign Language symbols and more. The included manual is very informative, with great examples of lesson plans and educational goals. *$39.95*
Windows/Mac

2517 Great Beginnings

Teacher Support Software
325 North Kirkwood Rd
St. Louis, MO 63122
888-726-8100
FAX 314-984-8063
http://www.gamco.com
e-mail: support@siboneylg.com
Robin Tinker, VP Marketing

From a broad selection of topics and descriptive words, students may create their own stories and illustrate them with colorful graphics. *$69.95*

2518 Language Experience Recorder Plus

Teacher Support Software
325 North Kirkwood Rd
St. Louis, MO 63122
888-726-8100
FAX 314-984-8063
http://www.gamco.com
e-mail: support@siboneylg.com
Robin Tinker, VP Marketing

This program provides students with the opportunity to read, write and hear their own experience stories. Analyzes student writing. Cumulative word list, word and sentence counts and readability estimate. *$99.95*

2519 Mega Dots

Duxbury Systems
270 Littleton Road
Westford, MA 01886
978-692-3000
800-347-9594
FAX 978-692-7912
http://www.duxburysystems.com
e-mail: info@duxsys.com
Joe Sullivan, President

MegaDots is a mature DOS braille translator with powerful features for the volume transcriber and producer. Its straightforward, style based system and automated features let you create great braille with only a few keystrokes, yet it is sophisticated enough to please the fussiest braille producers. You can control each step MegaDots follows to format, translate and produce braille documents. *$540.00*

2520 Once Upon a Time Volume I: Passport to Discovery

Compu-Teach
16541 Redmond Way
Redmond, WA 98052
425-885-0517
800-448-3224
FAX 425-883-9169
http://www.compu-teach.com
e-mail: info@compu-teach.com
David Urban, President

Features familiar objects associated with three unique themes. These graphic images offer limitless possibilities for new stories and illustrations. As children author books from one to hundreds of pages, they can either display them on screen or print them out. Themes: Farm Life; Down Main Street; and On Safari. *$59.95*
Ages 4-12

2521 Once Upon a Time Volume II: Worlds of Enchantment

Compu-Teach
16541 Redmond Way
Redmond, WA 98052
425-885-0517
800-448-3224
FAX 425-883-9169
http://www.compu-teach.com
e-mail: info@compu-teach.com
David Urban, President

Makes writing, reading and vocabulary skills easy to learn. While building their illustrations, children experiment with perspective and other spatial relationships. This volume features familiar objects associated with three unique themes: Underwater; Dinosaur Age; and Forest Friends. *$59.95*
Ages 4-12

2522 Once Upon a Time Volume III: Journey Through Time

Compu-Teach
16541 Redmond Way
Redmond, WA 98052
425-885-0517
800-448-3224
FAX 425-883-9169
http://www.compu-teach.com
e-mail: info@compu-teach.com
David Urban, President

Makes writing, reading and vocabulary skills easy to learn. With imagination as a youngster's only guide, the important concepts of story creation and illustration are naturally discovered. Themes: Medieval Times, Wild West and Outer Space. *$59.95*
Ages 4-12

2523 Once Upon a Time Volume IV: Exploring Nature

Compu-Teach
16541 Redmond Way
Redmond, WA 98052
425-885-0517
800-448-3224
FAX 425-883-9169
http://www.compu-teach.com
e-mail: info@compu-teach.com
David Urban, President

The latest in award-winning creative writing series. Kids just hear, click and draw as the state of the art graphics and digitized voice make writing, reading and vocabulary skills easy to learn. Themes: Rain Forest; African Grasslands; Ocean; Desert; and Forest. *$59.95*

2524 Read, Write and Type Learning System

Talking Fingers, California Neuropsych Services
830 Rincon Way
San Rafael, CA 94901
415-472-3103
800-674-9126
FAX 415-472-7812
http://www.readwritetype.com
e-mail: contact@talkingfingers.com
Jeannine Herron, President

A 40-level software adventure providing highly motivating instruction and practice in phonics, reading, writing, spelling and typing. This multisensory program includes 9 levels of assessment and reports. Classroom packs available.

2525 StartWrite Handwriting Software

Therapro
225 Arlington Street
Framingham, MA 01702
508-872-9494
800-257-5376
FAX 508-875-2062
http://www.theraproducts.com
e-mail: info@theraproducts.com
Therapro Staff, Author
Karen Conrad, President

With this easy-to-use software package, you can make papers and handwriting worksheets to meet individual student's needs. Type letters, words, or numbers and they appear in a dot format on the triple line guide. Change letter size, add shading, turn on or off guide lines and arrow strokes and place provided clipart. Fonts include Manuscript and Cursive, Modern Manuscript and Cursive and Italic Manuscript and Cursive. Useful manual included. *$39.95*

Windows/Mac

2526 Wish Writer

Consultants for Communication Technology
508 Bellevue Terrace
Pittsburgh, PA 15202
412-761-6062
FAX 412-761-7336
http://www.ConCommTech.com
e-mail: CCT@ConCommTech.com
Kathleen Miller PhD, Partner
Jaime Olivia, Partner

Wish Writer is a word processing program designed to be used by keyboard or single switch users. Word Prediction feature produces documents with fewer keystrokes. When used with the K, S, or multivoice synthesizers, text typed into the PC can be spoken or printed. *$300.00*

2527 Writing Trek Grades 4-6

Sunburst Technology
1550 Executive Drive
Elgin, IL 60123
888-492-8817
FAX 888-800-3028
http://www.sunburst.com
e-mail: Service@sunburst.com
Mark Sotir, CEO
Mike Gavelek, Senior Vice President of Marketi
Katie Birmingham, Office Manager

Enhance your students' experience in your English language arts classroom with twelve authentic writing projects that build students' competence while encouraging creativity.

2528 Writing Trek Grades 6-8

Sunburst Technology
1550 Executive Drive
Elgin, IL 60123
888-492-8817
FAX 888-800-3028
http://www.sunburst.com
e-mail: Service@sunburst.com
Mark Sotir, CEO
Mike Gavelek, Senior Vice President of Marketi
Katie Birmingham, Office Manager

Twelve authentic language arts projects, activities, and assignments develop your students' writing confidence and ability.

2529 Writing Trek Grades 8-10

Sunburst Technology
1550 Executive Drive
Elgin, IL 60123
888-492-8817
FAX 888-800-3028
http://www.sunburst.com
e-mail: Service@sunburst.com
Mark Sotir, CEO
Mike Gavelek, Senior VP Marketing
Katie Birmingham, Office Manager

Help your students develop a concept of genre as they become familiar with the writing elements and characteristics of a variety of writing forms.

General

2530 American Institute for Foreign Study
9 W Broad Street
Stamford, CT 06902
203-399-5000
FAX 203-399-5590
http://www.aifs.com
e-mail: info@aifs.com
William Gertz, President

Provides summer travel programs overseas and in the US ranging from one week to a full academic year.

2531 American Universities International Program
108 S Main Street
Winterville, GA 30683
706-742-9285
http://www.auip.com
e-mail: info@auip.com
One hundred colleges and universities throughout the USA and Canada that participate in exchange programs.

2532 Association for International Practical Training
10400 Little Patuxent Parkway
Columbia, MD 21044
410-997-2200
800-994-2443
FAX 410-992-3924
http://www.aipt.org
e-mail: aipt@aipt.org
Elizabeth Chazottes, CEO

With more than 55 years of experience and expertise, AIPT is the J-1 visa and work abroad provider that offers the most comprehensive array of programs.

2533 Earthstewards Network
PO Box 10697
Bainbridge Island, WA 98110
206-842-7986
800-561-2909
FAX 206-842-8918
http://www.earthstewards.org
e-mail: outreach@earthstewards.org
Beverly Boos, Vice President
Chuck Meadows, Manager

Hundreds of active, caring people in the US, Canada and other countries. Puts North American teenagers working alongside Northern Irish teenagers and more.

2534 Educational Foundation for Foreign Study
1 Education Street
Cambridge, MA 02141
617-619-1000
800-447-4273
FAX 617-619-1401
http://www.effoundation.org
Asa Fanelli, President
Louise Julian, CEO

Offers an opportunity to study and live for a year in a foreign country for students between the ages of 15 and 18.

2535 Higher Education Consortium for Urban Affairs
2233 University Avenue W
Saint Paul, MN 55114
651-646-8831
800-554-1089
FAX 651-659-9421
http://www.hecua.org
e-mail: info@hecua.org
Michael Eaton, Director of Enrollment Services
Judy , Assistant to Director
Phil Hatlie, Director of Operations
Consortium of 15 Midwest colleges and universities offering undergraduate, academic programs, both international and domestic that incorporate field study and internships in the examination of urban and global issues.

2536 International Homestays
620 SW 5th Avenue
Portland, OR 97204
503-274-1776
800-274-6007
FAX 503-274-9004
http://www.andeo.org
e-mail: info@andeo.org
Melinda Samis, Director
Patty Hayashi, Assistant Director

Formerly International Summerstays, an international network of families, students, teachers, independent travelers and homestay specialists who are dedicated to exploring cross-cultural friendship and understanding.
1981

2537 Lisle Fellowship
900 County Road
Leander, TX 78641
512-259-7621
800-477-1538
FAX 512-259-0392
http://www.lisleinternational.org
e-mail: lisle2@io.com
Mark Kinney, Executive Director

Educational organization which works toward world peace and a better quality of human life through increased understanding between persons of similar and different cultures.

2538 National Society for Experimental Education
c/o Talley Management Group
Mt. Royal, NJ 08061
856-423-3427
FAX 856-423-3420
http://www.nsee.org
e-mail: nsee@talley.com
Karen Roloff, President
Albert Cabral, President Elect
Jenny Keyser, Executive Director
A nonprofit membership association of educators, businesses, and community leaders. Also serves as a national resource center for the development and improvement of experimental education programs nationwide.
1971

2539 No Barriers to Study
Lock Haven University
401 N Fairview Street
Lock Haven, PA 17745
570-893-2011
800-223-8978
FAX 570-893-2659
Russell Jameson Jr, Resident Hall Director
Roger Johnson, Dean

A regional consortium committed to facilitating study abroad for college students with disabilities.

2540 People to People International
501 E Armour Boulevard
Kansas City, MO 64109
816-531-7231
FAX 816-561-7502
http://www.ptpi.org
e-mail: ptpi@ptpi.org
Mary Eisenhower, CEO
Marc Bright, Executive Vice President
Rosanne Rosen, Operations Senior VP
Nonpolitical, nonprofit organization working outside the government to advance the cause of international understanding through international contact.

2541 World Experience
2440 S Hacienda Boulevard
Hacienda Heights, CA 91745
626-330-5719
800-633-6653
FAX 626-333-4914
http://www.worldexperience.org
e-mail: weworld@weworld.com
Bobby Fraker, President
Marje Archambault, Vice President

Nonprofit organization which sponsors, develops and carries out international student exchange programs for study and service abroad.

2542 Youth for Understanding USA

6400 Goldsboro Road
Bethesda, MD 20817

240-235-2100
800-833-6243
FAX 240-235-2104
http://www.yfu-usa.org
e-mail: admissions@yfu.org

Mike Finnell, President
David Barber, Director Admissions/Registration

Nonprofit international exchange program, prepares young people for their responsibilities and opportunities in todays changing, interdependent world through homestay exchange programs. Offers year, semester, and summer study abroad and scholarship opportunities in 34 countries worldwide.

Federal

2543 ABLE DATA
USDE National Institution on Disability and Rehabi
8630 Fenton Street
Silver Spring, MD 20910
301-608-8998
800-227-0216
FAX 301-608-8958
TDY:301-608-8912
http://www.abledata.com
e-mail: abledata@orcmacro.com
Katherine Belknap, Project Director
Steve Lowe, Associate Project Manager

Sponsored by the National Institute on Disability and Rehabilitation Research (NIDRR) of the US Department of Education; provides information on more than 34,000 assistive technology products, including detailed descriptions of each product, price and company information.

2544 ADA Clearinghouse and Resource Center
National Center for State Courts
300 Newport Avenue
Williamsburg, VA 23185
800-616-6164
FAX 757-564-2022
http://www.ncsconline.org
e-mail: webmaster@ncsc.dni.us
Mary Campbell McQueen, President/CEO
Gwen W Williams, CFO/VP Finance & Administration
Robert N Baldwin, Executive VP/General Counsel
Disseminates information on ADA compliance to state and local court systems. Will develop a diagnostic checklist and strategies for compliance specifically relevant to the state and local courts.

2545 ADA Information Line
US Department of Justice
950 Pennsylvania Avenue NW
Washington, DC 20530
800-514-0301
FAX 202-307-1198
http://www.ada.gov
John L Wodatch, Chief

Answers questions about Title II (public services) and Title III (public accommodations) of the Americans with Disabilities Act (ADA). Provides materials and technical assistance on the provisions of the ADA.

2546 ADA Technical Assistance Programs
US Department of Justice
950 Pennsylvania Avenue NW
Washington, DC 20530
202-514-2000
800-514-0301
http://www.usdoj.gov
Federally funded regional resource centers that provide information and referral, technical assistance, public awareness, and training on all aspects of the Americans with Disabilities Act (ADA).
1991

2547 Civil Rights Division: US Department of Justice
Coordination and Review Section
950 Pennsylvania Avenue NW
Washington, DC 20530
202-307-2222
800-848-5306
FAX 202-307-0595
TDY:888-848-0383
http://www.usdoj.gov/crt
Merrily A Friedlander, Chief
Elizabeth Keenan, Deputy Chief
Christine Stoneman, Deputy Chief
The program institution within the federal government responsible for enforcing federal statutes prohibiting discrimination on the basis of race, sex, disability, religion, and national origin.

1957

2548 Clearinghouse on Adult Education and Literacy
US Department of Education
400 Maryland Avenue SW
Washington, DC 20202
800-872-5327
FAX 202-401-0689
TDY:800-437-0833
http://www.ed.gov
Anne Hancock

The Clearinghouse was established in 1981 to link the adult education community with existing resources in adult education, provide information which deals with state administered adult education programs funded under the Adult Education and Family Literacy Act, and provide resources that support adult education activities.

2549 Clearinghouse on Disability Information
Office of Special Education and Rehabilitative Svc
550 12th Street, SW
Washington, DC 20202
202-245-7307
FAX 202-245-7636
TDY:202-205-5637
http://www.ed.gov/about/offices/list/osers/codi
Carolyn Corlett, Contact

Provides information to people with disabilities, or anyone requesting information, by doing research and providing documents in response to inquiries. Information provided includes areas of federal funding for disability-related programs. Staff is trained to refer requests to other sources of disability-related information, if necessary.
1980

2550 Developmental Disability Services: US Department of Health & Human Services
200 Independence Avenue SW
Washington, DC 20201
202-619-0257
877-696-6775
FAX 202-690-7203
http://www.hhs.gov
Michael O Leavili, Secretary

Councils in each state provide training and technical assistance to local and state agencies, employers and the public, improving services to people with developmental disabilities.

2551 Employment Standards Administration: US Department of Labor
200 Constitution Avenue NW
Washington, DC 20210
866-487-2365
http://www.dol.gov
e-mail: esa-public@dol.gov
Elaine Chao, Secretary of Labor

Develops policy and implements legislation for all workers in the nation.

2552 Employment and Training Administration: US Department of Labor
Frances Perkins Building
200 Constitution Avenue NW
Washington, DC 20210
202-693-2700
877-872-5627
FAX 202-693-2725
http://www.doleta.gov
Emily Stover DeRocco, Assistant Secretary
Douglas F Small, Deputy Assistant Secretary
Mason Bishop, Deputy Assistant Secretary
Administers federal government job training and worker dislocation programs, federal grants to states for public employment service programs, and unemployment insurance benefits. These services are primarily provided through state and local workforce development systems.

2553 Equal Employment Opportunity Commission
1801 L Street NW
Washington, DC 20507
202-663-4900
800-669-4000
http://www.eeoc.gov
e-mail: info@ask.eeoc.gov

Naomi C Earp, Chair
Leslie E Silverman, Vice Chair
Stuart J Ishimaru, Commissioner
Enforces Section 501 which prohibits discrimination on the basis of disability in Federal employment, and requires that all Federal agencies establish and implement affirmative action programs for hiring, placing and advancing individuals with disabilities. Also oversees Federal sector equal employment opportunity complaint processing system.

2554 National Council on Disability
1331 F Street NW
Washington, DC 20004
202-272-2004
FAX 202-272-2022
http://www.ncd.gov
e-mail: ncs@ncs.gov

John R Vaugh, Chairman

An independent federal agency comprised of 15 members appointed by the President and confirmed by the Senate.
1978

2555 National Institute of Child Health and Human Development
National Institutes of Health
9000 Rockville Pike
Bethesda, MD 20892
301-496-4000
800-370-2943
FAX 301-496-7101
http://www.nichd.nih.gov
e-mail: NICHDInformationResourceCenter@mail.nih.gov
Elias Zerhouni MD, Director

Its mission is science in pursuit of fundamental knowledge about the nature and behavior of living systems and the application of that knowledge to extend healthy life and reduce the burdens of illness and disability.

2556 National Institute of Mental Health
Public Information & Communications Branch
6001 Executive Boulevard
Bethesda, MD 20892
301-443-4513
866-615-6464
FAX 310-443-4279
http://www.nimh.nih.gov
e-mail: nimhinfo@nih.gov

Dr Thomas Insel MD, Director

Mission is to diminish the burden of mental illness through research. This public health mandate demands that we harness powerful scientific tools to achieve better understanding, treatment and eventually prevention of mental illness.

2557 National Institute on Disability and Rehabilitation Research
US Department of Education
400 Maryland Avenue SW
Washington, DC 20202
202-245-7640
FAX 202-245-7323
http://www.ed.gov/offices
Richard Fisher, Acting Director/Deputy Director

Provides leadership and support for a comprehensive program of research related to the rehabilitation of individuals with disabilities. All of the programmatic efforts are aimed to improving the lives of individuals with disabilities from birth through adulthood.
1978

2558 National Library Services for the Blind and Physically Handicapped
Library of Congress
101 Independence Avenue, SE
Washington, DC 20540
202-707-8000
FAX 202-707-0712
http://www.loc.gov/nls
e-mail: nls@loc.gov

Kenneth E Lopez, Director

Administers a free program that loans recorded and braille books and magazines, music scores in braille and large print, and specially designed playback equipment to residents of the United States who are unable to read or use standard print materials because of visual or physical impairment.

2559 National Technical Information Service: US Department of Commerce
5285 Port Royal Road
Springfield, VA 22161
703-605-6000
http://www.ntis.gov
Dr John Regazzi, Chairperson

Serves the nation as the largest central resource for government-funded scientific, technical, engineering, and business related information available today.

2560 Office for Civil Rights: US Department of Health and Human Services
US Department of Health & Human Services
200 Independence Avenue SW
Washington, DC 20201
800-368-1019
TDY:800-537-7697
http://www.hhd.gov/ocr
e-mail: ocrmail@hhs.gov

Winston Wilkinson, Director

Promotes and ensures that peopl ehave equal access to an dopportunity to participate in and receive services from all HHS programs without facing unlawful discrimination, and that the privacy of their health information is protectec while ensuring access to care.

2561 Office of Civil Rights: US Department of Education
400 Maryland Avenue, SW
Washington, DC 20202
800-421-3481
FAX 202-245-6840
TDY:877-521-2172
http://www.ed.gov/ocr
e-mail: ocr@ed.gov
Stephanie Monroe, Assistant Secretary Civil Rights
David Black, Deputy Asst Secretary Enforcemt
Tonya M Johnson-Fitzpatrick, Deputy Asst Secretary for Policy
To ensure equal access to education and to promote educational excellence throughout the nation through vigourous enforcement of civil rights.

2562 Office of Disability Employment Policy
US Department of Labor
200 Constitution Avenue NW
Washington, DC 20210
866-633-7365
http://www.dol.gov/odep
Elaine Chao, Secretary of Labor
Howard M Radzely, Acting Deputy Secretary
Ruth D Knouse, Executive Secretariat Director
Provides national leadership by developine and influencing disability-related employment policy as well as practice affecting the employment of people with disabilities.

2563 Office of Federal Contract Compliance Programs: US Department of Labor
200 Constitution Avenue NW
Washington, DC 20210
202-693-0101
http://www.dol.gov/esa/ofccp
e-mail: ofccp-public@dol.gov
David Frank, Deputy Director
Charles E James Sr, Deputy Assistant Secretary

Responsible for ensuring that employers doing business with the Federal government comply with the laws and regulations requiring nondiscrimination and affirmative action in employment.

2564 Office of Personnel Management
Office of Human Resources & EEO
1900 E Street NW
Washington, DC 20415
202-606-1800
http://www.opm.gov
e-mail: general@opm.gov

Linda M Springer, Director

The central personnel agency of the federal government. Provides information on the selective placement program for persons with disabilities.

2565 **Office of Program Operations: US Department of Education**
400 Maryland Avenue SW
Washington, DC 20202
202-205-5413
800-872-5327
FAX 202-401-0689
http://www.ed.gov
e-mail: customerservice@inet.ed.gov
Programs in each state provide information and assistance to individuals seeking or receiving services under the Rehabilitation Act of 1973.

2566 **Protection & Advocacy System**
Comprehensive Advocacy, Inc (Co-Ad)
4477 Emerald Street
Boise, ID 83706
208-336-5353
866-262-3462
FAX 208-336-5396
TDY:208-336-5353
http://users.moscow.com/co-ad
e-mail: coadinc@cableone.net
James R Baugh, Executive Director

Comprehensive Advocacy, Inc is the designated Protection and Advocacy System for Idaho. Co-Ad provides advocacy for people with disabilities who have been abused/neglected; denied services or benefits; have experienced rights violations or discrimination because of their disability; or have voting accessibility problems. Co-Ad provides information 7 referral; negotitation & mediation; short term & technical assistance; legal advice/representation.

2567 **Rehabilitation Services Administration State Vocational Program**
US Department of Education
400 Maryland Avenue SW
Washington, DC 20202
202-401-2000
800-872-5327
FAX 202-401-0689
Margaret Spellings, CEO

State and local vocational rehabilitation agencies provide comprehensive services of rehabilitation, training and job-related assistance to people with disabilities and assist employers in recruiting, training, placing, accommodating and meeting other employment-related needs of people with disabilities.

2568 **Social Security Administration**
Office of Public Inquiries
Windsor Park Building
Baltimore, MD 21235
800-772-1213
http://www.socialsecurity.gov
e-mail: webmaster@ssa.gov
Michael J Astrue, Commissioner

Provides financial assistance to those with disabilities who meet eligibility requirements.

2569 **US Bureau of the Census**
4700 Silver Hill Road
Washington, DC 20233
301-763-4748
http://www.census.gov
e-mail: recruiter@census.gov
Jeri A Green, Chief, Census Advisory Committee

The principal statistical agency of the federal government. It publishes data on persons with disabilities, as well as other demographic data derived from censuses and surveys.

Alabama

2570 **Alabama Council for Developmental Disabilities**
RSA Union Building, 100 N Union St
Montgomery, AL 36130
334-242-3973
800-232-2158
FAX 334-242-0797
http://www.acdd.org
e-mail: addpc@mh.state.al.us
Elmyra Jones, Executive Director
Cheryl Bartlett PhD, Planning/Quality Assurance
Debra Florea, Information/Referral
Serves as an advocate for Alabama's citizens with developmental disabilities and their families; to empower them with the knowledge and opportunity to make informed choices and exercise control over their own lives; and to create a climate for positive social change to enable them to be respected, independent and productive integrated members of society.

2571 **Alabama Department of Industrial Relations**
649 Monroe Street
Montgomery, AL 36131
334-242-8990
FAX 334-242-3960
http://http://dir.alabama.gov
e-mail: director@dir.alabama.gov
Phyllis Kennedy, Director
Donald K Fisher, Assistant Director

To effectively use tax dollars to provide state and federal mandated workforce protection programs promoting a positive economic environment for Alabama employers and workers and to produce and disseminate information on the Alabama economy.

2572 **Alabama Disabilities Advocacy Program**
PO Box 870395
Tuscaloosa, AL 35487
205-348-4928
800-826-1675
FAX 205-348-3909
http://www.adap.net
e-mail: adap@adap.ua.edu
Ellen Gillespie, Director

To provide quality, legally-based advocacy services to Alabamians with disabilities in order to protect, promote and expand their rights.

2573 **Employment Service Division: Alabama**
Department of Industrial Relations
649 Monroe Street
Montgomery, AL 36131
334-242-8003
FAX 334-242-8012
http://dir.alabama.gov
e-mail: es@dir.alabama.gov
Steve Horton, Director

Alaska

2574 **Alaska Department of Labor: Employment Security Division**
Department of Labor
PO Box 115509
Juneau, AK 99811
907-465-2712
FAX 907-465-4537
http://http://labor.state.ak.us
e-mail: esd_director@labor.state.ak.us
Thomas Nelson, Director

Promotes employment, economic stability, and growth by operating a no-fee labor exchange that meets the needs of employers, job seekers, and veterans.

2575 **Alaska State Commission for Human Rights**
800 A Street
Anchorage, AK 99501
907-274-4692
FAX 907-278-8588
TDY:907-276-3177
http://www.gov.state.ak.us/aschr
Paula Haley, Executive Director
Anne Keene, Administrative Manager

2576 **Assistive Technology**
2217 E Tudor Road
Anchorage, AK 99507
907-563-2599
800-723-2852
FAX 907-563-0699
http://www.atla.biz
e-mail: kathy@atla.biz

Kathy Privratsky, Executive Director
Richard Sanders, Program Manager & AT

To enhance the quality of life for Alaskans through education, demonstration, consultation, acquisition and implementation of assistive technologies.

2577 **Center for Community**
700 Katlian Street
Sitka, AK 99835
907-747-6960
800-478-6970
FAX 907-747-4868

Margaret Andrews, Services Director
Connie Sipe, Executive Director

Center for Community is a multiservice agency that provides early intervention, respite, futures planning, functional skills training, and vocational assistance for people with disabilities.

2578 **Correctional Education Division: Alaska**
Department of Corrections/Division of Institutions
551 W 7th Avenue
Anchorage, AK 99501
907-269-7434
FAX 907-269-7420
http://www.correct.state.ak.us/
e-mail: anna.herzberger@alaska.gov

Anna Herberger, Criminal Justice Planner

2579 **Disability Law Center of Alaska**
3330 Arctic Boulevard
Anchorage, AK 99503
907-565-1002
800-478-1234
FAX 907-565-1000
http://www.dlcak.org
e-mail: akpa@dlcak.org

David Fleurant, Executive Director

An independent non-profit organization that provides legal advocacyservices for people with disabilities anywhere in Alaska. To promote and protect the legal and human rights of individuals with physical and/or mental disabilities.

2580 **State Department of Education & Early Development**
Department of Education
801 W 10th Street, Suite 200
Juneau, AK 99801
907-465-2800
FAX 907-465-4156
http://www.eed.state.ak.us/

Barbara Thompson, Interim Commissioner

Committed to develop, maintain and continuously improve a comprehensive, quality system to rpovide resources, data and world class support services that inspire quality learning for all.

2581 **State GED Administration: GED Testing Program**
Alaska Department of Education
801 W 10th Street
Juneau, AK 99801
907-465-2880
http://www.eed.state.ak.us/

Roger Samson, Commissioner
Karen Rehfeld, Executive Director
Barbara Thompson, TLS Director

2582 **State of Alaska Community & Regional Affairs Department: Administrative Services**
150 3rd Street
Juneau, AK 99801
907-465-4708
FAX 907-465-3519

Arizona

2583 **Arizona Center for Disability Law**
100 N Stone Avenue
Tucson, AZ 85701
520-327-9547
800-922-1447
FAX 520-884-0992
http://www.acdl.com
e-mail: center@azdisabilitylaw.org

Peri Jude Radecic, Executive Director

Advocates for the leagl rights of persons with disabilities to be free from abuse, neglect and discrimination; and to have access to education, healthcare, housing and jobs, and other services in order to maximize independence and achieve equality.

2584 **Arizona Center for Law in the Public Interest**
2205 E Speedway Boulevard
Tucson, AZ 85719
520-529-1798
FAX 520-529-2927
http://www.NAU.edu\~ihd/acdl.html
e-mail: info@aclpi.org

Leslie Cohen, Executive Director

2585 **Arizona Department of Economic Security**
Rehabilitation Services Administration
1789 W Jefferson Street 2NW
Phoenix, AZ 85007
602-542-3332
800-563-1221
FAX 602-542-3778
http://www.azdes.gov/rsa
e-mail: azrsa@azdes.gov

Tracy Wareing, Director
Sharon Sergent, Deputy Director

Promotes the safety, well-being, and self sufficiency of children, asults and families.
1972

2586 **Arizona Department of Education**
1535 W Jefferson Street
Phoenix, AZ 85007
602-542-5393
800-352-4558
http://www.ade.az.gov

Tom Horne, Superintendent, Public Instruct

To ensure academic excellence for all students.

2587 **Arizona Governor's Committee on Employment of the Handicapped**
ALS Association Arizona Chapter
4520 N Central Avenue
Phoenix, AZ 85012
602-297-3800
866-350-2572
http://www.alsaz.org
e-mail: ken@alsaz.org

Ken Brissa, Executive Director
Jo Tanzer, Patient Services Director
Kim Hughes, Patient Services Coordinator
To lead the fight to cure and treat ALS through global, cutting-edge research, and to empower people with Lou Gehrig's disease and their families to live fuller lives by providing them with compassionate care and support.

2588 **Correctional Education**
Arizona Department of Corrections
1601 W Jefferson Street
Phoenix, AZ 85007
602-542-5536
FAX 602-364-0259
e-mail: bkilian@adc.state.az.us

Dora Schriro, Manager

2589 **Division of Adult Education**
Arizona Department of Education
1535 W Jefferson Street
Phoenix, AZ 85007
602-258-2410
FAX 602-258-4986
http://www.ade.az.gov
e-mail: adulted@ade.az.gov
Karen Liersch, Adult Education

2590 **Fair Employment Practice Agency**
Office of the Arizona Attorney General
1275 W Washington Street
Phoenix, AZ 85007
602-542-5263
877-491-5742
FAX 602-542-8885
TDY:602-542-5002
http://www.azag.gov
e-mail: civilrightsinfo@azag.gov
Terry Goddard, Attorney General

2591 **GED Testing Services**
Arizona Department of Education
1535 W Jefferson Street
Phoenix, AZ 85007
602-258-2410
FAX 602-258-4977
http://www.ade.az.gov
e-mail: phxged@ade.az.gov
Karen Liersch, Adult Education

2592 **Governor's Council on Developmental Disabilities**
3839 N 3rd Street
Phoenix, AZ 85012
602-863-0484
866-771-9378
FAX 602-277-4454
http://www.azgcdd.org
e-mail: djohnson@azdes.gov
Dara Johnson, Acting Executive Director
Sue Miller, Administrative Assistant

To work in partnership with individuals with developmental disabilities and their families through systems change, advocacy and capacity building activities that promote indpendence, choice and the ability to pursue their own dreams.

Arkansas

2593 **Arkansas Deparment of Correction**
PO Box 8707
Pine Bluff, AR 71611
870-267-6999
http://www.arkansas.gov/doc
Larry B Norris, Director

To provide public safety by carrying out the mandates of the courts; provide a safe humane environment for staff and inmates; provide programs to strengthen the work ethic; and provide opportunities for spiritual, mental, and physical growth.

2594 **Arkansas Department of Education**
4 Capitol Mall
Little Rock, AR 72201
501-682-4475
http://arkansased.org
e-mail: ade.communications@arkansas.gov
T Kenneth James, Commissioner
Dr Diana Julian, Deputy Commissioner

Strives to ensure that all children in the state have acess to a quality education by providing educators, administrators anad staff with leadership, resources and training.

2595 **Arkansas Department of Human Services: Division of Rehabilitation Services**
PO Box 1437
Little Rock, AR 72203
501-682-1121
FAX 501-682-8679
http://www.state.ar.us/dhs
Marcia Harding, Associate Director
Barbara Pardue, Executive Director

2596 **Arkansas Department of Special Education**
1401 W Capitol Ave, Victory Bldg
Little Rock, AR 72201
501-682-4221
http://arksped.k12.ar.us
e-mail: spedsupport@arkansas.gov
Marcia Harding, Associate Director

2597 **Arkansas Department of Workforce Education**
Lither Hardin Building
Little Rock, AR 72201
501-682-1500
FAX 501-682-1509
http://dwe.arkansas.gov
e-mail: william.walker@arkansas.gov
William J Walker Jr, Director

To provide the leadership and contribute resources to serve the diverse and changing workforce training needs of the youth and adults in Arkansas.

2598 **Arkansas Employment Security Department**
PO Box 2981
Little Rock, AR 72203
501-682-3105
FAX 501-682-3748
TDY:501-296-1669
http://www.state.ar.us/esd
e-mail: ed.rolle.aesd@mial.state.ar.us
Albessie Thompson, Equal Opportunity Manager

2599 **Arkansas Governor's Developmental Disabilities Council**
5800 W 10th Street
Little Rock, AR 72204
501-661-2589
800-482-5400
FAX 501-661-2399
http://www.ddcouncil.org
e-mail: mary.edwards@arkansas.gov
Mary Edwards, Council Coordinator
Lee C Russell, Information Officer
Brenda L Mercer, Family Services Coordinator
Supports people with developmental disabilities in the achievement of independence, productivity, integration and inclusion in the community.

2600 **Assistive Technology Project**
Increasing Capabilities Access Network (ICAN)
26 Corporate Hill
Little Rock, AR 72205
501-666-8868
800-828-2799
FAX 501-666-5319
http://www.arkansas-ican.org
A consumer responsive statewide program promoting assistive technology devices and resources for persons of all ages and all disabilities.

2601 **Client Assistance Program (CAP): Arkansas Division of Persons with Disabilities**
Disability Rights Center
1100 N University Avenue
Little Rock, AR 72207
501-296-1775
800-482-1174
FAX 501-296-1779
http://www.arkdisabilityrights.org
e-mail: panda@arkdisabilityrights.org
Nan Ellen D East, Executive Director
Eddie Miller, CAP Director

The purpose of CAP is to protect the rights of persons receiving or seeking services funded under the federal Rehabilitation Act. According to thise law, CAP services are available for all clients or applicants of the following services: Vocational Rehabilitation Services, Independent Living Services, Supported Employment, Independent Living Centers, and Projects with Industry.

2602 Increasing Capabilities Access Network
26 Corporate Hill Drive
Little Rock, AR 72205
601-666-8868
800-828-2799
FAX 501-666-5319
TDY:501-666-8868
http://www.arkansas-ICAN.org
e-mail: bmvuletich@ars.state.ar.us
Barry Vuletich, Project Administrator

A federally funded program of Arkansas Rehabilitation Services, is designed to make technology available and accessible for all who need it. ICAN is a funding information resource and provides information on new and existing technology free to any person regardless of age or disability.

2603 Office of the Governor
State Capitol
Little Rock, AR 72201
501-682-2345
FAX 501-682-1382
http://www.governor.arkansas.gov
Mike Beebe, Governor

2604 Protection & Advocacy Agency
Disability Rights Center
1100 N University Avenue
Little Rock, AR 72207
501-296-1775
800-482-1174
FAX 501-296-1779
http://www.arkdisabilityrights.org
e-mail: panda@arkdisabilityrights.org
Nan Ellen D East, Executive Director

Carry out activities under several Federal programs to provide a range of services to adocate for and protect the rights of persons with disabilities throughout the state

2605 State GED Administration
Department of Workforce Education
Luther S Hardin Building
Little Rock, AR 72201
501-682-1978
FAX 501-682-1982
http://dwe.arkansas.gov
e-mail: janice.hanlon@mail.state.ar.us
Janice Hanlon, GED Test Administrator

California

2606 California Department of Fair Employment and Housing
2000 O Street
Sacramento, CA 95814
916-445-5523
800-884-1684
FAX 916-323-6092
http://www.dfeh.ca.gov
David Supkofl, Manager

To protect the people of California from unlawful discrimination in employment, housing and public accomodations, and from the perpetration of acts of hate violence.

2607 California Department of Rehabilitation
PO Box 944222
Sacramento, CA 94244
916-263-7365
FAX 916-263-7474
TDY:916-263-7477
http://www.rehab.cahwnet.gov
e-mail: publicaffairs@dor.ca.gov
Catherine Campisi, Director

Works in partnership with consumers and other stakeholders to provide services and advocacy resulting in employment, independent living and equality for individuals with disabilities.

2608 California Department of Special Education
1430 N Street
Sacramento, CA 95814
916-445-4613
FAX 916-327-3516
Mary Hudler, Director

2609 California Employment Development Department
800 Capitol Mall
Sacramento, CA 95814
916-654-8210
FAX 916-657-5294
http://www.edd.ca.gov
Patrick Henning, Director
Pam Harris, Chief Deputy Director

Promotes California's economic growth by providing services to keep employers, employees, and job seekers competitive.

2610 California State Board of Education
1430 N Street
Sacramento, CA 95814
916-319-0800
FAX 916-319-0175
http://www.cde.ca.gov/be
Roger Magyar, Executive Director
Gary Borden, Chief Deputy Director

The State Board of Education (SBE) is the governing and policy making body of the California Department of Education. The SBE sets K-12 education policy in the areas of standards, instructional materials, accessment, and accountability.

2611 California State Council on Developmental Disabilities
1507 21st Street
Sacramento, CA 95814
916-322-8481
866-802-0514
FAX 916-443-4957
TDY:916-324-8420
http://www.scdd.ca.gov
e-mail: council@dss.ca.gov
Sascha Bittner, Chair

Advocates, promotes and implements policies and practices that achieve self-determination, independence, productivity and inclusion in all aspects of community life for Californians with developmental disabilities and their families.

2612 Career Assessment and Placement Center Whittier Union High School District
9401 Painter Avenue
Whittier, CA 90605
562-698-8121
FAX 562-693-5354
Daniel Hubert

Provides job placement programs, remunerative work services and work adjustment training programs.

2613 Clearinghouse for Specialized Media
California Department of Education
1430 N Avenue
Sacramento, CA 95838
916-323-2202
FAX 916-323-9732
http://www.cde.ca.gov/re/pn/sm
e-mail: rbrawley@cde.ca.gov
Thomas Adams, Director
Rod Brawley, Clearinghouse Media Manager
Steven Parker, BSA
Supports access to general education curriculum by students with disabilities. This unit of the state curriculum framework and instructional resources division produces accessible versions of textbooks, workbooks, and literature books adopted for all public schools by the State Board of Education.

2614 Education & Inmate Programs Unit
PO Box 942883
Sacramento, CA 94283
916-445-8035
800-952-5544
FAX 916-324-1416
http://www.corr.ca.gov
Jan Stuter, Manager
Gary Sutherland, Federal Grand Administrator
Adrianne Johnson, Secretary

2615 Employment Development Department: Employment Services Woodland
800 Capitol Mall
Sacramento, CA 95814
530-661-2600
FAX 530-668-3152
http://www.edd.ca.gov
Bill Burke, Contact

The Employment Development Department promote's California's economic growth by providing services to keep employers, employees, and job seekers competitive.

2616 Employment Development Department: Employment Services W Sacramento
California Health and Human Services Agency
500 Jefferson Boulevard
W Sacramento, CA 95605
916-375-6288
FAX 916-375-6310
http://www.edd.ca.gov
Bill Burke, Contact

2617 Office of Civil Rights: California
50 Beale Street
San Francisco, CA 94105
415-486-5555
FAX 415-486-5570
TDY:877-521-2172
http://www.ed.gov/ocr
e-mail: ocr.sanfrancisco@ed.gov

2618 Pacific Disability and Business Technical Assistance Center
555 12th Street
Oakland, CA 94607
510-285-5600
800-949-4232
FAX 510-285-5614
http://www.pacdbtac.org
e-mail: info@pdbtac.com
Erica Jones, Executive Director

To build a partnership between the disability and business communities and to promote full and unrestricted participation in society for persons with disabilities through education and technical assistance.

2619 Protection & Advocacy
100 Howe Avenue
Sacramento, CA 95825
916-488-9955
http://www.pai-ca.org
Catherine Blakemore, Executive Director

Advancing the human and legal rights of people with disabilities.

2620 Region IX: US Department of Education
US Department of Education
50 United Nations Plaza
San Francisco, CA 94012
415-556-4120
FAX 415-437-7540
http://www.ed.gov
The Office of Federal Contract Compliance Programs is part of the US Department of Labor's Employment Standards Administration. It has a national network of six regional offices, each with district and area offices in major metropolitan centers.

2621 Region IX: US Department of Health and Human Services
50 United Nations Plaza
San Francisco, CA 94102
415-437-8500
FAX 415-437-8505
http://www.hhs.gov/region9
e-mail: thomas.lorentzen@hhs.gov
Tom Lorentzen, Regional Director
Michael Kruley, Regional Manager, Civil Rights

2622 Sacramento County Office of Education
10474 Mather Boulevard
Sacramento, CA 95827
916-228-2500
http://www.scoe.net
David Gordon, Superintendent

A customer-driven educational leader and agent got change in the country, region and state, is to support the preparation of students for a changing and global 21st century society, through a continuously improving system of aprtnerships and coordinated services for our diverse community.

Colorado

2623 Assistive Technology Partners
601 E 18th Avenue
Denver, CO 80203
303-315-1280
800-255-3477
FAX 303-837-1208
http://www.uchsc.edu/atp
Cathy Bodine, Director
Miya Adams, Administrative Assistant

Designed to support capacity building and advocacy activities, and to assist states in maintaining permanent, comprehensive statewide programs of technology related assistance for all people with disabilities living in Colorado.

2624 Colorado Civil Rights Division
1560 Broadway
Denver, CO 80202
303-894-2997
FAX 303-894-7830
http://www.dora.state.co.us/civil-rights/
e-mail: ccrd@dora.state.co.us
Wendell Pryor, Director

2625 Colorado Department of Labor and Employment
633 17th Street
Denver, CO 80202
303-318-8000
http://www.coworkforce.com
Donald J Mares, Executive Director

2626 Colorado Developmental Disabilities
3824 W Princeton Circle
Denver, CO 80236
303-866-7450
FAX 303-866-7470
http://www.colorado.gov
e-mail: cddpc@aol.com
Fred DeCrescentis, Executive Director
Barbara Ramsey, Assistant Director

2627 Correctional Education Division
Colorado Department of Corrections
2862 S Circle Drive
Colorado Springs, CO 80906
719-579-9580
FAX 719-226-4755
http://www.doc.state.co.us/programs.htm
e-mail: executive.director@doc.state.co.us
Joe Ortiz, Executive Director
Dr Anthony Romero, Asst Director, Educational Serv

To meet the diverse educational needs of inmates through the provision of quality academic, vocational, life skills, and transitional services whereby inmates can successfully integrate into society, gain and maintain employment and become responsible, productive individuals.

2628 Protection & Advocacy Agency
455 Sherman Street
Denver, CO 80203
303-722-0300
800-288-1376
FAX 303-722-0720
http://www.thelegalcenter.org
e-mail: tlcmail@thelegalcenter.org
An independent public interest non-profit specializing in civil rights and discrimination issues. Protects the human, civil and leagl rights of people with mental and physical disabilities, people with HIV, and older people throughout Colorado.

2629 Region VIII: US Department of Education
Office of Civil Rights
Cesar E Chavez Memorial Building
Denver, CO 80204
303-844-5695
FAX 303-844-4303
http://www.ed.gov
e-mail: ocr.denver@ed.gov

Helen Littlejohn, Manager
Lilian Gutierrez, Civil Rights Director
Nancy Haberkorn, Office Assistant
This office covers the states of Arizona, Colorado, New Mexico, Utah, and Wyoming.

2630 Region VIII: US Department of Health andHuman Services
Bryon G Rogers Federal Building
1961 Stout Street
Denver, CO 80294
303-844-3372
FAX 303-844-4545
http://www.hhs.gov/region8
e-mail: joe.nunez@hhs.gov

Joe Nunez, Regional Director
Velveta Howell, Regional Manager Civil Rights

2631 Region VIII: US Department of Labor-Office of Federal Contract Compliance
US Department of Labor
1809 California Street
Denver, CO 80202
303-844-1600
FAX 303-844-1616
These regional offices of agencies enforce laws prohibiting employment discrimination on the basis of disability.

2632 State Department of Education
201 E Colfax Avenue
Denver, CO 80203
303-866-6600
http://www.cde.state.co.us
e-mail: howerter_c@cde.state.co.us
William J Moloney, Commissioner

The administrative arm of the Colorado Board of Education. CDE serves colorado's 178 local school districts, providing them with leadership, consultation and administrative services on a statewide and regional basis.

Connecticut

2633 Assistive Technology Project
25 Sigourney Street
Hartford, CT 06106
860-424-4881
800-537-2549
FAX 860-424-4850
http://www.cttechact.com

Arlene Lugo, Coordinatior

To increase independence and improve the lives of individuals with disabilities through increased access to Assistive Technology for work, school and community living.

2634 Bureau of Special Education & Pupil Services
Department of Education
25 Industrial Park Road
Middletown, CT 06457
860-807-2005
FAX 860-807-2047
http://www.stat.ct.us/sde/
e-mail: george.dowaliby@po.state.ct.us
George Coleman, Manager

Offers information on educational programs and services. The Complaint Resolution Process Office answers and processes parent complaints regarding procedural violations by local educational agencies and facilities. The Due Process Office is responsible for the management of special education and due process proceedings which are available to parents and school districts.

2635 CHILD FIND of Connecticut
25 Industrial Park Road
Middletown, CT 06457
860-632-1485
800-445-2722
FAX 860-632-8870
http://www.ctserc.org

Marianne Kirner, Director
Carol Sullivan, Assistant Director
Sarah Barzee, Assistant Director
A service under the direction of The Connecticut State Department of Education and operated by the Special Education Resource Center. The primary goal is the identification, diagnosis and programming of all unserved disabled children.
1969

2636 Connecticut Bureau of Rehabilitation Services
State of Connecticut
25 Sigourney Street
Hartford, CT 06106
860-424-4844
800-537-2549
FAX 860-424-4850
TDY:860-424-4839
http://www.brs.state.ct.us
e-mail: evelyn.knight@ct.gov
Michael Starkowski, Commissioner
Brenda L Moore, Bureau Director

Offers vocational rehabilitation and independent living services to individuals who are physically or mentally disabled.

2637 Connecticut Department of Social Services
25 Sigourney Street
Hartford, CT 06106
800-842-1508
TDY:800-842-4524
http://www.ct.gov/dss
e-mail: pgr.dss@ct.gov
Michael P Starkowski, Commissioner

Provides a broad range of services to the elderly, disabled, families and individuals who need assistance in maintaining or achieving their full potential for self-director, self-reliance and independent living.

2638 Connecticut Office of Protection & Advocacecy for Handicapped & DD Persons
Office of Protection & Advocacy
60 W Street
Hartford, CT 06106
860-297-4300
800-842-7303
FAX 860-566-8714
TDY:860-566-2102
http://www.state.ct.us/opapd
e-mail: james.mcgaughey@po.state.ct.us
James Gaughey, Executive Director

Supports families and individuals who are affected by developmental disabilities.

2639 Connecticut State Department of Education
165 Capitol
Hartford, CT 06145
860-713-6543
http://www.state.ct.us/sde
Dr Mark K McQuillan, Commissioner

The adminstrative arm of the Connecticut State Board of Education. Through leadership, curriculum, research, planning, evaluation, assessment, data analyses and other assistance, the Department helps to ensure equal opportunity and excellence in education for all Connecticut students.

2640 Correctional Education Division: Connecticut
Unified School District #1
24 Wolcott Hill Road
Wethersfield, CT 06109 860-692-7536
FAX 860-692-7538
http://www.state.ct.us/doc/
e-mail: angela.jalbert@po.state.ct.us
William B Barber, Superintendent
Theresa C Lantz, Commissioner

Education continues to be one of the Department's more valuable assets in providing opportunities that will support an offender's successful community reintegration. Education programming is available to inmates through the Unified School District (USD)#l, a legally vested school district within the Department of Correction (DOC).

2641 Protection & Advocacy Agency
Office of P&A for Persons with Disabilities
60B Weston Street
Hartford, CT 06120 860-297-4300
800-842-7303
FAX 860-566-8714
http://www.ct.gov/opapd
James Gaughey, Executive Director

To advnace the cause of equal rights for persons with disabilities and their families.

2642 State GED Administration
Bureau of Adult Education and Training
25 Industrial Park Road
Middletown, CT 06457 860-807-2110
FAX 860-807-2112
e-mail: roberta.pawloski@po.state.ct.us
Paul F Flinter, Bureau Chief
Carl Paternostro, GED Administrator

The primary aid of the GED testing program in Connecticut is to provide a second opportunity for individuals to obtain their high school diplomas.

2643 State of Connecticut Board of Education & Services for the Blind
184 Windsor Avenue
Windsor, CT 06095 860-602-4000
FAX 860-602-4020
TDY:860-602-4221
http://www.ct.gov/besb
e-mail: besb@po.state.ct.us
Brian Signan, Executive Director
Keith Maynard, Plant Manager

Provide quality educational and rehabilitative service to all people who are legally blind or deaf-blind and children who are visually impaired at no cost to our clients or their families.

Delaware

2644 Client Assistance Program (CAP): Maryland Division of Persons with Disabilities
254 E Camden Wyoming Avenue
Camden, DE 19934 302-698-9336
800-640-9336
FAX 302-698-9338
http://www.protectionandadvocacy.com
e-mail: info@magpage.com
Melissa Shahun, Executive Director

Provides free services to consumers and applicants for projects, programs and facilities funded under the Rehabilitation Act.

2645 Correctional Education Division
Department of Corrections
245 McKee Road
Dover, DE 19904 302-739-5601
FAX 302-739-7215
http://www.state.de.us/correct/ddoc/default.htm
e-mail: johnj.ryan@state.de.us
Carl Danberg, Commissioner
Alexa Faucey, Contact Person
John Ryan, Associate

2646 Delaware Assistive Technology Initiative
University of DE/Alfred I duPont Hosp for Children
PO Box 269
Wilmington, DE 19899 302-651-6790
800-870-DATI
FAX 302-651-6793
TDY:302-651-6794
http://www.dati.org
Beth Mineo Mollica, Director

Connects Delawareans who have disabilities with the tools they need in order to learn, work, play, and participate in community life safely and independently. Also operates Assistive Technology Resource Centers that offer training as well as no-cost equipment demonstrations and loans. Also provide funding information, develop partnerships with state agenices and organizations and publish resource materials and event calendars.

2647 Delaware Department of Education
John G Townsend Building
401 Federal Street
Dover, DE 19901 302-735-4000
FAX 302-739-4654
http://www.doe.state.de.us
e-mail: dedoe@doe.k12.de.us
Valerie Woodruff, Secretary of Education
Nancy Wilson, Deputy Secretary of Education

Committed to promoting the highest quality education for every Delaware student by providing visionary leadership and superior service.

2648 Delaware Department of Labor
4425 N Market Street
Wilmington, DE 19802 302-575-7371
FAX 302-761-6621
http://www.delawareworks.com
e-mail: dlabor@state.de.us
Thomas B Sharp, Secretary of Labor

Connects people to jobs, resources, monetary benefits, workplace protections and labor market information to promote financial independence, workplace justice and a strong economy.

2649 Protection & Advocacy Agency
Community Legal Aid Society
Community Services Bldg, Suite 801
Wilmington, DE 19801 302-575-0660
FAX 302-575-0840
TDY:302-575-0696
http://www.declasi.org
Christopher W White, Executive Director

Community Legal Aid Society is a private, non-profit law firm dedicated to equal justice for all. Prodive civil legal services to assist clients in becoming self sufficient and meeting basic needs with dignity. Clients include members of the community who have low incomes, who have disabilities, or who are age 60 and over.

2650 State GED Administration: Delaware
Department of Education
35 Commerce Way
Dover, DE 19904 302-857-3340
FAX 302-739-1770
http://www.doe.k12.de.us
e-mail: mwhelan@doe.k12.de.us
Maureen Whelan, Director Adult Education
Valerie Woodruff, Secretary of Education

The primary aid of the GED testing program in Delaware is to provide a second opportunity for individuals to obtain their high school diplomas.

District of Columbia

2651 Client Assistance Program (CAP): District of Columbia
University Legal Services: Protection and Advocacy
220 I Street NE
Washington, DC 20002
202-547-0198
877-211-4638
FAX 202-547-2662
http://www.uls-dc.org
e-mail: jcooney@uls-dc.org
Jane M Brown Esq, Executive Director
Sandy Bernstein Esq, Legal Director
Joseph Cooney, CAP Program Director
A federally funded program authorized under the amended Rehabilitation Act of 1973. University Legal Services administers the CAP program i the District of Columbig under contract with the District of Columbia Rehabilitation Services Administration. The goal of CAP is to identify, explain, and resolve the problems residents of the District of Columbia may be having with the rehabilitation program as quickly as possible.

2652 DC Department of Employment Services
609 H Street NE
Washington, DC 20002
202-724-7000
FAX 202-673-6993
TDY:202-698-4817
http://www.does.dc.gov
e-mail: does@dc.gov
Summer Spencer, Director

The mission of the Department of Employment Services is to plan, develop and administer employment-related services to all segments of the Washington, DC metropolitan population. We achieve our mission through empowering and sstaining a diverse workforce, which enables all sectors of the community to achieve economic and social stability.

2653 District of Columbia Department of Corrections
1923 Vermont Avenue NW
Washington, DC 20001
202-673-7316
FAX 202-671-2063
http://www.dc.gov
Devon Brown, Director

Provides public safety by ensuring the safe, secure, and human confinement of pertrial detainees and sentenced misdemeanant prisoners.
1946

2654 District of Columbia Fair Employment Practice Agencies
DC Office of Human Rights
414 4th Street NW
Washington, DC 20001
202-727-4559
FAX 202-727-9589
http://www.ohr.dc.gov
e-mail: ohr@dc.gov
Gustavo F Velasquez, Director

The DC Office of Human Rights is an agency of the District of Columbia government that seeks to eradicate discrimination, increase equal opportunity, and protect human rights in the city. The Office is also the advocate for the practice of good human relations and mutual understanding among the various racial ethnic and religious groups in the District of Columbia.

2655 District of Columbia Office of Human Rights
441 4th Street NW
Washington, DC 20001
202-727-4559
FAX 202-727-9589
http://www.ohr.dc.gov
e-mail: ohr@dc.gov
Gustavo F Velasquez, Director

The DC Office of Human Rights is an agency of the District of Columbia government that seeks to eradicate discrimination, increase equal opportunity, and protect human rights in the city.

2656 Office of Civil Rights: District of Columbia
US Department of Education
1100 Pennsylvania Ave, NW
Washington, DC 20044
202-786-0500
FAX 202-208-7797
TDY:877-521-2172
http://www.ed.gov.ocr
e-mail: ocr.dc@ed.gov
This office covers the states of District of Columbia, North Carolina, South Carolina and Virginia.

2657 State Department of Adult Education
University of the District of Columbia
4200 Connecticut Avenue NW
Washington, DC 20008
202-274-7181
FAX 202-274-7188
http://www.literacydc.org
e-mail: cspinner@literacydc.org
C Vanessa Spinner, State Director
Tracy Winston, Administrative Assistant

To impact positively the quality of life an deconomic and workforce outcomes for all District of Columbia residents by expanding access to high quality education.

Florida

2658 Client Assistance Program (CAP): Florida Division of Persons with Disabilities
2728 Centerview Drive
Tallahassee, FL 32301
850-488-9071
800-342-0823
FAX 850-488-8640
TDY:800-346-4127
http://www.advocacycenter.org
e-mail: webmaster@advocacycenter.org
Gary Weston, Executive Director

A non-profit organizatio providing protection and advocacy services in the State of Florida. The Center's mission is to advance the dignity, equality, self-determination and expressed choices of individuals with disabilities.

2659 Florida Department of Labor and Employment Security

2571 Executive Center Drive
Tallahassee, FL 32301
850-414-4615
FAX 850-921-1459
Sandra Bell, Manager

2660 Florida Fair Employment Practice Agency
Florida Commission on Human Relations
2009 Apalachee Parkway
Tallahassee, FL 32301
850-488-7082
FAX 850-488-5291
http://www.fchr.state.fl.us
e-mail: fchrinfo@fchr.myflorida.com
Derick Daniel, Executive Director

To prevent unlawful discrimination by ensuring people in Florida are treated fairly and are given access to opportunities in employment, housing, and certain public accommodations; and to promote mutual respect among groups through education and partnerships.

Georgia

2661 Client Assistance Program (CAP): Georgia Division of Persons with Disabilities
123 N McDonough Street
Decatur, GA 30030
404-373-2040
800-822-9727
FAX 404-373-4110
http://www.georgiacap.com

Charles L Martin, Director
Tom Dennis, Assistant Director
Anil Lewis, Counselor
Provides free services to consumers and applicants for projects, programs and facilities funded under the Rehabilitation Act.

2662 Georgia Assistive Technology Project
Georgia DOL/VR/Tools for Life Program
1700 Century Circle
Atlanta, GA 30345
404-657-0698
800-497-8665
TDY:866-373-7778
http://www.gatfl.org
e-mail: info@gatfl.org
Christopher Lee, Contact

The Tools for Life lists local and national training opportunities coming to Georgia.

2663 Georgia Department of Technical & Adult Education
1800 Century Place NE
Atlanta, GA 30345
404-679-1610
FAX 404-679-6932
http://www.dtae.org
Ronald Jackson, Interim Commissioner

The Georgia Department of Technical and Adult Education oversees the state's system of technical colleges, the adult literacy program, and a host of economic and workforce development programs

2664 Governor's Council on Developmental Disabilities
2 Peachtree Street NW
Atlanta, GA 30303
404-657-2126
888-275-4233
FAX 404-657-2132
TDY:404-657-2133
http://www.gcdd.org
e-mail: eejacobson@dhr.state.ga.us
Eric Jacobson, Executive Director
Patricia D Nobbie, Deputy Director
Kim Person, Executive Assistant
To collaborate with Georgia citizens, public and private advocacy organizations, and policy makers to positively influence ppublic policies that enhance the quality of life for people with developmental disabilities and their families.

2665 Office of Civil Rights: Georgia
US Department of Education
61 Forsyth Street, SW
Atlanta, GA 30303
404-562-6350
FAX 404-562-6455
TDY:877-521-2172
http://www.ed.gov
e-mail: ocr.atlanta@ed.gov
This office covers the states of Florida, Georgia and Tennessee

2666 Protection & Advocacy Center
Georgia Advocacy Office
150 E Ponce de Leon Avenue
Atlanta, GA 30030
404-885-1234
800-537-2329
FAX 404-378-0031
http://www.thegao.org
e-mail: info@thegao.org
Ruby Moore, Executive Director

Our mission is to work with and for oppressed and vulnerable individuals in Georgia who are labeled as disabled of mentally ill of secure their protection and advocacy.

2667 Region IV: Office of Civil Rights
Sam Nun Atlanta Federal Center
61 Forsyth Street SW
Atlanta, GA 30303
404-562-7888
FAX 404-562-7899
http://www.hhs.gov/region4
e-mail: roosevelt.freeman@hhs.gov
Roosevelt Freeman, Regional Manager

2668 State Department of Education
Department of Technical and Adult Education
2051 Twin Towers E
Atlanta, GA 30334
404-657-7410
800-331-3627
FAX 404-657-6978
http://www.doe.k12.ga.us
e-mail: stateboard@doe.k12.ga.us
Jean DeVard-Kem MD, Assistant Commissioner

2669 State GED Administration: Georgia
Georgia Department of Technical and Adult Educatio
1800 Century Place NE
Atlanta, GA 30345
404-679-1621
FAX 404-679-4911
http://www.dtae.tec.ga.us
e-mail: klee@dtae.org
Kimberly Lee, Director GED

The primary aid of the GED testign program in Georgia is to provide a second opportunity for individuals to obtain their high school diplomas.

Hawaii

2670 Correctional Education
Department of Public Safety
919 Ala Moana Boulevard
Honolulu, HI 96814
808-587-1288
FAX 808-587-1280
e-mail: maureen@smsii.com
Maureen Tito, Program Manager

2671 Hawaii Disability Rights Center
900 Fort Mall
Honolulu, HI 96813
808-949-2922
FAX 808-949-2928
http://www.hawaiidisabilityrights.org
e-mail: gary@hawaiidisabilityrights.org
Gary Smith, President

2672 Hawaii State Council on Developmental Disabilities
919 Ala Moana Boulevard
Honolulu, HI 96814
808-586-8100
FAX 808-586-7543
http://www.hiddc.org
e-mail: council@hiddc.org
Waynette Cabral, Executive Administrator
Debbie Miyasaka Gushiken, Community/Legislative Liason
Susan Kawano, Secretary
To support people with developmental disabilities to control their own destiny and determine the quality of life they desire.

2673 State GED Administration: Hawaii
Community Education Section
1270 Queen Emma Street
Honolulu, HI 96813
808-594-0170
Iris Mizuguchi, GED Administrator

The primary aid of the GED testing program in Hawaii is to provide a second opportunity for individuals to obtain their high school diplomas.

Idaho

2674 Idaho Assistive Technology Project
129 W 3rd Street
Moscow, ID 83843
208-885-3557
800-432-8324
FAX 208-885-3628
http://www.idahoat.org
e-mail: rseiler@uidaho.edu
Ron Seiler, Project Director
Sue House, Information Specialist

The Idaho Assistive Technology Project)IATP) is a federally funded program managed by the Center on Disabilities and Human Development at the University of Idaho. The goal of IATP is to increase the availability of assistive technology devices and services for Idahoans with disabilities. The IATP offers free trainings and technical assistance, a low-interest loan program, assistive technology assessments for children and agriculture workers, and free informational materials.

2675 Idaho Department of Education
650 W State Street
Boise, ID 83720
208-332-6800
800-432-4601
FAX 208-334-2228
http://www.sde.state.id.us
e-mail: trluna@sde.state.id.us
Tom Luna, Superintendent

Determined to create a customer-driven education system that meets the needs of every student in Idaho and prepares them to live, work and succeed in the 21st century.

2676 Idaho Division of Vocational Rehabilitation
650 W State Street
Boise, ID 83720
208-334-3390
FAX 208-334-5305
http://www.vr.idaho.gov
e-mail: mgraham@vr.idaho.gov
Michael Graham, Administrator
Chuck Gullstrom, IT Resource Manager

A state-federal program whose goal is to assist people with disabilities to prepare for, secure, retain or regain employment.

2677 Idaho Fair Employment Practice Agency
Idaho Human Rights Commission
1109 Main Street
Boise, ID 83720
208-334-2873
888-249-7025
FAX 208-334-2664
http://www.state.id.us/ihrc
Leslie Goddard, Director

2678 Idaho Human Rights Commission
1109 Main Street, Suite 400
Boise, ID 83720
208-334-2873
888-249-7025
FAX 208-334-2664
TDY:208-334-4751
http://www.state.id.us/ihrc
e-mail: lgoddard@ihrc.idaho.gov
Leslie Goddard, Director

To administer state and federal andti-discrimination laws in Idaho in a manner that is fair, accurate, and timely; and to work towards ensuring that all people within the state are treated with dignity and respect in their places of employment, housing, education and public accommodations.

2679 State Department of Education: Special Education
Special Education Team
Idaho Department of Education
Boise, ID 83720
208-332-6918
FAX 208-332-2228
http://www.sde.idaho.gov/SpecialEducation/defau
e-mail: jetaylor@sde.idaho.gov; jshyatt@sde.idaho.gov
Jean Taylor, Co-Director, Special Education
Jacque Hyatt, Co-Director, Special Education

Our mission is to enable all students to achieve high academic standards and quality of life. The Special Education Team works collaboratively with districts, agencies, and parents to ensure students receive quality, meaningful, and needed services.

2680 State GED Administration: IdahoDepartment of Education
650 West State Street
Boise, ID 83720
208-334-3216
FAX 208-334-2365
http://www.sde.state.id.us/certification/adult
e-mail: tmruiz@sde.iadho.gov
Cheryl Engel, GED Administrator
Tina Ruiz, GED Transcipts/Information

The primary aid of the GED testing program in Idaho is to provide a second opportunity for individuals to obtain their high school equivalency certificate.

Illinois

2681 Board of Education of Chicago
125 S Clark Street
Chicago, IL 60603
773-553-1000
FAX 773-553-1501
http://www.cps.k12.il.us/
Rufus Williams, President

Offers instruction and information services, curriculum information and government relations advocacy.

2682 Client Assistance Program (CAP): Illinois Division of Persons with Disabilities
100 N First Street
Springfield, IL 62702
217-782-5374
800-641-3929
FAX 217-524-1790
http://www.dhs.state.il.us/ors/cap
e-mail: dhscap@dhs.state.il.us
Cathy Meadows, Director
Carol L Adams PhD, Secretary

Provides free services to consumers and applicants for projects, programs and facilities funded under the Rehabilitation Act.

2683 Correctional Education
Illinois Department of Corrections
1301 Concordia Court
Springfield, IL 62702
217-558-2200
800-546-0844
FAX 217-557-7902
http://www.idoc.state.il.us/
e-mail: webmaster@idoc.state.il.us
Roger Walker, Director

2684 Great Lakes ADA and Accessible IT Center
1640 W Roosevelt Road
Chicago, IL 60608
312-413-1407
800-949-4232
FAX 312-413-1856
TDY:312-413-1407
http://www.adagreatlakes.org
Robin Jones, Project Director
Peter Berg, Technical Assistance
Claudia Diaz, Project Coordinator
Great Lakes ADA Center provides information, materials, technical assistance and training on the Americans with Disabilities Act of 1990. Great Lakes ADA Center's AIT Initiative, encourages incorporation of accessible information technology in K-12 and post secondary school settings.

2685 Illinois Affiliation of Private Schools for Exceptional Children
Lawrence Hall Youth Services
4833 N Francisco Avenue
Chicago, IL 60625
773-769-3500
FAX 773-769-0106
http://www.lawrencehall.org
Mary Hollie, CEO
Sharri Demitrowicz, Education Vice President

2686 Illinois Assistive Technology
1 W Old State Capitol Plaza
Springfield, IL 62701
217-522-7985
800-852-5110
FAX 217-522-8067
http://www.iltech.org
e-mail: wgunther@iltech.org
Wilhelmina Gunther, Executive Director
Sherry Edwards, Information/Assistance Director

The primary focus is on education, employment, community living, information technology and telecommunications. The mission is to enable people iwth disabilities so they can fully participate in all aspects of life.

2687 Illinois Council on Developmental Disabilities
830 S Spring Street
Springfield, IL 62704
217-782-9696
FAX 217-524-5339
http://www.state.il.us
e-mail: sheila.romano@illinois.gov
Sheila Romano EdD, Director

2688 Illinois Department of Commerce and Community Affairs
JTPA Programs Division
620 E Adams Street
Springfield, IL 62701
217-782-7500
800-785-6055
FAX 800-785-6055
TDY:800-785-6055
http://www.commerce.state.il.us
Jack Labin, Director
Pam Donough, Manager

2689 Illinois Department of Employment Security
33 S State Street
Chicago, IL 60603
312-793-5700
TDY:800-622-3943
http://www.ides.state.il.us
James P Sledge, Director
Elizabeth Nicholson, Deputy Director Administration
Marlene Demuzio, Deputy Director Information Svcs
IDES helps job seekers find jobs and employers find workers. We also analyze and publish a gold mine of information on careers and the Illinois economy.

2690 Illinois Department of Human Rights
100 W Randolph Street
Chicago, IL 60601
312-814-6200
FAX 312-814-6251
http://www.state.il.us/dhr
Rocco Claps, Director

Administers the Illinois Human Rights Act, which prohibits discrimination because of race, color, religion, sex, natural origin, ancestry, citizenship status, age 40 and over, marital status, physical or mental handicap, military service, or unfavorable military discharge.

2691 Illinois Department of Rehabilitation Services
1026 E Jackson
Macomb, IL 61455
309-833-4573
FAX 309-837-1659
TDY:888-261-2867
http://www.dhs.state.il.us
e-mail: dhs.ors@illinois.gov
Karen Engstrom, Manager

2692 Illinois Office of Rehabilitation Services
Illinois Department of Human Services
100 S Grand Avenue E
Springfield, IL 62762
217-557-1601
e-mail: ors@dhs.state.il.us
Teyonda Wertz, Chief of Staff
Carol Adams, Manager
Rafael Diaz, Information Services Manager
DHS' Office of Rehabilitation Services is the state's lead agency serving individuals with disabilities.

2693 Illinois State Board of Education
100 N First Street
Springfield, IL 62777
212-782-4321
866-262-6663
http://www.isbe.state.il.us/
Jean Ladage, Board Services Coordinator
Christopher Koch MD, Superintendent

Provides leadership, advocacy, and support for the work of school districts, policymakers, and Illinois residents in making Illinois education second to none.

2694 Office of Civil Rights: Illinois
US Department of Education
Citigroup Center
Chicago, IL 60661
312-730-1560
FAX 312-730-1576
TDY:877-521-2172
http://www.ed.gov/ocr
e-mail: ocr.chicago@ed.gov
This office covers the states of Illinois, Indiana, Iowa, Minnesota, North Dakota, and Wisconsin.

2695 Protection & Advocacy Agency
Equip for Equality
20 N Michigan Avenue
Chicago, IL 60602
312-341-0022
800-537-2632
FAX 312-341-0295
http://www.equipforequality.org
e-mail: contactus@equipforequality.org
Zena Naiditch, President/CEO

The mission of Equip for Equality is to advance the human and civil rights of children and adults with physical and mental disabilities. The only state-wide cross-disability, comprehensive advocacy organization providing self-advocacy assistance, legal services, and disability rights education while also engaging in publi policy and legislative advocacy and conducting abuse investigation and other oversight activities.

2696 Region V: Civil Rights Office
US Department of Health & Human Services
233 N Michigan Avenue
Chicago, IL 60601
312-353-5160
FAX 312-353-4144
http://www.hhs.gov/region5
e-mail: lisa.simeone@hhs.gov
Lisa Simeone, Regional Manager

2697 Region V: US Department of Labor-Office of Federal Contract Compliance
US Department of Labor
230 S Dearborn Street
Chicago, IL 60604
312-886-6503
FAX 312-886-0934
http://www.dol.gov
Robert Jur, Director
Christopher Fox, Manager

These regional offices of agencies enforce laws prohibiting employment discrimination on the basis of disability.

2698 Region V: US Small Business Administration
500 W Madison Street
Chicago, IL 60661
312-353-4528
FAX 312-886-5688
http://www.sba.gov/il
Judith A Roussel, District Director
Ivan E Irizarry, Deputy District Director

These regional offices of agencies enforce laws prohibiting employment discrimination on the basis of disability.

2699 State Department of Adult Education
State Board of Education
100 N 1st Street
Springfield, IL 62777
217-782-4321
FAX 217-782-9224
http://www.isbe.net
e-mail: jll.lit@isbe.net
Randy Dunn MD, State Superintendent
Glen Max McGee, Administrator

Indiana

2700 Assistive Technology
5333 Commerce Square Drive
Indianapolis, IN 46241
800-528-8246
http://www.attaininc.org
e-mail: attaininfo@attaininc.org
Gary Hand, Executive Director
Mary Duffer, Executive Assistant

Provide direct service programs and creates structural change in the public and private sectors to promote the availability and use of Assistive Technology.

2701 Indiana ATTAIN Project
Indiana Family and Social Services Administration
PO Box 7083
Indianapolis, IN 46207
317-233-0800
http://www.in.gov/fssa
Mitch Robb, Director
John Clark, Secretary
Rita Anderson, Executive Director

2702 Indiana Department of CorrectionU
302 W Washington Street
Indianapolis, IN 46204
317-232-5715
http://www.in.gov/indcorrection/
e-mail: commissioner@doc.in.gov
J David Donahue, Commissioner

To maintain public safety and provide offenders with self improvement programs, job skills and family values in an efficient and cost effective manner for a successful return to the community as law-abiding citizens.

2703 Indiana Employment Services and Job Training Program Liaison
10 N Senate Avenue
Indianapolis, IN 46204
317-232-6702
FAX 317-233-1670
TDY:317-232-7560
http://www.in.gov/dwv/
e-mail: jhoward@dwd.state.in.us
Darian Patterson, Director of Human Resources
Joy Howard, Administrative Assistant

2704 Indiana Employment Services and Job Training Program Liaison
10 N Senate Avenue
Indianapolis, IN 46204
317-232-6702
FAX 317-233-1670
TDY:317-232-7560
http://www.in.gov/dwv/
e-mail: jhoward@dwd.state.in.us
Darian Patterson, Director of Human Resources

2705 Indiana Protection & Advocacy Services
4701 N Keystone Avenue
Indianapolis, IN 46205
800-622-4845
http://www.in.gov/ipas
e-mail: tgallagher@ipas.in.gov
Thomas Gallagher, Executive Director

Created to protect and advocate the rights of people with disabilities and is Indiana's federally designated Protection and Advocacy system and client assistance program. An independent state agency, which recieves no state funding and is independent from all service providers, as required by federal and state law.
1977

2706 State Department of Education
State House
Indianapolis, IN 46204
317-232-6665
800-527-4931
FAX 317-232-8004
http://www.doe.state.in.us
e-mail: sreed@doe.state.in.us
Suellen Reed, Superintendent

2707 State GED Administration
Indiana Department of Education
State House
Indianapolis, IN 46204
317-232-0522
FAX 317-233-0859
http://www.doe.state.in.us
e-mail: lwarner@doe.state.in.us
Linda Warner, Director
Nancy Waite, GED State Administrator

Iowa

2708 Client Assistance Program (CAP): Iowa Division of Persons with Disabilities
Lucas State Office Building
Des Moines, IA 50319
888-219-0471
FAX 515-242-6119
http://www.state.ia.us/government/dhr/pd
e-mail: dhr.disabilities@iowa.gov
Jill Fulitano-Avery, Administrator

Exists to promote the employment of Iowans with disabilities and reduce barriers to employment by providing information, referral, assessment and guidance, training and negotiation services to employers and citizens with disabilities.

2709 Governor's Council on DevelopmentalDisabilities
617 E 2nd Street
Des Moines, IA 50309
515-281-9082
800-452-1936
FAX 515-281-9087
http://www.state.ia.us/ddcouncil/
e-mail: fmorris@dhs.state.ia.us
Becky Harker, Executive Director

Identifies, develops and promotes public policy and support practices through capacity building, advocacy, and systems change activities. The purpose is to ensure that people with developmental disabilities and their families are included in planning, decision making, and development of policy related to services and supports that affect their quality of life and full participation in communities of their choice.

2710 Iowa Department of Education
Grimes State Office Building
Des Moines, IA 50319
515-281-3436
FAX 515-281-4122
http://www.state.ia.us/educate
e-mail: judy.jeffrey@iowa.gov
Judy Jeffrey, Director

Champion excellence in education through superior leadership and services. Committed to high levels of learning, achievement and performance for all students, so they will become successful members of their community and the workforce.

2711 Iowa Employment Service
1000 E Grand Avenue
Des Moines, IA 50319
515-281-9619
FAX 515-281-9650
http://www.state.ic.us/jobs/
e-mail: IWD.customerservice@iwd.state.ic.us

2712 Iowa Welfare Programs
Iowa Department of Human Services
Hoover State Building
Des Moines, IA 50319
515-281-5452
FAX 515-281-4940
TDY:800-735-2942
http://www.dhs.state.ia.us
e-mail: kconcan@dhs.state.ia.us
Kevin Concannon, Executive Director
Sally Cunningham, Deputy Director
Dan Gilbert, Administrator
To provide assistance to families in need in the Des Moines area.

2713 Iowa Workforce Investment Act
Department of Economic Development
200 E Grand Avenue
Des Moines, IA 50309
515-242-4700
FAX 515-242-4809
TDY:800-735-2934
http://www.iowalifechanging.com
e-mail: iowasmart@ided.state.ia.us
David Lyons, Executive Director
Mike Blouin, Director
Deb Townsend, Web Specialist
Job placement and training services. Especially for those workers who have been laid off, or have other barriers to steady employment.

2714 Learning Disabilities Association of Iowa
321 E 6th Street
Des Moines, IA 50329
515-280-8558
888-690-5324
FAX 515-243-1902
http://www.lda-ia.org
e-mail: kathylda@askresource.org
Dr Richard Owens, President
Kathy Specketer, Coordinator

Dedicated to identifying causes and promoting prevention of learning disabilities and to enhancing the quality of life for all individuals with learning disabilities and their families.

2715 Protection & Advocacy Services
950 Office Park Road
W Des Moines, IA 50265
515-278-2502
800-779-2502
FAX 515-278-0539
http://www.ipna.org
e-mail: info@ipna.org
Karen M Wilson, President

A federally funded program that will protect and advocate for the human and legal rights that ensure individuals with disabilities and/or mental illness a free, appropriate public education, employment opportunities and residence or treatment in the least restricitve environment or method and for freedom from stigma.

Kansas

2716 Client Assistance Program (CAP):Disability Rights Center of Kansas
635 SW Harrison Street
Topeka, KS 66603
785-273-9661
877-776-1541
FAX 785-273-9414
TDY:877-335-3725
http://www.drckansas.org
e-mail: info@drckansas.org
Rocky Nichols, Executive Director
Timothy Voss JD, Advocacy Director

Provides free services to consumers and applicants for projects, programs and facilities funded under the rehabilitation act.

2717 Kansas Adult Education Association
Barton County Community College
245 NE 30th Road
Great Bend, KS 67530
620-792-9340
800-748-7594
http://www.barton.cc.ks.us
Veldon Law, President
Todd Moore, Director for Admission
Cassandra Montoya, Student Work Services
The Kansas Adult Education Association has been the professional association for adult educators at community colleges, school districts, and non-profit organizations.

2718 Kansas Department of Labor
401 SW Topeka Boulevard
Topeka, KS 66603
785-296-5000
http://www.dol.ks.gov
Jim Garner, Secretary
Winona Ralston, Executive Secretary
John Polzar, Deputy Secretary/CAO
Formerly the Kansas Department of Human Resources, advances the economic well being of all Kansans through responsive workforce services.

2719 Kansas Department of Social and Rehabilittion Services

915 SW Harrison Street
Topeka, KS 66612
785-296-3959
FAX 785-296-2173
http://www.srskansas.org
Don Jordan, Secretary
Laura Howard, Assistant Secretary

To protect children and promote adult self-sufficiency.

2720 Kansas Human Rights Commission
900 SW Jackson Street
Topeka, KS 66612
785-296-3206
FAX 785-296-0589
http://www.khrc.net
e-mail: khrc@ink.org
William Minner, Director
Beth Montgomery, Office Manager

To prevent and eliminate discrimination and assure equal opportunities in all employment relations, to eliminate profiling in conjunction with traffic stops, to eliminate and prevent discrimination, segregation or separation, and assure equal opportunities in all places of public accommodations an in housing.

2721 Kansas State Department of Education
120 SE 10th Avenue
Topeka, KS 66612
785-296-3201
FAX 785-296-7933
http://www.ksde.org
e-mail: pplamann@ksde.org

Dr Alexa Posny, Commissioner

2722 Kansas State GED Administration Department of Education
Kansas Board of Regents
1000 SW Jackson Street
Topeka, KS 66612
785-296-3421
FAX 785-296-4526
http://www.kansasregents.org
e-mail: mhasman@ksbor.org
Kim Wilcox, Executive Director
Madison Hasman, State GED Administrator

Promotes adult education.

2723 Office of Disability Services
Witchita State University
1845 Fairmount Street
Wichita, KS 67260
316-978-3309
FAX 316-978-3114
TDY:316-978-3391
http://webs.wichita.edu/?u=disserv
e-mail: grady.landrum@witchita.edu
Grady Landrum, Director
Kathy Stewart, Services Coordinator
Mary Rice, Adminstrative Specialist
To enable students, staff, faculty and guests of Wichita State University to achieve their educational goals, both personal and academic, to the fullest of their abilities by providing and coordinating accessibility services which afford individuals with learning, mental or physical disabilities the equal opportunity to attain these goals.

2724 State Literacy Resource Center
Kansas Board of Regents, Adult Education
1000 SW Jackson Street
Topeka, KS 66612
785-296-0175
FAX 785-296-4526
http://www.kansasregents.org
e-mail: dglass@ksbor.org

Dianne Glass, Director
Michelle Carson, Associate Director
Reginald Robinson, President/CEO

2725 Western Kansas Community Service Consortiuum
348 NE Sr
Pratt, KS 67124
620-672-6251
http://www.wkcsc.org
e-mail: dedram@genmail.pcc.cc.ks.us
Dedra Manes, Executive Director

Mission is to provide cooperative community services to Western Kansas. Total service area includes 73 counties and nearly 3/4 of the state's geographic area.

Kentucky

2726 Assistive Technology Office
Charles McDowell Center
Louisville, KY 40242
502-429-4484
800-327-5287
FAX 502-429-7114
http://www.katsnet.org
e-mail: charles.forrester@ky.gov
Charles Forrester, Director
James Brown, Program Analyst/AT Coordinator

To make assistive technology information, devices and services easily obtainable for people of any age and/or disability.

2727 Client Assistance Program (CAP): Kentucky Division of Persons with Disabilities
209 Saint Clair Street
Frankfort, KY 40601
502-564-8035
800-633-6283
FAX 502-564-1566
http://kycap.ky.gov
e-mail: vickil.staggs@ky.gov
Vicki Staggs, Contact

Provides advocacy for persons with disabilities who are clients or applicants of the Office of Vocational Rehabilitation or the Office for the Blind and are having problems receiving services.

2728 Kentucky Department of Corrections
Health Services Building
275 E Main Street
Frankfort, KY 40602
502-564-4726
FAX 502-564-5037
http://www.corrections.ky.gov
John D Rees, Commissioner

To protect the citizens of the Commonwealth and to provide a safe, secure and human environment for staff and offenders in carrying out the mandates of the legislative and judicial processes; and to provide opportunities for offenders to acquire skills which facilitate non-criminal behavior.

2729 Kentucky Department of Education
500 Mero Street
Frankfort, KY 40601
502-564-4770
FAX 502-564-5680
http://www.education.ky.gov
Dr Barbara Erwin, Commisioner

2730 Learning Disabilities Association of Kentucky
2210 Goldsmith Lane
Louisville, KY 40218
502-473-1256
877-587-1256
FAX 502-473-4695
http://www.ldaofky.org
e-mail: LDAofky@aol.com
Tim Woods, Executive Director

2731 Protection & Advocacy Agency
100 Fair Oaks Lane
Frankfort, KY 40601
502-564-2967
800-372-2988
FAX 502-564-0848
TDY:502-372-2988
http://www.kypa.net
Maureen Fitzgerald, Executive Director

An independent state agency that was designated by the Governor as the protection and advocacy agency for Kentucky. To protect and promote the rights of Kentuckians with disabilities through legally based individuals and systemic advocacy, and education.

2732 State Department of Adult Education
1024 Capital Center Drive
Frankfort, KY 40601
502-573-5114
800-928-7323
FAX 502-573-5436
http://www.kyae.ky.gov
e-mail: reecied.stagnolia@mail.state.ky.us
Reecie Stagnolia, Associate Vice President

To provide a responsive and innovative adult education system that enables students to acheive and prosper.

Louisiana

2733 Client Assistance Program (CAP): Shreveport Division of Persons with Disabilities
Advocacy Center
2620 Centenary Boulevard
Shreveport, LA 71104
318-227-6186
800-839-7688
FAX 318-227-1841
http://www.advocacyla.org
e-mail: dmirvis@advocacyla.org
Diane Mirvis, Executive Director

Advocacy services for applicants and clients of Louisiana Rehabilitation Services (LRS) and American Indian Rehabilitation Services (AIRS). No fee.

2734 Client Assistance Program (CAP): Louisiana HDQS Division of Persons with Disabilities
Advocacy Center
1010 Common Street
New Orleans, LA 70112
504-522-2337
800-960-7705
http://www.advocacyla.org
e-mail: advocacycenter@advocacyla.org
Lois Simpson, Executive Director

Advocacy services to applicants and clients of Louisiana Rehabilitation Services (LRS) and American Indian Rehabilitation Services (AIRS). No fee. Committed to the belief in the dignity of every life and the freedom of everyone to experience the highest degree of self-determination. Exists to protect and advocate for human and legal rights of the elderly and disabled. Umbrella organization for Advocacy Centers in Baton Rouge, Lafayette, Shreveport, Monroe, Pineville, Jackson, and Mandeville.

2735 Correctional Education
Louisiana Department of Education
PO Box 94064
Baton Rouge, LA 70804
225-383-4761
877-453-2721
FAX 225-342-0193
http://www.doe.state.la.us
Cosby Joiner, Director
George Nelson, President

Promotes quality correctional education.

2736 Louisiana Assistive Technology Access Network
3042 Old Forge Drive
Baton Rouge, LA 70808
225-952-9500
800-270-6185
FAX 225-925-9560
http://www.latan.org
e-mail: cpourciau@latan.org
Julie Nesbit, President/CEO
Clara Pourciau, Assistant Director
Cyndi Mabry, Public Information Officer
Assists individuals with disabilities to achieve a higher quality of life and greater independence through increased access to assistive technology as part of their daily lives.

2737 State Department of Adult Education
Department of Education
PO Box 94064
Baton Rouge, LA 70804
225-342-3336
FAX 225-219-4439
http://www.doe.state.la.us
e-mail: customerservice@la.gov
Cecil Picard, Superintendent
Rodney Watson, Confidential Assistant

2738 State GED Administration
Louisiana Department of Education
PO Box 94604
Baton Rouge, LA 70804
225-383-4761
877-453-2721
FAX 225-342-0193
http://www.doe.state.la.us
Glen Gosett, Director
George Nelson, President

Promotes quality education.

Maine

2739 Adult Education Team
Maine Department of Education
23 State House Station
Augusta, ME 04333
207-624-6750
FAX 207-624-6731
http://www.maine.gov
e-mail: becky.dyer@maine.gov
Rebecca Dyer, Adult Education State Director

2740 Bureau of Rehabilitation Services
Department of Labor
150 State House Station
Augusta, ME 04333
800-698-4440
FAX 207-623-7965
http://www.maine.gov/labor
Penny Plourde, Director for Vocational Rehab

Works to bring about full access to employment, independence and community integration for people with disabilities.

2741 Consulting Advocacy Research Evaluation Services (CARES) and Client Assistance Program (CAP)
47 Water Street
Hallowell, ME 04347
207-622-7055
800-773-7055
FAX 207-621-1869
http://www.caresinc.org
e-mail: steve.beam@caresinc.com
Steve Beam, Program Director
G Dean Crocker, Executive Director

A federally funded program that provides information, assistance and advocacy to people with disabilities who are applying for or receiving services under the Rehabilitation Act.

2742 Developmental Disabilities Council
139 State House Station
Augusta, ME 04333
207-287-4213
800-244-3990
FAX 207-287-8001
http://www.maine.ddc.org
e-mail: jbell@maineddc.org
Julia Bell, Executive Director
Liza Collins, Policy/Research Analyst

A partnership of people with developmental disabilities, family memebers, and state and local agencies and organizations. The purpose is to assure that individuals with disabilities and their families participate in the design of, and have access to needed community services, individualized supports, and other forms of assistance thqat promote-self determination, independence, productivity, integration, and inclusion in all facets of family and community life.

2743 Maine Department of Labor: Employment Services
Bureau of Employment Security
20 Union Street
Augusta, ME 04330
207-287-2271
FAX 207-287-2947
John Dorrer, Manager

2744 Maine Human Rights Commission
51 State House Station
Augusta, ME 04333
207-624-6050
FAX 207-624-6063
http://www.maine.gov/mhrc
Patricia Ryan, Executtive Director

Holds the responsibility of enforcing Maine's anti-discrimination laws. The Commission investigates complaints of unlawful discrimination in employmen, housing, education, access to public accommodatoins, extension of credit, and offensive names.
1971

2745 Protection & Advocacy Agency
Disability Rights Center
PO Box 2007
Augusta, ME 04338
207-626-2774
800-452-1948
FAX 207-621-1419
http://www.drcme.org
e-mail: advocate@drcme.org
Kim Moody, Executive Director
Leeann Mosley, Operations Director

The Disability Rights Center is Maine's protection and advocacy agency for people with disabilities. To enhance and promote the equality, self-determination, independence, productivity, integratio, and inclusion of people with disabilities through education, strategoc advocacy and legal intervention.

Maryland

2746 Client Assistance Program (CAP): Maryland Division of Persons with Disabilities
2301 Argonne Drive
Baltimore, MD 21218
410-554-9361
800-638-6243
FAX 410-554-9362
TDY:410-554-9360
http://www.dors.state.md.us
e-mail: cap@dors.state.md.us
Beth Lash, Director

Helps individuals who have concerns or difficulties when applying or receiving rehabiliation services funded under the Rehabilitation Act.

2747 Correctional Education
State Department of Education
200 W Baltimore Street
Baltimore, MD 21201
410-767-0100
888-246-0016
FAX 410-333-6033
TDY:410-333-6442
http://www.marylandpublicschools.org
Nancy Garsmick, State Superintendent
Dr Mark Mechlinski, Director

Provides educational programs and library services to residents of the Division of Correction and the Patuxent Institution.

2748 Disability Law Center
The Walbert Building
Baltimore, MD 21201
410-727-6352
800-233-7201
FAX 410-727-6389
TDY:410-727-6387
http://www.mdlcbalto.org
Virginia Knowlton, Executive Director

A provate, non-profit organization staffed by attorneys and paralegals. MDLC is the Protection and Advocacy organization for Maryland. MDLC's mission is to endure that people with disabilities are accorded the full rights and entitlements afforded to them by state and federal law.

2749 Maryland Developmental Disabilities Council
217 E Redwood Street
Baltimore, MD 21202
410-767-3670
800-305-6441
FAX 410-333-3686
http://www.md-council.org
e-mail: brianc@md-council.org
Brian Cox, Executive Director
Catherine Lyle, Deputy Director
Stephanie Watkins, Family Networks, Resource Spec.
A public policy organization comprised of people with disabilities and family memebers who are joined by state officials, service providers an dother designated partners. Also an independent, self-governing organization that represents the interests of people with developmental disabilities and their families.

2750 Maryland Technology Assistance Program
2301 Argonne Drive
Baltimore, MD 21218
410-554-9230
800-832-4827
FAX 410-554-9237
TDY:866-881-7488
http://www.mdtap.org
e-mail: mdtap@mdtap.org
Michael Dalto, Executive Director
Jessica Vollmer, Office Manager

Provides tools to help people who are disabled or elderly enjoy the same rights and opportunities as other citizens.

2751 State Department of Education
200 W Baltimore Street
Baltimore, MD 21201
410-767-0100
888-246-0016
FAX 410-333-6033
TDY:410-333-6442
http://www.marylandpublicschools.org
Nancy Garsmick, State Superintendent

To provide leadership, support, and accountability for effective systems of public education, library services, and rehabilitation services.

Massachusetts

2752 Autism Support Center: Northshore Arc
6 Southside Road
Danvers, MA 01923
978-777-9135
800-728-8476
FAX 978-762-3980
http://www2.shore.net/~nsarc
e-mail: asc@nsarc.org
Gail Kastorf, Director
Jerry Carthy, Executive Director

Created to support parents and professionals who expressed a need for assistance finding information and support about autism, pervasive developmental disorder (PDD) and Asperger's Disorder. Empowers families who have a member with autism or related disorder by providing current, accurate, and unbiased information about autism, services, referrals, resources and research trends.
1991

2753 Department of Corrections
50 Maple Street
Milford, MA 01757
508-422-3300
FAX 508-422-3383
http://www.mass.gov
Kathleen M Dennehy, Commissioner

Promote public safety by incarcerating offenders while providing opportunities for participation in effective programs.

2754 Massachusetts Commission Against Discrimination
1 Ashburton Place
Boston, MA 02108
617-994-6000
FAX 617-994-6024
TDY:617-994-6196
http://www.mass.goc/mcad
Walter J Sullivan Jr, Chairman
Dorca I Gomez, Commissioner
Martin S Ebel, Commissioenr
The state's chief civil rights agency that works to eliminate discrimination on a variety of bases and areas, and strives to advance the civil rights of the people of the Commonwealth through law enforcement, outreach and training.

2755 Massachusetts Department of Education
GED Office
Malden, MA 02148
781-338-6625
http://www.doe.mass.edu/ged
e-mail: rderfler@doe.mass.edu
Jeff Nelhaus, Acting Commissioner of Education

Thirty-two test centers operate state-wide to serve the needs of the adult population in need of a high school credential.

2756 Massachusetts Office on Disability
1 Ashburton Place
Boston, MA 02108
617-727-7440
800-322-2020
FAX 617-727-0965
http://www.mass.gov/mod
e-mail: myra.berloff@massmail.stae.ma.us
Myra Berloff, Director
Phyllis Mitchell, Civil Rights Advocate

To bring about full and equal participation of people with disabilities in all aspects of life. It works to assure the advancement of legal rights and for the promotion of maximum opportunities, supportive services, accommodations and accessibility in a manner which fosters dignity and self determination.

2757 Massachusetts Rehabilitation Commission
27 Wormwood Street
Boston, MA 02210
617-204-3600
800-245-6543
FAX 617-727-1354
http://www.state.ma.us/mrc
Charles Carr, Commissioner

Promotes dignity for individuals with disabilities through employment and independent living in the community.

2758 Office of Civil Rights: Massachusetts
US Department of Education
33 Arch Street
Boston, MA 02110
617-289-0111
FAX 617-289-0150
TDY:877-521-2172
http://www.ed.gov/ocr
e-mail: ocr.boston@ed.gov
This office covers the states of Connecticut, Maine, Massachusetts, New Hampshire, Rhode Island and Vermont.

2759 Office of Federal Contract Compliance: Boston District Office
US Department of Labor
E235 JFK Federal Building
Boston, MA 02203
617-565-7000
FAX 617-624-6702
TDY:617-565-9869
http://www.dol.gov/dol/esa
e-mail: beatty.reba@dol.gov
Reba Beatty, District Director
Rhonda Aubn-Smith, Assistant Director

Enforces laws prohibiting employment discrimination on the basis of disability.

2760 Protection & Advocacy Agency
Disability Law Center
11 Beacon Street
Boston, MA 02108
617-723-8455
800-872-9992
FAX 617-723-9125
TDY:617-227-9464
http://www.dlc-ma.org
e-mail: mail@dlc-ma.org
Robert Whitney, President
Jonathan Delman, Vice President

A private, non-profit organization responsible for providing protection and advocacy for the rights of Massachusetts residents with disabilities.Provides legal advocacy on disability issues that promote the fundamental rights of all pepole with disabilities to participate fully and equally in the social and economic life of Massachusetts.

2761 Region I: Office for Civil Rights
US Department Health & Human Services
Government Center
Boston, MA 02203
617-565-1500
FAX 617-565-1491
http://www.hhs.gov/region1
e-mail: peter.chan@hhs.gov
Peter Chan, Regional Manager

2762 Region I: US Small Business Administration
Massachusetts District Office
10 Causeway Street
Boston, MA 02222
617-565-5590
FAX 617-565-5598
TDY:617-565-5797
http://www.sba.gov
e-mail: robert.coen@sba.gov
G Jean Sawyer, Acting District Director
Mark S Hayward, Acting New England Regional Admi

These regional offices of agencies enforce laws prohibiting employment discrimination on the basis of disability.

2763 State Department of Adult Education
Adult and Community Learning Services
350 Main Street
Malden, MA 02148
781-388-3300
FAX 781-388-3394
http://www.doe.mass.edu/acls/#
e-mail: acls@doe.mass.edu
Adult and Community Learning Services, a unit at the MA Department of Education, oversees and improves no-cost basic educational services (ABE) for adults in Masssachusetts. ACLS's mission is to provide each and every adult with opportunities to develop literacy skills needed to qualify for further education, job training, and better employment, and to reach his/her full potential as a family member, productive worker, and citizen.

Michigan

2764 Assistive Technology
Michigan Jobs Commission
119 Pere Marquette Drive
Lansing, MI 48912
517-485-4477
FAX 517-485-4488
http://www.publicpolicy.com/nyc.html
e-mail: ppa@publicpolicy.com
Jeffrey Padden, President
Nancy Hewat, Executive Director

2765 Client Assistance Program (CAP): Michigan Department of Persons with Disabilities
409 Legacy Parkway
Lansing, MI 48911
517-487-1755
800-292-0827
FAX 517-373-0565
http://www.mpas.org
e-mail: molson@mpas.org
Elmer Cerano, Executive Director
Manuela Kress-Shull, Manager

Assists people who are seeking or receiving services from Michigan Rehabilitation Services, Consumer Choice Programs, Michigan Commission for the Blind, Centers for Independent Living, and Supported Employment and Transition Programs.

2766 Michigan Assistive Technology: Michigan Rehabilitation Services
Michigan Jobs Commission
119 Pere Marquette Drive
Lansing, MI 48912
517-485-4477
FAX 517-485-4488
http://www.publicpolicy.com
e-mail: ppa@publicpolicy.com
Jeffrey Padden, President
Nancy Hewat, Executive Director

2767 Michigan Correctional Educational Division
Department of Corrections: Prisoner Education Prog
Grandview Plaza, 206 E Michigan Ave
Lansing, MI 48909
517-335-1426
FAX 517-335-0045
http://www.michigan.gov/corrections
e-mail: spencede@state.mi.us
Diane Spence, Director

The goal of the Michigan Department of Corrections is to provide the greatest amount of protection while making the most efficient use of the State's resources.

2768 Michigan Department of Community Health
Capitol View Building
Lansing, MI 48913
517-373-3740
FAX 517-334-7353
TDY:517-373-3573
http://www.michigan.gov/ddcouncil
e-mail: norris@michigan.gov

Janet Olszewski, Director
Ed Dore, Chief Deputy Director
T J Bucholtz, Public Information Officer
An advocacy organization that engages in advocacy, capacity building and systemic change activities that promote self-determination, independence, productivity, integration and inclusion in all facets of community life for people with developmental disabilities.

1989

2769 Michigan Employment Security Commission
7310 Woodward Avenue
Detroit, MI 48202
313-876-5000
FAX 313-876-5304
Sharon Bommarito, Manager

Brings people and jobs together.

2770 Michigan Protection and Advocacy Service
4095 Legacy Parkway
Lansing, MI 48911
517-487-1755
800-288-5923
FAX 517-487-0827
http://www.mpas.org
e-mail: molson@mpas.org
Elmer Cerano, Executive Director
Michele Brand, Finance Administrator

Advocates for people with disabilities and gives information and advice about their rights as a person with disabilities.

2771 State Department of Adult Education
Michigan Department of Labor & Economic Growth
Office of Adult Education
Lansing, MI 48913
517-373-8800
FAX 517-335-3630
http://www.michigan.gov/mdcd
e-mail: adulted@michigan.gov
Dianne Duthie, Director
Janice Vernon, Secretary

Promotes quality adult education.

2772 State GED Administration
Michigan Department of Labor & Economic Growth
Office of Adult Education
Lansing, MI 48913
517-241-2497
FAX 517-335-3461
http://www.michigan.gov/mdcd
e-mail: heckmana@michigan.gov
Ben Williams, GED State Administrator
Amy Heckman, Administrative Assistant

Promotes adult education.

Minnesota

2773 Assistive Technology
Minnesota STAR Program
50 Sherburne Avenue
Saint Paul, MN 55155
651-201-2640
888-234-1267
FAX 651-282-6671
http://www.starprogram.state.mn.us
e-mail: star.program@state.mn.us
Chuck Rassbach, Executive Director
Joan Gillum, Executive Assistant

STAR's mission is to help all Minnesotans with disabilities gain access to and acquire the assistive technology they need to live, learn, work and play. The Minnesota STAR Program is federally funded by the Rehabilitation Services Administration in assordance with the Assistive Technology Act of 1998.

2774 Minnesota Department of Children, Families & Learning
Department of Education
1500 Highway 36 W
Roseville, MN 55113
651-582-8200
FAX 651-582-8202
http://www.education.state.mn.us
e-mail: alice.seagren@state.mn.us
Alice Seagren, Commissioner
Chas Anderson, Deputy Commissioner

To improve educational achievement by establishing clear standards, measuring performance, assisting educators and increasing opportunities for life long learning.

2775 Minnesota Department of Human Rights
190 5th Street
Saint Paul, MN 55101
651-296-5663
800-657-3704
http://www.humanrights.state.mn.us
e-mail: webmaster@therightsplace.net
Velma Korbel, Commissioner

To make Minnesota discrimination free.

2776 Minnesota Governor's Council on Developmental Disabilities
370 Centennial Office Building
Saint Paul, MN 55155
651-296-4018
877-348-0505
FAX 651-297-7200
http://www.mncdd.org
e-mail: admin.dd@state.mn.us
Colleen Wieck PhD, Executive Director

To provide information, education, and training to build knowledge, develop skills, and change attitudes that will lead to increased independence, productivit, self determination, integration and inclusion for all people with developmental disabilities and their families.

2777 Minnesota Life Work Center
University of St. Thomas
1000 Lasalle Avenue
Minneapolis, MN 55403
651-962-4763
http://www.stthomas.edu/lifeworkcenter
e-mail: lifework@stthomas.edu
Brian Dusbiber, Director

Provides special services and resources to meet the unique needs of graduate students, education students (both graduate and undergraduate), and alumni/ae.

2778 Protection & Advocacy Agency
Minnesota Disability Law Center
430 1st Avenue N
Minneapolis, MN 55401
612-334-5784
800-292-4150
FAX 612-334-5755
TDY:612-332-4668
http://www.mnlegalservices.org/mdlc
e-mail: lcohen@midmnlegal.org
Pamela Hoopes, Manager
Lisa Cohen, Administrator

2779 State Department of Adult Education
Department of Education
1500 Highway 36 W
Roseville, MN 55113
651-582-8446
http://education.state.mn.us
e-mail: mde.abe@state.mn.us
Becky Lashner, Director

Offered through Minnesota's public school system, provides opportunities to obtain academic, interpersonal and problem-solving skills necessary to live self-sufficient lives.

Mississippi

2780 Client Assistance Program (CAP): Mississippi Division of Persons with Disabilities
500 G Woodrow Wilson Drive
Jackson, MS 39296
601-362-2585
800-362-2400
FAX 601-982-1951
http://www.mississippicap.com
Presley Posey, Director
Carla Thompson, CEO

A federal grant to the State of Mississippi to provide advocacy services for clients and client applicants of the Office of Vocational Rehabilitation, Vocational Rehabiliation for the Blind, and the Independent Living programs.

2781 Mississippi Department of Corrections
723 N President Street
Jackson, MS 39202
601-359-5600
http://www.mdoc.state.ms.us
e-mail: cepps@mdoc.state.ms.us
Christopher Epps, Commissioner

To provide and promote public safety through efficient and effective offender custody, care, control and treatment consistent with sound correctional prinicipals and constitutional standards.

2782 Mississippi Department of Employment Security
1235b Echelon Parkway
Jackson, MS 39215
601-321-6000
http://www.mdes.ms.gov
e-mail: internet@mdes.ms.gov
Brings people and jobs together.

2783 Mississippi Project START
PO Box 1698
Jackson, MS 39215
601-987-4872
800-852-8328
FAX 601-364-2349
http://www.msprojectstart.org
e-mail: contactus@msprojectstart.org
Dorothy Young, Project Director
Jywanza Goodman, Administrative Assistant

To ensure the provision of appropriate Technology-Related services for Mississippians with disabilities by increasing the awareness of and access to Assistive Technology and by helping the existing service systems to become more consumer repsonsive so that all Mississippians with disabilities will receive appropriate Technology-related services and devices.

2784 State Department of Adult Education
State Board for Community & Jr Colleges
PO Box 771
Jackson, MS 39205
601-359-3498
FAX 601-359-2198
http://www.mde.k12.ms.us
e-mail: dbowman@mdek12.state.ms.us
Melody Bounds, Executive Director
Paulette White, Bureau Director

Promotes adult education.

2785 State Department of Education
PO Box 771
Jackson, MS 39205
601-359-3498
FAX 601-359-2198
http://www.mde.k12.ms.us
e-mail: dbowman@mdek12.state.ms.us
Melody Bounds, Executive Director
Paulette White, Bureau Director

Promotes quality education.

Missouri

2786 Assistive Technology
4731 S Cochise Drive
Independence, MO 64055
816-373-5193
800-647-8557
FAX 816-373-9314
http://www.at.mo.gov
e-mail: matpmo@swbell.net
Diane Golden, Director

To increase access to assistive technology for Missourians with all types of disabilities, of all ages.

2787 Assistive Technology Project
University of Missouri-Kansas City
5100 Rockhill Road
Kansas City, MO 64110
816-235-1000
FAX 816-235-2662
http://www.umkc.edu
Elson Floyd, President
Stephen Lehmkuhle, Manager

Promotes independent living through technology.

2788 Correctional Education
Department of Corrections
2729 Plaza Drive
Jefferson City, MO 65102
573-751-2389
888-877-2389
FAX 573-571-4099
TDY:573-571-5984
http://www.corrections.state.mo.us/divis
Larry Crawford, Director
David Rost, Deputy Director

2789 EEOC St. Louis District Office
Robert A Young Federal Building
1222 Spruce Street
Saint Louis, MO 63103
800-669-4000
FAX 314-539-7894
http://www.eeoc.gov
James R Neely Jr, Director
Robert G Johnson, Regional Attorney

These regional offices of agencies enforce laws prohibiting employment discrimination on the basis of disability.

2790 Great Plains Disability and Business Technical Assistance Center (DBTAC)
100 Corporate Lake Drive
Columbia, MO 65203
573-882-3600
800-949-4232
FAX 573-884-4925
http://www.adaproject.org
e-mail: ada@missouri.edu
Jim de Jong, Director

To provide information, materials and technical assistance to individuals and entities that are covered by the Americans with Disabilities Act. In addition to the ADA, Great Plains ADA Center provides the ADA and disability-related legislation such as the Family Medical Leave Act, Workforce Investment Act and the Telecommunications Act.

2791 Missouri Protection & Advocacy Services
925 S Country Club Drive
Jefferson City, MO 65109
573-893-3333
800-392-8667
FAX 573-893-4231
TDY:800-735-2966
http://www.moadvocacy.org
e-mail: mopasjc@earthlink.net
Shawn Loyola, Executive Director

A federally mandated system in the state of Missouri which provides protection of the rights of persons with disabilities through leagally-based avocacy

1977

2792 **Office of Civil Rights: Missouri**
US Department of Education
8930 Ward Parkway
Kansas City, MO 64114
816-268-0550
FAX 816-823-1404
TDY:877-521-2172
http://www.ed.gov/ocr
e-mail: ocr.kansascity@ed.gov

This office covers the states of Kansas, Missouri, Nebraska, Oklahoma and South Dakota.

2793 **Protection & Advocacy Agency**
925 S Country Club Drive
Jefferson City, MO 65109
573-893-3333
800-392-8667
FAX 573-893-4231

Shawn Loyola, Executive Director
Lymette Scott, Secretary

Protects the rights of individuals with disabilities by providing advocacy and legal services.

2794 **Region VII: US Department of Health and Human Services**
Office For Civil Rights
601 E 12th Street
Kansas City, MO 64106
816-426-6367
FAX 816-426-3686
TDY:816-426-7065
http://www.hhs.gov/region7
e-mail: fred.laing@hhs.gov

Fred Laing, Regional Manager

Montana

2795 **Assistive Technology Project**
University of Montana Rural Institute
52 Corbin Hall
Missoula, MT 59812
406-243-5467
800-732-0323
FAX 406-243-4730
http://www.ruralinstitute.umt.edu
e-mail: rural@ruralinstitute.umt.edu

Marsha Katz, Project Director

This statewide program at the University of Montana promotes assistive devices and services for persons of all ages with disabilities.

2796 **Correctional Education**
Department of Corrections & Human Services
PO Box 201301
Helena, MT 59620
406-444-3930
FAX 406-444-4920
http://www.cor.state.mt.us/css/default.csp

Bill Slaughter, Director
Ted Ward, Administrative Support

2797 **Developmental Disabilities Planning and Advisory Council**
PO Box 526
Helena, MT 59624
406-443-4332
866-443-4332
http://www.mtcdd.org
e-mail: dswingley@state.mt.us

Deborah Swingley, Executive Director

The goal of the Council is to increase the indpendence, productivity, inclusion and integration into the community of people with developmental disabilities through systemic change, capacity building and advocacy activities.

2798 **MonTECH**
634 Eddy Ave
Missoula, MT 59812
406-243-5751
877-243-5511
http://montech.ruralinstitute.umt.edu
e-mail: montech@ruralinstitute.umt.edu

Kathy Laurin PhD CRC, Director
Leslie Mullette OTR/L ATP, MTAC Clinical Coordinator
Chris Clasby, MATP Coordinator

A program of the University of Montana Rural Institute: Center for Excellence in Disability, Education, Research and Service. Specialize in Assistive Technology and oversee a variety of AT related grants and contracts. The overall goal is to develop a comprehensive, statewide system of assistive technology related assistance.

2799 **Montana Department of Labor & Industry**
PO Box 1728
Helena, MT 59624
406-444-2840
FAX 406-444-1394
http://dli.mt.gov
e-mail: dliquestion@mt.gov

Keith Kelly, Commissioner

Promotes the well-being of Montana's workers, employers, an dcitixens, and upholds their rights and responsibilities. Committed to being responsive to communities and businesses at the local level.

2800 **Montana Office of Public Instruction**
PO Box 202501
Helena, MT 59620
406-444-3095
888-231-9393
http://www.opi.state.mt.us
e-mail: opisupt@mt.gov

Linda McCulloch, State Superintendent

Supports schools so that students acheive high standards.

2801 **Office of Adult Basic and Literacy Education**
Montana Office of Public Instruction
PO Box 202501
Helena, MT 59620
406-444-3095
888-231-9393
http://www.opi.state.mt.us

Linda McCulloch, Superintendent
Margaret Bowles, ABLE Specialist
David Strong, Adult Education Services Directo

Adult education programs include basic literacy, workplace literacy, family literacy, preparation for GED, English as a Second Language and other services that provide adults and out of school youth opportunities at enhancing skills, improving parenting, and youth assistance related to employment and self-sufficiency.

Nebraska

2802 **Answers4Families: Center on Children, Families, Law**
121 S 13th Street
Lincoln, NE 68588
402-472-0844
800-746-8420
http://www.answers4families.org
e-mail: clewis@answers4families.org

Charlotte Lewis, Director
Jessica Williams, Project Assistant

A project of the Center on Children, Families and Law at University of Nebraska. Mission is to provide info, opportunities, education and support to Nebraskans through Internet resources. The Center serves individuals with special needs and mental health disorders, foster families, caregivers, assisted living, and school nurses.

2803 **Assistive Technology Partnership**
5143 S 48th Street
Lincoln, NE 68516
402-471-0734
888-806-6287
FAX 402-471-6052
http://atp.ne.gov
e-mail: mark.schultz@atp.state.ne.us

Mark Schultz, Executive Director

Dedicated to helping Nebraskan's with disabilities, their families and professionals obtain assistive technology devices and services.
1989

2804 Client Assistance Program (CAP): Nebraska Division of Persons with Disabilities
Nebraska Department of Education
301 Centennial Mall S
Lincoln, NE 68508 402-471-3656
800-742-7594
http://www.cap.state.ne.us
e-mail: victoria.rasmussen@cap.ne.gov
Frank Lloyd, Executive Director

The Client Assistance Program helps individuals who have concerns or difficulties when applying for or receiving rehabilitation services funded under the Rehabilitation Act.

2805 Nebraska Advocacy Services
Center for Disability Rights, Law & Advocacy
134 S 13th Street
Lincoln, NE 68508 402-474-3183
800-422-6691
FAX 402-474-3274
http://www.nebraskaadvocacyservices.org
e-mail: info@nebraskaadvocacyservices.org
Timothy F Shaw, CEO

Created to assist individuals with disabilities and their families in protecting and advocating for their rights. From its beginning, NAS has promoted the principles of equality, self-determination, and dignity of persons with disabilities.
1977

2806 Nebraska Department of Labor
PO Box 94600
Lincoln, NE 68509 402-471-2600
FAX 402-471-9867
http://www.dol.state.ne.us/
e-mail: lme_ne@dol.state.ne.us
Philip Baker, Administrator

2807 Nebraska Equal Opportunity Commission
1313 Farnam Street
Omaha, NE 68102 402-595-2028
800-382-7820
http://www.neoc.ne.gov.
Anne Hobbs, Executive Director

To receive, investigate and make decisions on charges of unlawful employment, housing, and public accommodations practices occurring within the boundaries of the State of Nebraska.

2808 State Department of Education
301 Centennial Mall S
Lincoln, NE 68508 402-471-2295
FAX 402-471-0117
http://www.nde.state.ne.us
e-mail: doug.christensen@nde.ne.gov
Douglas D Christensen, Commissioner
Polly Feis, Deputy Commissioner

Organized into teams that interact to operate the agency and carry out the duties assigned by state and federal statutes and the policy directions of the State Board of Education.

2809 State GED Administration: Nebraska
Nebraska Department of Education
301 Centennial Mall S
Lincoln, NE 68509 402-471-4807
http://www.nde.state.ne.us
e-mail: vicki.bauer@nde.ne.gov
Vicki L Bauer, Director
Shirley Gruntorad, GED Staff Assistant

To provide educational opportunities for adults to improve their literacy skills to a level requisite for effective citizenship and productive employment. This includes preparation for and successful completion of the high school equivalency program.

2810 Vocational Rehabilitation Nebraska Department of Education
3335 W Capital Avenue
Grand Island, NE 68803 308-385-6200
800-632-3382
http://www.vocrehab.state.ne.us
e-mail: vr.grandisland@vr.ne.gov
Frank C Lloyd, Asst Commissioner of Education

The Nebraska Rehabilitation Program has people with disabilities join the workforce. Our team of experts provides direct services for employers and people with disabilities that lead to employment.
1921

Nevada

2811 Assistive Technology
Office of Community Based Services
3636 56th Research Way
Carson City, NV 89706 775-687-4452
FAX 775-687-3292
TDY:701-687-3388
http://www.dol.ks.gov/index.html
e-mail: kvogel@gov.mail.state.nv.us
Richard Weather, Head Director
Ken Vogel, Director
Todd Butterworth, Manager
Promotes independent living through technology.

2812 Client Assistance Program (CAP): Nevada Division of Persons with Disability
Department of Employment, Training and Rehabilitat
800 E St Louis
Las Vegas, NV 89104 702-486-6688
800-633-9879
http://www.detr.state.nv.us/rehab/reh_cap
e-mail: detrcap@nvdetr.org
Robin Hall-Walker, Director

To assist and advocate for clients and applicants in their relationships with projects, programs, and community rehabilitation programs that provide services under the Act. The program is also responsible for informing individuals with disabilities in Nevada, of the services and benefits available to them.

2813 Correctional Education and Vocational Training
Nevada Department of Corrections
5500 Snyder Avenue
Carson City, NV 89701 775-887-3285
FAX 775-687-6715
http://www.doc.nc.gov
e-mail: mhall@doc.nv.gov
Jackie Crawford, Director
Marta Hall, Education Coordinator

To continue and expand an educational training program which contains literacy, ESL, numeracy, community outreach, and vocational training that will provide long-term benefits to both inmates and the Nevada community in general.

2814 Department of Employment, Tranining and Rehabilitation
500 E 3rd Street
Carson City, NV 89713 775-684-3913
FAX 775-684-8681
http://www.detr.state.nv.us
Larry J Mosley, Director

Comprised of four divisions with numerous bureaus programs, and services housed in offices throughout Nevada to provide citizens the state's premier source of employment, training, and rehabilitative programs.

2815 Nevada Bureau of Disability Adjudication
1050 E William Street
Carson City, NV 89701 775-687-4430
http://detr.state.nv.us/rehab
e-mail: detrvr@nvdetr.org
Kraig Schutte, Manager

Evaluates applications from individuals with permanent disabilities to determine if they are eligible for federal Supplemental Security Income or Social Security Disability Insurance (SSDI).

2816 Nevada Disability and Law Center
6039 Eldora Avenue
Las Vegas, NV 89146
702-257-8150
888-349-3843
FAX 702-257-8170
http://www.ndalc.org
e-mail: ndalc@ndalclv.org
Jack Mayes, Executive Director
Lois Johnson, Manager

A private, nonprofit organization and serves as Nevada's federally mandated protection and advocacy system for the human, legal, and service rights of individuals with disabilities.
1995

2817 Nevada Employment Security Department
500 E 3rd Street
Carson City, NV 89713
775-684-3913
FAX 775-684-3910
http://www.nncdetr.org
e-mail: bakeresd@govmail.state.nv.us
Birgit Baker, Manager

2818 Nevada Equal Rights Commission
1515 E Tropicana Avenue
Las Vegas, NV 89119
702-486-7161
FAX 702-486-7054
TDY:702-486-7164
http://www.detr.state.nu.us/nerc
e-mail: detrcerc@nvdetr.org
Mary Mosley, Director

To foster the rights of all persons to seek, obtain and maintain employment, and to access services in places of public accomodation without discrimination, distinction, exclusion or restriction because of race, religion creed, color, age, sex (gender and/or orientation), disability, national origin, or ancestry.

2819 Nevada Governor's Council on Developmental Disabilities
3636 56th Research Way
Carson City, NV 89701
775-687-4452
http://www.nevadaddcouncil.org
e-mail: rweathermon@dhr.state.nv.us
Richard Weathermon, Executive Director

Tp provide resources at the community level which promote equal opportunity and life choices for people with disabilities through which they may positively contribute to Nevada society.

2820 Nevada State Rehabilitation Council
Nevada Rehabilitation Division
1370 S Curry Street
Carson City, NV 89703
775-684-3200
http://www.detr.state.nv.su
e-mail: pjjune@nvdetr.org
Pamela June, Chief-Office of, Disability Employment Policy

To help insure vocational rehabilitation programs are consumer oriented, driven and result in employment outcomes for Nevadans with disabilities. Funding for innovation and expansions grants

2821 State Department of Adult Education
Nevada Department of Education
700 E 5th Street
Carson City, NV 89701
775-687-9200
FAX 775-687-9101
http://www.nde.state.nv.us
e-mail: pdryden@doe.nv.gov
Phyllis Dryden, Director

To provide leadership and resources to enable all learners to gain knowledge and skills needed to achieve career and employment goals, meet civic duties and accomplish educational objective.

2822 State Department of Education
Carson City Main Location
700 E Fifth Street
Carson City, NV 89701
775-687-9200
FAX 775-687-9101
http://www.doe.nv.gov
e-mail: krheault@doe.nv.gov
Keith W Rheault, Superintendent
Gloria Dopf, Deputy Superintendent
James R Wells, Deputy Superintendent
The Nevada State Board of Education acts as an advocate and visionary for all children and sets the policy that allows every child equal access to educational services, provides the vision for a premier educational system and works in partnership with other stakeholders to ensure high levels of success for all in terms of job readiness, graduation, ability to be lifelong learners, problem solvers, citizens able to adapt to a changing world and contributing members of a society.

New Hampshire

2823 Disability Rights Center
18 Low Avenue
Concord, NH 03301
603-228-0432
800-834-1721
FAX 603-225-2077
TDY:800-834-1721
http://www.drcnh.org
e-mail: advocacy@drcnh.org
Richard Cohen, Executive Director
Joe Dickinson, Board President
Amy Messer, Legal Director
Dedicated to eliminating barriers existing in New Hampshire to the full an dequal enjoyment of civil and other legal rights by people with disabilities.

2824 Granite State Independent Living
21 Chenell Drive
Concord, NH 03301
603-228-9680
800-826-3700
FAX 603-225-3304
TDY:888-396-3459
http://www.gsil.org
Clyde Terry, Executive Director

A statewide non-profit, service and advocacy organization that provides tools for living life on your terms. To promote life with independence for people with disabilities through the four core services of advocacy, information, education and support.
1980

2825 Institute on Disability at theUniversity of New Hampshire
2 N Main Street
Concord, NH 03301
603-228-2084
FAX 603-271-5265
http://www.iod.unh.edu
Jan Nisbet, Director
Linda Bimbo, Deputy Director
Mary Schuh, Associate Director
Established to provide a coherent university-based focus for the improvement of knowledge, policies, and practices related to the lives of persons with disabilities and their families. Also advances policies and systems changes, promising practices, education, and research that strengthen communities and ensure full access, equal opportunities, and participation for all persons.

2826 New Hampshire Commission for Human Rights
2 Chenell Drive
Concord, NH 03301
603-271-2767
FAX 603-271-6339
http://www.nh.gov.hrc
e-mail: humanrights@nhsa.state.nh.us
Katharine Daly, Executive Director
Roxanne Juliano, Assistant Director

Established by RSA 354-A for the puropse of eliminating discrimination in employment, public accommodations and the sale or rental of housing or commercial property, because of age, sex, sexual orientation, race, creed, color, marital status, familial status, physical or mental disability or national origin.

2827 New Hampshire Developmental Disabilities Council
21 S Fruit Street
Concord, NH 03301
603-271-3236
800-852-3345
TDY:800-735-2964
http://www.nhddc.com
Gordon Allen, Executive Director
David Ouellette, Project Manager
Bonnie Addario, Program Specialist
A federally funded agency that supports public policies and initiative that remoce barriers and promote opportunities in all areas of life.

2828 New Hampshire Employment Security
32 S Main Street
Concord, NH 03301
603-224-3311
800-852-3400
http://www.nhes.state.nh.us
e-mail: webmaster@nhes.state.nh.us
Richard S Brothers, Commissioner

Refers individuals with disabilities to organizations and agencies that assist people with disabilities without charge.

2829 New Hampshire Governor's Commission on Disability
57 Regional Drive
Concord, NH 03301
603-271-2773
800-852-3405
FAX 603-271-2837
http://www.nh.gov/disability
e-mail: carol.nadeau@nh.gov
Carol Nadeau, Executive Director
Maureen Stimpson, Project Specialist

To remove barriers, architectural or attitudinal, which bar persons with disabilities from participating in the mainstream of society.

2830 Parent Information Center
PO Box 2405
Concord, NH 03302
603-224-7005
800-947-7005
FAX 603-224-4365
TDY:800-947-7005
http://www.parentinformationcenter.org
e-mail: picinfo@parentinformationcenter.org
Heather Thalheimer, Executive Director
Sylvia Abbott, Business Manager

A recognized leader in building strong family/school partnerships. PIC provides information, support, and educational programs for parents, family members, educators, and the community. PIC is a pioneer in promoting effective parent involvment in the special education process.

2831 ServiceLink
555 Auburn Street
Manchester, NH 03103
603-644-2240
866-634-9412
FAX 603-644-2361
http://www.servicelink.hailboroughcounty.org
Dennis Hett, Manager
Wendi Aultman, Program Coordinator

Provides community information and assistance to adults with disabilities in accessing services for caregiver support, financial and legal concerns, home care services, housing information, prescription drug options, recreational and social events, volunteer opportunities, wellness education. Offices in Laconia, Chocorua, Keene, Berlin, Littleton, Manchester, Lebanon, Nashua, Concord, Portsmouth, Rochester, Claremont and more satellites in each county, all reached through the toll-free number.

2832 State Department of Education: Division of Vocational Rehabilitation
21 S Fruit Street
Concord, NH 03301
603-271-3471
800-299-1647
FAX 603-271-7095
http://www.ed.state.nh.us
e-mail: pwheeler@ed.state.nh.us

Paul K Leather, Director

Provides services to both individuals with disabilities and employers. People with disabilities can work and take advantage of the opportunities available to the citizens of New Hampshire. A joint State/Federal program that seeks to empower people to make informed choices, build viable careers, and live more independently in the community.

New Jersey

2833 Assistive Technology
Assistive Technology Advocacy Center (ATAC)
210 S Broad Street
Trenton, NJ 08608
609-292-9742
800-922-7233
FAX 609-777-0187
http://www.njpanda.org
e-mail: advocate@njpanda.org
Sarah Mitchell, Manager
Jamie Prioli, Assistive Technology Technician

Serves as New Jersey's federally funded assistive technology project through a sub-contract with New Jersey's Department of Labor and Workforce Development. Its purpose is to assist individuals in overcoming barriers in the system and making assistive technology more accessible to individuals with disabilities throughout the state.

2834 New Jersey Department of Education: Special Education
Office of Special Education Programs
PO Box 500
Trenton, NJ 08625
609-292-0147
800-322-8174
FAX 609-984-8422
http://www.state.nj.us
Roberta Wohle, Director

The office is resonsible for administering all federal funds received for educating people with disabilities ages 3 through 21. Also monitors the delivery of special education programs operated under state authority, provides mediation services to parents and school districts, processes hearings and conducts complaint investigations. Also funds four learning resource centers (LRCs) that provide information, circulate materials, offer technical assistance/consultation and production services.

2835 New Jersey Department of Law and Public Safety
New Jersey Division on Civil Rights
31 Clinton Street, 3rd Floor
Newark, NJ 07101
973-648-2700
FAX 973-648-4405
http://www.njcivilrigths.org
J Frank Vespa-Papaleo, Director

The Division on Civil Rights enforces the New Jersey Law Against Discrimination which prohibits discrimination in employment, housing and public accommodations because of race, creed, color, national origin, ancestry, sex, affectional and sexual orientation, marital status, nationality or handicap.

2836 New Jersey Programs for Infants and Toddlers with Disabilities: Early Intervention System
New Jersey Department of Health
50 E State Street
Trenton, NJ 08625
609-777-7713
FAX 609-292-0296
http://www.state.nj.us/health/fhs/eiphome.htm
Terri Harrison, Coordinator
Mary Carnevale, Coordinator

Implements a statewide system of service for infants and toddlers, birth to age three, with developmental delays or disabilities. Maintains Services-Case Management in each county as entry into the system. Here a service coordinator talks with the family about their concerns and offers referral information if needed. If developmental evaluation is indicated, the coordinator will facilitate a multidisciplinary evaluation and assessment with no cost to the parents.

2837 Protection & Advocacy Agency (NJP&A)
210 S Broad Street
Trenton, NJ 08608
609-292-9742
800-922-7233
FAX 609-777-0187
http://www.njpanda.org
e-mail: advocate@njpanda.org
Sarah Mitchell, Executive Director
Joseph Young, Deputy Director
Marie Davis, Office Manager
To protect, advocate for and advance the rights of persons with disabilites in pursuit of a society in which persons with disabilities exercise self-determination and choice, and are treated with dignity.

2838 State Department of Adult Education
Department of Education
PO Box 500
Trenton, NJ 08625
609-984-5593
FAX 609-633-9825
http://www.state.nj.us/education
Arlene Roth, Director Adult Education

2839 State GED Administration: Office of Specialized Populations
New Jersey Department of Education
PO Box 500
Trenton, NJ 08625
609-292-8853
FAX 609-633-9825
http://www.state.nj.us/education
Arlene Roth, Director
Alfred Murray, Executive Director

New Mexico

2840 Client Assistance Program (CAP): New Mexico Protection and Advocacy System
1720 Louisiana Boulevard NE
Albuquerque, NM 87110
505-256-3100
800-432-4682
FAX 505-256-3184
http://www.nmpanda.org
James Jackson, Executive Director

Helps persons with disabilities who have concerns about agencies in New Mexico that provide rehabilitation or independent living services. The kind of help may be information or advocacy. For questions about Division of Vocational Rehabilitation, Commission for the Blind, Independent Living Centers and Preojects With Industsry CAP can help.

2841 New Mexico Department of Labor: Employment Services and Job Training Programs
PO Box 1928
Albuquerque, NM 87103
505-841-8409
FAX 505-841-8491
http://www3.state.nm.us/dol/dol_esd.html
Currently composed of two bureaus and under the supervision of a Division Director responsible for the design, administration, management and implementation of the Workforce Investment Act in New Mexico and any successor legislation. Within this capacity, the Division serves on behalf of the Governor with respect to statewide oversight and compliance, and as the principle support staff to the State Workforce Development Board.

2842 New Mexico Human Rights Commission Education Bureau
1596 Pacheco Street
Santa Fe, NM 87505
505-827-6838
800-566-9471
FAX 505-827-6878
http://www.user.gov/crd/cds_all.htm
Francie Cordova, Executive Director

2843 New Mexico Public Education Department
300 Don Gaspar Avenue
Santa Fe, NM 87503
505-827-5800
http://www.sde.state.nm.us
e-mail: askcommunityrealtions@state.nm.us
Dr Veronica Garcia, Secretary

To provide leadership, technical assistance and quality assurance to improve student performance and close the achievement gap.

2844 New Mexico State GED Testing Program
New Mexico Public Education Department
300 Don Gaspar Avenue
Santa Fe, NM 87501
505-827-6702
FAX 505-827-6616
http://www.ped.state.nm.us
Lisa G Salazar, GED Administrator

The primary aid of the GED testing program in New Mexico is to proive a second opportunity for individuals to obtain their high school diplomas.

2845 New Mexico Technology-Related Assistance Program
Department of Education
300 Don Gaspar Avenue
Santa Fe, NM 87503
505-827-6516
FAX 505-827-5066
e-mail: mlandazuri@ade.state.nm.us
Andrew Winnegar, Project Director

2846 Protection & Advocacy System
1720 Louisiana Boulevard NE
Albuquerque, NM 87110
505-256-3100
800-432-4682
FAX 505-256-3184
http://www.nmpanda.org
e-mail: info@nmpanda.org
James Jackson, Executive Director

Advocates working together with people who have disabilities in promoting and protecting their legal and service rights.

2847 State Department of Adult Education
Department of Education
300 Don Gaspar Avenue
Santa Fe, NM 87501
505-827-6516
FAX 505-623-8220
http://www.sde.state.nm.us
Patricia Chavez, Contact

New York

2848 Client Assistance Program
CAP Director, NY Commission on Quality of Care
99 Washington Avenue
Albany, NY 12210
518-473-7378
FAX 800-624-4143
Provides free services to consumers and applicants for projects, programs and facilities funded under the rehabilitation act.

2849 Department of Correctional Services
1220 Washington Avenue
Albany, NY 12226
518-474-8126
http://www.docs.state.ny.us
Brian Fischer, Commissioner

To provide for public protection by administering a network of correctional facilities that: retain inmates in safe custody until released by law; offer inmates an opportunity to improve their rmployment potential and their ability to function in a non-criminal fashion; offer staff a variety of opportunities for career enrichment and advancement; and, offer stable and humane community environments in which all participants, staff anf inmates can perform their required tasks.

2850 NYS Commission on Quality of Care/TRAID Program

1 Empire State Plaza
Albany, NY 12223
518-449-7860
800-522-4369
FAX 518-473-6005
http://www.cqcapd.state.ny.us
e-mail: lisa.rosano@cqcapd.state.ny.us
Lisa Rosano-Kaczkowski, Project Manager

A statewide systems advocacy program promoting assistive technology devices and services to persons of all ages with all disabilities.

2851 NYS Developmental Disabilities Planning Council

155 Washington Avenue
Albany, NY 12210
518-486-7505
800-395-3372
FAX 518-402-3505
TDY:800-395-3372
http://www.ddpc.state.ny.us
e-mail: ddpc@ddpc.state.ny.us
Sheila M Carey, Executive Director
Anna Lobosco, Deputy Executive Director
Thomas Lee, Public Information Officer
In partnership with individuals with developmental disabilities, their families and communities provides leadership by promoting policies, plans and practices.

2852 New York Department of Human Rights

1 Fordham Plaza
Bronx, NY 10458
718-741-8400
http://www.dhr.state.ny.su
Kumiki Gibson, Commissioner

To ensure that every individual has an equal opportunity to participate fully in the economic cultural and intellectual life of the State.

2853 New York Department of Labor: Employment Services & Job Training

State Office Building Campus
Albany, NY 12240
518-437-0027
FAX 518-485-1126
TDY:888-783-1370
http://www.labor.state.ny.us
e-mail: nysdol@labor.state.ny.us
Robert Lillpopp, Director Communications
Ruth Pillittere, Assistant Director
Monica Winters, Manager

2854 New York State Commission on Quality Care and Advocacy for Persons with Disabilities (CQCAPD)

One Empire State Plaza
Albany, NY 12223
518-474-2825
800-522-4369
FAX 518-473-6005
TDY:518-473-4231
http://www.cqcapd.state.ny.us
e-mail: rosemary.lamb@cqcapd.state.ny.us
Rosemary Lamb, Director Advocacy/Outreach
Gary O'Brien, Commissioner

Our mission is to improve the quality of life for persons with disabilities, to protect their rights, and to advocate needed changes by promoting the development of laws, policies and practices that advance the inclusion of all persons with disabilities into the rich fabric of our society.

2855 New York State Office of Vocational & Educational Services for Individuals with Disabilities

One Commerce Plaza
Albany, NY 12334
800-222-5627
http://www.vesid.nysed.gov
e-mail: vesidadm@mail.nysed.gov
Rebecca H Cort, Deputy Commissioner
Richard P Mills, Commissioner

To promote educational equity and excellence for students with disabilities while ensuring that they receive the rights and protection to which they are entitles; assure appropriate continuity between the child and adult services systems; and provide the highest quality vocational rehabilitation and independent living services to all eligible persons as quickly as those services are required to enable them to work and live independent, self-directed lives.

2856 Northeast ADA & IT Center

Employment and Disability Institute
Cornell Unversity
Ithaca, NY 14853
607-255-6686
800-949-4232
FAX 607-255-2763
http://www.ilr.cornell.edu
e-mail: northeastada@cornell.edu
S Antonio Ruiz-Quintanilla, Project Director
Hannah Rudstam, Training Director

We provide training, technical assistance and materials on the Americans with Disabilities Act and Accessible Information Technology throughout New York, New Jersey, Puerto Rico and the US Virgin Islands.

2857 Office of Civil Rights: New York

US Department of Education
32 Old Slip
New York, NY 10005
646-428-3900
FAX 646-428-3843
TDY:877-521-2172
http://www.ed.gov./ocr
e-mail: ocr.newyork@ed.gov
This office covers the states of New Jersey and New York.

2858 Office of Curriculum & Instructional Support

89 Washington Avenue
Albany, NY 12234
FAX 518-474-0319
http://www.emsc.nysed.gov/cis
e-mail: emscocis@mail.nysed.gov
Howard J Goldsmith, Executive Coordinator

2859 Programs for Children with Special Health Care Needs

Bureau of Child & Adolescent Health, Dept of Healt
Corning Tower Building
Albany, NY 12237
518-474-2084
FAX 518-474-5445
http://www.health.state.ny.us
e-mail: cak03@health.state.ny.us
Antonia C Novello MD MPH, Commissioner
Christopher Kus, Director

Our mission is to achieve a statewide system of care for CSHCN and their families that links them to appropriate health and related services, identifies gaps and barriers and assists in their resolution, and assures access to quality health care.

2860 Programs for Infants and Toddlers with Disabilities

Bureau of Early Intervention
Corning Tower Building
Albany, NY 12237
518-473-7016
800-577-2229
FAX 518-486-1090
http://www.health.state.ny.us
e-mail: blm01@health.state.ny.us
Barbara McTague, Acting Director

The Early Intervention Program offers a variety of therapeutic and support services to eligible infants and toddlers with disabilities and their families.

2861 **Protection & Advocacy Agency**
NY Commission on Quality of Care
99 Washington Avenue
Albany, NY 12210
518-487-7708
FAX 800-624-4143
Jonathan Nye, Director

2862 **Region II: US Department of Health and Human Services**
Office of Civil Rights
Jacob K Javits Federal Building
New York, NY 10278
212-264-3313
FAX 212-264-3039
TDY:212-264-2355
http://www.hhs.gov/region2
e-mail: michael.carter@hhs.gov
Michael Carter, Regional Manager

2863 **State GED Administration**
State Education Department
PO Box 7348
Albany, NY 12224
518-474-3852
FAX 518-474-3041
http://www.emsc.nysed.gov/workforce/ged
e-mail: ged@mail.nysed.gov
Richard Mills, Manager
Patricia Mooney, GED Administrator

Instruction and testing for those over the age of 16 to earn the General Educational Development diploma.

North Carolina

2864 **Assistive Technology Program**
1110 Navaho Drive
Raleigh, NC 27609
919-850-2787
FAX 919-850-2792
http://www.ncatp.org
e-mail: ldeese@ncatp.org
Lynne Deese, AT Consultant

A state and federally funded program that provides assistive technology services statewide to people of all ages and abilities.

2865 **Client Assistance Program (CAP): North Carolina Division of Persons with Disabilities**
2801 Mail Service Center
Raleigh, NC 27699
919-733-2850
800-215-2772
FAX 919-715-2456
e-mail: kathy.brack@ncmail.net
Kathy Brack, Director
Gloria Sims, Executive Director
Tamy Andrews, Administrative Assistant
The Client Assistance Program helps people understand and use rehabilitation services.

2866 **North Carolina Council on Developmental Disabilities**
3801 Lake Boone Trail
Raleigh, NC 27607
919-420-7901
800-357-6916
FAX 919-420-7917
TDY:800-357-6916
http://www.nc-ddc.org
Bob Rickelman, Council Chair
Holly Riddle, Executive Director

To ensure that people with developmental disabilities and their families participate in the design of and have access to culturally competent services and supports, as well as other assistance and opportunities, which promote inclusive communities.

2867 **North Carolina Division of Vocational Rehabilitation**
2801 Mail Services Center
Raleigh, NC 27699
919-855-3500
FAX 919-733-7968
http://dvr.dhhs.state.nc.us
e-mail: dvr.info@ncmail.net
Linda Harrington, Director

To promote employment and independence for people with disabilities through customer partnership and community leadership.

2868 **North Carolina Division of Workforce Services**
313 Chapanoke Road, Suite 12
Raleigh, NC 27699
919-661-6010
800-562-6333
FAX 919-662-4770
http://www.ncdet.com
Roger J Schackleford, Executive Director

2869 **North Carolina Employment Security Commission**
PO Box 27625
Raleigh, NC 27611
919-733-7522
http://www.ncesc.com
e-mail: harry.payne@ncmail.net
Harry Payne, Chairman
Tom Whitaker, Chief Legal Counsel
Manfred Emmrich, Director, Employment Services

2870 **North Carolina Office of Administrative Hearings: Civil Rights Division**
1200 Front Street
Raleigh, NC 27609
919-733-0431
FAX 919-733-4866
http://www.oah.state.nc.us
Edward Smith, Director
Rhonda Wright, Adminstrative Assistant

Responsible for charges alleging discrimination in the basis of race, color, sex, religion, age, national origin or disability in employment, or charges alleging retaliation for opposition to such discrimination brought by previous and current state employees or applicants for employment for positions covered by the State Personnel Act, including county government employees.

2871 **State Department of Adult Education**
North Carolina Community College System
5016 Mail Service Center
Raleigh, NC 27699
919-828-4387
FAX 919-807-7164
http://www.ncccs.cc.nc.us
e-mail: randyw@ncccs.cc.nc.us
Elizabeth Fentress, President
Randy Whitfield MD, Associate Vice President

North Dakota

2872 **Client Assistance Program (CAP): Nebraska Division of Persons with Disabilities**
1237 W Divide Avenue
Bismarck, ND 58501
701-328-8947
800-207-6122
FAX 701-328-8969
TDY:701-328-8968
http://www.nd.gov/cap
e-mail: cap@nd.state.gov
Dennis Lyon, Director

Assists clients and client applicants of North Dakota Vocational Rehabilitation services, Tribal Vocational Rehabilitation, or Independent Living services.

2873 **North Dakota Department of Human Services**
600 E Boulevard Avenue
Bismarck, ND 58505
701-328-2310
800-472-2622
FAX 701-328-8969
http://www.nd.gov.dhs
e-mail: dhseo@nd.gov
Carol K Olson, Executive Director

To provide quality, efficient, and effective human services, which improve the lives of people.

2874 **North Dakota Department of Labor: Fair Employment Practice Agency**
600 E Boulevard Avenue
Bismarck, ND 58505
701-328-2660
800-582-8032
FAX 701-328-2031
TDY:800-366-6888
http://www.nd.gov/labor
e-mail: labor@nd.gov; humanrights@nd.gov
Lisa Fair McEvers, Commissioner of Labor
Kathy Kulesa, Human Rights Director
Robin Bosch, Office Manager
Provides information and enforces laws related to labor standards and discrimination in employment, housing, public services, public accommodations and lending. The department also issues sub minimum wage certificates, verifies independent contractor status and licenses employment agencies.

2875 **North Dakota Department of Public Instruction**
600 E Boulevard Avenue
Bismarck, ND 58505
701-328-2260
FAX 701-328-2461
http://www.dpi.state.nd.us
Dr Wayne G Sanstead, Superintendent

To ensure a uniform, statewide system for effective learning.

2876 **North Dakota State Council on Developmental Disabilities**
ND Department of Human Services
600 E Boulevard Avenue
Bismarck, ND 58505
701-328-8953
FAX 701-328-8969
e-mail: sowalt@nd.gov
Tom Wallner, Executive Director

Ohio

2877 **Assistive Technology**
455 E Dublin-Granville Road
Worthington, OH 43085
614-293-3600
800-784-3425
FAX 614-293-0767
http://www.atohio.org
e-mail: atohio@osu.edu
William T Darling, Executive Director
Gaye Spetka, Program Coordinator

To help Ohioans with disabilities acquire assistive technology. Offer several programs and services to achieve that goal. Also keep up with current legislative activity that affects persons with disabilities.

2878 **Client Assistance Program (CAP): Ohio Division**
Ohio Legal Rights Service
50 W Broad Street
Columbus, OH 43215
614-466-7264
800-282-9181
FAX 614-644-1888
http://olrs.ohio.gov
Michael Kirkman, Executive Director

To protect and advocate, in partnership with people with disabilities, for their human, civil and legal rights.

2879 **Correctional Education**
Department of Rehabilitation & Correction
1050 Freeway Drive N
Columbus, OH 43229
614-752-1159
FAX 614-752-1086
http://www.drc.state.oh.us
e-mail: drc.publicinfo@odrc.state.oh.us
Terry J Collins, Director

Protects and supports Ohioans by ensuring that adult felony offenders are effectively supervised in environments that are safe, humane, and appropriately secure.

2880 **Office of Civil Rights: Ohio**
US Department of Education
600 Superior Avenue E
Cleveland, OH 44114
216-522-4970
FAX 216-522-2573
TDY:877-521-2172
http://www.ed.gov/ocr
e-mail: ocr.cleveland@ed.gov
This office covers the states of Michigan and Ohio.

2881 **Ohio Adult Basic and Literacy Education**
Office of Career-Technical & Adult Education
25 S Front Street
Columbus, OH 43215
614-466-5015
FAX 614-728-8470
http://www.ode.state.oh.us
e-mail: kathy.shibley@ode.state.oh.us
Kathy Shibley, Director
Denise L Pottmyer, Assistant Director
Joyce Sheets, Secretary
Provides quality leadership for the establishment, improvement an dexpansion of lifelong learning opportunities for adults in their family, community and work roles.

2882 **Ohio Civil Rights Commission**
Rhodes State Office Tower
Columbus, OH 43215
614-466-2785
FAX 614-466-7748
http://crc.ohio.gov
e-mail: paytonm@ocrc.state.oh.us
G Michael Payton, Executive Director
Beleta Ebron, Regional Director

TO enforce state laws against discrimination. OCRC receives and investigates charges of discrimination in employment, public accommodations, housing, credit and higher education on the bases of race, colo, religion, sex, national origin, disability, age, ancestry or familial status.

2883 **Ohio Developmental Disabilities Council**
8 E Long Street
Columbus, OH 43215
614-466-5205
800-766-7426
FAX 614-466-0298
http://ddc.ohio.gov
e-mail: david.zwyer@dmr.state.oh.us
David Zwyer, Director

To create change that improves independence, productivity and inclusion for people with developmental disabilities and their families in community life.

2884 **Ohio Governor's Office of Advocacy for People With Disabilities**
8 E Long Street
Columbus, OH 43266
614-466-9956
FAX 614-644-1888
TDY:614-728-2553
http://www.olrs.ohio.gov
e-mail: webmaster@olrs.state.oh.us
Carolyn Knight, Administrator
Jeffrey Folkerth, Administrative Services Director

Helps children and adults with disabilities.

2885 **Ohio Office of Workforce Development**
Ohio Department of Job & Family Services
4020 E 5th Avenue
Columbus, OH 43219
614-466-2115
FAX 614-995-1298
http://jfs.ohio.gov/owd
e-mail: workforce@odjfs.state.oh.us
Linda O'Connor, Deputy Director

The role of OWD is to work in partnership with the U.S. Department of Labor, Governor's Office and a variety of stakeholders in order to provide administration and operational management for several federal programs and to offer specific services in support of the programs. OWD's primary responsibility is to promote job creation and to advance Ohio's workforce.

2886 **Protection & Advocacy Agency**
Ohio Legal Rights Service
50 W Broad Street
Columbus, OH 43215
614-466-7264
800-282-9181
FAX 614-644-1888
http://olrs.ohio.gov
Michael Kirkman, Executive Director

To protect and advocate, in partnership with people with disabilities, for their human, civil and legal rights.

2887 **State Department of Education**
25 S Front Street
Columbus, OH 43215
614-995-1545
877-644-6338
FAX 614-728-2338
http://www.ode.state.oh.us
Susan Tave Zelman, Superintendent, Public Instructi

2888 **State GED Administration**
State Department of Education
25 S Front Street
Columbus, OH 43215
614-466-0224
FAX 614-728-2338
Sandra Miller, Manager
David Fischer, GED Administrator

Oklahoma

2889 **Assistive Technology**
Seretean OSU-Wellness Center
1514 W Hall of Fame
Stillwater, OK 74078
405-744-7414
FAX 405-744-2487
TDY:888-885-5588
http://www.okabletech.okstate.edu
e-mail: linda.jaco@okstate.edu
Ken Roberts, Manager
Linda Jaco, Interim Assoc. Sponsored Prog.

2890 **Client Assistance Program (CAP): Oklahoma Division**
Office of Handicapped Concerns
2401 NW 23rd Street
Oklahoma City, OK 73107
405-521-3756
800-522-8224
FAX 405-522-6695
TDY:405-522-6706
http://www.ohc.state.ok.us
e-mail: steven.stokes@ohc.state.ok.us
Steven Stokes, Director
Dalene Barton, Office Manager

The purpose of this program is to advise and inform clients and client applicants of all services and benefits available to them through programs authorized under the Rehabilitation Act of 1973. Assist and advocates for clients and client applicants in their relationships with projects, programs, and community rehabilitation programs providing services under the Act.

2891 **Correctional Education**
Department of Corrections
PO Box 11400
Oklahoma City, OK 73111
405-425-2500
FAX 405-425-2500
http://www.doc.state.ok.us
e-mail: justin.jones@doc.state.ok.us
Justin Jones, Director

2892 **Oklahoma State Department of Education**
2500 N Lincoln Boulevard
Oklahoma City, OK 73105
405-521-3301
FAX 405-521-6205
http://www.sde.state.ok.us
Sandy Garrett, State Superintendent

Improve student success through: service to schools, parents and students; leadership for education reform; and regulation/deregulation of state and federal laws to provide accountability while removing any barriers to student success.

2893 **Protection & Advocacy Agency**
Disability Law Center
2915 N Classen Boulevard
Oklahoma City, OK 73106
405-525-7755
800-880-7755
FAX 405-525-7759
http://www.oklahomadisabiltylaw.org
e-mail: kayla@okdlc.org
Kayla Bower, Executive Director

Helps people with disabilities achieve equality, inclusion in society and personal independence without regard to disabling conditions.

2894 **State Department of Adult Education**
Department of Education
2500 N Lincoln Boulevard
Oklahoma City, OK 73105
405-521-3301
800-405-0355
FAX 405-522-3503
http://www.sde.state.ok.us
e-mail: linda_young@mail.sde.state.ok.us
Linda Young, Director
Sandy Garrett, Administrator

2895 **State GED Administration**
State Department of Education
2500 N Lincoln Boulevard
Oklahoma City, OK 73105
405-521-4873
FAX 405-522-3503
http://www.sde.state.ok.us
Linda Young, Director

Oregon

2896 **Assistive Technology Program**
Access Technologies
3070 Lancaster Drive NE
Salem, OR 97305
503-361-1201
800-677-7512
FAX 503-370-4530
TDY:503-361-1201
http://www.accesstechnologiesinc.org
e-mail: info@accesstechnologiesinc.org
Laurie Brooks, Manager

A statewide program promoting services and assistive devices for people with disabilities.

2897 Department of Community Colleges and Workforce Development
255 Capitol Street NE
Salem, OR 97310
503-378-8648
FAX 503-378-8434
http://www.oregon.gov/ccwd
e-mail: ccwd.info@odccwd.state
Sharlene Walker, GED Administrator

Contribute leadership and resources to increase skills, knowledge and carrier opportunities.

2898 Oregon Advocacy Center
620 SW 5th Avenue
Portland, OR 97204
503-243-2081
800-452-1694
FAX 503-243-1738
TDY:800-556-5351
http://www.oradvocacy.org
Robert Joondeph, Executive Director
Barbara Printemps Hergeth, Director of Operations

An independent non-profit organization which provides legal advocacy services for people with disabilities anywhere in Oregon. OAC offers free legal assistance and other advocacy services to individuals who are considered to have physical or mental disabilities. OAC works only on legal problems which relate directly to the disability.

2899 Oregon Bureau of Labor and Industry: Fair Employment Practice Agency
800 NE Oregon Street
Portland, OR 97232
503-731-4200
FAX 503-731-4208
http://www.boli.state.or.us
e-mail: dan.gardner@boli.state.or.us
Dan Gardner, Commissioner
Annette Talbott, Deputy Commissioner

2900 Oregon Council on Developmental Disabilities
540 24th Place NE
Salem, OR 97301
503-945-9941
800-292-4154
FAX 503-945-9947
http://www.ocdd.org
e-mail: ocdd@ocdd.org
Bill Lynch, Executive Director

To create change that improves the lives of Oregonians with developmental disabilities.

2901 Oregon Department of Education: School-to-Work
255 Capitol Street NE
Salem, OR 97310
503-986-4614
FAX 503-378-5156
TDY:503-378-3825
http://www.ode.state.or.us
e-mail: ode.frontdesk@ode.state.or.us
Katy Coba, Executive Director
Patrick Burk, Education Policy Deputy Director
Robert Larson, Policy & Research Director
School-to-Work is a federally funded initiative that provides funding for state and local implementation of the Oregon Educational Act for the 21st Century.

2902 Oregon Department of Human Services: Children, Adults & Families Division
500 Summer Street NE
Salem, OR 97310
503-945-5944
FAX 503-378-2897
http://www.dhs.state.or.us
e-mail: dhr.info@state.or.us
Ramona Foley, Assistant Director

This group is responsible for administering self-sufficiency and child-protective programs. These include Jobs, Temporary Assistance for Needdy Families, Employment Related Day Care, Food Stamps, child-abuse investigation and intervention, foster care and adoptions.

2903 Oregon Employment Department
875 Union Street NE
Salem, OR 97311
877-517-5627
800-237-3710
FAX 503-947-1668
http://www.employment.oregon.gov
Laurie Warner, Director
Tom Fuller, Communications Director

Supports economic stability for Oregonians and communities during times of unemployment through the payment of unemployment benefits. Serves businesses by recruiting and referring the best qualified applicants to jobs, and provides resources to diverse job seekers in support of their employment needs.

2904 Vocational Rehabilitation Division
Department of Human Services
500 Summer Street NE
Salem, OR 97301
503-945-5600
877-277-0513
FAX 503-378-2897
http://www.dhs.state.or.us/vr/index.html
e-mail: info.vr@state.or.us
Gary Weeks, Executive Director
Stephanie Parrish-Taylor, Program Director

Helps Oregonians with disabilities to prepare for, finad and retain jobs.

Pennsylvania

2905 Client Assistance Program (CAP): Pennsylvania Division
1617 JFK Boulevard
Philadelphia, PA 19103
215-557-7112
888-745-2357
FAX 215-557-7602
TDY:215-577-7112
http://www.equalemployment.org
e-mail: info@equalemployment.org
Stephen Pennington, Executive Director
Jamie C Ray, Assistant Director

CAP is an advocacy program for people with disabilities administered by the Center for Disability Law and Policy. CAP helps people who are seeking services from the Office of Vocational Rehabilitation, Blindness and Visual Services, Centers for Independent Living and other programs funded under federal law. CAP services are provided at no charge.

2906 Disability Rights Network
1414 N Cameron Street
Harrisburg, PA 17103
717-236-8110
800-692-7443
FAX 717-236-0192
TDY:877-375-7139
http://drnpa.org
e-mail: arnpa.hbg@drnpa.org
Ilene Shane, Executive Director

A statewide, non-profit corporation designated as the federally-mandated organization to advance and protect the civil rights of adults and children with disabilities. DRN works with people with disabilities and their families, their organizations, and their advocates to ensure their rights to live in their communities with the services they need, to receive a full and inclusive education, to live free of discrimination, abuse and neglect.

2907 Office of Civil Rights: Pennsylvania
US Department of Education
100 Penn Square E
Philadelphia, PA 19107
215-656-8541
FAX 215-656-8605
TDY:877-521-2172
http://www.ed.gov/ocr
e-mail: ocr_philadelphia@ed.gov
This office covers the states of Delaware, Kentucky, Maryland, Pennsylvania and West Virginia.

2908 Pennsylvania Department of Corrections
2520 Lisburn Road
Camp Hill, PA 17001
717-975-4859
http://www.cor.state.pa.us
Jeffrey A Beard PhD, Secretary
John S Shaffer, Executive Deputy Secretary

To protect the public by confining persons committed to our custody in safe, secure facilities, and to provide opportunities for inmates to acquire the skills and values necessary to become productive law-abiding citizens; while respecting the rights of crime victims.

2909 Pennsylvania Developmental Disabilities Council
Commonwealth Avenue
Harrisburg, PA 17120
717-787-6057
FAX 717-772-0738
http://www.paddc.org
e-mail: info@paddc.org
Graham Mulholland, Executive Director

Engages in advocacy, systems change and capacity building for people with disabilities and their families in order to: support people with disabilities in taking control of their own lives; ensure access to goods, services, and supports; build inclusive communities; pursue a cross-disability agenda; and to change negative societal attitudes towards people with disabilities.

2910 Pennsylvania Human Rights Commission and Fair Employment Practice
301 Chestnut Street
Harrisburg, PA 17101
717-787-4410
FAX 715-214-0584
TDY:717-783-9308
http://www.phrc.state.pa.us
Homer Floyd, Executive Director

To administer and enforce the PHRAct and the PFEOA of the Commonwealth of the Pennsylvania for the identification and elimination of discrimination and the providing of equal opportunity for all persons.

2911 Pennsylvania Initiative on Assistive Technology
423 Ritter Annex
Philadelphia, PA 19122
215-204-1356
FAX 215-204-6336
TDY:215-204-1356
http://www.temple.edu/ins_disabilities
e-mail: dianeb@astro.ocis.temple.edu
Amy Goldman, Director

Mission to increase access to assistive technology for all Pennsylvanians with disabilities.

2912 Pennsylvania's Initiative on Assistive Technology
Institute on Disabilities at Temple University
1301 Cecil B Moore Avenue
Philadelphia, PA 19122
800-204-7428
FAX 215-204-9371
http://disabilities.temple.edu
e-mail: atinfo@temple.edu
Sandra McNally, Information/Referral Coordinator

Strives to enhance the lives of Pennsylvanians with disabilities, older Pennsylvanians, and their families, through access to and acquisition of assitive technology devices and services, which allow for choice, control and independence at home, work, school, play and in their neighborhoods

2913 Region III: US Department of Health and Human Services, Civil Rights Office
US Department of Health & Human Services
150 S Independence Mall W
Philadelphia, PA 19106
215-861-4441
800-368-1019
FAX 215-861-4431
http://www.hhs.gov/region3
e-mail: paul.cushing@hhs.gov
Paul Cushing, Regional Manager

2914 State Department of Adult Education
333 Market Street
Harrisburg, PA 17101
717-787-6458
FAX 717-783-0583
http://www.pde.psu.edu/able/index.html
e-mail: ckeenan@state.pa.us
Cheryl Keenan, Director
Pedro Cortes, Manager

2915 State Department of Education
333 Market Street
Harrisburg, PA 17101
717-787-5820
FAX 717-787-7222
http:// www.pde.state.pa.us
e-mail: pde@psupen.psu.edu
Francis Barnes, Manager
Donald Carroll, Secretary

2916 State GED Administration
Pennsylvania Department of Education
333 Market Street
Harrisburg, PA 17101
717-787-5820
FAX 717-787-7222
http://www.pde.state.pa.us
e-mail: pde@psupen.psu.edu
Lawrence Goodwin, Director
Francis Barnes, Manager

Rhode Island

2917 Correctional Education
Rhode Island Department of Corrections
PO Box 8312
Cranston, RI 02920
401-462-1000
FAX 401-464-2509
Timothy Murphy, Administrator Education Services

2918 Protection & Advocacy Agency
Rhode Island Disability Law Center
349 Eddy Street
Providence, RI 02903
401-831-3150
800-733-5332
FAX 401-274-5568
TDY:401-831-5335
http://www.ridlc.org
e-mail: info@ridlc.org
Raymond Bandusky, Executive Director

To assist people with differing abilities in their efforts to achieve full inclusion in society and to exercise their civil and human rights through the provision of legal advocacy.

2919 Rhode Island Commission for Human Rights
180 Westminster Street
Providence, RI 02903
401-222-2661
FAX 401-222-2616
http://www.richr.ri.gov
Michael D Evora, Executive Director

A state agency that enforces civil rights law.

2920 Rhode Island Department of Elementary and Secondary Education
Rhode Island Department of Education
255 Westminster Street
Providence, RI 02903
401-222-4600
http://www.ridoe.net
e-mail: todd.flaherty@ride.ri.gov

Peter McWalters, Commissioner
Todd Flaherty, Deputy Commissioner
David V Abbott, Deputy Commissioner

2921 Rhode Island Department of Labor & Training
Center General Complex
Cranston, RI 02920
401-462-8000
TDY:401-462-8006
http://www.dlt.state.ri.us
e-mail: mmadonna@dlt.ri.gov
Adelita S Orefice, Director

Providing workforce protection and development services with courtesy, responsiveness and effectiveness.

2922 Rhode Island Developmental Disabilities Council
400 Bald Hill Road
Warwick, RI 02886
401-732-1238
FAX 401-737-3395
http://www.riddc.org
e-mail: riddc@riddc.org
Christine Singleton, Chairperson
Mary Okero, Interim Executive Director

Promotes the ideas that will enhance the lives of people with developmental disabilities.

2923 State Department of Adult Education
200 Westminster Street
Providence, RI 02903
401-222-8991
FAX 701-222-4256
http://www.ridoe.net
Johan Uvin, State Director, Adult Education
Elizabeth Jardine, Adult Education Prog Specialist
Jacqueline Korengel, Adult Eduction Prog Specialist
Administer grant funded programs in Adult Basic Education, GED, and English for Speakers of Other Languages. Promote stronger families, upward mobility, and active citizenship through effective adult basic education services. The classes support adults who wish to advance their education towards a high school credential, training, and/or post secondary degrees.

South Carolina

2924 Assistive Technology Program
South Carolina Developmental Disabilities Council
1205 Pendleton Street
Columbia, SC 29201
803-734-0660
http://www.scddc.state.sc.us
e-mail: jjennings@oepp.state.sc.gov
Charles Lang, Executive Director
Peggy Rice-Cannon, Administrative Assistant
Jennifer Jennings, Program Information Coordinator
A statewide project established to provide an opportunity for individuals with disabilities to lead the fullest, most productive lives possible.

2925 Protection & Advocacy for People with Disabilities
3710 Landmark Drive
Columbia, SC 29204
803-782-0639
866-275-7273
FAX 803-790-1946
http://www.protectionandadvocacy-sc.org
e-mail: info@protectionandadvocacy-sc.org
Gloria Prevost, Executive Director

To protect the legal, civil, and human rights of people with disabilities in South Carolina by enabling individuals to advocate for themselves, speaking in their behalf when they have been discriminated against or denied a services to which they are entitled, and promoting policies and services which respect their choices.

2926 South Carolina Department of Corrections
PO Box 21787
Columbia, SC 29221
803-896-8555
FAX 803-896-1220
http://www.state.sc.us/scdc
e-mail: corrections.info@doc.state.sc.us
John Ozmint, Agency Director
Donna Hodges, Executive Assistant

Protects the citizens by confining offenders in controlled facilities and by providing rehabilitative, self-improvement opportunities to prepare inmates for their reintegration into society.

2927 South Carolina Developmental Disabilities Council
1205 Pendleton Street
Columbia, SC 29201
803-734-0660
http://www.scddc.state.sc.us
e-mail: jjennings@oepp.sc.gov
Charles Lang, Executive Director
Peggy A Rice-Cannon, Administrative Assistant
Jennifer Jennings, Program Information Coordinator
To provide leadership in advocating, funding and implementing initiatives which recognize the inherent dignity of each individual, and promote independence, productivity, respect and inclusion for all persons with disabilities and their families.

2928 South Carolina Employment Security Commission
1550 Gadsden Street
Columbia, SC 29202
803-737-2588
800-436-8190
FAX 803-737-0140
http://www.sces.org
e-mail: cfallaw@sces.org
Camille Fallaw, Program Coordinator
Martha Stephenson, Director, E&T Technical Services
Roosevelt Halley, Executive Director

2929 South Carolina Employment Services and Job Training Services
1550 Gadsden Street
Columbia, SC 29202
803-748-2588
800-436-8190
FAX 803-737-0140
http://www.sces.org
e-mail: cfallaw@sces.org
Camille Fallaw, Program Coordinator
Martha Stephensen, Director, E&T Technical Services
Roosevelt Halley, Executive Director

2930 South Carolina Human Affairs Commission
2611 Forest Drive, Suite 200
Columbia, SC 29204
803-737-7800
800-521-0725
FAX 803-253-4191
http://www.state.sc.us/schac/index.html
e-mail: information@schac.state.sc.us
Jessie Washington, Commissioner

To eliminate and prevent unlawful discrimination in: employment on the basis of race, color, national origin, religion, sex, age and disability; housing on the basis of race, color, national origin, religion, sex, familial status and disability; and public accommodations on the basis of race, color, national origin and religion.

2931 State Department of Adult Education
1429 Senate Street
Columbia, SC 29201
803-734-8071
FAX 803-734-3643
http://ed.sc.gov
e-mail: dstout@ed.sc.gov
David Stout, Interim Director

Provides the opportunity for adults with low literacy skills (less than eighth grade level), to work with materials to be taught in an environment conducive to their level, and to improve their reading, math, and writing skills.

2932 State GED Administration
Department of Education
1429 Senate Street
Columbia, SC 29201
803-734-8347
FAX 803-734-8336
http://ed.sc.gov
e-mail: dstout@ed.sc.gov
David Stout, GED Administrator

South Dakota

2933 Client Assistance Program (CAP): South Dakota Division
South Dakota Advocacy Services
221 S Central Avenue
Pierre, SD 57501
605-224-8294
800-658-4782
FAX 605-224-5125
http://www.sdadvocacy.com
e-mail: sdas@sdadvocacy.com
Robert Kean, Executive Director

Provides free services to consumers and applicants for projects, programs and facilities funded under the rehabilitation act.

2934 Department of Correction: Education Coordinator
3200 E Highway 34
Pierre, SD 57501
605-773-3478
FAX 605-773-3194
http://www.state.sd.us
Tim Reisch, Secretary

To protect the citizens of South Dakota by providing safe and secure facilities for juvenile and adult offenders committed to our custody by the courts, to provide effective community supervision upon their release.

2935 Easter Seals South Dakota
1351 N Harrison Avenue
Pierre, SD 57501
605-224-5879
FAX 605-224-133
http://sd.easterseals.com
Creates solutions that change the lives of children, adults and families with disabilities or other needs; to promote disability prevention and awareness.

2936 South Dakota Advocacy Services
221 S Central Avenue
Pierre, SD 57501
605-224-8294
800-658-4782
FAX 605-224-5125
http://www.sdadvocacy.com
e-mail: sdas@sdadvocacy.com
Robert Kean, Executive Director

To protect and advocate the rights of South Dakotans with disabilities through legal, administrative, and other remedies.

2937 South Dakota Council on Developmental Disabilities
Department of Human Services
3800 E Highway 34
Pierre, SD 57501
605-773-6369
800-265-9684
FAX 605-773-5483
http://dhs.sd.gov/ddc
Arlene Poncelet, Executive Director

To assist people with developmental disabilities to control their own destiny and to achieve the quality of life they desire.

2938 South Dakota Department of Labor: Employment Services & Job Training
700 Governors Drive
Pierre, SD 57501
605-773-3131
FAX 605-773-4211
http://www.state.sd.us/dol/dol.htm
e-mail: miker@dol.pr.state.sd.us
Michael Ryan, Administrator
Dorothy Leigl, Manager

Job training programs provide an important framework for developing public-private sector partnerships. We help prepare South Dakotans of all ages for entry or re-entry into the labor force.

2939 South Dakota Division of Human Rights
700 Governors Drive
Pierre, SD 57501
605-773-4493
FAX 605-773-6893
http://www.state.sd.us/dor/hr
e-mail: james.marsh@state.sd.us
James Marsh, Director

To promote equal opportunity through the administration and enforcement of the Human Relations Act of 1972. The act is designed to protect the public from discrimination because of race, color, creed, religion, sex, disability, ancestry or national origin.

2940 South Dakota Division of Special Education
Department of Education
700 Governors Drive
Pierre, SD 57501
605-773-3678
FAX 605-773-3782
http://doe.sa.gov
Ann Larsen, Special Education Programs Dir

The Office of Special Education advocates for the availability of the full range of personnel, programming, and placement options, including early intervention and transition services, required to assure that all individuals with disabilities are able to achieve maximum independence upon exiting from school.

2941 State GED Administration
Department of Labor
700 Governors Drive
Pierre, SD 57501
605-773-3681
FAX 605-773-6184
e-mail: roxie.thielen@state.sd.us
Pam Roberts, Manager
Marcia Hess, Adult Education/Literacy

Tennessee

2942 Council on Developmental Disabilities
Parkway Towers, Suite 130
Nashville, TN 37243
615-532-6615
FAX 615-532-6964
http://www.tennessee.gov/cdd
e-mail: wanda.willis@state.tn.us
Wanda Willis, Executive Director

A State office that promotes public policies to increase and support the inclusion of individuals with developmental disabilities in their communities.

2943 Department of Human Services: Division of Rehabilitation Services
400 Deaderick Street
Nashville, TN 37248
615-313-4700
FAX 615-741-4165
http://www.tennessee.gov/humanserv
e-mail: human-services.webmaster@state.tn.us
Virginia T Lodge, Commissioner

To improve the well-being of economically disadvantaged, disabled or vulnerable Tennesseans through a network of financial, employment, rehabilitative and protective services.

2944 State Department of Education
Andrew Johnson Tower
Nashville, TN 37243
615-741-2731
http://www.state.tn.us
e-mail: education.comments@state.tn.us
Lana C Seivers, Commissioner
Tim Webb, Deputy Commissioner

The department provides many services, and it is our responsibility to ensure equal, safe, and quality learning opportunities for all students, pre-kindergartern through 12th grade.

2945 **State GED Administration**
State Department of Education
710 James Robertson Parkway
Nashville, TN 37210
615-741-2731
800-531-1515
FAX 615-532-4791
http://www.state.tn.us
Phil White, Director

2946 **Tennessee Technology Access Project**
400 Deaderick Street
Nashville, TN 37248
615-313-5183
800-732-5059
FAX 615-532-4685
http://www.state.tn.us/humanserv/rehab.ttap.htm
e-mail: tn.ttap@state.tn.us
Kevin Wright, Executive Director

Texas

2947 **Advocacy**
7800 Shoal Creek Boulevard
Austin, TX 78757
512-454-4816
800-252-9108
FAX 512-323-0902
http://www.advocacyinc.org
e-mail: infoai@advocacyinc.org
Mary Faithfull, Executive Director
Jeff Garrison-Tate, Policy Services Manager

Protection & Rights Legal Organization for People with Disabilities

2948 **Learning Disabilities Association**
1011 W 31st Street
Austin, TX 78705
512-458-8234
800-604-7500
FAX 512-458-3826
http://www.ldat.org
e-mail: contact@ldat.org
Jean Kueker, President
Ann Robinson, State Coordinator

Promotes the educational and general welfare of individuals with learning disabilities.

2949 **Office of Civil Rights: Texas**
US Department of Education
1999 Bryan Street
Dallas, TX 75201
214-661-9600
FAX 214-661-9587
TDY:877-521-2172
http://www.ed.gov/ocr
e-mail: ocr.dallas@ed.gov
The Dallas office covers the states of Alabama, Arkansas, Louisiana, Mississippi and Texas.

2950 **Southwest Texas Disability & Business Technical Assistance Center: Region VI**
2323 S Shepherd Drive
Houston, TX 77019
713-520-0232
800-949-4232
FAX 713-520-5785
http://www.dlrp.org
e-mail: dlrp@ilru.org
Wendy Wilkinson, Project Director
Laurie Redd, Executive Director

One of ten DBTACs funded by the National Institute on Disability and Rehabilitation Research. The DBTAC serves a wide range of audiences who are interested in or impacted by these laws, including employers, businesses, government agencies, schools and people with disabilities.

2951 **State GED Administration**
Texas Education Agency
1701 Congress Avenue
Austin, TX 78701
512-463-9292
FAX 512-305-9493
http://www.tea.state.tx.us
e-mail: ged@tea.state.tx.us
G Paris Ealy, Administrator

To build capacity for consistent testing services throughout the state in order that all eligible candidates may have an pooportunity to earn high school equivalency credentials based on the General Educational Development (GED) Tests.

2952 **Texas Department of Assistive and Rehabilitative Services**
4800 N Lamar Boulevard
Austin, TX 78756
800-628-5115
http://www.dars.state.tx.us
e-mail: DARS.inquiries@dars.state.tx.us
Terry Murphy, Commissioner
Mary Elder, Deputy Commissioner

To work in partnership with Texans with disabilities and families with children who have developmental delays to improve the quality of their lives and to enable their full participation in society.

2953 **Texas Department of Criminal Justice**
PO Box 99
Huntsville, TX 77342
936-295-6371
http://www.tdcj.state.tx.us/
e-mail: webmaster@tdcj.state.tx.us
Brad Livingston, Executive Director
Christina Melton-Crain, Chairperson

To provide public safety, promote positive change in offender behavior, reintegrate offenders into society, and assist victims of crime.

2954 **Texas Education Agency**
1701 Congress Avenue
Austin, TX 78701
512-463-9734
http://www.tea.state.tx.us
e-mail: commissioner@tea.state.tx.us
Robert Scott, Chief Deputy Commissioner

To provide leadership, guidance, and resources to help schools meet the educational needs of all students.

2955 **Texas Employment Services and Job Training Program Liaison**
15th & Congress Avenue
Austin, TX 78778
512-463-2652

2956 **Texas Planning Council for Developmental Disabilities**
6201 E Oltorf Street
Austin, TX 78741
512-437-5432
800-262-0334
FAX 512-437-5434
http://www.txddc.state.tx.us
e-mail: roger.webb@tcdd.state.tx.us
Roger Webb, Executive Director

To create change so that all people with disabilities are fully included in their communities and exercise control over their own lives.

2957 **Texas Workforce Commission: Civil Rights Division**
1117 Trinity Street
Austin, TX 78778
512-463-2642
888-452-4778
FAX 512-463-2643
http://www.twc.state.tx.us
e-mail: robert.gomez@twc.state.tx.us
Robert Gomez, Director

Enforces the Texas Commission on Human Rights Act and the Texas Fair Housing Act. The Human Rights Act prohibits employment discrimination based on race, color, religion, sex, age, national origin, disability and retaliation. The Fair Housing Act prohibits housing discrimination based on race, color, religion, sex, national origin, mental or physical disability, familial status and retaliation.

2958 Texas Workforce Commission: Workforce Development Division
PO Box 12728
Austin, TX 78711 512-936-0697
http://www.twc.state.tx.us
e-mail: larry.jones@twc.state.tx.us
Larry Jones, Director

Provides oversight, coordination, guidance, planning, technical assistance and implementation of employment and training activities with a focus on meeting the needs of employers throughout the state of Texas. Also supports work conducted in local workforce development areas, provides assistance to boards in the achievement of performance goals, evaluates education and training providers, and promotes and develops partnerships with other agencies and institutions.

Utah

2959 Assistive Technology Center
1595 W 500 S
Salt Lake City, UT 84104 801-887-9500
800-866-5550
http://www.usor.utah.gov/ucat
Pete Miner, Director
Lynn Marcoux, Executive Secretary
Craig Boogaard, Manager
To enhance human potential through facilitating the application of assistive technologies for persons with disabilities.

2960 Assistive Technology Program
6588 Old Main Hill
Logan, UT 84322 435-797-3824
800-524-5152
FAX 435-797-2355
http://www.uatpat.org
Martin Blair, Director

Serve individuals with disabilities of all ages in Utah and the intermountain region. Provide AT devices and services, and train university students, parents, children with disabilities and professional services providers about AT. Also coordinate the services with community organizations and others who provide independence-related support to individuals with disabilities.

2961 Center for Persons with Disabilities
6800 Old Main Hall
Logan, UT 84322 435-797-1981
866-284-2821
FAX 435-797-3944
http://www.cpd.usu.edu
Sarah Rule, Director

Utah's University Center for excellence in developmental disabilities education, research, and services. We collaborate with partners to strengthen families and individuals across the lifespan through education, policy, research and services.

2962 Disability Law Center
205 N 400 W
Salt Lake City, UT 84103
800-662-9080
http://www.disabilitylawcenter.org
e-mail: mattknotts@disabilitylawcenter.org
Matt Knotts, Executive Director

A private non-profit organization designated as the Protection and Advocacy agency for the state of Utah to protect the rights of people with disabilities in Utah. To enforce and strengthen laws that protect the opportunities, choices and legal rights of people with disabilities in Utah.

2963 Utah Developmental Disabilities Council
155 E 300 W
Salt Lake City, UT 84101 801-533-3965
FAX 801-533-3968
http://uthaddc.org
e-mail: clairmantonya@utah.gov
Claire Mantonya, Executive Director

To be the states leading source of critical innovative and progressive knowledge, advocacy, leadership and collaboration to enhance the life of individuals with developmental disabilities.

2964 Utah Labor Commission for Anti-Discrimination
PO Box 146630
Salt Lake City, UT 84114 801-530-6801
800-222-1238
FAX 801-530-7609
TDY:801-530-7685
http://www.laborcommission.utah.gov
e-mail: paulinecarter@utha.gov
Sherrie Hayashi, Director
Anna Jensen, Executive Director
Harold Stephens, Case Manager for Employment
Investigates and resolves employment and housing discrimination complaints and enforces Utah's minimum wage, wage payment requirements, laws which protect youth in employment and the requirement that private employemnt agencies be licensed. The Division also conducts public awareness and educational presentations.

2965 Utah State Office of Education
250 E 500 S
Salt Lake City, UT 84114 801-538-7870
FAX 801-538-7868
http://www.schools.utah.gov
e-mail: mmeszaros@schools.utah.gov
Murray Meszaros, State GED Administrator

Promotes adult education and GED Testing in Utah.

2966 Utah Work Force
PO 45249
Salt Lake City, UT 84111 801-526-9675
FAX 801-526-9211
http://www.jobs.utah.gov
e-mail: dwscontactus@utah.gov
Kristen Cox, Executive Director

Provides employment and support services for our customers to improve their economic opportunities.

Vermont

2967 Learning Disabilities Association of Vermont
Learning Disabilities Association of America
PO Box 1041
Manchester Center, VT 05255 802-362-3127
FAX 802-362-3128
Christina Thurston, President

A nonprofit organization whose members are individuals with learning disabilities, their families, and the professionals who work with them.

2968 Protection & Advocacy Agency
141 Main Street
Montpelier, VT 05602 802-229-1355
800-834-7890
FAX 802-229-1359
TDY:802-229-2603
http://www.vtpa.org
e-mail: info@vtpa.org
Ed Paquin, Executive Director
Jason Whitney, President of the Board

Mission is to defend and advance the rights of people who have been labeled mentally ill.

2969 Protection and Advocacy Agency
141 Main Street
Montpelier, VT 05602
802-229-1355
800-834-7890
http://www.vtpa.org
e-mail: ed.paquin@vtpa.org
Ed Paquin, Executive Director

Dedicated to addressing problems, questions and complaints brought to it by Vermonters with disabilities. Mission is to promote the equality, dignity, and self-determination of people with disabilities. Provides information, referral and advocacy services, in cluding legal representation when appropriate, to individuals with disabilities throughout Vermont. Also advocates to promote positive systematic responses to issues affecting people with disabilities.

2970 REACH-UP Program: Department of Social Welfare
103 S Main Street
Waterbury, VT 05671
802-241-2800
800-287-0589
FAX 802-241-2830
http://www.dws.state.vt.us
Joseph Petrissi, Deputy Commissioner

2971 State GED Administration
Department of Education,Career & Lifelong Learning
120 State Street
Montpelier, VT 05620
802-828-3134
FAX 802-828-3146
e-mail: srobinson@doe.state.vt.us
Tracy Gallo, Director Life Long Learning

Promotes adult education.

2972 Vermont Agency of Human Services
Vocational Rehabilitation Division
103 S Main Street
Waterbury, VT 05671
802-241-2186
866-879-6757
http://vocrehab.vermont.gov
Diane Dalmasse, Executive Director

To assist Vermonters with disabilities to find and maintain meaningful employment in their communities.

2973 Vermont Department of Children & Families
103 S Main Street
Waterbury, VT 05671
802-241-2100
800-287-0589
http://www.dcf.state.vtus
Steve Dale, Commissioner

To promote the social, emotional, physical and economic well being and the safety of Vermont's children and families.

2974 Vermont Department of Education
120 State Street
Montpelier, VT 05620
802-828-3135
http://www.state.vt.us
e-mail: doe-edinfo@state.vt.us
Richard H Cate, Education Commissioner

Provide leadership and support to help all Vermont students achieve excellence.

2975 Vermont Department of Labor
5 Green Mountain Drive
Montpelier, VT 05601
802-828-4000
FAX 802-828-4022
TDY:802-828-4203
http://www.labor.vermont.gov
e-mail: pat.moulton.powden@state.vt.us
Patricia Moulton Powden, Commissioner
Tom Douse, Deputy Commissioner

To improve and enhance services to the public by combining under one department: employment security, employment-related services, labor market information, safety and training for Vermont workers, and employers, workers compensation, and wage and hour.

2976 Vermont Developmental Disabilities Council
103 S Main Street
Waterbury, VT 05671
802-241-2612
888-317-2006
FAX 802-241-2989
http://www.humanservices.vermont.gov/boards
e-mail: karen.schwartz@ahs.state.vt.us
Karen Schwartz, Executive Director

Statewide board that works to increase public awareness about critical issues affecting Vermonters with developmental disabilities and their families. 13 of the 21 board members are people with developmental disabilities or family members.

2977 Vermont Governor's Office
109 State Street, Pavilion
Montpelier, VT 05609
802-828-3333
FAX 802-828-3339
http://www.vermont.gov\governor
Jim Douglas, Governor

2978 Vermont Legal Aid Client Assistance Program and Disability Law Project
PO Box 1367
Burlington, VT 05402
802-863-2881
800-747-5022
FAX 802- 863- 71
Laura Philipps, Co-Director
Judy Dickson, Co-Director

Program assists people with disabilities seeking information on vocational rehabilitation and independent living services from state agencies. Offers advisement of employment rights and services available under the ADA.

2979 Vermont REACH-UP Program
Department of Social Welfare
103 S Main Street
Waterbury, VT 05671
802-241-2860
800-775-0506
FAX 802-241-2830
Linda Knosp, Manager

2980 Vermont Special Education
120 State Street
Montpelier, VT 05620
802-828-3130
FAX 802-828-3140
TDY:802-828-2755
http://www.state.vt.us\educ
e-mail: edinfo@education.state.vt.us
Karin Edward, Executive Director
Elaine Pickney, Deputy Director

Promotes the quality of special education.

Virginia

2981 Adult and Employment Training: Virginia Department of Education
Department of Education: Office of Adult Education
PO Box 2120
Richmond, VA 23218
804-225-2075
FAX 804-225-3352
http://www.pen.k12.va.us
Elizabeth Hawa, Director

Employment training for individuals in Virginia.

2982 Assistive Technology System
8004 Franklin Farms Drive
Richmond, VA 23288
804-662-9990
FAX 804-622-9478
http://www.vats.org
e-mail: ken.knorr@drs.virginia.gov
Ken Knorr, Project Director

To ensure that Virginians of all ages and abilities can acquire the appropriate, affordable assistive and information technologies and services they need to participate in society as active citizens.

2983 Department of Correctional Education
James Monroe Building, 7th Floor
Richmond, VA 23219
804-225-3310
FAX 804-225-3255
TDY:804-371-8647
http://dce.virginia.gov
e-mail: webmaster@dce.state.va.us
Walter Farlane, Manager
Sharon Trimmer, Director of Special Education

Provides quality educational programs that enable incarcerated youth and adults to become responsible, productive, tax-paying members of their community.

2984 State Department of Education
Department of Education: Office of Adult Education
PO Box 2120
Richmond, VA 23218
804-225-2075
FAX 804-225-3352
http://www.pen.k12.va.us
Lennox McLedon, Associate Director Adult Ed

Promotes quality education.

2985 State GED Administration
Department of Education: Office of Adult Education
PO Box 2120
Richmond, VA 23218
804-225-2075
FAX 804-225-3352
http://www.pen.k12.va.us
Patricia Ta'ani MD, Specialist

Promotes quality education for adults.

2986 Virginia Board for People with Disabilities
202 N 9th Street
Richmond, VA 23219
804-786-0016
FAX 804-786-1118
TDY:800-846-4464
http://www.vaboard.org
e-mail: heidi.lawyer@vbpd.virginia.gov
Heidi Lawyer, Executive Director
Sandra Smalls, Executive Assistant

To enrich the lives of Virginians with disabilities by providing a voice for their concerns.

2987 Virginia Office for Protection & Advocacy Agency
1910 Byrd Avenue
Richmond, VA 23250
804-225-2042
800-552-3962
FAX 804-662-7057
http://www.vopa.state.va.us
e-mail: general.vopa@vopa.virginia.gov
P Brent Brown, Chairman

Through zealous and effective advocacy and legal representation to: protect and advance legal, human, and civil rights of persons with disabilities; combat and prevent abuse, neglect, and discrimination; and to promote independence, choice, and self determination by persons with disabilities.

Washington

2988 Client Assistance Program (CAP): Washington Division

2531 Rainier Avenue S
Seattle, WA 98144
206-721-5999
800-544-2121
http://www.washingtoncap.org
e-mail: caprogram@qwest.net
Jerry Johnsen, Executive Director
Bob Huven, Rehabilitation Coordinator

Provides information and advocacy for persons seeking services from the Department of Services for the Blind and the Division of Vocational Rehabilitation. Approximately 25 percent of cases involve assistive technology issues.

2989 Correctional Education
Department of Corrections
PO Box 41100
Olympia, WA 98504
360-725-8213
FAX 360-586-6582
http://www.doc.wa.gov
e-mail: doccorrespondence@doc1.wa.gov
Harold Clarke, Secretary of Department

The Department of Corrections, in collaboration with its criminal justice partners, will contribute to staff and community safety and hold offenders accountable through administration of criminal sanctions and effective re-entry programs.

2990 Department of Personnel & Human Services
Department of Personnel & Human Services
614 Division Street
Port Orchard, WA 98366
360-337-7185
FAX 360-337-7187
http://www.kitsapgov.com/hr
Bert Furuta, Director
Steve Frazier, Manager of Human Services

Exists to serve the needs of elected County Officials, appointed department heads, County employees and the entire community through a variety of programs and processes. The employees of this department perform work in a wide variety of specialized areas, providing programs and services vital to the community and to Kitsap County as a unit of local government.

2991 Developmental Disabilities Council
2600 Martin Way, Suite F
Olympia, WA 98504
360-725-2870
800-634-4473
FAX 360-586-2424
TDY:800-634-4473
http://www.wa.gov/ddc
e-mail: edh@cted.wa.gov
Edward Holen, Executive Director

Holds that individuals with developmental disabilities, including those with the most severe disabilities, have the right to achieve independence, productivity, integration and inclusion into the community.

2992 Disability Rights Washington
315 5th Avenue S
Seattle, WA 98104
206-324-1521
800-562-2702
FAX 206-957-0729
http://www.disabilityrightswa.org
e-mail: wpas@wpas-rights.org
Mark Stroh, Executive Director

A private non-profit organization that protects the rights of people with disabilities statewide. To advance the dignity, equality, and self-determination of people with disabilities. Also work to pursue justice on matters related to human and legal rights.

2993 Region X: US Department of Education Office for Civil Rights
US Department of Education
915 2nd Avenue
Seattle, WA 98174
206-220-7900
FAX 206-220-7887
TDY:877-521-2172
http://www.ed.gov
e-mail: ocr.seattle@ed.gov
Donna Foxley, Secretary Regional Rep
Linda Powley, Administrative Assistant
Carla Nuxoll, Manager
This office covers the states of Alaska, Hawaii, Idaho, Montana, Nevada, Oregon, and Washington.

2994 **Region X: US Department of Health and Human Services, Office of Civil Rights**
US Department of Health & Human Services
2201 6th Avenue
Seattle, WA 98121
206-615-2010
FAX 206-615-2087
http://www.hhs.gov/region10
e-mail: james.whitfield@hhs.gov
James Whitfield, Regional Director

2995 **Region X: US Department of Labor Office of Federal Contract Compliance**
US Department of Labor
1111 3rd Avenue
Seattle, WA 98101
206-553-4543
FAX 206-553-0098

These regional offices of agencies enforce laws prohibiting employment discrimination on the basis of disability.

2996 **WA State Board for Community and Technical Colleges**

Office of GED for Washington State
PO Box 42495
Olympia, WA 98504
360-704-4321
FAX 360-704-4414
http://www.sbctc.ctc.edu/public/y_ged.aspx
e-mail: abruch@sbctc.edu
Alleyne Bruch, GED Program Administrator

Promotes adult education.

2997 **Washington Human Rights Commission**
711 S Capitol Way, #402
Olympia, WA 98504
360-753-6770
800-233-3247
FAX 360-586-2282
http://www.hum.wa.gov
e-mail: mbrenman@hum.wa.gov
Marc Brenman, Executive Director

2998 **Washington State Board for Community and Technical Colleges**
Office of Adult Basic Education
PO Box 42495
Olympia, WA 98504
360-704-4326
FAX 360-704-4419
http://www.sbctc.ctc.edu/college/e_abe.aspx
e-mail: imendoza@sbctc.edu
Israel David Mendoza, Director, Adult Basic Education

Promotes the quality of adult education.

2999 **Washington State Governor's Committee on Disability Issues & Employment**
PO Box 9046
Olympia, WA 98507
360-438-3168
FAX 360-438-3208
http://www.wa.gov/esd/gcde
Toby Olson, Director

Employment services and training programs provided to those working in Washington state.

West Virginia

3000 **Assistive Technology System**
955 Hartman Run Road
Morgantown, WV 26505
304-293-4692
800-841-8436
FAX 304-293-7294
http://www.cedwvu.org
e-mail: contact@cedwvu.org
Jamie L Hayhurst-Marshall, Assistive Technology Coordinator

Dedicated to increasing awareness of and accessibility to assistive technology for West Virginians of all ages and all types of disabilities.

3001 **Client Assistance Program (CAP): West Virginia Division**
West Virginia Advocates
Litton Building, Suite 400
Charleston, WV 25301
304-346-0847
800-950-5250
FAX 304-346-0867
http://www.wvadvocates.org
e-mail: wvainfo@wvadvocates.org
Susan Given, Program Director
Clarice Hausch, Executive Director

Mandated in 1984, to provide advocacy to individuals seeking services under the federal Rehabilitation Act (such as services from the West Virginia Division of Rehabilitation Services, Centers for Independent Living, supported employment programs and sheltered workshops).

3002 **Correctional Education**
State Department of Education
1900 Kanawha Boulevard E
Charleston, WV 25305
304-558-2000
FAX 304-558-5042
Frank Andrews, Superintendent
Tam Wright, Secretary
James Teets, Executive Director

3003 **State Department of Education**
1900 Washington Street E
Charleston, WV 25305
304-558-2000
FAX 304-558-0304
http://wvde.state.wv.us
Dr Steven L Paine, State Superintendent
Dr Jack McClanahan, Deputy Superintendent

Promotes quality education.

3004 **State GED Administration**
1900 Kanawha Boulevard E
Charleston, WV 25305
304-558-6315
FAX 304-558-4874
http://www.wvabe.org/ged/
e-mail: dkimbler@access.k12.wv.us
Debra Kimbler, GED Administrator

Our organization's goal is to provide reasonable accommodations to qualifying GED candidates.

3005 **West Virginia Adult Basic Education**
Department of Education
1900 Kanawha Boulevard E
Charleston, WV 25305
304-558-5616
FAX 304-558-3946
http://www.wvabe.org
e-mail: bwilcox@access.k12.wv.us
Bill Wilcox, Executive Director

To enable adult learners to be literate, productive, and successful in the workplace, home and community by delivering responsive adult education programs and services.

Wisconsin

3006 **Correctional Education**
Department of Corrections
3099 E Washington Ave
Madison, WI 53707
608-240-5000
FAX 608-240-3300
http://www.wi-doc.com
e-mail: docweb@doc.state.wi.us
Matthew Frank, Secretary
Rick Raemisch, Deputy Secretary
Susan Crawford, Executive Assistant

3007 Disability Rights Wisconsin
131 Wilson Street
Madison, WI 53703
608-267-0214
800-928-8778
FAX 608-267-0368
http://www.disabilityrightswi.org
e-mail: lynnb@wca.org
Lynn Breedlove, Executive Director

Serves people of all ages, including people with developmental disabilities, people with mental illness, people with physical or sensory disabilities, and people with traumatic brain injury.

3008 State Capitol
State of Wisconsin Department of Administration
PO Box 7863
Madison, WI 53707
608-266-2529
FAX 608-267-8983
http://www.wisgov.state.wi.us
e-mail: governor@wisconsin.gov
Claire Franz, Manager
Michael Stark, Bureau Director

3009 State Department of Education
Department of Public Instruction
125 S Webster Street
Madison, WI 53707
800-441-4563
http://dpi.wi.gov
Elizabeth Burmaster, State Superintendent

Promotes quality education.

3010 State GED Administration
Department of Public Instruction
125 S Weston Street
Madison, WI 53707
608-257-2275
800-441-4563
FAX 608-267-9275
http://dpi.wi.gov
e-mail: robert.enghagen@dpi.state.wi.us
Robert Enghagen, GED/HSED Administrator
Judy Stowell, GED/HSED Program Assistant

Promotes quality adult education.

3011 Wisconsin Council on Developmental Disabilities
201 W Washington Avenue
Madison, WI 53703
608-266-7826
888-332-1677
FAX 608-267-3906
TDY:608-266-6660
http://www.wcdd.org
e-mail: help@wcdd.org
Jennifer Ondrejka, Manager
John Shaw, Supervisor

Established to advocate on behalf of individuals with developmental disabilities, foster welcoming and inclusive communities, and improve the disability service system. To help people with developmental disabilities become independent, productive, and included in all facets of community life.

3012 Wisconsin Department of Workforce Development
PO Box 7946
Madison, WI 53707
608-266-3131
FAX 608-266-1784
http://www.dwd.state.wi.us
e-mail: dwdsec@dwd.state.wi.us
Roberta Gassman, Secretary
JoAnna Richard, Deputy Secretary
Janel Hanes, Executive Assistant
A state agency charged with building and strengthening Wisconsin's workforce in the 21st century and beyond. The Departmen's primary responsibilities include providing job services, training and employment assistance to people looking for work, at the same time as itworks with employers on finding the necessary workers to fill current job openings.

3013 Wisconsin Equal Rights Division
201 E Washington Avenue, Room A300
Madison, WI 53708
608-266-6860
FAX 608-267-4592
TDY:608-264-8752
http://www.dwd.wisconsin.gov
e-mail: jennnifer.ortiz@dwd.state.wi.us
Jennifer A Ortiz, Administrator

To protect the rights of all people in Wisconsin under the civil rights and labor standards laws we administer; to achieve compliance through education, outreach, and enforcement by empowered and committed employees; and to perform our responsibilities with reasonableness, efficiency, and fairness.

3014 Wisconsin Governor's Commission for People with Disabilities
1 W Wilson Street, Room 1150
Madison, WI 53709
608-266-7974
FAX 608-266-3386
http://www.dhfs.state.wi.us
e-mail: lincosj@dhfs.state.wi.us
Sarah Lincoln, Contact

Wyoming

3015 Adult Basic Education
Wyoming Community College Commission
2020 Carey Avenue
Cheyenne, WY 82002
307-777-3545
FAX 307-777-6567
http://www.commission.wcc.edu@wccc.ABE/
e-mail: kmilmont@commission.wcc.edu
Karen Milmont, Director

3016 Client Assistance Program (CAP): Wyoming Division
320 W 25th Street
Cheyenne, WY 82001
307-638-7668
FAX 307-638-0815
e-mail: wypanda@vcn.com
Lee Beidleman, Director
Kris Smith, Executive Director

Provides free services to consumers and applicants for projects, programs and facilities funded under the rehabilitation act.

3017 Correctional Education: Wyoming Women's Center
PO Box 20
Lusk, WY 82225
307-334-3693
FAX 307-334-2254
e-mail: cthaye@state.wy.us
Nola Blackburn, Warden
Melissa Bischner, Public Information Officer

The Wyoming Women's Center is a full service, secure correctional facility for female offenders and the sole adult female facility in the State of Wyoming. In October 2000, WWC opened a self-contained 16 bed intensive addiction treatment unit, a is highly structured long term 7-9 month program based upon the therapeutic community treatment model. It is tailored to provide gender specific services and is funded with a combination of state and federal resources.

3018 Protection & Advocacy Agency System
320 W 25th Street
Cheyenne, WY 82001
307-632-3496
FAX 307-638-0815
http://www.wypanda.vcn.com
e-mail: wypanda@vcn.com
Jeanne Thobro, Executive Director

3019 State Department of Education
2300 Capitol Avenue
Cheyenne, WY 82002
307-777-7690
FAX 307-777-6234
http://www.k12.wy.us
Dr Jim McBride, Superintendent

3020 State GED Administration
State Department of Education
2300 Capitol Avenue
Cheyenne, WY 82002
307-777-7363
FAX 307-777-6234
http://www.k12.wy.us
e-mail: nshels@educ.state.wy.us
Trent Blankensh MD, Superintendent
Nance Shelsta, Director for Special Education
Debbie Holdridge, Manager
Promotes quality adult education.

3021 Woming Dpeartment of Workforce Services
1510 E Pershing Boulevard
Cheyenne, WY 82002
307-777-3700
FAX 307-777-5870
http://www.wydoe.state.wy.us
Joan Evans, Director
Tony Moralles, Administration Administrator

Employment training for persons working in Wyoming.

National Programs

3022 Academic Institute
O'Shaughnessy & Associates
13400 NE 20th Street
Bellevue, WA 98005
425-401-6844
FAX 425-401-6323
http://www.academicinstitute.com
e-mail: sherrill@academicinstitute.com
Sherrill O'Shaughnessy, Director

Advising families and teens who have special needs.

3023 Adaptive Environments
Adaptive Environments
374 Congress Street
Boston, MA 02210
617-695-1225
800-949-4232
FAX 617-482-8099
TDY:617-695-1225
http://www.adaptiveenvironments.org
e-mail: info@adaptiveenvironments.org
Valerie Fletcher, Executive Director
Andy Washburn, Information Specialist

Adaptive Environments promotes design that works for everyone across the spectrum of ability and age and enhances human experience.

3024 American Association for Adult and Continuing Education
4380 Forbes Boulevard
Lanham, MD 20706
301-918-1913
FAX 301-459-6241
http://www.aaace.org
e-mail: aaace10@aol.com
Marjean Buckner, President
Cle Anderson, Association Manager

Mission is to provide leadership for the field of adult and continuing education: by expanding opportunities for adult growth and development; unifying adult educators; fostering the development and dissemination of theory, research, information and best practices; promoting identity and standards for the profession; and advocating relevant public policy and social change initiatives.

3025 American Literacy Council
148 W 117th Street
New York, NY 10026
212-663-4200
800-781-9985
http://www.americanliteracy.com
e-mail: support@americanliteracy.com
Edward Lias M.D., President

Provides resources and assistance to persons and organizations who are involved in the literacy crisis in America. The organization provides software and publications that seek to promote solutions to the problem of illiteracy in English speaking countries. One primary product of the Council is Sound-Write (TM), a Windows-based writing program with instant audiovisual feedback and a 25,000 word vocabulary.

3026 Association of Educational Therapists
100 Bush Street
San Francisco, CA 94104
415-982-2389
800-286-4267
FAX 415-982-9204
http://www.aetonline.org
e-mail: aet@aetonline.org
Tiffany Goeman, President

A national professional organization dedicated to establishing ethical professional standards, defining the roles and responsibilities of the educational therapist, providing opportunities for professional growth, and to studying techniques and technologies, philosophies and research related to the practice of educational therapy.

3027 Association on Higher Education and Disability
PO Box 540666
Waltham, MA 02454
781-788-0003
FAX 781-788-0033
http://www.AHEAD.org
e-mail: AHEAD@ahead.org
Stephan Smith, Executive Director
Richard Allegra, Assistant Executive

An international, muiticultural organization of professionals committed to full participation in higher education for persons with disabilities. The Association is a vital resource, promoting excellence through education, communication and training.

3028 Career College Association (CCA)
10 G Street NE
Washington, DC 20002
202-336-6700
FAX 202-336-6828
http://www.career.org
e-mail: cca@career.org
Nick Glakas, President

Represents more than 1,000 private for profit post secondary schools, institutes, colleges and universities.

3029 Center for the Improvement of Early Reading Achievement CIERA
University of Michigan School of Education
610 E University Avenue
Ann Arbor, MI 48109
734-647-6940
FAX 734-615-4858
http://www.ciera.org
e-mail: ciera@umich.edu
Karen Wixson, Director
Joanne Carlisle, Co Director

CIERA is a national center for research on early reading, representing a consortium of educators from five universities.

3030 Council for Educational Diagnostic Services
Council for Exceptional Children
1110 N Glebe Road
Arlington, VA 22201
703-245-0600
888-232-7733
FAX 703-264-9494
http://www.cec.sped.org
e-mail: cathym@cec.sped.org
Bruce Ramirez, Manager

The mission of the Council for Educational Diagnostic Services is: to promote the most appropriate education of children and youth through appraisal, diagnosis, educational intervention, implementation, and continuous evaluation of a prescribed educational program.

3031 Distance Education and Training Council (DETC)
1601 18th Street NW
Washington, DC 20009
202-234-5100
FAX 202-332-1386
http://www.detc.org
e-mail: detc@detc.org
Michael Lambert, Executive Director

Nonprofit educational association located in Washington, DC. DETC serves as a clearinghouse of information about the distance study/correspondence field and sponsors a nationally recognized accrediting agency called the Accrediting Commission of the Distance Education and Training Council.

3032 Division for Children's Communication Development
Council for Exceptional Children
1110 N Glebe Road
Arlington, VA 22201
703-245-0600
888-232-7733
FAX 703-264-9494
http://www.cec.sped.org
e-mail: service@cec.sped.org
Bruce Ramirez, Manager

Dedicated to improving the education of children with communication delays and disorders and hearing loss. Members include professionals serving individuals with hearing, speech and language disorders in the areas of receptive and expressive, verbal and nonverbal spoken, written and sign communication. Members receive a quarterly journal and newsletter three times a year.

3033 Division for Culturally and Linguistically Diverse Learners
Council for Exceptional Children
1110 N Glebe Road
Arlington, VA 22201
703-245-0600
888-232-7733
FAX 703-620-2521
http://www.cec.sped.org

Bruce Ramirez, Manager

Dedicated to advancing and improving educational opportunities for culturally and linguistically diverse learners with disabilites and/or who are gifted, their families and the professionals who serve them.

3034 Division for Research
Council for Exceptional Children
1110 N Glebe Road
Arlington, VA 22201
703-245-0600
888-232-7733
FAX 703-264-9494
http://www.cec.sped.org
e-mail: cathym@cec.sped.org

Bruce Ramirez, Manager

Devoted to the advancement of research related to the education of individuals with disabilities and/or who are gifted. Members include university, public and private school teachers, researchers, administrators, psychologists, speech/language clinicians, parents of children with special learning needs and other related professionals and service personnel. Members receive quarterly journal and newsletter three times a year.

3035 Educational Advisory Group
2222 E Lake Avenue E
Seattle, WA 98102
206-323-1838
FAX 206-267-1325
http://www.eduadvisory.com

Yvonne Jones, Owner
Paul Auchterlonie, Associate

Specializes in matching children with the learning environments that are best for them and works with families to help them identify concerns and establish priorities about their child's education.

3036 HEATH Resource Center: The George Washington University
2134 G Street NW
Washington, DC 20052
202-973-0904
http://www.heath.gwu.edu
e-mail: askheath@heath.gwu.edu

Donna Martinez, Director

An online clearinghouse on postsecondary education for individuals with disabilities. The HEATH Resource Center Clearinghouse has information for students with disabilities on educational disability support services, policies, procedures, adaptions, accessing college or univeristy campuses, career-technical schools, and other postsecondary training entities.

3037 Institute for Educational Leadership
4455 Court Avenue NW
Washington, DC 20008
202-822-8405
FAX 202-872-4050
http://www.iel.org
e-mail: iel@iel.org

Elizabeth Hale, President
Louise Clarke, Chief Administrator
Martin Blank, Principal

Mission is to improve education and the lives of children and their families through positive and visionary change. Everyday, we face that challenge by bringing together diverse constituencies and empowering leaders with knowledge and applicable ideas.

3038 Institute for the Study of Adult Literacy
Pennsylvania State Univ. College of Education
102 Rackley Building
University Park, PA 16802
814-865-1327
FAX 814-863-6108
http://www.ed.psu.edu/isal
e-mail: isal@psu.edu

Barbara Van Horn, Co-Director
Prins Co-Director, Co-Director
Sanford Thatcher, Executive Director

The Institute for the Study of Adult Literacy's goals include development and dissemination of sound conceptual and research base in the field of adult literacy; improvement of practice in the field of adult literacy; and leadership and coordination of a comprehensive approach to the delivery of adult literacy.

3039 International Dyslexia Association: National Headquarters
8600 Lasalle Road
Baltimore, MD 21286
410-296-0232
800-223-3123
FAX 410-321-5069
http://www.interdys.org
e-mail: MBIDA4@hotmail.com

Cathy Rosemond, President
Tom Biall, Director

Nonprofit, scientific and educational organization dedicated to the study and treatment of dyslexia. Focus is educating parents, teachers and professionals in the field of dyslexia in effective teaching methodologies. Programs and services include: information and referral; public awareness; medical and educational research; governmental affairs; conferences and publications.

3040 International Reading Association
PO Box 8139
Newark, DE 19714
302-731-1600
800-336-7323
FAX 302-737-0878
http://www.reading.org
e-mail: pubinfo@reading.org

Alan Farstrup, Executive Director
Mark Mullen, Assistant Director

A professional association with more than 80,000 members in nearly 100 countries dedicated to promoting higher achievement levels in literacy, reading and communications worldwide.

3041 Learning Resource Network
1130 Hostetler Drive
Manhattan, KS 66502
785-539-5376
800-678-5376
FAX 785-426-9558
http://www.lern.org
e-mail: info@lern.org

William Draves, President
Greg Marcelo, Coordinator
Rebel Rush, Executive Director

This network for educators provides resources to adult education and adult basic education service providers.

3042 Literacy Volunteers of America
Pro-Literacy Worldwide
1320 Jamesville Avenue
Syracuse, NY 13210
315-422-9121
888-528-2224
FAX 315-422-6369
http://www.proliteracy.org
e-mail: info@proliteracy.org

Robert Wedgeworth, President

Literacy Volunteers of America is a fully integrated national network of local, state, and regional literacy providers that give adults and their families the opportunity to acquire skills to be effective in their roles as members of their families, communities, and workplaces.

3043 National Adult Education Professional Development Consortium
444 N Capitol Street NW
Washington, DC 20001
202-624-5250
FAX 202-624-1497
http://www.naepdc.org

Lennox McLenoon, Executive Director

The Consortium, incorporated in 1990 by state adult education directors, provides professional development, policy analysis, and dissemination of information important to state staff in adult education.

3044 National Adult Literacy & Learning Disabilities Center (NALLD)
Academy for Educational Development
1825 Connecticut Avenue NW
Washington, DC 20009
202-884-8700
FAX 202-884-8400
http://www.aed.org
e-mail: admindc@aed.org

Stephen Mosley, President
Edward Russell, Chairman
Bill Smith, Vice President

The center is a national resource for information on learning disabilities in adults and on the relationship between learning disabilities and low-level literacy skills.

3045 National Association for Adults with Special Learning Needs
PO Box 716
Bryn Mawr, PA 19010
610-525-8336
888-562-2756
http://www.naasln.org

Joan Hudson-Miller, President

A nonprofit organization designed to organize, establish, and promote an effective national and international coalition of professionals, advocates, and consumers of lifelong learning for the purpose of educating adults with special learning needs.

3046 National Association of Private Special Education Centers
NAPSEC
1522 K Street NW
Washington, DC 20005
202-408-3338
FAX 202-408-3340
http://www.napsec.com
e-mail: napsec@aol.com

Sherry Kolbe, Executive Director
Alison Figi, Communications Coordinator
Rice President, President

A nonprofit association whose mission is to ensure access for individuals to private special education as a vital component of the continuum of appropriate placement and services in American education. The association consists solely of private special education schools that serve both privately and publicly placed children with disabilities.

3047 National Center for ESL Literacy
4646 40th Street NW
Washington, DC 20016
202-362-0700

Donna Christian, President

3048 National Center for Family Literacy
325 W Main Street
Louisville, KY 40202
502-584-1133
FAX 502-584-0172
http://www.famlit.org
e-mail: ncfl@famlit.org

Sharon Darling, President
Ken Middleton, Vice President

Provides leadership for family literacy development nationwide; promotes policies at the national and state level to support family literacy; designs, develops and demostrates new family literacy practices that addresses the need of families in a changing social, economic and political landscape; delivers high quality, dynamic, research-based training, staff development and technical assistance; conducts research to expand the knowledge base of family literacy.

3049 National Center for Learning Disabilities (NCLD)
National Center for Learning Disabilities
381 Park Avenue S
New York, NY 10016
212-545-7510
888-575-7373
FAX 212-545-9665
http://www.ncld.org
e-mail: help@ncld.org

Fredrick Poses, Chairman of the Board
James Wendorf, Executive Director
Marcia Griffith, Marketing Executive

Increases opportunities for all individuals with learning disabilities to achive their potential. NCLD accomplishes its mission by increasing public awareness and understanding of learning disabilities, conducting educational programs and services that promote research-based knowledge, and providing national leadership in shaping public policy. Provides solutions that help people with LD participate fully in society.

3050 National Center for the Study of Adult Learning & Literacy
Harvard Graduate School of Education
7 Appian Way
Cambridge, MA 02138
617-495-5828
FAX 617-495-4811
http://www.gse.harvard.edu
e-mail: ncsall@gse.harvard.edu

John P Comings MD, Director
Elizabeth Molle, Grant Administrator
Dhrue Taneja, Manager

The National Center for the Study of Adult Learning & Literacy both informs and learns from practice. Its rigorous, high quality research increases knowledge and gives those teaching, managing, and setting policy in adult literacy education a sound basis for making decisions.

3051 National Center on Adult Literacy (NCAL)
University of Pennsylvania
3910 Chestnut Street
Philadelphia, PA 19104
215-898-1548
FAX 215-898-9804
http://www.literacyonline.org
e-mail: editor@literacy.upenn.edu

Daniel A Wagner MD, Director
Denise Smiyth, Fiscal Coordinator

NCAL's mission incorporates three primary goals: to improve understanding of youth and adult learning; to foster innovation and increase effectiveness in youth and adult basic education and literacy work; and to expand access to information and build capacity for literacy and basic skills service.

3052 National Education Association (NEA)
1201 16th Street NW
Washington, DC 20036
202-833-4000
FAX 202-822-7974
http://www.nea.org

Reg Weaver, President
John Wilson, CEO

NEA is a volunteer-based organization supported by a network of staff at the local, state and national level. At the local level, NEA affiliates are active in a wide variety of activities, everything from conducting professional workshops on discipline and other issues that affect faculty and school support staff to bargaining contracts for school district employees. At the state level, NEA affiliate activities are equally wide-ranging.

3053 National Institute for Literacy (NIFL)
1775 I Street NW
Washington, DC 20006
202-233-2025
FAX 202-233-2050
TDY:877-576-7734
http://www.nifl.gov
e-mail: sbaxter@nifl.gov

Sandra Baxter, Manager
Steve Langley, Staff Assistant

NIFL's mission is to ensure that the highest quality of literacy services is available to adults. By fostering communication, collaboration, and innovation, NIFL works to build and strengthen a comprehensive, unified system for literacy in the US. NIFL maintains a database of over 7,000 literacy programs across the country and operates a hotline seven days a week.

3054 **National Lekotek Center**
3204 W Armitage Avenue
Chicago, IL 60647
773-276-5164
800-366-7529
FAX 773-276-8644
http://www.lekotek.org
e-mail: lekotek@lekotek.org
Dianna Nielander, Executive Director

The mission of the National Lekotek Center is driven by the philosophy that children learn best when play is a family-centered activity that includes all children, regardless of their abilities or disabilities, in family and community activities. We offer play-centered services to children with disabilities and supportive services to their families. We also offer computer play, parent support and national resources for families and professionals.

3055 **Office of Special Education Programs**
US Department of Education
330 C Street SW
Washington, DC 20202
202-208-5815
http://www.ed.gov/osers/osep/
Alex Posny, Director
John Sherrod, Executive Director

Administers programs and projects relating to the free appropriate public education of all children and young adults with disabilities, from birth through age 21; provides information and publications about disabilities and special education.

3056 **Reach for Learning**
1221 Marin Avenue
Albany, CA 94706
510-524-6455
FAX 510-524-5154
Corinne Gustafson, Executive Director

Educational center providing diagnosis, instruction, consultation for children, youth, adults with learning disabilities or under achievement.

3057 **Thinking and Learning Connection**
239 Whitclem Court
Palo Alto, CA 94306
650-493-3497
FAX 650-494-3499
http://www.php.com
Lynne Stietzel, Co-Director
Eric Stietzel, Co-Director

A group of independent associates committed to teaching students to learn new paths of knowledge and understanding. Our primary focus is working with dyslexic and dyscalculia. Individualized educational programs utilize extensive multisensory approaches to teach reading, spelling, handwriting, composition, comprehension, and mathematics. The students are actively involved in learning processes that integrate visual, auditory, and tactile techniques.

Alabama

3058 **Alabama Commission on Higher Education**
PO Box 302000
Montgomery, AL 36130
334-242-1998
FAX 334-242-0268
http://www.ache.state.al.us
e-mail: tvick@ache.state.al.us
Michael Malone, Executive Director
Tim Vick, Associate Executive Director
Deborah Nettles, Administrative Assistant
The Commission on Higher Education has the statutory responsibility for the overall statewide planning and coordination of higher education in Alabama, the administration of various student aid programs and the performance of designated regulatory functions.

3059 **North Baldwin Literacy Council**
PO Box 144
Bay Minette, AL 36507
251-937-1112
e-mail: nblc144@hotmail.com
Marilyn Waters, Contact

3060 **Northwest Alabama Reading Aides**
PO Box 391
Florence, AL 35631
256-766-5709
e-mail: litnara@aol.com
Anne Jackson, Contact

3061 **PLUS Tuscaloosa**
Box 179
Tuscaloosa, AL 35405
205-391-2671
e-mail: julia.chancy@sheltonstate.edu
Fran Turner, Contact

3062 **South Baldwin Literacy Council**
PO Box 1973
Foley, AL 36536
251-943-7323
FAX 251-970-3578
http://www.baldwinliteracy.com
e-mail: literacy@gulftel.com
Lynda Folks, Coordinator

Organization with an extensive library of supplementary audio, video and written materials for use by tutors and learners. Also publishes and illustrated version of the Alabama Driver's Manual for low-level readers, which is accompanied by an audio tape. Also, comes with a computer lab with a variety of software that is available for use by learners and their tutors.

3063 **The Literacy Council**
2301 First Avenue N
Birmingham, AL 35203
205-326-1925
888-448-7323
FAX 205-326-0538
http://www.literacy-council.org
e-mail: info@literacy-council.org
Jackie Wuska, Executive Director
Hannum Provider Services Memb, Provider Services Manager
Wheat Helpline Services Mana, Helpline Services Manager
Mission is to strengthen and support organizations that provide literacy services in Central Alabama.

3064 **Wallace State Community College Adult Education**
5565 Montgomery Highway
Dothan, AL 36303
334-983-2282
http://www.wallace.edu
e-mail: livey@wallace.edu
Lynn Ivey, Supervisor
Barefield Coordinator, Coordinator

Dedicated to preparing adults for a better future. Classes are free and each class is individualized and self-paced, and are available to anyone age 16 and over and no longer enrolled in school.

Alaska

3065 **Alaska Adult Basic Education**
SERRC
210 Ferry Way
Juneau, AK 99801
907-586-6806
FAX 907-463-3811
http://www.serrc.org
e-mail: info@serrc.org
Carin Smolin, Manager

The mission of the Adult Basic Education program is to provide instruction in the basic skills of reading, writing, and mathematics to adult learners in order to prepare them for transitioning into the labor market or higher academic or vocational training.

3066 **Alaska Literacy Program**
Nine Star Enterprises
125 W 5th Avenue
Fairbanks, AK 99705
907-279-7827
800-478-7587
FAX 907-279-3299
http://www.ninestar.com
e-mail: amyy@ninestar.com

Arva Carlson, Literacy Contact

Evaluates student needs and addresses those needs through specialized lesson plans, private tutoring and personal attention.

3067 Anchorage Literacy Project
1345 Rudakof Circle
Anchorage, AK 99508
907-338-8486
FAX 907-338-3105
http://http://anchorageliteracyproject.org
e-mail: alp@alaska.com
Steve Ponto, President
Smith Executive Director, Executive Director

Dedicated to improving the lives of adults and their families by helping to build their literacy skills. Offer direct literacy skills for adults-native born citizens and recent immigrants alike-through on-site classes and one-on-one tutoring.

3068 Arkansas Adult Basic Education
SERRC
210 Ferry Way
Juneau, AK 99801
907-586-5718
FAX 907-586-5971
e-mail: carins@serrc.org
Carin Smolin, Manager

The mission of the Adult Basic Education program is to provide instruction in the basic skills of reading, writing, and mathematics to adult learners in order to prepare them for transitioning into the labor market or higher academic or vocational training.

3069 Literacy Council of Alaska
Pro Literacy America
823 3rd Avenue
Fairbanks, AK 99701
907-456-6212
FAX 907-456-4302
http://www.literacycouncilofalaska.org
e-mail: lca@literacycouncilofalaska.org
Mike Donaldson, Executive Director

The Literacy Council of Alaska is a private, nonprofit educational agency. Our mission is to promote literacy for people of all ages in Fairbanks and the interior.

Arizona

3070 Adult Education Division of the Arizona Department of Education
1535 W Jefferson Street
Phoenix, AZ 85007
602-271-0945
800-352-4558
FAX 602-258-4986
http://www.ade.az.gov/adult-ed
e-mail: kliersc@ade.az.gov
Tom Horne, Superintendent
Wilda Theobald, Manager for Adult Education
Robert Horne, Manager
To ensure that learners 16 years of age and older have access to quality educational opportunities that will support them in their employment, job training, assist them in acquiring the knowledge and skills necessary for effective participation in society.

3071 American Evangelican Lutheran Church
1985 Scott Drive
Prescott, AZ 86301
928-445-4348
FAX 928-445-8343
http://www.americanlutheran.net
Evelyn Rappath, Contact

3072 Chandler Public Library Adult Basic Education
MS 601 PO Box 4008
Chandler, AZ 85244
480-782-2810
http://www.chandlerlibrary.org/core.htm
e-mail: marybeth.gardner@chandleraz.gov
Mary Beth Gardner, Contact

Provides adult basic education classes for learners who need to improve their basic skills in reading, writing, and math. Gives GED preparation classes to help students prepare to take the GED exam.

3073 Kingman Literacy Council
PO Box 4782
Hualapai, AZ 86412
928-692-7101
e-mail: terchar@npgcable.com
Charlene Haffner, Contact

3074 Lake Havasu Area Literacy Council
PO Box 2186
Lake Havasu, AZ 86405-2186
928-855-3468
e-mail: ralph@affinity4.net
Christine M Lupien, Contact

3075 Literacy Volunteers of America: MaricopaCounty
Literacy Volunteers of Maricopa County
500 E Thomas Road
Phoenix, AZ 85014
602-274-3430
FAX 602-274-5983
http://www.literacyvolunteers-maricopa.org
e-mail: lvmc@lvmc.net
Lynn Reed, Executive Director
Belinda Chron, Administrative Assistant

To ensure that learners 16 years of age and older have access to quality educational opportunities that will support them in their employment, job training, assist them in acquiring the knowledge and skills necessary for effective participation in society.

3076 Literacy Volunteers of America: Santa CruzCounty
Pro Literacy Worldwide
21 E Court Street
Nogales, AZ 85621
520-287-0111
FAX 520-287-0704
e-mail: lruiz@co.santa-cruz.az.us
Lizzette Ruiz, Director
Dora Rayon, Project Coordinator

Literacy Volunteers of America is a national organization with over 1000 chapters teaching adult literacy throughout the United States. The Santa Cruz County Chapter is run out of the Nogales-Santa Cruz County Public Library, and relies on the work of local volunteer tutors and Americorps volunteers.

3077 Literacy Volunteers of Coconino County
715 N Humphreys Street
Flagstaff, AZ 86001-3025
928-556-0313
e-mail: abeck@lvccreads.org
Ann Beck PhD, Contact

3078 Literacy Volunteers of Tucson
1948 E Allen Road
Tucson, AZ 85719
520-882-8006
FAX 520-882-4986
http://www.lovetoread.org
e-mail: info@lovetoread.org
Betty Stauffer, Executive Director
Senders Program Director, Program Director

Recruits, trains and matches tutors with adults (age 16 and up) in need of basic literacy (reading and writing) skills and/or English Language Acquisition for Adults (ELAA). Provide a friendly non-threatning environment that appeals to adult learners in all walks of life.

3079 Mesa Laubach Literacy Council
5136 E Evergreen Street
Mesa, AZ 85205
480-964-3833
e-mail: charleneaunti3@aol.com
Charlene Davidson, Contact

3080 Mohave Literacy Council
PO Box 21921
Bullhead City, AZ 86442
928-704-6539

Marty Cheney, Contact

3081 Prescott Valley Adult Literacy Group
7501 E Civic Circle
Prescott Valley, AZ 86314 928-759-3049
e-mail: jrkdrenner@earthlink.net
Joan Renner, Contact

3082 Southwest Valley Literacy Organization
PO Box 855
Avondale, AZ 85323 623-850-1118
http://www.southwestvalleyliteracy.org
e-mail: info@southwestvalleyliteracy.org
Agnes Franzen, Contact

3083 Yuma Reading Council
825 S Orange Ave
Yuma, AZ 85364 928-343-9363
FAX 928-539-1918
http://www.yumalibrary.org/yrc
e-mail: barbaras@firstinter.net
Barbara Sutton, Executive Director
Dannenberg President, President

Provides one to one tutoring for basic literacy and english as a second language, and converstaion classes for beginning, intermediate and advanced levels for English as a second language students.

Arkansas

3084 Arkansas Adult Learning Resource Center
3905 Cooperative Way
Little Rock, AR 72209 501-907-2490
800-832-6242
FAX 501-907-2492
http://www.aalrc.org
e-mail: info@aalrc.org
Marsha Taylor, Manager
Klaus Neu, Media Coordinator

The Arkansas Adult Learning Resource Center was established in 1990 to provide a source for identification, evaluation, and dissemination of materials and information to adult education/literacy programs within the state.

3085 Arkansas Literacy Council: ProLiteracy America
Arkansas Literacy Council
4942 W Markham Street
Little Rock, AR 72205 501-663-4321
800-264-7323
FAX 501-663-3041
http://www.arkansasliteracy.org
e-mail: marie@arkansasliteracy.org
Marie Bruno, Executive Director
Katie McManners, Director Development

Arkansas Literacy Council is a statewide 501 (c) (3) nonprofit agency on supporting local literacy councils that use trained volunteers to help adults improve reading skills.

3086 Carroll County Literacy Council
PO Box 740
Berryville, AR 72616 870-423-4500
e-mail: litbvar@hbeark.com
Ethel J Meyer, Contact

3087 Community Literacy Council
PO Box 1382
Mt Ida, AR 71957 870-867-2602
e-mail: communityliteracycouncil@yahoo.com
Tinas Geller, Contact

3088 Crawford County Literacy Council
513 Main Street
Van Buren, AR 72956 479-474-4594
e-mail: ccvl@mynewroads.com
Anita James, Contact

3089 Drew County Literacy Council
PO Box 534
Monticello, AR 71655-0534 870-367-7007
e-mail: mkjarrett71655@yahoo.com
Margaret Jarrett, Director

Formed by citizens that were concerned about the adult illiteracy rate reported in the 1980 census. Strives to recruit, train and match volunteer tutors with illiterate adults in the county using The Laubach Way to Reading and Laubach Way to English.

3090 Dumas Literacy Council
PO Box 364
Dumas, AR 71639 870-382-4983
FAX 870-382-6786
e-mail: daec@centurytel.net
Flora Simon, Contact

3091 Eastern Arkansas Literacy Project
East Arkansas Community College
1700 Newcastle Road
Forrest City, AR 72335 870-633-4480
e-mail: mriley@eacc.edu
Mary Ella Ray, Contact

3092 Faulkner County Literacy Council
PO Box 2106
Conway, AR 72033 501-329-7323
FAX 501-329-2018
e-mail: fclc@conwaycorp.net
Christine Rega, Contact

3093 Literacy Action of Central Arkansas
PO Box 900
Little Rock, AR 72203-0900 501-372-7323
e-mail: literacy@cals.lib.ar.us
Kathy Gattinger, Contact

3094 Literacy Council of Arkansas County
PO Box 94
Stuttgart, AR 72160 870-673-4551
e-mail: litarco@sbcglobal.net
Eddye Kay Hansen, Contact

3095 Literacy Council of Benton County
1140 N Walton Boulevard
Bentonville, AR 72712-0372 479-273-3486
e-mail: readlcbc@sbcglobal.net
Vicki Ronald, Contact

3096 Literacy Council of Crittenden County
Mid-South Community College
2000 W Broadway
West Memphis, AR 72301 870-733-6763
http://www.midsouthcc.edu
e-mail: bschultz@midsouthcc.edu
Bill Schultz, Contact

3097 Literacy Council of Garland County
119 Hobson Street
Hot Springs, AR 71901 501-624-7323
e-mail: lcgc@sbcglobal.net
Pat McClaren, Contact

3098 Literacy Council of Grant County
1685 Highwy 270 E
Sheridan, AR 72150-0432 870-942-5711
e-mail: literacy@alltel.net
Mary Frances Harper, Contact

3099 Literacy Council of Hot Spring County
PO Box 1485
Malvern, AR 72104 501-332-4039
e-mail: readhelp#sbcglobal.net
Jane Goodwin, Contact

Offers a variety of educational services at no charge that range from literacy for adults to peer-tutoring for children; English as a second language to Learning Differences screening.

3100 Literacy Council of Jefferson County
402 E 5th Street
Pine Bluff, AR 71601 870-536-7323
e-mail: literacy@cablelynx.com
Jennifer Hurst, Contact

3101 Literacy Council of Monroe County
234 W Cedar
Brinkley, AR 72021 870-734-3333
e-mail: folsom@futura.net
Martha Pineda, Contact

3102 Literacy Council of North Central Arkansas
PO Box 187
Leslie, AR 72645 870-447-3241
e-mail: catwoman26@excite.com
Susan Vorwald, Contact

3103 Literacy Council of St Francis County
1700 Newcastle Road
Forrest City, AR 72335 501-633-4480
Ann Harbin, Contact

3104 Literacy Council of Union County
2800 N College Avenue
El Dorado, AR 71730-5842 870-864-0101
e-mail: lcuc@cox-internet.com
Paula H Cotton, Contact

3105 Literacy Council of Western Arkansas
PO Box 423
Fort Smith, AR 72902-0423 479-783-2665
e-mail: helptoread@sbcglobal.net
Bruce A Singleton, Contact

3106 Literacy Council of White County
119 E Center
Searcy, AR 72143 501-279-2870
e-mail: acvneato@sbcglobal.net
Ann C Nieto, Contact

3107 Literacy League of Craighead County
301 S Main Street
Jonesboro, AR 72401 870-910-6511
877-910-6511
FAX 870-910-0552
e-mail: llcc@newsources.net
Thomas Templeton, Executive Director

Offering information and resources on literacy throughout the area.

3108 Little Red Literacy Council
102 E Main Street
Herber Springs, AR 72543 501-362-0640
e-mail: ucanread@arkansas.net
Sha;Ah Slayton, Contact

3109 Lonoke County Literacy Council
Box 234
Lonoke, AR 72086 501-676-7478
e-mail: lonokeliteracy@sbcglobal.net
Maria Turner, Contact

3110 Mississippi County Literacy Council
PO Box 682
Blytheville, AR 72316 870-763-0032
e-mail: lovieden@yahoo.com
Denise Hester, Contact

3111 Ozark Literacy Council
2596 N Keystone Crossing
Fayetteville, AR 72703 479-521-8250
FAX 479-582-0846
http://www.ozarkliteracy.org
e-mail: ozarklc@swbell.net
Jim Allen, Executive Director
Humphrey Director Program Devel, Director Program Development

Provides a quality literacy environment which enables individuals to learn the skills necessary for them to become contributing members of society and meet the challenges of an ever-changing world.

3112 Pope County Literacy Council
PO Box 1276
Russellville, AR 72811 479-967-7323
e-mail: popecoliteracy@tyler.net
Jennifer Benham, Contact

3113 Sharp County Literacy Council
PO Box 63
Cherokee Village, AR 72525 870-856-3038
e-mail: sclcread@centurytel.net
Amy Buckingham, Contact

3114 Southwest Arkansas Development Council
PO Box 574
Hope, AR 71802-0574 870-777-8892
e-mail: swadc@sbcglobal.net
Kristen Ambercrombie, Contact

3115 St. John's ESL Program
583 W Grand
Hot Springs, AR 71901 501-624-3171
e-mail: mermerlee@sbcglobal.net
Merlin Lee, Contact

3116 Twin Lakes Literacy Council
1322 Bradley Drive #7
Mountain Home, AR 72653 870-425-7323
e-mail: twinlakeslc@cox-internet.com
Nancy Tester, Contact

3117 Van Buren County Literacy Council
PO Box 897
Clinton, AR 72031 501-745-6440
e-mail: charlie@hypertech.net
Stella Sample, Contact

California

3118 Butte County Library Adult Reading Program
1820 Mitchell Avenue
Oroville, CA 95966
530-538-7525
FAX 530-538-7235
http://www.buttecounty.net/bclibrary/literacy.h
e-mail: literacy@buttecounty.net
Nancy Brower, Executive Director
Jean Lewis, Administrative Assistant

Tutoring at no charge in reading, writing and math. Participants will learn the basics and more with one-on-one tutoring. A volunteer tutor will meet with participants at any branch library in Butte County.

3119 California Association of Special Education & Services
CASES Executive Office
1722 J Street
Sacramento, CA 95814
916-447-7061
FAX 916-447-1320
http://www.capses.com
e-mail: info@capses.com
Janeth Serrano, Manager
Rita Celaya, Executive Administrative Assista

The purposes are to serve as a liaison between the public and private sectors and to lend support for a continuum of programs and objectives which improve the delivery of services provided to the exceptional individual.

3120 California Department of Education
Office of the Secretary for Education
1121 L Street
Sacramento, CA 95814
916-323-0611
http://www.ose.ca.gov
Jack O'Connell, Superintendent
Judy Tracy, Legislative Assistant

The Office of the Secretary for Education is responsible for advising and making policy recommendations to the Governor on education issues.

3121 California Literacy
PO Box 70916
Pasadena, CA 91117
626-395-9989
FAX 626-356-9327
http://www.caliteracy.org
e-mail: office@caliteracy.org
Lisa Bennett-Garrison, Interim Executive Director
Archana Carey, Operations Director

California Literacy was founded in 1956 and is the nation's oldest and largest statewide adult volunteer literacy organization. Its purpose is to establish literacy programs and to support them through tutor training, consulting, and ongoing education.

3122 Lake County Literacy Coalition
Pro Literacy Worldwide
1425 N High Street
Lakeport, CA 95453
707-263-7633
FAX 707-263-6796
http://www.co.lake.ca.us
e-mail: dianaf@co.lake.ca.us
Sookie Duncan, Administrative Assistant

We provide free, basic literacy instruction to adult learners through confidential one-on-one study sessions that are geared to what the student wants to learn.

3123 Literacy Program: County of Los Angeles Public Library
7400 Imperial Highway
Downey, CA 90242
562-940-8511
http://www.colapublib.org
e-mail: hilda@colapl.org
Margaret Donnellan, Librarian
Barbara Hirsch, Contact

The Literacy Centers of the County of Los Angeles Public Library offer a variety of literacy services for adults and families at no charge. Literacy services include one-to-one basic literacy tutoring, English as a Second Language group instruction, Family Literacy and self-help instruction on audio cassettes, videocassettes and computer-based training. The literacy program is an affiliate of Literacy Volunteers of America, Inc.

3124 Literacy Volunteers of America: ImperialValley
Pro Literacy Worldwide
2695 S 4th Street
El Centro, CA 92243
760-352-8541
FAX 760-352-7812
e-mail: lva_ivy@icoet.org
Norma Gomez, Director
MonaLisa Castleberry, Office Manager

Literacy Volunteers of America is affiliated with ProLiteracy of America and provides the opportunity to acquire skills to be effective in their roles as members of their families, communities and workplaces.

3125 Literacy Volunteers of America: WillitsPublic Library
390 E Commercial Street
Willits, CA 95490
707-459-5098
http://www.mendolibrary.org/willits
e-mail: lvawillits@pacific.net
Donna Kerr, Branch Librarian
Pamela Shilling, Contact

The Literacy program offers one-on-one reading, writing and tutoring for adults in the area.

3126 Marin Literacy Program
San Rafael Public Library
1100 E Street
San Rafael, CA 94901
415-485-3323
FAX 415-485-3112
http://www.marinliteracy.org
e-mail: marinliteracy@marinliteracy.org
Barbara Barwood, Director
Martha Haidet, Project Coordinator
David Dodd, Executive Director
The Marin Literacy Program offers reading, writing and English conversation through professionally trained volunteers to Marin County adults who skills are too low to be helped by other services in the county.

3127 Merced Adult School
50 E 20th Street
Merced, CA 95340
209-385-6524
FAX 209-385-6430
e-mail: croberds@muhsd.k12.ca.us
Carol Roberds, Principal

To empower and educate our adult students to discover their own unique, productive place in our dynamic world and encourage them to be lifelong learners.

3128 Metropolitan Adult Education Program
760 Hillsdale Avenue
San Jose, CA 95136
408-723-6400
http://www.metroed.net
e-mail: jmondo@metroed.net
Timothy Hallett, Administrator
Nancy Arnold, Principal

MetroED is the largest career-oriented educational organization in Santa Clara County. We provide vocational and adult education programs for the high school students and adults in their geographic areas.

3129 Mid City Adult Learning Center
Belmont Community Adult School
1510 Cambria Street
Los Angeles, CA 90017
213-483-8689
FAX 213-413-1356
e-mail: midcity@otan.dni.us
Barbara Menke, Manager
Helen Menke, Coordinator
Judy Griffin, Regional Center Manager
Provides adult education on ESL, basic reading, language and literacy programs.

3130 Newport Beach Public Library LiteracyServices
1000 Avocado Avenue
Newport Beach, CA 92660 949-717-3800
http://www.citynewportbeachlibrary.org
e-mail: literacy@city.newport-beach.ca.us
Linda Katsouleas, Executive Director
Sheila Tierney, Program Assistant
Diane Moseley, Program Coordinator
The mission of the Literacy Services Program is to help English-speaking adults improve their reading and writing skills.

3131 Pomona Public Library Literacy Services
Pro Literacy Worldwide
PO Box 2271
Pomona, CA 91769 909-620-2035
FAX 909-620-3713
TDY:909-620-3690
http://www.youseemore.com/pomona
e-mail: library@ci.pomona.ca.us
Muriel Spill, Library Director
Verna English, Administrative Assistant

The Pomona Literacy Service provides free adult literacy services to the City of Pomona. Volunteers provide tutorial programs to adults (16 years and older) who do not have basic literacy skills or whose literacy skills are so limited that they are not able to function independently in daily life or acquire employment or higher education.

3132 Recording for the Blind & Dyslexic: Los Angeles
5022 Hollywood Boulevard
Los Angeles, CA 90027 323-664-5525
800-732-8398
FAX 323-664-1881
http://www.rfbda.org/LA
e-mail: los_angeles@rfbda.org
Carol Smith, Executive Director
Stacey Eubank, Outreach Director

A national, nonprofit organization providing recorded textbooks, library services and other educational materials to students who cannot read standard print because of a visual, physical or learning disability. $50.00 registration fee and a $25.00 annual renewal fee. No fee for students whose schools are members.

3133 Recording for the Blind & Dyslexic: Northern California Unit
488 W Charleston Road
Palo Alto, CA 94306 650-493-3717
866-493-3717
FAX 650-493-5513
http://www.rfbd.org
Matt Ward, Production Director
Vallie Brown, Educational Outreach Director
Lynne Van Tilburg, Development Director
A national network of thirty three studios with headquarters in Princeton, NJ. The sole purpose is to provide educational materials in recorded and computerized formats at every academic level. The materials are for all people unable to read standard print because of a visual, perceptual (dyslexia), or other physical disability.

3134 Recording for the Blind and Dyslexic: Inland Empire-Orange County Unit
Orange County Studio
2021 E Fourth Street
Santa Ana, CA 92705 714-547-4171
FAX 714-547-4241
http://www.rfbd.org
e-mail: mdavis@rfbd.org
Mike Davis, Executive Director

Volunteers record texts on audio cassettes and computer disks for the visually, physically and perceptually disabled.

3135 Regional Resource Center for San Diego: Imperial Counties
6401 Linda Vista Road
San Diego, CA 92111 858-292-3556
FAX 858-268-9726
TDY:858-571-7273
Richard C Smith, Senior Director
Susan Yamate, Project Administrator

The center assists regional adult education and literacy providers as they work to provide high quality and effective services to adult learners.

3136 Sacramento Public Library Literacy Service
828 I Street
Sacramento, CA 95814 916-966-7323
800-561-4636
FAX 916-264-2755
http://www.saclibrary.org/literacy
e-mail: contact@saclibrary.org
Jackie Miller, Literacy Coordinator
Judith Alvi, Literacy Service Representative
Anne Gold, Executive Director
The Literacy Service is committed to helping adults attain the skills they need to achieve their goals and develop their knowledge and potential. Free one-on-one tutoring is provided to English speaking adults who want to improve their basic reading and writing skills.

3137 Sweetwater State Literacy Regional Resource Center
Adult Resource Center
458 Moss Street
Chula Vista, CA 91911 619-691-5624
FAX 619-425-8728
http://www.literacynet.org/slrc/sweetwater/home
e-mail: hurley@otan.dni.us
Alice Hurley, Regional Manager

The Sweetwater State Literacy Resource Center is located at the Adult and Continuing Education Division of the Sweetwater Union High School District. The Division is the fourth largest adult education program in the State of California, serving over 32,000 adult learners yearly.

3138 Vision Literacy of California
Pro Literacy Worldwide
540 Valley Way
Milpitas, CA 95035 408-262-1349
FAX 408-956-9384
http://www.visionliteracy.org
e-mail: info@visionliteracy.org
Patricia Lawson-North, Manager
Brenda Eitemiller, Associate Manager of Operations

Vision Literacy is dedicated to enriching the community in which we live by helping adults improve their literacy skills.

Colorado

3139 Adult Learning Center
PO Box 710
Ignacio, CO 81137 970-563-0681
e-mail: svisser@adult-learning-inc.com
Susan Visser, Contact

3140 Adult Literacy Program
PO Box 4856
Basalt, CO 81621 970-963-9200
e-mail: julie@englishinaction.org
Julie Fox-Rubin, Contact

3141 Archuleta County Education Center
PO Box 1079
Pagosa Springs, CO 81147-1066 970-264-2835
e-mail: llynch@pagosa.k12.co.us
Livia Cloman Lynch PhD, Contact

3142 Colorado Adult Education and Family Literacy
Colorado Department of Education
201 E Colfax Avenue
Denver, CO 80203 303-698-2121
FAX 303-830-0793
http://www.cde.state.co.us
e-mail: smith p@cde.state.co.us
Pamela Smith, State Director
Laura Reilly, CEO

To assist adults to become literate in English and obtain the knowledge and skills necessary for employment and self-sufficiency.

3143 Durango Adult Education Center
301 E 12th Street
Durango, CO 80488B 970-354-4354
FAX 970-385-7968
http://www.durangoaec.org
e-mail: info@durangoaec.org
Bob Harrington, President
Church Executive Director, Executive Director

Provides educational resources for adults, seniors and youth through fundraising, grants and partnerships with other organizations in order to provide affordable educational services to our community.

3144 Learning Disabilities Association of Colorado
4596 E Iliff Avenue
Denver, CO 80222 303-894-0992
FAX 303-830-1645
http://www.ldacolorado.org
e-mail: info@ldacolorado.com
Tim Carroll, Public Relations

A non-profit volunteer organization dedicated to advocacy and education of learning disabled children and adults.

3145 Literacy Coalition of Jefferson County
10125 W 6th Avenue
Lakewood, CO 80215 303-271-6387
http://www.literacyjeffco.org
e-mail: marcie.hanson@judicial.state.co.us
Slavica Olujic, Chair

The purpose of the organization is to promote and foster increased literacy in Jefferson County, Colorado.

3146 Literacy Volunteers of America: Colorado Literacy Outreach
Pro Literacy Worldwide
413 9th Street
Glenwood Springs, CO 81601 970-945-5282
FAX 970-945-7723
http://www.literacyvolunteers.org/who/states
e-mail: mfred@coloradomtn.edu
Martha Fredendall, Administrator
Bill Crymble, Coordinator

Literacy Volunteers of America is a fully integrated national network of local, state and regional literacy providers that give adults and their families the opportunity to acquire skills to be effective in their roles as members of their families, communities, and workplaces.

3147 Logan County Literacy Coalition
Sterling Public Library
425 N 5th Street
Sterling, CO 80751-2311 970-522-2023
e-mail: ament@sterlingcolo.com
Patty Ament, Contact

3148 The Learning Source
455 S Pierce Street
Lakewood, CO 80226 303-922-4683
FAX 303-742-9929
http://www.coloradoliteracy.org
e-mail: info@coloradoliteracy.org
Susan Lythgoe, Executive Director
Bratt Assistant Director, Pr, Assistant Director, Programs

Provides opportunities for motivated adult learners and families to attain their educational goals through adult and family literacy, GED preparation and English Language instruction.

3149 The Literacy Center
Mesa County Public Library
PO Box 20000-5019
Grand Junction, CO 81502-5019 970-245-5522
e-mail: apfennig@mcpld.org
Christi Williams, Contact

3150 The Literacy Project
PO Box 608
Miniturn, CO 81645 970-949-5026
e-mail: literacy@vail.net
Colleen Gray, Contact

Connecticut

3151 Connecticut Institute for Cultural Literacy and Wellness
60 Connolly Parkway
Hamden, CT 06514 203-248-0255
FAX 203-281-1386
Fredrick Chappelle, Executive Director

Offers adult education and literacy programs, as well as other programs that touch on other aspects of a well-rounded education.

3152 Connecticut Literacy Resource Center
CREC/ATDW
111 Charter Oak Avenue
Hartford, CT 06106 860-525-1556
FAX 860-246-3304
http://www.crec.org/lc/index.shtml
e-mail: atyskiewicz@crec.org
Marcy Slye, Executive Director
Colleen Palmer, Assistant Executive Director

The Literacy Center offers services that foster literacy development from early childhood to adult. Technical assistance and training are available in the following areas: School Readiness; k-12; and Family Literacy.

3153 LEARN: Connecticut Reading Association
44 Hatchetts Hill Road
Old Lyme, CT 06371 860-434-4800
FAX 860-434-4837
http://www.learn.k12.ct.us
e-mail: director@learn.k12.ct.us
Virginia Seccombe, Executive Director

LEARN initiates, supports and provides a wide range of programs and services that enhance the quality and expand the opportunities for learning in the educational community.

3154 Literacy Center of Milford
Fannie Beach Community Center
16 Dixon Street
Milford, CT 06460 203-792-8260
http://www.literacycenterofmilford.com
e-mail: literacyctrofmlfd@juno.com
Joy Stonier, Director

Serves people from other countries who want to learn the English language and it helps people in need of mastering basic reading, writing and math skills. Provides a quality program where people can find the help and support they require o meet their basic literacy needs.

3155 Literacy Volunteers On The Green
62 Bridge Street
New Milford, CT 06776 860-354-0185
e-mail: literacyvolunteersonthegreen@yahoo.com
Guaruglia Maitland, Contact

3156 Literacy Volunteers of America-Danbury
261 Main Street
Danbury, CT 06810-6606 203-792-8260
e-mail: lva-d@snet.net
Tom Pinkham, Contact

3157 Literacy Volunteers of Central Connecticut
20 High Street
New Britian, CT 06051-4226 860-229-7323
http://http://literacycentral.org
e-mail: director@literacycentral.org
Darlene Hurtado, Executive Director
Prairie Associate Director, Associate Director

Provide small group and one-on-one literacy tutoring to over 340 adults with flexible hours, individual attention, student centered learning, and high quality, caring volunteer tutors. Provide free, high quality training to adults who would like to become Literacy Volunteers.

3158 Literacy Volunteers of Eastern Connecticut
106 Truman Street
New London, CT 06320-5632 860-443-4800
http://www.englishhelp.org
e-mail: executivedirector@englishhelp.org
Susan Townsley, Executive Director

Mission is to improve literacy in our community, especially those organizations and civic, social, and religious groups that know first hand how valuable it is for their members or clients to gain increased literacy skills.

3159 Literacy Volunteers of Greater Hartford
30 Arbor Street
Hartford, CT 06106 860-233-3853
http://www.lvgh.org
e-mail: susan.roman@lvgh.org
Carol Hauss, Executive Director
George Demetrion, Outreach Manager

Literacy Volunteers of Greater Hartford has trained volunteers to provide free English literacy instruction to Hartford area adults.

3160 Literacy Volunteers of Greater Middletown
Russell Library
123 Broad Street
Middletown, CT 06457 860-347-0337
e-mail: lvgm@russekk.lioninc.org
Bruce Markot, Contact

3161 Literacy Volunteers of Greater New Haven
580 Ella Grasso Boulevard
New Haven, CT 06519 203-865-3867
FAX 203-562-7833
http://www.lvagnh.org
e-mail: info@lvagnh.org
Janet Ryan, President
Venema Executive Director, Executive Director

Trains, certifies and supports tutors to provide tutoring in basic literacy and english for speakers of other languages.

3162 Literacy Volunteers of Greater Waterbury
267 Grand Street
Waterbury, CT 06702 203-754-1164
e-mail: lva.greater.wby@snet.net
Tina Agati, Executive Director

3163 Literacy Volunteers of Northern Connecticut
Asnuntuck CC B-131
170 Elm Street
Enfield, CT 06082 860-253-3038
e-mail: info@lvanc.com
Brain J Mc Cartney, Executive Director

3164 Literacy Volunteers of Southeastern Fairfield County
177 State Street
Bridgeport, CT 06604 203-579-2208
e-mail: wayvalct@aol.com
Wayne Valaitis, Executive Director

3165 Literacy Volunteers-Stamford/Greenwich
141 Franklin Street
Stamford, CT 06901 203-324-5214
FAX 203-348-8917
e-mail: djr@lvsg.org
Diane Rosenthal, Director
Lawson Volunteer/Outreach Coo, Volunteer/Outreach Coordinator

A community-based organization that utilizes the services of trained volunteers to provide reading, writing and English language instruction to native and foreign born adults who are over the age of 18, out of school and whose literacy abilities make it difficult for them to function independently in society.

3166 Literacy Volunteers-Valley Shore
61 Goodspeed Road
Westbrook, CT 06498-1006 860-399-5428
e-mail: lvvs@snet.net
Mary Ellen Jewett, Executive Director

3167 Mercy Learning Center
637 Park Avenue
Bridgeport, CT 06604 203-334-6699
http://www.mercylearningcenter.org
e-mail: mercy.learning.cntr@snet.net
Jane Ferreira, President
Flinn Volunteer Coordinator, Volunteer Coordinator

Mission is to bring about a positive change to the problem of illiteracy; specifically, to provide basic literacy and life skills training using a 'holistic' approach within a compassionate , supportive community.

3168 Springs Learning Center
115 Blatchley Avenue
New Haven, CT 06513 203-787-1025
e-mail: springs115@aol.com
Sister Maryann Lawlor, Contact

Delaware

3169 Delaware Department of Education: Adult Community Education
Department of Public Instruction
PO Box 1402
Dover, DE 19903 302-739-3340
FAX 302-739-1770
http://www.doe.state.de.us
e-mail: ftracy-mumf@doe.k12.de.us
Fran Mumford, Director Adult Education
Valerie Woodruff, Education Secretary

Provides students with opportunities to develop skills needed to qualify for further education, job training, and better employment.

3170 Literacy Volunteers Serving Adults/Northern Delaware
PO Box 2083
Wilmington, DE 19899-2083 302-658-5624
http://www.wilmlib.org/lva.html
e-mail: litvolunteers@aol.com
Carmen A Knox, Executive Director

Trains volunteers to teach functionally illiterate adults to read, and to teach spoken English to foreigners.

3171 Literacy Volunteers of America: Wilmington Library
PO Box 2083
Wilmington, DE 19899 302-571-7400
http://www.wilmlib.org
e-mail: litvolunteers@aol.com
David Burdash, Executive Director

An organization of volunteers that provide a variety of services locally to enable people to achieve personal goals through literacy programs.

3172 MARK Literacy Center
430 New Castle Avenue
Dover, DE 19901 302-678-4952
e-mail: lynbaybyrd@aol.com
Lynne Baynard, Recruitment/Training Specialist
Showell Executive Director, Executive Director

3173 NEW START Adult Learning Program
Corbit-Calloway Memorial Library
115 High Street
Odessa, DE 19730-9999 302-378-3444
FAX 302-378-7803
http://www.corbitlibrary.org/newstart
e-mail: smenei@juno.com
Susan Menei, Coordinator

Educational organization with a mission to enable adults acquire the listening, speaking, reading, writing, mathematics and technology skills they need to solve problems they encounter in daily life; to take advantage of opportunities in their environment; and to participate in the transformation of their society.

3174 State of Delaware Adult and CommunityEducation Network
PO Box 639
Dover, DE 19903 302-739-5556
FAX 302-739-5565
http://www.acenetwork.org
e-mail: acedir@yahoo.com
Joanne Heaphy, Statewide Management Liaison
Meredith Mumford, Data Specialist

The ACE Network is a service agency that supports adult education and literacy providers through training and resource development.

District of Columbia

3175 Academy of Hope
1501 Columbia Road NW
Washington, DC 20009-4213 202-328-2029
http://www.aohdc.org
Anette Banks, Interim Executive Director
Hilfiker Co-Founder, Instructor, Co-Founder, Instructor

Provides educational empowerment to DC adults. We help students earn high school credentials, improve their math and reading skills, and learn how to use and apply computer technologies.

3176 Carlos Rosario School
1100 Harvard Street NW
Washington, DC 20009 202-797-4700
FAX 202-232-6442
http://www.carlosrosario.org
e-mail: info@carlosrosario.org
Sonia Guitierrez, Executive Director/Founder

Successfully trains and mainstreams the diverse workforce of the ation's capital. Highly qualified teachers and staff consistently provide new challenges, encouraging intensive learning and career development.

3177 District of Columbia Department of Education: Vocational & Adult Education
400 Maryland Avenue SW
Washington, DC 20202 202-842-0973
800-872-5327
FAX 202-205-8748
http://www.ed.gov/offices/OVAE
e-mail: ovae@ed.gov
Tassie Thompson, Manager

To help all people achieve the knowledge and skills to be lifelong learners, to be successful in their chosen careers, and to be effective citizens.

3178 District of Columbia Literacy Resource Center
Martin Luther King Memorial Library
901 G Street NW
Washington, DC 20001 202-727-1101
FAX 202-727-1129
e-mail: marcia_harrington@csgi.com
Francis Buckley Jr., Manager
Marcia Harrington, ABE Specialist

As part of the State Library, the State Resource Center provides electronic and print resources.

3179 District of Columbia Public Schools
825 N Capitol Street NE
Washington, DC 20202 202-842-0973
FAX 202-442-5517
http://www.k12.dc.us
e-mail: callcenter@k12.dc.us
Elfreda Massie MD, Superintendent
Tassie Thompson, Manager

The public school system is committed to constant improvements in the achievement of all students today in preparation for their world tomorrow.

3180 Friendship House Adult Education Program
619 D Street SE
Washington, DC 20003 202-675-9050
e-mail: lrucker@friendshiphouse.net
Lisa Gail Rucker, Contact

3181 Literacy Volunteers of the NationalCapital Area
PO Box 73275
Washington, DC 20056 202-387-1772
FAX 202-588-0724
http://www.lvanca.org
e-mail: dlewis@lvanca.org
Connie Bumbaugh, Executive Director

Literacy Volunteers of the National Capital Area is an affiliate of ProLiteracy Network and provides free tutoring to illiterate adults in the Washington, D.C./National Capital Area.

3182 Metropolitan/Delta Adult Literacy Council
2728 Sherman Avenue NW
Washington, DC 20001-3920 202-234-2665
FAX 202-234-1511
http://http://mdalc.org
e-mail: mdalc@mdalc.org
Artee J Milligan Jr, Contact

Mission is to enable adults, older youths, and families within the Washington D.C. vicinity to solve problems they encounter in their daily lives and to participate in and contribute to their community.

3183 Washington Literacy Council
1918 18th Street NW
Washington, DC 20009 202-387-9029
FAX 202-387-0271
http://www.washingtonliteracycouncil.org
e-mail: info@washlit.org
Elisabeth Liptak, Executive Director
Lubar Program Director, Program Director

Mission is to raise the literacy level of adult nonreaders in the nation's capital, and to be the standard-bearer for adult literacy instruction.

Florida

3184 Adult Literacy League
345 W Michigan Street
Orlando, FL 32806-4465
407-422-1540
FAX 407-422-1529
http://www,adultliteracyleague.org
e-mail: info@adultliteracyleague.org
Joyce Whidden, Contact

Provides free one-to-one & small group literacy instruction; recruits & refers adult learners & volunteers; trains literacy tutors; provides continuing education to tutors & students through mentoring, training, seminars & computer labs; provides scholarships for learning materials & curriculum; deliver family literacy services in partnership with Head Start; provides 'Reach Out & Read' pediatric family literacy service with Community Health Centers & increases public awareness of literacy

3185 Florida Coalition
Florida Literacy Coalition
934 N Magnolia Avenue
Orlando, FL 32803
407-246-7110
800-237-5113
FAX 407-246-7104
http://www.floridaliteracy.org
e-mail: info@floridaliteracy.org
Greg Smith, Executive Director
Kelley Jain, Education & Training Coordinator

A nonprofit organization funded through private and corporate donations, state of Florida grants, and a diverse membership.

3186 Florida Laubach Literacy Action
52 E Main Street
Apopka, FL 32703
407-889-0100
FAX 407-889-5576
Teresa McElwee, President
Sis McElwee, Owner

Laubach Literacy is a nonprofit educational corporation dedicated to helping adults of all ages improve their lives and their communities by learning reading, writing, math and problem solving skills.

3187 Florida Literacy Coalition
934 N Magnolia Avenue
Orlando, FL 32803
407-246-7110
800-237-5113
FAX 407-246-7104
http://www.floridaliteracy.org
e-mail: info@floridaliteracy.org
Greg Smith, Executive Director
Kelley Jain, Education/Training Coordinator

A nonprofit organization funded through private and corporate donations, state of Florida grants, and a diverse membership.

3188 Florida Literacy Resource Center
Adult & Community Educators of Florida
912 S Martin Luther King Jr Blvd
Tallahassee, FL 32301
850-922-5343
FAX 850-922-5352
http://www.ace-leon.org
e-mail: ace@aceofflorida.org
Veronica Sehrt, Project Manager
Barbara Camp, Principal

As part of the State Library, the State Resource Center provides electronic and print resources.

3189 Florida Protection & Advocacy Agency for Persons with Disabilities
2671 W Executive Center Circle
Tallahassee, FL 32301
850-488-9071
800-342-0823
FAX 850-488-8640
TDY:800-346-4127
http://www.advocacycenter.org
e-mail: hubertg@advocacy.org
Hubert Grissom, President
Sandy Evans, Administrative Assistant

Offers help for people with disabilities.

3190 Florida Vocational Rehabilitation Agency: Division of Vocational Rehabilitation
Florida Department of Education
2002 Old Saint Augustine Road
Tallahassee, FL 32301
850-488-6210
FAX 850-921-7217
http://www.rehabworks.org
Bill Palmer, Director
Linda Parnell, Manager
Amanda Grimes, Assistant
A statewide employment resource for businesses and people with disabilities that enables individuals with disabilities to obtain and keep employment.

3191 Learn To Read
2747 Art Museum Drive
Jacksonville, FL 32207
904-399-8894
FAX 904-399-2508
http://www.learntoreadinc.org
e-mail: info@learntoreadinc.org
Heather Corey, Executive Director

Trains and certifies community volunteers to teach reading skills to adults one-on-one or in a small group; offers classes and tutor support to students who are native speakers of other languages; and provides FREE innovative instruction in skills necessary to successfully function in today's society.

3192 Learning Disabilities Association of Florida
331 E Henry Street
Punta Gorda, FL 33950
941-637-8957
FAX 941-637-0617
http://www.lda-fl.org
e-mail: ldaf00@sunline.net
Cheryl Kron, Executive Secretary

The Learning Disabilities Association of Florida is a nonprofit volunteer organization of parents, professionals and LD adults.

3193 Literacy Florida
PO Box 672
Coca, FL 32923-0672
321-633-1809
http://www.literacyflorida.org
e-mail: sbuchanan@brev.org
Susan Buchanan, Contact
Jim Wilder, President

Provides information and services literacy volunteers and providersa in communications and networking, technical assistance and training, public affairs, advocacy, and student leadership.

Georgia

3194 Albany/Dougherty Certified Literate Community Program
Albany Area Chamber of Commerce
225 W Broad Avenue
Albany, GA 31701
229-434-8700
e-mail: hhollis@albanyga.com
Harriet Hollis Bradford, Contact

3195 Americus Literacy Action
Lake Blackshear Regional Library
307 E Lamar Street
Americus, GA 31709-3633
229-924-9010
e-mail: bbyram@lbrls.org
Bill Byram, Contact

3196 Effingham Literacy Fundamentals (ELF)
711 Zitterour Road
Rincon, GA 31326
912-826-3792
e-mail: eff@uwce.org

Glenda Bowers, Contact

3197 Gainesville/Hall County Alliance for Literacy
PO Box 58
Gainesville, GA 30503 770-531-4337
FAX 770-531-6406
http://http://allianceforliteracy.org
e-mail: contact@allianceforliteracy.org
Marci Hipp, Director
Dorothy Shinafelt, Executive Director

A nonprofit agency designed to SUPPORT the literacy providers of Hall County. The Alliance for Literacy promotes education for adults, ages 16 and older.

3198 Georgia Department of Education
Department of Technical & Adult Education
1800 Century Place NE
Atlanta, GA 30345 404-679-1600
FAX 404-679-1710
http://www.dtae.org
e-mail: mdelaney@dtae.org
Kimberly Hogan, Technical Education
Ron Jackson, Commissioner
Michael Vollmer, Manager
To oversee the state's system of technical colleges, the adult literacy program, and a host of economic workforce development programs.

3199 Georgia Department of Technical & Adult Education
Office of Adult Literacy
1800 Century Place NE
Atlanta, GA 30345 404-679-1600
FAX 404-679-1710
http://www.dtae.org
e-mail: mdelaney@dtae.org
Tony Bruehl, Director
Ron Jackson, Commissioner
Michael Vollmer, Manager
The Georgia Department of Technical and Adult Education oversees the state's system of technical colleges, the adult literacy program, and a host of economic and workforce development programs

3200 Georgia Literacy Resource Center: Office of Adult Literacy
1800 Century Place NE
Atlanta, GA 30345 404-679-1600
FAX 404-679-1630
http://www.dtae.org
e-mail: mdelaney@dtae.org
Tony Bruehl, Director
Ron Jackson, Commissioner
Michael Vollmer, Manager
The mission of the adult literacy programs is to enable every adult learner in Georgia to acquire the necessary basic skills in reading, writing, computation, speaking, and listening to compete successfully in today's workplace, strengthen family foundations, and exercise full citizenship.

3201 Literacy Volunteers Troup County
200 Main Street
La Grange, GA 30241 706-883-7837
e-mail: lvtc@charterinternet.com
Charlotte Anderson, Contact

3202 Literacy Volunteers of America: Forsyth County
PO Box 1097
Cumming, GA 30028 770-887-0074
http://www.litreacyforsyth.org
e-mail: focolit@sellsouth.net
Eddith DeVeau, Executive Director
Dianne Anth, Director

Dedicated to teaching adults to read in the Forsyth County region.

3203 Literacy Volunteers of America: Tift County
211 Chestnut Avenue
Tifton, GA 31794 229-382-0505
FAX 229-387-0442
e-mail: tiftlva@surfsouth.com
Mary Laster, Manager

3204 Literacy Volunteers of America: Troup County
PO Box 1087
Lagrange, GA 30241 706-883-7837
FAX 706-882-5114
e-mail: lvatc@mindspring.com
Charlotte Anderson, Executive Director

The Literacy Volunteers of America is a fully integrated national network of local, state and regional literacy providers that give adults and their families the opportunity to acquire skills to be effective in their roles as members of their families, communities and workplace.

3205 Literacy Volunteers of Atlanta
246 Sycamore Street
Decatur, GA 30030 404-377-7323
FAX 404-377-8662
http://www.lvama.org
e-mail: lva_ma@mindspring.com
Colette Duncan, Executive Director
Kelly Trotter, Program Manager

An organization dedicated to teaching adults to read in the Atlanta area.

3206 Nancy Hart Literacy Council of Georgia
PO Box 1294
Hartwell, GA 30643 706-376-5534
FAX 706-856-2655
Emily Gunnells, Manager

To organize volunteers for the purpose of improving literacy.

3207 Newton County Reads
8134 Geiger Street
Covington, GA 30014 770-787-2778
http://www.newtonreads.org
e-mail: newtoncountyreads@earthlink.net
Janet Hodges, Director

3208 North Georgia Technical College Adult Ed Dept
PO Box 65
Clarkesville, GA 30523 706-754-7700
FAX 706-754-7777
http://www.ngtcollege.org
e-mail: info@northgatech.edu
Barbara E Melichar, Contact

3209 Okefenokee Regional Library System
401 Lee Avenue
Waycross, GA 31501 912-287-4980
http://www.ware.public.lib.ga.us
e-mail: mgalantinesteis@yahoo.com
Midge Galentine-Steis, Contact

3210 Portal Adult Literacy Program
114 N First Avenue
Portal, GA 30450 912-865-5459
e-mail: wgmason@bulloch.net
Gary Mason, Contact

3211 Statesboro Regional Library Literacy Services
124 S Main Street
Statesboro, GA 30458 912-764-1345
e-mail: elainem@srls.public.lib.ga.us
Elaine H McDuffie, Contact

3212 **Toccoa/Stephens County Literacy Council**
PO Box 63
Toccoa, GA 30577
706-886-6082
FAX 706-282-7633
e-mail: mwalters3@yahoo.com
Michelle Austin, Manager
Maggie Walters, Tutor Coordinator

3213 **Volunteers for Literacy of Habersham County**
Po Box 351
Cornelia, GA 30531
706-776-4063
e-mail: literacy1@alltel.net
Teri Lewis, Contact

Hawaii

3214 **CALC/Hilo Public Library**
300 Waianuenue Avenue
Hilo, HI 96720
808-933-8893
FAX 808-933-8895
http://www.literacynet.org/calchilo
e-mail: calchilo@hawaiiantel.net
Kit Holz, Project Manager
Suttle Learner Services Coord, Learner Services Coordinator

Mission is to provide access to learning resources and tutoring services to help adults acquire and/or improve their skills in reading, writing, math, English as a Second Language and computer use.

3215 **Hawaii Laubach Literacy Action**
Hawaii Literacy
200 N Vineyard Boulevard
Honolulu, HI 96817
808-537-6706
FAX 808-528-1690
http://www.hawaiiliteracy.org
e-mail: info@hawaiiliteracy.org
Blune T Yokota, President
Katy Chen, Executive Director

Laubach Literacy Action is a nonprofit educational corporation dedicated to helping adult of all ages improve their lives and their communities by learning reading, writing, math and problem-solving skills.

3216 **Hawaii Literacy Resource Center**
Office of State Libraries
3225 Salt Lake Boulevard
Honolulu, HI 96818
808-831-6878
FAX 808-831-6882
http://www.literacynet.org/hawaii/home.html
e-mail: susann@lib.state.hi.us
Sue Berg, State Literacy Director

As part of the state library, the state resource center provides electronic and print resources.

3217 **Hui Malama Learning Center**
375 Mahalani Street
Wailuku, HI 96793
808-249-0111
e-mail: joanna.barnes@huimalama.org
Joanna Barnes, Contact

3218 **Kona Literacy Council**
Kailua Village Condomeniums
75-5766 Kuakini Highway #106A
Kailua Kona, HI 96745
808-329-1180
e-mail: konalit@msn.com
Brenda Natina, Contact

Idaho

3219 **ABE-College of Southern Idaho**
Adult Basic Education
PO Box 1238
Twin Flass, ID 83303-1238
208-732-6534
800-6800-CSI
FAX 208-736-3029
http://www.csi.edu/ip/adc/ABE/default.htm
e-mail: msteel@csi.edu
Marian Steel, Director

Designed to improve the educational level of adults, out-of-school youth and non-English speaking persons in our eight-county service area.

3220 **Idaho Adult Education Office**
Adult Education Office
PO Box 83720
Boise, ID 83720
208-332-6800
FAX 208-334-4664
http://www.sde.state.id.us
e-mail: Shoehler@sde.state.id.us
Mary Bostick, Manager

3221 **Idaho Coalition for Adult Literacy**
325 W State Street
Boise, ID 83702
208-334-2150
800-458-3271
FAX 208-334-4016
http://www.lili.org
e-mail: lili@libraries.idaho.gov
Peggy McClendon, Literacy Coordinator
Ann Joslin, Manager

An nonprofit organization which raise public awareness about the importance of a literate society.

3222 **Idaho Department of Corrections**
1299 N Orchard Street
Boise, ID 83706
208-658-2000
FAX 208-327-7496
http://www.corr.state.id.us
e-mail: inquire@corr.state.id.us
Tom Beauclair, Manager
Gale Cushman, Education Bureau Chief

The Education Bureau of the Idaho Department of Correction operates prison education programs in seven facilities across the state.

3223 **Idaho State Library**
325 W State Street
Boise, ID 83702
208-334-2150
800-458-3271
FAX 208-334-4016
http://www.lili.org
e-mail: lili@isL.state.id.us
Stephanie Bailey-White, Public Information Officer
Ann Joslin, Manager

Offers a history of pioneering new frontiers in library services.

3224 **Idaho Workforce Investment Act**
Idaho Department of Commerce & Labor
317 W Main Street
Boise, ID 83735
208-332-3570
FAX 208-334-6300
http://www.cl.idaho.gov
e-mail: cheryk,brush@cl.idaho.gov
Cheryl Brush, Bureau Chief
Cherly Ausman, Office of Workforce Policy

Provides vocational training services for economically disadvantaged adults and youth, dislocated workers and others who face significant employment barriers.

3225 **Learning Lab**
715 W Capitol Boulevard
Boise, ID 83702 208-344-1335
FAX 208-344-1171
http://www.learninglabinc.org
e-mail: gvanhole@learninglabinc.org
Gemma VanHole, Director

A computer-assisted learning center for adults and families with birth to six-year-old children. Students receive basic instruction including, mathematics, reading, writing, spelling, GED preparation and workplace skills in a comfortable, confidential environment.

Illinois

3226 **Adult Literacy at People's Resource Center**
201 S Naperville Road
Wheaton, IL 60187 630-682-5402
FAX 630-682-5412
http://www.peoplesrc.org
e-mail: mmilton@peoplesrc.org
Maryanna Milton, Co-Director
Knight Co-Director, Co-Director

Develops english as a second language ad adult basic academic skills, improves opportunities for employment and self-sufficiency, and strengthens family and community relationdships. Resulting in clients participating more effectively in the larger community and society.

3227 **Aquinas Literacy Center**
3525 S Hermitage Ave
Chicago, IL 60609 773-927-0512
http://www.aquinasliteracycenter.org
Joan Mary, Director

Offers individualized tutoring in the english language to residents of the McKinley Park and surrounding areas at no cost to the student. Provides an environment conducive to learning, and one which reverences and respects each individual person.

3228 **C.E.F.S. Literacy Program**
1805 S Banker Street
Effingham, IL 62401-0928 217-342-2193
FAX 217-342-4701
http://www.cefseoc.org
e-mail: cefs@effingham.net
Paul White, Chief Executive Officer
Schniederjon Director, Director

Helping people to achieve their full individual and economic potential. Develop, implement and evaluate social service programs to assist economically and socially disadvantaged people in their quest for greater self-sufficiency.

3229 **Carl Sandburg College Literacy Coalition**
C/O Carl Sandburg College
2400 Tom L Wilson Boulevard
Galesburg, IL 61401 309-341-5330
http://www.sandburg.edu
e-mail: kavalos@sandburg.edu
Gwen Koehler, Dean

3230 **Common Place Adult Literacy Programs**
514 S Shelley Street
Peoria, IL 61605-1837 309-674-3315
e-mail: cvoss04@sbcglobal.net
Connie Voss, Director

3231 **Dominican Literacy Center**
260 Vermont Avenue
Aurora, IL 60505-3100 630-898-4636
http://www.dominicanliteracycenter.org
e-mail: domlitctr@sbcglobal.net
Sister Kathleen Ryan OP, Contact
Ann Clennon Contact, Contact

A program for women that is a community based literacy program sponsored by the Dominican Sisters of Springfield, Illinois. Program is for women who cannot speak, read, and/or write english.

3232 **Illinois Library Association**
33 W Grand Avenue
Chicago, IL 60610 312-644-1896
FAX 312-644-1899
http://www.ila.org
e-mail: ila@ila.org
Robert Doyle, Executive Director

The Illinois Library Association is the voice for Illinois Libraries and the millions who depend on them. It provides leadership for the development, promotion, and improvement of library services in Illinois and for the library community.

3233 **Illinois Literacy Resource Center**
IL Network of Literacy/Adult Education Resources
431 S 4th Street
Springfield, IL 62701 217-785-6921
800-665-5576
FAX 217-785-6927
TDY:888-261-2709
Cyndi Coletti, Manager

As part of the State Library, the State Resource Center provides electronic and print resources.

3234 **Illinois Literacy Resource Development Center**
209 W Clark Street
Champaign, IL 61820 217-355-6068
FAX 217-355-6347
http://www.ilrdc.org
e-mail: ilrdc@ilrdc.org
Suzanne Knell, Executive Director
Janet Scogins, Associate Director

The Illinois Literacy Resource Development Center is dedicated to improving literacy policy and practice at the local, state, and national levels. It is a nonprofit organization supporting literacy and adult education efforts throughout Illinois and the nation. One key to its success has been its ability to build partnerships among the organizations, individuals and agencies working in the literacy arena from the local to the national level.

3235 **Illinois Office of Rehabilitation Services**
Illinois Department of Human Services
100 S Grand Avenue E
Springfield, IL 62762 217-557-1601
http://http://drs.dhs.state.il.us/owr
e-mail: ors@dhs.state.il.us
Teyonda Wertz, Chief of Staff
Rafael Diaz, Manager of Information Services
Carol Adams, Manager
DHS' Office of Rehabilitation Services is the state's lead agency serving individuals with disabilities.

3236 **Illinois Protection & Advocacy Agency:Equip for Equality**
11 E Adams Street
Chicago, IL 60603 312-341-0022
800-537-2632
FAX 312-341-0295
http://www.equipforequality.org
e-mail: hn6177@handsnet.org
Peter Grosz, Developmental Director

Equip for Equality is a not-for-profit Federally-funded organization that advocates for disability rights in the state of Illinois.

3237 **Literacy Chicago**
17 N State Street
Chicago, IL 60602 312-236-0341
FAX 312-870-4488
http://www.literacychicago.org
e-mail: info@literacychicago.org
Susan Kidder, Executive Director
Judy Klikun, Program Director

Literacy Chicago is dedicated to improving the literacy skills of Chicago-area adults and families.

3238 Literacy Volunteers of America: Illinois

30 E Adams Street
Chicago, IL 60603 312-857-1582
FAX 312-857-1586
http://www.literacyvolunteersillinois.org
e-mail: info@lvillinois.org

Dorothy Miaso, Executive Director
Dorish Rabinovitz, Program Coordinator

Literacy Volunteers of Illinois is a statewide organization committed to developing and supporting volunteer literacy programs that help families, adults and out-of-school teens increase their literacy skills.

3239 Literacy Volunteers of DuPage

24W500 Maple Avenue
Naperville, IL 60540-6057 630-416-6699
FAX 630-416-9465
http://www.literacyvolunteersdupage.org
e-mail: lvadupage@aol.com

Jacqueline Peterson, Executive Director
Thackeray Program Manager, Program Manager

Mission is to help adult learners achieve sufficient skills in english literacy so they may function independently in our communities.

3240 Literacy Volunteers of Fox Valley

St Charles Public Library
1 S 6th Avenue
Saint Charles, IL 60174-2105 630-584-4428
630-584-2811
http://www.lvfv.org
e-mail: info@lvfv.org

Peg Coker, Contact

Helping adults to improve their language and life skills so they can achieve their personal goals and participate more fully in the local business and social community.

3241 Literacy Volunteers of Western Cook County

125 N Marion Street
Oak Park, IL 60301-1067 708-848-8499
FAX 708-848-9564
http://www.lvwcc.org
e-mail: info@lvwcc.org

Angela West Blank, Director

Dedicated to improving the literacy skills of Western Cook County, Illinois. Mission is to empower each individual to reach reading independence and to actively involve each community in our drive toward higher literacy.

3242 Literacy Vounteers of Lake County

128 N County Road
Waukegan, IL 60085 847-623-2041
http://www.adultlearningconnection.org
e-mail: cmorris@waukeganpl.info

Carol Morris, Executive Director

Provides support and direction for individuals. Funded by the United Way of Lake County.

3243 Project CARE-Morton College

3801 S Central
Cicero, IL 60804 708-656-8000
http://www.morton.edu
e-mail: projectcare@morton.edu

Karen Latham-Williams, Co-Coordinator
Ficca Co-Coordinator, Co-Coordinator

3244 Project READ

5800 Godfrey Road
Godfrey, IL 62035 618-468-4144
866-433-5222
FAX 618-468-2387
http://www.lc.cc.il.us
e-mail: njohnson@lc.edu

Nancy Johnson, Coordinator Literacy Services

Goal is to increase literacy throughout the area with one-on-one tutoring. Project READ Community Service Coordinators are available to provide information to community groups, arrange free training for volunteers and distribute materials and support to tutor-learner pairs.

3245 The Literacy Connection

270 N Grove Avenue
Elgin, IL 60120 847-742-6565
FAX 847-742-6599
http://www.elginliteracy.org
e-mail: info@elginliteracy.org

Karen L Oswald, Executive Director
Orozco Program Coordinator, Program Coordinator

Non-profit, community-based organization helping local individuals acquire fundamental literacy skills. Helps thousands of area adults and youth acquire the skills they need to realize personal success and become fully functioning members of society.

3246 The Literacy Council

982 N Main Street
Rockford, IL 61103-7061 815-963-7323
FAX 815-963-7347
http://www.theliteracycouncil.org
e-mail: read@theliteracycouncil.org

Karen Scheffels, Director

Indiana

3247 Adult Literacy Program of Gibson County

PO Box 1134
Princeton, IN 47670 812-386-9100
http://www.gibsonadultliteracy.org
e-mail: literacy@gibsoncounty.net

Sharon Buyher, President

Mission is to provide an opportunity for any adult in Gibson County to attain basic English language literacy skills.

3248 Indiana Literacy & Technical Education Resource Center

Indiana State Library
140 N Senate Avenue
Indianapolis, IN 46204 317-232-3675
800-233-4572
FAX 317-232-3728
http://www.ciesck.k12.in.us/ilterc
e-mail: ilterc@statelib.lib.in.us

C Ewick, Manager

Provides literacy, technical, and career education resources to meet basic adult educational needs. Adult education materials include GED, learning disabilities and ESL resources. A thirty day loan period is provided to literacy, business and industry, goverment, schools and other adult education programs as well as to individual Indiana residents.

3249 Indiana Literacy Foundation

1920 W Morris Street
Indianapolis, IN 46221 317-639-6106
FAX 317-639-2782
http://www.indianaliteracy.org
e-mail: info@indianaliteracy.org

Robert Burgbacher, Executive Director

Indiana Literacy Foundation is a non-profit organization dedicated to strengthening basic skills among children and adults working with and through volunteer literacy programs across Indiana.

3250 Indiana Workforce Literacy

10 N Senate Avenue
Indianapolis, IN 46204 317-232-6702
FAX 317-232-1815
http://www.in.gov/dwd/information
e-mail: workone@dwd.in.gov

The Office of Workforce Literacy is dedicated to strengthening the skills of Indiana's workforce and to increasing the competitive edge of Indiana employers. Workforce Literacy grants provide on-site, customized, specific job related training. Employers and workers alike report that knowledge, skills, work attitudes, and productivity improves as a result of job-specific training.

3251 Indy Reads: Indianapolis/Marion County Public Library
PO Box 211
Indianapolis, IN 46206 317-269-1700
http://www.imcpl.org
e-mail: lgabrielson@imcpl.org
Linda Gabrielson, Manager
Laura Bramble, Executive Director

Indy Reads, a nationally recognized not-for-profit affiliate of the Indianapolis-Marion County Public Library, exists to improve the reading and writing skills of adults in Marion County who read at or below the sixth grade level.

3252 Literacy Volunteers of America: Cass County
PO Box 626
Logansport, IN 46947 574-722-6809
FAX 219-722-6810
Terri Marcellino, Manager

Literacy Volunteers of America is a fully integrated national network of local, state and regional literacy providers that gives adults and their families the opportunity to acquire skills to be effective in their roles as members of their families, communities, and workplaces.

3253 Literacy Volunteers of White County
1001 S Main Street
Monticello, IN 47960 574-583-0789
FAX 574-583-7982
Judy Hickman, Contact

A not-for-profit organization which provides a variety of free services to help people achieve personal goals through literacy.

3254 Morrisson/Reeves Library Literacy Resource Center
80 N 6th Street
Richmond, IN 47374 765-966-8291
FAX 765-962-1318
http://www.mrlinfo.org
e-mail: library@mrlinfo.org
Debra Clanahan, Manager

The Literacy Resource Center provides free training for volunteers to tutor adults in Wayne County who want to learn to read, write and do basic math.

3255 Steuben County Literacy Coalition
Community Center
317 S Wayne Street
Angola, IN 46703 260-665-1414
http://www.steubencountyliteracycoalition.org
e-mail: sclc@locl.net
Rebecca Fifer, President
Kathy Armstrong, Executive Director

The Steuben County Literacy Coalition helps adults and families develop their potential through improved literacy, education, and training.

3256 Three Rivers Literacy Alliance
Pro Literacy Worldwide
709 Clay Street
Fort Wayne, IN 46802 260-426-7323
FAX 260-424-0371
http://www.tria.org
e-mail: trlafw@yahoo.com
Kathleen Benson-Chaney, Literacy Coordinator
Judith Stabelli, Executive Director

Three Rivers Literacy Alliance addresses literacy issues with the adult population of Fort Wayne and the surrounding community.

Iowa

3257 Adult Literacy ProgramKirkwood Community College
Lincoln Learning Center
912 18th Ave SW
Cedar Rapids, IA 52404 319-366-0142
800-332-2055
http://www.kirkwood.edu
e-mail: lincoln@kirkwood.edu
Marlene Burns, Office Coordinator

Offers high school transfer courses, a high school completion program, and high school courses which will prepare you for career pathways.

3258 Iowa Bureau of Community Colleges
Department of Education
400 E 14th Street
Des Moines, IA 50319 515-281-5294
FAX 515-281-6544
http://www.state.ia.us/educate/commcoll.html
e-mail: helene.grossman@iowa.gov
Helene Grossman, Adult Literacy Consultant

3259 Iowa Department of Education: Iowa Literacy Council Programs
400 E 14th Street
Des Moines, IA 50319 515-281-5294
FAX 515-242-5988
http://www.state.ia.us/educate/commcoll
e-mail: sally.schroeder@ed.state.ia.us
Judy Jeffrey, Director
Ted Stilwater, Director, Family Literacy

Helps adults and families develop their potential through improved literacy, education, and training.

3260 Iowa JOBS Program: Division of Economic Assistance
Department of Human Services
Hoover State Building
Des Moines, IA 50319 515-286-3555
FAX 515-281-4940
Kevin Concannon, Executive Director
Jaili Cunningham, Manager

3261 Iowa Literacy Resource Center
Iowa Literacy Resource Center
415 Commercial Street
Waterloo, IA 50701 319-233-1200
800-772-2023
FAX 319-233-1964
http://www.readiowa.org
e-mail: riesberg@neilsa.org
Eunice Riefberg, Administrator
Denise Luppen, Administrative Assistant

The Center provides a link to resource materials in Iowa and at a regional and national level for adult literacy practitioners and students.

3262 Iowa Vocational Rehabilitation Agency
Department of Education
400 E 14th Street
Des Moines, IA 50319 515-281-5294
FAX 515-281-4703
TDY:515-242-5988
http://www.state.ia.us./educate/comcol
Steve Wooderson, Administrator
Judy Jeffrey, Director

3263 Iowa Workforce Investment Act
Department of Economic Development
200 E Grand Avenue
Des Moines, IA 50309 515-242-4700
FAX 515-242-4809
TDY:800-735-2934
http://www.iowalifechanging.com
e-mail: info@iowalifechanging.com

Mike Blouin, Director
David Lyons, Executive Director
Deb Townsend, Web Specialist
Job placement and training services. Especially for those workers who have been laid off, or have other barriers to steady employment.

3264 Learning Disabilities Association of Iowa
321 E 6th Street
Des Moines, IA 50329
515-280-8558
888-690-5324
FAX 515-243-1902
http://www.lda-ia.org
Vicki Goshon, President
Kathy Specketer, Coordinator

The Learning Disabilities Association of Iowa advances the education and general welfare of children and youth of normal, near-normal, and potentially normal intelligence who have learning disabilities.

3265 Library Literacy Programs: State Library of Iowa
1112 E Grand Avenue
Des Moines, IA 50319
515-281-4105
800-248-4483
FAX 515-281-6191
http://www.silo.lib.ia.us
Helen Dagley, Information Services
Mary Wegner, Manager

3266 Southeastern Community College-Literacy Program
127 N Main Street
Mt Pleasant, IA 52641
319-385-8012
http://www.scciowa.edu
e-mail: jcrull@scciowa.edu
Jennifer Crull, Director

Provides information to students who need to get their GED, and helps them to read and write.

3267 Western Iowa Tech Community CollegeAdult Literacy Program
4647 Stone Avenue
Sioux City, IA 51102-5199
712-274-8733
800-352-4649
Derek Albert, Coordinator
Chris Case, Coordinator

Website: www.witcc.edu/continuing_ed/literacy_program.cfm
Recruits volunteer mentors and adult learners throughout the year, and arranges for them to meet and work together.

Kansas

3268 Arkansas City Literacy Council
120 E 5th Avenue
Arkansas City, KS 67005
316-442-1280
e-mail: ligeracy@acpl.org
Michelle Swain, Director

A non-profit educational corporation dedicated to helping adults of all ages improve their lives and their communities by learning reading, writing, math and problem-solving skills.

3269 Butler County Community College Adult Basic Education/GED
901 S Haverhill Road
El Dorado, KS 67042
316-320-1689
http://www.butlercc.edu/abe_ged/index.cfm
Virginia Choens, Director

Mission is to produce students who make measurable gains in educational skills, workplace readiness, and technology skills.

3270 Client Assistance Program (CAP):Kansas Division of Persons with Disabilities
2914 SW Plass Court
Topeka, KS 66611
785-266-8193
800-432-2326
Mary Reyer, Director

Provides free services to consumers and applicants for projects, programs and facilities funded under the rehabilitation act.

3271 Emporia Literacy Program
620 Constitution Avenue
Emporia, KS 66801
620-343-4630
e-mail: dgladow@fhtc.net
Diane Gladow, Director

3272 Hutchinson Public LibraryLiteracy Resources
901 N Main
Hutchinson, KS 67501
620-663-5441
FAX 620-663-1583
http://http://hutchpl.org
e-mail: webmaster@hutchpl.org
Sandra Gustafson, Contact

3273 Kansas Adult Education Association
Barton County Community College
245 NE 30th Road
Great Bend, KS 67530
620-792-9340
800-722-6842
http://www.barton.cc.ks.us
Veldon Law, President
Todd Moore, Director for Admission
Cassandra Montoya, Student Work Service
The Kansas Adult Education Association has been the professional association for adult educators at community colleges, school districts, and non-profit organizations.

3274 Kansas Correctional Education
900 SW Jackson Street
Topeka, KS 66612
785-296-3317
888-317-8204
http://www.kdoc.dc.state.ks.us
Roger Haden, Secretary of Programs & Staff
Margaret Murdock, Administrative Assistant

The provision of correctional education programming to inmates.

3275 Kansas Department of Corrections
900 SW Jackson Street
Topeka, KS 66612
785-296-3317
888-317-8204
FAX 785-296-3317
http://www.kdoc.dc.state.ks.us
e-mail: jan.clausing@kdoc.dc.state.ks.us
Jan Clausing, Human Resource Director
Bill Noll, Information Technology Director

Correctional education programming to inmates.

3276 Kansas Department of Social & Rehabilitation Services
915 SW Harrison Street
Topeka, KS 66612
785-296-3959
FAX 785-296-2173
http://www.srskansas.org
Gary J Daniels, Secretary
Laura Howard, Assistant Secretary

To assist people with disabilities achieve suitable employment and independence.

3277 Kansas Laubach Literacy Action
120 E 5th Avenue
Arkansas City, KS 67005
316-442-1280
A non-profit educational corporation dedicated to helping adults of all ages improve their lives and their communities by learning reading, writing, math and problem-solving skills.

3278 Kansas Library Literacy Programs: Kansas State Library
PO Box 132
Independence, KS 67301
620-331-8218
FAX 620-331-9087
e-mail: vikkijo@kslib.info
Vikki Stewart, Management Coordinator

The goal of the Kansas Library Literacy Program is to provide Kansans with current volunteer management information to assist in their effort to use volunteers to meet a mission, e.g., libraries, literacy programs, etc. and to provide Kansans with current literacy information to assist in their effort to help adults and youth to read better, e.g., community-based literacy programs, traditional adult education, etc.

3279 Kansas Literacy Resource Center
Kansas Board of Regents/Literacy Resource Center
1000 SW Jackson Street
Topeka, KS 66612
785-296-3421
800-296-4526
FAX 785-296-0983
http://www.literacy.kent.edu
e-mail: dglass@ksbor.org
Dianne Glass, State Director Adult Education
Diane Whitley, Associate Director
Kim Wilcox, Executive Director
The Kansas Literacy Resource Center enhances systems, both private and public, that provide basic skills education across Kansas.

3280 Kansas Literacy Volunteers of America
Kansas State Library
State Capital Building
Topeka, KS 66612
785-296-3296
800-432-3919
FAX 785-296-6650
http://www.skyways.org
e-mail: KSST15LB@INK.ORG
Vikki Stewart, Literacy Program Director
Christie Brandau, Head of Library

To give adults and their families the opportunity to acquire skills to be effective in their roles as members of their families, communities and workplaces.

3281 Kansas State Department of Adult Education
120 SE 10th Avenue
Topeka, KS 66612
785-296-3201
FAX 785-296-7933
http://www.ksde.org
e-mail: atompkins@ksde.org
Karen Watney, Director
Dale Dennis, Deputy Commissioner
Andy Tompkins, Manager
To assist adults to become literate and obtain the knowledge and skills necessary for employment and self-sufficiency.

3282 Kansas State Literacy Resource Center: Kansas State Department of Education
1000 SW Jackson Street
Topeka, KS 66612
785-296-0175
FAX 785-296-0983
Dianne Glass, Director
Dianne Glass, Co-Director

The State Literacy Resource Center can assist adult education practitioners across the nation in locating and accessing the most current materials in their issue area.

3283 Preparing for the Future: Adult LearningServices
Dorothy Bramlage Public Library
230 W 7th Street
Junction City, KS 66441
785-238-4311
FAX 785-238-7873
http://www.jclib.org
e-mail: jclibrary@jclib.org
Susan Moyer, Director
Cheryl Jorgensen, Asst Dir for Adult Services
Patty Collins, Asst Dir for Youth Services

3284 Topeka Literacy Council
1119 SW 10th Avenue
Topeka, KS 66604-1105
785-234-2806
e-mail: topekaliteracy@juno.com
Kevin Koen, Director

Not for profit organization of volunteers who help adults learn to read & write effectively for the benefit of their economic advancement & self esteem.

3285 Western Kansas Community Service Consortiuum
348 NE Sr
Pratt, KS 67124
620-672-6251
http://www.wkcsc.org
e-mail: dedram@genmail.pcc.cc.ks.us
Dedra Manes, Executive Director

Mission is to provide cooperative community services to Western Kansas. Total service area includes 73 counties and nearly 3/4 of the state's geographic area.

Kentucky

3286 Ashland Adult Education
4818 Roberts Drive
Ashland, KY 41102
606-326-2440
http://www.ashlandboydadultedu.com
e-mail: joan.flanery@kctcs.edu
Joan Flanery, Program Director

Set up for any adult who wants to learn how to read or wants to improve his/her reading skills. They can choose to learn in a small group or to be tutored one-on-one with an individual instructor.

3287 Kentucky Laubach Literacy Action
Department for Adult Education & Literacy
1024 Capital Center Drive
Frankfort, KY 40601
502-573-5114
800-928-7323
FAX 502-573-5436
http://adulted.state.ky.us
e-mail: dvislisel@mail.state.ky.us
Dave Vislisel, Director
Reecie Stagnolia, Vice President

Dedicated to helping adults of all ages improve their lives and their communities by learning reading, writing, match and problem-solving skills.

3288 Kentucky Literacy Resource Center
Center for Adult Education & Literacy
1048 E Chestnut Street
Louisville, KY 40204
502-815-7000
800-win-net2
FAX 502-815-7001
http://www.win.net
e-mail: scallaway@mail.state.ky.us
Michael Tague, President

As part of the State Library, the State Resource Center provides electronic and print resources.

3289 Kentucky Literacy Volunteers of America
1024 Capital Center Drive
Frankfort, KY 40601
502-573-5114
FAX 502-573-5436
http://adulted.state.ky.us
e-mail: dvislsel@mail.state.ky.us
Dave Vislisel, Director
Reecie Stagnolia, Vice President

Promotes literacy for people of all ages.

3290 Operation Read
251 W 2nd Street
Lexington, KY 40507
859-254-9964
FAX 859-254-5834
http://www.opread.com
e-mail: opread@gx.net

Michelle Adomitis, Interim Executive Director
Morgan Salyer, Basic Adult Literacy/Tutor Cood

Helping adults learn to read to help imrove their lives, the lives of their children and the lives in their community.

3291 Simpson County Literacy Council
303 N High Street
Franklin, KY 42134 270-586-7234
FAX 270-598-0906
http://www.readtobefree.org
e-mail: read@readtobefree.org
Deborah Thompson, Director

Organization of volunteers, supported by a staff, which provides a variety of services that make it possible for adults to reach their personal goals-through literacy.

3292 Winchester/Clark County Literacy Council
Po Box 4023
Winchester, KY 40392-4023 859-744-1975
FAX 859-744-1424
http://www.clarkadulteducation.org
e-mail: literacyinfo@clarkeadulteducation.org
Jim Porter, Contact

Tutors provide one-on-one basic instruction to help improve your reading and writing skills.

Louisiana

3293 Adult Literacy Advocates of Baton Rouge
460 N 11th Street
Baton Rouge, LA 70802-4607 225-383-1090
FAX 225-387-5999
http://www.adultliteracyadvocates.org
e-mail: info@adultliteracyadvocates.org
Pamela Creighton, Executive Director
Susan Flowers, Instructor & Student Coordinator
Ann Ours, Instructor

3294 Literacy Council of Southwest Louisiana Lifelong Learning Center
809 Kirby Street
Lake Charles, LA 70601-5311 337-494-7000
800-393-READ
FAX 337-494-7915
http://www.literacyswla.org
e-mail: tsemien@literacyswla.org
Tommeka Semien, Executive Director
Falencia Bias, Director of Programs
Monica Orsot, ESL & Financial Literacy Cood
Offers free small group classes for adults in Workplace Essential Skills, Computer Basics, Financial Basic, Citizenship, English Language, Math and Family Reading programs. Also, has fully equipped computer learning lab where adults can do self-directed study.

3295 Literacy Volunteers of America: Centenary College Program
PO Box 41188
Shreveport, LA 71134 318-869-2411
FAX 318-869-2474
e-mail: lvacent@bellsouth.net
Sue Lee, Executive Director
Garcy Balton, Office Secretary

3296 Louisiana State Literacy Resource Center: State Department of Education
Office of School & Community Support
PO Box 94064
Baton Rouge, LA 70804 225-342-3340
877-453-2721
FAX 225-219-4439
http://www.louisianaschools.net
e-mail: mbryant@la.gov
Kim Fitch, Director Human Resources
Casper Dir Communications/Leg, Dir Communications/Legisl Svs

The Center provides a link to resource materials in Louisiana and at a regional and national level for adult literacy, practitioners and students.

3297 Reading Education for Adult Development(READ)
PO Box 1148
Oakdale, LA 71463 318-215-0490
866-367-7323
http://www.allen.lib.la.us/READ.htm
e-mail: read@wnonline.net
Nora K Duncan, Executive Director
Flora Currie, Literacy Coordinator
Sharon Dunn, READ Teacher

3298 VITA (Volunteer Instructors Teaching Adults)
905 Jefferson Street
Lafayette, LA 70501-6901 337-234-4600
FAX 337-234-4672
http://www.vitalaf.org
e-mail: vita@vitalaf.org
Jeanette F Barras, Contact

Specially trained volunteers learn to teach reading and writing using easy to follow manuals and to also provide goal-oriented, one on one or in small group. VITA provides the professional training, materials, and support that enable the volunteers to assist adults in acquiring basic reading and writing skills.

Maine

3299 Biddeford Adult Education
18 Maplewood Avenue
Biddeford, ME 04005 207-282-3883
FAX 207-286-9581
http://www.biddschools.org
e-mail: abeaulieu@biddschools.org
Anita W Findlen, Contact

3300 Center for Adult Learning and Literacy: University of Maine
Pro Literacy Worldwide
5749 Merrill Hall
Orono, ME 04469 207-581-2498
FAX 207-581-1517
http://www.umaine.edu/call
e-mail: evelyn.beaulieu@umit.maine.edu
Evelyn Beaulieu, Director
Carol Wynne, Project Coordinator

The Center for Adult Learning and Literacy offers quality, research-based professional development and resources, based on funded initiatives to improve the quality of services within the Maine Adult Education System.

3301 Literacy Volunteers of Androscoggin
277 Main Street
Auburn, ME 04210-5727 207-753-1772
http://www.avcnet.org/literacyvolunteers
e-mail: lvandro@midmaine.com
Tahlia Hope, Executive Director

Mission is to increase literacy for adults and their families, effectively utilizing and supporting volunteers in the delivery of their services, and provide research, training and technical assistance related to the various aspects of literacy.

3302 Literacy Volunteers of Aroostook County
PO Box 522
Limestone, ME 04750 207-325-3490
FAX 207-325-8916
http://www.lvmaine.org
Jo-Ellen Kelley, Executive Director
Al Menard, President

Volunteer-based organization, committed to enabling adults in need of basic literacy skills to achieve their potential through one-on-one or small group instruction.

3303 Literacy Volunteers of Bangor

200 Hogan Road
Bangor, ME 04401
207-947-8451
FAX 207-942-1391
http://http://lvbangor.org
Mary (Marin) Lyon, Executive Director
Allison Cote, President

Connects adults who want to improve their literacy (via learning how to read or speaking english) with trained, volunteer tutors. Focus is to serve those adults with the lowest literacy levels so that they can improve their economic, social and personal lives.

3304 Literacy Volunteers of Greater Augusta

295 Water Street
Augusta, ME 04330-4621
207-626-3440
FAX 207-626-7588
http://www.lva-augusta.org
e-mail: info@lva-augusta.org
Gail E Dyer, Coordinator

Mission is to promote and foster increased literacy for adults who have low literacy skills or those for whom English is not their native language through volunteer tutoring.

3305 Literacy Volunteers of Greater Portland

Po Box 8585
142 High Street
Portland, ME 04101
207-780-1352
http://www.lvaportland.org
e-mail: lvportland@gwi.net
Kristen Stevens, Executive Director

Offers free, confidential, student-centered, individual and small group tutoring to adults seeking to develop the literacy skills they need to reach important life goals like reading their first books, obtaining citizenship, helping their children with homework, taking care of personal bills and employment.

3306 Literacy Volunteers of Greater Saco/Biddeford

180 Main Street
Saco, ME 04072-1507
207-283-2954
http://www.sacoliteracy.com
e-mail: lvasaco@gwi.net
Kristen Stevens, Executive Director

Mission is to train volunteers to provide educational programs and services that improve reading, writing and related literacy skills, and to empower adults by enhancing their liffe skills in the area of family, work, health and community.

3307 Literacy Volunteers of Greater Sanford

883 Main Street
Sanford, ME 04073
207-324-2486
877-303-5899
http://www.sanfordliteracy.org
e-mail: lvgs@metrocast.net
Ann Gamble, Coordinator

Purpose is to support the literacy needs of adults (especially those reading below the ninth grade reading level) with free, confidential, one-on-one tutoring and small group instruction by trained adult volunteers.

3308 Literacy Volunteers of Maine

142 High Street
Portland, ME 04101-2228
207-773-3191
FAX 207-773-3191
http://www.lvmaine.org
e-mail: info@lvmaine.org
Stella Hernandez, Executive Director
Elaine Tselikis, Program Coordinator
Abbie Embry Turner, Program Coordinator
Dedicated to providing increased access to literacy services for Maine adults who wish to acquire or improve their literacy skills.

3309 Literacy Volunteers of Mid-Coast Maine

28 Lincoln Street
Rockland, ME 04841-2940
207-594-5154
FAX 207-594-5154
http://www.villagesoup.com/lvmcm
e-mail: bgifford@midcoast.com
Beth Gifford, Executive Director
Marianne Doyle, President

Assists adults in Knox xounty and the surrounding area to improve their reading, writing and related literacy skills.

3310 Literacy Volunteers of Waldo County

9 Field Street
Belfast, ME 04915-0234
207-338-2843
FAX 207-382-6267
http://http://waldolva.acadia.net
e-mail: waldolva@acadia.net
Frances L Walker, Program Coordinator

Works to improve reading, writing, and related literacy skills of adults and their families. Programs are free, private, and confidential. Trained volunteer tutors help learners identify needs and achieve their personal literacy goals.

3311 Maine Bureau of Applied Technical Adult Learning: Adult Career and Technical Education

Maine Department of Education
23 State House Station
Augusta, ME 04333
207-624-6600
FAX 207-624-6700
http://www.maine.gov/education
e-mail: yvonne.davis@maine.gov
Susan A Gendron, Commissioner
Yvonne Davis, Director

3312 Maine Literacy Resource Center

University of Maine
5749 Merrill Hall
Orono, ME 04469
207-581-1110
FAX 207-581-1517
http://www.umaine.edu
e-mail: evelyn.beaulieu@umit.maine.edu
Robert Kennedy, President
Carol Wynne, Project Coordinator
Evelyn Beaulieu, Director
As part of the State Library, the State Resource Center provides electronic and print resources.

3313 Maine Literacy Volunteers of America

PO Box 8585
Portland, ME 04104
207-780-1352
http://www.lvaportland.org
e-mail: lvportland@gwi.net
Kristian Stevens, Director
Suzanne Hunt, Manager

A non-profit organization that provides free tutoring to adults who cannot read and to adults whose native language is not English.

3314 Tri-County Literacy Volunteers

2 Sheridan Road
Bath, ME 04530
207-443-6384
877-885-7441
http://www.tricountyliteracy.org
e-mail: tricountyliteracy@tricountyliteracy.org
Darlene Marciniak, Executive Director
Emmy Kappler, Adult Literacy Coordinator

Maryland

3315 Anne Arundel County Literacy Council
80 W Street
Annapolis, MD 21041
410-269-4419
FAX 410-974-2023
http://www.icanread.org
e-mail: info@aaclc.org
Nancy Grigsby, President
Judy Mooney, Basic Lit. Tutor Training Super
Elsie Couper, ESL Training Supervisor
Serves the needs of functionally illiterate adults in Anne Arundel County. Offers free one-to-one educational assistance to non-reading adults in the community.

3316 Calvert County Literacy Council
PO Box 2508
Prince Frederick, MD 20678
410-535-3233
http://www.somd.lib.md.us/CALV/Literacy
e-mail: calvertliteracy@somd.lib.md.us
Maria Isle Birnkammer, Contact

Provides volunteers to help with one-on-one tutoring or small group tutoring.

3317 Center for Adult and Family Literacy: Community College of Baltimore County
7200 Sollers Point Road
Baltimore, MD 21222
410-285-9593
http://www.ccbcmd.edu/ceed/literacy.html
e-mail: gmcallister@ccbcmd.edu
Gayle McAllister, Director

Classes to provide training and instruction for adults with literacy problems.

3318 Charles County Literacy Council
3795 Leonardtown Road
Waldorf, MD 20601
301-870-5974
FAX 301-870-9106
http://www.charlescountyliteracy.org
e-mail: ccliteracy@ccboe.com
Danielle Fish, Director

Goal is to provide free help to adult non-readers throughout the county with one-on-one and small group tutoring.

3319 Howard University School of Continuing Education
1100 Wayne Avenue
Silver Spring, MD 20910
301-585-2296
FAX 301-585-8911
http://www.con-ed.howard.edu
e-mail: paberry@howard.edu
Peggy A Berry, Executive Director

Howard University Continuing Education was established in April 1986 to meet the education and training needs of professionals, administrators, entrepreneurs, technical personnel, paraprofessionals and other adults on an individual or group basis.

3320 Learning Bank of Coil
1200 W Baltimore Street
Baltimore, MD 21223
410-659-5452
FAX 410-576-0782
http://http://thelearningbank.org
e-mail: info@thelearningbank.org
J Carol Osgood, Director

Community-based adult education program in Southwest Baltimore.

3321 Literacy Council of Frederick County
110 Patrick Street
Frederick, MD 21701
301-694-2066
http://www.frederickliteracy.org
e-mail: info@frederickliteracy.org
Tracy Beidleman, Director

Non-profit, non-sectarian educational organization of volunteers dedicated to helping adult residents improve their language skills through our one-on-one or group tutoring.

3322 Literacy Council of Montgomery County
11701 Georgia Avenue
Wheaton, MD 20902
301-942-9292
http://www.literacycouncilmcmd.org
e-mail: info@literacycouncilmcmd.org
Pamela Saussy, Executive Director
Kim Brown, Deputy Director

Dedicated to helping adults in Montgomery COunty learn to speak, read, write and understand english.

3323 Literacy Council of Prince George's County
6532 Adelphi Road
Hyattsville, MD 20782-2008
301-699-9770
FAX 301-699-9707
http://www.literacycouncil.org
e-mail: info@literacycouncil.org
Gail Drake, Executive Director

Serves as the primary non-profit organization for the advocacy and implementation of literacy programs in the county. Provides services for adult learners in acquiring, improving and applying basic literacy skills including reading, writing, math and oral communication.

3324 Maryland Adult Literacy Resource Center
UMBC, Department of Education
1000 Hilltop Cir
Baltimore, MD 21228
410-455-6725
800-358-3010
FAX 410-455-1139
http://www.umbc.edu/alrc
e-mail: ira@umbc.edu

Katherine Ira, Director
Robert Somers, Manager

As part of the State Library, the State Resource Center provides resources and information for adult literacy providers and students in Maryland.

3325 Maryland Literacy Resource Center
UMBC, Department of Education
1000 Hilltop Cir
Baltimore, MD 21250
410-455-2665
800-358-3010
FAX 410-455-1139
http://www.umbc.edu
e-mail: help@umbc.edu

Katherine Ira, Director
Robert Somers, Manager

As part of the State Library, the State Resource Center provides resources and information for adult literacy providers and students in Maryland.

3326 Project Literacy
Howard County Library
10375 Little Patuxent Parkway
Columbia, MD 21044
410-313-7800
FAX 410-313-7811
TDY:410-313-7883
http://www.hclibrary.org
e-mail: ostendoe@hclibrary.org
Yu-Ching Ostendorp, Project Manager

3327 South Baltimore Learning Center
28 E Ostend Road
Baltimore, MD 21230-4209
410-625-4215
FAX 410-727-8316
http://www.southbaltimorelearns.org
e-mail: ssocha@southbaltimorelearns.org
Sonia Socha, Executive Director

A neighborhood based initiative providing tutoring to adults in the community and has since grown to serve hundreds of adults each year offering a variety of services.

Massachusetts

3328 A Legacy for Literacy
330 Homer Street
Newton, MA 02459
617-796-1364
e-mail: legacyforliteracy@yahoo.com
Susan Becam, ESL/Literacy Program Coordinator

www.newtonfreelibrary.net/Services/Literacy/literacy.htm

3329 Adult Center at PAL: Curry College
1071 Blue Hill Ave
Milton, MA 02186
617-333-0500
FAX 617-333-2114
http://www.curry.edu/pal
e-mail: pal@curry.edu
Jane Adelizzi PhD, Contact

The Adult Center at PAL (Program for Advancement of Learning) is the first program to offer academic and socio-emotional services to adults with LD/ADHD/Dyslexia in a college setting in the New England area. The ACD offers one-to-one academic tutorials; small support groups that meet weekly; and Saturday Seminars that explore issues that impact the lives of adults with LD/ADHD.

3330 ESL Center
43 Amity Street
Amherst, MA 01002
413-256-4090
http://http://joneslibrary.org
e-mail: esl@joneslibrary.org
Lynne Weintraub, Coordinator

Award winning program providing volunteer tutors, tutoring space, study materials, computer-assisted instruction, citizenship classes, English classes and referrals to adult immigrants in the Amherst area.

3331 Eastern Massachusetts Literacy Council
English At Large
400 High Street
Medford, MA 02155
781-395-2374
http://www.emlc.org
e-mail: volunteer@englishatlarge.org
Steven Reny, President
Christine Ellersick, Executive Director

The Eastern Massachusetts Literacy Council is a private non-profit affiliate of ProLiteracy Worldwide, the largest non-profit volunteer adult literacy organization in the world. The EMLC trains volunteers to assist adults who are learning English as another language and adults who wish to strengthen their basic reading skills.

3332 JOBS Program: Massachusetts Employment Services Program
Dept of Transitional Assistance/Office of Health
600 Washington Street
Boston, MA 02111
617-348-8400
http://www.state.ma.us/dta/index.htm
John Wagner, Manager
Julie Noble, Assistant to the Assistant Direc

The Employment Services Program is a joint federal and state funded program whose primary goal is to provide a way to self-sufficiency for TAFDC families ESP is an employment-oriented program that is based on a work-first approach.

3333 Literacy Network of South Berkshire
100 Main Street
Lee, MA 31238
413-243-0471
FAX 413-243-6754
http://www.litnetsb.org
e-mail: info@litnetsb.org
Tricia Farley-Bouvier, Director of Education
Mary Spina, Assoc. Director of Education

Serving the 15 towns of Southern Berkshire County in Massachusetts. Providing free one-on-one tutoring to adults in reading, GED preparation, English as a Second Language and Citizenship preparation.

3334 Literacy Volunteers of Greater Worcester
3 Salem Square
Worcester, MA 01608
508-754-8056
http://www.lvgw.org
e-mail: mail@lvgw.org
Michael Mills, President
Laurie D'Amico, Contact

Mission is to build a more literacte community by providing volunteers to help with tutoring adults in reading, writing, and other areas of need.

3335 Literacy Volunteers of Massachusetts
15 Court Square
Boston, MA 02108
617-367-1313
888-466-1313
FAX 617-367-8894
e-mail: catherinlvm@aol.com
Roberta Soolman, Executive Director
Catherine Ward, Coordinator

Literacy Volunteers of Massachusetts helps adults learn to read and write or speak English by matching them with trained volunteer tutors.

3336 Literacy Volunteers of Methuen
305 Braodway
Methuen, MA 01844
978-686-4080
FAX 978-686-8669
http://www.nevinslibrary.org
Kristen Underwood, Coordinator

Promotes and encourages literacy skills for both English language learners and native English speakers in the Methuen area through the use of trained volunteer tutors.

3337 Literacy Volunteers of the Montachusett Area
610 Main Street
Fitchburg, MA 01420
978-343-8184
FAX 978-343-4680
http://www.literacyvolunteersmontachusett.org
e-mail: literacy26@aol.com
Gloria Maybury, Program Coordinator

Promtoes and fosters increased literacy in the Montachusett area through trained volunteers tutoring and to empower adults for whom English is a second language. Encourages and aids individuals, groups or organizations desiring to increase literacy through voluntary programs.

3338 Massachusetts Correctional Education: Inmate Training & Education
Department of Correction
PO Box 43
Norfolk, MA 02056
508-660-3924
FAX 508-850-5214
http://www.state.ma.us
Carolyn Vicari, Director Program Services
Paul Ruane, Manager

To establish departmental policy regarding inmates' involvement in academic and vocational training programs.

3339 Massachusetts Family Literacy Consortium
State Government
350 Main Street
Malden, MA 02148
781-338-3300
FAX 781-338-3394
http://www.doe.mass.edu
e-mail: MFLC@doe.mass.edu
Kathy Rodriguez, MFLC Coordinator
Arlene Dale, State Coordinator

The Massachusetts Family Literacy Consortium is a statewide initiative with the mission of forging effective partnerships among state agencies, community organizations, and other interested parties to expand and strengthen family literacy and support.

3340 **Massachusetts GED Administration: Massachu setts Department of Education**
350 Main Street
Malden, MA 02148
781-338-6604
http://www.doe.mass.edu
e-mail: rderfler@doe.mass.edu
Ruth Derfler, Director

Thirty-three test centers operate state-wide to serve the needs of the adult population in need of a high school credential.

3341 **Massachusetts Job Training Partnership Act: Department of Employment & Training**
CF Hurley Building, 3rd Floor
19 Staniford Street
Boston, MA 02114
617-626-6600
FAX 617-727-0315
http://www.detma.org
e-mail: mstonge@detma.org
John O'Leary, Commissioner
Ed Malmborg, Executive Director

Supplies information on the local labor market and assists companies in locating employees.

3342 **Pollard Memorial Library Adult Literacy Program**
401 Merrimack Street
Lowell, MA 01852
978-970-4120
FAX 978-970-4117
TDY:978-970-4129
http://www.pollardml.org
Dora St Martin, Director

Offers free, confidential, private and flexibly scheduled tutoring to adults with little or no reading or writing skills, and those who wish to become more fluent English speakers, readers or writers.

Michigan

3343 **Genesee County Literacy Coalition**
Zimmerman Center
2421 Corunna Road
Flint, MI 48503
810-760-1853
FAX 810-760-1215
http://www.flint.lib.mi.us
Kimberly Pillen Brown, Literacy Provider
Pat Mrozek, Chairperson
Grace Tucker, Secretary
The Genesee County Literacy Coalition is a non-profit organization dedicated to promoting literacy in Genesee County.

3344 **Kent County Literacy Council**
111 Library Street NE
Grand Rapids, MI 49503-3219
616-459-5151
FAX 616-245-8069
http://www.kentliteracy.org
e-mail: info@kentliteracy.org
Susan Ledy, Executive Director
Mary Hassinger, Literacy Coordinator

Mission is to build a literate community and transform lives by strengthening reading and language skills.

3345 **Literacy Volunteers of America: Lansing Area Literacy Coalition**
1028 E Saginaw Street
Lansing, MI 48906
517-485-4949
FAX 517-485-1924
http://www.thereadingpeople.org
e-mail: mail@thereadingpeople.org
Lois Bader, Executive Director
Di Clark, Assistant Director

The Capital Area Literacy Coalition helps children and adults learn to read, write and speak English with an ultimate goal of helping individuals achieve self-sufficiency.

3346 **Literacy Volunteers of America: Sanilac Council**
Grace Temple
46 N Jackson Street
Sandusky, MI 48471
810-648-2200
Tony Parker, Administrator

Helps children and adults learn to read, write and speak English with self sufficiency as the ultimate goal.

3347 **Michigan Adult Learning & Technology Center**
Central Michigan University
219 Ronan Hall
Mount Pleasant, MI 48859
989-774-3686
FAX 989-714-7713
http://www.malt.cmich.edu
e-mail: malt@cmich.edu
Michael Kent, Special Projects Coordinator
Stan Shingles, Executive Director

A professional development center that extends support services and resources to adult education providers, volunteers, and students. These efforts include: disseminating research information; conducting and sponsoring training for tutors and educators; coordinating conferences; aiding in the utilization of technology in professional development and the classroom; providing grants or sponsoring research projects related to the field of education.

3348 **Michigan Assistive Technology: Michigan Rehabilitation Services**
Michigan Jobs Commission
119 Pere Marquette Drive
Lansing, MI 48912
517-485-4477
FAX 517-485-4488
http://www.publicpolicy.com
e-mail: ppa@publicpolicy.com
Jeff Padden, President
Nancy Hewat, Executive Director

Solves information and policy-development problems for clients.

3349 **Michigan Laubach Literacy Action**
2157 University Park Drive
Okemos, MI 48864
517-349-7511
FAX 517-349-6667
http://www.michiganliteracy.org
e-mail: mli@voyager.net
Levona Whitaker, Contact

Dedicated to advancing basic literacy skills throughout Michigan and beyond.

3350 **Michigan Libraries and Adult Literacy**
PO Box 30007
Lansing, MI 48909
517-373-1297
FAX 517-373-5853
TDY:517-373-1592
http://www.michigan.gov/libraryofmichigan
e-mail: librarian@michigan.gov
Nancy Robertson, State Librarian
Jenny Sipe, Administrative Assistant

3351 **Michigan State Department of Adult Education: Office of Extended Learning Services**
Department of Education
608 W Allegan Street
Lansing, MI 48933
517-373-3324
FAX 517-335-0592
http://www.michigan.gov
e-mail: kingsleym@michigan.gov
Jeremy Hughs, Manager
Lindy Buch, Director
Maria Kinglsey, Educational Consultant

3352 **Michigan Workforce Investment Act**
Michigan Jobs Commission
119 Pere Marquette Drive
Lansing, MI 48912
517-485-4477
FAX 517-485-4488
http://www.publicpolicy.com
e-mail: ppa@publicpolicy.com

Jeff Padden, President
Nancy Hewat, Executive Officer

Minnesota

3353 Alexandria Literacy Project
817 Fillmore Street
Alexandria, MN 56308-1739 320-762-0627
http://www.thealp.org
e-mail: sschroep@alexandria.k12.mn.us
Sandy Schroepfer, Contact

3354 English Learning Center
2315 Chicago Avenue S
Minneapolis, MN 55404 612-874-9963
FAX 612-871-0017
http://www.englishlc.org
e-mail: info@englishlc.org
Nicole Pettitt, Contact

Provides English as a Second Language, math,computer skills, and advocacy to immigrant and refugee families in the Phillips Neighborhood and Cedar Riverside areas for South Minnieapolis.

3355 Minnesota Department of Adult Education: Adult Basic Education
Department of Children, Families & Learning
1500 Highway 36 West
Roseville, MN 55113 651-582-8200
FAX 651-634-5154
http://www.education.state.mn.us
Alice Seagreen, Education Commissioner
Chas Anderson, Deputy Education Commissioner
Randy Wanke, Director Communications
Our mission is to improve educational achievement by establishing clear standards, measuring performance, assisting educators and increasing opportunities for lifelong learning.

3356 Minnesota Department of Employment and Economic Development
Minnesota Workforce Center
332 Minnesota Street
Saint Paul, MN 55101 651-296-6786
800-657-3858
http://www.mnwfc.org
e-mail: mdes.customerservice@state.mn.us
Bonnie Elsey, Director
Jack Stoehr, Manager

The Department of Employment and Economic Development is Minnesota's principal economic development agency, with programs promoting business expansion and retention, workforce development, international trade, community development and tourism.

3357 Minnesota GED Administration
550 Cedar Street
Saint Paul, MN 55101 612-296-2704
FAX 651-582-8458
Patrick Rupp, GED Director

State of Minnesota General Educational Development.

3358 Minnesota LDA Learning Disabilities Center
4301 Highway 7
Minneapolis, MN 55416 952-922-8374
FAX 952-922-8102
http://www.ldaminnesota.org
e-mail: info@ldaminnesota.org
Kitty Christiansen, Executive Director
Victoria Weinberg, Program Director

The LDA Learning Center maximizes the potential of children, youth and adults with learning disabilities or related learning difficulties so that they and their families lead more productive and fulfilled lives.

3359 Minnesota LINCS: Literacy Council
756 Transfer Road
Saint Paul, MN 55114 651-645-2277
800-225-7323
FAX 651-645-2272
http://www.mlc.org
Jason Brazier, MLC Tech Svs Specialist
Eric Nesheim, Executive Director

Makes information available to literacy and other educators throughout Minnesota. The system is a result of cooperation between numerous agencies and organizations in Minnesota that realize the benefit of using the internet to provide information to the public. The system allows literacy and other educators to locate information at one central site or follow links to connect to wherever the information resides.

3360 Minnesota Life Work Center
University of St. Thomas
1000 Lasalle Avenue
Minneapolis, MN 55403 651-962-4000
http://www.stthomas.edu
e-mail: lifework@stthomas.edu
Brian Dusbiber, Director
Sharon Ficher, Executive Director
Mary Kernan, Career Counselor
Supporting the educational goals, personal growth and career management needs of graduate students, education students, and alumni, through professional services and comprehensive resources.

3361 Minnesota Literacy Training Network
University of St. Thomas
1000 Lasalle Avenue
Minneapolis, MN 55403 651-962-4000
800-328-6819
FAX 651-962-4169
http://www.stthomas.edu
Deborah Simmons, Director
Sharon Ficher, Executive Director

Literacy Training Network offers noncredit learning opportunities for adult basic education and literacy training staff in Minnesota.

3362 Minnesota Vocational Rehabilitation Agency: Rehabilitation Services Branch
Department of Economic Security
390 Robert Street N
Saint Paul, MN 55101 651-296-3711
800-328-9095
FAX 651-297-5159
http://www.mnworkforcecenter.org
e-mail: Howard.Glad@state.mn.us
Howard Glad, Contact

Provides basic vocational rehabilitation services to consumers including vocational counseling, planning, guidance and placement, as well as certain special services based on individual circumstances.

3363 Minnesota Vocational Rehabilitation Agency
Department Employment and Economic Development
332 Minnesota Street
Saint Paul, MN 55101 651-296-3711
800-328-9095
FAX 651-297-5159
http://www.deed.state.mn.us
e-mail: kim.peck@state.mn.us
Kimberly Peck, RS Director

Provides basic vocational rehabilitation services to consumers including vocational counseling, planning, guidance and placement, as well as certain special services based on individual circumstances.

Mississippi

3364 Corinth-Alcorn Literacy Council
1023 Fillmore Street
Corinth, MS 38834-4100 662-286-9759
http://www.alcornliteracy.com

Dorothy Hopkins, Contact

3365 Grenada League for Adult Development(GLAD)

423 S Line Street
Grenada, MS 38668 662-429-2354

Mary Murphy, Contact

Provides free literacy services.

3366 Tunica County Literacy Council

5217 Old Moon Landing Road
Tunica, MS 38676 662-363-1296

Betty Jo H Dulaney, Conact

Provides tutoring, childcare and educational services for Tunica youth and adults in reading, math, writing, life-skills and ESL in a safe environment.

Missouri

3367 Joplin NALA Read

PO Box 447
Joplin, MO 64802 417-782-2646
http://www.joplinnala.org
e-mail: joplinnala@joplin.com

Marj Boudreaux, Contact

3368 Literacy Investment for Tommorrow: St Louis

815 Olive Street
St Louis, MO 63101 314-678-4443
800-729-4443
FAX 314-678-2938
http://www.lift-missouri.org
e-mail: todeawebster.edu

Timothy O'Dea, Executive Director
Sarah Beaman-Jones, Literacy Program Developer

Provides training, technical assistance, and materials for educators and family literacy programs. Also, helps to improve literacy services by integrating research-proven practices into the field.

3369 Literacy Investment for Tomorrow: Saint Ann

500 Northwest Plaza
Saint Ann, MO 63074 314-291-4443
800-729-4443
FAX 314-678-2938
http://www.literacy.kent.edu/~missouri/
e-mail: lift@icon-stl.net

Sarah Beaman-Jones, Literacy Program Developer
Timothy , Executive Director

LIFT develops and promotes resources to increase literacy skills of Missourians so all individuals can reach their personal and economic potential.

3370 Literacy Kansas City

Pro Literacy America
205 W 65th Street
Kansas City, MO 64113 816-333-9332
FAX 816-444-6628
http://www.literacykc.org
e-mail: info@literacykc.org

Janis Doty, Program Director
Dianne Daldudrup, Executive Director

Literacy Kansas City is a 501 (c) (3) not-for-profit organization that helps adults from greater metropolitan Kansas City improve their basic literacy skills.

3371 Literacy Roundtable

5078 Kendington
St Louis, MO 63108 314-367-5000
FAX 314-367-3057
http://www.literacyroundtable.org
e-mail: maryann.kramer@slps.org

Mary Ann Kramer, Coordinator

A consortium of literacy service providers from throughout the St. Louis-Metro East area.

3372 MVCAA Adult/Family Literacy

1415 S Odell Avenue
Marshall, MO 65340 660-886-7476
FAX 660-886-5868
http://www.mvcaa.net
e-mail: info@mvcaa.net

Ann Graff, Executive Director

3373 Parkway Area Adult Education

12657 Fee Fee Road
St Louis, MO 63146 314-415-7063
FAX 314-415-5050
http://www.pkwy.k12.mo.us/ael
e-mail: pkwyael@yahoo.com

Sally Sandy, Program Director
Carol Diehl, ESL Coordinator
Merle Oberman, Literacy Coordinator

3374 St Louis Public Schools Adult Education and Literacy

5078 Kensington Avenue
St Louis, MO 63108 314-367-5000
FAX 314-367-3057
http://www.slps.org/departments/services.htm
e-mail: robert.weng@slps.org

Robert Weng, Administrator

Provides opportunities for adults to participate in the GED; ESOL; Workforce Development; Life Skills; Literacy Enhancement and Family Literacy programs.

Montana

3375 LVA Richland County

121 3rd Avenue NW
Sidney, MT 59270-4025 406-480-1970
http://www.richlandlva.org
e-mail: info@richlandlva.org

Sue Zimmerman, Program Coordinator

Helps area adults meet individual learning goals using trained volunteers.

3376 Literacy Volunteers of America: Montana

Pro Literacy Worldwide
PO Box 244
Butte, MT 59703 406-723-7905
888-606-7905
FAX 406-723-6196
e-mail: lvabulit@in-tch.com

Paula Arneson, Executive Director
Vicki Mihelich, Assistant Director

We provide adults and their families the opportunity to acquire skills to be effective in their roles as members of their families, communitites, and workplaces.

3377 Montana Literacy Resource Center

Montana State Library
PO Box 201800
Helena, MT 59620 406-444-3016
FAX 406-444-0266
TDY:406-444-3005
http://www.msl.mt.gov
e-mail: dstaffeldt@mt.gov

Darlene Dstaffeldt, State Librarian
Kris Schmitz, Head of Administration
Karen Strege, Manager
A state-wide literacy support network.

Nebraska

3378 **Answers4Families: Center on Children, Families, Law**
121 S 13th Street
Lincoln, NE 68508
402-472-0844
800-746-8420
http://www.answers4families.org/nrrs
e-mail: chayek@answers4families.org
Charlie Lewis, Director
Sharon Bloechle, Omaha Parent Coordinator

A project of the Center on Children, Families and Law at University of Nebraska. Mission is to provide info, opportunities, education and support to Nebraskans through Internet resources. The Center serves individuals with special needs and mental health disorders, foster families, caregivers, assisted living, and school nurses.

3379 **Client Assistance Program (CAP): Nebraska Division of Persons with Disabilities**
Nebraska Department of Education
301 Centennial Mall S
Lincoln, NE 68508
402-471-3656
800-742-7594
FAX 402-471-0117
http://www.nde.state.ne.us
e-mail: victoria@cap.state.ne.us
Frank Lloyd, Executive Director

The Client Assistance Program helps individuals who have concerns or difficulties when applying for or receiving rehabilitation services funded under the Rehabilitation Act.

3380 **Lincoln Literacy Council**
745 S 9th Street
Lincoln, NE 68508
402-476-7323
FAX 402-476-2122
http://www.lincolnliteracy.org
e-mail: info@lincolnliteracy.org
Brett Harris, President

Mission is to assist all people of all cultures in our community by teaching and fostering literacy.

3381 **Literacy Center for the Midlands**
3615 Dodge Street
Omaha, NE 68131-3218
402-342-7323
FAX 402-345-9045
http://www.midlandsliteracy.org
e-mail: staff@midlandsliteracy.org
Terry E Patterson, Executive Director
Patrick Mahoney, Program Director
Laura Pfeffer, Program Assistant
Mission is to provide free and confidential learning opportunitiees for all Omaha area residents who lack basic literacy skills; using as its corps, community volunteers who are trained to provide tutoring in a caring, nuturing one-on-one relationship.

3382 **Platte Valley Literacy Association**
2504 14th Street
Columbus, NE 68601
402-564-5196
FAX 402-563-3378
http://www.megavision.net/literacy
e-mail: literacy@megavision.com
Jolene Hake, Executive Director
Kelly McGowan, Volunteer Coordinator
Theresa Wachal, Family Literacy Director
Organization that collaborates with Central Community College Adult Basic Education to respond to the educational needs of our community.

3383 **State Literacy Resource Center for Nebraska: Institute for the Study of Adult Literacy**
Department of Vocational and Adult Education
222 Bancroft Hall
Lincoln, NE 68588
402-472-5924
FAX 402-472-5907
http://www.literacy.kent.edu
e-mail: bsparks1@unl.edu
Barbara Sparks, Director
Qian Geng, Coordinator

As the State Literacy Resource Center for Nebraska, NISAL provides a central point of contact for researchers, decision makers and literacy providers in Nebraska and serves as a vital link between providers and user groups, community based organizations, state agencies and business and industry. The institute enhances existing practice by promoting and providing information and resources to enhance and encourage best practices.

Nevada

3384 **Nevada Department of Adult Education**
Nevada Department of Education
700 E 5th Street
Carson City, NV 89701
775-884-6125
FAX 775-687-9114
http://www.literacynet.org/adulted
Mary Katherine Moen, Director

Provides adult basic education and literacy services in order to assist adults to become literate and obtain the knowledge and skills necessary for employment and self-sufficiency.

3385 **Nevada Economic Opportunity Board: Community Action Partnership**
PO Box 270880
Las Vegas, NV 89127
702-647-1510
FAX 702-647-6639
http://www.eobcap.org
James Lester Murray, Executive Director
Salinas Director Program Opera, Director Program Operations

Located in one of the fastest growing and most diverse communities in the United States, the Economic Opportunity Board of Clark County is a highly innovative Community Action Agency. Our mission is to eliminate poverty by providing programs, resources, services, and advocacy for self-sufficiency and economic empowerment.

3386 **Nevada Literacy Coalition: State Literacy Resource Center**
Pro Literacy Worldwide
100 N Stewart Street
Carson City, NV 89701
775-684-3340
800-445-9673
FAX 775-684-3344
http://www.nevadaculture.org/docs/nsla/literacy
e-mail: sfgraf@clan.lib.nv.us
Susan Graf, Literacy Coordinator
Sara Jones, Library Administrator

The Nevada State Literacy Resource Center has books, newsletters and a wide variety of multi-media resources such as videos, audiotapes and games for literacy instruction and programs for literacy students, trainers and tutors.

3387 **Northern Nevada Literacy Council**
1400 Wedekind Road
Reno, NV 89512
775-356-1007
FAX 775-356-1009
http://www.nnlc.org
e-mail: director@nnlc.org
Vicki Newell, Executive Director

Provides a framework that assists Nevada's communities in addressing their literacy needs at the local level.

New Hampshire

3388 **New Hampshire Literacy Volunteers of America**
Manchester City Library
405 Pine Street
Manchester, NH 03104
603-624-6550
FAX 603-624-6559
http://www.manchesternh.gov

Elizabeth Sabol, Program Director
Gwen Brown, Assistant Director

This program is the only nationally accredited adult literacy program in New Hampshire. Provides free confidential one-to-one tutoring for adults who want to learn to write and read for lifelong learning.

3389 New Hampshire Second Start Adult Education
17 Knight Street
Concord, NH 03301
603-228-1341
FAX 603-228-3852
http://www.second-start.org
e-mail: ABE@second-start.org
Gerry Mitchell, Manager

Provides basic reading, writing and math skills for people who want to achieve educational goals, participate in the life of the community, gain independence and become lifelong learners.

New Jersey

3390 Jersey City Library Literacy Program
472 Jersey Avenue
Jersey City, NJ 07302-3456
201-547-4518
FAX 201-435-5746
http://www.jclibrary.org
e-mail: literacy@jclibrary.org
Nancy G Sambul, Executive Director
Darnelle Richardson, Program Coordinator

Offers free, confidential, one-on-one basic skills literacy instructions for Jersey City residents age 16 and older through the Literacy Program Office, which is affiliated with Pro Literacy America.

3391 LVA Camden County
203 Laurel Road
Voorhees, NJ 08043-2349
856-772-1636
http://http://lva.camden.lib.nj.us
e-mail: literacy@camden.lib.nj.us
Jackie Mintz, Coordinator

3392 Literacy Volunteers in Mercer County
3535 Quakerbridge Road
Hamilton, NJ 08619
609-587-6027
FAX 609-587-6137
http://www.princetonol.com/groups/lvamc
e-mail: lvmercer@verizon.net
June Vogel, Contact

Provides comprehensive training in the skills necessary to teach and motivate adult students.

3393 Literacy Volunteers of America Essex/Passaic County
303 University Avenue
Newark, NJ 07102
973-733-9404
http://www.lvanewark.org
e-mail: lvanewark@verizon.net
Robert Dicker, Contact

Provides free literacy services to adults who have been identified as needing instruction in reading and/or english conversation; and families who are experiencing literacy and/or learning difficulties.

3394 Literacy Volunteers of Cape-Atlantic
743 N Main Street
Pleasantville, NJ 08232
609-383-337-
FAX 609-383-0234
http://www.lvacapeatlantic.org
e-mail: lvatula@comcast.net
Tula Christopoulos, Executive Director

Teaching people how to read, and offering English as a Second Language program.

3395 Literacy Volunteers of Englewood Library
31 Engle Street
Englewood, NJ 07631
201-568-2215
http://www.englewoodlibrary.org
Donald Jacobsen, Director

Offers three tutor-training workshops each year with an extensive collection of books, workbooks, and cassettes for tutors and students to borrow with a current library card.

3396 Literacy Volunteers of Gloucester County
PO Box 1106
Turnersville, NJ 08012-0876
856-218-4743
http://www.literacyvgc.org
Joan McAllister, Executive Director

Serving adults with free tutoring offered by tutors who have gone through a class specifically geared to teaching adults that haven't learned the conventional way.

3397 Literacy Volunteers of Middlesex
11 Stephen Street
South River, NJ 08882-1240
732-432-8000
FAX 732-432-8189
http://www.lva-middlesex.org
e-mail: lvm24libs@aol.com
Mary Ellen Firestone, President
Christine Sienkielewski, Program Director

Trained volunteers that provide free tutoring services to adults with limited literacy skills, enabling them to achieve their personal goals and to enhance their contributions to the community.

3398 Literacy Volunteers of Monmouth County
213 Broadway
Long Branch, NJ 07740-7005
732-571-0209
http://www.lvmonmouthnj.org
e-mail: lvmonmouth@brookdalecc.edu
Rebecca Lucas, Contact

Mission is to promote increased literacy for adults in Monmouth County, through the effective use of volunteers and collaboration with individuals, groups and organizations desiring to foster increased literacy.

3399 Literacy Volunteers of Morris County
36 S Street
Morristown, NJ 07960
973-984-1998
FAX 973-971-0291
http://www.lvamorris.org
e-mail: lvamorris@yahoo.com
Beverly Shimada, Contact

Provides one-on-one or small group tutoring in basic literacy and english as a second language to adults in Morris COunty.

3400 Literacy Volunteers of Plainfield PublicLibrary
800 Park Avenue
Pplainfield, NJ 07060
908-755-7998
FAX 908-754-0063
http://www.plainfieldlibrary.info
e-mail: joseph.daroid.plfdpl.info
Joe Da Rold, Contact

Mission is to develop the literacy skills of adults with minimum reading skills.

3401 Literacy Volunteers of Somerset County
120 Finderne Avenue
Bridgewater, NJ 08807
908-725-5430
FAX 908-707-2077
http://www.lvscnj.org
e-mail: lvsc@optonline.net
Doryce L Wheeler, Contact

Promotes literacy through a network of community volunteers.

3402 **Literacy Volunteers of Union County**
201 W Grove Street E
Westfield, NJ 07090 908-518-0600
FAX 908-518-0601
http://www.lvaunion.org
e-mail: elizabeth@lvaunion.org
Elizabeth Gloeggler, Executive Director
Dawn Harrison, Field Services Coordinator
Claudia Freire, Outreach Coordinator
Committed to increasing literacy for adults and their families; effectively utilizing and supporting volunteers in delivery of services; and providing research, training and technical assistance related to the various aspects of literacy.

3403 **New Jersey Literacy Volunteers of America: Peoplecare Center**
Pro Literacy America
120 Finderne Avenue
Bridgewater, NJ 08807 908-203-4582
800-848-0048
FAX 908-203-4585
e-mail: lvanj@aol.com
Elissa Director, Executive Director
Mitch Heather, Administrative Assistant

Literacy Volunteers of America-New Jersey (LVA-NJ) is a non-profit, education organization providing training, technical assistance, communications, and program support to adult literacy organizations in New Jersey. It directs most of its services to its affiliated community based organizations located in twenty counties of the state.

New Mexico

3404 **Adult Basic Education Division of Dona Ana Community College**
PO Box 30001
Las Cruces, NM 88003-8001 505-527-7641
800-903-7503
FAX 505-527-7515
http://http://dabcc-www.nmsu.edu/comm/abe
e-mail: sdegiuli@nmsu.edu
Stephen DeGiulio, Coordinator, Literacy Services

3405 **Carlsbad Literacy Program**
Ann Wood Literacy Center
511 N 12th Street
Carlsbad, NM 88220 505-885-1752
FAX 505-885-7980
http://www.pccnm.com/customer/literacy
e-mail: literacy@pccnm.com
Delora C Elizondo, Coordinator
Jessie Morales, Literacy Assistant
Katie Dominquez, Literacy Assistant
An educational and charitable non-profit organization dedicated to reducing illiteracy in Carlsbad and surrounding areas.

3406 **Curry County Literacy Council**
417 Schepps Boulevard
Clovis, NM 88101 505-769-4095
http://www.clovis.edu/cclc
e-mail: curry.literacy@clovis.edu
Miranda Gerberding, Director

Goal is to provide one with a sense of security to gain employment, have life skills, and assist in language development.

3407 **Deming Literacy Program**
PO Box 1932
Deming, NM 88031 505-546-7571
FAX 505-546-1356
e-mail: dlp@zianet.com
Marisol Perez, Contact

The Literacy Home Mentoring and After School Project will encourage parents to read to their children at home, as well as provide mentors to help children with their reading skills after school.

3408 **Literacy Center of Albuquerque**
3113 Carlisle nE
Albuquerque, NM 87110
FAX 505-884-3129
http://www.lcbq.org
e-mail: lcabq@flash.net
Kathleen Salas, Program Coordinator

The Literacy Center of Albuquerque is a non-profit organization of students, tutors and supporters working together to enhance the lives of people with English as a Second Language and addresses literacy needs by providing programs through volunteers and community resources.

3409 **Literacy Volunteers of America: Cibola County**
Pro Literacy Worldwide
PO Box 306
Grants, NM 87020 505-285-5995
FAX 505-285-5995
http://www.7cities.net
e-mail: lvagrants@7cities.net
Barbara Wesley, Executive Director

Offers basic reading and ESL tutoring at no charge to adults in Cibola County.

3410 **Literacy Volunteers of America: Dona Ana County**
Dona Ana Branch Community College
3400 S Espina Street
Las Cruces, NM 88003 505-527-7540
800-903-7540
FAX 505-527-7515
http://http://dabcc-www.nmsu.edu/comm/abe
e-mail: sdegiuli@nmsu.edu
Sylvia Nickerson, Executive Director
Patricia Moncoya, Secretary

The Literacy Volunteers of America is designed to help people who cannot read or write the English language. This program gives adults a new opportunity to learn reading through the sixth-grade level.

3411 **Literacy Volunteers of America: Las Vegas, San Miguel**

PO Box 516
Las Vegas, NM 87701 505-454-8043
http://www.nmhu.edu
Ann Costello, Director

Las Vegas/San Miquel Literacy Volunteers are a part of the national non-profit organization Literacy Volunteers of America, which is dedicated to promoting literacy throughout the country.

3412 **Literacy Volunteers of America: Otero County**
New Mexico State University at Alamogordo
2400 Scenic Drive
Alamogordo, NM 88310 505-439-3600
FAX 505-439-3643
http://www.alamo.nmsu.edu
e-mail: raynor@nmsua.nmsu.edu
Anita Raynor, Director for Adult Basic Ed
Roger Bates, CEO
Angie Gorgensen, Bookstore Manager
Can provide volunteer tutors to work one-on-one with adult non-readers and non-English speaking adults. All these services are provided free of charge to adults.

3413 **Literacy Volunteers of America: Read West**
PO Box 44058
Rio Rancho, NM 87174 505-892-1131
FAX 505-892-1131
http://www.readwest.org
e-mail: readwest@earthlink.net
Susan Ryerson, Executive Director

Programs that assist adults in reading development. English as a second language program offered. Family literacy workshops for parents.

3414 Literacy Volunteers of America: Santa Fe
6401 S Richards Avenue
Santa Fe, NM 87508
505-428-1353
FAX 505-428-1237
http://www.lvsf.net
e-mail: lnaranjo@sfccnm.edu
Letty Naranjo, Executive Director
Catherine Johnson, Program Coordinator

Literacy Volunteers of Santa Fe was established to provide free tutoring services for adults in the Santa Fe area seeking to improve their reading skills or learn English as a second language.

3415 Literacy Volunteers of America: Socorro County
PO Box 1431
Socorro, NM 87801
505-835-4659
FAX 505-835-1182
e-mail: lva_socorro@hotmail.com
Joyce Aguilar, Executive Director

Promotes literacy for people of Socorro County.

3416 New Mexico Coalition for Literacy
3209 Mercantile Court
Santa Fe, NM 87507
505-982-3997
800-233-7587
FAX 505-982-4095
http://www.nmcl.org
e-mail: info@nmcl.org
Rena Paradis, Executive Director
Harry Pearson, President

The Coalition encourages and supports community-based literacy programs and is the New Mexico affiliate and coordinator for the national program of ProLiteracy America.

3417 Read West
2009 Grande Boulevard
Rio Rancho, NM 87174-4508
505-892-1131
FAX 505-896-3780
http://www.readwest.org
e-mail: readwest@earthlink.net
Susan Ryerson, Executive Director
Rosalie Romero, Volunteer Coordinator

Providing one-to-one tutoring by trained certified volunteers, FREE OF CHARGE.

3418 Roosevelt County Literacy Council
218 S Avenue B
Portales, NM 88130
505-356-8500
http://www.rclc.yucca.net
e-mail: rclc@yucca.net
Sue Alexander, Executive Director
Martha A Lemus, Coordinator

Mission is to provide literacy opportuinites to all residents of Roosevelt County, and to encourage citizen interest and community cooperation in the development of a totally literacte population.

3419 Roswell Literacy Council
609 W 10th Street
Roswell, NM 88201
505-625-1369
http://www.roswell-literacy.org
e-mail: literacy@dfn.com
Andrae England, Director

Dedicated to literacy development and to teaching English speakers of other languages in Roswell and the surrounding communities in Chaves County.

3420 Valencia County Literacy Council
Belen Public Library
280 La Entrada Road
Los Lunas, NM 87031
505-925-8926
FAX 505-864-7798
http://www.golibrary.org/vclc.htm
e-mail: joglesby@unm.edu
Jill Oglesby, Executive Director

Promotes and supports literacy in the area.

New York

3421 Literacy Volunteers of America: Middletown
Literacy Volunteers of Western County Incorporated
70 Fulton Street
Middletown, NY 10940
845-341-5460
FAX 845-343-7191
http://www.literacymiddletown.org
e-mail: baclvamdtn@frontiernet.net
Barbara Clifford, Executive Director
Rowena Reich, Program Coordinator

An organization of volunteers which provides a variety of services to enable people to achieve personal goals through literacy. We believe that the ability to read is critical to personal freedom and maintenance of a democratic society. These beliefs have led us to make the following commitments: the personal growth of our students; the effective use of our volunteers; the improvement of society and strengthening and improving our organization.

3422 Literacy Volunteers of Oswego County
100 E 1st Street
Oswego, NY 13126-2105
315-342-8839
http://www.lvoswego.org
e-mail: lvoswego@verizon.net
Jane Murphy, Contact

3423 Literacy Volunteers of Otsego/Delaware Counties
Oneonta Community Education Center
10 Market Street
Oneonta, NY 13820
607-433-3645
800-782-3858
FAX 607-433-3649
http://www.oneontaadulted.org
e-mail: jeanetcm@oneonta.edu
Cathy Jeanette, Contact

3424 New York Laubach Literacy International
ProLiteracy Worldwide
1320 Jamesville Avenue
Syracuse, NY 13210
315-422-9121
888-528-2224
FAX 315-422-6369
http://www.proliteracy.org
e-mail: info@proliteracy.org
Robert Wedgeworth, President

The Syracuse chapters of the world's two largest adult volunteer literacy organization merged and Laubach Literacy International and Literacy Volunteers of America became ProLiteracy Worldwide. This organization sponsors educational programs and services for adults and their families. These programs assist participants to acquire the literacy practices and skills needed to function more effectively in their daily lives and participate in their societies.

3425 New York Literacy Assistance Center
32 Broadway
New York, NY 10004
212-803-3300
FAX 212-785-3685
http://www.lacnyc.org
e-mail: elyser@lacnyc.org
Ira Yankwitt, Director of Adult Literacy
Elyse Rudolph, Executive Director

Founded in 1983, a not-for-profit organization that provides essential referral, training information and technical assistance services to hundreds of adult and youth literacy programs in New York. Our mission is to support and promote the expansion of quality literacy services in New York.

3426 New York Literacy Partners
30 E 33rd Street
New York, NY 10016
212-725-9200
FAX 212-725-9744
http://www.literacypartners.org
e-mail: susanne@literacypartners.org
Susan McLean, Executive Director
Doris Meister, Executive VP

Literacy Partners, is a not-for-profit organization, providing free community-based adult and family literacy programs to ensure that all adults have the access to quality education needed to fully realize their potential as individuals, parents, and citizens.

3427 New York Literacy Resource Center
State University of New York
135 Western Avenue
Albany, NY 12222
518-443-5662
800-331-0931
FAX 518-442-5021
http://www.albany.edu
Maritza Ramirez-Vallinas, Director

State Literacy Resource Center is a statewide literacy information network throughout the state.

3428 New York Literacy Volunteers of America
Literacy Volunteers of New York State
777 Maryvale Drive
Buffalo, NY 14225
716-631-5282
FAX 716-631-0657
http://www.lvanys.org
e-mail: cuddanee@aol.com
Janice Cuddahee, Associate Executive Director
Rosalinde Mecca, Program Director
Kevin Smith, CEO
Literacy Volunteers of America in New York State is a nonprofit educational organization that provides training and technical assistance to 48 local, community-based literacy programs in New York. In addition, LVA-NYS offers consultation services and support to literacy organizations nationally.

3429 Resources for Children with Special Needs
116 E 16th Street
New York, NY 10003
212-677-4650
FAX 212-254-4070
http://www.resourcesnyc.org
e-mail: info@resourcesnyc.org
Karen Schlesinger, Executive Director
Helene Crane, Associate Director

An independent, nonprofit organization that provides information and referral, case management and support, individual and systemic advocacy, parent and professional training and library services to New York City parents and caregivers of children with disabilities and special needs and to professionals who work with them. Our publications include: Camps 2003; After School and more; The Comprehensive Directory; and Schools for Children with Autisum Spectrum Disorders.

North Carolina

3430 Blue Ridge Literacy Council
PO Box 1728
Hendersonville, NC 28793
828-696-3811
FAX 828-696-3887
http://www.litcouncil.org
e-mail: info@litcouncil.org
Diane Bowers, Executive Director

The Blue Ridge Literacy Council provides Henderson County adult students the English communication and literacy skills they need to reach their full potential as individuals, parents, workers and citizens.

3431 Buncombe County Literacy Council
86 Victoria Road
Asheville, NC 28801
828-254-3442
FAX 828-254-1742
http://www.main.nc.us/literacy
e-mail: literacy@main.buncombe.nc.us
Amanda Edwards, Executive Director
Irma Khasanoza, Office Manager

Promotes increased adult literacy in Buncombe County through effective use of trained tutors; to provide support services for tutors and learners; and to collaborate with individuals, groups, or other community organizations desiring to foster increased adult literacy.

3432 Durham Literacy Center
1410 W Chapel Hill Street
Durham, NC 27701
919-489-8383
FAX 919-489-1456
http:// www.durhamliteracy.org
e-mail: info@durhamliteracy.org
Reginald Hodges, Executive Director
George Kariuki, Office Manager

The Durham Literacy Center provides training in adult basic education (including reading, writing and mathematics), English for Speakers of Other Languages, GED examination preparation, Family Literacy, workplace literacy, and technology.

3433 Gaston Literacy Council
116 S Marietta Street
Gastonia, NC 28052
704-868-4815
FAX 704-867-7796
http://www.gastonliteracy.org
e-mail: literacy@gaston.org
Kaye Gribble, Executive Director

The Gaston Literacy Council is dedicated to improving literacy throughout the Gastonia area.

3434 Gastonia Literacy Council
116 S Marietta Street
Gastonia, NC 28052
704-868-4815
FAX 704-867-7796
http://www.gastonliteracy.org
e-mail: literacy@gaston.org
Kaye Gribble, Executive Director

The Gaston Literacy Council is dedicated to improving literacy throughout the Gastonia area.

3435 Literacy Volunteers of America: Pitt County
504 Dexter Street
Greenville, NC 27834
252-353-6578
FAX 252-353-6868
e-mail: literacyvolunteers@geeksnet.com
Laura Smith, Executive Director

The mission of LVA-PC is to teach adults to read or improve their reading, writing or English speaking skills through free, confidential, and small group instruction by trained volunteers.

3436 North Carolina Literacy Resource Center
North Carolina Community College
200 W Jones Street
Raleigh, NC 27699
919-828-4387
FAX 919-807-7164
http://www.ncccs.cc.nc.us
e-mail: ALLENB@ncccs.cc.nc.us
Elizabeth Fentress, President
Bob Allen, Coordinator
Marge Young, Assistant
North Carolina Community College Literacy Resource Center collects and disseminates information about literacy resources and organizations.

3437 Reading Connections of North Carolina
122 N Elm Street
Greensboro, NC 27401
336-230-2223
FAX 336-230-2203
http://www.Readingconnections.org
e-mail: info@readingconnections.org
Jennifer Gore, Executive Director
Ira Williams, Program Coordinator

The mission of Reading Connections is to help adults live more independently by providing free and confidential basic literacy services, to increase community awareness of adult literacy needs and to serve as a resource for the provision of basic literacy services.

North Dakota

3438 North Dakota Adult Education and Literacy Resource Center
1609 4th Avenue NW
Minot, ND 58703
701-857-4467
FAX 701-857-4489
http://www.dpi.state.nd.us/adulted/
e-mail: deb.sisco@sendit.nodex.edu

Deb Sisco, Coordinator
Vicky Campbell, Director

The purpose of the North Dakota Adult Education Resource Center is to provide training for adult education staff and volunteer personnel engaged in programs designed to carry out the purposes of the National Literacy Act.

3439 North Dakota Department of Career and Technical Education
600 E Boulevard Avenue
Bismarck, ND 58505
701-328-2455
FAX 701-328-1255
http://www.state.nd.us
e-mail: cte@state.nd.us

Wayne Kutcer, Director
Bryan Klipfel, Manager

The mission of the Board for Vocational and Technical Education is to work with others to provide all North Dakota citizens with the technical skills, knowledge, and attitudes necessary for successful performance in a globally competitive workplace.

3440 North Dakota Department of Corrections
3100 Railroad Avenue
Bismarck, ND 58501
701-328-6372
FAX 701-328-6651
TDY:800-366-6888
http://www.state.nd.us
e-mail: elittle@state.nd.us

Elaine Little, Director
Michael Froemke, Manager
Jeannine Piatz, Administrative Assistant

Mission is to protect the public while providing a safe and humane environment for both adults and juveniles placed in the department's care and custody.

3441 North Dakota Department of Human Services:Welfare & Public Assistance
State Capitol
600 E Boulevard Avenue
Bismarck, ND 58505
701-328-2310
800-472-2622
FAX 701-328-2359
http://www.state.nd.us/humanservices
e-mail: dhseo@state.nd.us

Carol Olson, Executive Director
Yvonne Smith, Deputy Director

To provide services and support for poor, disabled, ill, elderly or juvenile clients in North Dakota.

3442 North Dakota Department of Public Instruction
600 E Boulevard Avenue
Bismarck, ND 58505
701-328-2260
FAX 701-328-2461
http://www.dpi.state.nd.us
e-mail: dpiweb@mail.dpi.state.nd.us

Wayne G Sanstead, Director
Jolli Marcellais, Administrative Assistant

This unit provides funding and technical assistance to local programs and monitors progress of each funded project. This unit is also responsible for the administration of the GED Testing Program.

3443 North Dakota Reading Association
2420 2nd Avenue SW
Minot, ND 58701
701-857-4642
FAX 701-857-8761
http://http://ndreadon.utma.com
e-mail: Paula.Rogers@sendit.nodak.edu

Joyce Hinman, IRA State Coordinator
Paula Rogers, VP

North Dakota Reading Association's mission is to provide a variety of professional development opportunities.

3444 North Dakota Workforce Development Council
North Dakota Department of Commerce
PO Box 2057
Bismarck, ND 58502
701-328-5300
FAX 701-328-5320
http://www.ndcommerce.com
e-mail: commerce@nd.gov

Paul Govig, Interim Director
Lee Peterson, Commissioner Department of Comme

The role of the North Dakota Workforce Development Council is to advise the Governor and the Public concerning the nature and extent of workforce development in the context of North Dakota's economic development needs, and how to meet these needs effectively while maximizing the efficient use of available resources and avoiding unnecessary duplication of effort.

3445 Project Advancing Literacy
2110 Library Circle
Grand Forks, ND 58201-6324
701-772-6344
FAX 701-772-1379
http://www.grandforksgov.com/readpal
e-mail: info@grandforksgov.com

Barbara J Knipe, Contact

Project Advancing Literacy (PAL) is a basic literacy support program among adults in the Greater Grand Forks area. PAL provides one-to-one tutoring support to those who have identified a need to increase basic literacy.

3446 Project Advancing Literacy in North Dakota
2110 Library Circle
Grand Forks, ND 58201
701-772-6344
FAX 701-772-1379
http://www.grandforksgov.com/readpal
e-mail: info@grandforksgov.com

Diane Bell, President
Dennis Page, Treasurer

Project Advancing Literacy (PAL) is a basic literacy support program among adults in the Greater Grand Forks area. PAL provides one-to-one tutoring support to those who have identified a need to increase basic literacy.

Ohio

3447 Central/Southeast ABLE Resource CenterOhio University
338 McCraken Hall
Athens, OH 45701
740-593-4419
800-753-1519
FAX 740-593-2834
http://www.able-ohiou.org
e-mail: fantine@ohio.edu

Jeff Fantine, Director
Tom Davis, Grant Administrator
Robbie James, Res Ctr Specialist/Prgm Liaison

Provides leadership and expertise in the areas of professional development and instructional resources for Adult Basic and Literacy Education (ABLE) staff.

3448 Clark County Literacy Coalition
137 E High Street
Springfield, OH 45502-1215
937-323-8617
FAX 937-328-6911
http://www.clarkcountyliteracy.org
e-mail: support@clarkcountyliteracy.org

Jeffery S Clouse, President
Priscilla Marshall, Contact

Composed of thirteen members and two honorary members united to support literacy issues, while others provide literacy education and other services to other Clark County individuals.

3449 Columbus Literacy Council
195 N Grant Avenue
Columbus, OH 43215 614-221-5013
http://www.columbusliteracy.com
e-mail: columbusliteracy@columbusliteracy.org
Tammy Wharton, Executive Director
LeRoy Boikai, Program Director

Modes of instruction include one-to-one tutoring, small group instruction and computer-assisted instruction.

3450 Family Learning Center
701 Wayne Street
Marietta, OH 45750 740-374-6548
FAX 740-376-2457
http://http://familylearningcenter.net
e-mail: ma_mkern@seovec.org
Mary Kern, Executive Director

Provides individualized and small group instruction in basic skills areas including reading, math,writing, computers, GED preparation, English as a Second Language, and U.S. Citizenship.

3451 Literacy Council of Clermont/Brown Counties
756 Old State Route 74
Cincinnati, OH 45245 513-943-3740
FAX 513-943-3002
http://www.clermontbrownliteracy.org
e-mail: susan.vilardo@clermontbrownliteracy.org
Susan Vilardo, Executive Director

Mission is to enable adults to acquire basic listening, speaking, reading and writing skills needed to participate fully in society, and to increase awareness of literacy needs in our community.

3452 Literacy Council of Medina County
Project Learn
222 S Broadway Street
Medina, OH 44256 330-723-1314
FAX 330-722-6033
http://www.projectlearnmedina.org
e-mail: dmorawski@zoominternet.net
Diane Morawski, Executive Director

Our program helps individuals 14 and older improve basic reading, writing, spelling and comprehensive skills necessary to meet the challenges they encounter in the workplace and other aspects of their daily lives. It provides the only one-on-one tutoring available free of charge to anyone interested in improving basic skills.

3453 Miami Valley Literacy Council
18 W 1st Street
Dayton, OH 45402-1249 937-223-4922
FAX 937-223-0271
http://www.discoverliteracy.org
e-mail: mvlc@discoverliteracy.org
Kathy Bohachek, Chief Executive Officer
Michelle Brown, Director Education & Programs

Promoting literacy and strengthening adult learners and children who are functioning at the lowest literacy levels through instruction, supportive services and resources.

3454 Ohio Literacy Network
6161 Busch Boulevard
Columbus, OH 43229 614-505-0716
FAX 614-505-0718
http://www.ohioliteracynetwork.org
e-mail: atoops@ohioliteracynetworking.org
Maureen O'Rourke, Executive Director

The Ohio Literacy Network is an association of organizations and individuals dedicated to helping adults achieve effectively in today's society, and to promote public awareness of adult literacy issues and needs.

3455 Ohio Literacy Resource Center
Kent State University
PO Box 5190
Kent, OH 44242 330-672-2497
800-765-2897
FAX 330-672-4841
http://www.literacy.kent.edu/oasis/
e-mail: olrc@literacy.kent.edu
Marty Ropog, Director
John Crawford, Manager

Mission is to stimulate joint planning and coordination of literacy services at the local, regional and state levels and to enhance the capacity of state and local organizations and services delivery systems.

3456 Project L.I.T.E
351 6th Street
Lorain, OH 44052 440-244-1192
800-322-READ
FAX 440-244-1733
http://www.lorain.lib.oh.us
e-mail: contact-lite@lorain.lib.oh.us
Linda Pierce, Contact

3457 Project LEARN of Summit County
60 S High Street
Akron, OH 44326 330-434-9461
866-866-7323
http://http://projectlearnsummit.org
e-mail: info@projectlearnsummit.org
Rick McIntosh, Executive Director
Kolter Kiess, Family Literacy Coordinator
Marquita Mitchell, Program Manager
Non-profit, community-based organization providing Summit County's nonreading adult population with free, confidential, small group classes and tutoring.

3458 Project Learn of Summit County
Pro Literacy America
60 S High Street
Akron, OH 44326 330-434-9461
866-866-7323
FAX 330-643-9195
http://www.projectlearnsummit.org
e-mail: info@projectlearnsummit.org
Rick McIntosh, Executive Director
Marquita Mitchell, Program Manager

Project LEARN is a nonprofit, community-based organization providing Summit County's nonreading adult population with free, confidential, small group classes and tutoring.

3459 Seeds of Literacy Project: St Colman Family Learning Center
2001 W 65th Street
Cleveland, OH 43624 216-651-4302
http://www.seedsforliteracy.org
e-mail: seedsofliteracy@hotmail.com
Bonnie Hogue Entler, Contact

Helping adults in need of assistance in reading, writing and mathematical skills and to improve their ability to function, compete, and advance in society in an atmosphere of Christian care and compassion.

Oklahoma

3460 Center for Study of Literacy: Northeastern Center
Po Box 549
Muskogee, OK 74402-0549 918-456-5511
FAX 918-781-5425
http://www.nsuok.edu/literacy/index.html
e-mail: mcelroyt@nsuok.edu
Tim McElroy, Director

Mission is to provide the illiterate or undereducated adult with training, provide instructional support for the Northwestern State University's faculty and pre-service teachers participate in computer literacy training to gain an understanding of computer assisted instruction. To serve as a resource for other social agencies, teachers, administrators and public school students, to serve as the clearinghouse for literacy for the state of Oklahoma, and to initiate reasearch on literacy.

3461 Community Literacy Center
3707 Blackwelder Avenue
Oklahoma City, OK 73146 405-524-7323
http://www.communityliteracy.com
e-mail: okread@aol.com
Becky O'Dell, Executive Director
Shelley Anderson, Education Program Coordinator

Using private contributions we apply sound educational principles with a business perspective to create the most innovative, cost efficient means to teach thousands to read inexpensively.

3462 Creek County Literacy Program
Sapulpa Public Library
27 W Dewey Avenue
Sapulpa, OK 74066 918-224-5624
FAX 918-224-3546
http://www.cityofsapulpa.net
e-mail: creeklit@yahoo.com
Barbara Belk, Executive Director
Bessie Krajicek, Manager

Free one-on-one tutoring services for those residents of Creek County who wish to improve reading skills.

3463 Great Plains Literacy Council: Southern Prairie Library System
421 N Hudson Street
Altus, OK 73521 580-477-2890
http://www.spls.lib.ok.us
e-mail: literacy1@spls.lib.ok.us
Katherine Hale, Director

Helps to increase the awareness of the illiteracy problem and offers a viable solution. Recruits, dedicated humanitarian tutors who help to motivate those who are considered illiterate and give them the opportunity to become contributing members of the community.

3464 Guthrie Literacy Program
201 N Division Street
Guthrie, OK 73044 405-282-0050
http://www.guthrie.okpls.org
e-mail: hefjek@swbell.net
Melody Kellogg, Contact
Jeanne Kuhlman, Contact

Utilizes curriculum that focuses on the individual student's interests and needs, then tutors help the student set the goals and work with them to achieve those goals.

3465 Junior League of Oklahoma City
1001 NW Grand Boulevard
Oklahoma City, OK 73118 405-843-5668
FAX 405-843-0994
http://www.jloc.org
e-mail: info@jloc.org
Betsy Mantor, President
Ann-Clare Duncan, Contact

Organization of women committed to promoting volunteerism, developing the potential of women and to improving the community through the effective action and leadership of trained volunteers. The purpose is exclusively educational and charitable.

3466 Literacy & Evangelism International
1800 S Jackson Avenue
Tulsa, OK 74107 918-585-3826
http://www.literacyevangelism.org
e-mail: general@literacyevangelism.org
John Taylor, Contact

A missionary fellowship, Chirstians from various nations and denominations, drawn together by a passion for God and compassion for people who cannot yet read the Word of God.

3467 Literacy Volunteers of America: Tulsa City County Library
400 Civic Center
Tulsa, OK 74103 918-596-7977
FAX 918-596-7907
http://www.tulsalibrary.org/central
e-mail: jgreb@tccl.lib.ok.us
Linda Saferite, Executive Director
Richard Parker, Deputy Director

We offer one-on-one tutoring to adults and young adults who wish to improve their reading and writing skills.

3468 Muskogee Area Literacy Council
Muskogee Public Library
801 W Okmulgee Street
Muskogee, OK 74401-6800 908-682-6657
888-291-8152
FAX 918-682-9466
http://www.eok.lib.ok.us
e-mail: loetaa@eok.lib.ok.us
Loeta Adams, Literacy Coordinator
Janette Rose, Contact

3469 Northwest Oklahoma Literacy Council
1500 Main Street
Woodward, OK 73801 580-254-8582
FAX 580-254-8546
e-mail: nwoklitcouncil@woodward.lib.ok.us
Cathy Johnson, Contact
Patty McGuire, Contact

Mission is to break the intergenerational cycle of illiteracy by broadening the learner and service base to include family members. Services include literacy and parenting instruction, as a compliment to ESL, adult basic education, and learning disabilities programs.

3470 Oklahoma Literacy Council
300 Park Avenue
Oklahoma City, OK 73102-3600 405-232-3780
FAX 405-236-5219
http://www.literacyokc.org
e-mail: literacycouncil@metrolibrary.org
Millonn B Lamb, Contact

3471 Oklahoma Literacy Resource Center
Oklahoma Department of Libraries
200 NE 18th Street
Oklahoma City, OK 73105 405-521-2502
800-522-8116
FAX 405-525-7804
http://www.odl.state.ok.us/literacy
e-mail: lgelders@oltn.state.ok.us
Leslie Gelders, Literacy Coordinator
Colleen Woolery, Family Literacy Coordinator
Susan Vey, Executive Director
Dedicated to supporting Oklahoma's library and community based literacy programs and their volunteer tutors. The office has been serving the literacy community in Oklahoma since 1983, first as the ODL Literacy Office, and now as the Oklahoma Literacy Resource Office.

3472 Opportunities Industrialization Center of Oklahoma County
400 N Walnut Avenue
Oklahoma City, OK 73104 405-235-2651
FAX 405-235-2653
http://http://oicofoklahomacounty.org
e-mail: oicoc@sbcglobal.net
Patricia Kelly, Executive Director
Shannon Carter, Literacy Instructor
Dickie Johnson, ABE/GED Instructor
Providing individualized services, education, and skills training to anyone who would need a special place-and a special staff-that could help make their dreams of a better, more prepared future come true.

3473 **Pontotoc County Literacy Coalition**
124 S Rennie Street
Ada, OK 74820
580-436-5443
http://www.adalit.okpls.org
e-mail: pclc@ada.lib.ok.us
Mary Ellen Davenport, President
Dell Harris, Program Director

3474 **Pushmataha County Literacy Council**
PO Box 8
Snow, OK 74567
580-298-5365
http://http://geocities.com/pushliteracycouncil
e-mail: pushliteracycouncil@yahoo.com
Fred Kimball, Contact

Volunteers that help adults who want to read and write better by tutoring them one-on-one.

Oregon

3475 **Benton Literacy Council**
1745 Menlo Drive
Corvallis, OR 97330
541-754-8615
http://www.oregonliteracy.org/bentonliteracy
e-mail: bentonliteracy@copper.net
Perry E Niskanen, Director

Goal is to improve the basic literacy skills of county residents.

3476 **Literacy Council of Eugene/Springfield**
51 W Broadway
Eugene, OR 97401-3254
541-344-3949
e-mail: literacy.e@juno.com
Gail Weathers, Program Coordinator
Marjorie Smith, Director

Recruits volunteers from the community to tutor, one-to-one, adult learners in basic skills (reading, writing, math) or to teach them to speak English , with no charge for the service.

3477 **Oregon Department of Corrections**
2575 Center Street NE
Salem, OR 97301
503-945-9090
FAX 503-373-1173
http://www.oregon.gov/ddc/
e-mail: DOCinfo@doc.state.or.us
Max Williams, Executive Director
Mitch Morrow, Deputy Director

The Oregon Department of Corrections is responsible for the management and administration of all adult correctional institutions and other functions related to state programs for adult corrections.

3478 **Oregon Department of Education: School-to-Work**
255 Capitol Street NE
Salem, OR 97310
503-986-4614
FAX 503-378-2892
TDY:503-378-2892
http://www.ode.state.or.us
e-mail: rob.larson@state.or.us
Katy Coba, Executive Director
Patrick Burk, Education Policy Deputy
Robert Larson, Policy & Research Director
School-to-Work is a federally funded initiative that provides funding for state and local implementation of the Oregon Educational Act for the 21st Century.

3479 **Oregon Department of Human Resource Adult & Family Services Division**
500 Summer Street NE
Salem, OR 97310
503-945-5944
FAX 503-378-2897
http://www.dhs.state.or.us
e-mail: dhr.info@state.or.us
Ramona Foley, Assistant Director
Gary Weeks, Director
Bruce Goldberg, Executive Director

This group combines programs from the former Adult & Family Services Division and the State Office for Services to Children and Families.

3480 **Oregon Employment Department**
875 Union Street NE
Salem, OR 97311
503-947-1394
800-237-3710
FAX 503-947-1668
http://www.workinoregon.com
Laurie Warner, Director
Greg Hickman, Deputy Director

Supports economic stability for Oregonians and communities during times of unemployment through the payment of unemployment benefits. Serves businesses by recruiting and referring the best qualified applicants to jobs, and provides resources to diverse job seekers in support of their employment needs.

3481 **Oregon GED Administrator: Office of Community College Services**
255 Capitol Street NE
Salem, OR 97310
503-378-8648
FAX 503-378-3365
http://www.oregon.gov/ccwd
e-mail: Sharlene.WALKER@state.or.us
Deborah Lares, GED Administrator

Mission is to contribute leadership and resources to increase the skills, knowledge and career opportunities of Oregonians.

3482 **Oregon Literacy**
1001 SW 5th Avenue
Portland, OR 97204
503-244-3898
800-322-8715
FAX 503-244-9147
http://www.oregonliteracy.org
e-mail: info@oregonliteracy.org
John Toorock, Director For Community Developme
Elizabeth Raymond, Executive Director

Mission is to increase the capacity and effectiveness of literacy services through partnerships with community-based programs across the state.

3483 **Oregon Office of Education and Workforce Policy**
900 Court Street NE
Salem, OR 97301
503-378-4582
FAX 503-378-4863
http://www.arcweb.sos.state.or.us
e-mail: annette.talbott@state.or.us
Annette Talbott, Workforce Policy Coordinator
Danny Santos, Education Policy Coordinator

The Governor's Office of Education and Workforce Policy was established to assist the Governor in examining education and workforce efforts with a view to supporting and strengthening what is working well. The goal is to have Oregonians prepared to meet the education and workforce needs of Oregon businesses rather than having to recruit from outside the state to fill quality jobs.

3484 **Oregon State Library**
250 Winter Street NE
Salem, OR 97310
503-378-4243
FAX 503-588-7119
TDY:503-585-8059
http://www.oregon.gov/osl
e-mail: leann.bromeland@state.or.us
Jim Scheppke, Manager
LeAnn Bromeland, Volunteer Coordinator

Mission is to provide quality information services to Oregon state government, to provide reading materials to blind and print-disabled Oregonians, and to provide leadership, grants, and other assistance to improve local library service for all Oregonians.

3485 Oregon State Literacy Resource Center
Department of Community Colleges & Workforce
255 Capitol Street NE
Salem, OR 97310
503-378-8648
FAX 503-378-8434
http://www.oregon.gov/ccwd
e-mail: ric.latour@state.or.us
Karen Madden, GED Administrator
Sharlene Walker, Unit Leader

To contribute leadership and resources to increase the skills, knowledge and career opportunities of Oregonians.

3486 Project Literacy Douglas County
1945 SE Stephens Street
Roseburg, OR 97470
541-957-9072
FAX 541-957-9072
e-mail: PLUR@rosenet.net
Eva Reynolds, Manager

3487 Salem Literacy Council
4485 River Road S
Salem, OR 97302
503-588-0307
FAX 503-588-0307
http://www.angelfire.com/or/salemliteracy/

Pennsylvania

3488 Delaware County Literacy Council
2217 Providence Avenue
Chester, PA 19013
610-876-4811
FAX 610-876-5414
http://www.delcolif.org
e-mail: delcolit@erols.com
Patricia Gaul, Executive Director

The Delaware County Literacy Council is a private, nonprofit, educational agency that provides one-on-one, free literacy instruction to non- and low-reading adults through a county-wide network of trained volunteer tutors. It is unique among the limited options available to adult residents of Delaware County who require help with their basic reading and writing skills in that it remains the only organization whose sole mission is adult literacy.

3489 Learning Disabilities Association: Pennsylvania
PO Box 208
Uwchland, PA 19480
610-458-8193
FAX 412-344-0224
http://www.ldanatl.org
e-mail: info@ldaamerica.org
Charlie Giglio, President
Reynolds Meeting Manager/Board, Meeting Manager/Board Cood.

LDAP is a nonprofit organization whose purpose is to advance the education and general well-being of persons with normal, potentially normal or above normal intelligence who have learning disabilities.

3490 Literacy Council of Lancaster/Lebanon
38 W King Street
Lancaster, PA 17603
717-295-5523
FAX 717-295-5342
http://www.adultlit.org
e-mail: info@adultlit.org
Mary Hohensee, Executive Director

Mission is to promote literacy for adults and children.

3491 Pennsylvania Adult Literacy
110 E Bald Eagle Street
Lock Haven, PA 17745
570-893-4038
FAX 570-748-1598
http://www.wbtc.ciu10.com
e-mail: vedmonst@lhup.edu
Mary Zigman, Special Project Facilitator II

3492 Pennsylvania Literacy Resource Center
ADVANCE Resource Center
333 Market Street
Harrisburg, PA 17126
717-783-9192
800-992-2283
FAX 717-783-5420
http://www.able.state.pa.us/advance
e-mail: ra-advancee@state.pa.us
Evelyn Werner, Director
Eileen Kocher, Librarian

As part of the State Library, the State Resource Center provides electronic and print resources.

3493 Project Literacy US (PLUS) in Pennsylvania
4802 5th Ave
Pittsburgh, PA 15213
412-622-1492
FAX 412-622-1492
http://www.dyslexia-add.org/plus.htm
Margot Woodwell, Project Director
Herb Stein, Assistant Director

PLUS promotes adult literacy. A joint project of the Public Broadcasting Service and the American Broadcasting Corporation, PLUS uses media to increase awareness of literacy issues and to recruit individuals into literacy training programs.

3494 York County Literacy Council
800 E King Street
York, PA 17403
717-845-8719
FAX 717-843-4082
http://www.yorkliteracy.org
e-mail: exec.dir@yorkliteracy.org
Joanne Olejowski, Executive Director

Provides literacy services to adults and families of York County. Define literacy as the ability to read, write and speak English in everyday life.

Rhode Island

3495 Family Independence Program of Rhode Island
Department of Human Services
600 New London Avenue
Cranston, RI 02920
401-462-1000
FAX 401-462-6504
TDY:401-462-3363
http://www.dhs.ri.gov
Ronald Label, Director
Christine Ferguson, Executive Director

Helps to improve the lives and economic conditions of Rhode ISalnd's families. Implemented according to law under the Family Independence Act on May 1, 1997. the program is part of Rhode Island's comprehensive reformation of the old Aid to Families with Dependent Children (AFDC) program.

3496 Learning Disabilities Association: Rhode Island
PO Box 6685
Providence, RI 02940
401-232-3822
Norma Veresko, President

Provides information and resources.

3497 Literacy Volunteers of America: Rhode Island
260 W Exchange Street
Providence, RI 02903
401-861-0815
FAX 401-861-0863
http://www.literacyvolunteers.org
e-mail: lvaricindy@aol.com
Yvette Kenner, Executive Director

The mission of LVA-RI is to advance adult literacy in Rhode Island by: providing training and support services to local LVA-RI affiliates, volunteer tutors and adult literacy services; providing the state with information about adult literacy and with appropriate referral services; collaborating with other organizations to promote adult literacy in Rhode Island.

3498 Literacy Volunteers of Kent County
1672 Flat River Road
Coventry, RI 02816-8909 401-822-9103
http://www.coventrylibrary.org/lva1.htm
e-mail: lvkc@coventrylibrary.org
Michele L Baluch, Executive Director

Receive intensive tutor training through a series of workshops that will prepare you to teach one-on-one or in small groups.

3499 Literacy Volunteers of Providence County
260 W Exchange Street
Providence, RI 02903-1000 401-351-0511
http://www.lvari.org
e-mail: chris@lvari.org
Christine Hedenberg, Executive Director

Provides critical support services to local literacy volunteer affiliates, volunteer tutors and adult literacy students; collaborating with organizations to promote adult literacy in Rhode Island; partnering with companies and employers to improve workforce literacy skills; and acting as a state-wide resource for awareness and information about adult literacy, and for adult learner referrals to educational programs.

3500 Literacy Volunteers of South County
c/o South County Community Office
1935 Kingstown Road
Wakefield, RI 02879 401-225-1068
e-mail: ionag_2002@yahoo.com
Iona Gardiner, Program Coordinator
David Henley, President

Volunteer-based literacy agent that provides services in Narragansett, North Kingstown and South Kingstown. Provides free, one-on-one tutoring to sdults who request Basic English Skills or English as a Second Language.

3501 Literacy Volunteers of Washington County
44 Broad Street
Westerly, RI 02891 401-596-9411
http://www.literacywashingtoncounty.org
e-mail: litwashcty@verizon.net
Mary Lou C Gentz, Executive Director
Susan M Dumouchel, President

Assists adults interested in improving their literacy skills through free programs based on a participant's individual goals.

3502 Literary Resources Rhode Island
Brown University
PO Box 1974
Providence, RI 02912 401-863-1000
FAX 401-863-3094
http://www.brown.edu
e-mail: janet_isserlis@brown .edu
Howard Dooley Jr., Director
Jim Miller, Manager

Literacy Resources Rhode Island was established in 1997. Its goals include: expand existing professional capacity within the state's adult education community; increase educator and learner capacity to use and interact with online technology; and assist in improving delivery of services to adult learners, thereby strengthening adult education provision across the state.

3503 Rhode Island Department of Employment and Training
1511 Pontiac Avenue
Cranston, RI 02920 401-462-8000
Sandra Powell, Manager

3504 Rhode Island Department of Human Services
600 New London Ave
Cranston, RI 02920 401-421-7005
http://www.dhs.state.ri.us
e-mail: rcarroll@ors.state.ri.us
Raymond Carroll, Administrator

3505 Rhode Island Department of State Library Services
1 Capitol Hill
Providence, RI 02908 401-222-2000
FAX 401-222-2083
Robert Carl Jr., Executive Director

3506 Rhode Island Human Resource Investment Council
Governor's Workforce Board
1511 Pontiac Avenue
Cranston, RI 02920 401-462-8860
FAX 401-462-8865
http://www.rihric.com
e-mail: larnodd@dlt.state.ri.us
Adelita Orefice, Director
Marshia , Administrative Assistant

3507 Rhode Island Vocational and Rehabilitation Agency
Rhode Island Department of Human Services
40 Fountain Street
Providence, RI 02903 401-421-7005
FAX 401-222-3574
TDY:401-421-7016
http://www.ors.ri.gov
e-mail: rcarroll@ors.state.ri.us
Raymond Carroll, Administrator
Steven Brunero, Deputy Administrator

Assists people with disabilities to become employed and to live independently in the community. In order to achieve this goal, we work in partnership with the State Rehabilitation Council, our customers, staff and community.

3508 Rhode Island Workforce Literacy Collaborative
Literacy Volunteers of Rhode Island
260 W Exchange Street
Providence, RI 02903 401-861-0815
FAX 401-861-0863
http://www.literacyvolunteers.org
e-mail: LVARIYVETT@aol.com
Yvette Kenner, Executive Director

Mission is to create a framework for an ongoing, comprehensive, seamless system for delivering adult workforce literacy services in Rhode Island.

South Carolina

3509 Greater Columbia Literacy Council
2728 Devine Street
Columbia, SC 29205-2412 803-765-2555
FAX 803-799-8417
http://www.literacycolumbia.org
e-mail: literacycolumbia@bellsouth.net
Deborah W Yoho, Executive Director

Mission is to enable adults, through customized learning programs, to improve English language and reading skills.

3510 Greenville Literacy Association
225 S Pleasantburg Drive
Greenville, SC 29607 864-467-3456
FAX 864-467-3558
http://www.greenvilleliteracy.org
e-mail: info@greenvilleliteracy.org
Jane Thomas, Executive Director
Nancy Renn, Program Director
Linda Brooks, Administrative Assistant
Recruits and trains community volunteers to provide instruction for adults who request assistance.

3511 Greenwood Literacy Council
PO Box 1467
Greenwood, SC 29648 864-223-1303
FAX 864-223-0475
e-mail: sowens@greenwood.net
Sandra Owens, Executive Director

Provides ongoing, comprehensive adult literacy programs in Greenwood, for illiterate adults and their families.

3512 Literacy Volunteers of the Lowcountry
Pro Literacy America
9 Town Center Court
Hilton Head, SC 29928
843-686-6655
FAX 843-686-6949
http://www.lowcountryliteracy.org
e-mail: nwilliams@lowcountryliteracy.org
Nancy Williams, Executive Director

3513 Oconee Adult Education
615 N Townville Street
Seneca, SC 29678
864-885-5014
FAX 864-985-1779
http://www.oconee.k12.sc.us
e-mail: swillis@oconee.k12.sc.us
Steve Willis, Director

3514 Resource Center for Literacy Technology & Parenting
South Carolina Department of Education
1429 Senate Street
Columbia, SC 29201
803-734-8500
FAX 803-734-8624
Inez Tenenbaum, Manager

Combines literacy programs with parenting instruction.

3515 South Carolina Adult Literacy Educators
PO Box 185
Blackville, SC 29817
803-284-4424
FAX 803-284-1444
http://www.barnwell19.k12.sc.us
Lindsey Toomer, Contact

3516 South Carolina Department of Education
1429 Senate Street
Columbia, SC 29201
803-734-8815
FAX 803-734-3389
http://www.myscschools.com
e-mail: tstokes@sde.state.sc.us
Inez Tenenbaum, Superintendent
Terri Stokes, Administrative Assistant

3517 South Carolina Literacy Resource Center
3710 Landmark Drive
Columbia, SC 29204
803-749-5466
800-277-READ
FAX 803-929-2571
http://http://tlrc.tamu.edu/s.carolina
e-mail: info@sclrc.org
Peggy May, Director

The mission of the South Carolina Resource Center is to provide leadership in literacy to South Carolina's adults and their families, in conjunction with state and local public and private nonprofit efforts. The Center serves as a site for training for adult literacy providers, as a reciprocal link with the National Institute for Literacy for the purpose of sharing information to service providers, and as a clearinghouse for state-of-the-art literacy materials and technology.

3518 Trident Literacy Association
5416-B
North Charleston, SC 29406
843-747-2223
FAX 843-744-2970
http://www.tridentlit.org
e-mail: echepenik@trident.org
Eileen Chepenik, Director

Mission is to increase literacy in Charleston, Berkeley and Dorchester counties by offering instruction, using a self-paced, individualized curriculum in reading, writing, mathematics, English as a Second Language, GED preparation and basic computer use.

South Dakota

3519 Adult Education and Literacy Program
SD Department of Labor
700 Governors Drive
Pierre, SD 57501
605-773-3101
FAX 605-773-6184
http://www.state.sd.us./dol/abe/index.html
e-mail: marcia.hess@state.sd.ed.us
Marcia Hess, State Administrator

Adult Education & Literacy instruction is designed to teach persons 16 years of age or older to read and write English and to substantially raise their educational level. The purpose of the program is to expand the educational opportunities for adults and to establish programs that will enable all adults to acquire basic skills necessary to function in society and allow them to continue their education to at least the level of completion of secondary school.

3520 South Dakota Literacy Council
816 Samara Avenue
Volga, SD 57071
605-627-5138
http://www.readsd.org
e-mail: bettyvz@readsd.org
Betty Vander Zee, Contact

Goal is to help people receive educational help in a confidential setting.

3521 South Dakota Literacy Resouce Center
800 Governors Drive
Pierre, SD 57501
605-773-3101
800-423-6665
FAX 605-773-6969
http://www.state.sd.us/deca/literacy/
e-mail: dan.boyd@state.sd.us
Marcia Hess, AEO & GED Program Specialist

The mission of the SD Literary Resource Center is to establish a state wide on-line computer catalog of all existing literacy materials within South Dakota and a South Dakota Literacy Resource Center home page with links to other literacy sites within South Dakota, regionally and nationally.

3522 South Dakota Literacy Resource Center
800 Governors Drive
Pierre, SD 57501
605-773-3101
800-423-6665
FAX 605-773-6969
http://www.state.sd.us/deca/literacy/
e-mail: dan.boyd@state.sd.us
Marcia Hess, AEO & GED Program Specialist

The mission of the SD Literary Resource Center is to establish a state wide on-line computer catalog of all existing literacy materials within South Dakota and a South Dakota Literacy Resource Center home page with links to other literacy sites within South Dakota, regionally and nationally.

Tennessee

3523 Better Tomorrows Adult Education Center
908 Meridian Street
Nashville, TN 37207
615-228-6225
http://www.better-tomorrows.com
e-mail: info@better-tomorrows.com
Mary Keen, Contact

Offers GED preparation, computer and office skills, learning how to read and write, bible study, finders/keepers, and Parenting: From Diapers to Diplomas.

3524 Blount County Literacy Council
1500 Jett Road
Maryville, TN 37809-9120
865-982-8998
FAX 865-982-8848
http://www.blountliteracycouncil.org
e-mail: info@blountliteracycouncil.org

Carol Ergenbright, Contact

Serving as an advocate for adult literacy by partnering with Adult Education programs and staff; promoting community involvement and providing assistance with funding.

3525 Center for Literary Studies Tennessee
University of Tennessee: Knoxville
600 Henley Street
Knoxville, TN 37996 865-974-4109
FAX 865-974-3857
http://www.cls.coc.utk.edu
e-mail: mziegler@utk.edu
Jean Stevens, Director
Peggy Robert, Administrative Assistant

The Center for Literacy Studies strengthens adult literacy education in order to equip adults with the knowledge and skills they need to be lifelong learners and effective members of their families, communities and workplaces. The Center links theory and practice through research, professional development, partnerships, and building and sharing the knowledge of the field.

3526 Claiborne County Adult Reading Experience
Claiborne County Schools
PO Box 800
Tazewell, TN 37879 423-626-7979
FAX 423-626-5945
http://www.claibornecountyschools.com/adulted/
e-mail: hansardr@kiztn.net
Susan Essary, Administrator
Roger Hansard, Adult Education Supervisor

3527 Collierville Literacy Council
167 Washington Street
Collierville, TN 38017-2678 901-854-0288
http://http://collierville literacy.org
e-mail: colliervilleliteracy@earthlink.net
Karen Ray, Contact

Offering Adult Basic Education, General Education Diploma preparation, and English as a Second Language.

3528 Department of Human Services: Division of Rehabilitation Services
400 Deaderick Street
Nashville, TN 37248 615-313-4700
FAX 615-741-4165
TDY:800-270-1349
http://www.state.tn.us/humanserv/rehabilitation
e-mail: carlbrown@mail.state.tn.usa
Carl Brown, Assistant Commissioner
Karen Wayson, Secretary
Gina Lodge, Manager
Agency takes an active leadership role in removing the barriers to employment due to disabilities.

3529 Literacy Council of Kingsport
326 Commerce Street
Kingsport, TN 37660 423-392-4643
http://www.literacycouncilofkingsport.org
e-mail: ltrcy@yahoo.com
Kris Mueller, Contact

Missionis to provide tutoring for adults and qualified children to improve their reading and writing skills and to be an advocate for literacy within the greater Kingsport community.

3530 Literacy Council of Sumner County
260 W Main Street
Hendersonville, TN 37075 615-822-8112
FAX 615-822-3665
http://www.literacysumner.org
e-mail: info@literacysumner.org
Margie Anderson, Director
Susan Stone, Program Coordinator
Carol Seals, E.S.L. Development Coordinator
Mission is to resources, counseling and tutoring to children, youth and adults to enhance their skills in all academic areas.

3531 Memphis Literacy Council
902 S Cooper Street
Memphis, TN 38104-5603 901-327-6000
http://www.memphisliteracycouncil.org
e-mail: gayjohnston@memphisliteracycouncil.org
Gay M Johnston, Executive Director
John Devin, Adult Learning
Wilson McCloy, Family Literacy
Provides programs for low-literate adults and disadvantaged families.

3532 Nashville Adult Literacy Council (NALC): Cohn Adult Learning Center
4805 Park Avenue
Nashville, TN 37209 615-298-8060
FAX 615-298-8444
http://www.nashvilleliteracy.org
e-mail: info@nashvilleliteracy.org
Meg Nugent, Director

Teaches reading to U.S.-born adults and English skills to adult immigrants.

3533 Nashville READ
PO Box 331988
Nashville, TN 37203 615-255-4982
FAX 615-255-4783
e-mail: literacy@nashvilleread.org
Carol Thigpin, Contact

3534 Opportunity for Adult Reading
833 N Oceoee Street
Cleveland, TN 37311 423-478-1117
FAX 423-478-1153
http://www.oar.ebradley.net
e-mail: info@oar.ebradley.net
Debra Conner, Contact

Funded by the United Way of Bradley County and free to adults and families who need to improve literacy skills.

3535 Protection and Advocacy Agency: Tennessee
PO Box 121257
Nashville, TN 37212 615-298-1080
800-342-1660
FAX 615-298-2046
TDY:901-343-4241
Shirley Shea, Executive Director
Gabriel Wood, Secretary

3536 Read To Succeed
1734 Somerset Drive
Murfreesboro, TN 37129 615-867-0581
http://www.readtosucceed.org
e-mail: info@readtosucceed.org
Ronni Shaw, Contact

A community partnership created to promote reading in Rutherford County, with emphasis on family literacy.

3537 Tennessee Department of Education
710 James Robertson Parkway
Nashville, TN 37243 615-741-2731
800-531-1515
FAX 615-532-4899
http://www.state.tn.us
e-mail: education.comments@state.tn.us
Lana C Seivers, Commissioner
Brewer Deputy Commissioner, Deputy Commissioner

Mission is to take Tennessee to the top in education. Guides administration of the state's K-12 public schools.

3538 Tennessee Department of Labor & Workforce Development: Office of Adult Education
500 James Robertson Parkway
Nashville, TN 37243 615-741-0466
FAX 615-532-4899

Phil White, Administrator
Haticile Buchanan, Manager

Grants funds that provide educational opportunities for those adults seeking basic skills upgrades, General Educational Development (GED) exam preparation, English for Speakers of Other Languages (ESOL) and basic workplace computer skills.

3539 Tennessee Literacy Coalition
1 Vantage Way
Nashville, TN 37228
615-259-3700
800-323-6986
FAX 615-248-6545
http://www.tnliteracy.org
e-mail: tnliteracy@yahoo.com

Established to serve as a organizational leader in creating a fully literate Tennessee. Acts as an advocate for 1.3 million adult Tennesseans who have limited skills; brokers adult literacy information and reosurces to providers, learners, volunteers and businesses; serves as a advisor to State and Federal legislators, business, and professional organizations.

3540 Tennessee School-to-Work Office
Andrew Johnson Tower
Nashville, TN 37243
615-741-2731
http://www.state.tn.us
e-mail: awilks@mail.state.tn.us
Alberta Wilks, Consultant

3541 Tennessee State Library and Archives
State Department of Education
403 7th Ave N
Nashville, TN 37243
615-741-3158
FAX 615-532-2472
http://www.state.tn.us/sos/statelib
Tricia Bengel, Special Projects Coordinator

Texas

3542 Adult Literacy Council of Tom Green County
3111 SW Boulevard
San Angelo, TX 76904
915-947-1536
FAX 915-947-1875
e-mail: adlitl@gte.net
Mary Cochran, Contact

Promote adult literacy.

3543 Commerce Library Literacy Program
PO Box 308
Commerce, TX 75429
903-886-5279
FAX 903-886-7239
e-mail: commerce@koyote.com
Pricilla Donovan, Contact

3544 Greater Orange Area Literacy Services
PO Box 221
Orange, TX 77631
409-886-4311
FAX 409-886-0149
e-mail: goalsliteracy@sbcglobal.net
Beth Schreiber, Executive Director

3545 Irving Public Library Literacy Program
440 S Nursery Road
Irving, TX 75060
972-721-3776
http://www.irvinglibrary.org
e-mail: rsalinas@irvinglibrary.org
Robert Salinas, Contact

Promotes literacy among people of all ages.

3546 Literacy Austin
2222 Rosewood Avenue
Austin, TX 78702
512-478-7323
FAX 512-479-7323
TDY:512-478-7323
http://www.literacyaustin.org
e-mail: info@literacyaustin.org
Gail Harmon, Executive Director
Hector Hernandez, Office Manager

Mission is to provide instruction for basic literacy and English as a Second Language (ESL) to adults, age 17 and older, who read below the fifth-grade leve. Vision is to improve the quality of an adult's life through improved literacy skills.

3547 Literacy Center of Marshall: Harrison County
700 W Houston Street
Marshall, TX 75670
903-935-0962
e-mail: joycehammer@hotmail.com
Joyce Hammers, Executive Director
Patricia Jersild, Assistant Director

3548 Literacy Council of Bowie/Miller Counties
PO Box 1111
Texarkana, TX 75504
903-838-8521
FAX 870-774-2078
e-mail: RMagee@cableone.net
Robbye Magee, Contact

3549 Literacy Volunteers of America: Bastrop
1201 Church Street
Bastrop, TX 78602
512-321-6686
e-mail: suemunster@aol.com
Sue Steinbring

Provides literacy training and pre-GED for students, English as a Second Language, tutoring and tutor training.

3550 Literacy Volunteers of America: Bay City Matagorda County
1921 5th Street
Bay City, TX 77414
979-244-9544
FAX 979-244-9566
e-mail: lva_me@hotmail.com
Linda Brown, Manager

Promotes literacy for people of all ages.

3551 Literacy Volunteers of America: Beaumont Public Library
PO Box 3827
Beaumont, TX 77704
409-835-7324
FAX 409-838-6734
e-mail: bbeard@bpls.lib.tx.us
Barbara Bear, Contact

3552 Literacy Volunteers of America: Brazos Valley
PO Box 3387
Bryan, TX 77805
979-595-2801
http://www.literacybrazosvalley.org
e-mail: lva@bvcog.org
Bobbee Pennington, Contact

Provides tutors for 18+ adults in reading, writing, math, and computer literacy. Lessons are one on one, free of charge.

3553 Literacy Volunteers of America: Cleburne
212 E Chambers Street
Cleburne, TX 76031
817-641-3187
FAX 817-556-3444
e-mail: dlajean@juno.com
Eduardo Ortiz, Education Manager

Promotes literacy for people of all ages.

3554 Literacy Volunteers of America: Houston
Heights Learning Center
1111 Lawrence Street
Houston, TX 77008
713-868-9600
FAX 713-802-2527
e-mail: sajaha7@aol.com
Sabrina Haselhorst Gould, Contact

Promotes literacy for people of all ages.

3555 Literacy Volunteers of America: Laredo
PO Box 6531
Laredo, TX 78042
956-724-5207
FAX 956-725-4253
e-mail: lvlaredo@grandecom.net
Doroteo Sandoval, Executive Director

Promotes literacy for people of all ages.

3556 Literacy Volunteers of America: Montgomery County
PO Box 2704
Conroe, TX 77305
936-494-0635
e-mail: literacymc@yahoo.com
Linda Ricketts, Contact

As part of the national literacy organization, combats illiteracy in Montgomery County through volunteer tutoring.

3557 Literacy Volunteers of America: Port Arthur Literacy Support
4615 9th Avenue
Port Arthur, TX 77642
409-982-7257
FAX 409-985-5969
http://www.pap.lib.tx.us/pap_pals
e-mail: rcline@pap.lib.tx.us
Ray Cline, Manager

A library based umbrella group which works with three primary programs: ono-on-one tutoring for those who cannot read or read at a very low level; GED Computer Lab assistance for adults who are striving to get their General Equivalency Diploma - in cooperation with Port Arthur Independent School District; and English-as-a-Second Language (ESL) in cooperation with the Port Arthur Independent School District.

3558 Literacy Volunteers of America: Wimberley Area
PO Box 135
Wimberley, TX 78676
512-847-8953
e-mail: trailsend@anvilcom.com
Linda Mueller, Contact
Linda Mueller, Accreditation Manager

Nonprofit, volunteer organization which exists to improve the reading, writing, speaking, cultural and life skills of adults reading at or below the sixth grade level and/or those for whom English is not their native language. Provides GED instruction. All services are free.

3559 Texas Center for Adult Literacy & Learning
College of Education
College Station, TX 77843
979-845-6615
800-441-7323
FAX 979-845-0952
http://www.tcall.tamu.edu
e-mail: tcall@coe.tamu.edu
Dominique Chlup, Director
Morris Contact, Contact

Created with the purpose of helping to reduce the incidence of adult literacy in Texas. Mission has evlved into responding to the needs of those who provide literacy services to Texas' adult literacy and family literacy learners.

3560 Texas Families and Literacy
110 W Barnett Street
Kerrville, TX 78028
830-896-8787
FAX 830-896-3639
e-mail: famlit@maverickbbs.com
Jimmy Sparks, Executive Director

3561 Texas Family Literacy Center
Vaughn Gross Ctr for Reading/Language Arts
College of Education SZB 228
Austin, TX 78712-0365
512-232-6030
FAX 512-232-2322
http://www.texasfamilyliteracy.org
e-mail: pbmorris@mail.utexas.edu
Pam Bell Morris PhD, Director
Taylor Executive Assistant, Executive Assistant

Mission is to strengthen family literacy programs and enhance the knowledge skills, instructional practices and resources available to family literacy educators statewide.

3562 Victoria Adult Literacy
Pro-literacy America
802 E Crestwood Drive
Victoria, TX 77901
361-573-7323
FAX 361-582-4348
e-mail: valctx@yahoo.com
Donna Bentley, Executive Director
Patt Polley, Administrative Assistant

3563 Victoria Adult Literacy Council
Pro-literacy America
802 E Crestwood Drive
Victoria, TX 77901-3309
361-573-7323
FAX 361-582-4348
e-mail: valctx@yahoo.com
Donna Bentley, Executive Director

3564 Weslaco Public Library
525 S Kansas Ave
Weslaco, TX 78596
956-968-4533
FAX 956-969-4069
http://www.weslaco.lib.tx.us
e-mail: webmaster@weslaco.lib.tx.us
Michael Fisher, Executive Director

Utah

3565 Bridgerland Literacy
255 N Main
Logan, UT 84321-3914
435-716-9141
http://www.bridgerlandliteracy.org
e-mail: literacy@loganutah.org
Sherrie Mortensen, Contact

Maximizing efforts by providing students with a quality trained program, tutor, excellent materials and effective support.

3566 Literacy Volunteers of America: Wasatch Front
English Skills Learning Center
175 N 600 W
Salt Lake City, UT 84116
801-328-5608
FAX 801-328-5637
http://http://eslcenter.org
e-mail: info@eslcenter.org
Barabra Fish, Contact

3567 Project Read
c/o Provo City Library
550 N University Avenue
Provo, UT 84601
801-852-6654
FAX 801-852-7663
http://www.provo.lib.ut.us/projread
e-mail: project_read@provo.lib.ut.us
Shauna K Brown, Director
Joy Glaus, Program Coordintor

Provides one-on-one tutorial program to enable functionally non-literate adults to improve their reading and writing skills sufficiently to meet their personal goals, function well in society, and become more productive citizens.

3568 Utah Literacy Action Center
3595 S Main Street
Salt Lake City, UT 84115
801-265-9081
FAX 801-265-9643
http://www.literacyactioncenter.org
e-mail: lac@netutah.net
Deborah Young, Executive Director

3569 Utah Literacy Resource Center
State Office of Education
PO Box 144200
Salt Lake City, UT 84114
801-538-7824
800-451-9500
FAX 801-538-7882
http://www.school.utah.gov
e-mail: dsteele@usoe.k12.ut.us
David Steele, Coordinator
Sandra Grant, Specialist
Shauna South, Specialist
As part of the State Library, the State Resource Center provides electronic and print resources.

Vermont

3570 ABE Career and Lifelong Learning: Vermont Department of Education
120 State Street
Montpelier, VT 05620
802-828-3134
FAX 802-828-3146
e-mail: srobinson@doe.state.vt.us
Sandra Robinson, Director
Tracy Gallo, Director Life Long Learning

Promotes quality education.

3571 Central Vermont Adult Basic Education
46 Washington Street
Barre, VT 05641
802-476-4588
http://www.cvabe.org
Mary H Leahy, Contact

Serves adults with less than a twelfth grade education. Student sinclude adults in the workforce, those moving from welfare to work, school droputs, single parent families, families in transition and immigrants.

3572 Learning Disabilities Association of Vermont
PO Box 1041
Manchester Center, VT 05255
802-362-3127
FAX 802-362-3128
Christina Thurston, President

A nonprofit organization whose members are individuals with learning disabilities, their families, and the professionals who work with them.

3573 Tutorial Center
208 Pleasant Street
Bennington, VT 05201
802-447-0111
FAX 802-442-7607
http://http://tutorialcenter.org
e-mail: info@tutorialcenter.org
Jack Glade, Contact

Most comprehensive educational support center in the state, serving children and adults with a wide variety of educational programming.

3574 Vermont Assistive Technology Project: Department of Aging and Disabilities
Agency of Human Services
103 S Main Street
Waterbury, VT 05671
802-241-2620
800-750-6355
FAX 802-241-2174
TDY:802-241-1464
http://www.dad.state.vt.us/atp
e-mail: atinfo@dad.state.vt.us
Julie Tucker, Project Director
Ross Administrative Assista, Administrative Assistant

Funded to increase statewide access of assistaive technology to people of all ages and abilities.

3575 Vermont Department of Corrections
103 S Main Street
Waterbury, VT 05671
802-241-2288
FAX 802-241-2565
TDY:800-241-1457
http://www.doc.state.vt.us
Robert Lucenti, Superintendent Education Service
Robert Hofmann, Commissioner
Maria Salem, Manager
Supports safe communities by providing leadership in crime prevention, repairing the harm done, addressing the needs of crime victims, ensuring offenders accountability for criminal acts and manageing the risk posed by offenders.

3576 Vermont Department of Welfare
Economics Services Division
103 S Main Street
Waterbury, VT 05671
802-241-2450
800-287-0589
FAX 802-241-2830
TDY:888-834-7898
http://www.path.state.vt.us
Joseph Patrissi, Deputy Commissioner
Dianne Carmenti, Welfare Director
Tony Morgan, Manager

3577 Vermont Human Resources Investment Council
Vermont Department of Employment & Training
PO Box 488
Montpelier, VT 05601
802-828-3273
FAX 802-828-4022
http://www.det.state.vt.us
e-mail: aevans@pop.det.state.vt.us
Bob Ware, Director for Jobs and Training
Anne Ginevan, Commissioner
Francis Woods, Manager

3578 Vermont Literacy Resource Center: Department of Education
120 State Street
Montpelier, VT 05602
802-828-5148
FAX 802-828-0573
http://www.state.vt.us/educ/vlrc/
e-mail: wross@doe.state.vt.us
Wendy Ross, Director Literacy Board

The Vermont Literacy Resource Center links Vermont to national, regional, and state literacy organizations, provides staff development and serves as a clearinghouse for the literacy community. The Vermont Literacy Resource Center is located at the Vermont Department of Education.

3579 Vermont REACH-UP Program
Department of Social Welfare
103 S Main Street
Waterbury, VT 05671
802-241-2860
800-775-0506
FAX 802-241-2830
Linda Knosp, Manager

3580 Vermont Workforce Reinvestment Act
Vermont Department of Employment & Training
PO Box 488
Montpelier, VT 05601
802-828-4000
FAX 802-828-4181
http://www.det.state.vt.us
e-mail: mcalcagni@det.state.vt.us
Anne Ginevan, Commissioner
Bob Ware, Director for Jobs and Training
Patricia Donald, Manager
Vocational training and job listings for displaced workers or others with difficulty finding regular employment.

3581 VocRehab Vermont
Agency of Human Services
103 S Main Street
Waterbury, VT 05671
802-241-2186
866-879-6757
FAX 802-241-3359
TDY:802-241-2186
http://http://humsanservices.vermont.gov
Diane Dalmasse, Executive Director
Cynthia D LaWare, Secretary
Wendy Hanifan, Administrative Assistant
Works in close partnership with the Vermont Association of Business and Industry Rehabilitation to assist Vermonters with disabilities and maintain meaningful employment in their communities.

Virginia

3582 Adult Learning Center
4160 Virginia Beach Boulevard
Virginia Beach, VA 23452
757-306-0991
FAX 757-306-0999
http://www.adultlearning.vbschools.com
e-mail: bmizenko@vbschools.com
Bonnie Mizenko, Director

Mission is to respond to the needs of the adult population by offering a comprehensive educational program to the community.

3583 Benedictine Educational Assistance
BEACON
9535 Linton Hall Road
Bristow, VA 20136
703-361-0106
FAX 703-361-0254
http://www.benedictinesistersofvirginia.org
e-mail: beacon2000@hotmail.com
Cecilia Dwyer, Prioress
Vicki Ix, Director of Vocation Ministry
Dana Pfeifer, Director of Development

3584 Charlotte County Literacy Program
395 Thomas Jefferson Highway
Charlotte Court House, VA 23923
434-542-5782
e-mail: charcolit@linkabit.com
Tonya Pulliam, Manager

Offers basic and family literacy programs, ESL and computer, parenting and work skills.

3585 Citizens for Adult Literacy & Learning
258 Second Street
Amherst, VA 24521
434-929-2630
http://www.callamherst.org
e-mail: feedback@callamherst.org
Marcia Swain, Program Coordinator

Free one-on-one help with reading, writing, math and GED preparation.

3586 Department of Correctional Education
James Monroe Bldg
101 N 14th Street
Richmond, VA 23219
804-225-3314
http://www.dce.state.va.us
e-mail: gwsisson@dce.state.va.us
Win Sisson, Contact

3587 Eastern Shore Literacy Council
PO Box 104
Belle Haven, VA 23306
757-442-6637
FAX 757-442-6517
http://www.shoreliteracy.org
e-mail: esliteracy@verizon.net
Janet Booth, Program Director
Linda Richardson, Administrative Director

Providing literacy tutoring without charge to adult residents of the Eastern Shore so they may acquire the skills needed to improve their particiaption in society and enrich their lives.

3588 Highlands Educational Literacy Program
PO Box 2044
Abingdon, VA 24212
276-676-4355
FAX 276-676-0677
e-mail: garretsj@jaxs.net
Sallie Garrett, Executive Director

Provides free one-on-one tutoring for adults 18 and older with a fourth grade reading level or below who desire to improve their reading/writing skills and/or who desire to learn basic computer skills.

3589 Literacy Council of Northern Virginia
2855 Annandale Road
Falls Church, VA 22042
703-237-0866
FAX 703-237-2863
http://www.lcnv.org
e-mail: info@lcnv.org
Patricia Donnelly, Executive Director

Recruits and trains volunteers to teach adults who need help reading, writing, speaking, and understanding English speaking.

3590 Literacy Volunteers of America: Fishersville
26 John Lewis Road
Fishersville, VA 22939
540-949-6134
FAX 540-245-5115
e-mail: lvaaa.cfw.com
Candida Clark

Provides free and confidential one-to-one tutoring in basic reading and ESL to persons not in the school system.

3591 Literacy Volunteers of America: Gloucester
PO Box 981
Gloucester, VA 23061
804-693-1306

3592 Literacy Volunteers of America: Louisa County
2128 S Lakeshore Drive
Louisa, VA 23093
540-967-1051
FAX 540-967-1051
e-mail: lv-louisa@cstone.net
Terry McElhone, Contact

3593 Literacy Volunteers of America: Nelson County
PO Box 422
Lovingston, VA 22949
434-263-8228
e-mail: nanamump@aol.com
Charles Strauss, Manager

3594 Literacy Volunteers of America: New River Valley
195 W Main Street
Christiansburg, VA 24073
540-382-7262
FAX 540-382-7262
e-mail: lvanrv@verizon.net
E Wertz, Executive Director

The empowerment of every adult in the New River Valley through the provision of opportunities to achieve independence through literacy.

3595 Literacy Volunteers of America: Prince William
4326 Dale Boulevard
Woodbridge, VA 22193
703-670-5702
FAX 703-583-0703
http://www.ivapw.org
e-mail: lvapw@aol.com
Kim Sells, Executive Director

Promotes literacy for adults living or working in Prince William County. We teach adults to read, write, and/or speak English.

3596 Literacy Volunteers of America: Shenandoah County
PO Box 303
Woodstock, VA 22664
540-459-2446
e-mail: pagould@adelphia.net

Paula A Gould, Contact

3597 Literacy Volunteers of Charlottesville/Albemarle
418 7th Street NE
Charlottesville, VA 22902 434-977-3838
http://www.avenue.org/lva
e-mail: lva@avenue.net
Mary Mullen, Program Director
Dutchie A Kidd, Contact

Offers free, confidential, individualized basic literacy and ESL instruction to adults.

3598 Literacy Volunteers of Roanoke Valley
5002 Williamson Road 2A
Roanoke, VA 24012-1727 540-265-9339
877-582-7323
FAX 540-265-4814
http://www.lvarv.org
e-mail: info@lvarv.org
Annette Loschert, Executive Director
Susie Boxley, Adult Education Program Manager

Mission is to teach English literacy skills to adults and to raise literacy awareness through the Roanoke Valley.

3599 Literacy Volunteers: Campbell County Public Library
684 Village Highway
Lynchburg, VA 24588 434-332-9561
FAX 434-332-9697
http://www.tlc.library.net/campbell
e-mail: ccothran@campbell.k12.us
Carolyn Cothran, Program Manager
Linda Owens, Director

Provides tutoring for basic literacy and English as a second language.

3600 Loudoun Literacy Council
PO Box 1932
Leesburg, VA 20177 703-777-2205
FAX 703-777-7260
http://www.loudounliteracy.org
e-mail: info@loudounliteracy.org
Barbara Notar, Executive Director
Kathy Fetzer, Adult Literacy Tutor Coordinator
Adrienne Miller, Family Literacy Program Manager
Values and supports education as a lifelong process. Programs include English as a Second Language, Basic Literacy, TOEFL preparation, GED preparation, workplace literacy program, family literacy program, and a sweet dreams program.

3601 Northern Neck Regional Adult Education Program
2172 Northumberland Highway
Lottsburg, VA 22511 804-529-5840
FAX 804-580-3152
Tonya Creasy, Regional Program Manager
Marjorie Lampkin, Lead Teacher
Jamie Blake, Administrator
Servcies Town of Colonial Beach, and Westmoreland, Richmond, Northumberland, and Lancaster Counties. Library adult basic ed, GED prep, GED Fast Track and ESL clinics.

3602 One-on-One Literacy Program: Wythe and Grayson Counties
PO Box 905
Independence, VA 24348 276-228-5225
e-mail: joanbolduc@ls.net
Joan Bolduc, Director

3603 Peninsula READS
393 Denbigh Boulevard
Newport News, VA 23608 757-283-5776
FAX 757-283-5779
http://www.peninsulareads.org
e-mail: learn@peninsulareads.org
Meghan Foster, Executive Director
Susan Clemens, Basic Literacy Coordinator

Teaching adults through personalized instruction, the literacy skills they need to particiapte fully in society.

3604 READ Center Reading & Education for Adult Development
1605 Monument Avenue
Richmond, VA 23220-2906 804-353-1587
FAX 804-355-7127
http://www.readcenter.org
e-mail: read@readcenter.org
Carol J Holmquist, Executive Director

Trains volunteer tutors to work with adult learners to meet their individual literacy goals.

3605 Skyline Literacy Coalition
PO Box 9
Dayton, VA 22821 540-879-2933
FAX 540-879-2517
http://www.skylineliteracy.org
e-mail: skylitbeth@aol.com
Jay Morgan-Bungar, Executive Director

3606 Virginia Adult Learning Resource Center
PO Box 842037
Richmond, VA 23284 804-828-6521
800-237-0178
FAX 804-828-7539
http://www.valrc.org
e-mail: vdesk@vcu.edu
George Bailey, Assistant Manager
Lauren Ellington, Adult LD Specialist
Barbara Gibson, Manager
We provide adult education and literacy resources, information, and professional development in Virginia.

3607 Virginia Council of Administrators of Special Education
Council for Exceptional Children
1110 N Glebe Road
Arlington, VA 22201 703-245-0600
800-224-6830
FAX 703-264-9494
TDY:703-620-3660
http://www.cec.sped.org
e-mail: service@cec.sped.org
Bruce Ramirez, Manager

The Virginia Council of Administrators of Special Education is organized to promote professional leadership, provide opportunity for the study of problems common to its members, and to communicate through discussions and publications information that will develop improved services for children with disabilities.

3608 Virginia Literacy Coalition
11503 Allecingie Parkway
Richmond, VA 23235 804-225-8777
FAX 804-225-1859
Jean Proffitt, Organizational Liaison

3609 Virginia Literacy Foundation
413 Stuart Circle
Richmond, VA 23220 804-237-8909
FAX 804-237-8901
http://www.virginialiteracy.org
e-mail: contact@virginialiteracy.org
Jeannie P Baliles, Founder/Chairman
Emblidge Executive Director, Executive Director

Provides funding and technial support to private, volunteer literacy organizations throughout Virginia via challenge grants and direct consultation.

Washington

3610 Division of Vocational Rehabilitation
PO Box 45340
Olympia, WA 98504
360-725-3636
800-737-0617
FAX 360-407-8007
http://www.dshs.wa.gov
e-mail: ruttllm@dshs.wa.gov
Lynnea Ruttledge, Manager
Lee Ruddy, Office Assistant

3611 Literacy Council of Kitsap
612 5th Street
Bremerton, WA 98337
360-377-3955
FAX 360-373-6859
e-mail: literacy@krl.org
Olga Fedorovski, Executive Director

3612 Literacy Council of Seattle
811 Fifth Avenue, FUMC
Seattle, WA 98104
206-233-9720
http://www.literacyseattle.org
e-mail: info@literacyseattle.org
Sharon S Victor, President
Sara Elefson, Program Coordinator

Volunteers teach adults the English skills they need to be successful in their jobs, families, and the community.

3613 Literacy Network of Washington
Literacy NOW Tacoma Community House
1314 S L Street
Tacoma, WA 98405
253-383-3951
FAX 253-597-6687
http://www.literacynow.info
e-mail: literacynow@tchonline.org
Marilyn Bentson, Training Coordinator
Steve Christensen, Program Assistant
Lisa Schubert, Public Relations Coordinator
Offers a statewide telephone hotline and website directory, adult literacy and ESL tutoring, conferences, workshops, and materials, technical assistance, and advocacy tools and training.

3614 Literacy Source: Community Learning Center
720 N 35th Street
Seattle, WA 98103
206-782-2050
FAX 206-781-2583
http://www.literacy-source.org
e-mail: info@literacy-source.org
Anne L Helmholz, Executive Director

Provides unique and responsive adult literacy services. Services include English as a Second Language (ESL), tutoring and conversation classes, computer literacy, workplace basic skills, Citizenship and civic classes, immigrant and refugee beginning ESL and the Newcomer Network, and an individualized adult high school diploma program.

3615 Mason County Literacy Council
133 W Railroad Avenue
Shelton, WA 98584
360-426-9733
FAX 360-426-9789
http://www.masoncountyliteracy.org
e-mail: lbusacca@masoncountyliteracy.org
Lynn Busacca, Executive Director
Angela Holley, Adult Service Coordinator

One-on-one and small group tutoring in basic skills is provided by trained volunteers and MCL instructors.

3616 Multi-Service Center
1200 S 336th Street
Federal Way, WA 98003
253-838-6810
FAX 253-874-7831
TDY:253-661-7827
http://www.multi-servicecenter.com
e-mail: stephaniep@multi-servicecenter.com
Stephanie Parson, Adult Education Supervisor
Dini Duclos, CEO

3617 Northwest Regional Literacy Resource Center
PO Box 42496
Seattle, WA 98195
360-704-4326
FAX 360-586-3529
http://www.sbctc.ctc.edu/oal
e-mail: imendoza@sbctc.ctc.edu
Israel David Mendoza, Director
Christy Lowder, Administrative Assistant

Provides resources and technical support to adult basic skills instructors in Alaska, Idaho, Oregon, Montana, Washington and Wyoming.

3618 People's Learning Center of Seattle
PO Box 28084
Seattle, WA 98118
206-325-8308
Georgia Rogers

3619 South King County Multi-Service Center
1200 S 336th Street
Federal Way, WA 98003
253-838-6810
FAX 253-874-7831
TDY:253-661-7827
http://www.multi-servicecenter.com
Dini Duclos, CEO
Stephanie Parson, Adult Education Supervisor

3620 St. James ESL Program
St. James Cathedral
804 9th Avenue
Seattle, WA 98104-1265
206-382-4511
FAX 206-622-5303
http://www.stjames-cathedral.org/esl
e-mail: ckoehler@stjamescatherdral.org
Christopher Koehler, Program Director
Michael Ryan, Religious Leader

Helps promote literacy among the community.

3621 Washington Department of Corrections
PO Box 41100
Olympia, WA 98504
360-236-4018
FAX 360-586-3676
http://www.doc.wa.gov
Maxine Hayes MD, Director

3622 Washington Laubach Literacy Action
Washington Literacy
220 Nickerson Street
Seattle, WA 98109
206-284-4399
FAX 206-284-7895
http://www.waliteracy.org
e-mail: WALT@aol.com
Brenda Gray, Executive Director

3623 Whatcom Literacy Council
PO Box 1292
Bellingham, WA 98227-1292
360-647-3264
FAX 360-752-6770
http://www.whatcomliteracy.org
e-mail: staff@whatcomliteracy.org
Rachel Myers, Contact

Funded through its own efforts and with the support of local groups. Donations are used chiefly to provide tutor training and materials for tutor and student use. All WLC services for students are provided free of charge.

West Virginia

3624 Division of Technical & Adult Education Services: West Virginia
State Department of Education
1900 Kanawha Boulevard E
Charleston, WV 25305
304-558-2000
FAX 304-558-3946
http://http://careertech.k12.wv.us
Stan Hopkins, Assistant Superintendent
Louise Miller, Coordinator
James Teets, Executive Director
Promotes the quality of adult education.

3625 Laubach Literacy Action: West Virginia
501 22nd Street
Dunbar, WV 25064
304-766-7655
800-642-2670
FAX 304-766-7915
e-mail: lwilcox@access-k12.wv.us
Laura Wilcox, Contact
Copher Contact, Contact

3626 W Virginia Regional Education Services
RESA III/Nitro-Putnam
501 22nd Street
Dunbar, WV 25064
304-766-7655
800-642-2670
FAX 304-766-2824
http://www.nuemedia.net
e-mail: cshank@access.k12.wv.us
Charles Nichols, Executive Director
Linda Andersen, Administrative Assistant

Offers services for literacy and adult basic education including literacy hotline, networks newsletter, resources for English as a second language, beginning literacy, learning disabilities and other special learning needs.

3627 West Virginia Department of Education
1900 Kanawha Boulevard E
Charleston, WV 25305
304-558-0549
800-642-2670
FAX 304-558-3946
http://www.wvde.state.wv.us
Preston Browning, Assistant Director
Sarah Hamrick, Executive Director

3628 West Virginia Literacy Volunteers of America
501 22nd Street
Dunbar, WV 25064
304-766-7655
800-642-2670
FAX 304-766-7915
David Greenstreet, Director

Wisconsin

3629 ADVOCAP Literacy Services
W911 State Road 44
Markesan, WI 53946
920-398-3907
800-631-6617
FAX 920-398-2103
http://www.advocap.org
e-mail: cheriew@advocap.org
Cherie Witkowski, Contact

3630 Fox Valley Literacy Coalition
103 E Washington Street
Appleton, WI 54911-5466
920-991-9840
FAX 920-991-1012
http://www.focol.org/literacy
e-mail: foxvalleylit@milwpc.com
Rosemary Burns, Executive Director
John Erchul, ABE Program Coordinator

Provides free, confidential literacy services. Works to meet the diverse needs of area learners and provides both basic education and English as a Second Language training. Offer flexible tutoring times for students and tutors as well as a variety of tutoring locations.

3631 Jefferson County Literacy Council
621 W Racine Street
Jefferson, WI 53549
920-675-0500
FAX 920-675-0510
http://www.jclc.us
e-mail: info@jclc.us
Jill Ottow, Director

Committed to building communities that are strong in literacy, language and cultural understandings through information and resource sharing, referral, assessment and instructional services.

3632 Laubach Literacy Action: Wisconsin
Literacy Plus-Grant County
PO Box 447
Lancaster, WI 53813
608-723-2136
FAX 608-723-4834
Arlene Siss, Co-Director
John Angeli, Manager
Leanne Smith, Office Assistant
Includes Grant County.

3633 Literacy Council of Brown County
424 S Monroe Avenue
Green Bay, WI 54301-4054
920-435-2474
FAX 920-435-2203
http://www.lcbc.org
e-mail: info@lcbc.org
Tori Rader, Executive Director
Kathy Cornell, Program Coordinator

Teaches reading, writing, listening and speaking to adults with families with limited basic skills and limited proficiency in English in order to help them improve the quality of their lives.

3634 Literacy Council of Greater Waukesha
217 Wisconsin Avenue
Waukesha, WI 53186-4946
262-547-READ
http://www.waukeshaliteracy.org
e-mail: drunning@waukeshaliteracy.org
Debra Running, Executive Director

Provides confidential, one-on-one tutoring and mentoring services to individuals who need help with reading, writing, spelling, math and English as a second language.

3635 Literacy Services of Wisconsin
2724 W Wells Street
Milwaukee, WI 53208
414-344-5878
FAX 414-344-1061
http://www.literacyservices.org
e-mail: barb@literacyservices.org
Barbara Felix, Exeuctive Director
Karen Horst, Program Manager
Kerry Nikutta, Program Manager
Providing literacy education to motivated adults through the efforts of dedicated volunteers , the gifts of private contributors and the use of specialized curriculum to meet individual and community needs.

3636 Literacy Volunteers of America: ChippewaValley
West Riverside Office Building
221 W Madison Street
Eau Claire, WI 54703-4417
715-834-0222
FAX 715-834-2546
e-mail: lfisher@lvcv.org
Heidi Fisher, Executive Director

Promotes literacy for people of all ages.

3637 Literacy Volunteers of America: Eau Claire
221 W Madison Street
Eau Claire, WI 54703 715-834-0222
FAX 715-834-2546
e-mail: info@lvacv.org
Carol Gabler, Director
Heidi Fisher, Executive Director

Promotes literacy for people of all ages.

3638 Literacy Volunteers of America: Marquette County
PO Box 671
Montello, WI 53949 608-297-8900
FAX 608-297-2673
e-mail: vjhawk@maqs.net
Vicki Huffman, Executive Director

Promotes literacy for people of all ages.

3639 Madison Area Literacy Council
1118 S Park Street
Madison, WI 53715 608-244-3911
FAX 608-244-3899
http://www.madisonarealiteracy.org
e-mail: greg@madisonarealiteracy.org
Lisa Schubert, Executive Director

Promotes literacy for people of all ages.

3640 Marathon County Literacy Council
300 N 1st Street
Wausau, WI 54403-5405 715-261-7292
FAX 715-261-7232
http://http://wvls.lib.wi.us/marathonliteracy
e-mail: cesolrud@mail.co.marathon.wi.us
Corinne Solsrud, Executive Director

Offering tutoring services for all Marathon COunty adults and all residents' families that need help.

3641 Milwaukee Achiever Literacy Services
1512 W Pierce Street
Milwaukee, WI 53204 414-643-5108
FAX 414-643-8804
http://http://milwaukeeachiever.org
e-mail: tknutson@milwaukeeachiever.org
Peg Palmer, Executive Director

Organizaed to provide adult literacy education to economically and educationally disadvantaged adults living in the Milwaukee area.

3642 Price County Area Literacy Council
211 N Lake Avenue
Phillips, WI 54555 715-339-2833
FAX 715-339-3909
e-mail: rgstueber@yahoo.com
Rudy Haubert, Manager

3643 Racine Literacy Council
734 Lake Avenue
Racine, WI 53403-1208 262-632-9495
FAX 262-632-9502
http://www.racineliteracy.com
e-mail: rlc@racineliteracy.com
Kay Gregor, Executive Director
Joyce Springmann, Educational Director

Providees free and confidential one-to-one tutoring by trained volunteer tutors. In addition to the instructional programs, the Council promotes awareness of literacy issues through its Speaker's Bureau and seeks support from the community to develop literacy programs.

3644 Walworth County Literacy Council
1000 E Centralia
Elkhorn, WI 53121 262-741-5278
http://www.walworthcoliteracy.com
e-mail: wclc@walworthcoliteracy.com
Judith Stone, Executive Director

Provides student-centered instruction in basic literacy skills and English as a second language. Primary focus is confidential and free tutoring by trained volunteer tutors.

3645 Western Wisconsin Literacy Services
113 Sillmore Street
Black River Falls, WI 54615 715-284-3361
FAX 715-284-9681
http://www.wwls.org
e-mail: jacksonlva@hotmail.com
Sandy Quance, Executive Director

3646 Winnebago County Literacy Council
106 Washington Avenue
Oshkosh, WI 54901-4985 920-236-5185
FAX 920-236-5227
http://www.winlit.org
e-mail: ellis@winlit.org
Lisa Ellis, Executive Director
Kari Uselman, Program Educator

Promotes literacy awareness; publicizes literacy services; recruits and trains volunteer tutors; facilitates the matching of students and tutors; provides one-on-one tutoring opportunities to clients; provides an administrative center that includes tutoring and training facilities and materials; and seeks funding from private and government sources

3647 Wisconsin Literacy
1118 S Park Street
Madison, WI 537 608-257-1655
FAX 608-244-3899
http://www.wisconsinliteracy.org
e-mail: info@wisconsinliteracy.org
Lisa Schubert, Executive Director

3648 Wisconsin Literacy Resource Center
Board of Vocational, Technical & Adult Education
1118 S Park Street
Madison, WI 53715 608-244-3899
FAX 608-257-1655
http://www.wisconsinliteracy.orgs
e-mail: mvellej@boardtec.wi.us
Mark Johnson, Director

As part of the state library, the State Resource Center provides electronic and print resources.

Wyoming

3649 Literacy Volunteers of Casper
125 College Drive
Casper, WY 82601 307-268-2230
FAX 307-268-3021
e-mail: lmixer@caspercollege.edu
Lisa Mixer, Executive Director

3650 Literacy Volunteers of Douglas
203 N 6th Street
Douglas, WY 82633 307-358-5622
FAX 307-358-5629
http://www.dwc.wy.edu
e-mail: slunsford@ewc.cc.wy.edu
Shannon Lunsford, Director
Connie Woehl, Executive Director
Carrie Frey, Administrative Assistant
Promotes adult literacy among the people in the community.

3651 Literacy Volunteers of Powell North College
231 W 6th Street
Powell, WY 82435 307-754-6280
FAX 307-754-6700
e-mail: bushnelr@nwc.cc.wy.us
Rom Bushnell, Director

Promotes literacy for people of all ages.

3652 Literacy Volunteers of Sheridan/Northern Wyoming

102 S Connor Street
Sheridan, WY 82801
307-673-2813
FAX 307-672-6157
e-mail: lva@fiberpipe.net

Dave Marshall, Director
Diane Marshall, Administrator

Promotes literacy for people of all ages.

3653 Teton Literacy Program

1465 Gregory Lane
Jackson, WY 83001
307-733-9242
FAX 307-733-9086
http://www.tetonliteracy.org
e-mail: info@tetonliteracy.org

Kari Belton, Executive Director

Provides literacy education and resources to open doors to individuals and families to achieve their personal, professional, and academic goals, as contributing members of our community.

3654 Wyoming Literacy Resource Center

Division of Lifelong Learning & Instruction
PO Box 3374
Laramie, WY 82071
307-766-3970
FAX 307-766-6668
e-mail: dstithem@uwyo.edu

Diana Stithem, Director

As part of the state library, the State Resource Center provides electronic and print resources.

Adults

3655 A Miracle to Believe In
Option Indigo Press
2080 S Undermountain Road
Sheffield, MA 01257 413-229-8727
800-562-7171
FAX 413-229-8727
http://www.optionindio.com
e-mail: indigo@bcn.net

Barry Neil Kaufman, Author
Melissa Rothvoss, Assistant Manager

A group of people from all walks of life come together and are transformed as they reach out, under the direction of Kaufman, to help a little boy the medical world had given up as hopeless. This heartwarming journey of loving a child back to life will not only inspire, but presents a compelling new way to deal with life's traumas and difficulties. *$7.99*

379 pages Yearly 1987
ISBN 0-449201-08-2

3656 All Kinds Of Minds: Young Student's BookAbout Learning Disabilities & Disorders
Educator's Publishing Service, Inc.
PO Box 9031
Cambridge, MA 02139 617-547-6706
800-225-5750
http://www.epsbooks.com

Gunnar Voltz, President

Written by Melvin Levine, and published in 1992. Helps children with learning disabilities to come to terms with it. Shows them how to get around or just work out any problems with their disabilities.

3657 Closer Look: Perspectives & Reflections on College Students with LD
Curry College Bookstore
1071 Blue Hill Avenue
Milton, MA 02186 617-333-2322
FAX 617-333-2018
http://www.curry.edu
e-mail: dgoss@curry.edu

Jane Adelizzi, Diane Goss, Author
Diane Goss, Editor
Jane Adelizzi, Editor

This book is a collection of personal accounts by teachers and learners. It's a sensitive portrayal of the real world of teaching and learning, particularly as it impacts on those with learning differences. Topics include connections between theory and practice, emotions and learning disabilities, classroom trauma, learning disabilities and social deficits, metacognitive development, ESL and learning disabilities, models for inclusion and practical strategies. *$ 24.95*

240 pages
ISBN 0-964975-20-3

3658 Dyslexia in Adults: Taking Charge of Your Life
Taylor Publishing
1550 W Mockingbird Lane
Dallas, TX 75235 214-637-2800
800-677-2800
FAX 214-819-8580
http://images.amazon.com

Kathleen Nosek, Author
Don Percenti, CEO

Adult dyslexics are experts at hiding reading, writing, and spelling difficulties long after high school. Dyslexia in Adults is a perfect guidebook for adult dyslexias to use in coping with day-to-day problems that are complicated by their learning disability. *$12.95*

192 pages Paperback
ISBN 0-878339-48-5

3659 Faking It: A Look into the Mind of a Creative Learner
Heinemann/Boynton Cook Publishers
361 Hanover Street
Portsmouth, NH 03801 603-431-7894
800-541-2086
FAX 800-354-2004
http://www.heinemann.com
e-mail: custserv@heinemann.com

Christopher Lee, Author
Rosemary Jackson, Author

Engage in professional dialog with Heinemann's celebrated authors and colleagues!

181 pages paperback
ISBN 0-867092-96-3

3660 How to Get Services by Being Assertive
Family Resource Center on Disabilities
20 E Jackson Boulevard
Chicago, IL 60604 312-939-3513
800-952-4199
FAX 312-939-7297
http://www.ameritech.net/users/frcdptiil
e-mail: FRCDPTIIL@ameritech.net

Charlotte Jardins, Executive Director

A 100 page manual that demonstrates positive assertiveness techniques. Price includes postage & handling. *$12.00*

3661 Language in Motion: Exploring the Nature of Sign
Harris Communications
15155 Technology Drive
Eden Prairie, MN 55344 952-906-1180
800-825-6758
FAX 952-906-1099
TDY:952-906-1198
http://www.harriscomm.com
e-mail: mail@harriscomm.com

David A Stewart, Author
Jerome D Schein, Author
Robert Harris, Owner
Bill Williams, National Sales Manager

Explore the nature of American Sign Language and its relationship to other sign languages and sign systems used around the world. An enlightening book about deaf people and their culture and a useful guide to interacting and communicating with deaf and hard-of-hearing people. *$24.95*

221 pages Hardcover

3662 Myth Of Laziness
Simon & Schuster
1230 Avenue of the Americas
New York, NY 10020 212-698-7000
http://www.simonsays.com
e-mail: shop.feedback@simonsays.com

Jack Romanos, CEO

Written by Melvin Levine and published in 2003. It shows parents how to nurture their children's strength's and improve their classroom productivity. Also, it shows how correcting these problems early will help children live a fulfilling and productive adult life.

3663 New Horizons Information for the Air Traveler with a Disability
Office of Aviation Enforcement and Proceedings
400 7th Street SW
Washington, DC 20590
http://www.airconsumer.ost.dot.gov

This guide is designed to offer travelers with disabilities a brief but authoritative source of information about Air Carrier Access rules; the accommodations, facilities, and services that are now required to be available.

3664 No Easy Answer
Bantam Partners
1745 Broadway
New York, NY 10019 212-782-9000
http://www.randomhouse.com/bantamdell/index.htm
e-mail: bdpublicity@randomhouse.com

Sally Smith, Author

Parents and teachers of learning disabled children have turned to No Easy Answer for information, advice, and comfort. This completely updated edition contains new chapters on Attention Deficit Disorder and Attention Deficit Hyperactivity Disorder, and on the public laws that guarantee an equal education for learning disabled children. *$23.00*

416 pages 1995

ISBN 0-553354-50-7

3665 One Mind At A Time

Simon & Schuster
1230 Avenue of the Americas
New York, NY 10020 212-698-7000
http://www.simonsays.com
e-mail: shop.feedback@simonsays.com
Jack Romanos, CEO

Written by Melvin Levine, and published in 2003. It shows parents and others how to identify the individual learning patterns, explaining how to strenghten a child's abilities and either bypasss or overcome the child's weakness, producing positive results instead of reapeated frustration and failure.

3666 Out of Darkness

Connecticut Assoc. for Children and Adults with LD
25 Van Zant Street
Norwalk, CT 06855 203-838-5010
FAX 203-866-6108
http://www.CACLD.org
Beryl Kaufman, Executive Director

Article by an adult who discovers at age 30 that he has ADD. *$1.00*

4 pages

3667 Painting the Joy of the Soul

Learning Disabilities Association of America
4156 Library Road
Pittsburgh, PA 15234 412-341-1515
FAX 412-344-0224
http://www.ldanatl.org
e-mail: ldanatl@usaor.net

The first comprehensively researched and written book on the art and life of America's beloved artist, P. Buckley Moss, whose passion for painting is equal only to her passion for people, especially those with learning disabilities. Inspirational book about a woman who succeeded not in spite of her disability, but because of it. Contains 168 full color pages, over 100 art images. *$50.00*

168 pages $5.00 postage

3668 Son-Rise: The Miracle Continues

Option Indigo Press
2080 S Undermountain Road
Sheffield, MA 01257 413-229-8727
800-562-7171
FAX 413-229-8727
http://www.optionindio.com
e-mail: indigo@bcn.net

This book documents Raun Kaufman's astonishing development from a lifeless, autistic, retarded child into a highly verbal, lovable youngster with no traces of his former condition. It includes details of Raun's extraordinary progress from the age of four into young adulthood. It also shares moving accounts of five families that successfully used the Son-Rise Program to reach their own special children. An awe-inspiring reminder that love moves mountains. *$14.95*

ISBN 0-915811-61-8

3669 Succeeding with LD

Free Spirit Publishing
217 5th Avenue N
Minneapolis, MN 55401 612-338-2068
800-735-7323
FAX 612-337-5050
http://www.freespirit.com
e-mail: help4kids@freespirit.com
Jill Lauren, MA, Author
Judy Galbraith, Owner
Betsy Gabler, Sales Manager

Twenty talented adults and children with LD share their stories, struggles, achievements, and tips for success. *$14.95*

160 pages Illustrated

ISBN 1-575420-12-0

3670 The Eight Ball Club: Ocean of Fire

ESOL Publishing LLC
10305 Colony View Drive
Fairfax, VA 22032 703-250-7097
http://www.theeightballclub.com
e-mail: esolpublishing@cox.net; mcpuginvodas@aol.com
MC Pugin-Rodas, Author
Melanie Rodas, President

Publisher of novels designed for Special Ed and ESL students and activity books that go with the novel. These novels can be enjoyed by mainstream students as well. The Eight Ball Club: Ocean of Fire has vocac words in bold print, photographic illustrations, academic science terms, and a glossary. It's a teen-interest, easy reading adventure. *$18.95*

144 pages

3671 You Don't Outgrow It: Living with Learning Disabilities

Academic Therapy Publications
20 Commercial Boulevard
Novato, CA 94949 415-883-3314
800-422-7249
FAX 415-883-3720
http://www.atpub.com
Marnell L. Hayes, Author
Anna Arena, President

Offers information to help the learning disabled adult. Uses strengths creatively to work around learning disabilities to reach a goal, get and hold a job, etc. Comprehensive glossary, related readings and recommended resources. *$6.00*

ISBN 0-878799-67-2

Children

3672 123 Sign with Me

Harris Communications
15155 Technology Drive
Eden Prairie, MN 55344 952-906-1180
800-825-6758
FAX 952-906-1099
TDY:952-906-1198
http://www.harriscomm.com
e-mail: info@harriscomm.com
Mary Pat Moeller MS, Brenda Schick PhD, Author
Robert Harris, Owner
Lori Foss, Marketing Director

The Sign with Me number book is a book for all children. It is designed to teach basic counting skills, the numerals 1-10, and their manual counterparts in sign language. The book offers a unique opportunity to introduce sign language to young children through the natural process of reading. *$12.00*

24 pages Paperback

ISBN 0-939849-01-1

3673 Adam Zigzag

Bantam Doubleday Dell
1540 Broadway
New York, NY 10036 212-782-5290
800-323-9872
FAX 212-302-7985
Barbara Barrie, Author

Dyslexia affects Adam's self-esteem and the lives of his family.

ISBN 0-385311-72-9

3674 An Alphabet of Animal Signs

Harris Communications
15155 Technology Drive
Eden Prairie, MN 55344 952-906-1180
800-825-6758
FAX 952-906-1099
TDY:952-906-1198
http://www.harriscomm.com
e-mail: info@harriscomm.com

S Harold Collins, Author
Robert Harris, Owner
Lori Foss, Marketing Director

A fun sign language starter book that presents an animal sign for each letter of the alphabet. *$5.95*
13 pages Paperback

3675 Basic Vocabulary: American Sign LanguageBasic Vocabulary: American Sign Language for Parents
Harris Communications
15155 Technology Drive
Eden Prairie, MN 55344
952-906-1180
800-825-6758
FAX 952-906-1099
TDY:952-906-1198
http://www.harriscomm.com
e-mail: info@harriscomm.com
Terrence J O'Rourke, Author
Robert Harris, Owner
Lori Foss, Marketing Director

A child's first dictionary of signs. Arranged alphabetically, this book incorporates developmental lists helpful to both deaf and hearing children with over 1,000 clear illustrations. *$8.95*
228 pages Paperback
ISBN 0-932666-00-0

3676 Beginning Signing Primer
Harris Communications
15155 Technology Drive
Eden Prairie, MN 55344
952-906-1180
800-825-6758
FAX 952-906-1099
TDY:952-906-1198
http://www.harriscomm.com
e-mail: info@harriscomm.com
Robert Harris, Owner
Lori Foss, Marketing Director

A set of 100 cards designed especially for beginning signers. The cards present seven topics with words and signs. The topics: Color; Creatures; Family; Months; Days; Time and Weather. *$5.95*

3677 Best Way Out
Harcourt Brace Jovanovich
6277 Sea Harbor Drive
Orlando, FL 32887
407-345-2000
FAX 407-352-1318
http://www.harcourtcollege.com
Karyn Follis Cheatham, Author
Patrick Tierrey, CEO
John D Benson, Vice President

A fictional story of thirteen-year-old Haywood Romby who faces the same real life academic and social problems faced daily by teenagers with learning disabilities.
168 pages

3678 Christmas Bear
Teddy Bear Press
3639 Midway Drive
San Diego, CA 92110
858-560-8718
FAX 619-255-2158
http://www.teddybearpress.net
e-mail: fparker@teddybearpress.net
Fran Parker, President

An 11x17 big book with color illustrations and a large print format uses the same simple sentence structure fount in I Can Read and Reading Is Fun programs. This story adds seasonal words to the developing sight vocabulary found in our reading programs. *$25.95*
12 pages
ISBN 1-928876-11-0

3679 Don't Give Up Kid
Verbal Images Press
46 Duncott Road
Fairport, NY 14450
585-377-3807
800-888-4741
FAX 716-377-5401
Jeanne Gehret, MA, Author
Victoria Harmison, Marketing Director

A picture book for children with dyslexia and other learning differences gives a clear understanding of their difficulties and the necessary courage to live with them. Young Alex finds in his hero, Thomas Edison, the strength to keep trying and to experiment with different ways to learn. Recommended by LDA and CHADD. *$9.95*
40 pages Paperback
ISBN 1-884281-10-9

3680 Fundamentals of Autism
Slosson Educational Publications
PO Box 280
East Aurora, NY 14052
716-652-0930
800-828-4800
FAX 800-655-3840
http://www.slosson.com
e-mail: slosson@slosson.com
Steven Slosson, President
Georgina Moynihan, TTFM

A handbook for those who work with children diagnosed as autistic.

3681 Funny Bunny and Sunny Bunny
Teddy Bear Press
3639 Midway Drive
San Diego, CA 92110
858-560-8718
FAX 619-255-2158
http://www.teddybearpress.net
e-mail: fparker@teddybearpress.net
Fran Parker, President

An 11x17 big book with color illustrations and a large print format uses the same simple sentence structure fount in I Can Read and Reading Is Fun programs. This story adds seasonal words to the developing sight vocabulary found in our reading programs. *$25.95*
17 pages
ISBN 1-928876-14-5

3682 Halloween Bear
Teddy Bear Press
3639 Midway Drive
San Diego, CA 92110
858-560-8718
FAX 619-255-2158
http://www.teddybearpress.net
e-mail: fparker@teddybearpress.net
Fran Parker, President

An 11x17 big book with color illustrations and a large print format uses the same simple sentence structure fount in I Can Read and Reading Is Fun programs. This story adds seasonal words to the developing sight vocabulary found in our reading programs. *$25.95*
13 pages
ISBN 1-928876-15-3

3683 Handmade Alphabet
Harris Communications
15155 Technology Drive
Eden Prairie, MN 55344
952-906-1180
800-825-6758
FAX 952-906-1099
TDY:952-906-1198
http://www.harriscomm.com
e-mail: info@harriscomm.com
Laura Rankin, Author
Robert Harris, Owner
Lori Foss, Marketing Director

An alphabet book which celebrates the beauty of the manual alphabet. Each illustration consists of the manual representation of the letter linked with an item beginning with that letter. *$16.99*
32 pages Hardcover 1991Grade Range: age 7
ISBN 0-803709-74-9

3684 I Can Read Charts
Teddy Bear Press
3639 Midway Drive
San Diego, CA 92110
858-560-8718
FAX 619-255-2158
http://www.teddybearpress.net
e-mail: fparker@teddybearpress.net
Fran Parker, President

Designed to accompany the I Can Read program is an 11x17 big book containing 54 charts which can be used to assist in introducing new words to students. These charts also provide review for previously taught words with either individual student or a small group. *$54.95*

54 pages

3685 I Can Sign My ABC's

Harris Communications
15155 Technology Drive
Eden Prairie, MN 55344
952-906-1180
800-825-6758
FAX 952-906-1099
TDY:952-906-1198
http://www.harriscomm.com
e-mail: info@harriscomm.com

Robert Harris, Owner
Lori Foss, Marketing Director

The Sign with Me alphabet book is a book for all children. It is designed to teach the 26 letters of the alphabet and the corresponding manual alphabet in sign language. The book provides early exposure to letter recognition plus a unique opportunity to introduce sign language to young children. *$11.95*

32 pages Paperback
ISBN 0-939849-00-3

3686 Josh: A Boy with Dyslexia

Waterfront Books
85 Crescent Road
Burlington, VT 05401
802-658-7477
800-639-6063
FAX 802-860-1368
http://www.waterfrontbooks.com
e-mail: helpkids@waterfrontbooks.com

Caroline Janover, Author
Sherrill N Musty, President

This is an adventure story for kids with a section in the back of facts about learning disabilities and a list of resources for parents and teachers. *$7.95*

100 pages Paperback
ISBN 0-914525-18-2

3687 Jumpin' Johnny Get Back to Work: A Child's Guide to ADHD/Hyperactivity

Connecticut Association Children & Adults with LD
25 Van Zant Street
Norwalk, CT 06855
203-838-5010
FAX 203-866-6108
http://www.CACLD.org
e-mail: cacld@juno.com

Michael Gordon PhD, Author
Beryl Kaufman, Executive Director
Marie Armstrong, Information Specialist

Written primarily for elementary age youngsters with ADHD, this book helps them to understand their disability. Also valuable as an educational tool for parents, siblings, friends and classmates. The author's text reflects his sensitivity toward children with ADHD. *$12.50*

$2.50 shipping

3688 Leo the Late Bloomer

Connecticut Assoc. for Children and Adults with LD
25 Van Zant Street
Norwalk, CT 06855
203-838-5010
FAX 203-866-6108
http://www.CACLD.org
e-mail: cacld@juno.com

Robert Kraus, Author
Beryl Kaufman, Executive Director
Marie Armstrong, Information Specialist

A wonderful book for the young child who is having problems learning. Children follow along with Leo as he finally blooms. *$6.50*

$2.50 shipping

3689 Mandy

Harris Communications
15155 Technology Drive
Eden Prairie, MN 55344
952-906-1180
800-825-6758
FAX 952-906-1099
TDY:952-906-1198
http://www.harriscomm.com
e-mail: info@harriscomm.com

Barbar D Booth, Author
Robert Harris, Owner
Lori Foss, Marketing Director

This book is presented in a lively, picture-book format and will give readers an understanding of the joys of sound and what it would be like not to be able to hear. Mandy, a young deaf girl, shares her perception of the world and her wonder of what sound actually is. Mandy is a fluent speechreader but also uses sign language occasionally in the text. *$5.35*

32 pages Hardcover 1991

3690 My Brother Matthew

Woodbine House
6510 Bells Mill Road
Bethesda, MD 20817
301-897-3570
800-843-7323
FAX 301-897-5838
http://www.woodbinehouse.com
e-mail: info@woodbinehouse.com

Mary Thompson, Author
Mary Thompson, Illustrator
Irv Shapell, Owner

Narrated by a young boy who describes the ups and downs of day-to-day life as he and his family adjust to his new brother, Matthew, who is born with a disability. *$14.95*

28 pages Hardcover
ISBN 0-933149-47-6

3691 My First Book of Sign

Harris Communications
15155 Technology Drive
Eden Prairie, MN 55344
952-906-1180
800-825-6758
FAX 952-906-1099
TDY:952-906-1198
http://www.harriscomm.com
e-mail: info@harriscomm.com

Pamela J Baker, Author
Robert Harris, Owner
Lori Foss, Marketing Director

This book is an excellent source to teach children and even adults sign language. The illustrations are accurate in their representation of sign. It is colorful and visually attractive which makes it easy to read. The black and white manual alphabet, the fingerspelling, and aspects of sign provide exellent directions and pointers to signing correctly. The sign descriptions are a great supplement to the illustrations. *$11.96*

76 pages Hardcover 1986

3692 My Signing Book of Numbers

Harris Communications
15155 Technology Drive
Eden Prairie, MN 55344
952-906-1180
800-825-6758
FAX 952-906-1099
TDY:952-906-1198
http://www.harriscomm.com
e-mail: info@harriscomm.com

Patricia Bellan Gillen, Author
Robert Harris, Owner
Lori Foss, Marketing Director

Learn signs for numbers 0 through 20, and 30 through 100 by tens. *$14.95*

56 pages Hardcover 1988

3693 **Rosey: The Imperfect Angel**
Special Needs Project
324 State Street
Santa Barbara, CA 93101
805-962-8087
800-333-6867
FAX 805-962-5087
e-mail: books@specialneeds.com
Sandra Lee Peckinpah, Author
Trisha Moore, Illustrator

Rosie, an angel with a cleft palate, works hard in her heavenly garden after the Boss Angel declares her disfigured mouth as lovely as a rose petal. Her reward is to be born on earth, as a baby with a cleft. *$15.95*

3694 **Scare Bear**
Teddy Bear Press
3639 Midway Drive
San Diego, CA 92110
858-560-8718
FAX 619-255-2158
http://www.teddybearpress.net
e-mail: fparker@teddybearpress.net
Fran Parker, President

An 11x17 big book with color illustrations and a large print format uses the same simple sentence structure fount in I Can Read and Reading Is Fun programs. This story adds seasonal words to the developing sight vocabulary found in our reading programs. *$25.95*
13 pages
ISBN 1-928876-16-1

3695 **Signing is Fun: A Child's Introduction to the Basics of Sign Language**
Harris Communications
15155 Technology Drive
Eden Prairie, MN 55344
952-906-1180
800-825-6758
FAX 952-906-1099
TDY:952-906-1198
http://www.harriscomm.com
e-mail: info@harriscomm.com
Mickey Flodin, Author
Robert Harris, Owner
Lori Foss, Marketing Director

The author of Signing for Kids offers children their first glimpse at a whole new world. Starting with the alphabet and working up to everyday phrases, this volume uses clear instructions on how to begin using American Sign Language and features an informative introduction to signing and its importance. One hundred and fifty illustrations. *$9.00*
95 pages Paperback 1995

3696 **Sixth Grade Can Really Kill You**
Penquin Putnam Publishing Group
375 Hudson Street
New York, NY 10014
212-366-2000
800-788-6262
FAX 212-366-2666
Barthe DeClements, Author

Helen's learning difficulties cause her to act up and are threatening to keep her from passing sixth grade. *$4.60*
Paperback
ISBN 0-670806-56-0

3697 **Snowbear**
Teddy Bear Press
3639 Midway Drive
San Diego, CA 92110
858-560-8718
FAX 619-255-2158
http://www.teddybearpress.net
e-mail: fparker@teddybearpress.net
Fran Parker, President

An 11x17 big book with color illustrations and a large print format uses the same simple sentence structure fount in I Can Read and Reading Is Fun programs. This story adds seasonal words to the developing sight vocabulary found in our reading programs. *$25.95*
13 pages
ISBN 1-928876-12-9

3698 **Someone Special, Just Like You**
Special Needs Project
324 State Street
Santa Barbara, CA 93101
805-962-8087
800-333-6867
FAX 805-962-5087
e-mail: books@specialneeds.com
Tricia Brown, Author
Fran Ortiz, Photographer

A handsome photo-essay including a range of youngsters with disabilities at four preschools in the San Francisco Bay area. *$6.25*
19 pages

3699 **Study Skills: A Landmark School Student Guide**
429 Hale Street
Prides Crossing, MA 01965
978-236-3000
Chris Murphy, Principal

3700 **Unicorns Are Real!**
Learning Disabilities Association of America
4156 Library Road
Pittsburgh, PA 15234
412-341-1515
FAX 412-344-0224
http://www.ldanatl.org
e-mail: ldanatl@usaor.net
This mega best-seller provides 65 practical, easy-to follow-lessons to develop the much ignored right brain tendencies of children. These simple yet dramatically effective ideas and activities have helped thousands with learning difficulties. Includes an easy-to-administer screening checklist to determine hemisphere dominance, engaging instructional activities that draw on the intuitive, nonverbal abilities of the right brain, a list of skills associated with each brain hemisphere and more. *$14.95*

3701 **Valentine Bear**
Teddy Bear Press
3639 Midway Drive
San Diego, CA 92110
858-560-8718
FAX 619-255-2158
http://www.teddybearpress.net
e-mail: fparker@teddybearpress.net
Fran Parker, President

An 11x17 big book with color illustrations and a large print format uses the same simple sentence structure fount in I Can Read and Reading Is Fun programs. This story adds seasonal words to the developing sight vocabulary found in our reading programs. *$25.95*
13 pages
ISBN 1-928876-13-7

3702 **Zipper, the Kid with ADHD**
Woodbine House
6510 Bells Mill Road
Bethesda, MD 20817
301-897-3570
800-843-7323
FAX 301-897-5838
http://www.woodbinehouse.com
e-mail: info@Woodbinehouse.com
Caroline Janover, Author
Rick Powell, Illustrator
Irv Shapell, Owner

Readers will enjoy this middle-grade novel's amusing but realistic portrayal of the effect of attention deficit hyperactivity disorder on a young person's life. Zipper, the Kid with ADHD will encourage other kids to find ways to manage their behavior, and give their friends a look at what it's like to have this disorder. *$11.95*

108 pages Paperback
ISBN 0-933149-95-6

Law

3703 ADA Quiz Book: 3rd Edition

Rocky Mountain Dis. & Bus. Technical Assistance
3630 Sinton Road
Colorado Springs, CO 80907
719-522-0195
800-949-4232
FAX 719-444-0269
http://www.adainformation.org
e-mail: regionviii@mtc-inc.com

Jana Copeland, Editor
Bob Cook, Religious Leader

A collection of puzzles, quizzes, questions and case studies on the Americans with Disabilities Act of 1990 and accessible information technology. Features sections on ADA basics, employment, state and local governments, public accommodations, architectural accessibility, disability etiquette, effective communication, and electronic and information technology. *$9.95*
81 pages 4.00 shipping

3704 Americans with Disabilities Act Management Training Program

RPM Press
PO Box 31483
Tucson, AZ 85751
520-886-1990
888-810-1990
FAX 520-886-1990
http://www.rpmpress.com/

Paul McCray, President
Jan Stonebraker, Operations Manager

Provides authoritative information on the Americans with Disabilities Act and compliance requirements for employers, schools and other entities which provide employment, education or related opportunities to persons with disabilities. *$142.95*

3705 Approaching Equality: Education of the Deaf

T-J Publishers
2544 Tarpley Road
Carrollton, TX 75006
972-416-0800
800-999-1168
FAX 301-585-5930
TDY:301-585-4440
e-mail: tjpubinc@aol.com

Frank Bowe, Author
Angela K Thames, President
Jerald A Murphy, VP

Public education laws guarantee special education for all deaf and learning disabled children, but many find the special education system confusing, or are unsure of their rights under current laws. For anyone with interest in education, advocacy and the disabled community, this book reviews dramatic developments in education of special children, youth and adults. *$12.95*
112 pages
ISBN 0-932666-39-6

3706 Attention Deficit Disorder and the Law

JKL Communications
2700 Virginia Avenue NW
Washington, DC 20037
202-333-1713
FAX 202-333-1735
http://www.lathamlaw.org
e-mail: plath@lathamlaw.org

Peter S Latham and Patricia Horan Latham, Author

$29.00
ISBN 1-883560-09-8

3707 Discipline

Special Education Resource Center
25 Industrial Park Road
Middletown, CT 06457
860-632-1485
FAX 860-632-8870

Marianne Kirner, Executive Director

A general analysis of the problems encountered in the discipline of students with disabilities. Discussion of the legal principles of discipline that have evolved pursuant to Public Law 94-142.

3708 Dispute Resolution Journal

American Arbitration Association
335 Madison Avenue
New York, NY 10017
212-716-5800
FAX 212-716-5906
http://www.adr.org
e-mail: zuckermans@adr.org

Susan Zuckerman, Author
Susan Zuckerman, Editor
William Slate Ii, CEO

Provides information on mediation, arbitration and other dispute resolution alternatives. *$150.00*
96 pages Quarterly

3709 Documentation and the Law

JKL Communications
2700 Virginia Avenue NW
Washington, DC 20037
202-223-5097
FAX 202-223-5096
http://www.lathamlaw.org
e-mail: plath3@his.com

$29.00

3710 Education of the Handicapped: Laws

William Hein & Company
1285 Main Street
Buffalo, NY 14209
716-882-2600
800-828-7871
FAX 716-883-8100
http://www.wshein.com/

Bernard D Reams Jr, Author
Kevin Marmion, President

Focuses on elementary and secondary Education Act of 1965 and its amendment, Education For All Handicapped Children Act of 1975 and its amendments and acts providing services for the disabled.

3711 Ethical and Legal Issues in School Counseling

American School Counselor Association
1101 King Street
Alexandria, VA 22314
703-683-2722
800-306-4722
FAX 703-683-1619
http://www.schoolcounselor.org
e-mail: asca@schoolcounselor.org

Richard Wong, Executive Director
Stephanie Will, Office Manager

Perhaps the increase in litigation involving educators and mental health practitioners is a factor. Certainly the laws arc changing or at least are being interpreted differently, requiring counselors to stay up-to-date. The process of decision-making and some of the more complex issues in ethical and legal areas are summarized in this digest. *$40.50*

ISBN 1-556200-55-2

3712 Individuals with Disabilities: Implementing the Newest Laws

Corwin Press
2455 Teller Road
Thousand Oaks, CA 91320
805-499-9734
800-818-7243
FAX 805-499-5323
http://www.corwinpress.com
e-mail: order@corwinpress.com

Patricia F First & Joan L Curcio, Author
Kimberly Gonzales, Marketing Director
Robb Clouse, Senior Acquisitions Editor

Aimed at school administrators, this highly readable book covers the three major pieces of legislation: Americans with Disabilities Act of 1990; Individuals with Disabilities Education Act; and the Rehabilitation Act of 1973. Suitable for lay public use, anyone needing an overview of the laws affecting education and disabilities. *$12.95*

64 pages
ISBN 0-803960-55-7

3713 **Learning Disabilities and the Law**
JKL Communications
2700 Virginia Avenue NW
Washington, DC 20037
202-223-5097
FAX 202-223-5096
http://www.lathamlaw.org
e-mail: plath3@his.com

$29.00

3714 **Least Restrictive Environment**
Special Education Resource Center
25 Industrial Park Road
Middletown, CT 06457
860-632-1485
FAX 860-632-8870
Marianne Kirner, Executive Director

A general discussion and analysis of the mandate to educate students with disabilities to the maximum extent appropriate with nondisabled students.

3715 **Legal Notes for Education**
Oakstone Legal and Business Publishing
6801 Cahaba Valley Road
Birmingham, AL 35242
205-991-5188
800-365-4900
FAX 205-995-1926
e-mail: info@andrewspub.com
Nancy McMeekin, CEO

Summaries of court decisions dealing with education law. *$122.00*

3716 **Legal Rights of Persons with Disabilities: An Analysis of Federal Law**
LRP Publications
PO Box 980
Horsham, PA 19044
215-784-0912
800-341-7874
FAX 215-784-9639
TDY:215-658-0938
http://www.lrp.com
e-mail: custserv@lrp.com
Bonnie P Tucker & Bruce A Goldstein, Author
Kenneth Kahn, President
Honora McDowell, Product Group Manager

This book will provide professionals working with the disabled a comprehensive analysis of the rights accorded individuals with disabilities under federal law. *$185.00*
2226 pages +$7.50
ISBN 0-934753-46-6

3717 **New Directions**
Association of State Mental Health Program Direct.
66 Canal Center Plaza
Alexandria, VA 22314
703-739-9333
FAX 703-548-9517
http://www.nasddds.org
Robert Glover, Executive Director

A newsletter offering information on laws, amendments, and legislation affecting the disabled. *$55.00*

3718 **New IDEA Amendments: Assistive Technology Devices and Services**
Special Education Resource Center
25 Industrial Park Road
Middletown, CT 06457
860-632-1485
FAX 860-623-8870
Marianne Kirner, Executive Director

A discussion of new mandates created by the 1990 Amendments to Public Law 94-142. An overview of the requirement for the provision of assistive technology devices and services as well as a discussion on the transition services that are to be provided to disabled adolescents.

3719 **Numbers That Add Up to Educational Rights for Children with Disabilities**
Children's Defense Fund
25 E Street NW
Washington, DC 20001
202-628-8787
FAX 202-662-3510
http://www.childrensdefense.org
David Hornback, President

Information on the laws 94-142 and 504.

3720 **Parent's Guide to the Social Security Administration**
Eden Services
1 Eden Way
Princeton, NJ 08540
609-987-0099
FAX 609-987-0243
http://www.members.aol.com/edensvcs
e-mail: info@edenservices.org
David L Holmes EdD, Executive Director/President
Anne Holmes, Director Outreach Support Svcs
Tom Cool, President
A parents' guide to the Social Security Administration and Social Security Work Incentive Programs. *$16.00*

3721 **Procedural Due Process**
Special Education Resource Center
25 Industrial Park Road
Middletown, CT 06457
860-632-1485
FAX 860-632-8870
JJ Jennings
CL Weatherly

Analyzes the importance of the procedural safeguards afforded to parents and their children with disabilities by the Public Law 94-142. Safeguards are discussed and possible legal implications are addressed.

3722 **Public Law 94-142: An Overview**
Special Education Resource Center
25 Industrial Park Road
Middletown, CT 06457
860-632-1485
FAX 860-632-8870
Marianne Kirner, Executive Director

An overview of the general provisions of the Individuals with Disabilities Education Act, commonly referred to as Public Law 94-142. Designed to provide the less-experienced viewer with a fundamental understanding of the Public Law and its significance.

3723 **Purposeful Integration: Inherently Equal**
Federation for Children with Special Needs
1135 Tremont Street
Roxbury Crossing, MA 02120
617-236-7210
800-331-0688
FAX 617-572-2094
TDY:617-236-7210
http://www.fcsn.org
e-mail: fcsninfo@fcsn.org
Richard Robison, President

This publication covers integration, mainstreaming, and least restrictive environments. *$8.00*
55 pages

3724 **Section 504 of the Rehabilitation Act**
Special Education Resource Center
25 Industrial Park Road
Middletown, CT 06457
860-632-1485
FAX 860-632-8870
Marianne Kirner, Executive Director

A general overview of the legal implications of the Rehabilitation Act and its implementing regulations, a law that is often forgotten in the process of appropriately educating children with disabilities.

Monthly

3725 Section 504: Help for the Learning Disabled College Student

Connecticut Assoc. for Children and Adults with LD
25 Van Zant Street
Norwalk, CT 06855
203-838-5010
FAX 203-866-6108
http://www.CACLD.org
e-mail: cacld@juno.com

Joan Sedita, Author
Beryl Kaufman, Executive Director
Marie Armstrong, Information Specialist

Provides a review of Section 504 of the Vocational Rehabilitation Act as it relates specifically to the learning disabled. *$3.25*
$2.50 shipping

3726 So You're Going to a Hearing: Preparing for Public Law 94-142

Learning Disabilities Association of America
4156 Library Road
Pittsburgh, PA 15234
412-341-1515
FAX 412-344-0224
http://www.ldanatl.org
e-mail: ldanatl@usaor.net

A public informational source offering legal advice to children and youth with learning disabilities. *$5.50*

3727 Special Education Law Update

Data Research
4635 Nicols Road
Eagan, MN 55122
651-452-8267
800-365-4900
FAX 651-452-8694
http://www.dataresearchinc.com

Bruce Montgomery

Monthly newsletter service. Cases, legislation, administrative regulations and law review articles dealing with special education law. Annual index and binder included. *$159.00*

3728 Special Education in Juvenile Corrections

Council for Exceptional Children
1110 N Glebe Road
Arlington, VA 22201
703-245-0600
888-232-7733
FAX 703-264-9494
http://www.cec.sped.org/

Peter E Leone, Author
Robert B Rutherford Jr., Author
Bruce Ramirez, Manager

This topic is of increasing concern. This book describes the demographics of incarcerated youth and suggests some promising practices that are being used. *$8.90*
26 pages
ISBN 0-865862-03-6

3729 Special Law for Special People

Smith, Howard & Ajax
3333 Peachtree Road NE
Atlanta, GA 30326
404-266-6300
FAX 404-239-1930

Lafon Dees, Senior VP
Charles L Weatherly, Contact
Lafon

A ten-tape video series that is designed to assist in educating regular education personnel as to the legal requirements of IDEA and Section 504.

3730 Statutes, Regulations and Case Law

Center for Education and Employment Law
PO Box 3008
Malvern, PA 19355
800-365-4900
FAX 610-647-8089
http://www.ceelonline.com

Curt Brown Esq, Group Publisher
Steve McEllistrem Esq, Senior Editor

Provides summaries of recent court cases impacting disability issues as well as reports on legislation and administrative regulations that are of importance to you. *$259.00*

3731 Stories Behind Special Education Case Law

Special Needs Project
324 State Street
Santa Barbara, CA 93101
805-962-8087
800-333-6867
FAX 805-962-5087
e-mail: books@specialneeds.com

Ree Martin, Author

The personal stories behind ten leading court cases that shaped the basic principles of special education law. *$12.95*
150 pages

3732 Students with Disabilities and SpecialEducation

Center for Education and Employment Law
PO Box 3008
Malvern, PA 19355
800-365-4900
FAX 610-647-8089
http://www.ceelonline.com

Curt Brown Esq, Group Publisher
Steve McEllistrem Esq, Senior Editor

A desk reference that helps you determine if your program conforms to IDEA statutes and regulations in a comprehensive and concise format. We bring you analyses of recent court cases across the country that will help you safeguard your legal rights, and educate your colleagues in the law so they too are better qualified to identify and deal with developing legal issues. *$294.00*
500+ pages Annual
ISBN 0-939675-44-7

3733 Technology, Curriculum, and ProfessionalDevelopment

Corwin Press
2455 Teller Road
Thousand Oaks, CA 91320
805-499-9774
800-818-7243
FAX 805-499-0871
http://www.corwinpress.com
e-mail: order@corwinpress.com

John Woodward, Larry Cuban, Author
Robb Clouse, Editorial Director
Kimberly Gonzales, Director Marketing

Adapting schools to meet the needs of students with disabilities. The history of special education technologies, the requirements of IDEA'97, and the successes and obstacles for special education technology implementation. *$34.95*
264 pages
ISBN 0-761977-43-0

3734 Testing Students with Disabilities

Corwin Press
2455 Teller Road
Thousand Oaks, CA 91320
805-499-9774
800-818-7243
FAX 805-499-0871
http://www.corwinpress.com
e-mail: order@corwinpress.com

Martha Thurlow, Judy Elliott, James Ysseldyke, Author
Robb Clouse, Editorial Director
Kimberly Gonzales, Director Marketing

Practical strategies for complying with district and state requirements. Helps translate the issues surrounding state and district testing of students with disabilities, including IDEA, into what educators need to know and do. *$ 34.95*
296 pages
ISBN 0-803965-52-4

3735 US Department of Justice: Disabilities Rights Section

Civil Rights Division, DRS-NYA
Washington, DC 20530
800-514-0301
FAX 202-514-0404
http://www.ada.gov

Information concerning the rights people with learning disabilities have under the Americans with Disabilities Act.

3736 **US Department of Justice: Disability Rights Section**
950 Pennsylvania Avenue NW
Washington, DC 20530
202-514-2000
800-514-0301
FAX 202-307-1198
http://www.usdoj.gov/crt/ada/adahoml.htm
e-mail: askdoj@usdoj.gov
Alberto R Gonzales, Attorney General
Paul J McNulty, Deputy Attorney General

The primary goal of the Disability Rights Section is to achieve equal opportunity for people with disabilities in the United States by implementing the Americans with Disabilities Act (ADA).

Parents & Professionals

3737 **125 Brain Games for Babies**
Therapro
225 Arlington Street
Framingham, MA 01702
508-872-9494
800-257-5376
FAX 508-875-2062
http://www.theraproducts.com
e-mail: info@theraproducts.com
Jackie Silberg, Author
Karen Conrad, Owner

Packed with everyday opportunities to enhance brain development of children from birth to 12 months. Each game includes notes on recent brain research in practical terms.

3738 **A Miracle to Believe In**
Option Indigo Press
2080 S Undermountain Road
Sheffield, MA 01257
413-229-8727
800-562-7171
FAX 413-229-8727
http://www.optionindio.com
e-mail: indigo@bcn.net
Barry Neil Kaufman, Author

A group of people from all walks of life come together and are transformed as they reach out, under the direction of Kaufman, to help a little boy the medical world had given up as hopeless. This heartwarming journey of loving a child back to life will not only inspire, but presents a compelling new way to deal with life's traumas and difficulties. *$7.99*

ISBN 0-449201-08-2

3739 **A Practical Parent's Handbook on TeachingChildren with Learning Disabilities**
Charles C Thomas Publisher
2600 S 1st Street
Springfield, IL 62704
217-789-8980
800-258-8980
FAX 217-789-9130
http://www.ccthomas.com
e-mail: books@ccthomas.com
Shelby Holley, Author
Michael Thomas, President

Gives enough information for an adult with no previous teaching experience to design and implement an effective remedial program. Books sent on approval. This book is out of print. Available by specialorders only - must order in quantities of ten or more and they are non-returnable.
308 pages Cloth
ISBN 0-398059-03-9

3740 **ADHD in Adolescents: Diagnosis andTreatment**
Guilford Publications
72 Spring Street
New York, NY 10012
212-431-9800
800-365-7006
FAX 212-966-6708
http://www.guilford.com
e-mail: info@guilford.com
Arthur L Robin, Author
Bob Matloff, President

Here Dr. Robin teaches us not only about the facts of the disorder, but also about its nature and the proper means of clinically evaluating it. Includes numerous reproducible forms for clinicians and clients, among them rating scales and detailed checklists for psychological testing, interviewing, treatment planning, and school and family interventions. *$46.95*
461 pages Hardcover
ISBN 1-572303-91-3

3741 **About Dyslexia: Unraveling the Myth**
Connecticut Assoc. for Children and Adults with LD
25 Van Zant Street
Norwalk, CT 06855
203-838-5010
FAX 203-866-6108
http://www.CACLD.org
Priscilla Vail, Author
Beryl Kaufman, Executive Director

This book focuses on the communication patterns of strength and weaknesses in dyslexic people from early childhood through adulthood. *$7.95*
49 pages
ISBN 0-935493-34-4

3742 **Absudities of Special Education: The Best of Ants....Flying and Logs**
Peytral Publicatons
PO Box 1162
Minnetonka, MN 55345
952-949-8707
877-739-8725
FAX 952-906-9777
http://www.peytral.com
e-mail: help@peytral.com
Michael F Giangreco, Author
Peggy Hammeken, President

Now available in this full color edition. Create beautiful transperances or use in PowerPoint presentations for staff development. Also a great gift for parents of educators. *$39.95*
114 pages
ISBN 1-890455-40-7

3743 **Access Aware: Extending Your Reach to People with Disabilities**
Alliance for Technology Access
1304 Southpoint Boulevard
Petaluma, CA 94954
707-765-2080
FAX 707-765-2080
http://www.ataccess.org
e-mail: atainfo@ataccess.org
Mary Lester, Executive Director

This easy-to-use manual is designed to help any organization become more accessible for people with disabilities. *$45.00*
219 pages
ISBN 0-897933-00-1

3744 **Activities for a Diverse Classroom**
PEAK Parent Center
611 N Weber Street
Colorado Springs, CO 80903
719-531-9400
800-284-0251
FAX 719-531-9452
TDY:719-531-5403
http://www.peakparent.org
e-mail: info@peakparent.org
Leah Katz, Caren Sax, Douglas Fisher, Author

A valuable resource for elementary teachers, this book helps begin the sometimes difficult conversation about diversity in the classroom. With the 18 fun, enriching, and do-it-tomorrow activities outlined in this text, teachers can help create a sense of community in the classroom as they introduce students to new ways of thinking about the need for friendships and the acceptance of others. *$10.00*

80 pages
ISBN 1-884720-20-X

3745 Activity Schedules for Children with Autism: A Guide for Parents and Professionals
Woodbine House
6510 Bells Mill Road
Bethesda, MD 20817 301-897-3570
800-843-7323
FAX 301-897-5838
http://www.woodbinehouse.com
e-mail: info@woodbinehouse.com
Lynn E McClannahan PhD, Author
Patricia J Krantz PhD, Author
Irv Shapell, Owner
Detailed instructions and examples help parents prepare their child's first activity schedule, then progress to more varied and sophisticated schedules. The goal of this system is for children with autism to make effective use of unstructured time, handle changes in routine, and help them choose among an established set of home, school, and leisure activities independently. *$14.95*

117 pages Paperback
ISBN 0-933149-93-X

3746 Alternate Assessments for Students with Disabilities
Corwin Press
2455 Teller Road
Thousand Oaks, CA 91320 805-499-9774
800-818-7243
FAX 805-499-0871
http://www.corwinpress.com
e-mail: order@corwinpress.com
Sandra Thompson, Rachel Quenemoen, Martha Thurlow, Author
Robb Clouse, Editorial Director
Kimberly Gonzales, Director Marketing

Distinguished group of experts in a landmark book, co-published with the Council for Exceptional Children show you how to shift to high expectations for all learners, improve schooling for all. *$29.95*
168 pages
ISBN 0 761977 71 0

3747 American Sign Language Concise Dictionary
Harris Communications
15155 Technology Drive
Eden Prairie, MN 55344 952-906-1180
800-825-6758
FAX 952-906-1099
TDY:952-906-1198
http://www.harriscomm.com
e-mail: info@harriscomm.com
Martin Sternberg, Author
Robert Harris, Owner
Lori Foss, Marketing Director

A portable version containing 2,000 of the most commonly used words and phrases in ASL. Illustrated with easy-to-follow hand, arm and facial movements. *$11.95*
737 pages Paperback 1994

3748 American Sign Language Dictionary: A Comprehensive Abridgement
Harris Communications
15155 Technology Drive
Eden Prairie, MN 55344 952-906-1180
800-825-6758
FAX 952-906-1099
TDY:952-906-1198
http://www.harriscomm.com
e-mail: info@harriscomm.com
Martin Sternberg, Author
Robert Harris, Owner
Lori Foss, Marketing Director

An abridged version of American Sign Language. A comprehensive dictionary with 4,400 illustrated signs. It has 500 new signs and 1,500 new illustrations. Third edition. *$24.00*

772 pages Paperback 1998

3749 American Sign Language: A Comprehensive Dictionary
Harris Communications
15155 Technology Drive
Eden Prairie, MN 55344 952-906-1180
800-825-6758
FAX 952-906-1099
TDY:952-906-1198
http://www.harriscomm.com
Martin Sternberg, Author
Robert Harris, Owner
Lori Foss, Marketing Director

Contains over 5,000 entries and cross-references, an extensive bibliography and seven foreign language indexes. Contains clear illustrations and easily understood directions for forming and using each sign. *$75.00*
1132 pages

3750 Another Door to Learning
Crossroad Publishing
481 8th Avenue
New York, NY 10001 212-868-1801
FAX 212-868-2171
e-mail: sales@crossroadpublishing.com
Judy Schwartz, Author
John Jones, Executive Manager
Gwendolin Herder, Owner

Stories of eleven atypical learners who got the help they needed to make a lasting difference in their lives.

ISBN 0-824513-85-1

3751 Answers to Distraction
Pantheon Books
201 E 50th Street
New York, NY 10022 212-751-2600
800-638-6460
FAX 212-572-8700
Edward M Hallowell, Author
John Ratey, Author

Responses to common questions the authors' audiences have asked, organized by topic.

ISBN 0-679439-73-0

3752 Ants in His Pants: Absurdities and Realities of Special Education
Peytral Publication
PO Box 1162
Minnetonka, MN 55345 952-949-8707
877-739-8725
FAX 612-906-9777
http://www.peytral.com
e-mail: help@peytral.com
Michael F Giangreco, Author
Peggy Hammeken, President

With wit, humor, and profound one liners, this book will transform your thinking as you take a lighter look at the often comical and occcasionally harsh truth in the field of special education. This carefully crafted collection of 101 cartoons can be made into transparencies for staff development and training. *$19.95*
128 pages
ISBN 1-890455-42-3

3753 Assessment & Instruction of Culturally & Linguistically Diverse Students
Books on Special Children
PO Box 3378
Amherst, MA 01004 845-638-1236
FAX 845-638-0847
http://www.boscbooks.com/
e-mail: irene@boscbooks.com
Rita Brusca-Vega, Virginia Gonzalez, Thomas Yawkey, Author

Appropriate assessments and educational models and practices are discussed. Also, educational environment and how to help problems, understanding diversity and disability, legal aspects. *$88.20*

254 pages Hardcover
ISBN 0-205156-29-0

3754 Attention-Deficit Hyperactivity Disorder
Slosson Educational Publications
PO Box 280
East Aurora, NY 14052
716-652-0930
800-828-4800
FAX 800-655-3840
http://www.slosson.com
e-mail: slosson@slosson.com
Sue Larson, Author
Steven Slosson, President

The book addresses issues of theory and practice quickly, with compassion and practicality and, most importantly, is very effective. Well-grounded answers and suggestions which would facilitate behavior, learning, social-emotional functioning, and other factors in preschool and adolescence are discussed.

3755 Attention-Deficit Hyperactivity Disorder: A Handbook for Diagnosis and Treatment, 2nd Edition
Guilford Publications
72 Spring Street
New York, NY 10012
212-431-9800
800-365-7006
FAX 212-966-6708
http://www.guilford.com
e-mail: info@guilford.com
Russell A Barkley, Author
Bob Matloff, President

Incorporates the latest findings on the nature, diagnosis, assessment, and treatment of ADHD. Clinicians, researchers, and students will find practical and richly referenced information on nearly every aspect of the disorder. *$ 55.00*
628 pages

3756 Autism and the Family: Problems, Prospects and Coping with the Disorder
Charles C Thomas Publisher
2600 S 1st Street
Springfield, IL 62704
217-789-8980
800-258-8980
FAX 217-789-9130
David E Gray, Author
Michael Thomas, President

The object of this work is to explore aspects of the family's experience of autism, and in this regard, it offers a sociological account of what it is like to be parents of an autistic child. This text serves as an excellent resource for parents, families, therapists, professionals and those who work with autistic children. Paperback, ISBN: 0-398-06843-7, 38.95. *$52.95*
210 pages Hardcover 1998
ISBN 0-398068-42-9

3757 Backyards & Butterflies: Ways to Include Children with Disabilities
Brookline Books
PO Box 1209
Brookline, MA 02445
617-734-6772
800-666-BOOK
FAX 617-734-3952
http://www.brooklinebooks.com
e-mail: brbooks@yahoo.com
Doreen Greenstein, PhD, Author

This colorful, profusely illustrated book shows parents and others who work with disabled children how to design and build simple, inexpensive assistive technology devices that open up the world of outdoor experiences for these children. *$14.95*
72 pages Paperback 1995
ISBN 1-571290-11-7

3758 Behavior Management Applications for Teachers and Parents
Livrenoir Books
10 Jay Street
Brooklyn, NY 11201
718-243-1207
Thomas J Zirpoli, Kristine J Melloy, Author

A clear, extensive presentation of the technical basis and appropriate implementation strategies for managing behavior in classrooms, day care centers, even at home. *$30.64*
512 pages Paperback 1996
ISBN 0-135205-37-9

3759 Behavior Technology Guide Book
1 Eden Way
Princeton, NJ 08540
609-987-0099
FAX 609-987-0243
http://www.edenservices.org
e-mail: info@edenservices.org
David L Holmes, Executive Director/President
Anne Holmes, Director Outreach Support Svcs
Tom Cool, President
Techniques for increasing and decreasing behavior using the principles of applied behavior analysis and related teaching strategies — discrete trial, shaping, task analysis and chaining. *$50.00*

3760 Beyond the Rainbow
Learning Disabilities Association of America
4156 Library Road
Pittsburgh, PA 15234
412-341-1515
FAX 412-344-0224
http://www.ldanatl.org
e-mail: ldanatl@usaor.net
Patricia Dodds, Author

A guide for parents with children with dyslexia and other disabilities. *$16.00*

3761 Bridges to Reading
Parents & Educators Resource Center
1660 South Amphlett Boulevard
San Mateo, CA 94402
650-655-2411
800-471-9545
FAX 650-655-2411
http://www.schwablearning.org
e-mail: perc@perc-schwabfdn.org
PERC provides services to parents and educators to help students with learning differences succeed. Services include a lending library and Bridges-to-Reading, a step-by-step guide to understanding, identifying, and addressing reading problems. *$20.00*

3762 Building Healthy Minds
CDS
1094 Flex Drive
Jackson, TN 38301
731-423-1973
800-343-4499
Stanley Greenspan, MD, Author
Pete Dubuisson, Plant Manager

Explains what sorts of games, conversations and other interactions foster cognitive, emotional and moral development. *$17.00*
398 pages Paperback
ISBN 0-738203-56-4

3763 Building a Child's Self-Image: A Guide for Parents
Learning Disabilities Association of America
4156 Library Road
Pittsburgh, PA 15234
412-341-1515
FAX 412-344-0224
http://www.ldanatl.org
e-mail: ldanatl@usaor.net

$9.25

3764 Care of the Neurologically Handicapped Child
Special Needs Project
324 State Street
Santa Barbara, CA 93101
805-962-8087
800-333-6867
FAX 805-962-5087
e-mail: books@specialneeds.com
Arthur Prensky, Author

This book describes normal and abnormal development, what to expect from the various specialists parents may consult, and seven of the most common neurological disorders. *$32.95*

331 pages

3765 **Caring for Your Baby and Young Child: Birth to Age 5**

Bantam
400 Hahn Road
Westminster, MD 21157
800-726-0600
FAX 800-659-2436
http://www.randomhouse.com/bantamdell
e-mail: bdpublicity@randomhouse.com
Sponsored by the American Academy of Pediatrics, Author

Offers reassuring advice on child rearing that covers everything from preparing for childbirth to toilet training to nuturing your child's self esteem. Here is an indispensable guide to recognizing and solving common childhood health problems, plus detailed instructions for coping with emergency medical situations. *$20.00*

784 pages Paperback
ISBN 0-553110-45-4

3766 **Children with Autism**

Special Needs Project
324 State Street
Santa Barbara, CA 93101
805-962-8087
800-333-6867
FAX 805-962-5087
e-mail: books@specialneeds.com
Michael Powers, Author

Recommended as the first book that parents should read, this book provides a complete introduction to autism, while easing a family's fears and concerns as they adjust and cope with their child's disorder. *$14.95*

368 pages

3767 **Children with Cerebral Palsy: A Parent's Guide**

Therapro
225 Arlington Street
Framingham, MA 01702
508-872-9494
800-257-5376
FAX 508-875-2062
http://www.theraproducts.com
e-mail: info@theraproducts.com
Elaine Geralis, Editor
Karen Conrad, Owner

This book explains what cerebral palsy is, and discusses its diagnosis and treatment. It also offers information and advice concerning daily care, early intervention, therapy, educational options and family life.

3768 **Children with Special Needs: A Resource Guide for Parents, Educators, Social Workers...**

Charles C Thomas Publisher
2600 S 1st Street
Springfield, IL 62704
217-789-8980
800-258-8980
FAX 217-789-9130
Karen L Lungu, Author
Michael Thomas, President

Writing from her own experience as the parent of a special needs child and with the background of both a therapist and educator, the author presents a most readable text discussing developmental disabilities, emotional and intellectual challenges, neurological disabilities, communication and learning disorders, attention deficit disorders and more. Paperback, ISBN: 0-398-06934-4, 42.95. *$57.95*

234 pages Cloth 1999
ISBN 0-398069-33-6

3769 **Children with Tourette Syndrome**

Woodbine House
6510 Bells Mill Road
Bethesda, MD 20817
301-897-3570
800-843-7323
FAX 301-897-5838
http://www.woodbinehouse.com
e-mail: info@Woodbinehouse.com
Tracy Haerle, Editor
Irv Shapell, Owner

A guide for parents of children and teenagers with Tourette syndrome. Covers medical, educational, legal, family life, daily care, and emotional issues, as well as explanations of related conditions. *$14.95*

352 pages Paperback
ISBN 0-933149-39-5

3770 **Classroom Success for the LD and ADHD Child**

Therapro
225 Arlington Street
Framingham, MA 01702
508-872-9494
800-257-5376
FAX 508-875-2062
http://www.theraproducts.com
e-mail: info@theraproducts.com
Suzanne H Stevens, Author
Karen Conrad, Owner

Helpful book for parents and therapists who work with children with learning disabilities. It addresses specific issues such as organization, homework and concentration. Stevens offers practical suggestions on adjusting teaching techniques, adapting texts, adjusting classroom management procedures and testing and grading fairly.

Revised

3771 **Common Ground: Whole Language & Phonics Working Together**

Modern Learning Press
PO Box 9067
Cambridge, MA 02139
609-397-2214
800-627-5867
FAX 888-558-7350
http://www.modlearn.com
e-mail: customer_service@epsbooks.com
Priscilla L Vail, Author

Offers guidelines for reading instruction in the primary grades that combines whole language with multisensory phonics instruction. *$8.95*

ISBN 0-935493-27-1

3772 **Common Sense About Dyslexia**

Special Needs Project
324 State Street
Santa Barbara, CA 93101
805-962-8087
800-333-6867
FAX 805-962-5087
e-mail: books@specialneeds.com
Ann Marshall Huston, Author

Offers important, need-to-know information about dyslexia. *$16.95*

300 pages

3773 **Communication Skills in Children with Down Syndrome**

Woodbine House
6510 Bells Mill Road
Bethesda, MD 20817
301-897-3570
800-843-7323
FAX 301-897-5838
http://www.woodbinehouse.com
e-mail: info@Woodbinehouse.com
Libby Kumin, PhD, CCC-SLP, Author
Irv Shapell, Owner

Accessible information, advice and practical home activities for children and adolescents with Down syndrome. *$14.95*

256 pages Paperback
ISBN 0-933149-53-0

3774 **Complete IEP Guide: How to Advocate for Your Special Ed Child**

NOLO
950 Parker Street
Berkeley, CA 94710
510-549-1976
800-955-4775
FAX 510-548-5902
http://www.nolo.com
Attorney Lawrence M Siegel, Author
David Rothenberg, CEO
Susan McConnell, Sales Director
Maira Dizgalvis, Trade Customer Service Manager

This book has all the plain-English suggestions, strategies, resources and forms to develop an effective IEP. *$17.47*
300 pages paperback
ISBN 0-873376-07-2

3775 Complete Learning Disabilities Resource Library
Slosson Educational Publications
PO Box 280
East Aurora, NY 14052
716-652-0930
800-828-4800
FAX 800-655-3840
http://www.sloss.com
e-mail: slosson@slosson.com
Joan M Harwell, Author
Steven Slosson, President

These volumes provide easy-to-use tips, techniques, and activities to help students with learning disabilities at all grade levels. *$29.95*

3776 Computer & Web Resources for People with Disabilities: A Guide to...
Alliance for Technology Access
1304 Southpoint Boulevard
Petaluma, CA 94954
707-765-2080
FAX 707-765-2080
http://www.ataccess.org
e-mail: atainfo@ataccess.org
Mary Lester, Executive Director

This highly acclaimed book includes detailed descriptions of software, hardware and communication aids, plus a gold mine of published and online resources. *$20.75*
364 pages

3777 Conducting Individualized Education Program Meetings that Withstand Due Process
Charles C Thomas Publisher
2600 S 1st Street
Springfield, IL 62704
217-789-8980
800-258-8980
FAX 217-789-9130
http://www.ccthomas.com
e-mail: books@ccthomas.com
James N Hollis, Author
Michael Thomas, President

Written to help parents, school administrators, teachers and assessment professionals meet basic requirements of conducting an IEP team meeting in a way that produces defensible IEP decisions in a litigious environment. Paperback, ISBN: 0-398-06847-X - 28.95. This book is out of print. Available by special orders only - must order in quantities of ten or more and they are non-returnable. *$41.95*
180 pages Cloth
ISBN 0-398068-46-1

3778 Connecting Students: A Guide to Thoughtful Friendship Facilitation
PEAK Parent Center
611 N Weber Street
Colorado Springs, CO 80903
719-531-9400
800-284-0251
FAX 719-531-9452
http://www.peakparent.org
e-mail: info@peakparent.org
C Beth Schaffner, and Barbara Buswell, Author

Offers real-life examples of how friendship facilitation can be implemented in natural ways in schools, neighborhoods, and communities. Perfect for anyone working to build classrooms and schools that ensure caring, acceptance and belonging for ALL students.

3779 Contemporary Intellectual Assessment: Theories, Tests and Issues
Guilford Publications
72 Spring Street
New York, NY 10012
212-431-9800
800-365-7006
FAX 212-966-6708
http://www.guilford.com
e-mail: info@guilford.com
Bob Matloff, President
Judy L Genshaft, Editor
Patti L Harrison, Editor

This unique volume provides a comprehensive conceptual and practical overview of the current state of the art of intellectual assessment. The book covers major theories of intelligence, methods of assessing human cognitive abilities, and issues related to the validity of current intelligence test batteries. *$60.00*
597 pages

3780 Controversial Issues Confronting Special Education
Books on Special Children
PO Box 305
Congers, NY 10920
845-638-1236
FAX 845-638-0847
http://www.boscbooks.com/
e-mail: irene@boscbooks.com
William Stainback, Susan Stainback, Author

The book has divergent perspectives from many contributors on twelve important controversial issues. Inclusive education, talented and gifted, classification and labeling, assessments, classroom management, research, adult services and more. *$59.00*
384 pages softcover
ISBN 0-205182-66-6

3781 Deciding What to Teach and How to Teach It Connecting Students through Curriculum and Instruction
PEAK Parent Center
611 N Weber Street
Colorado Springs, CO 80903
719-531-9400
800-284-0251
FAX 719-531-9452
http://www.peakparent.org
e-mail: info@peakparent.org
E Castagnera, D Fisher, K Rodifer, C Sax, Author

Provides exciting and practical resource tips to ensure that all students participate and learn successfully in secondary general education classrooms. Leads the reader through a step-by-step process for accessing general curriculum, making accommodations and modifications, and providing appropriate supports. Planning grids and concrete strategies make this an essential tool for both secondary educators and families. Support strategies are enhanced in this second edition *$ 13.00*

3782 Defiant Children
Guilford Publications
72 Spring Street
New York, NY 10012
212-431-9800
800-365-7006
FAX 212-966-6708
http://www.guilford.com
e-mail: info@guilford.com
Russell A Barkley, Author
Christine M Benton, Author
Bob Matloff, President
This book is written expressly for parents who are struggling with an unyielding or combative child, helping them understand what causes defiance, when it becomes a problem, and how it can be resolved. Its clear eight-step program stresses consistency and cooperation, promoting changes through a system of praise, rewards, and mild punishment. Filled with helpful sidebars, charts, and checklists. *$35.00*
255 pages Hardcover
ISBN 1-572301-23-6

3783 Developing Fine and Gross Motor Skills
Therapro
225 Arlington Street
Framingham, MA 01702
508-872-9494
800-257-5376
FAX 508-875-2062
http://www.theraproducts.com
e-mail: info@theraproducts.com
Donna Staisiunas Hurley, Author
Karen Conrad, Owner

This new home exercise program has dozens of beautifully illustrated, reproducible handouts for the parent, therapists, health care and child care workers. Each interval of 3 to 6 months in the child's development is divided into a fine motor and a gross motor section. Each section has several exercise sheets that guide parents in ways to develop specific motor skills that typically occur at that age level. Also includes practical information on how to guide parents when doing the exerecises.

Ages Birth-3

3784 Diamonds in the Rough
Slosson Educational Publications
PO Box 280
East Aurora, NY 14052
716-652-0930
888-756-7766
FAX 800-655-3840
http://www.slosson.com
e-mail: slosson@slosson.com

Peggy Strass Dias, Author
Steven Slosson, President
John Slosson, Vice President

An invaluable multidisciplinary reference guide to learning disabilities. It is an indispensable resource for educators, health specialists, parents and librarians. The author has printed a clear picture of the archetypical learner with a step-by-step view of the learning disabled child. *$53.00*

3785 Dictionary of Special Education & Rehabilitation: 4th Editon
Love Publishing
9101 East Kenyon Avenue
Denver, CO 80237
303-221-7333
FAX 303-221-7444
http://www.lovepublishing.com
e-mail: lpc@lovepublishing.com
Glenn A Vergason, M L Anderegg, Author

This updated edition of one of the most valuable resources in the field is over six years in the making incorporates hundreds of additions. It provides clear, understandable definitions of more than 2,000 terms unique to special education and rehabilitation. *$34.95*
210 pages Paperback 1997
ISBN 0-891082-43-3

3786 Directive Group Play Therapy: 2nd Edtion
Books on Special Children
PO Box 305
Congers, NY 10920
845-638-1236
FAX 845-638-0847
http://www.boscbooks.com/
e-mail: irene@boscbooks.com

Norma Leben, Author

Morning Glory Treatment Center for Children is a licensed therapeutic foster group home of about 10 children of ages 5-17. These games are played as part of therapy milieu. Each game contains objectives, supplies used. *$28.00*
96 pages spiralbound

3787 Directory for Exceptional Children
Porter Sargent Publishers
11 Beacon Street
Boston, MA 02108
617-523-1670
800-342-7470
FAX 617-523-1021
http://www.potersargent.com
e-mail: info@portersargent.com

Dan McKeever, Senior Editor
John Yonce, Manager
Leslie A Weston, Production Editor
A comprehensive survey of 3000 schools, facilities and organizations across the USA, serving children and young adults with developmental, emotional, physical and medical disabilities. An invaluable aid to parents and professionals. *$75.00*
1152 pages Triannual 1954Grade Range: K-12+
ISBN 0-875581-50-1

3788 Directory for Exceptional Children: 15th Edition
Porter Sargent Publishers
11 Beacon Street
Boston, MA 02108
617-523-1670
800-342-7470
FAX 617-523-1021
http://www.potersargent.com
e-mail: info@portersargent.com

Porter Sargent Staff, Author
Dan McKeever, Senior Editor
John Yonce, Manager
Leslie Weston, Production Editor

A comprehensive survey of 3000 schools, facilities and organizations across the USA, serving children and young adults with developmental, emotional, physical and medical disabilities. An invaluable aid to parents and professionals. *$75.00*
1152 pages Trienniel 1954Grade Range: K-Post Graduate
ISBN 0-875581-50-1

3789 Dr. Larry Silver's Advice to Parents on AD-HD
Learning Disabilities Association of America
4156 Library Road
Pittsburgh, PA 15234
412-341-1515
FAX 412-344-0224
http://www.ldanatl.org
e-mail: ldanatl@usaor.net

Dr. Larry B Silver, Author

Offers information on parenting children with Attention Deficit and Hyperactivity Disorders. *$19.95*

3790 Early Childhood Special Education: Birth to Three
Connecticut Assoc. for Children and Adults with LD
25 Van Zant Street
Norwalk, CT 06855
203-838-5010
FAX 203-866-6108
http://www.CACLD.org

J Jordan, Author
Beryl Kaufman, Executive Director

Resources on early childhood education.

3791 Educating Deaf Children Bilingually
Harris Communications
15155 Technology Drive
Eden Prairie, MN 55344
952-906-1180
800-825-9187
FAX 952-906-1099
TDY:952-906-1198
http://www.harriscomm.com
e-mail: info@harriscomm.com

Shawn Neal Mahshie, Author
Robert Harris, Owner
Lori Foss, Marketing Director

Perspectives and practices in educating deaf children with the goal of grade-level achievement in fluency in the languages of the deaf community, general society and of the home are discussed in this book. *$16.95*
262 pages

3792 Educating Students Who Have Visual Impairments with Other Disabilities
Brookes Publishing Company
PO Box 10624
Baltimore, MD 21285
410-337-9580
800-638-3775
FAX 410-337-8539
http://www.info@pbrookes.com
e-mail: custserv@brookespublishing.com

Sharon Z Sacks PhD, Editor
Rosanne K Silberman EdD, Editor
Paul Brooks, Owner
This text provides techniques for facilitating functional learning in students with a wide range of visual impairments and multiple disabilities. *$49.95*
552 pages Paperback
ISBN 1-557662-80-0

3793 Effective Instructions for Students withLearning Difficulties
Books on Special Children
PO Box 305
Congers, NY 10920
845-638-1236
FAX 845-638-0847
http://www.boscbooks.com/
e-mail: irene@boscbooks.com

PT Cegelka, Author

The book is designed to help teach students and prevent academic failure. Overview of effective education: identify; measure; then manage behavior. Classroom structure to meet individual needs and teach reading, spelling written language skills, math. How to plan transition to adulthood. Each chapter has objectives outline and summary charts and forms. *$68.00*

469 pages softcover
ISBN 0-205162-68-1

3794 **Effective Teaching Methods for Autistic Children**
Charles C Thomas Publisher
2600 S 1st Street
Springfield, IL 62704
217-789-8980
800-258-8980
FAX 217-789-9130
e-mail: books@ccthomas.com
Rosalind C Oppenheim, Author
Michael Thomas, President

This book is out of print. Available by special orders only - must order in quantities of ten or more and they are non-returnable. *$21.25*
124 pages Cloth
ISBN 0-398028-58-3

3795 **Emergence-Labeled Autistic**
Therapro
225 Arlington Street
Framingham, MA 01702
508-872-9494
800-257-5376
FAX 508-875-2062
http://www.theraproducts.com
e-mail: info@theraproducts.com
Temple Grandin, PhD as told by Margaret Scariano, Author
Karen Conrad, Owner

In this autobiography, Temple tells the story of her emergence from her fear-gripped, autistic childhood to becoming a successful professional. This astonishing, true story will give new insight into autism and show it from the'inside'.
180 pages

3796 **Emergence: Labeled Autistic**
Academic Therapy Publications
20 Commercial Boulevard
Novato, CA 94949
415-883-3314
800-422-7249
FAX 415-883-3720
http://www.academictherapy.com
e-mail: sales@academictherapy.com
Jim Arena
Joanne Urban

A recovered autistic individual shares her history, and includes her own suggestions for parents and professionals. Technical Appendix, which overviews recent treatment methods and more.

3797 **Essential ASL: The Fun, Fast, and Simple Way to Learn American Sign Language**
Harris Communications
15155 Technology Drive
Eden Prairie, MN 55344
952-906-1180
800-825-6758
FAX 952-906-1099
TDY:952-906-1198
http://www.harriscomm.com
e-mail: info@harriscomm.com
Martin LA Sternberg, EdD, Author
Robert Harris, Owner
Lori Foss, Marketing Director

This pocket version contains more than 700 frequently used signs with 2,000 easy-to-follow illustrations. Also, 50 common phrases. *$7.95*
322 pages Paperback 1996

3798 **Evaluation of the Association for Children with Learning Disabilities**
National Center for State Courts
300 Newport Avenue
Williamsburg, VA 23185
757-253-2000
FAX 757-220-0449
http://www.ncsconline.org
e-mail: webmaster@ncsc.dni.us
Final report on children with learning disabilities training institute. *$6.96*

3799 **Family Communication**
Harris Communications
15155 Technology Drive
Eden Prairie, MN 55344
952-906-1180
800-825-6758
FAX 952-906-1099
TDY:952-906-1198
http://www.harriscomm.com
Robert Harris, Owner

A broad range of topics that affect communication in the home and classroom, including support for families, and ways parents and school can work together toward language literacy development. *$10.95*
62 pages

3800 **Family Guide to Assistive Technology**
Federation for Children with Special Needs
1135 Tremont Street
Roxbury Crossing, MA 02120
617-236-7210
800-331-0688
FAX 617-572-2094
http://www.fcsn.org
e-mail: fcsninfo@fcsn.org
Richard Robison, President

This guide is intended to help parents learn more about assistive technology and how it can help their children. Includes tips for getting started, ideas about how and where to look for funding and contact information for software and equipment. *$10.00*
143 pages

3801 **Family Place in Cyberspace**
Alliance for Technology Access
1304 Southpoint Boulevard
Petaluma, CA 94954
707-765-2080
FAX 707-765-2080
http://www.ataccess.org
e-mail: atainfo@ataccess.org
Mary Lester, Executive Director

Includes We Can Play, a variety of suggestions and ideas for making play activities accessible to all. Available in English and Spanish. Access in Transition. Information and resources for students with disabilities who are facing the transition from public school to the next stage in life. Includes links and resources. Assistive Technology in K-12 Schools gives a range of information about integrating assistive technology into schools.

3802 **Fine Motor Skills in Children with Downs Syndrome: A Guide for Parents and Professionals**
Therapro
225 Arlington Street
Framingham, MA 01702
508-872-9494
800-257-5376
FAX 508-875-2062
http://www.theraproducts.com
e-mail: info@theraproducts.com
Maryanne Bruni B.Sc., OT(C), Author
Karen Conrad, Owner

Fine motor skills are the hand skills that allow us to do the things like hold a pencil, cut with scissors, eat with a fork, and use a computer. This practical guide shows parents and professionals how to help children with Downs syndrome from infancy to 12 years improve fine motor functioning. Includes many age appropriate activities for home or school, with step by step instructions and photos. Invaluable for families and professionals.

3803 **Fine Motor Skills in the Classroom: Screening & Remediation Strategies**
Therapro
225 Arlington Street
Framingham, MA 01702
508-872-9494
800-257-5376
FAX 508-875-2062
http://www.theraproducts.com
e-mail: info@theraproducts.com
Jayne Berry, OTR/L, Author
Karen Conrad, Owner

The Give Yourself a Hand program, revised. Developed as a tool to facilitate consultation in the classroom. The manual consists of training modules, a screening to administer to an entire class, report formats for teachers and parents, and classroom and home remediation activities. The program is designed to include everyone involved in the education process and to make them aware of the opportunites offered by occupational therapy in the classroom.

96 pages

3804 Flying By the Seat of Your Pants: More Absurdities and Realities of Special Education

Peytral Publication
PO Box 1162
Minnetonka, MN 55345
952-949-8707
877-739-8725
FAX 952-906-9777
http://www.peytral.com
e-mail: help@peytral.com

Michael F Giangreco, Author
Peggy Hammeken, President

In the sequel to Ants in His Pants, Giangreco continues to stimulate the reader to think differently about some of our current educational practices and raise questions about specific issues surrounding special education. Whether an educator, parent or advocate for persons with disabilities, you will smile, laugh aloud and ponder the hidden truths playfully captured in these carefully crafted cartoons. Transparencies may be created directly from the book. *$19.95*

126 pages
ISBN 1-890455-41-5

3805 For Parents and Professionals: Down Syndrome

LinguiSystems
3100 4th Avenue
East Moline, IL 61244
309-755-2300
800-776-4332
FAX 800-577-4555
http://www.linguisystems.com
e-mail: service@linguisystems.com

Linda Bowers, Co-Owner/Co-Founder
Rosemary Huisingh, Co-Owner/Co-Founder

This comprehensive resource gives you valuable information, helpful tips, and great activities to share with parents, teachers, and other caregivers. Packed with examples and activities, chapters cover: getting to know the child with Down syndrome; applying teaching and learning strategies, oral-motor and feeding skills, impact on overall communication skills, getting through the school years and more.

3806 Gross Motor Skills Children with Down Syndrome: A Guide For Parents and Professionals

Therapro
225 Arlington Street
Framingham, MA 01702
508-872-9494
800-257-5376
FAX 508-875-2062
http://www.theraproducts.com
e-mail: info@theraproducts.com

Patricia C Winders, PT, Author
Karen Conrad, Owner

Children with Down syndrome master basic gross motor skills, everything from rolling over to running, just as their peers do, but may need additional help. This guide describes and illustrates more than 100 easy to follow activities for parents and professionals to practice with infants and children from birth to age six. Checklists and statistics allow readers to track, plan and maximize a child's progress.

3807 Guide for Parents on Hyperactivity in Children Fact Sheet

Learning Disabilities Association of America
4156 Library Road
Pittsburgh, PA 15234
412-341-1515
FAX 412-344-0224
http://www.ldanatl.org
e-mail: ldanatl@usaor.net

Klaus K Minde, Author

Describes difficulties faced by a child with ADHD. Elaborates on types of management and ends with a section called 'A Day With a Hyperactive Child: Possible Problems'. *$2.00*

23 pages

3808 Guidelines and Recommended Practices for Individualized Family Service Plan

Education Resources Information Center
7910 Woodmont Avenue
Bethesda, MD 20814
FAX 301-986-4553

Mary J McGonigel, Author

Presents a growing consensus about best practices for comprehensive family-centered early intervention services as required by Part H of the Individuals with Disabilities Education Act.
$15.00

208 pages

3809 Handbook for Implementing Workshops for Siblings of Special Needs Children

Special Needs Project
324 State Street
Santa Barbara, CA 93101
805-962-8087
800-333-6867
FAX 805-962-5087
e-mail: books@specialneeds.com

Donald Meyer, Author

Based on three years of professional experience working with siblings ages 8 through 13 and their parents, this handbook provides guidelines and technologies for those who wish to start and conduct workshops for siblings. *$40.00*

65 pages

3810 Handbook of Research in Emotional and Behavioral Disorders

Guilford Press
72 Spring Street
New York, NY 10012
212-431-9800
800-365-7006
FAX 212-966-6708
http://www.guilford.com
e-mail: info@guilford.com

Robert B Rutherford Jr, Mary Magee Quinn, Author
Sarup R Mathur, Editor

Integrates current knowledge on emotional and behavioral disorders in the school setting. Also, emphasizes the importance of interdisciplinary collaboration in service provision and delineates best-practice guidelines for research. *$76.00*

622 pages August 2004
ISBN 1-593850-56-5

3811 Handling the Young Child with Cerebral Palsy at Home

Therapro
225 Arlington Street
Framingham, MA 01702
508-872-9494
800-257-5376
FAX 508-875-2062
http://www.theraproducts.com
e-mail: info@theraproducts.com

Nancie R Finnie, Author
Karen Conrad, Owner

This guide for parents remains a classic book on handling their cerebral palsied child during all activities of daily living. It has been said that its message is so important that it should be read by all those caring for such children including doctors, therapists, teachers and nurses. Many simple line drawings illustrate handling problems and solutions.

3rd Edition

3812 Help Build a Brighter Future: Children at Risk for LD in Child Care Centers

Learning Disabilities Association of America
4156 Library Road
Pittsburgh, PA 15234
412-341-1515
FAX 412-344-0224
http://www.ldanatl.org
e-mail: ldanatl@usaor.net

Offers information for parents and professionals caring for the learning disabled child. *$3.00*

3813 Help Me to Help My Child
Little Brown & Company
3 Center Plaza
Boston, MA 02108
617-227-0730
FAX 617-263-2871

Jill Bloom, Author

Contains nontechnical information on testing, advocacy, legal issues, instructional practices, and social-emotional development, as well as a resource list and bibliography.

ISBN 0-316099-82-1

3814 Help for the Hyperactive Child: A Good Sense Guide for Parents
Learning Disabilities Association of America
4156 Library Road
Pittsburgh, PA 15234
412-341-1515
FAX 412-344-0224
http://www.ldanatl.org
e-mail: ldanatl@usaor.net

A practical guide; offering parents of ADHD children alternatives to Ritalin. *$16.95*

3815 Help for the Learning Disabled Child
Slosson Educational Publications
PO Box 280
East Aurora, NY 14052
716-652-0930
800-828-4800
FAX 800-655-3840
http://www.slosson.com
e-mail: slosson@slosson.com

Lou Stewart, Author
Steven Slosson, President
John Slosson, Vice President

An easy-to-read text describes observable behaviors, offers remediation techniques, materials, and specific test to assist in further diagnosis. *$38.00*

3816 Helping Your Child Achieve in School
Academic Therapy Publications
20 Commercial Boulevard
Novato, CA 94949
415-883-3314
800-422-7249
FAX 415-883-3720
http://www.apub.com

Betty Lou Kratoville, Editor
Anna Arena, President

A wealth of simple and enjoyable at-home educational activities. Special emphasis is given to developing reading skills in primary-aged children and to building comprehension skills of middle-grade children. *$12.50*
264 pages
ISBN 0-878794-65-4

3817 Helping Your Child with Attention-Deficit Hyperactivity Disorder
Learning Disabilities Association of America
4156 Library Road
Pittsburgh, PA 15234
412-341-1515
FAX 412-344-0224
http://www.ldanatl.org
e-mail: ldanatl@usaor.net

M Fowler, Author

$12.95

3818 Helping Your Hyperactive Child
Connecticut Assoc. for Children and Adults with LD
25 Van Zant Street
Norwalk, CT 06855
203-838-5010
FAX 203-866-6018
http://www.CACLD.org

John Taylor, Author
Beryl Kaufman, Executive Director

A large, comprehensive book for parents, covering everything from techniques pertaining to sibling rivalry to coping with marital stresses. Contains thorough discussions of various treatments: nutritional, medical and educational. Also is an excellent source of advice and information for parents of kids with ADHD. *$2195.00*
483 pages

3819 Hidden Child: Linwood Method for Reaching the Autistic Child
Therapro
225 Arlington Street
Framingham, MA 01702
508-872-9494
800-257-5376
FAX 508-875-2062
http://www.theraproducts.com
e-mail: info@theraproducts.com

Jeanne Simmons and Sabine Oiski, PhD, Author
Karen Conrad, Owner

This book provides an explanation of autism, then a step-by-step analysis of the Linwood method of establishing relationships, patterning good behavior, overcoming compulsions, developing skills, and fostering social and emotional development. This guidebook for teachers and therapists also has a message for parents.

3820 Higher Education Services for Students with LD or ADD a Legal Guide
JKL Communications
2700 Virginia Avenue NW
Washington, DC 20037
202-223-5097
FAX 202-223-5096
http://www.lathamlaw.org
e-mail: plath3@his.com

$29.00

3821 How the Special Needs Brain Learns
Corwin Press
2455 Teller Road
Thousand Oaks, CA 91320
805-499-9774
800-818-7243
FAX 805-499-0871
http://www.corwinpress.com
e-mail: order@corwinpress.com

David A Sousa, Author
Robb Clouse, Editorial Director
Kimberly Gonzales, Director Marketing

Research on the brain function of students with various learning challenges. Practical classroom activities and strategies, such as how to build self-esteem, how to work in groups, and strategies for engagement and retention. Focuses on the most commmon challenges to learning for many students. *$34.95*
248 pages
ISBN 0-761978-51-8

3822 How to Get Services by Being Assertive
Family Resource Center on Disabilities
20 E Jackson Boulevard
Chicago, IL 60604
312-939-3513
800-952-4199
FAX 312-939-7297
TDY:312-939-3519

Family Resource Center on Disabilities, Author
Charolotte Jardins, Executive Director

A manual that demonstrates positive assertiveness techniques for staffing, IEP meetings, due process hearings and other special education meetings. *$10.00*
100 pages

3823 How to Organize Your Child and Save Your Sanity
Learning Disabilities Association of America
4156 Library Road
Pittsburgh, PA 15234
412-341-1515
FAX 412-344-0224
http://www.ldanatl.org
e-mail: ldanatl@usaor.net

Brown/Connelly, Author

$3.00

3824 How to Organize an Effective Parent-Advocacy Group and Move Bureaucracies
Family Resource Center on Disabilities
20 E Jackson Boulevard
Chicago, IL 60604
312-939-3513
800-952-4199
FAX 312-939-7297
TDY:312-939-3519

Charlotte Desjardins, Author
Charlotte Jardins, Executive Director

A 100-page handbook that gives step-by-step directions for organizing parent support groups from scratch. *$10.00*
100 pages

3825 How to Own and Operate an Attention Deficit Disorder
Learning Disabilities Association of America
4156 Library Road
Pittsburgh, PA 15234
412-341-1515
FAX 412-344-0224
http://www.ldanatl.org
e-mail: ldanatl@usaor.net
Clear, informative and sensitive introduction to ADHD. Packed with practical things to do at home and school, the author offers her insight as a professional and mother of a son with ADHD. *$8.95*
43 pages

3826 Hyperactive Children Grown Up
Guilford Publications
72 Spring Street
New York, NY 10012
212-431-9800
800-365-7006
FAX 212-966-6708
http://www.guilford.com
e-mail: info@guilford.com
Gabrielle Weiss, Author
Lily Trokenberg Hechtman, Author
Bob Matloff, President
Long considered a standard in the field, this book explores what happens to hyperactive children when they grow into adulthood. Updated and expanded, this second edition describes new developments in ADHD, current psychological treatments of ADHD, contemporary perspectives on the use of medications, and assessment, diagnosis and treatment of ADHD adults. *$26.00*
473 pages Paperback
ISBN 0-898625-96-3

3827 If it is to Be, It is Up to Me to Do it!
AVKO Educational Research Foundation
3084 W Willard Road
Clio, MI 48420
810-686-9283
FAX 810-686-1101
http://www.avko.org/upto.htm
e-mail: DonMcCabe@aol.com
Don McCabe, Author
Don Cabe, Executive Director

This is a tutors' book that can be used by anyone who can read this paragraph. It also contains the student's response pages. It is especially good to use to help an older child or adult. It uses the same basic format as Sequential Spelling I except it has the sentences to be read along with the word to be spelled. The students get to correct their own mistakes immediately. This way they quickly learn that mistakes are opportunities to learn. *$19.95*
96 pages
ISBN 1-564007-42-1

3828 In Their Own Way: Discovering and Encouraging Your Child's Learning
Special Needs Project
324 State Street
Santa Barbara, CA 93101
805-962-8087
800-333-6867
FAX 805-962-5087
e-mail: books@specialneeds.com
Dr. Thomas Armstrong, Author

An unconventional teacher has written a very popular book for a wide audience. It's customary to be categorical about youngsters who learn conventionally/are normal/are OK — and those who don't/who need special ed/are learning disabled. *$8.37*
224 pages Paperback

3829 In Time and with Love
Special Needs Project
324 State Street
Santa Barbara, CA 93101
805-962-8087
800-333-6867
FAX 805-962-5087
e-mail: books@specialnedds.com
Play and parenting techniques for children with disabilities. *$12.95*
19 pages

3830 In the Mind's Eye
Prometheus Books
59 John Glenn Drive
Amherst, NY 14228
716-691-0133
800-421-0351
FAX 716-691-0137
http://www.prometheusbooks.com
e-mail: mrogers@prometheusbooks.com
Thomas West, Author
Marcia Rogers, Sales Manager

Visual thinkers, gifted people with learning difficulties, computer images, and the ironies of creativity. Be concerned with results, not uniformity of learning style. *$29.00*
397 pages 1997
ISBN 1-573921-55-6

3831 Inclusion: A Practical Guide for Parents
Peytral Publication
PO Box 1162
Minnetonka, MN 55345
952-949-8707
877-739-8725
FAX 952-906-9777
http://www.peytral.com
e-mail: help@peytral.com
Lorraine O Moore, Author
Peggy Hammeken, President

This comprehensive resource answers parent questions related to inclusive education and provides the tools to promote and enhance their child's learning. This publication includes practical strategies, exercises, questionnaires and do-it-yourself graphs to assist parents with their child's learning. Beneficial for parents, psychologists, social workers, and educators. *$19.95*
192 pages
ISBN 0-964427-13-3

3832 Inclusion: Strategies for Working with Young Children
Peytral Publication
PO Box 1162
Minnetonka, MN 55345
952-949-8707
877-739-8725
FAX 952-906-9777
http://www.peytral.com
e-mail: help@peytral.com
Lorraine O Moore, Author
Peggy Hammeken, President

Developed for early childhood through grade two educators and parents, this comprehensive developmentally focused publication focuses on the whole child. Hundreds of developmentally-based strategies help young children learn about feelings, empathy, resolving conflicts, communication, large/small motor development, prereading, writing and math strategies are included, plus much more. Excellent training tool. *$21.95*
185 pages
ISBN 0-964427-13-3

3833 Inclusive Elementary Schools
PEAK Parent Center
611 N Weber Street
Colorado Springs, CO 80903
719-531-9400
800-284-0251
FAX 719-531-9452
http://www.peakparent.org
e-mail: info@peakparent.org
Douglas Fisher, Nancy Frey, Caren Sax, Author

Walks readers through a state of the art, step-by-step process to determine what and how to teach elementary school students with disabilities in general education classrooms. Highlights strategies for accommodating and modifying assignments and activities by using core curriculum. Complete with user-friendly sample forms and creative support strategies, this is an essential text for elementary educators and parents. *$13.00*

3834 Innovations in Family Support for People with Learning Disabilities
Brookes Publishing Company
PO Box 10624
Baltimore, MD 21285
800-638-3775
FAX 410-337-8539
http://www.pbrookes.com
e-mail: custserv@pbrookes.com
Barbara Coyne Cutler, EdD, Author
Paul H Brooks, President
Melissa A Behm, Executive Vice President
George Stamathis, Vice President/Publisher
272 pages Paperback $22.00
ISBN 1-870335-15-5

3835 Interventions for ADHD: Treatment in Developmental Context
Guilford Publications
72 Spring Street
New York, NY 10012
212-431-9800
800-365-7006
FAX 212-966-6708
http://www.guilford.com
e-mail: info@guilford.com
Phyllis Anne Teeter, Author
Bob Matloff, President

This book takes a lifespan perspective on ADHD, dispelling the notion that it is only a disorder of childhood and enabling clinicians to develop effective and appropriate interventions for preschoolers, school-age children, adolescents, and adults. The author reviews empirically-and clinically-based treatment interventions including psychopharmacology, behavior management, parent/teacher training, and self-management techniques. *$40.00*
378 pages Hardcover
ISBN 1-572303-84-0

3836 Invisible Disability: Understanding Learning Disabilities in the Context of Health & Edu.
Learning Disabilities Association of America
4156 Library Road
Pittsburgh, PA 15234
412-341-1515
FAX 412-344-0224
http://www.ldanatl.org
e-mail: ldanatl@usaor.net
Pasquale Accardo, Author

$9.00
ISBN 0-937846-39-2

3837 It's Your Turn Now
Harris Communications
15155 Technology Drive
Eden Prairie, MN 55344
952-906-1180
800-825-6758
FAX 952-906-1099
TDY:952-906-1198
http://www.harriscomm.com
e-mail: info@harriscomm.com
Cindy Bailes, Author
Robert Harris, Owner
Lori Foss, Marketing Director

Using dialogue journals with deaf students help the students learn to enjoy communicating ideas, information, and feelings through reading and writing. The book reviews teacher's questions and answers, frustrations and successes. *$14.95*
130 pages

3838 Key Concepts in Personal Development
Marsh Media
8082 Ward Parkway Plaza
Kansas City, MO 64114
816-523-1059
800-821-3303
FAX 866-333-7421
http://www.marshmedia.com
e-mail: info@marshmedia.com
Joan Marsh, Owner
Liz Sweeney, Editorial Assistant

Puberty Education for Students with Special Needs. Comprehensive, gender-specific kits and supplemental parent packets address human sexuality education for children with mild to moderate developmental disabilities.

3839 Ladders to Literacy: A Kindergarten Activity Book
Brookes Publishing Company
PO Box 10624
Baltimore, MD 21285
410-337-9580
800-638-3775
FAX 410-337-8539
http://www.info@pbrookes.com
e-mail: sales@pbrookes.com
Rollanda E O'Connor, PhD, et. al., Author
Paul Brooks, Owner

The kindergarten activities are designed for higher developmental levels, focusing on preacademic skills, early literacy development, and early reading development. Goals and scaffolding are more intense as children learn to recognize letters, match sounds with letters, and develop phonological awareness and the alphabetic principle. *$32.16*
272 pages Spiral bound
ISBN 1-557663-18-1

3840 Ladders to Literacy: A Preschool Activity Book
Brookes Publishing Company
PO Box 10624
Baltimore, MD 21285
410-337-9580
800-638-3775
FAX 410-337-8539
http://www.info@pbrookes.com
e-mail: sales@pbrookes.com
Angela Notari-Syverson, PhD, et. al., Author
Paul Brooks, Owner

The preschool activity book targets basic preliteracy skills such as orienting children toward printed materials and teaching letter sounds. It also provides professionals (and parents) with developmentally appropriate and ecologically valid assessment procedures — informal observation guidelines, structured performance samples, and a checklist — for measuring children's learning. *$34.96*
352 pages Spiral bound
ISBN 1-557663-17-3

3841 Landmark School's Language-Based TeachingGuides
Landmark School
429 Hale Street
Prides Crossing, MA 01965
978-236-3000
FAX 978-927-7268
http://www.landmarkoutreach.org
e-mail: outreach@landmarkschool.org
Joan Sedita, Author
Dan Ahearn, Director
Trish Newhall, Associate Director
Chris Murphy, Principal
Landmark School's Language-Based Teaching Guides provide research-based practical teaching strategies for teachers and parents working with students who have learning disabilities. Topics inlcude study skills, expressive langage skills, writing, mathematics. *$30.00*
125 pages
ISBN 0-962411-90-6

3842 Language and Literacy Learning in Schools
Guilford Publications
72 Spring Street
New York, NY 10012
212-431-9800
800-365-7006
FAX 212-966-6708
http://www.guilford.com
e-mail: info@guilford.com
Elaine R Stillman, Louise C Wilkinson, Author

Interweaves the voices of classroom teachers, speech-language pathologists whos children learning to become literate in English as a first or second language, and researchers from multiple disciplines. *$40.00*

366 pages October 2004
ISBN 1-593850-65-4

3843 Language-Related Learning Disabilities
Brookes Publishing Company
PO Box 10624
Baltimore, MD 21285
800-638-3775
FAX 410-337-8539
http://www.pbrookes.com
e-mail: custserv@pbrookes.com
Adele Gerber, MA, Author
Paul H Brooks, President
Melissa A Behm, Executive Vice President
George Stamathis, Vice President/Publisher
384 pages Paperback $47.00
ISBN 1-557660-53-0

3844 Learning Difficulties and Emotional Problems
Temeron Books
PO Box 896
Bellingham, WA 98227
FAX 360-738-4016
http://www.temerondetselig.com
e-mail: temeron@telusplanet.net
Roy Brown, Maurice Chazan, Author
Ted Giles
May Misfeldt

International authorities shed light on recent research. *$18.95*
239 pages Paperback
ISBN 0-920490-89-1

3845 Learning Disabilities & ADHD: A Family Guide to Living and Learning Together
John Wiley & Sons
10475 Crosspoint Boulevard
Indianapolis, IN 46256
317-572-3000
FAX 800-597-3299
http://www.wiley.com
Betty B Osman, Author
Lou Peragallo, Manager

228 pages paperback $14.95
ISBN 0-471155-10-1

3846 Learning Disabilities A to Z
Simon and Schuster
PO Box 11071
Des Moines, IA 50336
515-282-0205
800-223-2348
FAX 515-284-2607
http://www.simonandschuster.com
Smith, Corinne and Lisa Strick, Author
Harry Simon, Owner

Brings the best of recent research and educational experience to parents, teachers and caregivers who are responsible for children with information processing problems. Corinne Smith and Lisa Strick provide a comprehensive guide to the causes, identification and treatment of learning disabilities. You will learn how these subtle neurological disorders can have a major impact on a child's development, both in and out of school. *$25.00*
416 pages
ISBN 0-684827-38-7

3847 Learning Disabilities: Lifelong Issues
Brookes Publishing Company
PO Box 10624
Baltimore, MD 21285
410-337-9580
800-638-3775
FAX 410-337-8539
http://www.info@pbrookes.com
e-mail: sales@pbrookes.com
Shirley C Cramer, Editor
William Ellis, Editor
Paul Brooks, Owner
Based on the diverse, representative viewpoints of educators, practitioners, policy makers, and adults with learning disabilities, this volume sets forth an agenda for improving the educational and ultimately, social and economic, futures of people with learning disabilities. *$36.00*

352 pages Paperback
ISBN 1-557662-40-1

3848 Learning Disabilities: Literacy, and Adult Education
Brookes Publishing Company
PO Box 10624
Baltimore, MD 21285
410-337-9580
800-638-3775
FAX 410-337-8539
http://www.info@pbrookes.com
e-mail: sales@pbrookes.com
Susan A Vogel PhD, Editor
Stephen Reder PhD, Editor
Paul Brooks, Owner
This book focuses on adults with severe learning disabilities and the educators who work with them. *$49.95*
400 pages Paperback
ISBN 1-557663-47-5

3849 Learning Disabilities: Theories, Diagnosis and Teaching Strategies
Houghton-Mifflin
222 Berkeley Street
Boston, MA 02116
617-351-5000
FAX 617-351-1119
http://www.houghtonmifflinbooks.com
J Lerner, Author
Tony Lucki, CEO

Theories on learning disabilities.

ISBN 0-395796-85-7

3850 Learning Journey
PO Box 896
Bellingham, WA 98227
FAX 360-738-4016
http://www.temerondetselig.com
e-mail: temeron@telusplanet.net
Malcom Jeffreys, Robert Gall, Author

Enhancing lifelong learning and self-determination for people with special needs, this book presents a detailed view of emerging trends and models of service that promise a better future in terms of self-determination for the developmentally disabled. *$18.95*
204 pages Paperback
ISBN 1-550591-22-3

3851 Learning Outside The Lines: Two Ivy LeagueStudents with Learning Disabilities and Adhd
Fireside

Edward M Hallowell, Jonathan Mooney, David Cole, Author

Takes you on a personal empowerment and profound educational change, proving once again that rules sometimes need to be broken. *$14.00*
288 pages September 2000
ISBN 0-684865-98-X

3852 Legacy of the Blue Heron: Living with Learning Disabilities
Oxton House Publishers
PO Box 209
Farmington, ME 04938
207-779-1923
800-539-7323
FAX 207-779-0623
http://www.oxtonhouse.com
e-mail: info@oxtonhouse.com
William Berlinghoff PhD, Managing Editor
Bobby Brown, Marketing Director

This book is available as in soft cover or as a six-cassette audiobook. It is engaging personal account by a severe dyslexic who became a successful engineer, business, boat builder, and president of the Learning Disabilities Association of America. Drawing on his life experiences, the author presents a rich array of wise, common-sense advice for dealing with learning disabilities.

3853 Let's Learn About Deafness
Harris Communications
15155 Technology Drive
Eden Prairie, MN 55344
952-906-1180
800-825-6758
FAX 952-906-1099
TDY:952-906-1198
http://www.harriscomm.com
e-mail: info@harriscomm.com
Rachel Stone, Author
Robert Harris, Owner
Lori Foss, Marketing Director

Hands-on activities, games, bulletin board displays, surveys, quizzes, craft projects, and skits used to help teachers and their students become more aware of deafness and its implications are included in this book. *$16.95*
82 pages

3854 Life Beyond the Classroom: Transition Strategies for Young People with Disabilities
Brookes Publishing
PO Box 10624
Baltimore, MD 21285
410-337-9580
800-638-3775
FAX 410-337-8539
http://www.brookespublishing.com
e-mail: custserv@brookespublishing.com
Paul Wehman, PhD, Author
Paul H Brookes, President
Melissa A Behm, Vice President

Community living, leisure activities, personal relationships as well as employment. Planning with community, individualized, state and local governments, curriculum for transition, job development and placement, independent living plans for people with mild MR, severe disabilities, LD, physical and health impairments, and traumatic brain injury. *$74.95*
752 pages softcover
ISBN 1-557662-48-7

3855 Living with a Learning Disability
Southern Illinois University Press
PO Box 3697
Carbondale, IL 62902
618-453-5348
800-346-2680
FAX 800-346-2681
http://www.siu.edu/nsiupress
e-mail: townsend@siu.edu
Barbara Cordoni, Author
Arron Stearn, Manager
Larry Townsend, Director Sales/Marketing

This book presents the kinds of adaptations needed for educating, communicating with, and parenting the child, the adolescent, and the young adult with learning disabilities. Deals with such issues as relationships, the legal process, implications for the professional, juvenile delinquency, and the future.
17.5 pages
ISBN 0-809316-68-4

3856 Making Sense of Sensory Integration
Therapro
225 Arlington Street
Framingham, MA 01702
508-872-9494
800-257-5376
FAX 508-875-2062
http://www.theraproducts.com
e-mail: info@theraproducts.com
Koomar, Szklut, Cermak and Silver, Author
Karen Conrad, Owner

A discussion for parents and caregivers about sensory integration (SI), how it affects children throughout their lives, how diagnosis is made, appropriate treatment, recognizing red flags, and how SI difficulties affect child and family in their everyday lives. Informative 33 page book included. 75 minute audio tape.
Audio Tape

3857 Making the Writing Process Work: Strategies for Composition & Self-Regulation
Brookline Books
34 University Road
Brookline, MA 02445
617-734-6772
800-666-BOOK
FAX 617-734-3952
http://www.brooklinebooks.com
e-mail: brooklinebks@delphi.com
Karen R Harris, Steve Graham, Author

Presents cognitive strategies for writing sequences of specific steps which make the writing process clearer and enable students to organize their thoughts about the writing task. *$24.95*
Paperback 1995
ISBN 1-571290-10-9

3858 McGraw Hill Companies
2 Penn Plaza
New York, NY 10121
212-904-2000
FAX 212-904-5974
http://www.mcgraw-hill.com
e-mail: elizabeth_schacht@mcgraw-hill.com
Henry Hirschberg, President

Corrective reading program, helps students master the essential decoding and comprehension skills.

3859 Me! A Curriculum for Teaching Self-Esteem Through an Interest Center
Connecticut Assoc. for Children and Adults with LD
25 Van Zant Street
Norwalk, CT 06855
203-838-5010
FAX 203-866-6108
http://www.CACLD.org
e-mail: cacld@juno.com
Jo Ellen Hartline, Author
Marie Armstrong, Information Specialist
Beryl Kaufman, Executive Director

A curriculum for the professional. *$18.50*
$2.50 shipping

3860 Meeting the Needs of Students of ALL Abilities
Corwin Press
2455 Teller Road
Thousand Oaks, CA 91320
805-499-9774
800-818-7243
FAX 805-499-0871
http://www.corwinpress.com
e-mail: order@corwinpress.com
Colleen Capper, Elise Frattura, Maureen Keyes, Author
Robb Clouse, Editorial Director
Kimberly Gonzales, Director Marketing

Step-by-step handbook offers practical strategies for administrators, teachers, policymakers and parents who want to shift from costly special learning programs for a few students, to excellent educational services for all students and teachers, and adapting curriculum and instruction. *$32.95*
224 pages
ISBN 0-761975-01-2

3861 Misunderstood Child
Connecticut Assoc. for Children and Adults with LD
25 Van Zant Street
Norwalk, CT 06855
203-838-5010
FAX 203-866-6108
http://www.CACLD.org
LB Silver, Author
Beryl Kaufman, Executive Director

A guide for parents of learning disabled children. *$8.95*

3862 Moving Violations, A Memoir: War Zones, Wheelchairs, and Declarations of Independence
Books on Special Children
PO Box 305
Congers, NY 10920
845-638-1236
FAX 845-638-0847
http://www.boscbooks.com/
e-mail: irene@boscbooks.com

John Hockenberry, Author

He is a newspaper man, out to get his story, wherever. What sets him apart is his inability to move his legs. He does what he must in a wheelchair. This is his remarkable story, told with humor and without self-pity. *$26.95*

416 pages hardcover
ISBN 0-786881-62-3

3863 Negotiating the Special Education Maze 3rd Edition

Woodbine House
6510 Bells Mill Road
Bethesda, MD 20817
301-897-3570
800-843-7323
FAX 301-897-5838
http://www.woodbinehouse.com
e-mail: info@woodbinehouse.com

Irv Shapell, Owner
Stephen Chitwood, Author
Deidre Hayden, Author

Now in its third edition, Negotiating the Special Education Maze isone of the best tools available to parents and teachers for developing an effective special education program for their child or student. Every step is explained, from eligibility and evaluation to the Individualized Education Program and beyond. *$16.95*

264 pages Paperback 7x10
ISBN 0-933149-72-7

3864 New Language of Toys

Woodbine House
6510 Bells Mill Road
Bethesda, MD 20817
301-897-3570
800-843-7323
FAX 301-897-5838
http://www.woodbinehouse.com
e-mail: info@woodbinehouse.com

Irv Shapell, Owner
Joan E Heller Miller EdM, Author
Sue Schwartz PhD, Author

This revised and updated edition presents a fun, hands-on approach to developing communication skills in children with disabilities using everyday toys. There's a fresh assortment of toys and books, as well as newe chapters on computer technology and language learning, videotapes and television. *$16.95*

209 pages Paperback 7x10
ISBN 0-933149-73-5

3865 No One to Play with: The Social Side of Learning Disabilities

Connecticut Assoc. for Children and Adults with LD
25 Van Zant Street
Norwalk, CT 06855
203-838-5010
FAX 203-866-6108
http://www.CACLD.org
e-mail: cacld@juno.com

Betty Osman, Author
Marie Armstrong, Information Specialist
Beryl Kaufman, Executive Director

Your child suffers from a learning disability and you have read reams on how to improve on her academic skills and now want to address his or her social needs. *$13.00*

$2.50 shipping

3866 Nobody's Perfect: Living and Growing with Children who Have Special Needs

Brookes Publishing
PO Box 10624
Baltimore, MD 21285
410-337-9580
800-638-3775
FAX 410-337-8539
http://www.brookespublishing.com
e-mail: custserv@brookespublishing.com

Nancy B Miller, PhD, Author
Paul H Brookes, President
Melissa A Behm, Vice President

Study of four families with children who have special needs. How they all adapted in surviving, how they care for the child, family, parents and siblings. How families react and relate. What it is like in community and extended family? Basic issues dicussed: self-esteem, separating parent from the adult with special needs and other issues. *$23.00*

352 pages Paperback 1994
ISBN 1-557661-43-X

3867 Opening Doors: Connecting Students to Curriculum, Classmate, and Learning, Second Edition

PEAK Parent Center
611 N Weber Street
Colorado Springs, CO 80903
719-531-9400
800-284-0251
FAX 719-531-9452
http://www.peakparent.org
e-mail: info@peakparent.org

Barbara Buswell, Beth Schaffner, Alison B Seyler, Author

This innovative text contains practical how-to's for inculding and supporting students with disabilities in the general education classroom. It explores the processes, thinking, and approaches that successful implementers of inclusion have used. Written for educators and parents of both elementary and secondary students, topics include instructional strategies, curriculum modifications, behavior, standards, literacy, and providing support. *$13.00*

ISBN 0-884720-12-9

3868 Optimizing Special Education: How Parents Can Make a Difference

Insight Books
233 Spring Street
New York, NY 10013
212-620-8000
800-221-9369
FAX 212-807-1047
http://www.plenum.com
e-mail: info@plenum.com

N Wilson, Author
Rudiger Gebauer, Owner

The author shows families how to use education laws to increase services or change services to suit a child's needs. Book contains personal anecdotes and balanced viewpoint of parent and professional relationships. *$26.50*

300 pages
ISBN 0-306443-23-6

3869 Out of Sync Child: Recognizing and Coping with Sensory Integration Dysfunction

Therapro
225 Arlington Street
Framingham, MA 01702
508-872-9494
800-257-5376
FAX 508-875-2062
http://www.theraproducts.com
e-mail: info@theraproducts.com

Carol Stock Kranowitz, MA, Author
Karen Conrad, Owner

Finally, a parent-friendly book about sensory integration (SI) clearly written to explain SI dysfunction from the perspective of a teacher who has worked extensively with an OT. Part I deals with recognizing SI dysfunction. Part II addresses coping with SI dysfunction.

3870 Out of the Mouths of Babes: Discovering the Developmental Significance of the Mouth

Therapro
225 Arlington Street
Framingham, MA 01702
508-872-9494
800-257-5376
FAX 508-875-2062
http://www.theraproducts.com
e-mail: info@theraproducts.com

Frick, Frick, Oetter and Richter, Author
Karen Conrad, Owner

Help children who have difficulty with focusing, staying alert, or being calm with these simple techniqes and activities. Learn how behavior is affected by suck/swallow/breathe (SSB) synchrony with suggestions for correcting specific problems. This informal writing style and many illustrations make it a great resource for parents, teachers and therapists.

3871 Parent Manual
Federation for Children with Special Needs
1135 Tremont Street
Roxbury Crossing, MA 02120
617-236-7210
800-331-0688
FAX 617-572-2094
TDY:617-236-7210
http://www.fcsn.org
e-mail: fcsninfo@fcsn.org
Richard Robison, President

Outlines parents' and children's rights in special education as guaranteed by Chapter 766, the Massachusetts special education law, and the Individuals with Disabilities Education Act (IDEA), the federal special education law *$ 25.00*
75 pages

3872 Parent's Guide to Developmental Delays
Perigee Trade

Laurie LeComer, Author
John Duff, Publisher, VP & Senior Editor

Provides parents with essential information about important topics and uncomfortable questions on issues as spotting the 'red flasgs' of abnormal development; getting a diagnosis and treatment plan; obtaining the best treatment options, education, and help; and the keys to a successful, fulfilling life for every developmentally delayed child. *$14.95*
304 pages January 2006
ISBN 0-399532-31-5

3873 Parenting Children with Special NeedsPractical Parenting Series
AGC/United Learning
1560 Sherman Avenue
Evanston, IL 60201
888-892-3484
FAX 847-328-6706
http://www.unitedlearning.com
e-mail: info@unitedlearning.com
Bill Wagonseller, Author
Ron Reed, President
Joel Altschul, Chief Executive Officer
Coni Rechner, VP Marketing
This program deals exclusively with the subject of parenting children with mental or physical disabilities. Particular emphasis is placed on children from infancy through early childhood. The content includes important topics such as: Birth and diagnosis of a child with disabilities Impact on the family system Psychological stages that most parents of children with disabilities will experience Importance of early intervention programs. VHS #2541. *$79.00*
Video, 28 min 1995Grade Range: Grade 9-Adult

3874 Parenting to Make a Difference: Your One to Four Year-Old
Therapro
225 Arlington Street
Framingham, MA 01702
508-872-9494
800-257-5376
FAX 508-875-2062
http://www.theraproducts.com
e-mail: info@theraproducts.com
Brenda Hussey-Gardner, MA, MPH, Author
Karen Conrad, Owner

Covers twelve key topics to help parents foster the developmental growth of their young children.

3875 Physical Side of Learning
Therapro
225 Arlington Street
Framingham, MA 01702
508-872-9494
800-257-5376
FAX 508-875-2062
http://www.theraproducts.com
e-mail: info@theraproducts.com

Leela C Zion, Author
Karen Conrad, Owner

Assist preschool, elementary and special children with academic subjects by utilizing simple physical activities that are fun, easy to understand, and perform, all of which are clearly illustrated in this book. Explains the connection between movement/perception and learning, with special attention to promoting body awareness, directionality, balance, body concept, self-esteem and body mastery in general. Help prepare children for success in school through physical activities.

3876 Play Therapy
Books on Special Children
PO Box 3378
Amherst, MA 01004
413-256-8164
FAX 413-256-8896
http://www.boscbooks.com/
e-mail: irene@boscbooks.com
Kevin John O'Connor, Author
Irene Slovak, Founder

Leading authorities present various theoretical models of play therapy treatment and application. Case studies on how various treatments are applied. *$44.95*
350 pages Hardcover 1991
ISBN 0-471106-38-0

3877 Positive Self-Talk for Children
Books on Special Children
PO Box 305
Congers, NY 10920
845-638-1236
FAX 845-638-0847
http://www.boscbooks.com/
e-mail: irene@boscbooks.com
D Bloch, Author

This book teaches positive talk and ideas to achieve positive self-esteem. Use this as a refererence in specific situations: ie: fears on 1st day of school, doctor's visit. Covers cases, includes specific dialogue. *$12.95*
331 pages softcover
ISBN 0-553351-98-2

3878 Practical Parent's Handbook on Teaching Children with Learning Disabilities
Charles C Thomas Publisher
2600 S 1st Street
Springfield, IL 62704
217-789-8980
800-258-8980
FAX 217-789-9130
http://www.ccthomas.com
e-mail: books@ccthomas.com
Shelby Holley, Author
Michael Thomas, President

Helps children who learn differently and who have been failing or underachieving in school by enabling adults with no previous teaching experience to design and implement an effective remedial program. Helps parents make realistic changes in the physical and emotional environment at home and at school, gives simple objective tests that show what a child knows and what he needs to learn and shows how to use the test findings. *$65.95*
308 pages Cloth
ISBN 0-398059-03-9

3879 Raising Your Child to be Gifted: Successful Parents
Brookline Books
34 University Road
Brookline, MA 02445
617-734-6772
FAX 617-734-3952
http://www.brooklinebooks.com
James R Campbell, PhD, Author

Moving beyond the usual genetic eplanations for giftedness, Dr. James Campbell presents powerful evidence that it is parental involvement- very specific methods of working with and nurturing a child which increases the child's chances of being gifted. *$21.95*
275 pages Paperback
ISBN 1-571290-94-X

3880 Reading Writing & Rage: The Terrible Price Paid By Victims of School Failure
RWR Press
16800 Adlon Road
Encino, CA 91436
818-784-6561
FAX 818-906-2158
e-mail: dotrwr@earthlink.net

Dorothy Ungerleider, Author
Dorothy Ungerleider, Director

Offers the story of seeking help through the words and perceptions of one learning disabled teen, his parents, teachers and professionals. It reveals an often over-looked source of potential violence: pent-up rage from feeling powerless and misunderstood, school failure and ineffective interventions. *$19.95*
219 pages 2nd Ed. 1996
ISBN 0-965025-20-9

3881 Right from the Start: Behavioral Intervention for Young Children with Autism: A Guide
Therapro
225 Arlington Street
Framingham, MA 01702
508-872-9494
800-257-5376
FAX 508-875-2062
http://www.theraproducts.com
e-mail: info@theraproducts.com
Mary Jane Weiss, PhD,BCBA & Sandra Harris, PhD, Author
Karen Conrad, Owner

This informative and user-friendly guide helps parents and service providers explore programs that use early intensive behavioral intervention for young children with autism and related disorders. Within these programs, many children improve in intellectual, social and adaptive functioning, enabling them to move on to regular elementary and preschools. Benefits all children, but primarily useful for children age five and younger.
215 pages

3882 SMARTS: A Study Skills Resource Guide
Connecticut Assoc. for Children and Adults with LD
25 Van Zant Street
Norwalk, CT 06855
203-838-5010
FAX 203-866-6108
http://www.CACLD.org
e-mail: cacld@juno.com
Susan Custer, Author
Marie Armstrong, Information Specialist
Beryl Kaufman, Executive Director

A comprehensive teachers handbook of activities to help students develop study skills. *$20.50*
$2.50 shipping

3883 School-Based Home Developmental PE Program
Therapro
225 Arlington Street
Framingham, MA 01702
508-872-9494
800-257-5376
FAX 508-875-2062
http://www.theraproducts.com
e-mail: info@theraproducts.com
Barbara Wood, Author
Karen Conrad, Owner

A wire bound flip book. Comprehensive developmental physical education program indentifies and improves motor ability right down to the specific sensory and perceptual motor areas for children. Has what you need: assessment; parent involvement; understandable directions; examples; and sample letters to parents. Includes fun sheets that parents/professionals can use with children. Activities are for vestibular integration, body awareness, eye-hand coordination, and fine motor manipulation.

3884 Seeing Clearly
Therapro
225 Arlington Street
Framingham, MA 01702
508-872-9494
800-257-5376
FAX 508-875-2062
http://www.theraproducts.com
e-mail: info@theraproducts.com
Lois Hickman, MS, OTR FAOTA & Rebecca Hutchins, OD, Author
Karen Conrad, Owner

This booklet is chock-full of great information regarding vision andvisual perceptual problems and activities designed to improve visual skills of both adults and children. Begins with an overview of the development of vision with a checklist of warning signs of vision problems. 25 eye game activities are divided into those for Eye Movements, Suspended Ball, Chalkboard and Visualization (e.g. Pictures in your Mind, Spelling Comprehension, etc.)

3885 Sensory Defensiveness in Children Aged 2 to 12: An Intervention Guide for Parents/Caretakers
Therapro
225 Arlington Street
Framingham, MA 01702
508-872-9494
800-257-5376
FAX 508-875-2062
http://www.theraproducts.com
e-mail: info@theraproducts.com
Patricia Wilbarger and Julia Wilbarger, Author
Karen Conrad, Owner

This booklet defines and describes the symptoms and behaviors related to sensory defensiveness, treatment approaches and the rationale behind treatment strategies. Recommended for everyone administering the Wilbarger Protocol Pressure Program.

3886 Sensory Integration and the Child
Therapro
225 Arlington Street
Framingham, MA 01702
508-872-9494
800-257-5376
FAX 508-875-2062
http://www.theraproducts.com
e-mail: info@theraproducts.com
A Jean Ayres, PhD, Author
Karen Conrad, Owner

Designed to educate parents, students, and beginning therapists in sensory integration treatment.

3887 Sensory Integration: Theory and Practice
Therapro
225 Arlington Street
Framingham, MA 01702
508-872-9494
800-257-5376
FAX 508-875-2062
http://www.theraproducts.com
e-mail: info@theraproducts.com
Fisher, Murray, and Bundy, Author
Karen Conrad, Owner

This is the very latest in sensory integration theory and practicc.The entire volume achieves an admirable balance between theory and practice, covering sensory integration theory, various kinds of sensory integrative dysfunction and comprehensive discussions of assessment, direct treatment, consultation and continuing research issues.

3888 Siblings of Children with Autism: A Guide for Families
Therapro
225 Arlington Street
Framingham, MA 01702
508-872-9494
800-257-5376
FAX 508-875-2062
http://www.theraproducts.com
e-mail: info@theraproducts.com
Sandra Harris, PhD, Author
Karen Conrad, Owner

An invaluable guide to understanding sibling relationships, how they are affected by autism, and what families can do to support their other children while coping with the intensive needs of the child with autism.

3889 Simple Steps: Developmental Activities for Infants, Toddlers & Two Year Olds
Therapro
225 Arlington Street
Framingham, MA 01702
508-872-9494
800-257-5376
FAX 508-875-2062
http://www.theraproducts.com
e-mail: info@theraproducts.com
Karen Miller, Author
Karen Conrad, Owner

300 activites linked to the latest research in brain development. Outlines a typical developmental sequence in 10 domains: social/emotional, fine motor, gross motor, language, cognition, sensory, nature, music & movement, creativity and dramatic play. Chapters on curriculum development and learning environment also included.

3890 Social Perception of People with Disabilities in History

Learning Disabilities Association of America
4156 Library Road
Pittsburgh, PA 15234
412-341-1515
FAX 412-344-0224
http://www.ldanatl.org
e-mail: ldanatl@usaor.net

Herbert C Covey, Author

Shows how historical factors shape some of our current perceptions about disability. Of interest to special educators, historians, students of the humanities and social scientists. *$62.95*

324 pages Cloth
ISBN 0-398068-37-2

3891 Son Rise: The Miracle Continues

Option Indigo Press
2080 S Undermountain Road
Sheffield, MA 01257
413-229-8727
800-562-7171
FAX 413-229-8727
http://www.optionindio.com
e-mail: indigo@bcn.net

Barry Neil Kaufman, Author
Melissa Rothvoss, Assistant Manager

This book documents Raun Kaufman's astonishing develpment from a lifeless, autistic, retarded child into a highly verbal, lovable youngster with no traces of his former condition. It details Raun's extraordinary progress from the age of four into young adulthood. It also shares moving accounts of five families that successfully used the Son-Rise Program to reach their own special children. An awe-inspiring reminder that love moves mountains. A must for any parent, professional or teacher. *$14.95*

346 pages Bi-Annually 1994
ISBN 0-915811-61-8

3892 Source for Dysarthria

LinguiSystems
3100 4th Avenue
East Moline, IL 61244
309-755-2300
800-776-4332
FAX 800-577-4555
http://www.linguisystems.com
e-mail: service@linguisystems.com

Linda Bowers, Co-Owner/Co-Founder
Rosemary Huisingh, Co-Owner/Co-Founder

You'll reach for this book as a therapy tool again and again. This outstanding manual gives you information on types of dysarthria, evaluation and treatment planning options, axamples of documentation, and much more.

Adults

3893 Special-Needs Reading List

Woodbine House
6510 Bells Mill Road
Bethesda, MD 20817
301-897-3570
800-843-7323
FAX 301-897-5838
http://www.woodbinehouse.com
e-mail: info@woodbinehouse.com

Wilma Sweeney, Author
Irv Shapell, Owner

In one easy-to-use volume, The Special-Needs reading List reviews and recommends the best books, journals, newsletters, organizations, and other information sources on children with disabilities. *$18.95*

300 pages Paperback
ISBN 0-933149-74-3

3894 Study Skills: A Landmark School Teaching Guide

Landmark School
429 Hale Street
Prides Crossing, MA 01965
978-236-3216
FAX 978-927-7268
http://www.landmarkoutreach.org
e-mail: outreach@landmarkschool.org

Joan Sedita, Author
Dan Ahearn, Program Director
Trish Newhall, Associate Director

Designed to help all students learn to comprehend and organize the information they must learn in school, Study Skills: A Landmark School Student Guide offers instruction in how to apply specific comprehension and study skills including multiple exercises to practice each skill. Intended for reading levels of middle school and beyond. *$25.00*

104 pages 1989Grade Range: Middle-Second
ISBN 0-962411-96-5

3895 Stuttering and Your Child: Questions and Answers

Stuttering Foundation of America
PO Box 11749
Memphis, TN 38111
901-452-7343
800-992-9392
FAX 901-452-3931
http://www.stutteringhelp.org
e-mail: infor@stutteringhelp.org

Jane Fraser, President
Anne Edwards, Office Coordinator

Provides help, information, and resources to those who stutter, their families, schools day care centers, and all others who need help for a stuttering problem. *$2.00*

64 pages 1999Grade Range: Preschool-Elem
ISBN 0-933388-43-8

3896 Substance Use Among Children and Adolescents

John Wiley & Sons
10475 Crosspoint Boulevard
Indianapolis, IN 46256
877-762-2974
FAX 800-597-3299
http://www.wiley.com

Anne Marie Pagliaro, Louis A Pagliaro, Author
William J Pesce, President/CEO

Exposure and use among infants, children and adolescents. Impact on mental and physical health. Ingestion of substances during pregnancy and effects on fetus and neonate. Drug abuse effects on learning, memory.. Preventing and treating children and adolescents. Available only as a print on demand title. *$132.00*

416 pages Hardcover 1996
ISBN 0-471580-42-2

3897 Success with Struggling Readers: The Benchmark School Approach

Guilford Publications
72 Spring Street
New York, NY 10012
212-431-9800
800-365-7006
FAX 212-966-6708
http://www.guilford.com
e-mail: info@guilford.com

Irene West Gaskins, Author

Presents a proven approach for helping struggling students become fully engaged readers, learners, thinkers, and problem solvers. Demonstrates ways to teach effective strategies for decoding words and understanding concepts, and to give students the skills to apply these strategies across the curriculum based on their individual cognitive styles and the specific demands of the task at hand. *$30.00*

264 pages May 2005
ISBN 1-593851-69-3

3898 Supporting Children with Communication Difficulties In Inclusive Settings

Special Needs Project
324 State Street
Santa Barbara, CA 93101
800-333-6867
FAX 805-962-5087
http://www.specialneeds.com

Linda McCormick, Diane Frome Loeb, Author
Hod Gray, Founder/President

A collaboration of professionals and parents can achieve language communication competence in classroom and other settings. Essential background material, assessment and intervention and needs of special populations are discussed. Contains sectional headings and marginal comments, chapter summary. *$75.00*

530 pages Paperback
ISBN 0-023792-72-8

3899 Surface Counseling

Edge Enterprises
PO Box 1304
Lawrence, KS 66044
785-749-1473
FAX 785-749-0207
e-mail: edge@midusa.net
Joe N Crank, Donald D Deshler, Jean B Schumaker, Author
Jacqueline Schafer, Managing Editor
Sue Vernon, Manager

Details a set of relationship-building skills necessary for establishing a trusting, cooperative relationship between adults and youths and a problem-solving strategy that youths can learn to use by themselves. Includes study guide questions, model dialogues and role-play activities. Useful for any adult who has daily contact with children and adolescents. *$8.00*
60 pages Paperback

3900 Survival Guide for Kids with LD

Therapro
225 Arlington Street
Framingham, MA 01702
508-872-9494
800-257-5376
FAX 508-875-2062
http://www.theraproducts.com
e-mail: info@theraproducts.com
Gary Fisher, PhD & Rhonda Cummings, EdD, Author
Karen Conrad, Owner

Popular book that is highly reccommended. Contains vital information, practical advice, step-by-step strategies, and encouragement for children labeled Learning Disabled.

3901 Tactics for Improving Parenting Skills (TIPS)

Sopris West
4093 Specialty Place
Longmont, CO 80504
303-651-2829
800-547-6747
FAX 303-776-5934
Bob Algozzine, Author
Jim Ysseldyke, Author

Perhaps best described as a compliation of one-page parenting brochures, this helpful resource represents volumes of ideas and suggestions on topics of concern in today's families.
202 pages
ISBN 1-570350-35-3

3902 Tales from the Workplace ADD & LD

JKL Communications
2700 Virginia Avenue NW
Washington, DC 20037
202-223-5097
FAX 202-223-5096
http://www.lathamlaw.org
e-mail: plath3@his.com

$15.00

3903 Teach Me Language

Slosson Educational Publications
PO Box 280
East Aurora, NY 14052
716-652-0930
800-828-4800
FAX 800-655-3840
http://www.sloss.com
e-mail: slosson@slosson.com
Joan M Harwell, Author
Steven Slosson, President

Teach Me Language is designed for teachers, therapists, and parents, and includes a step-by-step how to manual with 400 pages of instructions, explanations, examples, and games and cards to attack language weaknesses common to children with peravasive developmental disorders. *$29.95*

3904 Teaching Developmentally Disabled Children

Slosson Educational Publications
PO Box 280
East Aurora, NY 14052
716-652-0930
800-828-4800
FAX 800-655-3840
http://www.slosson.com
e-mail: slosson@slosson.com
O Ivar Lovaas, Author
Steven Slosson, President

This instrructional program for teachers, nurses, and parents is clear and concisely shows how to help children who are developmentally disabled function more normally at home, in school, and in the community. *$34.00*
250 pages

3905 Teaching Old Logs New Tricks: Absurdities and Realities of Education

Peytral Publications
PO Box 1162
Minnetonka, MN 55345
952-949-8707
877-739-8725
FAX 952-906-9777
http://www.peytral.com
e-mail: help@peytral.com
Michael F Giangreco, Author
Kevin Ruelle, Illustrator
Peggy Hammeken, President

If you enjoyed Ants in His Pants and Flying by the Seat of your Pants - you'll love this book. This publication contains 100+ carefully crafted cartoons which may be reproduced as transparencies for staff development and training. This book is the third book in a series of three. *$19.95*
112 pages Educators
ISBN 1-890455-43-1

3906 Teaching Reading to Children with Down Syndrome

Woodbine House
6510 Bells Mill Road
Bethesda, MD 20817
301-897-3570
800-843-7323
FAX 301-897-5838
http://www.woodbinehouse.com
e-mail: info@woodbinehouse.com
Patricia Logan Oelwein, Author
Irv Shapell, Owner

Teach your child with Down syndrome to read using the author's nationally recognized, proven method. From introducing the alphabet to writing and spelling, the lessons are easy to follow. The many pictures and flash cards included appeal to visual learners and are easy to photocopy! *$16.95*
392 pages Paperback
ISBN 0-933149-55-7

3907 Teaching Students with Mild Disabilities

Books on Special Children
PO Box 305
Congers, NY 10920
845-638-1236
FAX 845-638-0847
http://www.boscbooks.com/
e-mail: irene@boscbooks.com
William N Bender, Author

Specific strategies for effective instruction in special ed. Basis for effective instruction, specialized instructional areas, strategies for curriculum content areas, information on indirect instructional responsibilities. Chapters have objectives, key words, chapter headings, interest boxes, tables, photos, sample questionaires. *$66.00*
388 pages softcover
ISBN 0-138927-20-0

3908 Teaching of Reading: A Continuum from Kindergarten through College

AVKO Educational Research Foundation
3084 W Willard Road
Clio, MI 48420
810-686-9283
FAX 810-686-1101
http://www.avko.org/teaching_of_reading.htm
e-mail: avkoemail@aol.com
Don McCabe, Author
Don Cabe, Executive Director

This book covers concepts, techniques, and practical diagnostic tests not normally taught in regular college courses on reading. It is designed to be used by teachers, parents, tutors, and college reading instructors willing to try new approaches to old problems. *$49.95*

364 pages
ISBN 1-564006-50-6

3909 Teaching the Dyslexic Child
Slosson Educational Publications
PO Box 280
East Aurora, NY 14052
716-652-0930
800-828-4800
FAX 800-655-3840
http://www.slosson.com
e-mail: slosson@slosson.com
Anita N Griffiths, Author
Steven Slosson, President

Teaching the Dyslexic Child talks about the frustrations that the dyslexic youngsters and their parents encounter in the day to day collisions with life's demand. *$12.00*
128 pages

3910 Understanding Learning Disabilities: A Parent Guide and Workbook, Third Edition
York Press
PO Box 504
Timonium, MD 21094
410-560-1557
800-962-2763
FAX 410-560-6758
http://www.yorkpress.com
e-mail: york@abs.net
Mary Louise Trusdell & Inge Horowitz, Author
Elinor Hartwig, President

An invaluable resource for parents who are new to the field of learning disabilities. Easy to read and overflowing with helpful information and advice. *$25.00*
380 pages
ISBN 0-912752-67-X

3911 Understanding and Teaching Children with Autism
John Wiley & Sons
10475 Crosspoint Boulevard
Indianapolis, IN 46256
877-762-2974
FAX 800-597-3299
http://www.wiley.com
Rita Jordan, Stuart Powell, Author
William J Pesce, President/CEO

The triad of impairment: social, language and communication and thought behavior aspects of development discussed. Difficulties in interacting, transfer of learning and bizarre behaviors are syndome. Many LD are associated with autism. *$175.00*
188 pages Hardcover 1995
ISBN 0-471958-88-3

3912 Unlocking the Mysteries of Sensory Dysfunction
Therapro
225 Arlington Street
Framingham, MA 01702
508-872-9494
800-257-5376
FAX 508-875-2062
http://www.theraproducts.com
e-mail: info@theraproducts.com
Elizabeth Anderson & Pauline Emmons, Author
Karen Conrad, Owner

A must-read for therapists, parents and educators. Written by parents, this book is informative and insightful regarding children with sensory integration problems. The autors offer practical suggestions dealing with the often complex realities of living with a child who has sensory issues. A good explanation of sensory integration therapy and advice about how to access it.

3913 What to Expect: The Toddler Years
Workman Publishing
708 Broadway
New York, NY 10003
212-254-5900
800-722-7202
FAX 800-521-1832
http://www.workman.com
Arlene Eisenberg, et al., Author
Peter Workman, President
Jerry Mandel, Special Markets Director

They guided you through pregnancy, they guided you through baby's first year, and now they'll guide you through the toddler years. In a direct continuation of What to Expect When You're Expecting and What to Expect the Frist Year, American's best-selling pregnancy and childcare authors turn their uniquely comprehensive, lively, and reassuring coverage to years two and three. *$15.95*
928 pages Paperback

3914 When Your Child Has LD
Free Spirit Publishing
217 5th Avenue N
Minneapolis, MN 55401
612-338-2068
800-735-7323
FAX 612-337-5050
http://www.freespirit.com
e-mail: help4kids@freespirit.com
Rhoda Cummings and Gary Fisher, Author
Judy Galbraith, Owner
Betsy Gabler, Sales Manager

Clear, reassuring advice and essential information for parents of children ages five and up who have a learning difference. *$12.95*

160 pages
ISBN 0-915793-87-3

Young Adults

3915 Assertive Option: Your Rights and Responsibilities
Research Press
PO Box 9177
Champaign, IL 61826
217-352-3273
800-519-2707
FAX 217-352-1221
http://www.researchpress.com
e-mail: rp@researchpress.com
Dr. Patricia Jakubowski, Dr. Arthur J Lange, Author
Russell Pence, President

A self instructional assertiveness book, with many exercises and self tests. *$24.95*
348 pages
ISBN 0-878221-92-1

3916 Behavior Survival Guide for Kids
Free Spirit Publishing
217 5th Avenue N
Minneapolis, MN 55401
612-338-2068
800-735-7323
FAX 612-337-5050
http://www.freespirit.com
e-mail: help4kids@freespirit.com
Thomas McIntyre PhD, Author
Judy Galbraith, Owner
Patricia Goodrich, Sales Associate

Up-to-date information, practical strategies, and sound advice for kids with general behavior problems and those with diagnosed behavior problems (BD, ED, EBD) so they can help themselves. *$14.95*
176 pages 1903Grade Range: 3-8
ISBN 1-575421-32-1

3917 Delivered form Distraction: Getting the Most out of Life with Attention Deficit Disorder
Ballantine Books

http://www.randomhouse.com
Edward M Hallowell, John J Ratey, Author

416 pages January 2004 $25.95
ISBN 0-345442-30-X

3918 Education of Students with Disabilities: Where Do We Stand?
National Council on Disability
1331 F Street NW
Washington, DC 20591
202-272-2004
FAX 202-272-2022
http://www.ncd.gov
e-mail: mquigley@ncd.ogv

Ethel D Briggs, Acting Executive Director
Brenda Bratton, Executive Secretary

The council reviews the education of students with disabilities as a critical priority. Success in education is a predictor of success in adult life. For students with disabilities, a good education can be the difference between a life of dependence and nonproductivity and a life of independence and productivity.

3919 Keeping Ahead in School: A Students Book About Learning Disabilities & Learning Disorders
Educators Publishing Service
PO Box 9031
Cambridge, MA 02139
617-547-6706
800-225-5750
FAX 617-547-0412
http://www.epsbooks.com
e-mail: eps@epsbooks.com
Mel Levine, Author
Gunnar Voltz, President

Written for students 9 to 15 years of age with learning disorders. This book helps students gain important insights into their problems by combining realism with justifiable optimism. *$24.75*

ISBN 0-838820-09-7

3920 Modern Consumer Education: You and the Law
Educational Design
345 Hudson Street
New York, NY 10014
800-221-9372
FAX 866-805-5723
http://www.triumphlearning.com
Buz Traugot, Sales Representative

An instructional program to teach independent living, with emphasis on legal resources and survival skills. *$59.00*

3921 Phonemic Awareness: Lessons, Activities & Games
Peytral Publicatons
PO Box 1162
Minnetonka, MN 55345
952-949-8707
877-739-8725
FAX 952-906-9777
http://www.peytral.com
e-mail: help@peytral.com
Victoria Groves Scott, Author
Peggy Hammeken, President

Help struggling readers with Phonemic Awareness training. This all inclusive book iuncludes 48 scripted lessons. May be used as a prerequisite to reading or for stuggling students. Includes 49 reproductible masters. May be used with individual students or with groups. *$27.95*
176 pages

3922 Reading Is Fun
Teddy Bear Press
3639 Midway Drive
San Diego, CA 92110
858-560-8718
FAX 619-255-2158
http://www.teddybearpress.net
e-mail: fparker@teddybearpress.net
Fran Parker, President

Introduces 55 primer level words in six reading books and accompanting activity sheets. This easy to use reading program provides repition, visual motor, visual discrimination and word comprehension excersies. The manual and placement test. *$85.00*

ISBN 1-928876-01-3

3923 Succeeding in the Workplace
JKL Communications
2700 Virginia Avenue NW
Washington, DC 20037
202-223-5097
FAX 202-223-5096
http://www.lathamlaw.org
e-mail: plath3@his.com

$29.00

3924 Survival Guide for Kids with ADD and ADHD
Free Spirit Publishing
217 5th Avenue N
Minneapolis, MN 55401
612-338-2068
800-735-7323
FAX 612-337-5050
http://www.freespirit.com
e-mail: help4kids@freespirit.com
John F Taylor PhD, Author
Judy Galbraith, Owner
Patricia Goodrich, Sales Associate

Free Spirit's newest survival guide helps kids with ADD and ADHD know they're not alone and offers practical strategies for taking care of oneself. modifying behavior, enjoying school, having fun, and dealing (when needed) with doctors, counselors, and medication. Includes real-life scenarios, quizzes, and a special message for parents. *$13.95*
128 pages 1906Grade Range: 2-6
ISBN 1-575421-95-X

3925 Survival Guide for Kids with LD
Free Spirit Publishing
217 5th Avenue N
Minneapolis, MN 55401
612-338-2068
800-735-7323
FAX 612-337-5050
http://www.freespirit.com
e-mail: help4kids@freespirit.com
Gary Fisher PhD, Rhonda Cummings EdD, Author
Judy Galbraith, Owner
Patricia Goodrich, Sales Associate

Explains lD in terms kids can understand, describes the different kinds of LD, discusses LD programs, and emphasizes that kids with LD can be winners. *$10.95*
112 pages 1902Grade Range: 2-6
ISBN 1-575421-19-4

3926 Survival Guide for Teenagers with LD
Free Spirit Publishing
217 5th Avenue N
Minneapolis, MN 55401
612-338-2068
800-735-7323
FAX 612-337-5050
http://www.freespirit.com
e-mail: help4kids@freespirit.com
Gary Fisher PhD, Rhoda Cummings EdD, Author
Judy Galbraith, Owner
Patricia Goodrich, Sales Associate

Clear, comprehensive, and matter-of-fact, this guide helps young people with LD succeed in school and prepare for life as adults. It explains what LD is and how kids get into LD programs, clarifies readers' legal rights and responsibilities, and covers other vital topics including assertiveness, jobs, friends, dating, self-sufficieny, and responsible citizenship. *$12.95*
200 pages 1993Grade Range: 6 and up
ISBN 0-915793-51-2

3927 Who I Can Be Is Up To Me: Lessons in Self-Exploration and Self-Determination
Research Press
Department 26W
Champaign, IL 61826
217-352-3273
800-519-2707
FAX 217-352-1221
http://www.researchpress.com
e-mail: rp@researchpress.com
Gloria D Campbell-Whatley, Author

127 pages April 2004 $24.95
ISBN 0-878224-84-X

3928 Winning at Math: Your Guide to Learning Mathematics Through Successful Study Skills
Academic Success Press
6023 26th Street W
Bradenton, FL 34207
941-746-1645
800-444-2524
FAX 941-753-2882
http://www.academicsuccess.com
e-mail: pnolting@ad.com

Paul Nolting, Author
Paul Nolting, Owner

A guide that helps people with learning disabilities learn math easier. *$24.95*

3929 Winning the Study Game

Peytral Publicatons
PO Box 1162
Minnetonka, MN 55345
952-949-8707
877-739-8725
FAX 952-906-9777
http://www.peytral.com

Lawrence J Greene, Author
Peggy Hammeken, President

A comprehensive study skills program for students with learning differences in grades 6-11. The student book has 16 units which will help students learn to study better, take notes, advance their thinking skills while stregthening their reading and writing. The student version is available in a reproducible or consumable format. Teachers guide sold separately. *$34.95*

2500 pages
ISBN 1-890455-48-2

3930 You Don't Have to be Dyslexic

Melvin-Smith Learning Center
7230 S Land Park Drive
Sacramento, CA 95831
916-392-6415
800-50L-EARN
FAX 916-392-6453

Joan M Smith, Author

Dr. Smith has designed this user-friendly book to: Demystify the area of learning that is emotionally charged for many people, Provide teaching methods for teachers, professionals and parents. Depict actual case studies, describing various dyslexic learning styles. And use real-life cases which show excellent examples of how to remediate learning issues. *$19.95*

205 pages

General

3931 A Student's Guide to Jobs
NICHCY
PO Box 1492
Washington, DC 20013
202-884-8200
800-695-0285
FAX 202-884-8441
http://www.nichcy.org
e-mail: nichcy@aed.org
Susan Ripley, Manager

Young people with mental retardation speak freely about their job-related experiences. *$2.00*
8 pages

3932 A Student's Guide to the IEP
NICHCY
PO Box 1492
Washington, DC 20013
202-884-8200
800-695-0285
FAX 202-884-8441
http://www.nichcy.org
e-mail: nichcy@ace.org
Susan Ripley, Manager

A guide for students that features other students discussing their experiences as active members on their IEP team. *$2.00*
12 pages

3933 Accessing Parent Groups
NICHCY
PO Box 1492
Washington, DC 20013
202-884-8200
800-695-0285
FAX 202-884-8441
http://www.nichcy.org
e-mail: nichcy@ace.org
Susan Ripley, Information Specialist

Helps parents locate support groups where they can share information, give and receive emotional support, and address common concerns. *$2.00*
12 pages

3934 Accessing Programs for Infants, Toddlers and Preschoolers
NICHCY
PO Box 1492
Washington, DC 20013
202-884-8200
800-695-0285
FAX 202-884-8441
http://www.nichcy.org
e-mail: nichcy@ace.org
Susan Ripley, Manager

This guide helps locate intervention services for infants and toddlers with disabilities. Also answers questions about educational programs for preschoolers. *$2.00*
20 pages

3935 Advocacy Services for Families of Children in Special Education
Arizona Department of Education
1535 W Jefferson Street
Phoenix, AZ 85007
602-271-0945
800-352-4558
FAX 602-542-5440
http://www.ade.state.az.us
e-mail: ADE@ade.az.gov
Robert Plummer, Manager

Information provided to families that have children in special education.

3936 Assessing Children for the Presence of a Disability
NICHCY
PO Box 1492
Washington, DC 20013
202-884-8200
800-695-0285
FAX 202-884-8441
http://www.nichcy.org
e-mail: nichcy@ace.org
Susan Ripley, Manager

Describes the criteria and process preformed by school systems to determine if a child has a learning disabilty. *$4.00*
28 pages

3937 Assessing the ERIC Resource Collection
NICHCY
PO Box 1492
Washington, DC 20013
202-884-8200
800-695-0285
FAX 202-884-8441
http://www.nichcy.org
e-mail: nichcy@ace.org
Susan Ripley, Manager

A nationwide network that gives access to education literature, this document explains how to search and retrieve documents from ERIC. Also explains how to find information about children with disabilites. *$2.00*
8 pages

3938 Complete Set of State Resource Sheets
NICHCY
PO Box 1492
Washington, DC 20013
202-884-8200
800-695-0285
FAX 202-884-8441
http://www.nichcy.org
e-mail: nichcy@ace.org
Susan Ripley, Manager

Provides a sheet for every state and territory in the United States. *$10.00*
200 pages

3939 Directory of Organizations
NICHCY
PO Box 1492
Washington, DC 20013
202-884-8200
800-695-0285
FAX 202-884-8441
http://www.nichcy.org
e-mail: nichcy@ace.org
Susan Ripley, Manager

Lists many organizations and services *$4.00*
28 pages

3940 Education of Children and Youth with Special Needs: What do the Laws Say?
NICHCY
PO Box 1492
Washington, DC 20013
202-884-8200
800-695-0285
FAX 202-884-8441
http://www.nichcy.org
e-mail: nichcy@ace.org
Susan Ripley, Manager

Provides an overview of 3 laws that aid disabled children; 1. Section 504 of the Rehabilitation Act of 1973, 2. the Individuals with Disabilities Education Act, and 3. the Carl P. Perkins Vocational Educational Act. *$4.00*
16 pages

3941 Ethical and Legal Issues in School Counseling
American School Counselor Association
1101 King Street
Alexandria, VA 22314
703-683-2722
800-306-4722
FAX 703-683-1619
http://www.schoolcounselor.org
e-mail: asca@schoolcounselor.org
Richard Wong, Executive Director
Stephanie Will, Office Manager

Contains answers to many of the most controversial and challenging questions school counselors face every day. *$40.50*

ISBN 1-556200-55-2

3942 **Fact Sheet: Attention Deficit Hyperactivity Disorder**

Learning Disabilities Association of America
4156 Library Road
Pittsburgh, PA 15234
412-341-1515
FAX 412-344-0224
http://www.ldanatl.org
e-mail: ldanatl@usaor.net

A pamphlet offering factual information on ADHD.

3943 **Fundamentals of Autism**

Slosson Educational Publications
PO Box 280
East Aurora, NY 14052
716-652-0930
800-828-4800
FAX 800-655-3840
http://www.slosson.com
e-mail: slosson@slosson.com

Sue Larson, Author
Steven Slosson, President
John Slosson, Vice President

Provides a quick, user friendly effective and accurate approach to help in identifying and developing educationally related program objectives for children diagnosed as Autistic. These materials have been designed to be easily and functionally used by teachers, therapists, special education/learning disability resource specialists, psychologists, and others who work with children diagnosed with similar disabilites.

3944 **General Information about Autism**

NICHCY
PO Box 1492
Washington, DC 20013
202-884-8200
800-695-0285
FAX 202-884-8441
http://www.nichcy.org
e-mail: nichcy@ace.org

Susan Ripley, Manager

Offers information about autism.

3945 **General Information about Disabilities**

NICHCY
PO Box 1492
Washington, DC 20013
202-884-8200
800-695-0285
FAX 202-884-8841
http://www.nichcy.org
e-mail: nichcy@ace.org

Susan Ripley, Manager

A fact sheet offering information on the Education of the Handicapped Act.
2 pages

3946 **General Information about Speech and Language Disorders**

NICHCY
PO Box 1492
Washington, DC 20013
202-884-8200
800-695-0285
FAX 202-884-8841
http://www.nichcy.org
e-mail: nichcy@ace.org

Susan Ripley, Manager

Offers characteristics, educational implications and associations in the area of speech and language disorders.

3947 **IDEA Amendments**

NICHCY
PO Box 1492
Washington, DC 20013
202-884-8200
800-695-0285
FAX 202-884-8441
http://www.nichcy.org
e-mail: nichcy@ace.org

Susan Ripley, Manager

Examines the important changes that have occured in the Individuals Education Act, amended in June of 1997. *$4.00*
40 pages

3948 **If Your Child Stutters: A Guide for Parents**

Stuttering Foundation of America
PO Box 11749
Memphis, TN 38111
901-452-7343
800-992-9392
FAX 901-452-3931
http://www.stuttersfa.org
e-mail: stutter@vantek.net

Anne Edwards, Coordinator
Jane Fraser, President

A guide that enables parents to provide appropriate help to children who stutter. *$1.00*

3949 **Individualized Education Programs**

NICHCY
PO Box 1492
Washington, DC 20013
202-884-8200
800-695-0285
FAX 202-884-8441
http://www.nichcy.org
e-mail: nichcy@ace.org

Susan Ripley, Manager

Provides guidance regarding the legal requirement for beginning a student's IEP. *$2.00*
32 pages

3950 **Interventions for Students with Learning Disabilities**

NICHCY
PO Box 1492
Washington, DC 20013
202-884-8200
800-695-0285
FAX 202-884-8441
http://www.nichcy.org
e-mail: nichcy@ace.org

Susan Ripley, Manager

A document that examines 2 different interventions for students who have learning disabilities; the first deals with strategies and the second with phonological awareness. *$4.00*
16 pages

3951 **National Resources**

NICHCY
PO Box 1492
Washington, DC 20013
202-884-8200
800-695-0285
FAX 202-884-8441
http://www.nichcy.org
e-mail: nichcy@ace.org

Susan Ripley, Manager

Lists different organizations that provide information about different disabilities.
6 pages

3952 **National Toll-free Numbers**

NICHCY
PO Box 1492
Washington, DC 20013
202-884-8200
800-695-0285
FAX 202-884-8441
http://www.nichcy.org
e-mail: nichcy@ace.org

Susan Ripley, Manager

Gives the names of organizations with toll-free numbers who specialize in different disabilities.
6 pages

3953 **Parenting a Child with Special Needs: A Guide to Reading and Resources**

NICHCY
PO Box 1492
Washington, DC 20013
202-884-8200
800-695-0285
FAX 202-884-8441
http://www.nichcy.org
e-mail: nichcy@ace.org

Susan Ripley, Manager

Provides information to families whose child has been diagnosed with a disability. Also gives insight on how disabilities can in turn affect the family. *$4.00*
24 pages

3954 Parents Guide
NICHCY
PO Box 1492
Washington, DC 20013
202-884-8200
800-695-0285
FAX 202-884-8841
http://www.nichcy.org
e-mail: nichcy@ace.org

Lisa Kupper, Editor
Susan Ripley, Manager

Talks directly to parents about specific disability issues.

3955 Planning a Move: Mapping Your Strategy
NICHCY
PO Box 1492
Washington, DC 20013
202-884-8200
800-695-0285
FAX 202-884-8441
http://www.nichcy.org
e-mail: nichcy@ace.org

Susan Ripley, Manager

This guide helps to make moving to a new place easier for parents and their children by listing available services in the new area and compiling educational and medical records. *$2.00*
12 pages

3956 Planning for Inclusion: News Digest
NICHCY
PO Box 1492
Washington, DC 20013
202-884-8200
800-695-0285
FAX 202-884-8441
http://www.nichcy.org
e-mail: nichcy@ace.org

Susan Ripley, Manager

Provides a general guide to raising children with learning disabilities in an educational setting. *$4.00*
32 pages

3957 Problem Sensitivity: A Qualitative Difference in the Learning Disabled
National Clearinghouse of Rehabilitation Materials
206 W 6th Street
Stillwater, OK 74078
405-744-2001
FAX 405-744-2000
http://www.nchrtm.okstate.edu

Presenting information that can be used in modifying the cognitive structure at the Problem Sensitivity level, this paper looks at the learning disabled adult from the viewpoint of cognitive psychology. Behavior is considered significantly deviant when a person's approach to a task is at a qualitatively different level than expected at the person's age.
21 pages

3958 Promising Practices and Future Directions for Special Education
NICHCY
PO Box 1492
Washington, DC 20013
202-884-8200
800-695-0285
FAX 202-884-8441
http://www.nichcy.org
e-mail: nichcy@ace.org

Susan Ripley, Manager

Examines different research regarding the educational methods for children with learning disabilities. *$4.00*
24 pages

3959 Public Agencies Fact Sheet
NICHCY
PO Box 1492
Washington, DC 20013
202-884-8200
800-695-0285
FAX 202-884-8841
http://www.nichcy.org
e-mail: nichcy@ace.org

Susan Ripley, Manager

General information on public agencies that serve the disabled individual.
2 pages

3960 Questions Often Asked about Special Education Services
NICHCY
PO Box 1492
Washington, DC 20013
202-884-8200
800-695-0285
FAX 202-884-8841
http://www.nichcy.org
e-mail: nichcy@ace.org

Susan Ripley, Manager

Offers information regarding special education.

3961 Questions Often Asked by Parents About Special Education Services
NICHCY
PO Box 1492
Washington, DC 20013
202-884-8200
800-695-0285
FAX 202-884-8441
http://www.nichcy.org
e-mail: nichcy@ace.org

Susan Ripley, Manager

A publication to help parents learn about the Individuals with Disabilities Education Act. Also discusses how student access special education and other related services.
12 pages

3962 Questions and Answers About the IDEA News Digest
NICHCY
PO Box 1492
Washington, DC 20013
202-884-8200
FAX 202-884-8441
http://www.nichcy.org
e-mail: nichcy@ace.org

Susan Ripley, Manager

Covers the more commonly asked questions from families and professionals about the IDEA. *$4.00*
28 pages

3963 Related Services for School-Aged Children with Disabilities
NICHCY
PO Box 1492
Washington, DC 20013
202-884-8200
800-695-0285
FAX 202-884-8441
http://www.nichcy.org
e-mail: nichcy@ace.org

Susan Ripley, Manager

Examines the different services offered to children with disabilities such as speech-language pathology, transportation, occupational and physical therapy and special health services. *$4.00*
24 pages

3964 Resources for Adults with Disabilities
NICHCY
PO Box 1492
Washington, DC 20013
202-884-8200
800-695-0285
FAX 202-884-8441
http://www.nichcy.org
e-mail: nichcy@ace.org

Susan Ripley, Manager

Helps adults with disabilities find organizations that will help them find employment, education, recreation and independent living. *$2.00*
16 pages

3965 Serving on Boards and Committees
NICHCY
PO Box 1492
Washington, DC 20013
202-884-8200
800-695-0285
FAX 202-884-8441
http://www.nichcy.org
e-mail: nichcy@ace.org
Susan Ripley, Manager

Part of the Parent's Guide series, this publication examines the different boards and committees on which parents of children with disabilities often serve. Also suggests ways to go about becoming involved with such organizations. *$2.00*
8 pages

3966 Special Education and Related Services: Communicating Through Letterwriting
NICHCY
PO Box 1492
Washington, DC 20013
202-884-8200
800-695-0285
FAX 202-884-8441
http://www.nichcy.org
e-mail: nichcy@ace.org
Susan Ripley, Manager

Identifies the rights of parents and their children with disabilities and explains when and how to notify the school in writing about such conditions. *$2.00*
20 pages

3967 State Capitals
PO Box 7376
Alexandria, VA 22307-7376
703-768-9600
800-876-2545
FAX 703-768-9690
http://www.statecapitals.com
e-mail: newsletters@statecapitals.com
Briefing on important selected state activities.

3968 State Resource Sheet
NICHCY
PO Box 1492
Washington, DC 20013
202-884-8200
800-695-0285
FAX 202-884-8441
http://www.nichcy.org
e-mail: nichcy@ace.org
Susan Ripley, Manager

List numbers of different organizations that deal with disabilities by state.

3969 Underachieving Gifted
Council for Exceptional Children
1110 N Glebe Road
Arlington, VA 22201
703-245-0600
888-232-7733
FAX 703-264-9494
http://www.cec.sped.org/
Bruce Ramirez, Manager

A collection of annotated references from the ERIC and Exceptional Child Evaluation Resources (171 abstracts). Note: Abstracts only. Not the complete research. *$1.00*

3970 What Every Parent Should Know about Learning Disabilities
Connecticut Assoc. for Children and Adults with LD
25 Van Zant Street
Norwalk, CT 06855
203-838-5010
FAX 203-866-6108
http://www.CACLD.org
CL Bete, Author
Beryl Kaufman, Executive Director

What to do with a child with a learning disability.

3971 Who's Teaching Our Children with Disabilities?
NICHCY
PO Box 1492
Washington, DC 20013
202-884-8200
800-695-0285
FAX 202-884-8441
http://www.nichcy.org
e-mail: nichcy@ace.org
Susan Ripley, Manager

Takes a detailied look at the people who are teaching children with disabilities. *$4.00*
24 pages

3972 Your Child's Evaluation
NICHCY
PO Box 1492
Washington, DC 20013
202-884-8200
800-695-0285
FAX 202-884-8441
http://www.nichcy.org
e-mail: nichcy@ace.org
Susan Ripley, Manager

This document describes the steps that the school system will use to determine if you child has a learning disability. *$2.00*
4 pages

Adults

3973 Community Education Journal
National Community Education Association
3929 Old Lee Highway
Fairfax, VA 22030
703-359-8973
FAX 703-359-0972
http://www.ncea.com
e-mail: ncea@ncea.com
Beth Robertson, Executive Director

A quarterly publication for people with disabilities. *$25.00*
Quarterly

3974 Correctional Education Quarterly News: US Department of Education
Office of Correctional Education
400 Maryland Avenue SW
Washington, DC 20202
202-205-5621
FAX 202-401-2615
e-mail: oce@inet.ed.gov
Provides information about correctional education and the activities of the Office of Correctional Education in the US Department of Education. Free.

3975 International Dyslexia Association: Illinois Branch Newsletter
751 Roosevelt Road
Glen Ellyn, IL 60137
630-469-6900
FAX 630-469-6810
http://www.readibida.org
e-mail: info@readibida.org
Jo Ann Paldo, President
Kathleen L Wagner, Executive Director

3976 International Dyslexia Association: Louisiana Branch Newsletter
2125 Coliseum Street
New Orleans, LA 70130
504-876-0034
FAX 504-595-8848
Marqua Brunette, President

3977 Moving Forward
1186 E Avenue
Napa, CA 94559
707-251-8603
FAX 510-934-9022
http://www.iser.com/movingforward-CA.html
e-mail: aia1@aol.com
Paul Aziz, Publisher/Editor
Agena Aziz, Publisher/Business Manager
Donna Feingold, Executive Director
A national newspaper for persons with disabilities offering convention information, book reviews, assistive technology, law and legislation information and more. *$11.50*

3978 NAASLN Newsletter
Nat'l Assn. of Adults with Special Learning Needs
8182 Lark Brown Road
Elkridge, MD 21075
888-562-2756
http://www.nassln.org
e-mail: lrsjhm@aol.com
Robyn Rennick MS, President
Joan Hudson-Miller, Communications/Newsletter/Websit

Newsletter focusing on issues related to teaching adults with special learning needs.

3979 NICHCY News DigestNat'l Dissemination Center For Children W/ Disabilities
NICHCY
PO Box 1492
Washington, DC 20013
202-884-8200
800-695-0285
FAX 202-884-8841
http://www.nichcy.org
e-mail: nichcy@ace.org
Lisa Kupper, Editor
Susan Ripley, Manager

Addresses a single disability issue in depth.

3980 Rural Education Forum
161 College Court
Manhattan, KS 66506
785-532-5560
FAX 785-532-5637
e-mail: wberryd@dce.ksu.edu
Provides information about rural education programs resources, research and events.

Children

3981 Calliope
Cobblestone Publishing Company
30 Grove Street
Peterborough, NH 03458
603-924-7209
800-821-0115
FAX 603-924-7380
http://www.cobblestonepub.com
Rosalie Baker, Editor

Kid's world history magazine, written for kids ages 9 to 14, goes beyond the facts to explore provoactive issues. *$29.95*
52 pages 9 times anually
ISSN 1050-7086

3982 KIND News
NAHEE
PO Box 362
East Haddam, CT 06423
860-434-8666
FAX 860-434-9579
http://www.nahee.org
e-mail: nahee@nahee.org
Lesia Winiarskyj, Director Publications
Cathy Vincenti, Managing Editor
William Rosa, President
Four-page color newspaper with games, puzzles and entertaining, informative articles designed to install kindness to people, animals, and the enviroment and to make reading fun. *$30.00*
4 pages 9x school year 1983Grade Range: K-6
ISSN 1050-9542

3983 KIND News Jr: Kids in Nature's Defense
Kind News
PO Box 362
East Haddam, CT 06423
860-434-8666
FAX 860-434-6282
http://www.kindnews.org
e-mail: nahee@nahee.org
Lesia Winiarsky, Director Publications
Cathy Vincenti, Managing Editor
William Rosa, President
Short, easy-to-read items on the environment and animal world with puzzles, contests and cartoons. Many illustrations, pictures.

3984 KIND News Primary: Kids in Nature's Defense
Kind News
PO Box 362
East Haddam, CT 06423
860-434-8666
FAX 860-434-6282
http://www.kindnews.org
e-mail: nahee@nahee.org
Lesia Winiarsky, Director Publications
Cathy Vincenti, Managing Editor
William Rosa, President
Short, easy-to-read items on the environment and animal world with puzzles, pictures to color and cartoons. Many illustrations, pictures.

3985 **KIND News Sr: Kids in Nature's Defense**
NAHEE
PO Box 362
East Haddam, CT 06423
860-434-8666
FAX 860-434-6282
http://www.kindnews.org
e-mail: nahee@nahee.org
Lesia Winiarsky, Director Publications
Cathy Vincenti, Managing Editor
William Rosa, President
Publication put out by the National Association for Humane and Environmental Education, KIND News Sr. is intended for children between grades 5 through 6. The magazine covers different pet issues such as how to care for,feed and play with pets.

3986 **Koala Club News**
San Diego Zoo Membership Department
PO Box 120551
San Diego, CA 92112
619-231-1515
FAX 619-231-0249
http://www.sandiegozoo.org
Georgeanne Irvine, Editor
Douglas Meyers, CEO

A magazine about animals going to kids who are members of the Zoological Society of San Diego Koala Club. *$9.00*

3987 **Let's Find Out**
Scholastic
555 Broadway
New York, NY 10012
212-343-6100
Jean Marzollo, Editor
Richard Robinson, CEO

Get your PreK and K classes off to a great start with Free-trail copies of Let's Find Out, and bring all this to your teaching program: monthly seasonal themes in 32 colorful weekly issues, activity pages to develop early reading and math skills. *$4.25*

3988 **National Association for Humane and Environmental Education**
PO Box 362
East Haddam, CT 06423
860-434-8666
FAX 860-434-6282
http://www.nahee.org
e-mail: nahee@nahee.org
Lesia Winiarsky, Director Publications
Cathy Vincenti, Managing Editor
William Rosa, President

3989 **Ranger Rick**
National Wildlife Foundation/Membership Services
11100 Wildlife Center Drive
Reston, VA 20190
703-438-6000
800-822-9919
FAX 703-438-6039
http://www.nuf.org
Gerry Bishop, Editor
Mark Putten, CEO

A magazine for children ages 6-12 that is dedicated to helping students gain a greater understanding and appreciation of nature. *$15.00*

3990 **Sibling Forum**
Family Resource Associates
35 Haddon Avenue
Shrewsbury, NJ 07702
732-747-5310
FAX 732-747-1896
Susan Levine, Editor
Nancy Phalanukorn, Manager

Newsletter for siblings aged 10 through teens with brothers or sisters with disabilities. Includes library information, special definitions and feedback from readers. Each issue also has a Focusing on Feelings discussion. A useful tool for siblings, parents, educators, and special workers. *$12.00*

12 pages 4 Times/Sibling

3991 **Stone Soup, The Magazine by Young Writers& Artists**
Children's Art Foundation
PO Box 83
Santa Cruz, CA 95063
831-426-5557
800-447-4569
FAX 831-426-1161
http://www.stonesoup.com
e-mail: editor@stonesoup.com
Gerry Mandel, Editor
William Rubel, Editor

A literary magazine publishing fiction, poetry, book reviews and art by children through age 13. ISSN: 0094 579X. *$34.00*
48 pages 6x/year 1973Grade Range: 3-8

Parents & Professionals

3992 **ALL Points Bulletin: Department of Education**
Division of Adult Education and Literacy
600 Independence Avenue SW
Washington, DC 20202
FAX 202-205-8973
The quarterly newsletter of the division of adult education and literacy. Issues focus on selected areas of interest in the field of adult education, current research, new publications, and upcoming events. Special sections concentrate on ESL and workplace literacy issues.

3993 **Adult Basic Education: An Interdisciplinary Journal for Adult Literacy Educators**
Commission on Adult Basic Education (COABE)
Piedmont College
Demorest, GA 30535
706-778-3000
FAX 706-778-2811
http://www.206.75.28/journal/abe.html
e-mail: kmelichar@piedmnt.edu
Ken Melichar, Editor
Ray Cleere, President

Adult Basic Education: An Interdisciplinary Journal for Adult Literacy Educators is a double-blind, peer review, scholarly journal with a practical intent devoted to improving the efforts of adult educators working with low-literally disadvantaged, and educationally oppressed people. *$25.00*
3x/year

3994 **Association of Higher Education Facilities Officers Newsletter**
1643 Prince Street
Alexandria, VA 22314
703-684-1446
FAX 703-549-2772
http://www.appa.org
E Medlin, Executive VP

A newsletter whose purpose is to promote excellence in the administration, care, operation, planning, and development of higher education facilities.

3995 **Cable in the Classroom Magazine**
CCI/Crosby Publishing
86 Elm Street
Peterborough, NH 03458
202-775-1040
800-216-2225
FAX 603-924-6838
http://www.ciconline.org
e-mail: ckirwin@cciweb.com
Stephen P Crosby, Publisher
Judy Campbell, Associate Publisher
Helen Soule, Executive Director
CIC fosters the use of cable content and technology to expand and enhance learning for children and youth nationwide. ISSN: 1545-603X *$27.95*
28 pages Monthly 1989

3996 **Children and Families**
National Head Start Association
1651 Prince Street
Alexandria, VA 22314
703-739-0875
FAX 703-739-0878

Sarah Greene, CEO

The magazine of the National Head Start Association.

3997 Connections: A Journal of Adult Literacy
Adult Literacy Resource Institute
100 William T Morrissey Boulevard
Dorchester, MA 02125 617-782-8956
FAX 617-782-9011
http://www.alri.org

Connections is primarily intended to provide an opportunity for adult educators in the Boston area to communicate with colleagues.

3998 Council for Exceptional Children
1110 N Glebe Road
Arlington, VA 22201 703-245-0600
888-232-7733
FAX 703-264-9494
http://www.cec.sped.org
e-mail: cathym@cec.sped.org

Bruce Ramirez, Manager
Dave Edyburn, Editor
Nancy Safer, Executive Director

3999 Education Funding News
Education Funding Research Council
1725 K Street NW
Washington, DC 20006 202-872-4000
800-876-0226
FAX 800-926-2012
http://www.grantsandfunding.com

Emily Lechy, Editor
Phil Gabel, CEO

Provides the latest details on funding opportunities in education.
$298.00
50 pages

4000 Exceptional Children
Council for Exceptional Children
1110 N Glebe Road
Arlington, VA 22201 703-245-0600
888-232-7733
FAX 703-264-9494
http://www.cec.sped.org

Bruce Ramirez, Manager

Peer review journal publishing original research on the education and development of toddlers, infants, children and youth with exceptionality and articles on professional issues of concern to special educators. Published quarterly.

4001 Exceptional Parent Magazine
551 Main Street
Johnstown, PA 15901
877-372-7368
http://www.eparent.com
e-mail: epar@kable.com

Rick Rader, Editor-in-Chief
Nikki Prevenslik, Managing Editor
Joseph M Valenzano, Jr, President/CEO/Publisher

EP is the magazine for exceptional parents with exceptional children. Each month EP provides a forum to network with others who are providing a richer life for themselves and for their children. ISSN: 0046-9157. *$39.95*
92 pages Monthly 1971

4002 Federation for Children with Special Needs Newsletter
1135 Tremont Street
Roxbury Crossing, MA 02120 617-236-7210
FAX 617-572-2094
http://www.fcsn.org
e-mail: fcsninfo@fcsn.org

Rich Robison, Executive Director

The mission of the Federation is to provide information, support, and assistance to parents of children with disabilities, their professional partners, and their communities. Major services are information and referrals and parent and professional training.

4003 International Dyslexia Association Quarterly Newsletter: Perspectives
40 York Road
Baltimore, MD 21204 410-296-0232
800-ABC-D123
FAX 410-321-5069
http://www.interdys.org
e-mail: jdallam@interdys.org

Joanna Dallan, Information & Referral

Leading resource for individuals with dyslexia, their families, teachers, and educational professionals around the world. A non-profit organization dedicates to the study and treatment of dyslexia, we encourage you to join our mission and become a member. You will receive regular information about managing dyslexia, access to an international network of professionals in the field, discounts on conference fees and publications, quarterly and biannual publications
50-56 pages Free to Members

4004 International Dyslexia Association: Illinois Branch Newsletter
751 Roosevelt Road
Glen Ellyn, IL 60137 630-469-6900
FAX 630-469-6810
http://www.readibida.org
e-mail: info@readibida.org

Jo Ann Paldo, President
Kathleen L Wagner, Executive Director

4005 International Dyslexia Association: Louisiana Branch Newsletter
2125 Coliseum Street
New Orleans, LA 70130 504-876-0034
FAX 504-595-8848

Marqua Brunette, President

4006 International Dyslexia Association: Philadelphia Branch Newsletter
PO Box 251
Bryn Mawr, PA 19010 610-527-1548
FAX 610-527-5011

Jann Glider, President
Amy Ress, Manager

An international 501(c)(3) nonprofit, scientific and educational organization dedicated to the study and treatment of dyslexia. All branches hold at least one public meeting, workshop or conference per year.

4007 International Reading Association Newspaper: Reading Today
800 Barksdale Road
Newark, DE 19714 302-731-1600
800-336-7323
FAX 302-731-1057
http://www.reading.org
e-mail: customerservice@reading.org

Alan Farstrup, Executive Director

The International Reading Association is a professional membership organization dedicated to promoting high levels of literacy for all by improving the quality of reading instruction, disseminating research and information about reading, and encouraging the lifetime reading habit. Our members include classroom teachers, reading specialistsss, consultants, administrators, supervisors, university faculty, researchers, psychologists, librarians, media specialists, and parents.
Bi-monthly

4008 Journal of Physical Education, Recreation and Dance
1900 Association Drive
Reston, VA 20191 703-476-3400
FAX 703-476-9537
http://www.aahperd.org

Michael T Shoemaker, Editor
Courtney Schmidt, Associate Editor

Most frequently published, and most wide-ranging periodical reaching over 20,000 members and providing information on a greater variety of HPERD issues than any other publication. ISSN NUMBER: 0730-3084 *$9.00*
80 pages monthly

4009 LDA Alabama Newsletter
Learning Disabilities Association Alabama
PO Box 11588
Montgomery, AL 36111
334-277-9151
FAX 334-284-9357
http://www.ldaal.org
e-mail: alabama@ldaal.org
Debbie Gibson, President

Educational, support, and advocacy group for individuals with learning disabilities and ADD.

4010 LDA Georgia Newsletter
Learning Disabilities Association Georgia
PO Box 1337
Roswell, GA 30077
678-461-4471
FAX 678-461-4472
http://www.accessatlanta.com/community/groups/
e-mail: ldaga@aol.com
Vicki Hansberger, Executive Director

Information and helpful articles on learning disabilities. Mailed free four times a year to members. Members also receive National Association newsletter four times a year *$40.00*

4011 LDA Illinois Newsletter
Learning Disabilities Association Illinois
10101 S Roberts Road
Palos Hills, IL 60465
708-430-7532
FAX 708-430-7592
http://www.idanatl.org/illinois
Sharon Schussler, Manager

A non profit organization dedicated to the advancement of the education and general welfare of children and youth of normal or potentially normal intelligence who have perceptual, conceptual, coordinative or related learning disabilities.

4012 Learning Disabilities Association of Texas Newsletter
1011 W 31st Street
Austin, TX 78705
512-458-8234
800-604-7500
FAX 512-458-3826
http://www.ourworld.compuserve.com/homepages/LD
e-mail: LDAT@compuserve.com
Ann Robinson, State Coordinator
Jean Kueker, President

Provides information, referral for services and support to those with learning disabilities.

4013 Link Newsletter
Parent Information Center of Delaware
5570 Kirkwood Highway
Wilmington, DE 19808
302-999-7394
888-547-4412
FAX 302-999-7637
e-mail: picofdel@picofdel.org
Marie-Anne Aghazadian, Executive Director
Kathie Herel, Assistant Director

20 pages quarterly $12.00

4014 Literacy News
National Institute for Literacy
1775 I Street NW
Washington, DC 20006
202-233-2025
FAX 202-233-2050
http://www.novel.nifl.gov
Sandra Baxter, Manager

Provides current information on what the Institute is doing and its progress.

4015 Louisiana State Planning Council on Developmental Disabilities Newsletter
PO Box 3455
Baton Rouge, LA 70821
225-342-6804
800-922-DIAL
FAX 225-342-1970
Sandee Winchell, Executive Director
Shelia Bridgewater, DIAL Coordinator

To improve circumstances, programs, and systems for people with developmental disabilities.

4016 Louisiana State Planning Council on Developmental Disabilities Newsletter
PO Box 3455
Baton Rouge, LA 70821
225-342-6804
800-922-DIAL
FAX 225-342-1970
Sandee Winchell, Executive Director
Sheila Bridgewater, DIAL Coordinator

To improve circumstances, programs, and systems for people with developmental disabilities.

4017 OSERS Magazine
Office of Special Education & Rehabilitative Svcs.
303 C Street SW
Washington, DC 20202
202-727-6436
800-433-3243
http://www.ed.gov
Provides information, research and resources in the area of special learning needs.
Quarterly

4018 Resources in Education
US Government Printing Office
710 N Capitol Street NW
Washington, DC 20401
202-512-0132
FAX 202-512-1355
http://www.access.gpo.gov
e-mail: www.admine@gpo.gov
Patricia Simmons, Manager

A monthly publication announcing education related documents.

4019 TASKS's Newsletter
100 W Cerritos Ave
Anaheim, CA 92805
714-533-8275
FAX 714-533-2533
e-mail: taskca@yahoo.com
Marta Anchondo, Executive Director
Brenda Smith, Deputy Director

TASK's mission is to enable children with disabilities to reach their maximum potential by providing them, their families and the professionals whoserve them, with training, support information resources and referrals. and by providing community awarness programs.
28 pages TASK members

4020 TESOL Journal
Teachers of English to Speakers of Other Languages
706 S Washington Street
Alexandria, VA 22314
703-836-0774
FAX 703-836-7864
http://www.tesol.org
e-mail: TJ@tesol.org
Charles Amorosino, Executive Director

TESOL Journal articles focus on teaching and classroom research for classroom practitioners. The journal includes articles about adult education and literacy in every volume year. Subscriptions available to members only.

4021 TESOL Newsletter
Teachers of English to Speakers of Other Languages
700 S Washington Street
Alexandria, VA 22314
703-836-0774
FAX 703-836-7864
e-mail: info@tesol.org
Charles Amorosino, Executive Director

TESOL produces the Adult Education Interest Section Newsletter and the Refugee Concerns Interest Section Newsletter. They provide news, ideas, and activities for ESL instructors. Subscriptions are available to members only.

4022 TESOL Quarterly
Teachers of English to Speakers of Other Languages
700 S Washington Street
Alexandria, VA 22314
703-836-0774
FAX 703-836-7864
http://www.tesol.edu
e-mail: info@tesol.org
Charles Amorosino, Executive Director

TESOL Quarterly is a referred interdisciplinary journal teachers of English to speakers of other languages. Subscriptions available to members.

Young Adults

4023 Get Ready to Read!
National Center for Learning Disabilities
381 Park Ave S
New York, NY 10016
212-545-7510
888-575-7373
FAX 212-545-9665
http://www.ld.org
e-mail: help@ncld.org
Amber Eden, Assistant Director Online Comm.
Hal Stucker, Managing Editor

Quarterly

4024 LD Advocate
National Center for Learning Disabilities
381 Park Ave S
New York, NY 10016
212-545-7510
888-575-7373
FAX 212-545-9665
http://www.ld.org
e-mail: help@ncld.org
Marcia Griffith, Marketing Executive
Hal Stucker, Managing Editor

Monthly

4025 LD News
National Center for Learning Disabilities
381 Park Ave S
New York, NY 10016
212-545-7510
888-575-7373
FAX 212-545-9665
http://www.ld.org
e-mail: help@ncld.org
Marcia Griffith, Marketing Executive
Hal Stucker, Managing Editor

Monthly

4026 Literary Cavalcade
Scholastic
555 Broadway
New York, NY 10012
212-343-6100
Richard Robinson, CEO

Every issue makes literature come alive with captivating reading students will love, and skill-building activities that meet your teaching needs. *$8.95*
48 pages

4027 National Geographic World
1145 17th Street NW
Washington, DC 20036
202-857-7000
800-647-5463
FAX 202-429-5712
Susan M Tejada, Editor
John Fahey, CEO

Features factual stories on outdoor adventures, natural history, sports, science and history. Special features include posters, games, crafts and mazes. *$17.95*
32 pages

4028 Our World
National Center for Learning Disabilities
381 Park Ave S
New York, NY 10016
212-545-7510
888-575-7373
FAX 212-545-9665
http://www.ld.org
e-mail: help@ncld.org
Marcia Griffith, Marketing Executive
Hal Stucker, Managing Editor

Quarterly

4029 Scholastic Action
Scholastic
555 Broadway
New York, NY 10012
212-343-6100
Patrick Daley, Editor
Richard Robinson, CEO

Motivate your grades 7-12 below-level readers to read and improve their language arts skills with FREE-trial copies of Scholastic Action. *$7.95*
32 pages

4030 Sibling Forum
Family Resource Associates
35 Haddon Ave
Shrewsbury, NJ 07702
732-747-5310
FAX 732-747-1896
Susan Levine, Editor
Nancy Phalanukorn, Manager

Newsletter for siblings aged 10 through teens with brothers or sisters with disabilities. Includes library information, special definitions and feedback from readers. Each issue also has a Focusing on Feelings discussion. A useful tool for siblings, parents, educators, and special workers. *$12.00*
12 pages 4 Times/Sibling

General

4031 ABC's of ADD
JKL Communications
2700 Virginia Ave NW
Washington, DC 20037
202-333-1713
FAX 202-333-1735
http://www.lathamlaw.org
e-mail: lathamlaw@gmail.com
Peter S Latham JD, Director
Patricia Horan Latham JD, Director

Childhood to adulthood. Packed with understandable information provided by experts. Library Journal(February 15, 1994) considered this video's one hour version an outstanding tape, highly recommended for your adults with ADD and those who care for them. *$29.00*
30 minutes
ISBN 1-883560-04-7

4032 ADD and the Law
JKL Communications
2700 Virginia Ave NW
Washington, DC 20037
202-333-1713
FAX 202-333-1735
http://www.lathamlaw.org
e-mail: lathamlaw@gmail.com
Peter S Latham JD, Director
Patricia Horan Latham JD, Director

Dr Sam Goldstein, Neurology Learning & Behavior Center, says of ADD and the Law: excellent, presented in a straight forward, understandable and extremely readable format. *$29.00*

ISBN 1-883560-09-8

4033 Academic Communication Associates
Educational Book Division
PO Box 4279
Oceanside, CA 92052
760-722-9593
888-758-9558
FAX 760-722-1625
http://www.acadcom.com
e-mail: acom@acadcom.com
Dr. Larry Mattes, Founder/President

Publishes hundreds of speech and language products, educational books and assessment materials for children and adults with speech, language, and hearing disorders, learning disabilities, developmental disabilities, and special learning needs. Products include books, software programs, learning games, augmentative communication materials, bilingual/multicultural materials, and special education resources.

4034 Academic Success Press
6023 26th Street W
PO Box 132
Bradenton, FL 34207
888-822-6657
http://www.academicsuccess.com
e-mail: info@academicsuccess.com
Paul D Nolting PhD, Learning Specialist
Kimberly Nolting, VP of Marketing & Research

Publishes books and materials in the interest of making the classroom learning experience less difficult, while improving student learning, to transform the classroom into a more successful environment where educators and students can use inventive learning techniques based on sound academic research.

4035 Academic Therapy Publications
20 Commercial Boulevard
Novato, CA 94949
415-883-3314
800-422-7249
FAX 415-883-3720
http://www.academictherapy.com
e-mail: sales@academictherapy.com
Anna Arena, President
Jim Arena, Vice President

Publishes supplementary education materials for people with reading, learning and communication disabilities; features professional texts and reference books, curriculum materials, teacher/parent resources, and visual/perceptual training aids.

4036 Active Parenting Publishers
1955 Vaughn Road NW
Kennesaw, GA 30144
770-429-0565
800-825-0060
FAX 770-429-0334
http://www.activeparenting.com
e-mail: cservice@activeparenting.com
Michael Popkin PhD, President
Susan Hopkins, Educational Consultant
Susan Reed, Director of Training
Publishes materials that teach parenting skills. Offers video-based training and program packages that include captioned videos, guidebooks, and additional items.

4037 American Guidance Service
PO Box 99
Circle Pines, MN 55014
651-287-7220
800-328-2560
FAX 800-471-8457
http://www.agsnet.com
e-mail: agsmail@agsnet.com
Produces assessments, textbooks, and instructional materials for people with a wide range of needs; publishes individually administered tests to measure cognitive ability, achievement, behavior, speech and language skills, and personal and social adjustment.

4038 American Printing House for the Blind
PO Box 6085
Louisville, KY 40206
502-895-2405
800-233-1839
FAX 502-899-2274
http://www.aph.org
e-mail: info@aph.org

Tuck Tinsley III, President
Fred Gissoni, Customer Support
Tony Grantz, Business Development Manager
Promotes independence of blind and visually impaired persons by providing specialized materials, products, and services needed for education and life.

4039 American Psychological Association
750 1st Street NE
Washington, DC 20002
202-336-5500
800-374-2722
FAX 202-336-5633
http://www.apa.org/psycinfo
e-mail: psycinfo@apa.org
Norman Anderson, CEO

Publishes periodicals, including PsycSCAN, a quarterly print abstract that provides citations to the journal literature on Learning Disorders and Mental Retardation, including theories, research, assessment, treatment, rehabilitation, and educational issues. Also publishes Psychological Abstracts, a monthly print reference tool containing summaries of journal articles, book chapters and books in the field of psychology and related disciplines.

4040 Associated Services for the Blind
919 Walnut Street
Philadelphia, PA 19107
215-627-0600
FAX 215-922-0692
http://www.asb.org
e-mail: asbinfo@asb.org
Lauren M Drinker, Public Relations Officer
Patricia Johnson, CEO

Promotes self-esteem, independence, and self determination in people who are blind or visually impaired. ASB accomplishes this by providing support through education, training and resources, as well as through community action and public education, serving as a voice for the rights of all people who are blind or visually impaired.

4041 At-Risk Youth Resources
Sunburst Visual Media
PO Box 9120
Plainview, NY 11803
800-431-1934
FAX 888-803-3908
http://www.at-risk.com

Publisher of life-skills educational media for the K-12 market. In addition, we also produce science and social studies programs for students in grades K-8
78 pages 1972

4042 Bethany House Publishers
11400 Hampshire Avenue S
Minneapolis, MN 55438
952-829-2500
800-877-2665
FAX 616-676-9576
http://www.bethanyhouse.com
e-mail: orders@bakerbooks.com

Gary Johnson, President
Teresa Fogarty, General Publicist

Publishes books in large-print format for the learning disabled.

4043 Blackwell Publishing
350 Main Street
Malden, MA 02148
781-388-8250
FAX 781-388-8210
http://www.blackwellpublishing.com
e-mail: dpeters@bos.blackwellpublishing.com

Gordan Iii, President
Rene Olivieri, Chief Executive
Dawn Peters, Media Contact

Publishes books and journals for the higher education, research and professional markets, including several journals on topics relating to learning disabilities.

4044 Brookes Publishing
PO Box 10624
Baltimore, MD 21285
410-337-9580
800-638-3775
FAX 410-337-8539
http://www.brookespublishing.com
e-mail: custserv@brookespublishing.com

Paul Brooks, Owner
Melissa Behm, Vice President

Publishes books, texts, curricula, videos, tools and a newsletter based on research in disabilities, education and child development, including learning disabilities, ADHD, communication and language, reading and literacy, and special education.

4045 Brookline Books/Lumen Editions
PO Box 1209
Brookline, MA 02445
617-734-6772
800-666-2665
FAX 617-734-3952
http://www.brooklinebooks.com
e-mail: milt@brooklinebooks.com

Milton Budoff, Executive Director

Publishes books on education, learning and topics relating to disabilities.

4046 Charles C Thomas Publisher
2600 S 1st Street
Springfield, IL 62704
217-789-8980
800-258-8980
FAX 217-789-9130
http://www.ccthomas.com
e-mail: books@ccthomas.com

Michael Thomas, President

Publishes books on education and special education for the blind and visually impaired, the gifted and talented, the developmentally disabled, and people with learning disabilities.

4047 Chess with Butterflies
Oxton House Publishing
PO Box 209
Farmington, ME 04938
207-779-1923
800-539-7323
FAX 207-779-0623
http://www.oxtonhouse.com
e-mail: info@oxtonhouse.com

Dion, Author
William Berlinghoff, Owner
Bobby Brown, Marketing Director

This is a phoneticaly controlled sequel to 'Fishing with Balloons.' It continues the adventures of the main character as it develops more sophisticated word families. Lists for those word families and notes on using them for reading instruction are included in the back of the book. Suggested for Classroom Resources section, Reading. *$5.95*
66 pages 1905Grade Range: 4-7
ISBN 1-881929-43-4

4048 City Creek Press
PO Box 8415
Minneapolis, MN 55408
612-823-2500
800-585-6059
FAX 612-823-5380
http://www.citycreek.com

Judy Liautaud, Owner

Publishes books and products offering a literature-based method of learning, such as books, clue cards, posters, magnetic math story boards, workbooks and audio tapes; the program is multisensory, interactive, and appeals to the visual, auditory and tactile learning styles.

4049 Concept Phonics
Oxton House Publishers
PO Box 209
Farmington, ME 04938
207-779-1923
800-539-7323
FAX 207-779-0623
http://www.oxtonhouse.com
e-mail: info@oxtonhouse.com

Phyllis E Fischer PhD, Author
William Burlinghoff PhD, Owner
Bobby Brown, Marketing Director

This is a remarkably effective, research-based, multisensory program for teaching reading to students with learning disabilities at any age or grade level. Its 13 component pieces include a book on understanding phonics, detailed teacher's guides, and sets of contrast cards, speed drills, worksheets, visual teaching aids, and comprehensive word lists. Suggested for Classroom Resources section, Reading. *$315.00*
1997
ISBN 1-881929-36-1

4050 Connecticut Association for Children and Adults with Learning Disabilities
25 Van Zant Street
Norwalk, CT 06855
203-838-5010
FAX 203-866-6108
http://www.cacld.org
e-mail: cacld@optonline.net

Beryl Kaufman, Executive Director

Offers over 300 books and titles to ensure access to the resources needed to help children and adults with learning disabilities and attention disorders achieve their full potential.

4051 Corwin Press
Sage Publications
2455 Teller Road
Thousand Oaks, CA 91320
805-499-0721
800-818-7243
FAX 800-583-2665
http://www.corwinpress.com
e-mail: webmaster@sagepub.com

Blaise Simqu, CEO

Publishes books and products for all learners of all ages and their educators, including subjects such as classroom management, early childhood education, guidance and counseling, higher/adult education, inclusive education, exceptional students, student assessment, as well as behavior, motivation and discipline.

4052 **Decoding Automaticity Materials for ReadinDecoding Automaticity Materials for Reading Fluency**

Oxton House Publishers
PO Box 209
Farmington, ME 04938
207-779-1923
800-539-7323
FAX 207-779-0623
http://www.oxtonhouse.com
e-mail: info@oxtonhouse.com

Phyllis E Fischer PhD, Author
William Burlinghoff PhD, Owner
Bobby Brown, Marketing Director

This six-part set is designed to bring students from decoding to fluency in reading words. The two sets of worksheets train the brain's visual processor to recognize letter units in words; the contrast cards train the brain's speech processor to say the sounds for the letter units; and the speed drills put these two tasks together for reading whole words automatically. Also included are comprehensive sets of lists of one-and two syllable words for designing customized materials. *$150.00*

1997Grade Range: All
ISBN 1-881929-37-X

4053 **Documentation and the Law**

JKL Communications
2700 Virginia Avenue NW
Washington, DC 20037
202-333-1713
FAX 202-333-1735
http://www.lathamlaw.org
e-mail: lathamlaw@gmail.com

Peter S Latham JD, Director
Patricia Horan Latham JD, Director

This text provides a legal overview of documentation requirements and a practical guide to writing diagnostic reports covering LD and ADD in today's medical/legal environment. *$29.00*

ISBN 1-883560-07-1

4054 **Edge Enterprises**

PO Box 1304
Lawrence, KS 66044
785-749-1473
FAX 785-749-0207
e-mail: edgeenterprises@alltel.net

Jean B Schumaker, President
Sue Vernon, Manager
Jacqueline Schafer, Managing Editor

A research, development and publishing company addressing the needs of at-risk learners. Offers research-based instructor's manuals and videotapes for teachers and parents in the areas of learning strategies, math strategies, self advocacy, social skills, cooperative thinking strategies and community building. Catalogue available upon request. Training required associated with some products.

4055 **Educators Publishing Service**

PO Box 9031
Cambridge, MA 02139
617-547-6706
800-435-7728
FAX 888-440-2665
http://www.epsbooks.com
e-mail: epsbooks@epsbooks.com

Dr. Mel Levine, Author
Gunnar Voltz, President

Publishes vocabulary, grammar and language arts materials for students from kindergarten through high school, and specializes in phonics and reading comprehension as well as materials for students with learning differences.

4056 **Federation for Children with Special Needs**

1135 Tremont Street
Roxbury Crossing, MA 02120
617-236-7210
800-331-0688
FAX 617-572-2094
http://www.fcsn.org
e-mail: fcsinfo@fcsn.org

Pat Blake, Associate Executive Director
Sara Miranda, Associate Executive Director
Rich Robison, Executive Director

The mission of the Federation is to provide information, support, and assistance to parents of children with disabilities, their professional partners, and their communities. Major services are information and referrals and parent and professional training.

4057 **Fishing with Balloons**

Oxton House Publishing
PO Box 209
Farmington, ME 04938
207-779-1923
800-539-7323
FAX 207-779-0623
http://www.oxtonhouse.com
e-mail: info@oxtonhouse.com

Dion, Author
William Burlinghoff PhD, Owner
Bobby Brown, Marketing Director

This is a phonetically controlled chapter book about a 10 year old who learns how his physical disability need not be a barrier to his aspirations. As the story holds the reader's interest, it also emphasizes certain families of words. Lists for those word families and notes on using them for reading instruction are included in the back of the book. Suggested for Classroom Resources section, Reading. *$5.95*

68 pages 1904Grade Range: 3-5
ISBN 1-881929-34-5

4058 **Free Spirit Publishing**

217 5th Avenue N
Minneapolis, MN 55401
612-338-2068
800-735-7323
FAX 612-337-5050
http://www.freespirit.com
e-mail: help4kids@freespirit.com

Judy Galbraith, Owner

Publishes non-fiction materials which empower young people and promote self-esteem through improved social and learning skills. Topics include self-awareness, stress management, school success, creativity, friends and family, and special needs such as gifted and talented learners and children with learning differences.

4059 **Gander Publishing**

412 Higuera Street
San Luis Obispo, CA 93401
805-541-5523
800-554-1819
FAX 805-782-0488
http://www.ganderpub.com

Wendy Cook, Marketing Manager
Rod Bell, Manager

Books, kits, videos and CD-ROMs used to train educators and parents in specific programs for helping people with learning disabilities.

4060 **Gordon Systems & GSI Publications**

PO Box 746
Dewitt, NY 13214
315-446-4849
800-550-2343
FAX 315-446-2012
http://www.gsi-add.com
e-mail: info@gsi-add.com

Michael Gordon PhD, Founder

Publishes books for parents, teachers, ADHD children and their siblings.

4061 **Great Potential Press**

PO Box 5057
Scottsdale, AZ 85261
602-954-4200
877-954-4200
FAX 602-954-0185
http://www.giftedpsychologypress.com
e-mail: info@giftedbooks.com

James Webb PhD, President

Specializes in education books for parents, teachers and educators of gifted, talented and creative children. Offers nearly forty products, including books and videos.

4062 **Guidance Channel**

PO Box 9120
Plainview, NY 11803-9020
800-999-6884
FAX 800-262-1886
http://www.guidancechannel.com
e-mail: info@guidancechannel.com

Jennifer Brady, Editor

Publishes educational products, media and resources available on the Internet and through direct mail catalogs. Offers multimedia programs, videos, curricula, information handouts, therapeutic games, prevention-awareness items, play therapy resources, newsletters and other publications.

4063 Guilford Publications
72 Spring Street
New York, NY 10012
212-431-9800
800-365-7006
FAX 212-966-6708
http://www.guilford.com
e-mail: info@guilford.com
Seymour Weingarten, Editor-in-Chief
Chris Jennison, Senior Editor, Education
Robert Matloff, President
Publishes books for education on the subjects of literacy, general education, school psychology and special education. Also offers books, videos, audio cassettes and software, as well as journals, newsletters, and AD/HD resources.

4064 Harcourt Achieve
6277 Sea Harbor Drive
Orlando, FL 32887
800-531-5015
FAX 800-699-9459
http://www.harcourtachieve.com
Tim McEwen, President/CEO
Joel Zucker, Chief Operating Officer

Produces learning solutions and materials to help young and adult learners, based on a development philosophy that assesses learner's skills, matches them to appropriate content, and accelerates the ability of learners to meet and exceed expectations.

4065 Hazelden Publishing and Educational Services
CO3, PO Box 11
Center City, MN 55012-0011
651-213-4200
800-257-7810
FAX 651-213-4577
http://www.hazelden.org
e-mail: info@hazelden.org

Nick Motu, VP/Publisher
Christine Anderson, Media Specialist

Publishes real-world resources that are accessible for all experience levels and learning styles, including audio and video formats, manuals for educators, workbooks for students, and a catalog of products.

4066 Heinemann-Boynton/Cook
361 Hanover Street
Portsmouth, NH 03801
603-431-7894
800-225-5800
FAX 603-431-2214
http://www.boyntoncook.com
e-mail: custserv@heinemann.com
George Goldberg, VP Human Resources

Publishes professional resources and provides educational services for teachers, and offers nearly 100 titles related to learning disabilities.

4067 High Noon Books
20 Commercial Boulevard
Novato, CA 94949
800-422-7249
FAX 888-287-9975
http://www.academictherapy.com
e-mail: sales@academictherapy.com
Features over 35 sets of high-interest, low-level books written on a first through fourth grade reading level, for people with reading difficulties, ages nine and up.

4068 Higher Education Services for Students with LD or ADD
JKL Communications
2700 Virginia Avenue NW
Washington, DC 20037
202-333-1713
FAX 202-333-1735
http://www.lathamlaw.org
e-mail: lathamlaw@gmail.com

Peter S Latham JD, Director
Patricia Horan Latham JD, Director

Offers a review of legal requirements and discussion of cases in a clear and understandable style. *$29.00*

ISBN 1-883560-10-1

4069 Holt, Rinehart and Winston
Language Arts Catalog
6277 Sea Harbor Drive
Orlando, FL 32887
800-225-5425
FAX 800-269-5232
http://www.hrw.com
e-mail: holtinfo@hrw.com
Publishes secondary educational material including curriculum-based textbooks, CD-ROMs, videodiscs, and other support and reference materials.

4070 JKL Communications
2700 Virginia Avenue NW
Washington, DC 20037
202-333-1713
FAX 202-333-1735
http://www.lathamlaw.org
e-mail: lathamlaw@gmail.com
Peter S Latham JD, Director
Patricia Horan Latham JD, Director

Publishes books and videos on learning disabilities and ADD with a focus on legal issues in school, higher education and employment.

4071 Jewish Braille Institute of America
110 E 30th Street
New York, NY 10016
212-889-2525
800-433-1531
FAX 212-689-3692
http://www.jewishbraille.org
e-mail: eisler@jbilibrary.org

Dr. Ellen Isler, President
Israel Taub, Associate Director
Sandra Radinsky, Director of Development
Publishes magazines, a newsletter, and special resources available to the reading disabled who are themselves print-handicapped in varying degrees. Seeks the integration of Jews who are blind, visually impaired and reading disabled into the Jewish community and society.

4072 LD/ADD Law Update
JKL Communications
2700 Virginia Avenue NW
Washington, DC 20037
202-333-1713
FAX 202-333-1735
http://www.lathamlaw.org
e-mail: lathamlaw@gmail.com
Peter S Latham JD, Director
Patricia Horan Latham JD, Director

A case update to all JKL publications. *$15.00*

ISBN 1-883560-13-6

4073 Learning Disabilities Association of America
4156 Library Road
Pittsburgh, PA 15234
412-341-1515
FAX 412-344-0224
http://www.ldanatl.org
e-mail: info@ldaamerica.org

Marianne Toombs, President
Suzanne Fornaro, First VP
Connie Parr, Second VP
Maintains a large inventory of publications, videos and other materials related to learning disabilities, and publishes two periodicals available by subscription as well as various books, booklets, brochures, papers and pamphlets on topics related to learning disabilities.

4074 Learning Disabilities Resources
6 E Eagle Road
Havertown, PA 19083
610-446-6126
800-869-8336
FAX 610-446-6129
http://www.learningdifferences.com
e-mail: rcooper-ldr@comcast.net
Dr. Richard Cooper, Owner

Offers a variety of resources to help teach the learning disabled, including alternative ways to teach math, language, spelling, vocabulary, and also how to organize and study. Available in books, videos, and audio tapes.

4075 Learning Disabilities and the Law
JKL Communications
2700 Virginia Avenue NW
Washington, DC 20037
202-333-1713
FAX 202-333-1735
http://www.lathamlaw.org
e-mail: lathamlaw@gmail.com
Peter S Latham JD, Director
Patricia Horan Latham JD, Director

Deals with Issues in education and employment. Covers: Section 504, the IDEA, and ADA. Reviews court cases. *$29.00*

ISBN 1-883560-11-X

4076 Library Reproduction Service
14214 S Figueroa Street
Los Angeles, CA 90061
310-354-2610
800-255-5002
FAX 310-354-2601
http://www.lrs-largeprint.com
e-mail: lrsprint@aol.com
Joan Miller, Owner

Offers large print reproductions to special needs students in first grade through post-secondary, as well as adult basic and continuing education programs; also produces an extensive collection of large print classics for all ages as well as children's literature.

4077 LinguiSystems
3100 4th Avenue
East Moline, IL 61244
309-755-2300
800-776-4332
FAX 800-577-4555
TDY:800-933-8331
http://www.linguisystems.com
e-mail: service@linguisystems.com
Linda Bowers, CEO
Rosemary Huisingh, Co-Owner

Publishes a newsletter and speech-language materials for learning disabilities, ADD/ADHD, auditory processing and listening, language skills, fluency and voice, reading and comprehension, social skills and pragmatics, vocabulary and concepts, writing, spelling, punctuation and other specialized subjects.

4078 Love Publishing Company
9101 E Kenyon Avenue
Denver, CO 80237
303-221-7333
FAX 303-221-7444
http://www.lovepublishing.com
e-mail: lpc@lovepublishing.com
Stan Love, Owner

Publishes titles for use in special education, counseling, social work, and individuals with learning differences.

4079 Magination Press
750 1st Street NE
Washington, DC 20002-4242
202-336-5510
800-374-2721
FAX 202-336-5502
http://www.maginationpress.com
e-mail: magination@apa.org
Publishes special books for children's special concerns, including starting school, learning disabilities, and other topics in psychology, development and mental health.

4080 Maing Handwriting Flow
Oxton House Publishing
PO Box 209
Farmington, ME 04938
207-779-1923
800-539-7323
FAX 207-779-0623
http://www.oxtonhouse.com
e-mail: info@oxtonhouse.com
Phyllis E Fischer PhD, Author
William Burlinghoff PhD, Owner
Bobby Brown, Marketing Director

This packet inlcudes a 16-page booklet, 'Using Models and Drills for Fluency,' and 28 pages of tracing models of numerals, whole words, phrases, and sentences for both manuscript and cursive handwriting, along with a chart for tracking student progress. Suggested for Classroom Resources section, Writing. *$24.95*

1901Grade Range: K-3
ISBN 1-881929-15-9

4081 Marsh Media
8025 Ward Parkway Plaza
Kansas City, MO 64114
816-523-1059
800-821-3303
FAX 866-333-7421
http://www.marshmedia.com
e-mail: info@marshmedia.com
Joan Marsh, Owner

Puberty education for special needs students. Offers educational videos, storybooks and language-intensive teaching guides with a focus on key character-building concepts, health and guidance.

4082 Mindworks Press
4019 Westerly Place
Newport Beach, CA 92660
949-266-3700
FAX 949-266-3770
http://http://amenclinics.com/ac/
e-mail: contact@amenclinic.com
Daniel G Amen MD, Medical Director & CEO

Features books, audio, video, and CD-ROMs addressing a range of disorders, including anxiety, depression, obsessive-compulsiveness and ADD.

4083 Modern Learning Press
PO Box 9067
Cambridge, MA 02139
800-627-5867
FAX 888-558-7350
http://www.modlearn.com
e-mail: mlp@epsbooks.com
Publishes materials to help students, teachers and parents with literacy, school readiness and other important aspects of education and childhood.

4084 Multi-Sequenced Speed Drills for FluencyMulti-Sequenced Speed Drills for Fluency in Decoding
Oxton House Publishing
PO Box 209
Farmington, ME 04938
207-779-1923
800-539-7323
FAX 207-779-0623
http://www.oxtonhouse.com
e-mail: info@oxtonhouse.com
Phyllis E Fischer PhD, Author
William Burlinghoff PhD, Owner
Bobby Brown, Marketing Director

This 179-page set of reading speed drills are carefully constructed to promote decoding automaticity and the fluent recognition of words. They follow the traditional Orton-Gillingham spelling and sound sequences. The set also includes eight pages of teaching advice and a master chart fro tracking student programs. Suggested for Classroom Resources section, Reading. *$29.95*

195 pages 1995Grade Range: All
ISBN 1-881929-14-0

4085 Music Section: National Library Service for the Blind and Physically Handicapped
Library of Congress
1291 Taylor Street NW
Washington, DC 20542
202-707-5100
800-424-8567
FAX 202-707-0712
TDY:202-707-0744
http://www.loc.gov/nls/music
e-mail: nlsm@loc.gov
John Hanson, Department Head
Frank Cylke, Executive Director

Offers a special music collection consisting of more than 30,000 braille and large print music scores, texts, and instructional recordings about music and musicians on cassette and audio disc.

4086 National Association for Visually Handicapped
22 W 21st Street
New York, NY 10010
212-889-3141
FAX 212-727-2931
http://www.navh.org
e-mail: staff@navh.org
Lorraine Marchi, CEO

Publishes information about sight and sight problems for adults and children. Offers a product line of low-vision aids, a collection of articles about eye conditions, causes and treatment modalities, and a newsletter issued four times a year with information to assist people in dealing with low vision.

4087 National Bible Association
1865 Broadway
New York, NY 10023
212-408-1390
FAX 212-408-1448
http://www.nationalbible.org
e-mail: nba@nationalbible.org
Thomas May, President
Tamara Collins, VP Reading Program

Publishes Read it! A Journal for Bible Readers, which is issued three times a year. Also offers many versions of the Bible, including large-print editions and the easy-to-read Contemporary English Version.

4088 Nimble Numeracy: Fluency in Counting andNimble Numeracy: Fluency in Counting and Basic Arithmet
Oxton House Publishers
PO Box 209
Farmington, ME 04938
207-779-1923
800-539-7323
FAX 207-779-0623
http://www.oxtonhouse.com
e-mail: info@oxtonhouse.com
Phyllis E Fischer PhD, Author
William Burlinghoff PhD, Owner
Bobby Brown, Marketing Director

This is a richly detailed handbook for teachers, tutors, and parents who want to help children develop fluent arithmetric skills. It provides explicit techniques for teaching counting and basic arithmetic, with special emphasis on the language of our base-ten, place-value system for speaking about and writing numbers. Suggested for Classroom Resources section, Math.
$19.95
136 pages 1902Grade Range: K-up
ISBN 1-881929-19-1

4089 Northwest Media
326 W 12th Avenue
Eugene, OR 97401
541-343-6636
800-777-6636
FAX 541-343-0177
http://www.sociallearning.com
e-mail: nwm@northwestmedia.com
Lee White, President
Susan Larson, Marketing Director

Publishes material with a focus on independent living and foster care products. Training resources for parents: www.fosterparentcollege.com and for teens: www.vstreet.com.

4090 Oxton House Publishers
PO Box 209
Farmington, ME 04938
207-779-1923
800-539-7323
FAX 207-779-0623
http://www.oxtonhouse.com
e-mail: info@oxtonhouse.com
William Burlinghoff PhD, Owner
Bobby Brown, Marketing Director

Publishes high quality, innovative, affordable materials for teaching, reading and mathematics and for dealing with learning disabilities.

4091 PEAK Parent Center
611 N Weber Street
Colorado Springs, CO 80903
719-531-9400
800-284-0251
FAX 719-531-9452
http://www.peakparent.org
e-mail: info@peakparent.org
Barbara Bushwell, Executive Director
Kent Willis, President, Board of Directors

A federally-designated Parent Traning and Information Center (PTI). As a PTI, PEAK supports and empowers parents, providing them with information and strategies to use when advocating for their children with disabilities by expanding knowledge of special education and offering new strategies for success.

4092 Performance Resource Press
1270 Rankin Drive
Troy, MI 48083
248-588-7733
800-453-7733
FAX 800-499-5718
http://www.prponline.net
e-mail: customerservice@prponline.net
George Watkins, President

Publishes over 600 products, including catalogs, journals, digests, newsletters, books, videos, posters and pamplets with a focus on behavioral health.

4093 Peytral Publications
PO Box 1162
Minnetonka, MN 55345
952-949-8707
877-739-8725
FAX 952-906-9777
http://www.peytral.com
e-mail: help@peytral.com
Peggy Hammeken, President

Publishes and distributes special education materials which promote success for all learners.

4094 Phillip Roy Catalog
Phillip Roy
13064 Indian Rocks Road
Largo, FL 33774
727-593-2700
800-255-9085
FAX 727-595-2685
http://www.philliproy.com
e-mail: info@philliproy.com
Ruth Bragman PhD, President
Phillip Roy, Manager

Publishes educational materials written for students of any age with different learning abilities. Offers an alternative approach to traditional education. Free catalog upon request.

4095 Reader's Digest Partners for Sight Foundation
Reader's Digest Road
Pleasantville, NY 10570
914-244-4900
800-877-5293
http://www.rd.com
e-mail: partnersforsight@rd.com
Susan Olivo, VP/General Manager
Dianna Kelly-Naghizadeh, Program Manager
Thomas Ryder, CEO
Offers large type editions of select books and large print editions of Readers Digest Magazines, as well as a foundation newsletter, Sightlines, which is published in large format with large type.

4096 Research Press Catalog

PO Box 9177
Champaign, IL 61826
217-352-3273
800-519-2707
FAX 217-352-1221
http://www.researchpress.com
e-mail: rp@researchpress.com
Russell Pence, President
Dennis Wiziecki, Marketing

Research Press provides user-friendly research-based prevention and intervention materials.

4097 Riggs Institute

21106 479th Avenue
White, SD 57276
503-646-9459
800-200-4840
FAX 503-644-5191
http://www.riggsinst.org
e-mail: riggs@riggsinst.org
Myrna McCulloch, Founder/Director/Author

Publishes materials to help remedial students using the Orton method, a multisensory approach to learning. Offers a catalog of products, including teacher's editions, phonogram cards, audio CDs for students, student materials and classroom materials.

4098 Scholastic

557 Broadway
New York, NY 10012
212-343-6100
800-246-2986
http://www.scholastic.com
Richard Robinson, CEO
Barbara A Marcus, VP/President Children's Books
Richard M Spaulding, Executive VP Marketing

Produces educational materials to assist and inspire students of all ages, including a range of special education books, software, and other products.

4099 Schwab Learning

1650 S Amphlett Boulevard
San Mateo, CA 94402
650-655-2410
800-230-0988
FAX 650-655-2411
http://www.schwablearning.org
e-mail: media@schwablearning.org
Catherine Ericson, Marketing Executive

Provides information, guidance, support and materials that address the emotional, social, practical and academic needs and concerns of children with learning difficulties, and their parents.

4100 Slosson Educational Publications

PO Box 280
East Aurora, NY 14052
716-652-0930
888-756-7766
FAX 800-655-3840
http://www.slosson.com
e-mail: slosson@slosson.com
Steven Slosson, President

Publishes and distributes educational materials in the areas of intelligence, aptitude, developmental disabilities, school screening and achievement, speech-language and assessment therapy, emotional/behavior, and special needs. Offers a product line of testing and assessment materials, books, games, videos, cassettes and computer software intended for use by professionals, psychologists, teachers, counselors, students and parents.

4101 Sounds and Spelling Patterns for Engilish;Sounds and Spelling Patterns for English; Phonics for

Oxton House Publishing
PO Box 209
Farmington, ME 04938
207-779-1923
800-539-7323
FAX 207-779-0623
http://www.oxtonhouse.com
e-mail: info@oxtonhouse.com
Phyllis E Fischer PhD, Author
William Burlinghoff PhD, Owner
Bobby Brown, Marketing Director

This book is a clear, concise, practical, jargon-free overview of the sounds that make up the English languate and the symbols that we use to represent them in writing. It includes an explanatory chapter on phonological and phonemic awareness and a broad range of strategies for helping beginning readers develop fluent decoding skills. Suggested for Classroom Resources section, Reading *$24.95*

140 pages 1993Grade Range: K-up
ISBN 1-881929-01-9

4102 Speed Drills for Arithmetric Facts

Oxton House Publishers
PO Box 209
Farmington, ME 04938
207-779-1923
800-539-7323
FAX 207-779-0623
http://www.oxtonhouse.com
e-mail: info@oxtonhouse.com
Phyllis E Fischer PhD, Author
William Burlinghoff PhD, Owner
Bobby Brown, Marketing Director

This looseleaf packet is a set of 48 pages of carefully constructed exercises to promote automaticity and fluency with basic arithmetic facts. The worksheets reinforce the interrelationship of three numbers in addition/subtraction and multiplication/division statements. Also included are six pages of detailed teaching advice and a chart template for tracking student progress. Suggested for Classroom Resources section, Math. *$24.95*

54 pages 1901Grade Range: 1-4
ISBN 1-881929-16-7

4103 Stories from Somerville

Oxton House Publishers
PO Box 209
Farmington, ME 04938
207-779-1923
800-539-7323
FAX 207-779-0623
http://www.oxtonhouse.com
e-mail: info@oxtonhouse.com
Kimberly Ramsey, Author
William Burlinghoff PhD, Owner
Bobby Brown, Marketing Director

This set of two readers and three workbooks contains a total of 75 separate but interconnected, phonetically-controlled stories that follow a careful pattern of skill development. They are compatible with most phonics-based reading programs. The realistic personal interactions of the characters also provide opportunities for rich class discussion about various social skills that may be troublesome for students with learning disabilities. Suggested for Classroom Resources section, Reading. *$69.95*

1902Grade Range: 2-5
ISBN 1-881929-40-4

4104 Succeeding in the Workplace

JKL Communications
2700 Virginia Avenue NW
Washington, DC 20037
202-333-1713
FAX 202-333-1735
http://www.lathamlaw.org
e-mail: lathamlaw@gmail.com
Peter S Latham JD, Director
Patricia Horan Latham JD, Director

Comprehensive review: understanding disabilities, how to find and get the right job, how to succeed on the job, strategies, job accommodations, legal rights and personal experiences. *$29.00*

ISBN 1-883560-03-9

4105 Succeeding in the Workplace (30 Minute Video)

JKL Communications
2700 Virginia Avenue NW
Washington, DC 20037
202-333-1713
FAX 202-333-1735
http://www.lathamlaw.org
e-mail: lathamlaw@gmail.com
Peter S Latham JD, Director
Patricia Horan Latham JD, Director

This fast paced video covers legal rights, accommodations and strategies to promote success for individuals with LD or ADD in the workplace. Includes personal stories. *$29.00*

30 minutes
ISBN 1-883560-06-3

4106 Succeeding in the Workplace (56 Minute Video)
JKL Communications
2700 Virginia Avenue NW
Washington, DC 20037 202-333-1713
FAX 202-333-1735
http://www.lathamlaw.org
e-mail: lathamlaw@gmail.com
Peter S Latham JD, Director
Patricia Horan Latham JD, Director

This (VHS) video offers more comprehensive information than the 30 minute video. *$49.00*
56 minutes
ISBN 1-883560-05-5

4107 Tales from the Workplace
JKL Communications
2700 Virginia Avenue NW
Washington, DC 20037 202-333-1713
FAX 202-333-1735
http://www.lathamlaw.org
e-mail: lathamlaw@gmail.com
Peter S Latham JD, Director
Patricia Horan Latham JD, Director

Easy to read. Explores through stories: What is the right job match? Should I disclose my disability? What are the signs of job trouble? John A Ratey, MD says a great how to book. *$15.00*

ISBN 1-883560-08-X

4108 Teaching Comprehension: Strategies for StoTeaching Comprehension: Strategies for Stories
Oxton House Publishing
PO Box 209
Farmington, ME 04938 207-779-1923
800-539-7323
FAX 207-779-0623
http://www.oxtonhouse.com
e-mail: info@oxtonhouse.com
Phyllis E Fischer PhD, Author
William Burlinghoff PhD, Owner
Bobby Brown, Marketing Director

This handbook gives teachers a richly detailed roadmap for providing students with effective strategies for comprehending and remembering stories. It inlcudes story-line masters for helping students to organize their thinking about a story and to accurately depict characters and sequence events. Suggested for Classroom Resources, Reading. *$24.95*
62 pages 1902Grade Range: Teachers, All
ISBN 1-881929-27-2

4109 Teddy Bear Press
3639 Midway Drive
San Diego, CA 92110 858-560-8718
FAX 619-255-2158
http://www.teddybearpress.net
e-mail: fparker@teddybearpress.net
Fran Parker, Author

Publishes books and reading materials designed with the beginning reader in mind, written and illustrated by a special education teacher specializing in elementary education, learning disabilities, and education for the emotionally and mentally challenged.

4110 Therapro
225 Arlington Street
Framingham, MA 01702 508-872-9494
800-257-5376
FAX 508-875-2062
http://www.theraproducts.com
e-mail: info@theraproducts.com
Karen Conrad, Owner

Offers specialty products and publications for all ages in the field of occupational therapy, including assistive technology, evaluations, handwriting programs, sensory-motor awareness and alerting products, oral motor products, early learning products, and perception, cognition and language resources.

4111 Thomas Nelson Publishers
PO Box 141000
Nashville, TN 37214 615-248-2110
800-889-9000
FAX 615-391-5225
http://www.thomasnelson.com
e-mail: publicity@thomasnelson.com
Thomas Nelson, Owner
Michael S Hyatt, Executive VP/Group Publisher
Phil Stoner, Executive VP/Group Publisher
Publishes books and other resources for the learning disabled.

4112 Thomas T Beeler, Publisher
PO Box 310
Rollinsford, NH 03869 603-794-0392
800-818-7574
FAX 888-222-3396
http://www.beelerpub.com
e-mail: tombeeler@beelerpub.com
Thomas T Beeler, Publisher
David W O'Connor, President
Traci Watson, Editor
Publishes and distributes hardcover, large print editions of popular titles for all ages, printed in 16-point type on acid-free paper and bound in sturdy, library-grade sewn binding with full color covers. Also offers audiobooks.

4113 Thorndike Press
295 Kennedy Memorial Drive
Waterville, ME 04901 207-859-1000
800-223-1244
FAX 800-558-4676
http://www.galegroup.com/thorndike
Debbie Ludden, Director Marketing
Jill Leckta, Publisher

Publishes and distributes over 900 new large-print editions per year, with an emphasis on bestsellers and genre fiction, as well as nonfiction titles.

4114 Transaction Publishers
Rutgers University
35 Berrue Circle
Piscataway, NJ 08854 732-445-3020
888-999-6778
FAX 732-445-3138
http://www.transactionpub.com
e-mail: trans@transactionpub.com
Irving Louis Horowitz, Chairman
Mary E Curtis, President
Scott B Bramson, President Express Book Division
Publishes over 70 books in large print, including new large print titles, as well as selections from the best of the company's backlist, with many classic titles from well-known American authors. The large print format makes selection easy for visually impaired readers.

4115 Ulverscroft Large Print Books
PO Box 1230
West Seneca, NY 14224 716-674-4270
800-955-9659
FAX 716-674-4195
http://www.ulverscroft.com
e-mail: enquiries@ulverscroft.co.uk
Janice Gowan, Executive Director

Publishes large print books and audio products for people hard of seeing.

4116 Volta Voices
Alexander Graham Bell Association for the Deaf and
3417 Volta Place NW
Washington, DC 20007 202-337-5220
866-37-5226
FAX 202-337-8314
http://www.agbell.org
e-mail: publications@agbell.org
Dawn Scarola, Managing Editor, Author
Todd Houston PhD, Executive Director
Jessica Ripper, Sr Dir Marketing/Communications
Jennifer Vernon, Coordinator Production/Editing
Publishes and distributes books, brochures, instructional materials, videos, CDs and audiocassettes relating to hearing loss. *$62.00*

64 pages Bimonthly

4117 Wadsworth Publishing Company

10 Davis Drive
Belmont, CA 94002
650-598-9757
800-354-9706
FAX 650-637-7544
http://www.wadworth.com
e-mail: dory.schaeffer@thomsonlearning.com

Dan Alpert, Acquisitions Editor
Dory Schaeffer, Marketing Manager

Publishes books on a wide range of topics in special education, including behavior modification, language disorders and development, and learning disabilities.

4118 Waterfront Books

85 Crescent Road
Burlington, VT 05401
800-639-6063
http://www.waterfrontbooks.com
e-mail: helpkids@waterfrontbooks.com

Sherrill N Musty, President

Publishes and distributes informative books and materials serving professionals and parents who are concerned with children at home, at school and in the workplace. Topics include overcoming barriers to learning, family support and parenting, personal safety, learning differences and special needs.

4119 Woodbine House

6510 Bells Mill Road
Bethesda, MD 20817
301-897-3570
800-843-7323
FAX 301-897-5838
http://www.woodbinehouse.com
e-mail: info@woodbinehouse.com

Irv Shapell, Owner

Specializes in books about children with special needs; publishes sixty-five titles within the Special Needs Collection, covering AD/HD, learning disabilities, special education, communication skills, and other disabilities, for use by parents, children, therapists, health care providers and teachers.

4120 Xavier Society for the Blind

154 E 23rd Street
New York, NY 10010
212-473-7800

Kathleen Lynch, Manager
Gina Ballero, Secretary to Director

Provides resources for the visually impaired, including large-print, braille, and audio products.

4121 York Press

PO Box 504
Timonium, MD 21094
800-962-2763
FAX 410-560-6758
http://www.yorkpress.com
e-mail: info@yorkpress.com

Publishes books about language development and disabilities, especially dyslexia, and about hearing impairment.

Classroom Resources

4122 ADD From A to Z
Connecticut Assoc. for Children and Adults with LD
25 Van Zant Street
Norwalk, CT 06855 203-838-5010
FAX 203-866-6108
http://www.CACLD.org
e-mail: cacld@juno.com
Edward Hallowell MD, Presenter
Beryl Kaufman, Executive Director

Dr. Hallowell, child and adult psychiatrist on the faculty of the Harvard Medical School, is widely regarded as a leading authority on the subject of Attention Deficit Disorder. This video version of one of his classic lectures provides a comprehensive overview of this complicated and often misunderstood subject. Topics include symptoms to look for, how to tell if it is not ADD, twenty steps to diagnosis, methods of treatment (medical and nonmedical) and the Ritalin controversy. *$34.95*
$5.00 shipping

4123 ASCD Cooperative Learning Series
Assoc. for Supervision/Curriculum Development
1250 N Beauregard Street
Alexandria, VA 22311 703-549-9110
800-933-ASCD
FAX 703-575-5400
http://www.ascd.org
RE Slavin, Author

A facilitator's manual, book and five videotapes focusing on: providing a fundamental knowledge of cooperative learning and the benefits derived from its use, providing a basic understanding of how to plan and teach cooperative lessons and providing resources.

4124 Arts Express
KET, The Kentucky Network Enterprise Division
600 Cooper Drive
Lexington, KY 40502 859-258-7000
800-354-9067
FAX 859-258-7396
Virginia Fox, Executive Director

A delightful way to introduce elementary students to the visual arts, music and dance. Twenty 15 minute video programs available individually or onfive videotapes of four programs each. *$320.00*
price/set

4125 Becoming a Proficient Cuer
Harris Communications
15155 Technology Drive
Eden Prairie, MN 55344 952-906-1180
800-825-6758
FAX 952-906-1099
TDY:952-906-1198
http://www.harriscomm.com
Robert Harris, Owner

Video lessons are combined with workbook drills to describe and teach Cued Speech, and prevent and eliminate errors. Designed for hearing people at all levels of Cued Speech proficiency. *$49.95*
19 pages 108-min. Video

4126 Collaboration in the Schools: The Problem-Solving Process
Pro-Ed
8700 Shoal Creek Boulevard
Austin, TX 78757 512-451-3246
800-897-3202
FAX 512-451-8542
http://www.proedinc.com
L Idol, Author
Donald Hamill, Owner

An inservice/preservice video that demonstrates the stages of the consultative/collaborative process, as well as many of the various communicative/interactive skills and collaborative problem solving skills. *$106.00*

4127 College Transition
Central Piedmont Community College
PO Box 35009
Charlotte, NC 28235 704-330-2722
FAX 704-330-6136
http://www.cpcc.cc.nc.us
Tony Zeise, President

A video developed for facilitators to show to audiences of high school students, college transfer students and college freshman.

4128 Cooperative Discipline: Classroom Management Promoting Self-Esteem
AGS
PO Box 99
Circle Pines, MN 55014 763-786-4343
800-328-2560
FAX 763-786-9077
http://www.agsnet.com
e-mail: agsmail@agsnet.com
L Albert, Author
Kevin Brueggeman, Manager

A leader's guide, teacher's guide, set of 23 blackline masters, 2 scripts and 2 videotapes comprise this comprehensive discipline training program that helps teachers achieve control and order in their classroom. *$495.00*

4129 Educational Evaluation
Stern Center for Language and Learning
135 Allen Brook Lane
Williston, VT 05495 802-878-2332
800-544-4863
FAX 802-878-0230
http://www.sterncenter.org
e-mail: learning@sterncenter.org
Blanche Podhajski, President

The evaluation is an assessment of intelligence, academic achievement, language, and emotional and behavioral issues related to learning and includes pre- and post- evaluation conferences with parents and/ or students as well as an extensive written report detailing results and recommendations.

4130 Fundamentals of Reading Success
Educators Publishing Service
PO Box 9031
Cambridge, MA 02139 617-547-6706
800-225-5750
FAX 617-547-0412
http://www.epsbooks.com
e-mail: eps@epsbooks.com
Arlene W Sonday, Author
Gunnar Voltz, President

This Orton-Gillingham-based video series teaches a phonic or code-emphasis approach to reading, spelling, and handwriting, and provides the foundation for a multisensory phonics curriculum. May be used by teachers and tutors. *$ 480.00*

ISBN 0-838872-52-2

4131 Harcourt Achieve
6277 Sea Harbor Drive
Orlando, FL 32887
800-531-5015
FAX 800-699-9459
http://www.harcourtachieve.com
e-mail: eha@harcourt.com
Tim McEwen, President/CEO
Susan Canizares, Sr. VP Publisher
Lee Wilson, Marketing VP
Harcourt Achieve provides educational materials that fundamentally and positively change the lives of learners. Through the Rigby, Saxon, and Steck-Vaughn imprints, Harcourt Achieve provides a wide array of both core and supplemental products to meet the needs of learners of all ages in all content areas.

4132 **Individual Instruction**
Stern Center for Language and Learning
135 Allen Brook Lane
Williston, VT 05495
802-878-2332
800-544-4863
FAX 802-878-0230
http://www.sterncenter.org
e-mail: learning@sterncenter.org
Blanche Podhajski, President

Individualized instruction to help students develop literacy skills and achieve academic success, building on learning strengths and compensating for areas of difficulty.

4133 **Instructional Strategies for Learning Disabled Community College Students**
Graduate School and University Center
365 5th Avenue
New York, NY 10016
212-817-7000
FAX 212-817-1503
http://www.gc.cuny.edu
Frances Degenhorowitz, President

For working with a cross-section of types of individuals with learning problems. *$47.50*

4134 **Key Concepts in Personal Development**
Marsh Media
8082 Ward Parkway Plaza
Kansas City, MO 64114
816-523-1059
800-821-3303
FAX 866-333-7421
http://www.marshmedia.com
e-mail: info@marshmedia.com
Joan Marsh, Owner
Liz Sweeney, Editorial Assistant

Puberty Education for Children with Special Needs. Comprehensive, gender-specific kits and supplemental parent packets address human sexuality for children with miild to moderate developmental disabilities.

4135 **Living With Attention Deficit Disorder**
Aquarius Health Media Care
18 N Main Street
Sherborn, MA 01770
508-650-1616
888-440-2963
FAX 508-650-1665
http://www.aquariusproductions.com
e-mail: aquarius@aquariusproductions.com
Leslie Kussmann, President

This video presents tips for teachers and students how to deal with ADD, including how to adapt school structures and classes. *$125.00*
Video, 22 mins

4136 **New Room Arrangement as a Teaching Strategy**
Teaching Strategies
PO Box 42243
Washington, DC 20015
202-362-7543
800-637-3652
FAX 202-364-7273
http://www.TeachingStrategies.com
e-mail: info@TeachingStrategies.com
Diane Trister-Dodge, Owner

A manual and video present the impact of the early childhood classroom environment on how children learn, how they relate to others and how teachers teach. *$35.00*

4137 **Now You're Talking: Extend Conversation**
Educational Productions
PO Box 957
Hillsboro, OR 97123
503-297-6393
800-950-4949
FAX 503-297-6395
http://www.edpro.com
e-mail: custserv@edpro.com
Linda Freedman, Owner

Video. Teachers in a language-based preschool and speech-language pathologists model effective techniques that focus and extend conversations of young children. *$295.00*

4138 **Phonemic Awareness: Lessons, Activities and Games**
Peytral Publication
PO Box 1162
Minnetonka, MN 55345
952-949-8707
877-739-8725
FAX 612-906-9777
http://www.peytral.com
e-mail: help@peytral.com
Victoria Groves Scott, Author
Peggy Hammeken, President

Exceptional field tested guide to help educators who want to reach phonemic awareness as a prerequisite to reading, and/or to supplement the current curriculum. Special educators and speech clinicians will find this practical guide especially helpful as research indicates that deficits in phonemic awareness is often a major contributor to reading disabilities. This book contains fifty-eight scripted lessons, forty-nine reproducible blackline master and progress charts. Video also available *$27.95*
176 pages
ISBN 1-890455-28-8

4139 **Planning Individualized Education Programs for Language-Impaired Children**
Purdue University Continuing Education
1586 Stewart Center
West Lafayette, IN 47907
765-494-7231
800-359-2968
FAX 765-494-0567
Nickola Wolf Nelson, PhD, Author

Stresses the need to select different kinds of intervention strategies and content for different types of language disorders. Includes general consideration regarding the identification, writing and implementing of goals and short-term objectives. *$81.00*

4140 **Professional Development**
Stern Center for Language and Learning
135 Allen Brook Lane
Williston, VT 05495
802-878-2332
800-544-4863
FAX 802-878-0230
http://www.sterncenter.org
e-mail: learning@sterncenter.org
Blanche Podhajski, President

Staff development programs for preschool through grade 12 designed in response to requests from teachers and administrators for cutting-edge information about different kinds of learners and the teaching strategies most successful for them.

4141 **Professional Development, Reference and Educational Materials for Speech-Language Pathologists**
American Speech-Language-Hearing Association
10801 Rockville Pike
Rockville, MD 20852
301-897-5700
888-498-6699
FAX 301-897-7358
http://www.asha.org
Leslie Katz, Brand Director
Arlene Pietranton, Executive Director

$104.00

4142 **Purdue University Speech-Language Clinic**
Grant Street
West Lafayette, IN 47907
765-494-7231
800-359-2968
FAX 765-494-0567
http://www.cla.purdue.edu
Mary Walker, Program Coordinator

The Speech-Language Clinic provides opportunities for individuals with communication problems to receive individual and group diagnostic evaluations, screenings and therapy services. The clinic provide services for children and adults with mild to severe speech sound problems and/or impaired oral-motor control, language problems associated with autism, language-learning disabilities, hearing impairment, stuttering, and voice problems. *$81.00*

4143 Restructuring America's Schools
Association for Supervision/Curriculum Development
1703 N Beauregard Street
Alexandria, VA 22311
703-578-9600
FAX 703-549-3891
http://www.ascd.org

M D'Arcangelo, Author
Gene Carter, Executive Director

A leader's guide and videotape designed for administrators, teachers, parents, school board members, and community leaders.

4144 Skillstreaming Video: How to Teach Students Prosocial Skills
Research Press
PO Box 9177
Champaign, IL 61826
217-352-3273
800-519-2707
FAX 217-352-1221
http://www.researchpress.com
e-mail: rp@researchpress.com

Dr. AP Goldstein And Dr. Ellen McGinness, Author
Russell Pence, President

A video and two books providing an overview of a training procedure for teaching elementary and secondary level students the skills they need for coping with typical social and interpersonal problems. *$365.00*

4145 Spelling Workbook Video
Learning Disabilities Resources
PO Box 716
Bryn Mawr, PA 19010
610-525-8336
800-869-8336
FAX 610-525-8337
http://www.ldonline.org

An instructional video which works through the spelling workbooks for teachers and students. *$16.00*

4146 Strategic Planning and Leadership
Assoc. for Supervision/Curriculum Development
1703 N Beauregard Street
Alexandria, VA 22311
703-578-9600
800-933-2723
FAX 703-575-5400
http://www.ascd.org

Gene Carter, Executive Director

Designed to explain and illustrate effective approaches to dealing with change through strategic planning.

4147 Strategies Intervention Program
Special Education Resource Center
25 Industrial Park Road
Middletown, CT 06457
860-632-1485
FAX 860-632-8870

A Marks, Author
Marianne Kirner, Executive Director

A video illustrating through an interview with five eighth grade students, the effectiveness of a program designed to develop specific learning strategies for adolescents with learning disabilities.

4148 Teaching Adults with Learning Disabilities
Stern Center for Language and Learning
135 Allen Brook Lane
Williston, VT 05495
802-878-2332
800-544-4863
FAX 802-878-0230
http://www.sterncenter.org
e-mail: bpodhajski@sterncenter.org

Blanche Podhajski, President

A videotape training program and companion guide designed to help adult literacy teachers identify and instruct adults with learning disabilities. The focus of this five hour video series is on teaching basic reading and spelling skills. *$199.95*

4149 Teaching Math
Learning Disabilities Resources
PO Box 716
Bryn Mawr, PA 19010
610-525-8336
800-869-8336
FAX 610-525-8337
http://www.ldonline.org

A video for educational professionals teaching math to disabled children. *$12.00*

4150 Teaching People with Developmental Disabilities
Research Press
PO Box 9177
Champaign, IL 61826
217-352-3273
800-519-2707
FAX 217-352-1221
http://www.researchpress.com
e-mail: rp@researchpress.com

Russell Pence, President

A set of four videotapes and accompanying participant workbooks designed to help teachers, staff, volunteers, or family members master task analysis, prompting, reinforcement and error correction. *$595.00*

4151 Teaching Strategies Library: Research Based Strategies for Teachers
Assoc. for Supervision/Curriculum Development
1250 N Pitt Street
Alexandria, VA 22314
703-549-9110
FAX 703-549-3891
http://www.ascd.org

HF Silver, Author

A trainer's manual and five videotapes designed for inservice education of teachers K-12 focusing on four different types of learning expected of students: mastery, understanding, synthesis and involvement.

4152 Teaching Students Through Their Individual Learning Styles
St. John's University, Learning Styles Network
8000 Utopia Parkway
Jamaica, NY 11439
718-990-6201
FAX 718-990-1882
http://www.learningstyles.net

R Dunn, Author
James Benson, Executive Director

A set of six videotapes introducing the Dunn and Dunn learning styles model. Explains the environmental, emotional, sociological, physical and psychological elements of style.

4153 Telling Tales
KET, The Kentucky Network Enterprise Division
600 Cooper Drive
Lexington, KY 40502
859-258-7000
800-354-9067
FAX 859-258-7396

Virginia Fox, Executive Director

Resource for teachers,librarians and drama departments at all levels of instruction. Telling Tales can be used to encourage creativity and self expression and help students understand their cultural and language arts skills, and develop openess to diverse cultures, build self confidence and leadership skills, improve communication and language arts skills and develop oral history projects. *$30.00*

4154 Word Feathers
KET, The Kentucky Network Enterprise Division
600 Cooper Drive
Lexington, KY 40502
859-258-7000
800-354-9067
FAX 859-258-7396

Virginia Fox, Executive Director

An activity-oriented language arts video series.

Parents & Professionals

4155 **3 R'S for Special Education: Rights, Resources, Results**
Brookes Publishing Company
PO Box 10624
Baltimore, MD 21285
410-337-9580
800-638-3775
FAX 410-337-8539
http://www.pbrookes.com
e-mail: sales@pbrookes.com
Paul Brooks, Owner

This video helps parents navigate the steps of the special education system and work towards securing the best education and services for their children. *$49.95*
Video

4156 **A Child's First Words**
Orange County Learning Disabilities Association
PO Box 25772
Santa Ana, CA 92799
714-547-4206
http://www.oclda.org
e-mail: info@oclda.org
Shows the importance of not waiting until your child is older to worry about their speech. *$20.00*
Catalog #7353

4157 **A Culture Undiscovered**
Fanlight Productions
4196 Washington Street
Boston, MA 02131
617-469-4999
FAX 617-439-3379
http://www.fanlight.com
e-mail: fanlight@fanlight.com
Ben Achtenberg, Owner
Nicole Johnson, Publicity Coordinator

Explores the needs and experiences of college students, from diverse racial and/or thnic backgrounds, who have learning disabilities.
Video, 36 min

4158 **A Mind of Your Own**
Fanlight Productions
4196 Washington Street
Boston, MA 02131
617-469-4999
800-937-4113
FAX 617-469-3379
http://www.fanlight.com
e-mail: fanlight@fanlight.com
Ben Achtenberg, Owner
Nicole Johnson, Publicity Coordinator

New video on learning disabilities from the National Film Board of Canada, follows four learning disabled students through their struggles academically and socially as well as their successes in learning to cope with their disabilities and develop their own unique talents. Amtec Award of Merit. 37 minutes. *$199.00*
Rental $60/day
ISSN DD29-0

4159 **ABC's of ADD**
JKL Communications
2700 Virginia Avenue NW
Washington, DC 20037
202-223-5097
FAX 202-223-5096
http://www.lathamlaw.org
e-mail: plath3@his.com

$29.00

4160 **ABC's of Learning Disabilities**
American Federation of Teachers
555 New Jersey Avenue NW
Washington, DC 20001
202-879-4400
FAX 202-879-4597
http://www.aft.org
e-mail: online@aft.org

Sandra Feldman, President

This film illustrates the case histories of four learning disabled students with various learning disabilities.

4161 **ADHD**
Brookes Publishing Company
PO Box 10624
Baltimore, MD 21285
800-638-3775
FAX 410-337-8539
http://www.pbrookes.com
e-mail: custserv@pbrookes.com
Paul H Brooks, President
Melissa A Behm, Executive Vice President
George Stamathis, Vice President/Publisher
This video shows methods for helping students who have ADHD increase attention to tasks, improve listening skills, become better organized, and boost work production. *$99.00*
Video
ISBN 1-557661-15-4

4162 **ADHD in Adults**
Guilford Publications
72 Spring Street
New York, NY 10012
212-431-9800
800-365-7006
FAX 212-966-6708
http://www.guilford.com
e-mail: info@guilford.com
Bob Matloff, President

This program integrates information on ADHD with the actual experiences of four adults who suffer from the disorder. Representing a range of professions, from a lawyer to a mother working at home, each candidly discusses the impact of ADHD on his or her daily life. These interviews are qugmented by comments from family members and other clinicians who treat adults with ADHD *$95.00*
36-min VHS

4163 **ADHD in the Classroom: Strategies for Teachers**
Guilford Publications
72 Spring Street
New York, NY 10012
212-431-9800
800-365-7006
FAX 212-966-6708
http://www.guilford.com
e-mail: info@guilford.com
Bob Matloff, President

Viewers see the problems teachers encounter with children who suffer with ADHD, as well as instructive demonstrations of effective behavior management techbiques including color charts and signs, point system, token economy, and turtle-control technique. Also includes a Leader's Guide and a 42-page Manual. *$95.00*
36-min. VHS

4164 **ADHD: What Can We Do?**
Guilford Publications
72 Spring Street
New York, NY 10012
212-431-9800
800-365-7006
FAX 212-966-6708
http://www.guilford.com
e-mail: info@guilford.com
Bob Matloff, President

A video program that introduces teachers and parents to a variety of the most effective techniques for managing ADHD in the classroom, at home, and on gamily outings. Includes Leader's Guide and 30-page Manual. *$95.00*

ISBN 0-898629-72-1

4165 **ADHD: What Do We Know?**
Guilford Publications
72 Spring Street
New York, NY 10012
212-431-9800
800-365-7006
FAX 212-966-6708
http://www.guilford.com
e-mail: info@guilford.com
Bob Matloff, President

An introduction for teachers and special education practitioners, school psychologists and parents of ADHD children. Topics outlined in this videoinclude the causes and prevalence of ADHD, ways children with ADHD behave, otherconditions that may accompany ADHD and long-term prospects for children with ADHD. *$95.00*
Video

4166 Adapting to Your Child's Personality
Aquarius Health Media Care
18 N Main Street
Sherborn, MA 01770
508-650-1616
888-440-2963
FAX 508-650-1665
http://www.aquarisproductions.com
e-mail: aquarius@aquarisproductions.com
Leslie Kussmann, President

Join a child behavioral specialist, two moms and their toddlers (with different personalities!) to find out how to mold your own responses so that you can more effectively influence your child. VHS: A-KIDSPERSONAL also on DVD. *$ 145.00*
Video, 30 mins

4167 Adults with Learning Problems
Learning Disabilities Resources
PO Box 716
Bryn Mawr, PA 19010
610-525-8336
800-869-8336
FAX 610-525-8337
http://www.ldonline.org
Educational materials for adults with a learning disability.

4168 All Children Learn Differently
Orange County Learning Disabilities Association
PO Box 25772
Santa Ana, CA 92799
714-547-7206
http://www.oclda.org
e-mail: info@oclda.org
Covers cognitive, perceptual, nutritional, optometric, speech and language motor aspects. *$29.95*
Catalog #6812

4169 American Sign Language Phrase Book Videotape Series
Harris Communications
15155 Technology Drive
Eden Prairie, MN 55344
952-906-1180
800-825-6758
FAX 952-906-1099
TDY:952-906-1198
http://www.harriscomm.com
Robert Harris, Owner

Includes book and three videotapes, each 60 minutes long. In Volume 1 you will find everyday expressions, signing and deafness, getting acquainted, health and water; in Volume 2 you will find family, school, food and drink, clothing, sports and recreation; and in Volume 3 you will find travel, animal, colors, civics, religion, numbers, time, dates and money. *$134.95*

4170 Andreas: Outcomes of Inclusion
Center on Disability and Community Inclusion
499c Waterman Building
Burlington, VT 05401
802-651-9050
FAX 802-656-1357
http://www.uvm.edu/zvapvt/timfox
e-mail: syuan@zoo.uvm.edu
Mitch Cantor, Executive Director

Video portrays the academic, occupational, and social inclusion of a high school student with severe disabilities. Includes commentary of parents, administrators, teachers, support personnel, classmates.

4171 Anger Within Programs 1-4: Walking Through the Storm Life Space Crisis Intervention
NAK Production Associates
4304 EW Highway
Bethesda, MD 20814
301-654-4777
FAX 301-654-7772
e-mail: NAK@makprod.com
NA Klotz, Author
Norman Klotz, Owner

Videos focusing on parental and professional perspectives, understanding of children's feelings, treatment models and techniques and skills for working with students with emotional problems.

4172 Around the Clock: Parenting the Delayed ADHD Child
Guilford Publications
72 Spring Street
New York, NY 10012
212-431-9800
800-365-7006
FAX 212-966-6708
http://www.guilford.com
e-mail: info@guilford.com
Bob Matloff, President

This videotape provides both professionals and parents a helpful look at how the difficulties facing parents of ADHD children can be handled. *$150.00*
45-min. VHS

4173 Art of Communication
United Learning
1560 Sherman Avenue
Evanston, IL 60201
847-328-6700
800-424-0362
FAX 847-647-0918
http://www.unitedlearning.com
e-mail: info@unitedlearning.com
B Wagonseller, Author
Ronald Reed, Vice President

Designed for parents and professionals, this video focuses on: effective parent-child communication; nonverbal communication in children; effective listening; effects of negative and critical messages; and deterrents limiting child/parent communication. *$99.00*

4174 Attention Deficit Disorder
Pro-Ed
8700 Shoal Creek Boulevard
Austin, TX 78757
512-451-3246
800-897-3202
FAX 512-451-8542
http://www.proedinc.com
DR Jordan, Author
Donald Hamill, Owner

A video and book providing helpful suggestions for both home and classroom management of students with attention deficit disorder. *$60.00*
Yearly

4175 Augmentative Communication Without Limitations
Prentke Romich Company (PRC)
1022 Heyl Road
Wooster, OH 44691
330-262-1984
800-262-1984
FAX 330-263-4829
http://www.prentrom.com
Dave Moffatt, President
Cherie Weaver, Marketing Coordinator

Prentke Romich Company (PRC) is a worldwide leader in the development and manufacture of augmentative communication devices, computer access products, and other assistive technology for people with severe disabilities.

4176 Autism
Aquarius Health Media Care
18 N Main Street
Sherborn, MA 01770
888-440-2963
FAX 508-650-1665
http://www.aquariusproductions.com
e-mail: orders@aquariusproductions.com
Leslie Kussmann, President/Producer

Through therapeutic horseback riding a young boy emerges from his isolated world. He finds a connection with his horse when he isn't able to talk to adults. A teenage girl gains social confidence as she leads her llama at a local fair. This film explores the power animals can have on helping someone with autism to connect. This film is great for anyone working the autistic and their families. VHS: A-DISHWAA also on DVD. *$125.00*

Video, 30 mins

4177 Autism is a World

Syracuse Univ./Facilitated Communication Institute
370 Huntington Hall
Syracuse, NY 13244
315-443-9657
FAX 315-443-9218
http://www.soeweb.syr.edu/thefci
e-mail: fcstaff@syr.edu
Gerardine Wurzburg, Director/Producer

This is a documentary about Sue who is autistic and a look into her world.

40-min/Video

4178 Avenues to Compliance

New England ADA Technical Assistance Center
374 Congress Street
Boston, MA 02210
617-695-0085
800-949-4232
FAX 617-482-8099
http://www.adaptenu.org/neada/defaultasp
Oce Harrison, Executive Director

This training video provides information on the requirements of a Title II entity to provide program access (as required by the Americans with Disabilities Act).

4179 Behind the Glass Door: Hannah's Story

Fanlight Productions
4196 Washington Street
Boston, MA 02131
617-469-4999
800-937-4113
FAX 617-469-3379
http://www.fanlight.com
e-mail: fanlight@fanlight.com
Karen Pascal, Producer
Ben Achtenberg, Owner

New video, produced in association with Vision TV, follows the Shepard family through five years of struggle, hardship and bittersweet success in raising their child, Hannah, who was diagnosed with autism. Offers insight into the stress families and educators face as they tackle this mysterious disorder. Offers hope and inspiration to parents. Recipient of Silver Screen Award; US International Film and Video Festival. *$245.00*

Rental $50/day
ISBN 1-572952-92-1

4180 Beyond the ADD Myth

Brookes Publishing Company
PO Box 10624
Baltimore, MD 21285
410-337-9580
800-638-3775
FAX 410-337-8539
http://www.pbrookes.com
e-mail: custerv@pbrookes.com
Dr. Thomas Armstrong, Author
Paul H Brooks, President
Melissa A Behm, Executive Vice President
George Stamthis, Vice President/Publisher

This video builds on the theory that many of the behaviors associated with attention deficit disorder are not solely due to neurological dysfunction but actually result from a wide range of social, psychological, and educational causes. *$22.00*

Video
ISBN 1-557661-15-4

4181 Characteristics of the Learning Disabled Adult

Special Education Nazareth
4245 E Avenue
Rochester, NY 14618
585-389-2700
800-462-3944
FAX 585-389-2826
Gary Fisher, Manager

An awareness interactive video recognizing characteristics and instructional needs of learning disabled adults.

4182 Child Who Appears Aloof: Module 5

Educational Productions
PO Box 957
Hillsboro, OR 97123
503-297-6393
800-950-4949
FAX 503-297-6395
http://www.edpro.com
e-mail: custserv@edpro.com
Linda Freedman, Owner

A 30 minute video and 60 page facilitation packet focusing on children who pull back, who avoid social contact. Teaches strategies to understand and support these children. Part of the Hand-in-Hand Series. *$295.00*

4183 Child Who Appears Anxious: Module 4

Educational Productions
PO Box 957
Hillsboro, OR 97123
503-297-6393
800-950-4949
FAX 503-297-6395
http://www.edpro.com
e-mail: custserv@edpro.com
Linda Freedman, Owner

A 35 minute video and 60 page training facilitation packet examining the issues of anxious children and how a supporting adult can help bring them into play. Part of the Hand-in-Hand Series. *$295.00*

4184 Child Who Dabbles: Module 3

Educational Productions
PO Box 957
Hillsboro, OR 97123
503-297-6393
800-950-4949
FAX 503-297-6395
http://www.edpro.com
e-mail: custserv@edpro.com
Linda Freedman, Owner

A 30-minute video and 60-page training facilitation guide that compares dabbling to quality, invested play and offers various strategies for adultsto help children build play skills. Part of Hand-in-Hand Series. *$295.00*

4185 Child Who Wanders: Module 2

Educational Productions
PO Box 957
Hillsboro, OR 97123
503-297-6393
800-950-4949
FAX 503-297-6395
http://www.edpro.com
e-mail: custserv@edpro.com
Linda Freedman, Owner

A 30-minute video and 67-page training facilitation packet showing how to identify children who cannot engage in play so wander about the room. Shows creative interventions to help teach new skills. Part of Hand-in-Hand Series.

4186 Child Who is Ignored: Module 6

Educational Productions
9000 SW Gemini Drive
Beaverton, OR 97008
503-644-7000
800-950-4949
FAX 503-350-7000
http://www.edpro.vom
Linda Freedman, Owner
Molly Krumm, Marketing Director

A 30 minute video and 60 page facilitation guide illustrating the children who are ignored by others and offering several interventions for them to learn social skills. Part of the Hand-in-Hand Series. *$295.00*

4187 Child Who is Rejected: Module 7

Educational Productions
PO Box 957
Hillsboro, OR 97123
503-297-6393
800-950-4949
FAX 503-297-6395
http://www.edpro.com
e-mail: custserv@edpro.com
Linda Freedman, Owner

A 35-minute video and 60-page facilitation packet with strategies to help children whose behavior and/or appearance causes them to be rejected by other children. Part of Hand-in-Hand Series.

4188 **Concentration Video**
Center for Alternative Learning
6 E Eagle Road
Havertown, PA 19083
610-446-6126
800-204-7667
FAX 610-446-6129
http://www.learningdifferences.com
e-mail: rcooper-ldr@comcast.net
Dr. Richard Cooper, Director/Founder/Author

A 53 minute instructional video provides an optimistic perspective about attention problems ADD. Dr. Cooper discusses different types of attention problems causes and solutions. The second part of the video contains concentration exercises to help children and adults with attention problems. *$16.00*
53 Mins/Video

4189 **Degrees of Success: Conversations with College Students with LD**
New York University
240 Greene Street
New York, NY 10003
212-387-8205
FAX 212-995-4114
http://www.nyu.edu/osl/csd

A new video which features college students with learning disabilities speaking in their own words about: making the decision to attend college, developing effective learning strategies, coping with frustrations and utilizing college support services. Includes resource packet with suggested discussion questions and list of other resources. *$49.95*

4190 **Developing Minds: Parent's Pack**
Learning Disabilities Resources
PO Box 2284
So. Burlington, VT 05407
800-542-9714
FAX 802-864-9846
http://www.ldonline.org
e-mail: ldonline@weta.com
Dr. Mel Levine, Author
Lia Salza, Editorial Associate

Created especially for parents, this video set provides an overview of why some children struggle with learning. The programs offer strategies for supporting kids' learning differences, based on the work of Dr. Mel Levin and his neurodevelopmental view on how to help children and adolescents become successful learners. *$59.90*
2 Videos

4191 **Developing Minds: Teachers's Pack**
Learning Disabilities Resources
PO Box 2284
So. Burlington, VT 05407
800-542-9714
FAX 802-864-9846
http://www.ldonline.org
e-mail: ldonline@weta.com
Dr. Mel Levine, Author
Lia Salza, Editorial Associate

Created especially for educators, this video set provides an overview of why some children struggle with learning. The programs offer strategies for supporting kids' learning differences, based on the work of Dr. Mel Levin and his neurodevelopmental view on how to help children and adolescents become successful learners. *$59.90*
2 Videos

4192 **Dyslexia: A Different Kind of Learning**
Aquarius Health Media Care
18 N Main Street
Sherborn, MA 01770
508-650-1616
888-440-2963
FAX 508-650-1665
http://www.aquarisproductions.com
e-mail: aquarius@aquarisproductions.com
Leslie Kussmann, President

Part of the Prescription for Learning Series. This programs shows us what it's like to grow up with dyslexia and the challenge people with dyslexia face in school. The video presents tips for teachers and students on how to deal with it, including how to adapt school structures and classes. VHS: A-TISDYSLEXIA *$125.00*
Video, 24 mins

4193 **Early Childhood STEP: Systematic Training for Effective Parenting**
AGS
PO Box 99
Circle Pines, MN 55014
763-786-4343
800-328-2560
FAX 763-786-9077
http://www.agsnet.com
e-mail: agsmail@agsnet.com
Kevin Brueggeman, Manager

Parenting young children can be ususally rewarding, occasionally difficult, and always a challenge. The updated Early Childhood STEP can help parents meet the challenge. It adapts and expands the proven principles and techniques of STEP while vividly illustrating how they can be applied to babies, toddlers, and preschoolers. *$229.95*

4194 **Enhancing the Communicative Abilities of Disabled Infants and Toddlers**
Purdue University Continuing Education
1586 Stewart Center
West Lafayette, IN 47907
765-494-7231
800-359-2968
FAX 765-494-0567
http://www.continuinged.purdue.edu/
Jeanne Wilcox, Author
Ivan Spencer, Director
Robert Showalter, Project Director

Discusses the communicatively handicapped child, traditional theraputic approaches, and the need to focus on the particular behaviors of the partners in facilitating communicative development and to measure enhancement. *$64.00*
105 min/Video

4195 **FAT City**
Connecticut Assoc. for Children and Adults with LD
25 Van Zant Street
Norwalk, CT 06855
203-838-5010
FAX 203-866-6108
http://www.CACLD.org
e-mail: cacld@juno.com
Beryl Kaufman, Executive Director
Marie Armstrong, Information Specialist

Nationally acclaimed video designed to sensitize adults to the frustration, anxiety and tension that the learning disabled child experiences daily. Add $5.00 for shipping and handling. *$49.95*

4196 **First Steps Series: Supporting Early Language Development**
Educational Productions
PO Box 957
Hillsboro, OR 97123
503-297-6393
800-950-4949
FAX 503-297-6395
http://www.edpro.com
e-mail: custserv@edpro.com
Linda Freedman, Owner

Four 20-minute videos used in early intervention efforts for training staff and parents. Teach how to support language acquisition and model responsive, connected adult-child relationships foundational for all development and learning

4197 **Getting Started With Facilitated Communication**
Syracuse Univ./Facilitated Communication Institute
370 Huntington Hall
Syracuse, NY 13244
315-443-9657
FAX 315-443-9218
http://www.soeweb.syr.edu/thefci
e-mail: fcstaff@syr.edu
Annegret Schubert, Producer/Director

Details on the getting started process, including discussion of candidacy, facilitator attitude, materials and equipment, and the components involved in a first session. Several first sessions are excerpted, showing a child, a teenager, a person with challenging behavior, and a child with significant but not fully functional speech.
14-min/Video

4198 Getting Started with Facilitated Communication
Syracuse University, Institute on Communication
370 Huntington Hall
Syracuse, NY 13244
315-443-9657
FAX 315-443-2274
http://www.soeweb.syr.edu/thefci
e-mail: fcstaff@syr.edu
Annegret Schubert, Author

This videotape describes the details of the getting started process, including discussion of candidacy, facilitator attitude, materials and equipment, and the components involved in a first session.

4199 Going to School with Facilitated Communication
Syracuse University, School of Education
805 S Krouse
Syracuse, NY 13244
315-443-4485
FAX 315-443-2562
D Biklen, Author
Raymond Colton, Manager

A video in which students with autism and/or severe disabilities illustrate the use of facilitated communication focusing on basic principles fostering facilitated communication.

4200 Help! This Kid's Driving Me Crazy!
Pro-Ed
8700 Shoal Creek Boulevard
Austin, TX 78757
512-451-3246
800-897-3202
FAX 512-451-8542
http://www.proedinc.com
L Adkins, Author
Donald Hamill, Owner

Designed for parents and professionals working with children up to five years old, this videotape and booklet offers information about the nature, special needs, and typical behavioral characteristics for young children with attention deficit disorder. *$5.00*

4201 How Difficult Can This Be?
Learning Disabilities Resources
PO Box 2284
So. Burlington, VT 05407
800-542-9714
FAX 802-864-9846
http://www.ldonline.org
e-mail: ldonline@weta.com
Richard Lavoie, Author
Lia Salza, Editorial Associate

This program looks at the world through the eyes of a child with learning disabilities by taking you to a unique workshop attended by parents, educators, psychologists, and social workers. There they join in a series of classroom activities that cause frustration, anxiety and tension - emotions all too familiar to the student with a learning disability. *$49.95*
70 mins/Video

4202 I Want My Little Boy Back
BBC - Autism Treatment Center of America
2080 S Undermountain Road
Sheffield, MA 01257
413-229-2100
800-714-2779
FAX 413-229-8931
http://www.autismtreatment.com
e-mail: autism@option.org
Tracy Baisden, Marketing Associate

This BBC documentary follows an English family with a child with autism before, during, and after their time at the Son-Rise Program. It uniquely captures the heart of the Son-Rise Program and is extremely useful in understanding its techniques. *$20.00*

4203 I'm Not Stupid
Learning Disabilities Association of America
4156 Library Road
Pittsburgh, PA 15234
412-341-1515
FAX 412-344-0224
http://www.ldanatl.org
e-mail: ldanatl@usaor.net

This video depicts the constant battle of the learning disabled child in school. *$22.00*

4204 Identifying Learning Problems
Center for Alternative Learning
6 E Eagle Road
Havertown, PA 19083
610-446-6126
800-204-7667
FAX 610-446-6129
http://www.learningdifferences.com
e-mail: rcooper-ldr@comcast.net
Dr. Richard Cooper, Director/Founder/Author

A presentation made to adult educators and volunteer tutors discusses what to look for in a student who has difficulty learning. The red flags (common behaviors and errors) are described. *$16.00*
1hr 40mins

4205 Inclusion Series
Comforty Mediaconcepts
2145 Pioneer Road
Evanston, IL 60201
847-475-0791
FAX 847-475-0793
e-mail: comforty@comforty.com
Jacky Comforty, Owner

A series of video programs on inclusive education and community life. Titles include: Choices, providing instruction for all audiences to the inclusion process; Inclusion: Issues for Educators, focusing on particular teachers and administrators in Illinois schools; Families, Friends, Futures, emphasizing the need for early inclusion; and Together We're Better, providing an overview of this comprehensive program. Videos available separately or as a set.

4206 Inside The Edge: A Journey To Using Speech Through Typing
Syracuse Univ./Facilitated Communication Institute
370 Huntington Hall
Syracuse, NY 13244
315-443-9657
FAX 315-443-9218
http://www.soeweb.syr.edu/thefci
e-mail: fcstaff@syr.edu
Jamie Burke, Writer/Narrator

A documentary written and narrated by a 15 year old high school student with autism. In this video he tells of his personal experiences with the use of facilitated communication, developing speech, and inclusive schooling.
18-min/Video

4207 International Professional Development Training Catalog
Center for Alternative Learning
6 E Eagle Road
Havertown, PA 19010
610-446-6126
800-204-7667
FAX 610-446-6129
http://www.learningdifferences.com
e-mail: scooper-ldr@comcast.net
Richard Cooper, Ph.D, Author
Dr. Richard Cooper Ph.D, Director/Founder/Author

Training session details how individuals with learning differences, problems and disabilities think and learn.

4208 Language Therapy
Purdue University Continuing Education
1586 Stewart Center
West Lafayette, IN 47907
765-494-7231
800-359-2968
FAX 765-494-0567
Laura L Lee, MA, Author

Discusses the clinical description of the typical preschool child manifesting a language disorder and observations that should be made by the clinician. *$64.00*

4209 Language and the Retarded Child
Purdue University Continuing Education
1586 Stewart Center
West Lafayette, IN 47907
765-494-7231
800-359-2968
FAX 765-494-0567
Herold Lillywhite Ph.D, Author

Describes the speech and language functions of the mentally retarded child; demonstrates problems in hearing, speech, language, cognition, and general motor development. *$64.00*
1hr 50mins

4210 Latest Technology for Young Children
Western Illinois University: Macomb Projects
27 Horrabin Hall
Macomb, IL 61455
309-298-1955
FAX 309-298-2305
http://www.mprojects.wiu.edu
e-mail: PL-Hutinger@wiu.edu
Patricia Hutinger EdD, Director
Joyce Johanson, Coordinator
Amanda Silberer, Manager
This 25 minute videotape focuses on the Macintosh LC and adaptations for young children and includes a discussion of the features and advantages of the Macintosh LC, software demonstrations, footage of child applications, and ideas for off-computer activities. Videotape and written materials available. *$40.00*
16-20 pages

4211 Learn to Read
KET, The Kentucky Network Enterprise Division
600 Cooper Drive
Lexington, KY 40502
859-258-7000
800-354-9067
FAX 859-258-7396
Virginia Fox, Executive Director

Offers 30 half-hour programs tailored for the adult student.

4212 Learning Disabilities and Discipline: Rick Lavoie's Guide to Improving Children's Behavior
Connecticut Assoc. for Children and Adults with LD
25 Van Zant Street
Norwalk, CT 06855
203-838-5010
FAX 203-866-6108
http://www.CACLD.org
e-mail: cacld@juno.com
Beryl Kaufman, Executive Director

In this video, Richard Lavoie, a nationally known expert on learning disabilities, offers practical advice on dealing with behavioral problems quickly and effectively. Shows how preventive discipline can anticipate many problems before they start. Explains how teachers and parents can create stable, predictable environments in which children with learning disabilities can flourish. 62 minutes. *$49.95*
$5.00 shipping

4213 Learning Disabilities and Self-Esteem
Connecticut Assoc. for Children and Adults with LD
25 Van Zant Street
Norwalk, CT 06855
203-838-5010
FAX 203-866-6108
http://www.CACLD.org
e-mail: cacld@juno.com
Beryl Kaufman, Executive Director

The 60 minute Teacher video contains program material for building self-esteem in the classroom. The 60 minute Parent video contains program material for building self-esteem in the home. A 16 page Program Guide accompanies each video. Dr. Robert Brooks, a clinical psychologist, renowned speaker and nationally known expert on learning disabilities, is on the faculty at Harvard Medical School and is the author of The Self-Esteem Teacher. *$49.95*
$5.00 shipping

4214 Learning Disabilities and Social Skills: Last One Picked..First One Picked On
Connecticut Assoc. for Children and Adults with LD
25 Van Zant Street
Norwalk, CT 06855
203-838-5010
FAX 203-866-6108
http://www.CACLD.org
e-mail: cacld@juno.com
Beryl Kaufman, Executive Director

Nationally recognized expert on learning disabilities, Richard Lavoie, gives examples on how to help LD children succeed in everyday social situations. Lavoie helps students dissect their social errors to learn correct behavior. Mistakes are seen as opportunities for learning. Available in parent (62 min.) or teacher (68 min.) version. *$49.95*
$5.00 shipping

4215 Learning Disabilities: A Complex Journey
Aquarius Health Media Care
18 N Main Street
Sherborn, MA 01770
888-440-2963
FAX 508-650-1665
http://www.aquariusproductions.com
e-mail: orders@aquariusproductions.com
Leslie Kussmann, President/Producer

Does your child have trouble reading? Does your daughter seem to have more difficulty with schoolwork than you would expect, even though she's trying her hardest? Is your son avoiding school, claiming illness a little to often, insisitng that he's stupid when you know that's not really true? If so, your child may have a learning disability— a neurological problem processing information that he's actually smart enough to understand. How do you find out? VHS: A-KIDSLD also on DVD. *$125.00*
Video, 26 mins

4216 Learning Problems in Language
Center for Alternative
6 E Eagle Road
Havertown, PA 19083
610-446-6126
800-204-7667
FAX 610-446-6129
http://www.learningdifferences.com
e-mail: rcooper-ldr@comcast.net
Dr. Richard Cooper Ph.D, Founder/Director/Author

This video was recorded at the National Laubach Conference in 1992 for reading tutors and teachers. In the video, Dr. Cooper discusses ideas for teaching reading and other academic skills to adults. *$16.00*
2hr, 50 mins

4217 Legacy of the Blue Heron: Living with Learning Disabilities
Oxton House Publishers
PO Box 209
Farmington, ME 04938
207-779-1923
800-539-7323
FAX 207-779-0623
http://www.oxtonhouse.com
e-mail: info@oxtonhouse.com
William Berlinghoff PhD, Managing Editor
Bobby Brown, Marketing Director

Thi book is available as a soft cover or as a six-cassette audiobook. It is an engaging personal account by a servere dyslexic who became a successful engineer, businesman, boat builder, and president of the Learning Disabilities Association of America. Drawing on his life experiences, the author presents a rich array of wise, common-sense advice for dealing with learning disabilities.

4218 Letting Go: Views on Integration
Iowa University Affiliated Programs
100 Hawkins Drive
Iowa City, IA 52242
319-353-6390
800-272-7713
FAX 319-356-8284
http://www.healthcare.uiowa.edu
e-mail: disability-library@uiowa.edu

Three parents share their thoughts regarding the struggle between protecting their children with disabilities verses allowing the same freedom as other children. *$25.00*
19 mins/Video

4219 **Lily Videos : A Longitudinel View of Lily with Down Syndrome**
Davidson Films
735 Tank Farm Road
San Luis Obispo, CA 93401
805-594-0422
888-437-4200
FAX 805-594-0532
http://www.davidsonfilms.com
e-mail: dfi@davidsonfilms.com
Elaine Taunt, Manager
Fran Davidson, Owner

1. Lily: A Story About a Girl Like Me 2. Lily: A Sequal 3. Lily: At Thirty.

4220 **Lost Dreams & Growth: Parents' Concerns**
Resource Networks
Evanston, IL 60204
847-328-7774
K Moses, Author
Kenneth Moses Ph.D, Manager

A video designed for professionals and parents of children with developmental disabilities.

4221 **Motivation to Learn: How Parents and Teachers Can Help**
Assoc. for Supervision/Curriculum Development
1703 N Beauregard Street
Alexandria, VA 22311
703-578-9600
800-933-2723
FAX 703-575-5400
http://www.ascd.org
Gene Carter, Executive Director

Two videos intended for all those concerned about how educators and families can develop student motivation to learn, solve motivational problems, and effectively participate in parent-teacher conferences.

4222 **Normal Growth and Development: Performance Prediction**
Love Publishing Company
PO Box 22353
Denver, CO 80222
303-221-7333
FAX 303-221-7444
http://www.lovepublishing.com
e-mail: lovepublishing@compuserve.com
Dan Love, Director
Stan Love, Owner

Teaches the age at which skills are normally achieved by children ages 0 to 48 months. *$140.00*
Video

4223 **Oh Say What They See: Language Stimulation**
Educational Productions
9000 SW Gemini Drive
Beaverton, OR 97008
503-644-7000
800-950-4949
FAX 503-350-7000
http://www.edpro.com
e-mail: custserv@edpro.com
Linda Freedman, Owner
Molly Krumm, Marketing Director

A complete video training program illustrating indirect language stimulation techniques to teachers, parents, students, child care staff, and other adult caregivers working with children.

4224 **Parent Teacher Meeting**
Learning Disabilities Resources
PO Box 716
Bryn Mawr, PA 19010
610-525-8336
800-869-8336
FAX 610-525-8337
http://www.ldonline.org
Discusses learning differences and instructional techniques. *$12.00*

4225 **Phonemic Awareness: The Sounds of Reading**
Peytral Publicatons
PO Box 1162
Minnetonka, MN 55345
952-949-8707
877-739-8725
FAX 952-906-9777
http://www.peytral.com
e-mail: help@peytral.com
Victoria Groves Scott, Author
Peggy Hammeken, President

This staff development video may be used with paraprofessionals and teachers to learn the techniques of teaching pnomemic awareness. *$59.95*
Video
ISBN 1-890455-29-6

4226 **Puberty Education for Students with Special Needs**
Marsh Media
PO Box 8082
Shawnee Mission, KS 66208
802-821-3303
FAX 866-333-7421
http://www.marshmedia.com
e-mail: info@marshmedia.com
Liz Smith, Liz Sweeney, Author

Two gender-specific kits include an instructional video, a comprehensive teaching guide and packets of 10 student booklets. These reassuring titles are clear, practical and positive and are intended for the following special populations: Students with developmental disabilities or delays, Intrusive behavior or mental illness, Down Syndrome, Autism Spectrum Disorder, Learning disabilities, Behavioral disabilities, Communicative disorders.
36 pages 1904Grade Range: 3-6

4227 **Regular Lives**
WETA-TV, Department of Educational Activities
2775 S Quincy Street
Arlington, VA 22206
703-998-2600
FAX 703-998-3401
http://www.weta.com
e-mail: info@weta.com
DP Biklen, Author
Sharon Rockefeller, President

Designed to show the successful integration of handicapped students in school, work and community settings. Demonstrates that sharing the ordinary routines of learning and living is essential for people with disabilities.

4228 **STEP/Teen: Systematic Training for Effective Parenting of Teens**
AGS
PO Box 99
Circle Pines, MN 55014
763-786-4343
800-328-2560
FAX 763-786-9077
http://www.agsnet.com
e-mail: agsmail@agsnet.com
D Dinkmeyer, Author
Kevin Brueggeman, Manager

A parent training program designed to help parents of teenagers in the following areas: understanding misbehavior; improving communication and family relationships; understanding and expressing emotions and feelings and discipline. *$229.50*

4229 **Sign Songs: Fun Songs to Sign and Sing**
Harris Communications
15155 Technology Drive
Eden Prairie, MN 55344
952-906-1180
800-825-6758
FAX 952-906-1099
TDY:952-906-1198
Robert Harris, Owner

Features performers John Kinstler, formerly with the National Theater of the Deaf, signing along to the lyrics of eleven kids' songs written and performed by Ken Lonnquist. Includes Public Performance rights and 10 lyric sheets for schools and public libraries. No captions. *$49.95*

29-min. video

4230 Someday's Child: Special Needs Families
Educational Productions
9000 SW Gemini Drive
Beaverton, OR 97008
503-644-7000
800-950-4949
FAX 503-350-7000

LL Pletcher, Author
Linda Freedman, Owner
Molly Krumm, Marketing Director

A complete training video for parents and professionals working with young children with special needs: the personal accounts of three families with young children of their adjustment to and advocacy for their children. *$250.00*

4231 Speech Therapy: Look Who's Not Talking
Aquarius Health Media Care
18 N Main Street
Sherborn, MA 01770
508-650-1616
888-440-2963
FAX 508-650-1665
http://www.aquariusproductions.com
e-mail: aquarius@aquarisproductions.com
Leslie Kussmann, President

A Keeping Kids Healthy Series. Your child is old enough to be talking - other children are by this age - but for some reason, your child just can't put the words together. When should you step in to help? And what, exactly, can you do? VHS: A-KIDSSPEECH. Also available on DVD. *$125.00*
Video, 14 mins

4232 Strengths and Weaknesses: College Students with Learning Disabilities
Altschul Group
2832 S Wentworth Avenue
Chicago, IL 60616
312-326-6700
FAX 312-326-6793

Eddie Lau, Owner

Four students share their feelings and four professionals explore possible adjustment and compensation relative to learning disabilities.

4233 Student Directed Learning: Teaching Self Determination Skills
Beech Center on Disability, University of Kansas
1200 Sunnyside Avenue
Lawrence, KS
785-864-7600
FAX 785-864-7605
http://www.beachcenter.org
e-mail: wehmeyer@ku.edu

M. Agran, C. Cole, Author
Mike Wehmeyer, Associate Director

Written for educators and service providers who seek a comprehensive understanding of the process of helping students develop self-determination skills. The text follows academic principles and clearly is geared to professionals rather than to families. An educator seeking to understand technical self-determination concepts will find this organizational structure effective. *$73.00*

ISBN 0-534159-42-7

4234 Study Skills: How to Manage Your Time
Guidance Associates
100 S Bedford Road
Mount Kisco, NY 10549
914-244-1055
800-431-1242
FAX 914-666-5319
http://www.guidanceassociates.com
e-mail: info@guidanceassociates.com
Fred Gaston, Owner

Describes how to create a personal schedule that will help users get more accomplished each day and waste less time. *$61.00*

Video

4235 Teach an Adult to Read
KET, The Kentucky Network Enterprise Division
600 Cooper Drive
Lexington, KY 40502
859-258-7000
800-354-9067
FAX 859-258-7396
Virginia Fox, Executive Director

A video series for reading tutors and tutor trainers that will help your program solve problems and give insight on how to teach an adult to read.

4236 Testing Your Child and Teen for LearningDiasabilities
Grey Eyes Media
29000 S Western Avenue
Rancho Palos Verdes, CA 90275
310-514-2200
866-791-2108
FAX 310-833-7746
http://www.greyeyesmedia.com
Claudia R McCulloch, Author

Identifies the true nature of your child or teen's learning difficulties and how to recognize red flags associated with learning disabilities, gives the limitations of school-based evaluations and how to obtain optimal results for your learning disabled student, recognize weaknesses or omissions of your child's school-based evaluation, step-by-step guide for understanding the comprehensive assessment and how critical to your student's success, and how to find an experienced evaluator.

4237 The Power of Positive Communication
Educational Productions
PO Box 957
Hillsboro, OR 97123
503-297-6393
800-950-4949
FAX 503-297-6395
http://www.edpro.com
e-mail: custserv@edpro.com
Linda Freedman, Owner

A complete three-session training on CD-ROM teaches how and why to use clear, positive language to help children to follow expectations and learn. Emphasizes strategies that assist both children with special needs and English language learners.

4238 Time Together: Adults Supporting Play
Educational Productions
PO Box 957
Hillsboro, OR 97123
503-297-6393
800-950-4949
FAX 503-297-6395
http://www.edpro.com
e-mail: custserv@edpro.com
Linda Freedman, Owner

A complete video training program for beginning childhood teachers,aides and parents illustrating when to join a child's play, how to enhance and extend the play, and when to step back.

4239 Tomorrow's Children
Vallejo City Unified School District
211 Valle Vista Avenue
Vallejo, CA 94590
707-556-8921
FAX 707-556-8820
http://www.uallejo.k12.ca.us
E Brower, Author
Richard Damelio, Administrator

Addresses the needs for early intervention and comprehensive services for high risk and handicapped infants and preschool children.

4240 TrainerVision: Inclusion, Focus on Toddlers and Pre-K
Educational Productions
PO Box 957
Hillsboro, OR 97123
503-297-6393
800-950-4949
FAX 503-297-6395
http://www.edpro.com
e-mail: custserv@edpro.com

Linda Freedman, Owner

Instructive video clips focus on non-typically developing toddlers and pre-K children. Shows how to gently support skill building, independence and social competence. The clips are ideal to enrich training, classes and online courses.

4241 Treatment of Children's Grammatical Impairments in Naturalistic Context
Purdue University Continuing Education
1586 Stewart Center
West Lafayette, IN 47907
765-494-7231
800-830-0269
FAX 765-494-0567
http://www.continuinged.purdue.edu/media/speech
Marc Fey, Presenter

The basic assumption is challenged that language intervention which takes place in naturalistic settings will be more effective than intervention that occurs in settings that are more heavily constrained by a clinician or other intervention agent. The concept of naturalness will be described as a continuum that is influenced by a number of factors that can be manipulated by clinicians. Several effective intervention approaches that reflect different levels of naturalness are presented. *$50.00*
1hr:42 mins 1991

4242 Understanding Attention Deficit Disorder
Connecticut Assoc. for Children and Adults with LD
25 Van Zant Street
Norwalk, CT 06855
203-838-5010
FAX 203-866-6108
http://www.CACLD.org
e-mail: cacld@juno.com
Beryl Kaufmann, Executive Director

A video in an interview format for parents and professionals providing the history, symptoms, methods of diagnosis and three approaches used to ease the effects of attention deficit disorder. A comprehensive general introduction to ADHD. 45 minutes. *$20.00*
Video

4243 United Learning
1560 Sherman Avenue
Evanston, IL 60201
888-892-3494
FAX 847-328-6706
http://www.unitedlearning.com
e-mail: crechner@unitedlearning.com
Ronald Reed, President
Joel Altschul, Vice President
Coni Rechner, Vice President
United Learning is a provider of audio-visual materials that inform and educate people of all ages. It helps teachers teach more effectively and to help students learn more efficiently. Offering videos, cd's, dvd's, and now delivery of video clips and text via the internet.

4244 What Every Teacher Should Know About ADD
United Learning
1560 Sherman Avenue
Evanston, IL 60201
888-892-3484
FAX 847-328-6706
http://www.unitedlearning.com
e-mail: info@unitedlearning.com
Ronald Reed, President
Mark Zinselmeier, Operations VP/General Manager
Coni Rechner, Marketing VP
This program is for teachers, paraprofessionals, administrators, and special educators because it separates clearly fact from fiction and is written specifically for and about educators who deal with disruptive, inattentive, and hyperactive pre-school and elementary age children on a daily basis. *$79.00*
28-min. video

4245 When a Child Doesn't Play: Module 1
Educational Productions
PO Box 957
Hillsboro, OR 97123
503297639300
800-950-4949
FAX 503-297-6395
http://www.edpro.com
e-mail: custserv@edpro.com
Linda Freedman, Owner

A 30 minute video with 100 pages of facilitation materials presentsdramatic footage of children with play problems and how they miss critical opportunities to learn. Illustrates supportive strategies for adults. Foundation program for Hand-in-Hand Series. *$350.00*

Vocational

4246 College: A Viable Option
HEATH Resource Center
2121 K Street NW
Washington, DC 20037
202-337-7600
800-544-3284
FAX 202-973-0908
http://gopher://bobcat-ace.nche.edu
e-mail: heath@ace.nche.edu
Janine Heath, Manager
Dan Gardner, Information Specialist

A video discussing what a learning disability is, learning strategies and compensatory techniques. *$23.00*

4247 Different Way of Learning
Brookes Publishing Company
PO Box 10624
Baltimore, MD 21285
800-638-3775
FAX 410-337-8539
http://www.pbrookes.com
e-mail: custserv@pbrookes.com
Paul H Brooks, President
Melissa A Behn, Executive Vice President
George Stamthis, Vice President/Publisher
This video prepares students with learning disabilities for the transition from school to the workplace. *$49.00*
Video
ISBN 1-557663-49-1

4248 Direct Link, May I Help You?
Direct Link for the Disabled
PO Box 1036
Solvang, CA 93464
805-688-1603
FAX 805-686-5285
Introduces Direct Link and demonstrates practical ideas to include those with disabilities in the work force. *$25.00*

4249 Employment Initiatives Model: Job Coach Training Manual and Tape
Young Adult Institute
460 W 34th Street
New York, NY 10001
212-273-6100
FAX 212-629-4113
http://www.yai.org
e-mail: ahorowitz@yai.org
Philip Levy, Manager
Thomas A Dern, Assoc. Executive Director
Aimee Horowitz, Project Specialist
Video and manual providing an overview and orientation for staff members involved in transition services to ensure that they are well-grounded inthe concepts, responsibilities, and activities that are required to provide quality supported employment services.

4250 First Jobs: Entering the Job World
Educational Design
345 Hudson Street
New York, NY 10014
800-221-9372
FAX 212-675-8922
Career/vocational education with emphasis on job search skills, job interviews and survival skills. *$139.00*

4251 How Not to Contact Employers
Nat'l Clearinghouse of Rehab. Training Materials
206 W 6th Street
Stillwater, OK 74078
405-744-2000
FAX 405-744-2001
http://www.nchrtm.okstate.edu/
e-mail: index_3.html
A single vignette of what not to do when visiting perspective employers to secure positions for clients. *$10.00*

4252 Job Coaching Video Training Series
RPM Press
PO Box 31483
Tucson, AZ 85751
520-886-1990
888-810-1990
FAX 520-886-1990
Jan Stonebraker, Operations Manager
Paul McCray, President

Multi-media professional training program designed for training educators, counselors, vocational rehabilitation personnel, employment specialists and paraprofessional staff in job coaching methods such as speed training, time sampling, fading, behavior observation and other methods. *$225.00*

4253 Job Interview Reality Seminar
Department of Assistive & Rehabilitative Services
4800 N Lamar Boulevard
Austin, TX 78756
512-377-0500
FAX 512-459-2682
http://www.dars.state.tx.us
e-mail: dars.inquiries@dars.state.tx.us
Terrell I Murphy, Commissioner
Mary Elder, Deputy Commissioner

These tapes include job interview and feedback to the interviewee about his/her performance. *$20.00*

4254 KET Basic Skills Series
KET, The Kentucky Network Enterprise Division
600 Cooper Drive
Lexington, KY 40502
859-258-7000
800-354-9067
FAX 859-258-7396
Virginia Fox, Executive Director

Offers an independent learning system for workers who need retraining or help with basic skills.

4255 KET Foundation Series
KET, The Kentucky Network Enterprise Division
600 Cooper Drive
Lexington, KY 40502
859-258-7000
800-354-9067
FAX 859-258-7396
Virginia Fox, Executive Director

A highly effective basic skills series that is tailor-made for the needs of proprietary and vocational schools.

4256 KET/GED Series
KET, The Kentucky Network Enterprise Division
600 Cooper Drive
Lexington, KY 40502
859-258-7000
800-354-9067
FAX 859-258-7396
Virginia Fox, Executive Director

This nationally acclaimed instructional series helps adults prepare for the GED test.

4257 KET/GED Series Transitional Spanish Edition
KET, The Kentucky Network Enterprise Division
600 Cooper Drive
Lexington, KY 40502
859-258-7000
800-354-9067
FAX 859-258-7396
Virginia Fox, Executive Director

This award-winning series offers ESL students effective preparation for the GED test.

4258 Life After High School for Students with Moderate and Severe Disabilities
Beech Center on Disability, University of Kansas
3111 Haworth Hall
Lawrence, MA
785-864-7600
FAX 785-864-7605
http://www.beachcenter.org
A set of three videotapes and a participant handbook document, and a teleconference in which family members, people with disabilities, teachers, rehabilitation specialists, program administrators and policy makers focus on improving the quality of services in high school and supported employment programs.

4259 On Our Own Transition Series
Young Adult Institute
460 W 34th Street
New York, NY 10001
212-273-6100
FAX 212-629-4113
http://www.yai.org
e-mail: ahorowitz@yai.org
Philip Levy, Manager
Thomas A Dern, Assoc. Executive Director
Aimee Horowitz, Project Specialist
Designed for parents and professionals, this series of 15 videotapes examines innovative transitional approaches that help create marketable skills, instill self-esteem and facilitate successful transition for individuals with developmental disabilities.

4260 Social Skills on the Job: A Transition to the Workplace for Special Needs
AGS
PO Box 99
Circle Pines, MN 55014
763-786-4343
800-328-2560
FAX 763-786-9077
http://www.agsnet.com
e-mail: agsmail@agsnet.com
Kevin Brueggeman, Manager

Presents 28 simulations to help students learn and practice 14 basic social skills that will allow them to compete successfully with their peers in the job market. *$299.95*

4261 Succeeding in the Workplace
JKL Communications
2700 Virginia Avenue NW
Washington, DC 20037
202-223-5097
FAX 202-223-5096
http://www.lathamlaw.org
e-mail: plath3@his.com

$49.00

4262 Tools for Transition: Preparing Students with Learning Disabilities
AGS
PO Box 99
Circle Pines, MN 55014
763-786-4343
800-328-2560
FAX 763-786-9077
http://www.agsnet.com
e-mail: agsmail@agsnet.com
EP Aune, Author
Kevin Brueggeman, Manager

Designed for learning disabled high school juniors and seniors, this program will prepare them for postsecondary education by focusing on: learningstyles, study skills, learning accommodations, self advocacy, career exploration, interpersonal relationships and choosing and applying to postsecondary schools. *$124.95*

General

4263 **www.abcparenting.com**

Information and resources related to learning disabilities.

4264 **www.adhdnews.com/sped.htm**

Guidance in writing IEPs, TIEPs for special education services.

4265 **www.ajb.dni.us**
America's Job Bank

Useful both for job seekers and employers; offers job announcements, talent banks and information about getting a job.

4266 **www.ala.org/roads**
Roads to Learning

Run by the American Library Association, this site works to raise public awareness about learning disabilities.

4267 **www.allaboutvision.com**
All About Vision

Vision information and resources, including articles on learning disabilities.

4268 **www.apa.org/psycinfo**
PsycINFO Database

An online abstract database that provides access to citations to the international serial literature in psychology and related disciplines from 1887 to present. Available via PsycINFO Direct at www.psycinfo.com.

4269 **www.ataccess.org**
Alliance for Technology Access

Not sure where to begin your search for assistive technology information and tools? A wealth of information can be found here. ATA is a national network of assistive technology center, vendors, community based organizations, and individuals committed to increasing the use of technology by people with disabilities and junctioned invitations.

4270 **www.autismtreatment.com**
Autism Treatment Center of America

Since 1983, the Autism Treatment Center of America, has provided innovative training programs for parents and professionals caring for children challenged by Autism, Autism Spectrum Disorders, Pervasive Developmental Disorders (PDD) and other developmental difficulties. The Son-Rise Program teaches a specific yet comprehensive system of treatment and education designed to help families and caregivers enable their children to dramatically improve in all areas of learning.

4271 **www.babycenter.com**

Includes an easy-to-follow milestone chart, advice on when to call the doctor, chat rooms and an immunization scheduler.

4272 **www.career.com**
Career Connections

Posts a job announcement and an online application form, and hosts cyber job fairs.

4273 **www.childdevelopmentinfo.com**
Child Development Institute

Provides online information on child development, psychology, parenting, learning, health and safety as well as childhood disorders such as attention deficit disorder, dyslexia and autism. Provides comprehensive resources and practical suggestions for parents.

4274 **www.childparenting.about.com**

Information, research and resources for the learning disabled.

4275 **www.disabilityinfo.gov**
Disability Direct

Provides one-stop online access to resources, services, and information available throughout the federal government to Americans with disabilities, their families, employers and service providers; also promotes awareness of disability issues to the general public.

4276 **www.disabilityresources.org**

Information about learning disabilities and related subjects.

4277 **www.discoveryhealth.com**

Information on conditions that impact learning.

4278 **www.dmoz.org**
DMOZ Open Directory Project

Information on special education and learning disabilities.

4279 **www.doleta.gov/programs/adtrain.asp**
O'Net: Department of Labor's Occ. Information

Useful for job seekers, employers and teachers; has career information and links to government resources.

4280 **www.drkoop.com**
Former Surgeon-General Dr. C Everett Koop

Information on health and conditions that affect learning.

4281 **www.dyslexia.com**
Davis Dyslexia Association

Links to internet resources for learning. Includes dyslexia, Autism and Asperger's Syndrome, ADD/ADHD and other learning disabilities.

4282 **www.familyvillage.wisc.edu**
University of Wisconsin-Madison

A global community that integrates information, resources and communication opportunities on the Internet for all those involved with cognitive and other disabilities.

4283 **www.funbrain.com**
Quiz Lab

Internet education site for teachers and kids. Access thousands of assessment quizzes online. Assign paperless quizzes that are graded automatically by email. Teaching tools are free and easy to use.

4284 **www.geocities.com**

A site that informs and educates about common misconceptions associated with learning disabilities.

4285 **www.healthanswers.com**

Health information, including learning disabilities, etc.

4286 **www.healthatoz.com**
Medical Network

Health information, including ADD, ADHD, etc.

4287 **www.healthcentral.com**

Information and products for a healthier life. Includes conditions that impact learning.

4288 **www.healthymind.com**

Information on ADD and learning disabilities.

4289 **www.hood.edu/seri/serihome.htm**
Special Education Resources on the Internet

Contains links to information about definitions, legal issues, and teaching and learning related to learning disabilities.

4290 **www.iamyourchild.org**

From Rob Reiner's I Am Your Child Foundation, featuring information on child development.

4291 **www.icpac.indiana.edu/infoseries/is-50.htm**
Finding Your Career: Holland Interest Inventory

Includes information on self-assessing one's skills and matching them to careers.

4292 **www.intelihealth.com**

Includes information on learning disabilities.

4293 **www.irsc.org**
Internet Research for Special Children

Attention deficit and hyperactivity disorder help website, created so information, support and ADD coaching are available without having to pour over all 531,136 links that come up on a net search.

4294 **www.jobhunt.org/slocareers/resources.html**
Online Career Resources

Contains assessment tools, tutorials, labor market information, etc.

4295 **www.kidsdirect.net/pd**

Information on education and learning disabilities.

4296 **www.ld-add.com**
Attention Deficit Disorder (ADD or ADHD)

Do you think that you or your child has ADHD with or without learning disabilities? If the answer is yes, this webpage is for you.

4297 **www.ldonline.org**
Learning Project at WETA

Learning disabilities information and resources.

4298 **www.ldpride.net**
LD Pride Online

Inspired by Deaf Pride, a site developed as an interactive community resource for youth and adults with learning disabilities and ADD.

4299 **www.ldresources.com**

Resources for people with learning disabilities.

4300 **www.ldteens.org**
Study Skills Web Site

Run by the New York State Chapter of the International Dyslexia Association; a site for students, created by students; provides helpful tips and links.

4301 **www.marriottfoundation.org**
Marriott Foundation

Provides information on job opportunities for teenagers and young adults with disabilities.

4302 **www.my.webmd.com**
Web MD Health

Medical website with information which includes learning disabilities, ADD/ADHD, etc.

4303 **www.ntis.gov**
National Techinical Information Service

A worldwide database for research, development and engineering reports on a range of topics, including architectural barrier removal, employing individuals with disabilities, alternative testing formats, job accommodations, school-to-work transition for students with disabilities, rehabilitation engineering, disability law and transportation.

4304 **www.ocde.K12.ca.us/PAL/index2.html**
Peer Assistance Leadership (PAL)

A California-based outreach program for elementary, intermediate and high school students.

4305 **www.oneaddplace.com**
One A D D Place

A virtual neighborhood of information and resources relating to ADD, ADHD and learning disorders.

4306 **www.optimums.com**
JR Mills, MS, MEd

Information on learning disabilities.

4307 **www.pacer.org**
Does My Child Have An Emotional Disorder

Our mission is to expand opportunities and enhance the quality of life of children and young adults with disabilities and their families, based on the concept of parents helping parents.

4308 **www.parentpals.com**
Ameri-Corp Speech and Hearing

Offers parents and professionals special education support, teaching ideas and tips, special education continuing education, disability-specific information and more.

4309 **www.parentsplace.com**

Shares the adventure of parenting through articles, newsletters, questions and answers and polls.

4310 **www.peer.ca/peer.html**
Peer Resources Network

A Canadian organization that offers training, educational resources, and consultation to those interested in peer helping and education. Their resources section has information on books, articles and videos.

4311 www.petersons.com
Peterson's Education and Career Center

Contains postings for full-and part-time jobs as well as summer job opportunities.

4312 www.schwablearnig.org

A parent's guide to helping kids with learning differences.

4313 www.son-rise.org
Autism Treatment Center of America

Since 1983, the Autism Treatment Center of America, has provided innovative training programs for parents and professionals caring for children challenged by Autism, Autism Spectrum Disorders, Pervasive Developmental Disorders (PDD) and other developmental difficulties. The Son-Rise Program teaches a specific yet comprehensive system of treatment and education designed to help families and caregivers enable their children to dramatically improve in all areas of learning.

4314 www.specialchild.com
Resource Foundation for Children with Challenges

Variety of information for parents of children with disabilities, including actual stories, family and legal issues, diagnosis search, etc.

4315 www.specialneeds.comSpecial Needs Project

A place to get books about disabilities.

4316 www.therapistfinder.net

Locate psychologists, psychiatrists, social workers, family counselors, and more specializing in disorders.

4317 www.wrightlaw.com
Wrightslaw

Provides information about advocacy.

4318 www4.gvsu.edu
Grand Valley State University

Information and resources for the learning disabled.

Counseling & Psychology

4319 American Psychologist
American Psychological Association
750 1st Street NE
Washington, DC 20002
202-336-5510
800-374-2721
FAX 202-336-5502
TDY:202-336-6123
http://www.apa.org
e-mail: journals@apa.org
Norman Anderson, Editor

Contains archivel documents and articles covering current issues in psychology, the science and practice of psychology, and psychology's contribution to public policy.

4320 Case Manager
Elsevier
6277 Sea Harbor Drive
Orlando, FL 32887
407-345-4020
877-839-7126
FAX 407-363-1354
http://www.elsevier.com
e-mail: cmullahy@optionsunlimited.org
Catherine M Mullahy, Editor

Targeted to medical case managers and other related professionals who create and manage patient care in hospital, home, long-term care, rehabilitation, mental health, and managed care settings. Articles, columns, and departments provide the latest information in the field though coverage of the profession's hottest topics, including outcomes management, guidelines and standards of practice, reimbursement, trends in managed care, and ethical/ legal issues. *$45.00*
Bi-Monthly

4321 Center Focus
Nat'l Center for Research in Vocational Education
University of California Berk
Berkeley, CA 94720
510-642-348/
FAX 510-642-4803
Each issue provides a brief but thorough distillation of research, development, evaluation and practice knowledge about a specific topic.
Quarterly

4322 Educational Therapist Journal
Association of Educational Therapists
11300 W Olympic Boulevard
Los Angeles, CA 90064
310-909-1490
800-286-4267
FAX 310-437-0585
http://www.aetonline.org
e-mail: aet@aetonline.org
Jane Adelizzi PhD, Editor

A multidisciplinary publication, that publishes articles and reviews on clinical practice, research, and theory. In addition, it serves to inform the reader of AET activities and business and presents issues relevant to the practice of educational therapy.
3x a year

4323 Journal of Social and Clinical Psychology
Guilford Press
72 Spring Street
New York, NY 10012
800-365-7006
FAX 212-966-6708
http://www.guilford.com
e-mail: info@guilford.com
James E Maddux, Editor

Discusses theory, research and research methodology from personality and social psychology toward the goal of enhancing the understanding of human well-being and adjustment. Also covers a wide range of areas, including intimate relationships, attributions, stereotyping, social skills, depression research, coping strategies, and more. It fosters interdisciplinary communication and scholarship among students and practitioners of social/personality and clinical/counseling/health psychology. *$150.00*
10x a year
ISSN 0736-7236

4324 Learning Disabilities: Research and Practice
Lawrence Erlbaum Associates
10 Industrial Avenue
Mahwah, NJ 07430
201-236-9500
800-926-6579
FAX 201-236-0072
Margo Mastropieri, Co-Editor
Thomas Scruggs, Co-Editor
Lawrence Erlbaum, Owner
Because learning disabilities is a multidisciplinary field of study, this important journal publishes articles addressing the nature and characteristics of learning disabled students, promising research, program development, assessment practices, and teaching methodologies from different disciplines. In so doing, LDRP provides information of great value to professionals involved in a variety of different disciplines including school psychology, counseling, reading and medicine. *$45.00*

ISSN 0938-8982

4325 School Psychology Quarterly: Official Journal of Div. 16 of the American Psychological Assoc
Guilford Publications
72 Spring Street
New York, NY 10012
212-431-9800
800-365-7006
FAX 212-966-6708
http://www.guilford.com
e-mail: info@guilford.com
Michael Gordon, Editor
Shelby Keiser, Editor
Bob Matloff, President
This journal advances the latest research, theory, and practice and features a new book review section. Strengthening the relationship between school psychology and broad-based psychological science. *$35.00*
4 issues/year
ISSN 1045-3830

General

4326 ASCD Update
Assoc. for Supervision/Curriculum Development
1703 N Beauregard Street
Alexandria, VA 22311
703-578-9600
800-933-2723
FAX 703-575-5400
http://www.ascd.org
e-mail: update@ascd.org
Gene R Carter, Executive Director

Explores a wide array of education topics concerning school leadership, curriculum, classroom practices and student achievement. Also provides news specific to the ASCD community.
12x a year

4327 Adult Basic Educaion and Literacy Journal
ProLiteracy America
1320 Jamesville Avenue
Syracuse, NY 13210
315-422-9121
FAX 315-422-6369
http://www.coabe.org
e-mail: journaleditor@literacyprogram.org
Linda Church, Interim Editor
Barbara Mangicaro, Subscriptions Manager

Co-published by the Commission on Adult Basic Education and ProLiteracy America, provides a place where scholarly researchers and frontline practitioners can feel at home and learn from each other. Ptovides a forum for sharing research, information, theory, commentary, and practical experiences that will omprove the quality of services for adult basic education, literacy, and numeracy learners. *$25.00*

3x/year

4328 American Journal of Occupational Therapy
American Occupational Therapy Association
4720 Montgomery Lane
Bethesda, MD 20824
301-652-2682
FAX 301-652-7711
TDY:800-377-8555
http://www.aota.org
e-mail: ajotsis@aota.org

Liz Holcomb, Managing Editor
Mary Binderman, Manager

An official publication of the American Occupational Therapy Association, inc. This peer reviewed journal focuses on research, practice, and health care issues in the field of occupational therapy. Also publishes articles that are theoretical and conceptual and that represent theory-based research, research reviews, and applied research realted to innovative program approaches, educational activities, and professional trends. *$50.00*

6x a year

4329 American School Board Journal
National School Boards Association
1680 Duke Street
Alexandria, VA 22314
703-838-6722
FAX 703-549-6719
http://www.asbj.com

Marilee C Rist, Publisher
Glenn Cook, Editor-in-Chief
Kathleen Vail, Managing Editor

American School Board Journal chronicles change, interprets issues, and offers readers — some 40,000 school board members and school administrators — practical advice on a broad range of topics pertinent to school go9vernance and management, policy making, student achievement, and the art of school leadership. In addition, regular departments cover education news, school law, research, and new books. *$54.00*

Monthly

4330 Annals of Otology, Rhinology and Laryngology
Annals Publishing Company
4507 Laclede Avenue
Saint Louis, MO 63108
314-367-4987
FAX 314-367-4988
http://www.annals.com
e-mail: manager@annals.com

Kenneth A Cooper Jr, President

Offers original manuscripts of clinical and research importance in otolaryngology - head and neck surgery, audiology, speech pathology, head and neck oncology and surgery, and related specialties. All papers are peer-reviewed *$ 179.00*

112 pages Monthly

4331 Autism Research Review International
Autism Research Institute
4182 Adams Avenue
San Diego, CA 92116
619-281-7165
FAX 619-563-6840
http://www.autism.com

Stephen M Edelson PhD, Director

Covering biomedical and educational advances in autism research. *$18.00*

Quarterly 1987

4332 CABE Journal
Connecticut Association of Boards of Education
81 Wolcott Hill Road
Wethersfield, CT 06109
860-571-7446
800-317-0033
FAX 860-571-7452
http://www.cabe.org
e-mail: bcarney@cabe.org

Bonnie Carney, Senior Staff Associate
Robert Rader, Executive Director

Reaches virtually all board members, superintendents and business managers in Connecticut. It's the only publication which does so on a regular basis. It is designed to encompass all material in an easy-to-read fashion. Readers if the journal find a wide range of topics covered in each issue.

11x a year

4333 CEC Today
Council for Exceptional Children
1110 N Glebe Road
Arlington, VA 22201
703-245-0600
888-232-7733
FAX 703-264-9494
http://www.cec.sped.org
e-mail: service@cec.sped.org

Lynda Voyles, Editor
Drew Albritten M.D., President
Bruce Ramirez, Manager

An online member newsletter that keeps you up-to-date on professional and legal developments.

4x per year

4334 Chalk Talk
Fresno Teachers Association
5334 N Fresno Street
Fresno, CA 93710
559-224-8430
FAX 559-224-1571
http://www.fresnoteachers.org
e-mail: larry@fresnoteachers.org

Larry Moore, President
Gary Alford, Associate Director
Brenda Amerson, Associate Director

Improvement in public education and the condition of the working environment of public school teachers. *$2.00*

6 pages

4335 Child Assessment News
Guilford Publications
72 Spring Street
New York, NY 10012
212-431-9800
800-365-7006
FAX 212-966-6708
http://www.guilford.com
e-mail: info@guilford.com

Michael Gordon, Editor
Shelby Keiser, Editor
Bob Matloff, President

Offers the easiest and most effective way possible for busy professionals to learn about: the hottest news in child assessment, brand new test materials, groundbreaking research developments, helpful clinical techniques, expertopinions of well-known and respected researchers and clinicians, important legislation, and software updates. *$75.00*

Bimonthly
ISSN 1055-0518

4336 Creative Classroom Magazine
170 5th Avenue
New York, NY 10010
212-243-5750
FAX 212-242-5628
http://www.creativeclassroom.org
e-mail: ccmag@inch.com

Meg Bozzone, Editor
Robin Bromley, Associate Editor

Classroom ideas, lesson suggestions, materials listings, advice and articles on teaching students current events such as environmental issues. Covers all subjects and includes a calendar of special events and suggestions for projects.

Bimonthly

4337 Diagnostique
Council for Exceptional Children
1110 N Glebe Road
Arlington, VA 22201
703-245-0600
888-232-7733
FAX 703-264-9494
TDY:703-620-3660
http://www.cec.sped.org/
e-mail: service@cec.sped.org

Bruce Ramirez, Manager

Offers information on preparation for postsecondary success. *$28.00*

4338 Disability Compliance for Higher Education
LRP Publications
360 Hiatt Drive
Pal Beach Gardens, FL 33418
561-622-6520
FAX 561-622-0757
http://www.lrp.com

Cynthia Gomez, Author
Kenneth Kahn, CEO
Erin Gonzalez, Product Group Manager

Combines insightful analyses of disability laws with details of innovative accomodations for your students and staff. *$198.00*
Monthly

4339 Division for Children with Communication Disorders Newsletter
Council for Exceptional Children
1110 N Glebe Road
Arlington, VA 22201
703-245-0600
888-232-7733
FAX 703-264-9494
http://www.cec.sped.org/
e-mail: service@cec.sped.org

Penny Griffith, Editor
Drew Albritten MD, President
Bruce Ramirez, Manager
Information concerning the education and welfare of children and youth with communication disorders; reports on division committee activities, highlights current research and programs.
12 pages

4340 Education Digest
College of Education
University of Illinois
Urbana, IL 61801
217-333-0260
http://www.ed.uiuc.edu

4341 Education Technology News
Business Publishers
2601 University Boulevard W
Silver Spring, MD 20902
301-587-6300
800-274-0122
FAX 301-585-9075

Howard Fields, Editor
Adam Goldstein, President

Full coverage of innovations in technology that can be implemented in the classroom, including those which enhance learning for children with disabilities. Focus is on computer use in the classroom, and related subjects such as teacher training, new software, research findings, grants and other funding issues. *$267.00*

4342 Education Week
Editorial Projects in Education Inc.
6935 Arlington Road
Bethesda, MD 20814
301-280-3100
800-346-1834
FAX 301-280-3100
http://www.edweek.org

Paul Hyland, Executive Producer
Jeanne McCann, Managing Editor

Offers articles of interest to educators, teachers, professionals and special educators on the latest developments, laws, issues and more in the various fields of education. *$69.94*

4343 Educational Leadership
Assoc. for Supervision/Curriculum Development
1703 N Beauregard Street
Alexandria, VA 22311
703-578-9600
800-933-2723
FAX 703-575-5400
http://www.ascd.org
e-mail: el@ascd.org

Marge Scherer, Editor in Chief
Deborah Perkins-Gough, Senior Editor/Book Review Editor
Amy Azzam, Senior Associate Editor
ASCD's flagship publication, acknowledged throughout the world as an authoritative source of information about teaching and learning, new ideas and practices relevant to practicing educators, and the latest trends and issues affecting prekindergarten through higher education.
8x a year

4344 Educational Researcher
American Educational Research Association
1430 17th Street NW
Washington, DC 20005
202-238-3200
FAX 202-238-3250
http://www.aera.net

Patricia B Elmore, Co-Editor
Gregory Camilli, Co-Editor

Received by all members of AERA, contains scholarly articles that come from a wide range of dosciplines and are of general significance to the education research community.
9x a year
ISSN 0013-189X

4345 Educational Technology
Educational Technology Publications
700 Palisade Avenue
Englewood Cliffs, NJ 07632
201-871-4007
800-952-BOOK
FAX 201-871-4009
http://www.asianvu.com/bookstoread/etp
e-mail: edtecpubs@aol.com
Lawrence Lipsitz, Senior Editor

The world's leading periodical publication covering the entire field of educational technology, an area pioneered by the magazine's editors in the early 1960s. *$159.00*
6x annually

4346 Faculty Inservice Education Kit
Association on Higher Education and Disability
PO Box 540666
Waltham, MA 02454
781-788-0003
FAX 781-788-0033
http://www.ahead.org
e-mail: ahead@postbox.acs.ohio-state.edu
Lists all the handouts and documentation necessary to conduct inservice training for the postsecondary community regarding the inclusion of students with disabilities in campus life. *$45.95*

4347 GED Items
GED Testing Services
1 Dupont Circle NW
Washington, DC 20036
202-223-2318
800-626-9433
FAX 202-775-8578
http://www.acenet.edu/programs/calec/ged/home
e-mail: ged@ace.nche.edu
Nancy Segal, Executive Director
Lyn Schaeser, Project Manager/ Director
Lisa Hone, Special Projects Manager
A newsletter for GED examiners and teachers as well as other adult education professionals. It provides information about GED policies and best practices.
5x/year

4348 Gifted Child Today
Prufrock Press
PO Box 8813
Waco, TX 76714
254-756-3337
800-998-2208
FAX 254-756-3339
http://www.prufrock.com
e-mail: info@prufrock.com
Joel McIntosh, Publisher/Marketing Director
Susan Johnson, Editor

Offers teachers information about teaching gifted children. Offers parents information about raising a gifted child, how to tell if your child is gofted, and effective strategies for parenting a gifted child. *$29.95*

4349 InfoTech Newsletter
InfoTech
University of Iowa
Iowa City, IA 52242
319-353-8777
800-331-3027

Jane Gay, Executive Director

A free publication covering topics relating to assistive technology, including announcements from Iowa's IPAT Program and from Minnesota's S.T.A.R. Program as well as Used Equipment Referral Service listing.

4350 Journal of Learning Disabilities
Pro-Ed
8700 Shoal Creek Boulevard
Austin, TX 78757
512-451-3246
800-897-3202
FAX 512-451-8542
http://www.proedinc.com
e-mail: info@proedinc.com

H Lee Swanson, Editor

Recognized internationally as the oldest and most authoritative journal in the area of learning disabilities. The editorial board reflects the international, multidisciplinary nature of JLD, comprising researchers and practitioners in numerous fields, including education, psychology, neurology, medicine, law and counseling.

Bimonthly
ISSN 0022-2194

4351 Journal of Postsecondary Education and Disability
Association on Higher Education and Disability
107 Commerce Center Drive
Huntersville, NC 28078
704-947-7779
FAX 704-948-7779
http://www.ahead.org
e-mail: ahead@ahead.org

James Martin PhD, Executive Editor

Serves as a resource to members and other professionals dedicated to the advancement of full participation in higher education for persons with disabilities. Is also the leading forum for scholarship in the field of postsecondary disability support services.

4352 Journal of Rehabilitation
National Rehabilitation Association
633 S Washington Street
Alexandria, VA 22314
703-836-0850
888-258-4295
FAX 703-836-0848
http://www.nationalrehab.org
e-mail: info@nationalrehab.org

Linda Winslow, Executive Director
David Strauser, Editor
Carol Hamilla, Managing Editor

The Journal of Rehabilitation publishes articles by leaders in the fields of rehabilitation. The articles are written for rehabilitation professionals and students studying in the fields of rehabilitation *$18.00*

ISSN 0022-4154

4353 Journal of School Health
American School Health Association
7263 State Route 43
Kent, OH 44240
330-678-1601
FAX 330-678-4526
http://www.ashaweb.org
e-mail: asha@ashaweb.org

Susan Wooley, Executive Director
Thomas Reed, Manager

Committed to communicating information regarding the role of schools and school personnel in facilitating the development and growth of healthy youth and healthy school environments.

4354 Journal of Secondary Gifted Education
Prufrock Press
PO Box 8813
Waco, TX 76714
254-756-3337
800-998-2208
FAX 254-756-3339
e-mail: periodical@prufrock.com

Joel McIntosh, Owner
Susan Johnsen, Editor

Publishes research and critical theory related to the education of adolescent gifted and talented students. *$35.00*

4355 Journal of Special Education Technology
Peabody College, Box 328
Vanderbilt University
Nashville, TN 37203
615-322-7311
FAX 615-322-8236
http://www.vanderbilt.edu/

Herbert Rieth, Editor
Paulette Jackson, Administrative Assistant
Harry Jacobson, Plant Manager

Quarterly $40.00

4356 KDDWB Variety Family Center
University of Minnesota
200 Oak Street SE
Minneapolis, MN 55455
612-626-2820
800-276-8642
FAX 612-624-0997
http://www.allaboutkids.umn.edu
e-mail: lib-web@tc.umn.edu

Karen Stutelberg, Manager

A University Community partnership that provides family-centered services that promote physical, emotional, psychological and social health and well-being for children and youth at risk, including children and youth with disabilities.

4357 LD Online
WETA Public Television
2775 S Quincy Street
Arlington, VA 22206
FAX 703-998-2060
http://www.ldonline.org

Noel Gunther, Executive Director

The world'e leading we site on learning disabilities and ADHD, serving more than 200,000 parents, teachers, and other professionals each month. Seeks to help children and adults reach their full potential by providing accurate and up-to-date information and advice about learning disabilities and ADHD.

4358 LDA Alabama Newsletter
Learning Disabilities Association of Alabama
PO Box 11588
Montgomery, AL 36111
334-277-9151
FAX 334-284-9357

Debbie Gibson, President

Educational support and advocacy for those with learning disabilities and Attention Deficit Disorder.

4359 LDA Rhode Island Newsletter
Learning Disabilities Association of Rhode Island
PO Box 8128
Cranston, RI 02920
401-946-6968
FAX 401-946-6968
TDY:401-946-6968
http://www.ldanatl.org
e-mail: lindixx@email.com

Linda DiCecco, President

A nonprofit, volunteer organization whose members give their time and support to children with learning disabilities as well as share information with other parents, professionals and individuals with learning disabilities.

4360 Learning Disabilities Quarterly
Council for Learning Disabilities
11184 Antioch Road
Overland Park, KS 66210
913-491-1011
FAX 913-941-1012
http://www.cldinternational.org
e-mail: lnease@cldinternational.org

David Scanlon, Editor
Linda Nease, Executive Director

Presents scientifically-based research, and includes articles by nationally known authors.

4x a year

4361 Learning Disabilities Research & Practice
Council for Exceptional Children
1110 N Glebe Road
Arlington, VA 22201
703-245-0600
888-232-7733
FAX 703-264-9494
http://www.cec.sped.org/
e-mail: service@cec.sped.org

Drew Albritten MD, President
Bruce Ramirez, Manager

Scholarly journal providing current research in the field of learning disabilities of importance to teachers, educators and researchers.

4362 Learning Disabilities: A Multidisciplinary Journal
Learning Disabilities Association of America
4156 Library Road
Pittsburgh, PA 15234
412-341-1515
FAX 412-344-0224
http://www.ldaamerica.org
e-mail: info@ldaamerica.org

Janet Lerner PhD, Co-Editor
Frank Kline PhD, Co-Editor

A technical publication oriented toward professionals in the field of learning disabilities. *$30.00*
Quarterly

4363 Learning and Individual Differences
National Association of School Psychologists
4340 EW Highway
Bethesda, MD 20814
301-657-0270
866-331-6277
FAX 301-657-0275
TDY:301-657-4155
http://www.nasponline.org
e-mail: publications@naspweb.org

Susan Gorin, Executive Director

A multidisciplinary journal in education.

4364 Mainstream
Johnson Press
2973 Beech Street
San Diego, CA 92102
619-234-3138
FAX 619-234-3155

Cyndi Jones, President

4365 Media & Methods Magazine
502 Woodside Avenue
Narberth, PA 19072
215-563-6005
800-555-5657
FAX 215-587-9706
http://www.media-methods.com

Michele Sokoloff, Publisher
Danielle Dunn, Office Assistant

The education source magazine that features how to use instructional technologies with all learning abilities. Practical and hands on teaching ideas and expectional resources.

4366 Mental Health Report
Business Publishers
2601 University Boulevard W
Silver Spring, MD 20902
301-587-6300
800-274-6737
FAX 301-585-9075
http://www.dpinews.com
e-mail: adodson@dpinews.com

Ami Dodson, Editorial Director
Adam Goldstein, President

Covers issues of interest to mental health program administrators including treatment of children with mental disorders and other special populations, tracks federal agency regulation and funding for programs nationwide, as well as court cases and state/federal law. *$325.00*

4367 National Dissemination Center for Children
Academy for the Educational Development
PO Box 1492
Washington, DC 20013
202-884-8200
800-695-0285
FAX 202-884-8841
TDY:800-695-0285
http://www.nichcy.org
e-mail: nichcy@aed.org

Susan Ripley, Manager

A newsletter offering information, guides, books and reference sources for the learning disabled.

4368 National Organization on Disability
910 16th Street NW
Washington, DC 20006
202-293-5960
800-248-2253
FAX 202-293-7999
http://www.nod.org
e-mail: ability@nod.org

Michael Deland, President

A newsletter offering information and articles on the organization.

4369 OT Practice
American Occupational Therapy Association
4720 Montgomery Lane
Bethesda, MD 20824
301-652-2682
800-SAY-AOTA
FAX 301-652-7711
TDY:800-377-8555
http://www.aota.org
e-mail: otpractice@aota.org

Laura Collins, Editor
Frederick P Somers, Executive Director

The clinical and professional magazone of the AOTA. It serves as a comprehensive, authoritative source for practical information to help occupational therapists and occupational therapy assistants to succeed professionally. Provides professional news and information on all aspects of practice and encourages a dialogue among AOTA members on professional concerns and views.
64 pages

4370 Occupational Outlook Quarterly
US Department of Labor
200 Constitution Avenue
Washington, DC 20212
202-693-5000
FAX 202-693-6111
http://www.dol.gov

Elaine Chao, CEO

Information on new educational and training opportunities, emerging jobs, prospects for change in the work world and the latest research findings.

4371 Ohio State Comparative Education Review
University Center for International Education
1712 Neil Avenue
Columbus, OH 43210
614-292-6101
FAX 614-292-4275
http://www.oie.ohio-state.edu
e-mail: oie@osu.eud

John Greisberger, Director

A scholarly journal that examines the application of social science theories and methods to international issues of education.

4372 Publications from HEATH
HEATH Resource Center
2134 G Street NW
Washington, DC 20052
202-973-0904
FAX 202-994-3365
http://www.heath.gwu.edu
e-mail: askheath@gwu.edu

Donna Martinez, Director

A newsletter offering information on postsecondary education for individuals with disabilities.

4373 **Rehabilitation Grants and Contracts Monitor**
RPM Press
PO Box 31483
Tucson, AZ 85751
520-886-1990
888-810-1990
FAX 520-886-1990
http://www.rpmpress.com
e-mail: pmccray@theriver.com
Jan Stonebraker, Operations Manager
Paul McCray, President

Newsletter providing a listing of grants and contracts available in the areas of special education, education, voc-ed special needs, vocational rehabilitation, mental health, job training, housing, transportation and a variety of other human service fields. *$97.00*

4374 **Report on Disability Programs**
Business Publishers
2601 University Boulevard W
Silver Spring, MD 20902
301-587-6300
800-274-6737
FAX 301-589-8463
http://www.bpinews.com
Adam Goldstein, President

Public policy issues that affect people with disabilities, plus court cases, funding opportunities and national news. Focus is on laws including American with Disabilities Act, Rehabilitation Act, Fair Housing Amendments, Affirmative Action, Individuals with Disabilities Education Act, and other legislation. Also tracks education, housing, job training, rehabilitation, Social Security and SSI, Medicare, Medicaid, and more. Tracks court cases and news from 50 states as well as federal news. *$286.00*

4375 **Report on Education of the Disadvantaged**
Business Publishers
951 Pershing Drive
Silver Spring, MD 20910
301-587-6300
FAX 301-585-9075
Adam Goldstein, President
Clair Hill, Marketing Manager

Covers federal aid to education programs affecting the disadvantaged, including children with special education needs. Covers funding programs, court cases and national/local news. *$273.00*
8 pages

4376 **Self-Advocacy Resources for Persons with Learning Disabilities**
Learning Disabilities Association of America
4156 Library Road
Pittsburgh, PA 15234
412-341-1515
FAX 412-344-0224
http://www.ldanatl.org
e-mail: ldanatl@usaor.net
Jane Browning, Editor-in-Chief

A newsletter offering information on resources and programs for the learning disabled. *$1.50*

4377 **Teacher Magazine**
Editorial Project in Education
6935 Arlington Road
Bethesda, MD 20814
301-280-3100
FAX 301-280-3150
http://www.edweek.org
e-mail: tm@epe.org
Virginia B Edwards, Editor

Offers articles and information on the latest programs, software, books, classroom materials and more for the teaching professional. *$17.94*

4378 **Teaching Exceptional Children**
Council for Exceptional Children
1110 N Glebe Road
Arlington, VA 22201
888-232-7733
FAX 703-264-9494
http://www.cec.sped.org/
e-mail: service@cec.sped.org
Drew Albritten MD, President
Bruce Ramirez, Manager

Published specifically for teachers and administrators of children who are gifted. Features practical articles that present methods and materials for classroom use as well as current issues in special education teaching and learning. Brings together its readers the latest data on technology, assistive technology, and procedures and techniques with applications to students with exceptionalities. The focus of its practical content is on immediate application.
6x per year

4379 **Texas Key**
Learning Disabilities Association of Texas
1011 W 31st Street
Austin, TX 78705
512-458-8234
800-604-7500
FAX 512-458-3826
http://www.ldat.org
e-mail: contact@ldat.org
Ann Robinson, Editor
Jean Kueker, President

Quarterly newsletter providing information of intrest to parents and professionals in the field of learning.
16-24 pages

Language Arts

4380 **ASHA Leader**
American Speech-Language-Hearing Association
10801 Rockville Pike
Bethesda, MD 20852
301-897-5700
888-498-6699
FAX 301-897-7358
TDY:301-897-5700
http://www.asha.org
e-mail: leader@asha.org
Laurie Ward, Marketing Coordinator
Arlene Pietranton, Executive Director

Pertains to the professional and administrative activities in the fields of speech-language pathology, audiology and the American Speech-Language-Hearing Association.
24X/year

4381 **American Journal of Speech-Language Pathology: A Journal of Clinical Practice**
American Speech-Language-Hearing Association
10801 Rockville Pike
Rockville, MD 20852
301-897-5700
888-498-6699
FAX 301-897-7358
TDY:301-897-5700
http://www.asha.org
e-mail: journals@asha.org
Dr Jeanette Hoit MD, Editor

The journal pertains to all aspects of clinical practice in speech-language pathology. Articles address screening, assessment, and treatment techniques; prevention; professional issues; supervision; and administration, and may appear in the form of clinical forums, clinical reviews, letters to the editor, or research reports that emphasize clinical practice.
Quarterly
ISSN 1058-0360

4382 **Communication Outlook**
Michigan State University Artificial Language Lab
405 Computer Center
East Lansing, MI 48824
517-353-0870
FAX 517-353-4766
http://www.msu.edu
e-mail: artlang@pilot.msu.edu
Rebecca Ann Baird, Editor
Deanna Marie Hoopingarner, Associate Editor
Robert Smith, Circulation Manager
Quarterly journal which focuses on communication aids and techniques. Provides information also for blind and visually impaired persons.

32 pages

4383 **Journal of Speech, Language, and Hearing Research**
American Speech-Language-Hearing Association
10801 Rockville Pike
N Bethesda, MD 20852
301-897-5700
888-498-6699
FAX 301-897-7358
TDY:301-897-5700
http://www.asha.org
e-mail: journals@asha.org
Dr Craig Champlin, Hearing Section Editor
Dr Karla McGregor, Language Section Editor
Dr Katherine Verdolini, Speech Section Editor
Pertains broadly to the studies of the processes and disorders of hearing, language, and speech and to the diagnosis and treatment of such disorders. Articles may take any of the following forms: reports of original research, including single-study experiments; theoretical, tutorial, or review pieces; research notes; and letters to the editor.
Bi-Monthly
ISSN 1092-4388

4384 **Kaleidoscope, Exploring the Experience of Disability Through Literature and Fine Arts**
701 S Main Street
Akron, OH 44311
330-762-9755
FAX 330-762-0912
TDY:330-379-3349
http://www.udsakron.org
e-mail: mshiplett@udsakron.org
Gail Willmott, Editor-in-Chief, Author
Phyllis Boerner, Publication Director
Gary Knuth, Executive Director

Creatively focuses on the experience of disability through diverse forms of literature and the fine arts. An award-winning magazine unique to the field of disability studies, it is open to writers with or without disabilities. KALEIDOSCOPE strives to express how disability does or does not affect society and individuals feelings and reactions to disability. Its portrayals of disability reflect a conscious effort to challenge and overcome stereotypical and patronizing attitudes. *$6.00*
64 pages $10.00/year

4385 **Language Arts**
National Council of Teachers of English
1111 W Kenyon Road
Urbana, IL 61801
217-328-3870
877-369-6283
FAX 217-328-9645
http://www.ncte.org
e-mail: lbianchini@ncte.org
Kent Williams, Executive Director

4386 **National Council of Teachers of English**
National Council of Teachers of English
1111 W Kenyon Road
Urbana, IL 61801
217-328-3870
800-369-6283
FAX 217-278-3761
http://www.ncte.org
e-mail: lbianchini@ncte.org
Lori Bianchini, Communications Specialist
Kent Williamson, Executive Director

With 75,000 individual and institutional members worldwide, NCTE is dedicated to improving the teaching and learning of English and the language arts at all levels of education. Members include elementary, middle, and high school teachers, supervisors of English programs, college and university faculty, teacher educators, local and state agency English specialists, and professionals in related fields.

College Guides

4387 Assisting College Students with Learning Disabilities: A Tutor's Manual
Association on Higher Education and Disability
PO Box 540666
Waltham, MA 02454
781-788-0003
FAX 781-788-0033
http://www.ahead.org
e-mail: ahead@postbox.acs.ohio-state.edu
This manual is designed for use by service providers and tutors working with students with learning disabilities. *$26.00*

4388 Bridges to Career Success: A Model for Training Career Counselors
National Clearinghouse of Rehabilitation Materials
206 W 6th Street
Stillwater, OK 74078
405-744-2000
FAX 405-744-2001
http://www.nchrtm.okstate.edu
Jamie Satcher, Author

This training package consists of materials for a one-day training program including an agenda outline, instructions and resource materials. Content encompasses services typically offered by college and university programs andresources to aid in career planning and placement. *$6.40*
54 pages

4389 Guide to Community Colleges Serving Students with Learning Disabilities
National Clearinghouse of Rehabilitation Materials
202 W 6th Street
Stillwater, OK 74078
405-744-2000
FAX 405-744-2001
http://www.nchrtm.okstate.edu
e-mail: brookdj@okway.okstate.edu
Sonja Burnhan, Author
Jamie Satcher, Author

The guide lists two-year community colleges in Mississippi, Alabama, Georgia, Tennessee, and Florida and describes services and accommodations provided for students with learning disabilities.
18 pages

4390 National Association of Colleges & Employe
College Placement Council
62 Highland Avenue
Bethlehem, PA 18017
610-868-1421
800-544-5272
FAX 610-868-0208
http://www.naceweb.org
e-mail: cnader@naceweb.org
Marilyn Mackes, Executive Director
Cecilia Nader, Administrative Assistant

Gives hard data on practitioners, budgets, the college relations and recruitment function, entry-level hiring, on-campus recruitment, new hires and much much more. *$46.95*
100+ pages

4391 Project TAPE: Technical Assistance for Postsecondary Education
Northern Illinois University
Dekalb, IL 60115
815-753-1311
FAX 815-753-0355
Tina Berg, Manager

Includes intervention strategies for persons with learning disabilities attending two-year community colleges.

4392 Student Support Services
Western Carolina University
137 Killian Annex
Cullowhee, NC 28723
828-227-7127
FAX 828-227-7078
http://www.wcu.edu/cap/sss/sss.html
Carol Mellen, Director
Suzanne Baker, Academic Coordinator
Joshua Kaufman, Services Coordinator
Student Support Services is an academic support program provided to eligible students through Academic Affairs at WCU. Our program assists students in choosing and working toward their academic, career, and personal goals with programs tailored to specific needs. *$20.50*

Counseling & Psychology

4393 A Decision Making Model for Occupational Therapy in the Public Schools
Therapro
225 Arlington Street
Framingham, MA 01702
508-872-9494
800-257-5376
FAX 508-875-2062
http://www.theraproducts.com
e-mail: info@theraproducts.com
Wendy Drobnyk,MS,OTR/L & Sara Sicilliano,MS, OTR/L, Author
Karen Conrad, Owner

Designed to guide the often complex decision making process of initiating, continuing, and discontinuing occupational therapy in the public school. The first publication of its kind to describe entrance and exit criteria for students referred for occupational therapy services.

4394 Accommodations in Higher Education under the Americans with Disabilities Act (ADA)
Guilford Press
72 Spring Street
New York, NY 10012
800-365-7006
FAX 212-966-6708
http://www.guilford.com
e-mail: info@guilford.com
Michael Gordon, Editor
Shelby Keiser, Editor

This practical manual offers essential information and guidance for anyone involved with ADA issues in higher education settings. Fundamental principals and actual clinical and administrative procedures are outlined for evaluating, documenting, and accommodating a wide range of mental and physical impairments. *$27.00*
245 pages
ISBN 1-572303-23-9

4395 Affect and Creativity
Lawrence Erlbaum Associates
365 Broadway
Hillsdale, NJ 07642
201-666-4110
800-926-6579
FAX 201-666-2394
Sandra Walker Russ, Author
Judy Nam, President/Owner

This volume offers information on the role of affect and play in the creative process. Designed as a required or supplemental text in graduate level courses in creativity, children's play, child development, affective/cognitive development and psychodynamic theory. *$36.00*
160 pages
ISBN 0-805809-86-4

4396 Behavior Management System
Connecticut Assoc. for Children and Adults with LD
25 Van Zant Street
Norwalk, CT 06855
203-838-5010
FAX 203-866-6108
http://www.CACLD.org
e-mail: cacld@optonline.net
Ethyl Papa, Author
Beryl Kaufman, Executive Director
Marie Armstrong, Information Specialist

Offers information on behavior management for learning disabled students. *$5.95*

4397 Behavioral Technology Guidebook
Eden Services
1 Eden Way
Princeton, NJ 08540
609-987-0099
FAX 609-987-0243
http://www.edenservices.org
e-mail: info@edenservices.org
David Holmes Ed.D, Executive Director
Anne Holmes, Director Outreach Support
Tom Cool, President
Practical guide for behavior modification techniques. *$50.00*

4398 Best Practice Occupational Therapy: Community Service with Children and Families
Therapro
225 Arlington Street
Framingham, MA 01702
508-872-9494
800-257-5376
FAX 508-875-2062
http://www.theraproducts.com
e-mail: info@theraproducts.com
Winnie Dunn, PhD, OTR, FAOTA, Author
Karen Conrad, Owner

An invaluable resource for sudents and practitioners interested in working with children and families in early intervention programs and public schools. Includes screening, pre-assessment, the referral process, best practice assessments, designing best paractice services and examples of IEPs and IFSPs. Many of the forms (screenings, checklists for teachers, referral forms assessment planning guide, etc.) are reproducible. The case studies give good examples of reports.

4399 Cognitive-Behavioral Therapy for Impulsive Children: 2nd Edition
Guilford Press
72 Spring Street
New York, NY 10012
800-365-7006
FAX 212-966-6708
http://www.guilford.com
e-mail: info@guilford.com
Philip Kendall, Author
Lauren Braswell, Author

The first edition of this book has been used successfully by thousands of clinicians to help children reduce impulsivity and improve their self-control. Building on the procedures reviewers call powerful tools and of great value to professionals who work with children. This second edition includes treatments, assessment issues and procedures and information on working with parents, teachers and groups of children. *$39.00*
239 pages
ISBN 0-898620-13-9

4400 Collaborative Problem Solving
Edge Enterprises
PO Box 1304
Lawrence, KS 66044
785-749-1473
FAX 785-749-0207
e-mail: eeinfo@edgeenterprises
Knackendoffel, Robinson, Deshler and Schumaker, Author
Jacqueline Schafer, Managing Editor
Sue Vernon, Manager

Outlines the communication skills necessary for establishing a cooperative relationship between two parties and then shows how to incorporate these skills within a problem-solving process that can be used to structure meetings between professionals and parents or students. This is especially useful for professionals who are consulting with teachers about problems they are having in their classrooms. *$10.00*
74 pages Paperback

4401 Curriculum Based Activities in Occupational Therapy: An Inclusion Resource
Therapro
225 Arlington Street
Framingham, MA 01702
508-872-9494
800-257-5376
FAX 508-875-2062
http://www.theraproducts.com
e-mail: info@theraproducts.com
Karen Conrad, Owner

This book is a comprehensive guide to classroom based occupational therapy. The authors have compiled over 162 classroom activities developed to provide a strong linkage between educational and therapeutic goals. Each structured activity is categorized into standard curriculum subsections (reading, math, written language, etc.). Designed for a 3rd and 4th grade classroom, it can be modified for use in lower grades.

4402 Disabled and Their Parents: A Counseling Challenge
Slack Incorporated
6900 Grove Road
Thorofare, NJ 08086
856-848-1000
FAX 856-848-6091
http://www.slackinc.com
e-mail: rbellolio@slackinc.co
Leo Buscaglia, Author
Robin Bellolio, Human Resource Director
Peter Slack, President

Offers information on inclusion and counseling services for the learning disabled student. *$22.95*

4403 Emotional Disorders & Learning Disabilities in the Elementary Classroom
Corwin Press
2455 Teller Road
Thousand Oaks, CA 91320
805-499-9734
800-233-9936
FAX 805-499-5323
http://www.corwinpress.com
e-mail: order@corwinpress.com
Jean Cheng Gorman, Author

This unique book focuses on the interaction between learning disabilities and emotional disorders, fostering an understanding of how learning problems affect emotional well-being and vice-versa. This resource and practical classroom guide for all elementary school teachers includes an overview of common learning disabilities and emotional problems and a classroom-tested, research-based list of classroom interactions and interventions. *$29.95*
60 pages
ISBN 0-761976-20-2

4404 Emotionally Abused & Neglected Child: Identification, Assessment & Intervention 2nd Edition
10475 Crosspoint Blvd
Indianapolis, IN 46256
877-762-2974
FAX 800-597-3299
http://www.wiley.com
Dorota Iwaniec, Author

Describes emotional abuse and neglect and how it affects child's growth, development and well-being. Diagnosis, assessment and issues that should be addressed. May 2006 *$50.00*
424 pages Paperback
ISBN 0-470011-01-7

4405 Ethical Principles of Psychologists and Code of Conduct

American Psychological Association
750 1st Street NE
Washington, DC 20002
202-336-5500
800-374-2722
FAX 202-336-5633
TDY:202-336-6123
http://www.apa.org
e-mail: psycinfo@apa.org
Marion Harrell, Deport Manager
Norman Anderson, CEO

General ethical principles of psychologists and enforceable ethical standards.

4406 General Guidelines for Providers of Psychological Services
American Psychological Association
750 1st Street NE
Washington, DC 20002
202-336-5500
800-374-2722
FAX 202-336-5633
TDY:202-336-6123
http://www.apa.org
e-mail: psycinfo@apa.org

Marion Harrell, Deport Manager
Norman Anderson, CEO

Offers information for the professional in the area of psychology.

4407 HELP...at Home
Therapro
225 Arlington Street
Framingham, MA 01702
508-872-9494
800-257-5376
FAX 508-875-2062
http://www.theraproducts.com
e-mail: info@theraproducts.com
Stephanie Parks, MA, Author
Karen Conrad, Owner

Practical and convenient format covers the 650 assesment skills from the Hawaii Early Learning Profile, with each page formatted as a separate, reproducible activity sheet. Therapist annotates, copies and hands out directly to parents to facilitate their involvement.

4408 Handbook of Psychological and Educational Assessment of Children
Guilford Press
72 Spring Street
New York, NY 10012
800-365-7006
FAX 212-966-6708
http://www.guilford.com
e-mail: info@guilford.com
Cecil Reynolds, Editor
Randy Kamphaus, Editor

Provides practitioners, researchers, professors, and students with an invaluable resource, this unique volume covers assessment of intelligence, learning styles, learning strategies, academic skills, and special populations, and discusses special topics in mental testing. Chapter contributions are by eminent psychologists and educators in the field of assessment with special expertise in research or practice in their topic areas. *$89.00*
714 pages

4409 Helping Students Become Strategic Learners: Guidelines for Teaching
Brookline Books
34 University Road
Brookline, MA 02445
617-734-6772
FAX 617-734-3952
http://www.brooklinebooks.com
Karen Schneid, Author

A practical book that helps the beginning or experienced teacher translate skill-specific strategy methods into their classroom teaching. The author demonstrates how teachers can implement cognitive strategy instruction in their own classrooms. Each chapter includes an introduction to the principles of a given teaching strategy and a review of the skill area in question—namely reading, writing and mathematics. *$26.95*
Paperback
ISBN 0-914797-85-9

4410 Helping Students Grow
American College Testing Program
PO Box 168
Iowa City, IA 52243
319-337-1000
FAX 319-339-3021
TDY:319-337-1701
http://www.act.org
e-mail: sandy.schlote@act.org
James Humphrey, Author
Richard Ferguson, CEO
Sandy Schlote, Testing Coordinator

Designed to assist counselors in using the wealth of information generated by the ACT assessment.

4411 Overcoming Dyslexia in Children, Adolescents and Adults
Connecticut Assoc. for Children and Adults with LD
25 Van Zant Street
Norwalk, CT 06855
203-838-5010
FAX 203-866-6108
http://www.CACLD.org
e-mail: cacld@optonline.net
Dale Jordan, Author
Beryl Kaufman, Executive Director
Marie Armstrong, Information Specialist

This book describes some forms of dyslexia in detail and then relates those problems to the social, emotional and personal development of dyslexic individuals. *$30.25*

4412 Pathways to Change: Brief Therapy Solutions with Difficult Adolescents
Guilford Press
72 Spring Street
New York, NY 10012
800-365-7006
FAX 212-966-6708
http://www.guilford.com
e-mail: info@guilford.com
Matthew D. Selekman, Author

This innovative, practical guide presents an effective brief therapy model for working with challenging adolescents and their families. The solution-oriented techniques and strategies so skillfullly presented in the original volume are now augmented by ideas and findings from other therapeutics traditions, with a heightened focus on engagement and relationship building. *$36.00*
292 pages
ISBN 1-572309-59-8

4413 Practitioner's Guide to Dynamic Assessment
Guilford Press
72 Spring Street
New York, NY 10012
800-365-7006
FAX 212-966-6708
http://www.guilford.com
e-mail: info@guilford.com
Carol S. Lidz, Author

A hands-on guide that is degined specifically for practitioners who engage in diagnostic assessment related to the functioning of children in school. It reviews and critiques current models of dynamic assessment and presents the research available on these existing models. *$29.00*
210 pages Paperback
ISBN 0-898622-42-5

4414 Prescriptions for Children with Learning and Adjustment Problems: A Consultant's Desk Reference
Charles C Thomas Publisher
2600 S 1st Street
Springfield, IL 62704
217-789-8980
800-258-8980
http://www.ccthomas.com
e-mail: books@ccthomas.com
Ralph F Blanco, David F Bogacki, Author

264 pages Paperback $39.95
ISBN 0-398060-22-0

4415 Problems in Written Expression: Assessment and Remediation
Guilford Press
72 Spring Street
New York, NY 10012
800-365-7006
FAX 212-966-6708
http://www.guilford.com
e-mail: info@guilford.com
Sharon Bradley-Johnson, Author
Jusi Lesiak, Author
Bob Matloff, President
A great resource for speech-language pathologists, counselors, resource specialists and other special educators. *$20.95*

178 pages Paperback

4416 **Reading and Learning Disability: A Neuropsychological Approach to Evaluation & Instruction**
Charles C Thomas Publisher
2600 S 1st Street
Springfield, IL 62704
217-789-8980
800-258-8980
http://www.ccthomas.com
e-mail: books@ccthomas.com
Estelle L Fryburg, Author

This text utilizes the current knowledge of neuropsychology (brain-behavior relationships) and the concepts of cognitive psychology to provide an understanding of reading and learning disability which has a practical application to education. The primary goal of the book is to provide teachers, psychologists, physicians, concerned professionals, and parents with an interdisciplinary view of learning and schooling. *$74.95*

398 pages Paper
ISBN 0-398067-45-8

4417 **Reflections Through the Looking Glass**
Association on Higher Education and Disability
PO Box 540666
Waltham, MA 02454
781-788-0003
FAX 781-788-0033
http://www.ahead.org
e-mail: ahead@postbox.acs.ohio-state.edu

A must for new professionals offering a philosophical review of the nature of the field written in first person by charter member and former Association President Richard Harris of Ball State University. *$5.50*

4418 **Revels in Madness: Insanity in Medicine and Literature**
University of Michigan Press
839 Greene Street
Ann Arbor, MI 48104
734-764-4388
FAX 734-763-0456
http://www.press.umich.edu
Allen Thiher, Author

Revels in Madness offers a history of western culture's shifting understanding of insanity as evidenced in its literature and as influenced by medical knowledge. *$75.00*

368 pages Cloth
ISBN 0-472110-35-3

4419 **Self-Advocacy Handbook for High School Students**
Utah Department of Special Education
PO Box 144200
Salt Lake City, UT 84114
801-584-8543
FAX 801-538-7991
http://www.usoe.k12.ut.us/sans/
e-mail: mtaylor@usoe.k12.ut.us
Ann Jepsen, Author
Travis Cook, Director
Holly Balken, Manager

This manual teaches the students to advocate for themselves.

4420 **Self-Advocacy for Junior High School Students**
Utah Department of Special Education
PO Box 144200
Salt Lake City, UT 84114
801-584-8543
FAX 801-538-7991
http://www.usoe.k12.ut.us/sans/
e-mail: mtaylor@usoe.k12.ut.us
Travis Cook, Director
Holly Balken, Manager

A program designed to increase students' verbal expressive skills in discussing learning disabilities, ADD and related characteristics.

4421 **Self-Injurious Behavior: A Somatosensory Treatment Approach**
Therapro
225 Arlington Street
Framingham, MA 01702
508-872-9494
800-257-5376
FAX 508-875-2062
http://www.theraproducts.com
e-mail: info@theraproducts.com
Haru Hirama, EdD, OTR/L, Author
Karen Conrad, Owner

Practical account of treatment. Stimulation is given to counteract the somatosensory deprivation experienced by the self-injurious individual. Includes reviews/illustrations of the treatment.

4422 **Teaching Students with Learning and Behavior Problems**
Pro-Ed
8700 Shoal Creek Boulevard
Austin, TX 78757
512-451-3246
800-897-3202
FAX 512-451-8542
http://www.proedinc.com
e-mail: info@proedinc.com
Donald D Hammill, Nettie R Bartel, Author

Provides teachers with a comprehensive overview of the best practices in informal assessment and adaptive instruction. With the current trend od both regular and exceptional students will find this text a useful resource. *$63.00*

4423 **Treating Troubled Children and Their Families**
Guilford Press
72 Spring Street
New York, NY 10012
800-365-7006
FAX 212-966-6708
http://www.guilford.com
e-mail: info@guilford.com
Ellen F Wachtel, Author

Integrating systemic, psychodynamic, and cognitive-behavioral perspectives, this acclaimed book presents an innovative framework for therapeutic work. Shows how parents and children all too often get entangled in patterns that cause grief to both generations, and demonstrates ho to help being about change with a combinations of family-focused interventions. *$29.00*

320 pages Paperback
ISBN 1-593850-72-7

General

4424 **A History of Disability**
University of Michigan Press
839 Greene Street
Ann Arbor, MI 48104
734-764-4392
FAX 734-615-1540
http://www.press.umich.edu
Henri-Jacques Stiker, Author

A bold analysis of the evolution of western attitudes toward disability. The book traces the history of western cultural responses to disability, from ancient times to the present. *$23.95*

264 pages Paper
ISBN 0-472086-26-9

4425 **A Human Development View of Learning Disabilities: From Theory to Practice**
Charles C Thomas Publisher
2600 S 1st Street
Springfield, IL 62704
217-789-8980
800-258-8980
http://www.ccthomas.com
e-mail: books@ccthomas.com
Corrine E Kass and Cleborne D Maddux, Author

Presents a human development model for understanding and treating age-related deficits that seem to be characteristic of individuals with learning disabilities. *$35.95*

252 pages Paper
ISBN 0-398075-65-1

4426 **A Manual of Sequential Art Activities for Classified Children and Adolescents**
Charles C Thomas Publisher
2600 S 1st Street
Springfield, IL 62704
217-789-8980
800-258-8980
http://www.ccthomas.com
e-mail: books@ccthomas.com
Rocco AL Fugaro, Author

246 pages Spiral (paper) $48.95
ISBN 0-398050-85-6

4427 **A Practical Approach to RSP: A Handbook for the Resource Specialist Program**
Charles C Thomas Publisher
2600 S 1st Street
Springfield, IL 62704
217-789-8980
800-258-8980
FAX 217-789-9130
http://www.ccthomas.com
e-mail: books@ccthomas.com
Leslie A Williams and Lucile S Arntzen, Author
Michael Thomas, President

Valuable to resource specialists in training and in service, administrators and related professionals. Books sent on approval. *$33.95*
120 pages Cloth
ISBN 0-398059-08-X

4428 **Academic Skills Problems Workbook**
Guilford Press
72 Spring Street
New York, NY 10012
800-365-7006
FAX 212-966-6708
http://www.guilford.com
e-mail: info@guilford.com
Edward S Shapiro, PhD, Author

This user-friendly workbook offers numerous opportunities for practicing and mastering direct assessment and intervention procedures. The workbook also includes teacher and student interview forms; a complete guide to using the Behavioral Observation of Students in Schools (BOSS) Observation code, exercises on administering assessments and scoring, interpreting, and graphing the results; and much more. *$29.00*
147 pages
ISBN 1-572309-68-7

4429 **Academic Skills Problems: Direct Assessment and Intervention**
Guilford Press
72 Spring Street
New York, NY 10012
800-365-7006
FAX 212-966-6708
http://www.guilford.com
e-mail: info@guilford.com
Edward S Shapiro, PhD, Author

Provides comprehensive framework for the direct assessment of academic skills. Presented is a readily applicable, four-step approach for working with students experiencing a range of difficulties with reading, spelling, written language, or math. *$45.00*

370 pages
ISBN 1-572309-77-6

4430 **Academic Therapy Publications**
20 Commercial Boulevard
Novato, CA 94949
415-883-3314
888-287-9975
FAX 415-883-3720
http://www.atpub.com
e-mail: atpub@aol.com

Anna Arena, President
Jim Arena, Vice President

What goes into an Individual Education Plan for a special education student? This book gives detailed information.

ISBN 0-878790-72-1

4431 **Academic and Developmental Learning Disabilities**
Love Publishing Company
PO Box 22353
Denver, CO 80222
303-221-7333
FAX 303-221-7444
http://www.lovepublishing.com
e-mail: lovepublishing@compuserve.com
Samuel Kirk, Author
Stan Love, Owner

This text is intended to serve as a basis for classifying children and to help teachers diagnose and remediate children who have major disabilities in the learning process. *$39.95*
337 pages

4432 **Accessing the General Curriculum Including Students with Disabilities in Standards-Based Reform**
Corwin Press
2455 Teller Road
Thousand Oaks, CA 91320
805-499-9734
800-233-9936
FAX 805-499-5323
http://www.corwinpress.com
Victor Nolet, Margaret J McLaughlin, Author

Provides updated frameworkd and strategies-with invaluable examples and flowcharts for fitting special education into the frameworks created by national standards and assessments. This invaluable resource provides K-12 educators with the support necessaty to produce expected results from every learner. *$27.95*
144 pages
ISBN 1-412916-49-3

4433 **Adapted Physical Education for Students with Autism**
Charles C Thomas Publishers
2600 S 1st Street
Springfield, IL 62704
217-789-8980
800-258-8980
http://www.ccthomas.com
e-mail: books@ccthomas.com
Kimberly Davis, Author

This book shows the need for additional information. It describes autism and offers suggestions on assessment and programming for students with autism in adapted physical education/regular physical education classes. *$27.95*
142 pages Paper
ISBN 0-398060-85-5

4434 **Adapting Curriculum & Instruction in Inclusive Early Childhood Settings**
Indiana Institute on Disability and Community
2853 E Tenth Street
Bloomington, IN 47408
812-855-6508
FAX 812-855-9630
http://www.iidc.indiana.edu
e-mail: iidc@indiana.edu
David Mank, Director

Offers ideas and strategies that will be beneficial to all young children, including children with identified disabilities, children who are at risk, and students who need enriched curricular options. This is also an excellent resource for preservice training as well as inservice training for independent child care providers, center, and schools. *$11.00*

4435 **An Introduction to Learning Disabilities**
Scott Foresman Addison Wesley
1900 E Lake Avenue
Glenview, IL 60025
847-486-2616
FAX 847-729-8910
http://www.sf.aw.com

Howard Adelman, Author
Paul McFall, President
Judith Besterfeldt, Manager

This text is designed to introduce learning disabilities in a way that clarifies both instructional options and large educational issues.

354 pages

4436 An Introduction to the Nature and Needs of Students with Mild Disabilities
Charles C Thomas Publisher
2600 S 1st Street
Springfield, IL 62704
217-789-8980
800-258-8980
FAX 217-789-9130
http://www.ccthomas.com
e-mail: books@ccthomas.com
Carroll J Jones, Author
Michael Thomas, President

Mild mental retardation, behavior disorders, and learning disabilities are covered in this text. Designed as an introductory text for an undergraduate degree program in special education. Also included is information on the historical background of services in Europe, early-to-current services in the United States, landmark legislation, litigation relevant to each categorical area, with definitions and classification systems. *$50.95*
300 pages Cloth
ISBN 0-398067-11-2

4437 Annals of Dyslexia
International Dyslexia Association
40 York Road
Baltimore, MD 21204
410-296-0232
FAX 410-321-5069
http://www.interdys.org
Elaine Niefled, Publications Director

The Society's scholarly journal contains updates on current research and selected proceedings from talks given at each ODS international conference. Issues of Annals are available from 1982 through the present year.

4438 Art for All the Children: Approaches to Art Therapy for Children with Disabilities
Charles C Thomas Publisher
2600 S 1st Street
Springfield, IL 62704
217-789-8980
800-258-8980
http://www.ccthomas.com
e-mail: books@ccthomas.com
Frances E Anderson, Author

This edition is for art therapists in training and for in-service professionals in art therapy, art education and special education who have children with disabilities as a part of their case/class load. A major goal of this edition is to show the many ways that art can be adapted so that all children may have a meaningful encounter with art. The book will prepare the reader to understand children, their art, their disabilities and how to adapt art to meet their needs. *$ 56.95*
398 pages Paper
ISBN 0-398060-07-7

4439 Art-Centered Education & Therapy for Children with Disabilities
Charles C Thomas Publisher
2600 S 1st Street
Springfield, IL 62704
217-789-8980
800-258-8980
FAX 217-789-9130
http://www.ccthomas.com
e-mail: books@ccthomas.com
Frances E Anderson, Author
Michael Thomas, President

To help both the regular education, and art and special education teachers, pre- and in-service, better understand the issues and realities of providing education and remediation to children with disabilities. Offers the concept that we must live, learn and develop through art - that art belongs at the core of the public school curriculum. *$49.95*
284 pages Cloth
ISBN 0-398058-96-2

4440 Attentional Deficit Disorder in Children and Adolescents
Charles C Thomas Publisher
2600 S 1st Street
Springfield, IL 62704
217-789-8980
800-258-8980
FAX 217-789-9130
http://www.ccthomas.com
e-mail: books@ccthomas.com
Jack Fadely, Author
Virginia Hosler, Author
Michael Thomas, President
This book presents an analysis of case studies of children and adolescents with attentional deficits and hyperactivity. The focus is to demonstrate CAUSAL factors in this disorder and to suggest treatment strategies both in psychological and medical practice. *$56.95*
292 pages Cloth
ISBN 0-398057-92-3

4441 Atypical Cognitive Deficits
Lawrence Erlbaum Associates
365 Broadway
Hillsdale, NJ 07642
201-666-4110
800-926-6579
FAX 201-666-2394
Sarah Broman; Jordan Grafman, Author

This volume is based on a conference held to examine what was known about cognitive behaviors and brain structure and function in three syndromes. *$29.95*
352 pages
ISBN 0-805811-80-0

4442 Auditory Processes
Academic Therapy Publications
20 Commercial Boulevard
Novato, CA 94949
415-883-3314
888-287-9975
FAX 415-883-3720
http://www.atpub.com
e-mail: atpub@aol.com
Pamela Gillel, Author
Jim Arena
Joanne Urban

Explains how teachers, educational consultants and parents can identify auditory processing problems, understand their impact and implement appropriate instructional strategies to enhance learning. *$15.00*
120 pages
ISBN 0-878790-94-2

4443 Auditory Processes: Revised Edition
Therapro
225 Arlington Street
Framingham, MA 01702
508-872-9494
800-257-5376
FAX 508-875-2062
http://www.theraproducts.com
e-mail: info@theraproducts.com
Pamela Gillet, PhD, Author
Karen Conrad, Owner

This author clearly describes the sequence of auditory skill development as well as the symptomatic behavior of youngsters with auditory processing problems. Offers hundreds of tests and remedial exercises in areas such as auditory discrimination, auditory memory, auditiory perception deficit.

4444 Auditory Training
Harris Communications
15155 Technology Drive
Eden Prairie, MN 55344
952-906-1180
800-825-6758
FAX 952-906-1099
TDY:952-906-1198
http://www.harriscmm.com
e-mail: info@harriscmm.com
Norman P Erber, Author
Robert Harris, Owner

Written for parents, educators, and rehabilitative audiologists, who are concerned with auditory development of hearing impaired children. Auditory instruction strategies encourage children to learn to hear through whatever type of amplification device they are using. Covers research and developments in auditory training, speech perception, speech production, screening, training and practical suggestions. *$23.95*

197 pages Paperback

4445 Body and Physical Difference: Discourses of Disability

University of Michigan Press
839 Greene Street
Ann Arbor, MI 48104
734-764-4392
FAX 734-615-1540
http://www.press.umich.edu

David T Mitchell, Editor
Sharon L Synder, Editor

For years the subject of human disability has engaged those in the biological, social and cognitive sciences, while at the same time, it has been curiously neglected within the humanitites. The Body and Physical Difference seeks to introduce the field of disability studies into the humanities by exploring the fantasies and fictons that have crystallized around conceptions of physical and cognitive difference. *$65.00*

320 pages cloth
ISBN 0-472066-59-9

4446 Bridging the Family-Professional Gap: Facilitating Interdisciplinary Services

Charles C Thomas Publisher
2600 S 1st Street
Springfield, IL 62704
217-789-8980
800-258-8980
FAX 217-789-9130
http://www.ccthomas.com
e-mail: books@ccthomas.com

Billy Ogletree, Martin Fischer, Jane Schulz, Author
Michael Thomas, President

Facilitates family preparedness for interdisciplinary team functioning and promotes interdisciplinary professionals' awareness of family members' concerns and priorities. *$49.95*

300 pages Cloth
ISBN 0-398069-88-3

4447 Brief Intervention for School Problems: Outcome-Informed Strategies

Guilford Press
72 Spring Street
New York, NY 10012
800-365-7006
FAX 212-966-6708
http://www.guilford.com
e-mail: info@guilford.com

John Murphy, Barry Duncan, Author

This practical guide provides innovative strategies for resolving academic and behavioral difficulties by enlisting the strengths and resources of students, parents, and teachers. *$30.00*

204 pages
ISBN 1-593854-92-7

4448 Case Studies of Exceptional Students: Handicapped and Gifted

Charles C Thomas Publisher
2600 S 1st Street
Springfield, IL 62704
217-789-8980
800-258-8980
FAX 217-789-9130
http://www.ccthomas.com
e-mail: books@ccthomas.com

Carroll J. Jones, Author
Michael Thomas, President

Clear, concise, educationally relevant case studies. *$56.95*

272 pages Cloth
ISBN 0-398058-56-3

4449 Center Work

Center for Research in Vocational Education
2150 Shattuck Avenue
Berkeley, CA 94704
800-762-4093

Profiles the center's current work and contains articles about policy issues, computer resources, NCRVE publications, and ERIC/ACVE digests.

Quarterly-Free

4450 Children, Problems and Guidelines, Special Ed

Slosson Educational Publications
PO Box 280
East Aurora, NY 14052
716-652-0930
800-828-4800
FAX 800-655-3840
http://www.slosson.com
e-mail: slosson@slosson.com

LaDeane Casey, Author
Steven Slosson, President

A professional and responsible resource book which addresses many of the most common problems involving children and their homes or schools. *$45.00*

99 pages Ages 6-16

4451 Classroom Management for Elementary Teachers: 5th Editon

Books on Special Children
22 Webster Court
Amherst, MA 01002
845-638-1236
FAX 845-638-0847
http://www.boscbooks.com
e-mail: irene@boscbooks.com

Carolyn Evertson; Edmund Emmer; Murray Worsham, Author

Good classroom management just doesn't happen, it takes good planning and effective teachers organizing classroom rules and procedures, planning and conducting instructions. Appropriate student behavior, managing problem behavior and special groups are discussed. *$34.95*

244 pages Paperback
ISBN 0-205308-38-4

4452 Classroom Management for Secondary Teachers: 4th Editon

Books on Special Children
22 Webster Court
Amherst, MA 01002
845-638-1236
FAX 845-638-0847
http://www.boscbooks.com
e-mail: irene@boscbooks.com

ET Emmer, Author
Marcia Young, President

Good classroom management just doesn't happen, it takes good planning and effective teachers organizing classroom rules and procedures, planning and conducting instructions. Appropriate student behavior, managing problem behavior and special groups are discussed. *$34.95*

216 pages softcover
ISBN 0-205264-28-X

4453 Classroom Notetaker: How to Organize a Program Serving Students with Hearing Impairments

Harris Communications
15155 Technology Drive
Eden Prairie, MN 55344
952-906-1180
800-825-6758
FAX 952-906-1099
TDY:952-906-1198
http://www.harriscomm.com
e-mail: info@harriscmm.com

Jimmie Joan Wilson, Author
Robert Harris, Owner
Patty Johnson, Office Manager

Promotes classroom note taking and gives specifics on establishing a note taking program. Topics include proving the need for a note taking program, recruiting and training note takers, and the principles of note taking. *$25.95*

127 pages Paperback

4454 Cognitive Approach to Learning Disabilities

McGraw-Hill
2 Penn Plaza
New York, NY 10121
212-904-2000
877-833-5524
http://www.books.mcgraw-hill.com
e-mail: pbg.ecommerce_custserv@mcgraw-hill.com

D Kim Reid, Author
Philip Rupple, Group Publisher/VP
Jeffrey Krames, Publisher/Editor-in-Chief

This book is the first to bridge the gap between cognitive psychology and information processing theory in understanding learning disabilities. *$44.00*
686 pages Hardcover
ISBN 0-070517-68-1

4455 Cognitive Retraining Using Microcomputers
Lawrence Erlbaum Associates
365 Broadway
Hillsdale, NJ 07642
201-666-4110
800-926-6579
FAX 201-666-2394

Veronica Bradley, Author
John Welch, Author

This text reviews representative examples from the literature relating to the training of cognitive systems with the emphasis on studies describing the use of computerized methods. *$69.95*
304 pages
ISBN 0-863772-02-1

4456 Cognitive Strategy Instruction That Really Improves Children's Performance
Brookline Books
34 University Road
Manchester, NH 03101
617-734-6772
FAX 617-734-3952
http://www.brooklinebooks.com

Michael Pressley, Author

A concise and focused work that summarily presents the few procedures for teaching strategies that aid academic subject matter learning that are empirically validated and fit well with the elementary school curriculum. *$27.95*
203 pages
ISBN 0-914797-66-2

4457 Competencies for Teachers of Students with Learning Disabilities
Council for Exceptional Children
1110 N Glebe Road
Arlington, VA 22201
703-245-0600
888-232-7733
FAX 703-264-9494
http://www.cec.sped.org/
e-mail: service@cec.sped.org

Amme Graves, Author
Mary Landers, Author
Bruce Ramirez, Manager

Lists 209 specific professional competencies needed by teachers of students with learning disabilities and provides a conceptual framework for the ten areas in which the competencies are organized. *$5.00*
25 pages

4458 Comprehensive Assessment in Special Education: Approaches, Procedures and Concerns
Charles C Thomas Publisher
2600 S 1st Street
Springfield, IL 62704
217-789-8980
800-258-8980
FAX 217-789-9130
http://www.ccthomas.com
e-mail: books@ccthomas.com

Rotatori, Fox, Sexton and Miller, Author
Michael Thomas, President

Books sent on approval. Shipping charges: $5.50, $6.50 Canada. Prices subject to change without notice. *$104.95*
578 pages
ISBN 0-398056-45-5

4459 Computers in Head Start Classrooms
4156 Library Road
Pittsburgh, PA 15234
412-341-1515
FAX 412-344-0224
http://www.ldaamerica.com
e-mail: ldanatl@usaor.net

Jane Browning, Executive Director
Mary , Office Manager

4460 Cooperative Learning and Strategies for Inclusion
Brookes Publishing Company
PO Box 10624
Baltimore, MD 21285
410-337-9580
800-638-3775
FAX 410-337-8539
http://www.brookspublishing.com
e-mail: custserv@brookespublishing.com

JoAnne Putnam Phd, Editor

This book supplies educators, classroom support personnel, and administrators with numerous tools for creating positive, inclusive classroom environments for students from preschool through high school. *$29.95*
288 pages Paperback
ISBN 1-557663-46-7

4461 Creative Curriculum for Early Childhood
Teaching Strategies
PO Box 42243
Washington, DC 20015
202-362-7543
800-637-3652
FAX 202-364-7273
http://www.teachingstrategies.com
e-mail: info@teachingstrategies.com

DT Dodge And LJ Collier, Author
Diane Trister-Dodge, Owner
Angel White, President

Focuses on the developmentally appropriate program in early childhood education. Illustrates how preschool and kindergarten teachers set the stage for learning, and how children and teachers interact and learn in various interest areas. *$39.95*
390 pages
ISBN 1-879537-06-0

4462 Curriculum Development for Students with Mild Disabilities
Charles C Thomas Publisher
2600 S 1st Street
Springfield, IL 62704
217-789-8980
800-258-8980
http://www.ccthomas.com
e-mail: books@ccthomas.com

Carroll J Jones, Author

Many teachers of students with mild disabilities experience difficulty writing IEPs because they lack a foundation in the regular education curriculum of academic skills and sequences associated with each grade level. *$38.95*
258 pages Spiral (paper)
ISBN 0-398707-18-2

4463 Curriculum Models and Strategies for Educating Individuals with Disabilities
Charles C Thomas Publisher
2600 S 1st Street
Springfield, IL 62704
217-789-8980
800-258-8980
FAX 217-789-9130
http://www.ccthomas.com
e-mail: books@ccthomas.com

George Taylor, Author
Michael Thomas, President
Claire Slagler, Sales Manager

Curriculum skills units developed as a guide to assist educators instructing disabled individuals in the areas of communication, math and science, socially effective and psychomotor skills, as well as morals and character. Also helpful to those working in community agencies with disabled individuals. *$48.95*
260 pages Cloth
ISBN 0-398069-75-1

4464 Curriculum-Based Assessment: A Primer
Charles C Thomas Publisher
2600 S 1st Street
Springfield, IL 62704
217-789-8980
800-258-8980
http://www.ccthomas.com
e-mail: books@ccthomas.com

Charles H Hargis, Author

The use of curriculum-based assessment (CBA) to ensure learning disabled and low achieving students adequate educational opportunity is the focus of this book. CBA requires an intimate relationship between teaching and testing. The author presents examples and methods of implementation through reading and arithmetic activities and discusses at length the issues involved in test validity and grading. *$33.95*
174 pages Paperback
ISBN 0-398075-52-1

4465 Curriculum-Based Assessment: The Easy Way
Charles C Thomas Publisher
2600 S 1st Street
Springfield, IL 62704
217-789-8980
800-258-8980
http://www.ccthomas.com
e-mail: books@ccthomas.com
Carroll J Jones, Author

Practical and specific methods for developing and using CBA's in an educational setting. *$32.95*
176 pages Spiral (paper)

4466 Deal Me In: The Use of Playing Cards in Learning and Teaching
CT Association for Children and Adults with LD
25 Van Zant Street
Norwalk, CT 06855
203-838-5010
http://www.CACLD.org
e-mail: cacld@optonline.net
M Golick, Author

A book of how to play cards with your learning disabled child. *$10.95*

4467 Defects: Engendering the Modern Body
University of Michigan Press
839 Greene Street
Ann Arbor, MI 48104
734-764-4392
FAX 734-615-1540
http://www.press.umich.edu
Helen Deutsch, Editor
Felicity Nussbaum, Editor

Defects brings together essays on the emergence of the concept of monstrosity in the eighteenth century and the ways it paralleled the emergence of notions of sexual difference. *$27.95*
344 pages Paper
ISBN 0-472066-98-8

4468 Developmental Variation and Learning Disorders
Educators Publishing Service
PO Box 9031
Cambridge, MA 02139
800-435-7228
FAX 888-440-2665
http://www.epsbooks.com
e-mail: eps@epsbooks.com
Dr. Melvin Levine, Author

The Second Edition of this useful reference includes completely revised on attention, memory, and language, with significant modifications of the remaining chapters. Sections on educational skills have been expanded and updated; the chapter on causes and complications of learning disorders has been updated to include recent references and ongoing reserach efforts. *$69.00*

ISBN 0-838819-92-3

4469 Dictionary of Special Education and Rehabilitation
Love Publishing Company
9101 E Kenyon Avenue
Denver, CO 80237
303-221-7333
FAX 303-221-7444
http://www.lovepublishing.com
e-mail: lpc@lovepublishing.com
Glenn A Vergason, M L Anderegg, Author

This updated edition of one of the most valuable resources in the field is over six years in the making and incorporates hundreds of additions. It provides clear, understandable definitions of more than 2,000 terms unique to special education and rehabilitation. It also provides listing of professional organizations and resources, includes latest terms, and is a critical reference for anyone in the special education field. *$34.95*
210 pages Paperback
ISBN 0-891802-43-3

4470 Directory for Exceptional Children
Porter Sargent Publishers
11 Beacon Street
Boston, MA 02108
617-523-1670
800-342-7870
FAX 617-523-1021
http://www.portersargent.com
e-mail: info@portersargent.com
Daniel McKeever, Senior Editor
John Yonce, Manager
Leslie Weston, Production Editor
A comprehensive survey of 3000 schools, facilities, and organizations across the USA. Serving children and yound adults with developmental, physical, medical, and emotional disabilities. Aide to parents, consultants, educators, and other professionals. *$64.00*
1312 pages
ISBN 0-875581-31-5

4471 Disability Awareness in the Classroom: A Resource Tool for Teachers and Students
Charles C Thomas Publisher
2600 S 1st Street
Springfield, IL 62704
217-789-8980
800-258-8980
http://www.ccthomas.com
e-mail: books@ccthomas.com
Lorie and Isabelle St. Onge Levison, Author

The purpose of this book is to reduce the discomfort and alienation of teachers and students regarding people with disabilities through the use of written and photographic materials. It aims to dispel misconceptions that contribute to stereotyping and in general to blur the divisions between two segments of our society: those with disabilities and those without. *$45.95*
230 pages Spiral (paper)
ISBN 0-398069-53-7

4472 Eden Institute Curriculum: Adaptive Physical Education, Volume V
Eden Services
1 Eden Way
Princeton, NJ 08540
609-987-0099
FAX 609-987-0243
http://www.edenservices.org
e-mail: info@edenservices.org
Thomas P McCool EdD, President

This volume contains teaching programs in the area of sensory integration and adaptive physical education. *$50.00*

4473 Eden Institute Curriculum: Classroom Orienation, Volume II
Eden Services
1 Eden Way
Princeton, NJ 08540
609-987-0099
FAX 609-987-0243
http://www.edenservices.org
e-mail: info@edenservices.org
Thomas P McCool EdD, President

This volume is geard toward those students who have mastered some basic academic skills and are able to learn in a small group setting. The teaching programs include academics, domestics, and social skills. *$100.00*

4474 Eden Institute Curriculum: Core
Eden Services
1 Eden Way
Princeton, NJ 08540
609-987-0099
FAX 609-987-0243
http://www.edenservices.org
e-mail: info@edenservices.org
Thomas P McCool EdD, President

This volume encompasses teaching strategies for students agesthree through fourteen. It includes teaching programs in the areas of learning readiness, pre-academics, academics, occupational skills, social and play skills, as well as general information regarding behavioral teaching techniques. *$200.00*

4475 Eden Institute Curriculum: Speech and Language, Volume IV

Eden Services
1 Eden Way
Princeton, NJ 08540 609-987-0099
FAX 609-987-0243
http://www.edenservices.org
e-mail: info@edenservices.org
Thomas P McCool EdD, President

This volume contains teaching programs for students ages three through adult in the area of speech and language development. *$170.00*

4476 Educating All Students Together

Corwin Press
2455 Teller Road
Thousand Oaks, CA 91320 805-499-9734
800-818-7243
FAX 805-499-5323
http://www.corwinpress.com
e-mail: order@corwinpress.com
Leonard C Burrello, Carl Lashley, Edith Beatty, Author

A plan for unifying the separate and parallel systems of special and general education. Key concepts include: schools embracing special services personnel; the role of the community; program evaluation and incentives; brain and holographic design; collaboration between school administrators and teachers; and adapting curriculum; and instruction. *$32.95*

264 pages
ISBN 0-761976-98-1

4477 Educating Children with Multiple Disabilities, A Collaborative Approach Fourth Edition

Brookes Publishing
PO Box 10624
Baltimore, MD 21285-0624 410-337-9580
800-638-3775
FAX 410-337-8539
http://www.brookespublishing.com
e-mail: custserv@brookespublishing.com
Fred P Orelove, Editor
Dick Sobsey, Editor
Rosanne K Silberman, Editor

Gives undergraduate and graduate students up-to-the-minute research and strategies for educating children with severe and multiple disabilities. *$49.00*

672 pages Paperback
ISBN 1-557667-10-1

4478 Educator's Guide to Students with Epilepsy

Charles C Thomas Publisher
2600 S 1st Street
Springfield, IL 62704 217-789-8980
800-258-8980
FAX 217-789-9130
http://www.ccthomas.com
e-mail: books@ccthomas.com
Robert J Michael, Author
Michael Thomas, President

The purposes of the book are to: present relevant knowledge about epilepsy for the educator; create an awareness of and sensitivity to students with epilepsy; focus on the role of education with students with epilepsy; present the major educational issues associated with epilepsy; define the educator's responsibility to students with epilepsy; and present useful resources. *$44.95*

174 pages Cloth
ISBN 0-398065-37-3

4479 Educator's Publishing Service

Delta Corporation
PO Box 9031
Cambridge, MA 02139 617-547-6706
800-225-5750
FAX 617-547-0412
http://www.epsbooks.com
e-mail: eps@epsbooks.com
Gunnar Voltz, President

Written for both parents and teachers, this is based on the view that education should be a system of care that looks after the specific needs of individual students. Using case studies, it identifies and illustrates twenty-six common behaviors or phenomena that often inhibit or interfere with school performance. These are arranged according to six different themes and include behaviors related to poorly regulated attention, reduced remembering. *$28.00*

340 pages
ISBN 0-838814-87-7

4480 Ending Discrimination in Special Education

Charles C Thomas Publisher
2600 S 1st Street
Springfield, IL 62704 217-789-8980
800-258-8980
http://www.ccthomas.com
e-mail: books@ccthomas.com
Herbert Grossman, Author

For special educators, school administrators, pychologists and regular education teachers who need to acquire the competencies necessary to succeed with all disabled, gifted and talented students who will be included in their classrooms. Books sent on approval. Shipping charges: $5.50 US/&6.50 Canada. Prices subject to change without notice. *$23.95*

142 pages Paper
ISBN 0-398073-04-6

4481 Enhancing Self-Concepts & Achievement of Mildly Handicapped Students

Charles C Thomas Publisher
2600 S 1st Street
Springfield, IL 62704 217-789-8980
800-258-8980
FAX 217-789-9130
http://www.ccthomas.com
e-mail: books@ccthomas.com
Carroll J Jones, Author
Michael Thomas, President

The self concept theory is reviewed and examined from a chronological and developmental perspective, relating the impact of self concept on academic functioning. Includes approaches and techniques a teacher might choose, including interventions which are metacognitive, behavioral, social, or academic in nature. A valuable review of current best practices for understanding and intervening on behalf of mildly handicapped learners with emotionally fragile self-concepts. *$ 39.95*

294 pages Cloth
ISBN 0-398057-60-5

4482 Exceptional Children: An Introduction to Special Education 7th Edition

Pearson Education/Prentice Hall Publishers
One Lake Street
Upper Saddle River, NJ 07458 201-236-7000
http://www.pearsoned.com
e-mail: communications@pearsoned.com
William L Heward, Author

This comprehensive text, the first in Australia, covers all major special education topics. It features special contributions from professionals working with special disabilities. It has been edited to achieve a balance of substantive text (with medical and educational implications for each special need) as well as practical illustrative components and first-hand commentary from professionals and organizations in the field. *$93.00*

704 pages
ISBN 0-729503-72-0

4483 Exceptional Teacher's Handbook: First Year Special Education Teacher's Guide for Success 2nd Edit

Corwin Press
2455 Teller Road
Thousand Oaks, CA 91320 805-499-9734
800-818-7243
FAX 805-499-5323
http://www.corwinpress.com
e-mail: order@corwinpress.com
Carla F Shelton, Alice B Pollingue, Author

Provides a step-by-step management approach complete with planning checklists and other ready-to-use forms. Arranged sequentially, the book guides new teachers through the entire school year, from preplanning to post planning. *$ 34.95*

240 pages
ISBN 0-761931-96-6

4484 Fawcett Book Group on Learning Disabilities

Fawcett Book Group
1745 Broadway
New York, NY 10019
212-751-2600
FAX 212-572-8700
http://www.randomhouse.com
Lawrence Greene, Author
Betsy Czajka, Human Resource Associate

Case studies, anecdotal material and educational data are used to tell parents of children with learning disabilities how to recognize the symptoms of a learning problem and what steps to take to see that their children receive the remediation needed. *$12.00*
255 pages

4485 Focus on Exceptional Children

Love Publishing Company
9101 E Kenyon Avenue
Denver, CO 80237
303-221-7333
FAX 303-221-7444
http://www.lovepublishing.com
Stan Love, Owner

Published monthly except June, July, and August, get a constant flow of fresh teaching ideas-and keep up with the latest research-with this monthly newsletter that translates theory into strategies for action. Each issue focuses in depth on a single topic, such as assessment, cooperative learning, attention deficit disorders, inclusion, classroom management, discipline, and ohter timely issues. *$36.00*

4486 Frames of Reference for the Assessment of Learning Disabilities

Brookes Publishing Company
PO Box 10624
Baltimore, MD 21285
410-337-9580
800-638-3775
FAX 410-337-8539
http://www.pbrookes.com
e-mail: custserv@brookespublishing.com
G Lyon PhD, Editor

This valuable reference offers an in-depth look at the fundamental concerns facing those who work with children with learning disabilities — assessment and identification.
672 pages Hardcover
ISBN 1-557661-38-3

4487 HELP Activity Guide

Therapro
225 Arlington Street
Framingham, MA 01702
508-872-9494
800-257-5376
FAX 508-875-2062
http://www.theraproducts.com
e-mail: info@theraproducts.com
Setan Furuns, PhD, Author
Karen Conrad, Owner

Takes you easily beyond assesment to offer the important next step, thousands of practical, task-analyzed curriculum activities and intervention strategies indexed by the 650 HELP skills. With up to ten activities and strategies per skill, this valuable resource includes definitions for each skill, illustrations, cross-references to skills in other developmental areas and a glossary. *$28.00*
190 pages

4488 HELP for Preschoolers Assessment and Curriculum Guide

Therapro
225 Arlington Street
Framingham, MA 01702
508-872-9494
800-257-5376
FAX 508-875-2062
http://www.theraproducts.com
e-mail: info@theraproducts.com
Karen Conrad, Owner

Assessment procedure and instructional activities in one easy to use reference. Offers 6 sections of key information for each of the 622 skills: Definition, Materials, Assesment Procedures, Adaptions, Instructional Materials, and Instructional Activities.

4489 Handwriting: Not Just in the Hands

Therapro
225 Arlington Street
Framingham, MA 01702
508-872-9494
800-257-5376
FAX 508-875-2062
http://www.theraproducts.com
e-mail: info@theraproducts.com
Eileen Vreeland MS OTR/L, Author
Karen Conrad, Owner

Save time and provide professional services with this comprehensive resource and presentation manual! Reviews current literature and research providing an excellent knowledge base. Covers pre-writing skills, handwriting skills, handwriting instruction, ergonomics and informal assessment in the classroom, remedial and compensatory exercises. Compatible with any handwriting program, it includes reproducible handouts, ready-to-make overheads, group activities and more. *$ 80.00*
3 ring binder

4490 Helping Learning Disabled Gifted Children Learn Through Compensatory Active Play

Charles C Thomas Publisher
2600 S 1st Street
Springfield, IL 62704
217-789-8980
800-258-8980
FAX 217-789-9130
http://www.ccthomas.com
e-mail: books@ccthomas.com
James H Humphrey, Author
Michael Thomas, President

About three percent of the school population is gifted and 5-8 percent suffer from learning disabilities. These children experience a great deal more trauma than the normal child. This text will help educators deal with learning disabilities more effectively. *$36.95*
164 pages Cloth
ISBN 0-398056-95-1

4491 Helping Students Succeed in the Regular Classroom

Jossey-Bass
989 Market Street
San Francisco, CA 94103
415-433-1740
FAX 415-433-0499
http://www.josseybass.com
e-mail: dhunter@josseybass.com
Joseph Zins, Author
Debrah Hunter, President

The first book in a series from Jossey-Bass on psychoeducational interventions. Shows how to develop programs to help the learning disabled students integrate within the regular classroom situation and avoid costly and often ineffective special education classes. *$26.95*

4492 Hidden Youth: Dropouts from Special Education

Council for Exceptional Children
1110 N Glebe Road
Arlington, VA 22201
703-245-0600
888-232-7733
FAX 703-264-9494
http://www.cec.sped.org/
e-mail: service@cec.sped.org
Donald L MacMillan, Author
Drew Albritten MD, President
Bruce Ramirez, Manager

Examines the characteristics of students and schools that place students at risk for early school leaving. Discusses the accounting procedures used by different agencies for estimating graduation and dropout rates and cautions educators about using these rates as indicators of educational quality. *$8.90*

37 pages
ISBN 0-865862-11-7

4493 How Difficult Can This Be?
CT Association for Children and Adults with LD
25 Van Zant Street
Norwalk, CT 06855
203-838-5010
FAX 203-866-6108
http://www.CACLD.org
e-mail: caccld@optonline.net
Rick Lavoie, Presenter
Beryl Kaufman, Executive Director

FAT City Workshop video and discussion guide. Looks at the world through the eyes of a learning disabled child. Features a unique workshop attended by educators, psychologists, social workers, parents, siblings and a student with LD. They participate in a series of classroom activities which cause Frustration, Anxiety, and Tension-emotions all too familiar to the student with a learning disability. A discussion of topics ranging from school/home communication to social skills follows. *$49.95*
$5.00 shipping

4494 How Does Your Engine Run? A Leaders Guide to the Alert Program for Self Regulation
Therapro
225 Arlington Street
Framingham, MA 01702
508-872-9494
800-257-5376
FAX 508-875-2062
http://www.theraproducts.com
e-mail: info@theraproducts.com
Mary Sue Williams,OTR & Sherry Schellenberge,OTR, Author
Karen Conrad, Owner

Introduces the entire Alert Program. Explains how we regulate our arousal states and describes the use of sensorimotor strategies to manage levels of alertness. This program is fun for students and the adults working with them, and translates easily into real life.

4495 How Significant is Significant? A Personal Glimpse of Life with LD
Association on Higher Education and Disability
PO Box 540666
Waltham, MA 02454
781-788-0003
FAX 781-788-0033
http://www.ahead.org
e-mail: ahead@postbox.acs.ohio-state.edu
Carolee Reiling, Author

Provides a perspective not usually found in learning disability research material. *$3.50*

4496 Human Development View of Learning Disabilities: From Theory to Practice
Charles C Thomas Publisher
2600 S 1st Street
Springfield, IL 62704
217-789-8980
800-258-8980
http://www.ccthomas.com
e-mail: books@ccthomas.com
Corrine E Kass, Author
Cleborne Maddux, Author

Presents a human development model for understanding and treating age-related deficits that seem to be characteristic of individuals with learning disabilities. The ultimate purpose of this book is to present a strategy for designing day-to-day, individualized lessons for learning disabled students from kindergarten through adulthood. *$35.95*
252 pages Paper
ISBN 0-398075-65-1

4497 Implementing Cognitive Strategy Instruction Across the School: The Benchmark Manual for Teachers
Brookline Books
34 University Road
Brookline, MA 02445
617-734-6772
FAX 617-734-3952
http://www.brooklinebooks.com
Irene Gaskins, Author
Thorne Elliot, Author

Describes a classroom based program planned and executed by teachers to focus and guide students with serious reading problems to be goal oriented, planful, strategic and self-assessing. *$24.95*
Paperback
ISBN 0-914797-75-1

4498 Improving Test Performance of Students with Disabilities in the Classroom
Corwin Press
2455 Teller Road
Thousand Oaks, CA 91320
805-499-9734
800-818-7243
FAX 805-499-5323
http://www.corwinpress.com
e-mail: order@corwinpress.com
Judy L Elliott, Martha L Thurlow, Author
Kimberly Gonzales, Marketing Director
Robb Clouse, Senior Acquisitions Editor

Elliott and Thurlow, long-time colleagues at the National Center on Educational Outcomes build on their highly respected work in accountability and assessment of students with disabilities to focus now on improving test performance — with an emphasis throughout on practical application. Common learning disabilities and emotional problems and a classroom-tested, research-based list of classroom interventions. *$34.95*
232 pages Paperback
ISBN 1-412917-28-X

4499 Including Students with Severe and Multiple Disabilities in Typical Classrooms
Brookes Publishing Company
PO Box 10624
Baltimore, MD 21285
410-337-9580
800-638-3775
FAX 410-337-8539
http://www.pbrookes.com
e-mail: custserv@brookespublishing.com
Mary A Favey, PhD, Author
Reid Lyon PhD, Editor
Paul Brooks, Owner

This straightforward and jargon-free resource gives instructors the guidance needed to educate learners who have one or more sensory impairments in addition to cognitive and physical disabilities. *$32.95*
224 pages Paperback
ISBN 1-557662-39-8

4500 Inclusion: 450 Strategies for Success
Peytral Publications
PO Box 1162
Minnetonka, MN 55345
952-949-8707
877-739-8725
FAX 952-906-9777
http://www.peytral.com
e-mail: help@peytral.com
Peggy Hammeken, Owner

Commences with step-by-step guidelines to help develop, expand and improve the existing inclusive education setting. Hundreds of practical teacher tested ideas and accommodations are conveniently listed by topic and numbered for quick, easy reference. *$23.95*
192 pages Educators
ISBN 1-890455-25-3

4501 Inclusion: An Annotated Bibliography
National Clearinghouse of Rehabilitation Materials
206 W 6th Street
Stillwater, OK 74078
405-744-2000
800-223-5219
FAX 405-744-2001
TDY:405-624-3156
http://www.nchrtm.okstate.edu
e-mail: brookdj@okstate.edu
Caroline Moore, Susanne Carter, Author

This annotated bibliography is an initial compilation of recently published literature about what the special education community calls inclusion rather than mainstreaming. *$57.30*

563 pages Item # 262.007A

4502 Inclusion: An Essential Guide for the Paraprofessional
Peytral Publications
PO Box 1162
Minnetonka, MN 55345
952-949-8707
877-739-8725
FAX 952-906-9777
http://www.peytral.com
e-mail: help@peytral.com
Peggy Hammeken, President

This best-selling publication is developed specifically for paraprofessionals and classroom assistants. The book commences with a simplified introduction to inclusive education, handicapping conditions, due process, communication, collaboration, confidentiality and types of adaptations. Used by many schools and universities as a training tool for staff development. *$23.95*
205 pages Assistants
ISBN 1-890455-34-2

4503 Inclusive Elementary Schools
PEAK Parent Center
611 N Weber Street
Colorado Springs, CO 80903
719-531-9400
800-284-0251
FAX 719-531-9452
http://www.peakparent.org
e-mail: info@peakparent.org
Douglas Fisher, Nancy Frey, Caren Sax, Author

Walks readers through a state of the art, step-by-step process to determine what and how to teach elementary school students with disabilities in general education classrooms. Highlights strategies for accommodating and modifying assignments and activities by using core curriculum. Complete with user-friendly sample forms and creative support strategies, this is an essential text for elementary educators and parents. *$13.00*

4504 Individualizing Instruction for the Educationally Handicapped: Teaching Strategies
Charles C Thomas Publisher
2600 S 1st Street
Springfield, IL 62704
217-789-8980
800-258-8980
FAX 217-789-9130
http://www.ccthomas.com
e-mail: books@ccthomas.com
Jack Campbell, Author
Michael Thomas, President

Covers children that qualify for special education as well as those that are just on the cusp and do not. The author advocates that by clinically analyzing the child's learning ecology and modifying the instructional plan based on student performance, the teacher is able to design instruction appropriate for the unique needs of each child.
186 pages Cloth
ISBN 0-398069-01-8

4505 Instructional Methods for Secondary Students with Learning & Behavior Problems
Allyn & Bacon
75 Arlington Street
Boston, MA 02116
617-848-6000
http://www.ablongman.com
Patrick Schloss, Maureen Schloss, Cynthia Schloss, Author

This book presents teaching principles useful to general high school educators and special educators working with students demonstrating a variety of academic, behavioral, and social needs in secondary schools. *$89.40*
432 pages
ISBN 0-205442-36-6

4506 Intervention in School and Clinic
Pro-Ed
8700 Shoal Creek Boulevard
Austin, TX 78757
512-451-3246
800-897-3202
FAX 512-451-8542
http://www.proedinc.com
e-mail: info@proedinc.com
Randall Boone PhD, Editor
Kyle Higgins PhD, Editor

Equips teachers and clinicians with hands-on tips, techniques, methods and ideas for improving assessment, instruction, and management for individuals with learning disabilities or behavior disorders. Articles focus on curricular, instructional, social, behavioral, assessment, and vocational strategies and techniques that have a direct application to the classroom setting. This innovative and readable periodical provides educational information ready for immediate implementation
5 times a year
ISSN 1053-4512

4507 KDES Health Curriculum Guide
Harris Communications
15155 Technology Drive
Eden Prairie, MN 55344
952-906-1180
800-825-6758
FAX 952-906-1099
http://www.harriscomm.com
e-mail: info@harriscmm.com
Sara Gillespie, Author
Doris Schwartz, Author

This guide provides students with the information they need to make wise choices for healthy living. Divided into age-appropriate sections; preschool through middle school; the units cover four main areas: Health and Fitness, Safety and First Aid, Drugs, and Life. Asspendices provide resource lists and information on topics such as hygiene, street safety, teaching health.
125 pages

4508 LD Teacher's IDEA Companion (2BK Set)
LinguiSystems
3100 4th Avenue
East Moline, IL 61244
309-755-2300
800-776-4332
FAX 309-755-2377
TDY:800-933-8331
http://www.linguisystems.com
e-mail: service@linguisystems.com
Linda Bowers, Co-Owner/Co-Founder
Rosemary Huisingh, Co-Owner/Co-Founder

Help your special education students succeed in the regular classroom! Each book gives you page after page of goals and strategies to comply with current IDEA regulations. You'll get content standards, goals, benchmarks, and instructional modifications for several academic areas. You'll also get information on life skills and transition beyond high school.
Ages 5-18

4509 LD Teacher's IEP Companion
LinguiSystems
3100 4th Avenue
East Moline, IL 61244
309-755-2300
800-776-4332
FAX 309-755-2377
TDY:800-933-8331
http://www.linguisystems.com
e-mail: service@linguisystems.com
Molly Lyle, Author
Linda Bowers, Co-Owner/Co-Founder
Rosemary Huisingh, Co-Owner/Co-Founder

These IEP goals are organized developmentally by skill area with individual objectives and classroom activity suggestions. Goals and objectives cover these academic areas: math; reading; writing; literacy concepts; attention skills; study skills; classroom behavior; social interaction; and transition skills. *$39.95*
169 pages Ages 5-18

4510 Landmark School Resources
Landmark Foundation
PO Box 227
Prides Crossing, MA 01965
978-236-3216
FAX 978-927-7268
http://www.landmarkschool.org
e-mail: outreach@landmarkschool.com
Joan Steinberg, Editor
Robert Broudo, President

A compilation of 28 of the best articles available on learning disabilities and a collection of resources for parents and educators, including an annotated bibliography, sources for video and audio material, government resources, and parent/professional organizations. *$25.00*
150 pages
ISBN 0-962411-94-9

4511 Learning Disabilities in High School
Learning Disabilities Association of America
4156 Library Road
Pittsburgh, PA 15234
412-341-1515
FAX 412-344-0224
http://www.ldanatl.org
e-mail: ldanatl@usaor.net
Jane Browning, Editor-in-Chief

$3.00

4512 Learning Disabilities: Theoretical and Research Issues
Lawrence Erlbaum Associates
10 Industrial Avenue
Mahwah, NJ 07430
201-258-2200
800-926-6579
FAX 201-236-0072
http://www.erlbaum.com
H. Lee Swanson, Author
Barbara Keogh, Author

This volume has been developed as a direct result of a conference sponsored by the International Academy for Research in Learning Disabilities, held at the University of California at Los Angeles. The test provides a review and critique achievement, and subtyping as they relate to learning disabilities. *$110.00*
384 pages Hardcover
ISBN 0-805803-92-0

4513 Learning Disability: Social Class and the Construction of Inequality in American Education
Bergin & Gravey Greenwood
88 Post Road W
Westport, CT 06880
203-226-3571
800-225-5800
FAX 203-222-1502
http://www.greenwood.com
e-mail: dgoss@curry.edu
Diane Goss, Author
George Goldberg, Head of Human Resources
James Deegan, Facility Manager
Wayne Goldberg, President
In straightforward, empathic tones, authors sensitively offer support to parents of children with LD/ADD. *$22.50*
248 pages
ISBN 0-964975-20-3

4514 Mainstreaming Exceptional Students: A Guide for Classroom Teachers
Allyn & Bacon
160 Gould Street
Needham Heights, MA 02494
781-455-1250
800-852-8024
FAX 781-455-1220
http://www.ablongman.com
e-mail: exam.copies@ablongman.com
Schultz & Carpenter, Author
Bill Parke, President

Provides a clear overview of mainstreaming and public law.

4515 Making School Inclusion Work: A Guide to Everyday Practices
Brookline Books
34 University Road
Brookline, MA 02445
617-734-6772
FAX 617-734-3952
http://www.brooklinebooks.com
Katie Blenk, Author
Doris Fine, Author

Tells the reader how to conduct a truly inclusive school program that educates a diverse student body together, regardless of ethnic or racial background, economic level, or physical or cognitive ability. Indication given on what is ment by true inclusion, what inclusion is not, and who should not be conducting an inclusive program. *$24.95*
264 pages Paperback
ISBN 0-914797-96-4

4516 Meeting the Needs of Special Students: Legal, Ethical, and Practical Ramifications
Corwin Press/Sage Publications
2455 Teller Road
Thousand Oaks, CA 91320
805-499-9734
800-818-7243
FAX 805-499-5323
http://www.corwinpress.com
e-mail: order@corwinpress.com
Lawrence J Johnson & Anne M Bauer, Author
Douglas Rife, Publisher/President

School administrators in America are more likely to end up in court about a special education programme or student than for any other reason. This book gives administrators the information they need to know about the rights of students, federal guidelines, and case law and precedents and is filled with helpful hints based on experience with special students in a variety of educational settings. *$17.00*
96 pages
ISBN 0-803960-21-2

4517 Mentoring Students at Risk: An Underutilized Alternative Education Strategy...
Charles C Thomas Publisher
2600 S 1st Street
Springfield, IL 62704
217-789-8980
800-258-8980
http://www.ccthomas.com
e-mail: books@ccthomas.com
Gary Reglin, Author

Research clearly shows that mentoring is a powerful alternative education (dropout prevention) strategy for students at risk, and this text meets a demand from teachers and case workers in the juvenile justice systems for a comprehensive guide to establish mentoring programs. The book is teacher-friendly, easy to read, positive and sull of suggestions. *$20.95*
110 pages Paper
ISBN 0-398068-33-2

4518 Myofascial Release and Its Application to Neuro-Developmental Treatment
Therapro
225 Arlington Street
Framingham, MA 01702
508-872-9494
800-257-5376
FAX 508-875-2062
http://www.theraproducts.com
e-mail: info@theraproducts.com
Regi Boehme, OTR, Author
Karen Conrad, Owner

This fully illustrated resource provides the therapist with techniques to approach myofascial restrictions which are secondary to tonal dysfunction in children and adults with neurological deficits. The Neuro-Developmental Treatment approach is included in the illustrated treatment rationale.

4519 Narrative Prosthesis: Disability and the Dependencies of Discourse
University of Michigan Press
839 Greene Street
Ann Arbor, MI 48104
734-764-4392
FAX 734-615-1540
http://www.press.umich.edu
David T Mitchell, Sharon L Snyder, Author

This book develops a narrative theory of the pervasive use of disability as a device of characterization in literature and film. It argues that, while other marginalized identities have suffered cultural exclusion due to dearth of images reflecting their experience, the marginality of disabled people has occurred in the midst of the perpetual circulation of images of disability in print and visual media. *$65.00*

264 pages Cloth
ISBN 0-472097-48-7

4520 Otitis Media: Coping with the Effects in the Classroom
Harris Communications
15155 Technology Drive
Eden Prairie, MN 55344
952-906-1180
800-825-6758
FAX 952-906-1099
TDY:952-906-1198
http://www.harriscomm.com
e-mail: info@harriscmm.com
Dorinne S Davis, MA, CCC-A, Author
Robert Harris, Owner

Designed to alert teachers and specialists to the potential for communication difficulties associated with children who are prone to recurrent middle ear infections. Ideas are provided to be used to assist children toward appropriate language skill development. *$28.95*
137 pages Paperback

4521 Points of Contact: Disability, Art, and Culture
University of Michigan Press
839 Greene Street
Ann Arbor, MI 48104
734-764-4392
FAX 734-615-1540
http://www.press.umich.edu
Susan Crutchfield, Editor
Marcy Epstein, Editor

A richly diverse collection of essays, memoir, poetry and photography on aspects of disability and its representation in art. Brings together contributions by leading writers, artists, scholars, and critics to provide a remarkably broad and consistently engaging look at the intersection of disability and the arts. *$60.00*
312 pages Cloth
ISBN 0-472097-11-1

4522 Prescriptions for Children with Learning and Adjustment Problems: A Consultant's Desk Reference
Charles C Thomas Publisher
2600 S 1st Street
Springfield, IL 62704
217-789-8980
800-258-8980
http://www.ccthomas.com
e-mail: books@ccthomas.com
Ralph F Blanco, David F Bogacki, Author

264 pages Paper $37.95

4523 Preventing Academic Failure
Educators Publishing Service
PO Box 9031
Cambridge, MA 02139
617-547-6706
800-225-5750
FAX 617-547-0412
Phyllis Bertin, Eileen Perlman, Author
Gunnst Voltz, President

This multisensory curriculum meets the needs of children with learning disabilities in regular classrooms by providing a four-year sequence of written language skills (reading, writing and spelling). PAF has a handwriting and numerical program. *$42.00*

ISBN 0-838852-71-8

4524 Project Success: Meeting the Diverse Needs of Learning Disabled Adults
Richland College of the Dallas Community College
12800 Abrams Road
Dallas, TX 75243
972-238-6106
FAX 972-238-3799
http://www.rlc.dcocd.edu
Marcy Duarte, Secretary

4525 Project Upgrade: Working with Adults Who Have Learning Disabilities
Manhattan Adult Learning and Resource Center
801 Poyntz Avenue
Manhattan, KS 66502
785-539-9009
Candace White, Executive Director

4526 Promoting Postsecondary Education for Students with Learning Disabilities
Pro-Ed
8700 Shoal Creek Boulevard
Austin, TX 78757
512-451-3246
800-897-3202
FAX 512-451-8542
http://www.proedinc.com
e-mail: info@proedinc.com
Loring Brinckerhoff, Author

The second edition of this best selling book has been completely updated and expanded to include 8 entirely new chapters plus an accompanying CD-ROM appendix. These new chapters add in depth information on transition planning from high school to college; determining eligibility for services and testing accommodations; policy development; accommodation provision; service delivery options for college students with ADHD; the latest advances in assistive technology. *$54.00*
586 pages
ISBN 0-890798-72-9

4527 Rehabilitation of Clients with Specific Learning Disabilities
National Clearinghouse of Rehabilitation Materials
202 W 6th Street
Stillwater, OK 74078
405-744-2000
FAX 405-744-2001
http://www.nchrtm.okstate.edu
e-mail: brookdj@okstate.edu
Functional definitions on SLD that made adults eligible for vocational rehabilitation services are given. Three types of populations are examined and the implications for vocational rehabilitation are considered. Administrative issues are addressed to encourage rehabilitation professionals to think ahead and to develop policies for SLD. *$11.00*
100 pages

4528 Relationship of Learning Problems and Classroom Performance to Sensory Integration
Therapro
225 Arlington Street
Framingham, MA 01702
508-872-9494
800-257-5376
FAX 508-875-2062
http://www.theraproducts.com
e-mail: info@theraproducts.com
Norma Quirk, MS, OTR and Marie DiMatties, MS, OTR, Author
Karen Conrad, Owner

This is an invaluable resource written for therapists and teachers to explain how sensory integration deficits impact classroom performance.

4529 Resourcing: Handbook for Special Education RES Teachers
Council for Exceptional Children
1110 N Glebe Road
Arlington, VA 22201
888-232-7733
FAX 703-264-9494
http://www.cec.sped.org
e-mail: service@cec.sped.org
Mary Yeomans Jackson, Author
Drew Albritten MD, President
Bruce Ramirez, Manager

Be prepared to function at your best as a member of a school-based team. Resourcing wil help you take a leadership role as you work in collaboration with general classroom teachers and other practitioners. Assess your personal readiness for being a resource professional within your school. Includes many useful forms and checklists for conducting meetings and organizing your workday. *$12.00*

64 pages
ISBN 0-865862-19-2

4530 **School Age Children with Special Needs**

Special Needs Project
324 State Street
Santa Barbara, CA 93101
805-962-8087
800-333-6867
FAX 805-962-5087
e-mail: books@specialneeds.com
Dale Borman Fink, Author
Loraine Gray, Conference Coordinator

The most comprehensive survey to date of child care practice for school aged children with a wide range of disabilities. *$12.95*
148 pages

4531 **School-Home Notes: Promoting Children's Classroom Success**

Guilford Press
72 Spring Street
New York, NY 10012
800-365-7006
FAX 212-966-6708
http://www.guilford.com
e-mail: info@guilford.com
Mary Lou Kelley, Author

Describes common obstacles to parent and teacher communication and clearly explicates how these obstacles can be overcome. It provides a critical appraisal of the relevant literature on parent-and-teacher managed contingency systems and factors influencing the efficacy of the procedure. *$28.00*
198 pages Paperback
ISBN 0-898622-35-2

4532 **Scissors, Glue, and Concepts, Too!**

LinguiSystems
3100 4th Avenue
East Moline, IL 61244
309-755-2300
800-776-4332
FAX 309-755-2377
TDY:800-933-8331
http://www.linguisystems.com
e-mail: service@linguisystems.com
Linda Bowers, Co-Owner/Co-Founder
Rosemary Huisingh, Co-Owner/Co-Founder

Your young students will learn to follow directions and understand basic concepts in context. Concepts for each activity are grouped as they naturally occur in our language. Teach over 50 concepts including right/left, above/below, empty/full, and more.
Ages 5-8

4533 **Segregated and Second-Rate: Special Education in New York**

Advocates for Children of New York
151 W 30th Street
New York, NY 10001
212-947-9779
FAX 212-947-9790
http://www.advocatesforchildren.org
e-mail: info@advocatesforchildren.org
Diane K Autin Esq., Author

Highlights the fact that New York rates last among all states in inclusive education. *$15.00*

4534 **Self-Advocacy Strategy for Education and Transition Planning**

Edge Enterprises
PO Box 1304
Lawrence, KS 66044
785-749-1473
FAX 785-749-0207
e-mail: eeinfo@edgeenterprises
A Van Reusen, C Bos, J Schumaker, D Deshler, Author
Jacqueline Schafer, Managing Editor
Sue Vernon, Manager

This research-based instructor's manual features step-by-step instructions on how to teach students to advocate for themselves within the context of meetings with adults. Covered are the instruction of basic social skills, creating a personal inventory of strengths and weaknesses, creating a list of goals and using a strategy to communicate at the meeting. Individual Education Planning Conferences, Transition Planning conferences as well as other types of meetings are covered. *$15.00*
204 pages Paperback

4535 **Sensory Integration: Theory and Practice**

Therapro
225 Arlington Street
Framingham, MA 01702
508-872-9494
800-257-5376
FAX 508-875-2062
http://www.theraproducts.com
e-mail: info@theraproducts.com
Anne Fisher, Ann Bundy, Elizabeth Murray, Author
Karen Conrad, Owner

The very latest in sensory integration theory and practice. *$45.00*
418 pages

4536 **Social and Emotional Development of Exceptional Students**

Charles C Thomas Publisher
2600 S 1st Street
Springfield, IL 62704
217-789-8980
800-258-8980
FAX 217-789-9130
http://www.ccthomas.com
e-mail: books@ccthomas.com
Carroll J Jones, Author
Michael Thomas, President

Provides teachers with understandable information regarding the social and emotional development of exceptional students. *$41.95*
218 pages Cloth
ISBN 0 398057-81-8

4537 **Sopris West**

Cambium Learning
4093 Specialty Place
Longmont, CO 80504
303-651-2829
FAX 303-776-5934
http://www.sopriswest.com
Dave Cabalucci, President

IEP connections, IEP Tracker, Better IEP's, Self Directed IEP's

4538 **Source for Down Syndrome**

LinguiSystems
3100 4th Avenue
East Moline, IL 61244
309-755-2300
800-776-4332
FAX 309-755-2377
TDY:800-933-8331
http://www.linguisystems.com
e-mail: service@linguisystems.com
Linda Bowers, Co-Owner/Co-Founder
Rosemary Huisingh, Co-Owner/Co-Founder

Get in-depth information on working with students with Down sydrome. Packed with helpful tips and therapy techniques, chapters cover characteristics of Down syndrome, feeding and oral motor skills, language development and intervention, augmentative communication, motor and sensorimotor skills, and much more.

4539 **Source for Learning Disabilities**

LinguiSystems
3100 4th Avenue
East Moline, IL 61244
309-755-2300
800-776-4332
FAX 309-755-2377
TDY:800-933-8331
http://www.linguisystems.com
e-mail: service@linguisystems.com
Linda Bowers, Co-Owner/Co-Founder
Rosemary Huisingh, Co-Owner/Co-Founder

This is the definitive source for information on learning disabilities. Get new information about federal mandates, teaming, transitioning, and involving parents. You'll also have a thorough discussion of the social and emotional aspects of LD and a glossary of terms.

424 pages
ISBN 0-890795-40-1

4540 Source for Nonverbal Learning Disorders
LinguiSystems
3100 4th Avenue
East Moline, IL 61244
309-755-2300
800-776-4332
FAX 309-755-2377
TDY:800-933-8331
http://www.linguisystems.com
e-mail: service@linguisystems.com
Sue Thompson, Author
Linda Bowers, Co-Owner/Co-Founder
Rosemary Huisingh, Co-Owner/Co-Founder

Not sure if you have a student with nonverbal learning disorder? See if this description sounds familiar: ignores nonverbal cues such as facial expressions; is clumsy for no apparent reason; makes inappropriate social remarks; and has difficulty with visual-spatial-organizational tasks. This resource provides you with useful checklists, anecdotes, and methods for dealing with this little understood disorder through the lifespan. *$41.95*
Birth-Adult

4541 Source for Treatment Methodologies in Autism
LinguiSystems
3100 4th Avenue
East Moline, IL 61244
309-755-2300
800-776-4332
FAX 309-755-2377
TDY:800-933-8331
http://www.linguisystems.com
e-mail: service@linguisystems.com
Linda Bowers, Co-Owner/Co-Founder
Rosemary Huisingh, Co-Owner/Co-Founder

Get basic, factual information on the leading treatment methodologies for autism in one handy resource. You'll get clear, helpful information to share with parents and other professionals faced with treatment decisions.
Ages Birth-18

4542 Special Educators Guide to Regular Education
CT Association for Children and Adults with LD
25 Van Zant Street
Norwalk, CT 06855
203-838-5010
FAX 203-866-6108
http://www.CACLD.org
e-mail: cacld@optonline.net
L Lieberman, Author
Beryl Kaufman, Executive Director
Marie Armstrong, Information Specialist

Offers information on special education for learning disabled students. *$10.50*

4543 Strategy Assessment and Instruction for Students with Learning Disabilities
Pro-Ed
8700 Shoal Creek Boulevard
Austin, TX 78757
512-451-3246
800-897-3202
FAX 512-451-8542
http://www.proedinc.com
Lynn Meltzer, Author
Donald Hamill, Owner
Judith Voress Ph.D, Periodicals Director

The unifying theme of this volume is the view that strategic learning is a critical component of academic success and that inefficient strategy use characterizes many learning disabled students and prevents them from functioning at the level of their potential. *$41.00*

4544 Survival Guide for Kids with LD
Free Spirit Publishing
217 5th Avenue N
Minneapolis, MN 55401
612-338-2068
866-703-7322
FAX 612-337-5050
http://www.freespirit.com
Gary Fisher PhD, Rhoda Cummings EdD, Author

Has helped countless young people labeled learning disabled -and the adults who care about them. Meanwhile, laws have changed and technology has advanced. This revised and updated edition retains the best of the original edition: the warmth, affirmation, and solid information kids need to know they're smart and can learn, they just learn differently. *$12.95*
112 pages
ISBN 1-575421-19-4

4545 Take Part Art
CT Association for Children and Adults with LD
25 Van Zant Street
Norwalk, CT 06855
203-838-5010
http://www.CACLD.org
e-mail: cacld@optonline.net
Bob Gregson, Author

Offers information on art therapies and their inclusion in learning disabled environments. *$19.50*

4546 Teachers Ask About Sensory Integration
Therapro
225 Arlington Street
Framingham, MA 01702
508-872-9494
800-257-5376
FAX 508-875-2062
http://www.theraproducts.com
e-mail: info@theraproducts.com
Carol Kranowitz, Stacey Szkult and David Silver, Author
Karen Conrad, Owner

A narration and discussion for teachers and school professionals about how to teach children with sensory integration problems. 60 page book included, filled with checklists, idea sheets, sensory profiles and resorces. 86 minute audio tape.
Audio Tape

4547 Teaching Gifted Kids in the RegularClassroom CD-ROM
Free Spirit Publishing
217 5th Avenue N
Minneapolis, MN 55401
612-338-2068
800-735-7323
FAX 612-337-5050
http://www.freespirit.com
Susan Winebrenner, Author

All of the reproducibles from the book, plus many additional content organization and vocabulary charts covering study areas from art and music to math and science. Most forms are customizable. Macintosh and Windows compatible. *$ 17.95*

ISBN 1-575421-01-4

4548 Teaching Gifted Kids in the Regular Classroom
Free Spirit Publishing
217 5th Avenue N
Minneapolis, MN 55401
612-338-2068
800-735-7323
FAX 612-337-5050
http://www.freespirit.com
Susan Winebrenner, Author

A gold mine of practical, easy-to-use teaching methods, strategies, and tips, it helps teachers differentiate the curriculum in all subject areas to meet the needs of all learners - including those labeled 'slow,' 'remedial,' or 'LD,' students of poverty. English language learners, and others who struggle to learn. *$34.95*

256 pages
ISBN 1-575420-89-9

4549 Teaching Students Ways to Remember: Strategies for Learning Mnemonically

Brookline Books
34 University Road
Brookline, MA 02445
617-734-6772
FAX 617-734-3952
http://www.brooklinebooks.com
Margo Mastropieri MD, Author

This book was written in response to the enormous interest in mnemonic instruction by teachers and administrators, telling them how it can be used with their students. *$21.95*

ISBN 0-398074-77-7

4550 Teaching Visually Impaired Children

Charles C Thomas Publisher
2600 S 1st Street
Springfield, IL 62704
217-789-8980
800-258-8980
http://www.ccthomas.com
e-mail: books@ccthomas.com
Virginia E. Bishop, Author

This book provides a comprehensive resource for the classroom teacher who is working with a visually impaired child for the first time, as well as a systematic overview of education for the specialist in visual disabilities. It approaches instructional challenges with clear explanations and practical suggestions, and it addresses common concerns of teachers in a reassuring and positive manner. The book is organized into three sections: Vision, Learning, and Testing & Transitions. *$49.95*

352 pages Paper
ISBN 0-398065-95-0

4551 Technology in the Classroom: Communication Module

American Speech-Language-Hearing Association
10801 Rockville Pike
N Bethesda, MD 20852
301-897-5700
888-498-6699
FAX 301-897-7358
TDY:301-897-5700
http://www.asha.org
e-mail: epietrarton@asha.com
Laurie Ward, Marketing Coordinator
Arlene Pietranton, Executive Director

Provides a brief background of assistive technology and a detailed discussion on augmentative communication. Contains technology and strategies aimed at giving children who have disabilities, another way to communicate when speaking is difficult or impossible. *$40.00*

4552 Technology in the Classroom: Education Module

American Speech-Language-Hearing Association
10801 Rockville Pike
N Bethesda, MD 20852
301-897-5700
888-498-6699
FAX 301-897-7358
TDY:301-897-5700
http://www.asha.org
e-mail: randerson@asha.org
Laurie Ward, Marketing Coordinator
Rick Anderson, Marketing Director
Arlene Pietranton, Executive Director

Offers in-depth discussion as to how assistive technology can be used in educational settings. The technology is geared for children who have severe disabilities and provides a discussion of how to assess a child's needs for assistive technology in order to perform both pre-academic and academic tasks. *$40.00*

4553 Technology in the Classroom: Positioning, Access and Mobility Module

American Speech-Language-Hearing Association-ASHA
10801 Rockville Pike
N Bethesda, MD 20852
301-897-5700
888-498-6699
FAX 301-897-7358
TDY:301-897-5700
http://www.asha.org
e-mail: randerson@asha.org
Laurie Ward, Marketing Coordinator
Rick Anderson, Marketing Director
Arlene Pietranton, Executive Director

This manual emphasizes the importance of proper positioning that comfortably enables a child to perform activities of everyday life, and the technology which is available to help children move about when they are physically unable to do so. *$35.00*

4554 Test Accommodations for Students with Disabilities

Charles C Thomas Publisher
2600 S 1st Street
Springfield, IL 62704
217-789-8980
800-258-8980
FAX 217-789-9130
http://www.ccthomas.com
e-mail: books@ccthomas.com
Edward Burns, Author
Michael Thomas, President

The purpose here is to consider legal questions, theoretical issues, and practical methods for meeting the assessment needs of students with disabilities. The ultimate goal of this book is to consider a variety of concerns and to provide several ideas for conceptualizing and implementing valid test accommodations. *$66.95*

340 pages Cloth
ISBN 0-398068-44-5

4555 The Strangest Song

Prometheus Books
59 John Glenn Drive
Amherst, NY 14228
716-691-0133
800-421-0351
FAX 716-691-0137
http://www.prometheusbooks.com
e-mail: mrogers@prometheusbooks.com
Marcia Rogers, Sales Manager

The first book to tell the story of Williams syndrome and the extraordinary musicality of many of the people who have it. An insppiring blend of human interest and breakthrough science, offers startling insights into the mysteries of the brian and hope that science can find new ways to help the handicapped. *$24.00*

300 pages
ISBN 1-591024-78-1

4556 To Be Gifted and Learning Disabled: From Definitions to Practical Intervention Strategies

Creative Learning Press
PO Box 320
Mansfield Center, CT 06250
860-429-8118
888-518-8004
FAX 860-429-7783
http://www.creativelearningpress.com
e-mail: clp@neca.com
Susan M Baum, Steven V Owen, John Dixon, Author
Kristina Morgan, Executive Director

The gifted and learning disabled child exhibits remarkable talents in some areas and disabling weakness in others. Covers everything a classroom or enrichment teacher must know in order to address the needs of gifted learning disabled youngsters, including identification, learning styles, and more. *$16.95*

149 pages
ISBN 0-936386-59-2

4557 To Teach a Dyslexic

AVKO Educational Research Foundation
3084 W Willard Road
Clio, MI 48420
866-285-6612
FAX 810-686-1101
http://www.avko.org
e-mail: avkoemail@aol.com
Don McCabe, Author

Just as it takes a thief to catch a thief, this is an autobiography of a dyslexic who discovered how to teach dyslexics. Common sense, logical approach, valuable to all who teach in our nation's classrooms. *$14.95*

288 pages
ISBN 1-564000-04-4

4558 **Tools for Transition**

AGS
PO Box 99
Circle Pines, MN 55014
763-786-4343
800-328-2560
FAX 763-786-9077
http://www.agsnet.com
e-mail: agsmail@agsnet.com

Kevin Brueggenan, Manager

The materials in this kit offer a curriculum that is not always included in learning disabled programs. Comes with a teacher's manual, complete with instructions for each unit and a Student Workbook filled with skill-building activities. The accompanying video presents a variety of sciences to demonstrate plus an interview with college students who have learning disabilities.

4559 **Understanding & Management of Health Problems in Schools: Resource Manual**

Temeron Books
PO Box 896
Bellingham, WA 98227
FAX 360-738-4016
http://www.temerondetselig.com
e-mail: temeron@telusplanet.net

H Moghadam, Author

Intended as a supplement to information given by parents and physicians, this book is a valuable aid to teachers and other school personnel in regards to some of the primary health issues that affect children and adolescents. *$ 13.95*

152 pages
ISBN 1-550591-21-5

4560 **Understanding and Managing Vision Deficits**

Therapro
225 Arlington Street
Framingham, MA 01702
508-872-9494
800-257-5376
FAX 508-875-2062
http://www.theraproducts.com
e-mail: info@theraproducts.com

Mitchell Scheiman, OD, Author
Karen Conrad, Owner

This book is a unique and comprehensive collaboration from OT's and optometrists developed to increase the understanding of vision. Learn to screen for common visual deficits and effectively manage patients with vision disorders. Provides recommendations for direct intervention techniques for a variety of vision problems and supportive and compensatory stratagies for visual field deficits and visual neglect.

4561 **Working Memory and Severe Learning Difficulties**

Lawrence Erlbaum Associates
10 Industrial Avenue
Mahwah, NJ 07430
201-258-2200
800-926-6579
FAX 201-236-0072
http://www.erlbaum.com

Charles Hulme, Author
Judy Nam, Owner

This monograph considers the development of working memory skills in children with severe learning difficulties. These children have marked difficulties with a wide range of cognitive tasks. The studies reported show that they also experience profound difficulties on verbal working memory tasks. *$29.95*

160 pages
ISBN 0-863770-75-4

4562 **Working with Visually Impaired Young Students: A Curriculum Guide for 3 to 5 Year-Olds**

Charles C Thomas Publisher
2600 S 1st Street
Springfield, IL 62704
217-789-8980
800-258-8980
http://www.ccthomas.com
e-mail: books@ccthomas.com

Ellen Trief, Author

The purpose of this guide is to offer a curriculum model to preschool programs that provides services to visually impaired 3 to 5 year olds with emphasis on the need for psychological evaluations to establish the preschooler's cognitive and intellectual level of functioning, basic pre-braille concepts, orientation and mobility, activities that help facilitate speech and language learning, art therapy methods, and the application of music therapy to improve motor, language, and social skills. *$42.95*

208 pages Spiral Paper
ISBN 0-398068-75-2

Language Arts

4563 **Clinical Interview: A Guide for Speech-Language Pathologists/Audiologists**

American Speech-Language-Hearing Association
10801 Rockville Pike
N Bethesda, MD 20852
301-897-5700
888-498-6699
FAX 301-897-7358
TDY:301-897-5700
http://www.asha.org
e-mail: randerson@asha.org

Laurie Ward, Marketing Coordinator
Rick Anderson, Marketing Director
Arlene Pietranton, Executive Director

Integrates the components of the clinical interview within the context of the speech-language pathology and audiology helping process. *$9.00*

4564 **Closer Look: The English Program at the Model Secondary School for the Deaf**

Harris Communications
15155 Technology Drive
Eden Prairie, MN 55344
952-906-1180
800-825-6758
FAX 952-906-1099
TDY:952-906-1198
http://www.harriscomm.com
e-mail: info@harriscmm.com

MSSD English Teachers, Author
Robert Harris, Owner

Features research-supported principles for incorporating the whole language philosophy into classroom routines, highlighting student-centered activities. Strategies are outlined for determining student levels based largely on the degree of teacher guidance needed. Reading and writing objectives are provided for grades 8-12. *$9.95*

67 pages

4565 **Communication Skills for Visually Impaired Learners**

Charles C Thomas Publisher
2600 S 1st Street
Springfield, IL 62704
217-789-8980
800-258-8980
http://www.ccthomas.com
e-mail: books@ccthomas.com

Randall Harley, Mila B. Truan & LaRhea D. Sanford, Author

Designed to provide a foundation for a better understanding of teaching reading, writing, and listening skills to students with visual impairments from preschool age through adult levels. The plan of the book incorporates the latest research finding with the practical experiences learned in the classroom. *$57.95*

322 pages Paper
ISBN 0-398066-93-2

4566 **First Start in Sign Language**

Harris Communications
15155 Technology Drive
Eden Prairie, MN 55344
952-906-1180
800-825-6758
FAX 952-906-1099
http://www.harriscomm.com
e-mail: info@harriscmm.com

Amy J Strommer, Author

Fun pictures, stories, and activities are all included in this introduction to American Sign Language. Students first learn to sign words for people, animals, objects and actions. Then they learn to produce simple sentences and to sign stories. Reproducible activity pages are included throughout the book. For students in kindergarten through sixth grade. *$32.00*
190 pages Paperback

4567 From Talking to Writing: Strategies forScaffolding Expository Expression
Landmark School
429 Hale Street
Prides Crossing, MA 01965
978-236-3000
FAX 978-927-7268
http://www.landmarkoutreach.org
e-mail: outreach@landmarkschool.org
Terrill Jennings and Charles Haynes, Author

Designed for teachers who work with students who have difficulty with writing and/or expressive language skills, this book provides practical strategies for teaching expository expression at the word, sentence, paragraph, and short essay levels. *$25.00*
191 pages

4568 Helping Young Writers Master the Craft
Brookline Books
300 Bedford Street
Manchester, NH 03101
617-734-6772
FAX 603-922-3348
http://www.brooklinebooks.com
Karen R Harris, Author

This text for teachers will help the beginning writer, the unmotivated student and the learning disabled student to learn writing. *$24.95*

4569 Language Learning Everywhere We Go
Harris Communications
15155 Technology Drive
Eden Prairie, MN 55344
952-906-1180
800-825-6758
FAX 952-906-1099
TDY:952-906-1198
http://www.harriscomm.com
e-mail: info@harriscmm.com
Cecilia Casas, Author
Robert Harris, Owner

Students learn the vocabulary associated with each situation that they encounter on their travels with Bernardo Bear. Questions and vocabulary lists are included in English and Spanish for each picture. The 103 situational pictures may all be reproduced. *$34.00*
209 pages Paperback

4570 Making the Writing Process Work: Strategies for Composition & Self-Regulation
Brookline Books
34 University Road
Brookline, MA 02445
617-734-6772
FAX 617-734-3952
http://www.brooklinebooks.com
Karen Harris, Author
Steve Graham, Author

Presents cognitive strategies for writing sequences of specific steps which make the writing process clearer and enable students to organize their thoughts about the writing task. The strategies help students know how to turn thoughts into writing products. This is especially important for students having difficulty producing acceptable writing products, but all students benefit from learning these procedures. *$24.95*

ISBN 1-571290-10-9

4571 Multisensory Teaching Approach
Deta Corporation
PO Box 9031
Cambridge, MA 02139
617-547-6706
800-225-5750
FAX 617-547-0412
http://www.epsbooks.com
e-mail: eps@epsbooks.com
Margaret Taylor Smith, Author
Gunnar Voltz, President

MTA is a comprehensive, multisensory program in reading, spelling, cursive handwriting, and alphabet and dictionary skills for both regular and remedial instruction. Ungraded, MTA is based on the Orton-Gillingham techniques and Alphabetic Phonics.

4572 Problems in Written Expression: Assessment and Remediation
Guilford Press
72 Spring Street
New York, NY 10012
800-365-7006
FAX 212-966-6708
http://www.guilford.com
e-mail: info@guilford.com
Sharon Bradley-Johnson, Author
Jusi Lesiak, Author
Bob Matloff, President
A great resource for speech-language pathologists, counselors, resource specialists and other special educators. *$20.95*
178 pages Paperback

4573 Report Writing in the Field of Communication Disorders
American Speech-Language-Hearing Association
10801 Rockville Pike
N Bethesda, MD 20852
301-897-5700
888-498-6699
FAX 301-897-7358
TDY:301-897-5700
http://www.asha.org
e-mail: randerson@asha.org
Laurie Ward, Marketing Coordinator
Rick Anderson, Marketing Director
Arlene Pietranton, Executive Director
Stresses the summarization and interpretation of vital information and highlights matters of ethics, privacy and more. *$7.00*

4574 Signs of the Times
Harris Communications
15155 Technology Drive
Eden Prairie, MN 55344
952-906-1180
800-825-6758
FAX 952-906-1099
http://www.harriscomm.com
e-mail: info@harriscmm.com
Edgar H Shroyer, Author

Containing 1,185 signs in 41 lessons, this classroom text is an excellent beginning Pidgin or Contact Sign English book that fills the gap between sign language dictionaries and American Sign Language texts. Each lesson contains clearly illustrated vocabulary, English glosses and synonyms, sample sentences to defice vocabulary context, and sentences for practice. *$34.95*
433 pages Softcover

4575 Slingerland-Multisensory Approach to Language Arts for Specific Language Disability Children
Deta Corporation
PO Box 9031
Cambridge, MA 02139
617-547-6706
800-225-5750
FAX 617-547-0412
http://www.epsbooks.com
e-mail: eps@epsbooks.com
Beth H Slingerland, Author
Gunnar Voltz, President

This adaptation of the Orton-Gillingham approach for classroom teachers provides a phonetically structured introduction to reading, writing and spelling. Books 1 and 2 are for first and second grade, Book 3 for primary classrooms and older students. Numerous supplementary materials are available.

4576 Source for Processing Disorders
LinguiSystems
3100 4th Avenue
East Moline, IL 61244
309-755-2300
800-776-4332
FAX 309-755-2377
TDY:800-933-8331
http://www.linguisystems.com
e-mail: service@linguisystems.com

Linda Bowers, Co-Owner/Co-Founder
Rosemary Huisingh, Co-Owner/Co-Founder

This great resource helps you differentiate between language processing disorders and auditory processing disorders. Chapters cover: the neurology of processing and learning; the central auditory processing model; the language processing model; and a lot more!
Ages 5-Adult

4577 Source for Syndromes
LinguiSystems
3100 4th Avenue
East Moline, IL 61244
309-755-2300
800-776-4332
FAX 309-755-2377
TDY:800-933-8331
http://www.linguisystems.com
e-mail: service@linguisystems.com
Gail J Richard, Debra Reichert Hoge, Author
Linda Bowers, Co-Owner/Co-Founder
Rosemary Huisingh, Co-Owner/Co-Founder

Do you often wish someone would just tell you what to do with a specific youngster on your caseload? The Source for Syndromes can do just that. Learn about the speech-language characteristics for each sydrome with a focus on communication issues. This resource covers pertinent information for such sydromes such as Angelman, Asperger's, Autism, Rett's, Tourette's, Williams, and more. *$41.95*
117 pages Ages Birth-18

4578 Teaching Language-Deficient Children: Theory and Application of the Association Method
Educators Publishing Service
PO Box 9031
Cambridge, MA 02139
617-547-6706
800-225-5750
FAX 617-547-0412
http://www.epsbooks.com
e-mail: eps@epsbooks.com
N Etoile duBard and Maureen K Martin, Author
Gunnar Voltz, President

This revised and expanded edition of Teaching Aphasics and Other Language Deficient Children offers information on its theory, implementation of the method and sample curriculum.
$42.00
360 pages
ISBN 0-838823-40-8

4579 Thematic Instruction: Teacher's Primer for Developing Speaking & Writing Skill
Landmark Foundation
PO Box 227
Prides Crossing, MA 01965
978-236-3216
FAX 978-927-7268
http://www.landmarkschool.org
e-mail: outreach@landmarkschool.org
Terrill Jennings, Author
Charles Haynes, Author
Joan Sedita, Outreach Program
This book introduces teachers to a theme-centered approach to expressive language skills instruction. It is designed for classroom teachers who are teaching speaking and writing skills. It combines a structured, skills-based approach with thematic orientation. *$20.00*

4580 Visualizing and Verbalizing for Language Comprehension/Thinking
Academy of Reading
416 Higuera Street
San Luis Obispo, CA 93401
805-541-3836
800-233-1819
FAX 805-541-8756
Nanci Bell, Author
Nanci Bell, CEO

This book identifies the important sensory connection that imagery provides and teaches specific techniques. Specific steps and sample dialog are presented. Summary pages after each step make it easy to implement the program in the classroom.
284 pages
ISBN 0-945856-01-6

4581 Writing: A Landmark School Teaching Guide
Landmark School
429 Hale Street
Prides Crossing, MA 01965
978-236-3216
FAX 978-927-7268
http://www.landmarkoutreach.org
e-mail: outreach@landmarkschool.org
Jean Gudaitis Tarricone, Author

This book offers strategies for teaching writing at the paragraph and short essay levels. It emphasizees the integration of language and critical thinking skills within a five-step writing process. Sample templates and graphic organizers as well as exercises that teachers can use in their classrooms are included.
$25.00
92 pages

Math

4582 Landmark Method for Teaching Arithmetic
Landmark School
429 Hale Street
Prides Crossing, MA 01965
978-236-3000
FAX 978-927-7268
http://www.landmarkoutreach.org
e-mail: outreach@landmarkschool.org
Christopher Woodin, Author

This book is written for teachers who work with students having difficulty learning math. It includes practical strategies for teaching multiplication, division, word problems, and math facts. It also introduces the reader to two learning tools developed at Landmark — Woodin Ladders and Woodmark Icons. Sample templates and exercises are included. *$2.50*
145 pages

4583 Math and the Learning Disabled Student: A Practical Guide for Accommodations
Academic Success Press
PO Box 132
Bradenton, FL 34206
941-746-1645
800-444-2524
FAX 800-777-2525
P Nolting, Author
Mary Liscio, Editor
Paul Nolting, Owner

More and more learning disabled students are experiencing difficulty passing mathematics. The book is especially written for counselors and mathematics instructors of learning disabled students, and provides information on accommodations for students with different types of learning disabilities.
91 pages
ISBN 0-940287-23-4

4584 Moving Toward the Standards: A National Action Plan for Math Education Reform for the Deaf
Harris Communications
15155 Technology Drive
Eden Prairie, MN 55344
952-906-1180
800-825-6758
FAX 952-906-1099
TDY:952-906-1198
http://www.harriscomm.com
e-mail: info@harriscmm.com
Robert Harris, Owner

Offers help for teachers working with students who are deaf and hard of hearing by presenting the most current, practical approaches to math instruction.

750 pages

4585 Teaching Mathematics to Students with Learning Disabilities
Pro-Ed
8700 Shoal Creek Boulevard
Austin, TX 78757
512-451-3246
800-897-3202
FAX 512-451-8542
http://www.proedinc.com
Nancy Bley, Carol A Thornton, Author

Offers information on problem-solving, estimation and the use of computers in teaching mathematics to the child with learning disabilities. *$470.00*

Preschool

4586 Access for All: Integrating Deaf, Hard of Hearing, and Hearing Preschoolers
Harris Communications
15155 Technology Drive
Eden Prairie, MN 55344
952-906-1180
800-825-6758
FAX 952-906-1099
TDY:952-906-1198
http://www.harriscomm.com
e-mail: info@harriscmm.com
Gail Solit, Author
Robert Harris, Owner
Maral Taylor, Author
Covers basic information needed to establish a successful preschool program for deaf and hearing children; interagency cooperation, staff training, and parental involvement. *$29.95*
169 pages Video-90 min.

4587 Administrator's Policy Handbook for Preschool Mainstreaming
Brookline Books
34 University Road
Brookline, MA 02445
617-734-6772
FAX 617-734-3952
http://www.brooklinebooks.com
Barbara J Smith, Deborah Rose, Author

Prepared specifically for the public school administrator who is developing the policies and procedures to place young children with disabilities in mainstreamed settings. *$39.95*
150 pages

4588 KDES Preschool Curriculum Guide
Harris Communications
15155 Technology Drive
Eden Prairie, MN 55344
952-906-1180
800-825-6758
FAX 952-906-1099
TDY:952-906-1198
http://www.harriscomm.com
e-mail: info@harriscmm.com
Robert Harris, Owner

A complete, four-year program developed for preschool children who are deaf or hard of hearing. The guide offers a comprehensive scope and sequence of objectives, resource units and evaluation tools: a sample instructional unit; a bibliography; and a record-keeping system for student progress. Also contains general information for teachers and administrators, including how to modify the program for children with special needs.
327 pages

4589 When Slow Is Fast Enough: Educating the Delayed Preschool Child
Guilford Press
72 Spring Street
New York, NY 10012
800-365-7006
FAX 212-966-6708
http://www.guilford.com
e-mail: info@guilford.com
Joan F Goodman, Author

This bold and controversial book asks what we are accomplishing in early intervention programs that attempt to accelerate development in delayed young children. She questions the value of such programs on educational, psychological, and moral grounds, suggesting that in pressuring these children to perform more, and sooner, we undermine their capacity for independent development and deprive them of the freedom we insist upon for the nondelayed. *$29.00*
306 pages Paperback
ISBN 0-898624-91-6

Reading

4590 Gillingham Manual
Educators Publishing Service
PO Box 9031
Cambridge, MA 02139
617-547-6706
800-225-5750
FAX 617-547-0412
http://www.epsbooks.com
e-mail: eps@epsbooks.com
Anna Gillingham Bessie W Stillman, Author
Gunnar Voltz, President

This classic in the field of specific language disability has now been completely revised and updated. The manual covers reading, spelling, writing and dictionary technique. It may be used with individuals or small groups. *$60.00*
352 pages
ISBN 0-838802-00-1

4591 Phonic Remedial Reading Lessons
Academic Therapy Publications
20 Commercial Boulevard
Novato, CA 94949
415-883-3314
888-287-9975
FAX 415-883-3720
http://www.atpub.com
e-mail: atpub@aol.com
Jim Arena
Joanne Urban

A step-by-step program for teaching reading to children who failed to learn by conventional methods. Consistent sound-symbol relationships are presented and reinforced using a grapho-vocal method. *$15.00*
144 pages
ISBN 0-878795-08-1

4592 Phonology and Reading Disability
University of Michigan Press
839 Greene Street
Ann Arbor, MI 48104
734-764-4388
FAX 734-615-1540
http://www.press.umich.edu
Donald Shankweiler, Editor
Isabelle Y Liberman, Editor

Discusses the importance to the learning process of the phonological structures of words. *$52.50*
184 pages Cloth
ISBN 0-472101-33-7

4593 Preventing Reading Difficulties in Young Children
National Academies Press
PO Box 285
Washington, DC 20055
202-334-3313
800-624-6242
FAX 202-334-1891
http://www.nap.edu
Catherine Snow, Susan Burns, Peg Griffin, Author

Explores how to prevent reading difficulties in the context of social, historical, cultural, and biological factors. *$34.16*

448 pages Hardback
ISBN 0-309064-18-X

4594 Readability Revisited: The New Dale-Chall Readability Formula
Brookline Books
34 University Road
Brookline, MA 02445
617-734-6772
FAX 617-734-3952
http://www.brooklinebooks.com
Jeanne Chall, Author
Edgar Dale, Author

Information is given on reading difficulties in children with learning disabilities and how to overcome them. *$29.95*
168 pages
ISBN 1-571290-08-7

4595 Reading Problems: Consultation and Remediation
Guilford Press
72 Spring Street
New York, NY 10012
800-365-7006
FAX 212-966-6708
http://www.guilford.com
e-mail: info@guilford.com
PG Aaron, Author
R Malatesha Joshi, Author

Designed to both help school psychologists and reading specialists effectively assume the consultation role, this volume provides an overview of reading problems while serving as a guide to effective practice. *$42.00*
285 pages

4596 Reading Programs that Work: A Review of Programs From Pre-K to 4th Grade
Milken Family Foundation
1250 4th Street
Santa Monica, CA 90401
310-570-4800
FAX 310-570-4801
http://www.mff.org
Dr. John Schacter, Author

This publication tackles two questions, joining the research behind why children fail to read with research on effective solutions to reverse this failure. Included in the reading report are analyses of 35 different reading programs and their impact on student achievement.
72 pages

4597 Reading and Learning Disabilities: A Resource Guide
NICHCY
PO Box 1492
Washington, DC 20013
202-884-8200
800-695-0285
FAX 202-884-8841
TDY:800-695-0285
http://www.nichcy.org
e-mail: nichcy@aed.org
Donna Waghorn, Assistant Executive
Susan Ripley, Manager

12 pages

4598 Reading and Learning Disability: A Neuropsychological Approach to Evaluation & Instruction
Charles C Thomas Publisher
2600 S 1st Street
Springfield, IL 62704
217-789-8980
800-258-8980
http://www.ccthomas.com
e-mail: books@ccthomas.com
Estelle L Fryburg, Author

This text utilizes the current knowledge of neuropsychology (brain-behavior relationships) and the concepts of cognitive psychology to provide an understanding of reading and learning disability which has a practical application to education. This book's primary goal is to provide teachers, psychologists, physicians, concerned professionals, and parents with an interdisciplinary view of learning and schooling. *$74.95*
398 pages Paper
ISBN 0-398067-45-8

4599 Reading-Writing-Rage: The Terrible Price Paid by Victims of School Failure
Jalmar Press
PO Box 370
Fawnskin, CA 92333
310-816-3085
FAX 310-816-3092
http://www.jalmarpress.com
DF Ungerleider, Author

4600 Starting Out Right: A Guide to Promoting Children's Reading Success
National Academies Press
500 Fifth Street NW
Washington, DC 20055
202-334-3313
888-624-8373
FAX 202-334-2451
http://www.nap.edu
Susan Burns, Peg Griffin, Catherine Snow, Author

This book discusses how best to help children succeed in reading. This book also includes 55 activities yo do with children to help them become successful readers, a list of recommended children's books, and a guide to CD-ROMs and websites. A must read for specialists in primary education as well as pediatricians, childcare providers, tutors, literacy advocates, and parents. *$13.46*
192 pages
ISBN 0-309064-10-4

4601 Teaching Reading to Disabled and Handicapped Learners
Charles C Thomas Publisher
2600 S 1st Street
Springfield, IL 62704
217-789-8980
800-258-8980
http://www.ccthomas.com
e-mail: books@ccthomas.com
Harold D Love and Freddie W Litton, Author

A significant contribution in helping the many children, adolsescents, and adults who encounter difficulty with reading. Designed as a text for undergraduate and graduate students, it guides prospective and present special education teachers in assisting and teaching handicapped learners to read. The text integrates traditional methods with newer perspectives to provide an effective reading program in special education. *$43.95*
260 pages Paperback
ISBN 0-398062-48-4

4602 Teaching the Dyslexic Child
Academic Therapy Publications
20 Commercial Boulevard
Novato, CA 94949
415-883-3314
888-287-9975
FAX 415-883-3720
http://www.atpub.com
e-mail: atpub@aol.com
Anita Griffiths, Author
Jim Arena
Joanne Urban

Dyslexia can be crushing to a child's self-image. The author shows teachers and parents how to focus on the child's ability and become a partner inlearning to help restore a positive self-image. *$13.00*
128 pages
ISBN 0-878792-05-8

4603 Textbooks and the Students Who Can't Read Them
Brookline Books
34 University Road
Brookline, MA 02445
617-734-6772
FAX 617-734-3952
http://www.brooklinebooks.com
Jean Ciborowski, Author

This book proposes how to involve low readers more effectively in textbook learning. It presents instructional techniques to improve students' willingness to work in mainstream textbooks. *$21.95*

Paperback
ISBN 0-914797-57-3

4604 Why Wait for a Criterion of Failure?
Educators Publishing Service
PO Box 9031
Cambridge, MA 02139
617-547-6706
800-225-5750
FAX 617-547-0412
http://www.epsbooks.com
e-mail: eps@epsbooks.com
B Slingerland, Author
Gunnar Voltz, President

A monograph concerning the teaching of reading to learning disabled students using the multi-sensory approach, which is the crux of the Orton-Gillingham approach. This book describes structured lessons, with sample word lists, and reading lessons. *$6.00*
48 pages
ISBN 0-838802-43-5

Social Skills

4605 ADHD in the Schools: Assessment andIntervention Strategies
Guilford Press
72 Spring Street
New York, NY 10012
800-365-7006
FAX 212-966-6708
http://www.guilford.com
e-mail: info@guilford.com
George DuPaul, Gary Stoner, Author

This popular reference and text provides essential guidance for school-based professionals meeting the challenges of ADHD at any grade level. Comprehensive and practical, the book includes several reproducible assessment tools and handouts. *$29.00*
330 pages
ISBN 1-593850-89-1

4606 Behavior Change in the Classroom: Self-Management Interventions
Guilford Press
72 Spring Street
New York, NY 10012
800-365-7006
FAX 212-966-6708
http://www.guilford.com
e-mail: info@guilford.com
Edward Shapiro, Christine Cole, Author

This book presents practical approaches for designing and implementing self-management interventions in school settings. Rich with detailed instruction, the volume covers the conceptual foundation for the development of self-management from both contingency management and cognitive-behavioral perspectives. *$35.00*
204 pages
ISBN 0-898623-66-9

4607 Group Activities to Include Students with Special Needs

Corwin Press/Sage Publications
2455 Teller Road
Thousand Oaks, CA 91320
805-499-9734
800-233-9936
FAX 805-499-5323
http://www.corwinpress.com
e-mail: order@corwinpress.com
Julia Wilkins, Author

This hands-on resource offers 120 group activities emphasizing participation, cooperation, teamwork, mutual support, and improved self-esteem. This practical guide provides instant activities that can be used without preparation and incorporated into the daily routine with ease and confidence. Classroom games, gym and outdoor games, and ball games are designed to help your students gain the valuable skills they need to interact appropriately within the school setting. *$34.95*
240 pages
ISBN 0-761977-26-1

4608 Joy of Listening
Harris Communications
15155 Technology Drive
Eden Prairie, MN 55344
952-906-1180
800-825-6758
FAX 952-906-1099
TDY:952-906-1198
http://www.harriscomm.com
e-mail: info@harriscmm.com
Janice Baliker Light, Author
Robert Harris, Owner

Includes lessons that improve listening skills, auditory discrimination, attention span, and memory in hearing-impaired children and adults. Also recommended for learning-disabled children with auditory weaknesses. Many of the sections may be used for teaching lipreading skills. *$12.95*
148 pages Paperback

4609 Key Concepts in Personal Development
Marsh Media
8082 Ward Parkway Plaza
Kansas City, MO 64114
816-523-1059
800-821-3303
FAX 866-333-7421
http://www.marshmedia.com
e-mail: info@marshmedia.com
Joan Marsh, Owner
Liz Sweeney, Editorial Assistant

Puberty Education for Children with Special Needs. Comprehensive, gender-specific kits and supplemental parent packets address human sexuality education for children with mild to moderate developmental disabilities.

4610 Progress Program
Edge Enterprises
PO Box 1304
Lawrence, KS 66044
785-749-1473
FAX 785-749-0207
e-mail: eeinfo@edgeenterprises
Jean Schumaker, Melbourne Hovell, James Sherman, Author
Jacqueline Schafer, Managing Editor
Sue Vernon, Manager

Describes how teachers, administrators and parents can work together to use a Daily Report Card Program to control disruptive student behavior and improve the academic and social performance of students who are at-risk for failure. This program is carefully sequenced to move from extrinsic control to student (intrinsic) control of behavior. *$10.00*
96 pages Paperback

4611 Teaching Social Skills to Hearing Impaired Students
Harris Communications
15155 Technology Drive
Eden Prairie, MN 55344
952-906-1180
800-825-6758
FAX 952-906-1099
TDY:952-906-1198
http://www.harriscomm.com
e-mail: info@harriscmm.com
Robert Harris, Owner
Maureen Smith MA, Author

Provides teachers and parents with a comprehensive, hands-on program to develop important social skills in hearing-impaired children and young adults. *$24.95*
203 pages Paperback

4612 Training for Independent Living Curriculum
RPM Press
PO Box 31483
Tucson, AZ 85751
520-886-1990
888-810-1990
FAX 520-886-1990
Paul McCray, President
Jan Stonebraker, Operations Manager

Provides educators and rehabilitation personnel with a 400 page curriculum designed to help teach developmentally disabled and other severely challenged persons essential independent living skills including personal and social adjustment, money management, meal preparation, money handling, personal safety, grooming and more. *$79.95*

Publications

4613 **Above and Beyond**
AASCU
1 Dupont Circle NW
Washington, DC 20036 202-736-5800
FAX 202-833-4760
Jade Ann Gingerich, Author
V Barmore, Manager

Describes college services for students with learning disabilities. *$8.00*
32 pages

4614 **Assisting College Students with Learning Disabilities: A Tutor's Manual**
Association on Higher Education and Disability
PO Box 540666
Waltham, MA 02454 781-788-0003
FAX 781-788-0033
http://www.ahead.org
e-mail: ahead@postbox.acs.ohio-state.edu
This resource manual is for service providers who want to take concrete action toward integrating women with disabilities into the mainstream of college life. *$9.95*

4615 **Campus Opportunities for Students with Learning Differences**
Octameron Associates
PO Box 2748
Alexandria, VA 22301 703-836-5480
FAX 703-836-5650
http://www.octameron.com
Judith & Stephen Crooker, Author
Anna Leider, President
J Katz, Public Relations Director

A book about going to college for young adults with various types of learning disabilities. Details questions to ask in selecting a college. CAMPUS OPPORTUNITIES teaches how to be a self-advocate. *$5.00*
36 pages Biannual
ISBN 1-575090-52-X

4616 **Chronicle Financial Aid Guide**
Chronicle Guidance Publications
66 Aurora Street
Moravia, NY 13118 315-497-0330
800-622-7284
FAX 315-497-3359
http://www.chronicleguidance.com
e-mail: janet@chronicleguidance.com
Janet Seemann, Managing Editor
Gary Fickeisen, Vice President

Offers information on more than 1,950 financial aid programs, offering over 400,000 awards from current, verified sources. *$25.49*
460 pages Annual
ISBN 1-556313-33-0

4617 **College Placement Council Directory**
College Placement Council
62 Highland Avenue
Bethlehem, PA 18017 610-868-1421
800-544-5272
http://www.naceweb.org
Marilyn Mackes, Executive Director

Offers the who's who in the college placement/recruitment field. *$47.95*

4618 **Directory of Catholic Special EducationPrograms and Facilities**
National Catholic Education Association
1077 30th Street NW
Washington, DC 20007 202-337-6232
FAX 202-333-6706
http://www.ncea.org
e-mail: nceadmin@ncea.org
Michael Guerra, President

A valuable resource for anyone seeking appropriate placements in Catholic settings. *$8.00*
100 pages
ISBN 1-558330-11-9

4619 **Dispelling the Myths: College Students and Learning Disabilities**
National Center for Learning Disabilities
381 Park Avenue S
New York, NY 10016 212-545-7510
888-575-7373
FAX 212-545-9665
http://www..ld.org
e-mail: help@ncld.org
James Wendors, Director
Marcia Pauyo, Executive Assistant
Marcia Griffith, Marketing Executive
A monograph for students and educators that explains what learning disabilities are and what faculty members can do to help students with learning disabilities achieve success in college.

4620 **Four-Year College Databook**
Chronicle Guidance Publications
66 Aurora Street
Moravia, NY 13118 315-497-0330
800-622-7284
FAX 315-497-3359
http://www.ChronicleGuidance.com
e-mail: janet@chronicleguidance.com
Janet Seemann, Managing Editor
Nancy Carmody, Marketing
Gary Fickeisen, Vice President
Chronicle Four-Year College Databook contains two sections: The Four-Year College Majors section lists 2,160 institutions offering 790 four-year graduate and professional majors. *$24.99*

487 pages Annual
ISBN 1-556312-92-X

4621 **From Access to Equity**
Association on Higher Education and Disability
PO Box 540666
Waltham, MA 02454 781-788-0003
FAX 781-788-0033
http://www.ahead.org
e-mail: ahead@postbox.acs.ohio-state.edu
This resource manual is for service providers who want to take concrete action toward integrating women with disabilities into the mainstream of college life. *$9.95*

4622 **Getting LD Students Ready for College**
HEATH Resource Center
2121 K Street NW
Washington, DC 20037 202-337-7600
800-544-3284
FAX 202-973-0908
http://www.heath.gwu.edu
e-mail: askheath@askheath.gwu.edu
Janine Heath, Manager
Dan Gardner, Publications Manager
Carol Sullivan, Counselor
List offering parents, counselors, teachers and learning disabled students a reminder of helpful skills and necessary steps to take as a high school student with a learning disability moves toward college.

4623 **Guide to Colleges for Learning Disabled Students**
Academic Success Press
PO Box 132
Bradenton, FL 34206 941-746-1645
800-444-2524
FAX 800-777-2525

Mary Liscio, Editor
Paul Nolting, Owner

4624 Guide to Community Colleges Serving Students with Learning Disabilities
Mississippi State University/ Student Services
01 Montgomery
University, MS 38677
662-325-3335
FAX 662-325-8190
http://www.ms.state.edu
e-mail: dbaker@saffairs.ms.state.edu
Sonja Burnham, Author
Debbie Baker, Executive Director
Julie Berry, Assistant Director

A list by state of two-year community colleges in Mississippi, Alabama, Georgia, Tennessee and Florida, describing services and accommodations provided for students with learning disabilities. *$1.50*

4625 HEATH Resource Directory
National Clearinghouse on Postsecondary Education
2121 K Street NW
Washington, DC 20037
202-973-0904
800-544-3284
FAX 202-973-0908
http://www.heath.gwu.edu
e-mail: askheath@gwu.edu
Dan Gardner, Publications Manager

Annotated listings of over 150 national organizations which can provide additional information about postsecondary education and individuals with disabilities. *$1.00*
30 pages

4626 Higher Education Information Center
Boston Public Library
700 Boylston Street
Boston, MA 02116
617-247-8980
800-442-1171
FAX 617-266-4673
http://www.bpl.org
e-mail: hr@bpl.org
Willis Hulings, President
Ann Coles, Vice President
P D'Arbeloff, Executive Director
Offers information on colleges and universities, vocational/technical schools, financial aid and careers, counseling on school selection and paying for educational costs.

4627 How the Student with Hearing Loss Can Succeed in College
Harris Communications
15155 Technology Drive
Eden Prairie, MN 55344
952-906-1180
800-825-6758
FAX 952-906-1099
TDY:952-906-1198
http://www.harriscomm.com
e-mail: info@harriscmm.com
Robert Harris, Owner
Ron Leavitt MS, Editor

A handbook for students families and professionals. Includes information on academic, financial, technological, and support services. *$28.95*
278 pages Paperback

4628 How to Succeed in College: A Handbook for Students with Learning Disabilities
National Center on Employment and Disability
201 i U Willets Road
Albertson, NY 11507
516-747-5400
FAX 516-747-5378
TDY:516-746-5355
http://www.ncds.org
Jennifer Neft, Assistant Director

These two volumes demonstrate the advantages of cooperation between vocational rehabilitation and education. *$15.00*

4629 ISS Directory of International Schools
International Schools Services
PO Box 5910
Princeton, NJ 08543
609-452-0990
FAX 609-452-2690
http://www.iss.edu
e-mail: iss@iss.edu
John Nicklas, President

Comprehensive guide to over 550 American and international schools worldwide. *$45.95*
550 pages Plus S&H
ISBN 0-913663-17-5

4630 K&W Guide to Colleges for the Learning Disabled
HarperCollins Publishers
10 E 53rd Stret
New York, NY 10022
212-207-7000
800-242-8192
FAX 212-207-7145
http://www.harpercollins.com
Marybeth Kravets, Author
Imy Wax, Author
Jane Friedman, CEO
Offers information on support services for learning disabled college students. Includes learning disability services available, programs offered, college graduation requirements, admissions policies, costs, housing, tutorial help, learning resource centers and athletics.

4631 Learning to Care
Incorporation For National & Community Service
1201 New York Avenue NW
Washington, DC 20525
202-606-5000
FAX 202-565-2777
A national directory of student community service programs.

4632 National Association of Private Schools for Exceptional Children
NAPSEC
1522 K Street NW
Washington, DC 20005
202-408-3338
FAX 202-408-3340
http://www.napsec.com
e-mail: napsec@aol.com
Sherry Kolbe, Executive Director
Alison Figi, Communications Coordinator

A membership directory listing NAPSEC'S members. Information given includes: disabilities served, program descriptions, school profiles, admissions procedures and funding approval. *$32.00*
300 pages

4633 Peterson's Colleges with Programs for Students with Learning Disabilities or ADD
Peterson's
2000 Lenox Drive
Lawrenceville, NJ 08648
609-896-4530
800-338-3282
FAX 609-896-1811
http://www.petersons.com
e-mail: custsvce@petersons.com
Charles Mangrum II, Author
Mary Gatsch, Officer In Charge

Directs special-needs students to educational programs and services at 1,000 two-and four-year colleges and universities in the US and Canada. *$29.95*
672 pages Sixth Edition
ISBN 0-768904-55-2

4634 Questions to Aid in Selecting an Appropriate College Program for LD
CT Association for Children and Adults with LD
25 Van Zant Street
Norwalk, CT 06855
203-838-5010
FAX 203-866-6108
http://www.CACLD.org
e-mail: cacld@optonline.net
Marie Armstrong, Information Specialist
Beryl Kaufman, Executive Director

A collection of five one page information sheets, each from a different source. *$2.00*

$1.00 shipping

4635 Schoolsearch Guide to Colleges with Programs & Services for Students with LD
Schoolsearch Press
127 Marsh Street
Belmont, MA 02478
617-489-5785
FAX 617-489-5641
http://schoolsearch.com
e-mail: mlipkin@schoolsearch.com
Midge Lipkin, Owner

Lists more than 770 colleges and universities that offer programs and services to high school graduates with learning disabilities. *$39.95*
1660 pages 3rd Edition
ISBN 0-962032-67-0

4636 Two-Year College Databook
Chronicle Guidance Publications
66 Aurora Street
Moravia, NY 13118
315-497-0330
800-899-0454
FAX 315-497-3359
http://www.chronicleguidance.com
e-mail: janet@chronicleguidance.com
Janet Seemann, Managing Editor
Gary Fickeisen, Vice President

Comprehensive package offers students and counselors up-to-date information for selection colleges. The Chronical Two-Year Databook contains information on college majors, and on 2,432 institutions offering 760 occupational-career, associate, and transfer programs. *$24.97*
385 pages Annual
ISBN 1-556312-93-8

4637 Vocational School Manual
Chronicle Guidance Publications
66 Aurora Street
Moravia, NY 13118
315-497-0330
800-899-0454
FAX 315-497-3359
http://www.chronicleguidance.com
e-mail: janet@chronicleguidance.com
Janet Seemann, Managing Editor
Gary Fickeisen, Vice President

Offers information on occupational education programs currently available in the United States, Guam, and Puerto Rico. Programs consist of study or training leading to definite occupations. Prepares people for employment in recognized occupations, helps people make educated occupational choices, and upgrade and update their occupational skills. Includes data on vocational schools offering postsecondary occupational education. Accrediting associations are listed with contact information. *$24.96*
260 pages Annual
ISBN 1-556312-90-8

4638 World of Options: A Guide to International Education
Mobility International USA
PO Box 10767
Eugene, OR 97440
541-343-1284
FAX 541-343-6812
http://www.miusa.org
e-mail: info@miusa.org
Christa Bucks, Editor
Susan Sygall, Executive Director

Offers information on a wide variety of opportunities available to disabled participants including travel and international programs, and personal experience stories from people with disabilities who have had successful international experiences. *$35.00*
600 pages

Alabama

4639 Alabama Aviation and Technical College
Enterprise Ozark Community College
3405 S Us Highway 231
Ozark, AL 36360
334-774-5113
800-624-3468
FAX 334-774-6399
http://www.eocc.edu
Stafford Thompson, President
Terry Spicer, Vice President
Matthew Hughes, Manager
A public two-year college with 15 special education students out of a total of 600. Certified by the Federal Aviation Administration, and offers the only comprehensive aviation maintenance training program in the state of Alabama, with instruction in airframe, powerplant and avionics.

4640 Alabama Southern Community College
PO Box 2000
Monroeville, AL 36461
251-575-3156
http://www.ascc.edu
John Johnson, President

A public two-year college with 21 special education students out of a total of 1,127.

4641 Auburn University
Program for Students with Disabilities
1244 Haley Center
Auburn, AL 36849
334-844-2096
FAX 334-844-2099
http://www.auburn.edu/disability
e-mail: psd@auburn.edu
Kelly Haynes, Director

Provides reasonable accommodations and services for qualified students with documented disabilities who are attending Auburn University, enrolled in distance learning classes, or participating in programs sponsored by Auburn University.

4642 Auburn University at Montgomery
Center for Special Services
PO Box 244023
Montgomery, AL 36124
334-244-3631
FAX 334-244-3907
TDY:334-244-3754
http://www.aum.edu
e-mail: css@maqil.aum.edu
Tamara Massey-Garrett, Director
Keyonna Dailey, Student Services Coordinator

Offers a variety of services to students with disabilities including equipment, extended testing time, interpreting services, counseling services, and special accommodations.

4643 Birmingham-Southern College
900 Arkadelphia Road
Birmingham, AL 35254
205-226-4960
800-523-5793
FAX 205-226-4627
http://www.bsc.edu
Judith Cox, Director Academic Advising
Sara Hoover, Director Personal Counseling
Neal Berte, CEO
Offers a variety of services to students with disabilities including notetakers, extended testing time, counseling services, and special accommodations.

4644 Bishop State Community College
414 Stanton Road
Mobile, AL 36617
251-473-8692
http://www.bscc.cc.al.us
e-mail: info@bscc.cc.al.us
Carrie Moore, Counselor
Terry Hazzard, Manager

A public two-year college with 2 special education students out of a total of 2144.

4645 Chattahoochee Valley State Community College

2602 College Drive
Phenix City, AL 36869
334-291-4900
FAX 334-291-4944
http://www.cvcc.cc.al.us

Dr Blackwell, President
Jacquie Thacker, ADA Coordinator

Offers a variety of services to students with disabilities including note takers, extended testing time, counseling services and special accommodations.

4646 George County Wallace State Community College

PO Box 2530
Selma, AL 36702
334-876-9227
FAX 334-876-9250
http://www.wccs.edu

Gail May, Dean
James Mitchell, President

Offers a variety of services to students with disabilities including note takers, extended testing time, counseling services and special accommodations.

4647 H Councill Trenholm State Technical College

1225 Air Base Boulevard
Montgomery, AL 36108
334-420-4200
FAX 334-284-9357
http://www.trenholmtech.cc.al.us
e-mail: information@trenholmtech.cc.al.us

A public two-year college with 101 special education students out of a total of 800.

4648 Horizons School

2018 15th Avenue S
Birmingham, AL 35205
205-322-6606
800-822-6242
FAX 205-322-6605
http://www.horizonsschool.org
e-mail: jkcarter@horizonsschool.org

Jade K Carter MD, Director
Marie H McElheny, Assistant Director

Offers a non-degree transition program specifically designed to facilitate personal, social and career independence for students with specific learning disabilities and other handicappinf conditions.

4649 Jacksonville State University

700 Pelham Road
Jacksonville, AL 36265
256-782-5781
FAX 256-782-5121
http://www.jsu.edu
e-mail: lbedford@jsucc.jsu.edu

Daniel Miller, Director
William Meehan, CEO

Offers a variety of services to students with disabilities including notetakers, extended testing time, counseling services, and special accommodations.

4650 James H Faulkner State Community College

1900 S US Highway 31
Bay Minette, AL 36507
251-580-2100
800-231-3752
FAX 251-580-2226
http://www.faulknerstate.edu
e-mail: bkennedy@faulknerstate.edu

Brenda Kennedy EdD, Dean Student Development
Nancy Williams, College Receptionist
Gary Branch, President

A public two-year community college with approximately 125 students with disabilities out of a total student population of 4,350. Committed to the professional and cultural growth of each student without regard to race, color, qualified disability, gender, religion, creed, national origin, or age. Attempts to provide an educational environment that promotes development and learning through a wide variety of educational programs, adequate and comfortable facilities, and flexible scheduling.

4651 Lureen B Wallace Community College

PO Box 910
Opp, AL 36467
334-493-3573
FAX 334-493-7003
http://www.lbwcc.edu

Edward Meadows, President

A public two-year college with 102 special education students out of a total of 630. Provides postsecondary occupational education on a nondiscriminatory basis for individuals who desire to prepare for entry level employment, advancement, or retraining in a career field.

4652 Marion Military Institute

1101 Washington Street
Marion, AL 36756
334-683-2347
800-664-1842
FAX 334-683-2383
http://www.mairon-institue.org

James Benson, President
Col. P Carruthers, Admissions Director

An independent two-year college with an academic advantage program for students with learning difficulties and for a limited number with diagnosed learning disabilities.

4653 Northeast Alabama Community College

PO Box 159
Rainsville, AL 35986
256-638-4418
FAX 256-228-6861
http://www.nacc.cc.al.us

Elaine Hayden, Assistant Dean Instruction
David Campbell, President

A public two-year college with support services for students with special needs that is consistant with the mission of the Alambama College System: to provide accessible quality educational opportunities, promote economic growth, and enhance the quality of life for people in Alabama.

4654 Troy State University Dothan

PO Box 8368
Dothan, AL 36304
334-983-6556
FAX 334-983-6322
http://www.tsud.edu
e-mail: kseagle@tsud.edu

Barbara Alford, President
Keith Seagle, Counseling Services Director

Offers a variety of services to students with disabilities including notetakers, extended testing time, counseling services, and special accommodations.

4655 University of Alabama

PO Box 870132
Tuscaloosa, AL 35487
205-348-6010
FAX 205-348-9046
http://www.ua.edu

Cathy Hitt, Counselor
Karen Clayton, Manager Physical Disabilities
Malcolm Portera, CEO

A public four-year college with approximately 650 students identified with disabilities out of a total of 19,200.

4656 University of Alabama: Huntsville

301 Sparkman Drive
Huntsville, AL 35899
256-824-6070
FAX 256-824-6073
http://www.uah.edu
e-mail: admitme@email.uah.edu

Delois Smith, Director
Frank , President

Offers a variety of services and accommodations to assist students with disabilities in eliminating barriers they encounter in pursuing higher education.

4657 University of Montevallo

Station 6030
Montevallo, AL 35115
205-665-6000
FAX 205-665-6042
http://www.montevallo.edu

Elaine Elledge, Special Services
Robert Chesney, President

Offers a variety of services to students with disabilities including notetakers, extended testing time, counseling services, and special accommodations.

4658 University of North Alabama
PO Box 5008
Florence, AL 35630
256-765-4100
FAX 256-765-4904
http://www.una.edu
e-mail: jadams@unanov.una.edu
Jennifer Adams, Associate Director
Kim Greenway, Director
William Kale, President
Developmental services of UNA provides accommodation and supportive services to assist students with disabilities throughout their college expirence.

4659 University of South Alabama
182 Adminstration Building
Mobile, AL 36688
334-265-9920
FAX 251-460-7827
http://www.usouthal.edu
e-mail: admiss@jaguarl.usouthal.edu
Keith Ayers, Director
Happy Fulford, Executive Director
Diane Agee, Administrative Assistant
Offers a variety of services to students with disabilities including note takers, extended testing time, counseling services, and special accommodations.

Alaska

4660 Alaska Pacific University
Disabled Student Services
4101 University Drive
Anchorage, AK 99508
907-564-8345
FAX 907-564-8806
http://www.alaskapacific.edu
e-mail: tamera@alaskapacific.edu
Tamera Randolph, Coordinator Disability Support

Four-year college offering special services to students that are learning disabled.

4661 Juneau Campus: University of Alaska Southeast
11120 Glacier Highway
Juneau, AK 99801
907-465-6462
877-465-4827
FAX 907-465-6365
http://www.uas.alaska.edu
e-mail: uas.info@uas.alaska.edu
Dolores Graver, Administrative Assistant
Joel Milsat, Director

Offers a variety of services to students with disabilities including notetakers, extended testing time, counseling services, and special accommodations.

4662 Ketchikan Campus: University of Alaska Southeast
2600 7th Avenue
Ketchikan, AK 99901
907-225-4722
FAX 907-225-3624
http://www.ketch.alaska.edu
e-mail: info@uas.alaska.edu
L Naugen, Assistant Professor
Kathleen Wiechelman, Manager

Offers a variety of services to students with disabilities including note takers, extended testing time, counseling services and special accommodations.

4663 University of Alaska Anchorage: Disability Support Services
3211 Providence Drive
Anchorage, AK 99508
907-786-1800
FAX 907-786-4888
http://www.uaa.alaska.edu
e-mail: ayenrol@alaska.edu
Lyn Stoller, Director
Edward Gorsuch, CEO

Provides equal opportunites for students who experience disabilities.

4664 University of Alaska: Fairbanks
PO Box 757480
Fairbanks, AK 99775
907-474-7211
FAX 907-474-5379
http://www.uaf.edu
e-mail: admission@uaf.edu
Nancy Dix, Director Admissions
Marshall Lind, CEO
Stacey Howdeshell, Office Manager
A public four-year college. Services provided to students with learning disabilities include: assistance determining accommodations, advocacy, testing accommodations, books on tape, peer support groups and individual counseling.

Arizona

4665 Arizona State University
PO Box 870112
Tempe, AZ 85287
480-965-2376
FAX 480-965-3610
TDY:480-965-1234
http://www.asu.edu
e-mail: upgradingones@asu.edu
Tedde Scharf, Director
Michael Crow, President

Four-year college that offers support to students with learning disabilities.

4666 Eastern Arizona College
615 N Stadium Avenue
Thatcher, AZ 85552
928-428-8233
800-678-3808
http://www.eac.edu
Beverly Teague, Student Services
Mark Bryce, President

Offers a variety of services to students with disabilities including note takers, extended testing time, counseling services and special accommodations.

4667 Glendale Community College
6000 W Olive Avenue
Glendale, AZ 85302
623-845-3000
FAX 623-845-3329
http://www.gc.maricopa.edu
Phil Randolph, President
Nancy Oreshack, LD Specialist
Mark Ferris, Disability Service Coordinator
A public two-year college with 212 special education students out of a total of 15,200.

4668 Grand Canyon University
PO Box 11097
Phoenix, AZ 85061
602-249-3300
800-800-9776
FAX 602-589-2580
http://www.gcu.edu
e-mail: admiss@gcu.edu
Jane Castillo MD, Instructor Education
Brent Richardson, President
Michael Clifford, Manager
Offers a variety of services to students with disabilities including note takers, extended testing time, counseling services, and special accommodations.

4669 Mesa Community College
1833 W Southern Avenue
Mesa, AZ 85202
480-461-7000
FAX 480-461-7139
http://www.mc.maricopa.edu
Judith Taussig, Special Services
Larry Christiansen, President

Offers a variety of services to students with disabilities including note takers, extended testing time, counseling services and special accommodations.

4670 Northern Arizona University

PO Box 4084
Flagstaff, AZ 86011
928-523-9011
FAX 928-523-7486
http://www.nau.edu
e-mail: undergraduate.admissions@nau.edu
Marsha Fields, Director
John Haeger, President

A public four-year college.

4671 Phoenix College

1202 W Thomas Road
Phoenix, AZ 85013
602-285-7500
FAX 602-285-7700
TDY:602-285-7477
http://www.pc.maricopa.edu
Anna Solley, President
Mitra Mehraban, Special Services

A public two-year college with 23 special education students out of a total of 14,327.

4672 Pima Community College

2202 W Anklam Road
Tucson, AZ 85709
520-206-6821
FAX 520-206-6071
http://www.pima.edu
Eric Morrison, Facility Advisor
Carolyn Reynolds, Administrator
Joseph Labuda, Manager

A public two-year college offering special education classes for students with disabilities.

4673 Scottsdale Community College

9000 E Chaparral Road
Scottsdale, AZ 85256
480-423-6651
FAX 480-423-6200
TDY:480-423-6377
http://www.scc.maricopa.edu
e-mail: donna.young@sccmail.maricopa.edu
Donna Young, Director
Becky Jaco, Program Adviser
Karen Biglin, Executive Director

Student Services office works closely with learning disabled students to provide the best accommodations possible.

4674 South Mountain Community College

7050 S 24th Street
Phoenix, AZ 85042
602-243-8000
FAX 602-243-8118
http://www.smc.maricopa.edu
e-mail: winkharnar@smcmail.maricopa.edu
Wink Harnar, Special Service Director
Janet Denson, Student Cooperative Director
Ken Atwater, President

Offers a variety of services to students with disabilities including note takers, extended testing time, counseling services and special accommodations.

4675 Spring Ridge Academy

13690 S Burton Road
Spring Valley, AZ 86333
928-632-4602
http://www.springridgeacademy.edu
e-mail: sraemail@northlink.com
Joe Gubbins, Principal
Jean Courtney, Administrator

4676 Strategic Alternative Learning Techniques(SALT)

SALT Center, University of Arizona
PO Box 210136
Tucson, AZ 85721
520-621-1242
http://www.salt.arizona.edu
Dr Jeff Orgera, Director
Dr Diane C Quinn, Director of Development

Students receive individualized educational planning and monitoring, assistance from trained tutors with course work, and an array of workshops geared toward the individual academic needs of these students.

4677 University of Advancing Computer Technology

2625 W Baseline Road
Tempe, AZ 85283
602-383-8228
800-658-5744
FAX 602-383-8222
http://www.uact.edu
e-mail: admissions@uat.edu
Randall Mertz, Senior Vice President
Daniel Edwards, National Admissions Director

The University of Advancing Computer Technology has a program for you. Areas of study include digital animation production, game design, digital video production, interactive media, web design, graphic design, application development, computer programming, database programming, Internet development and administration, network engineering, game programming, network security, web site production, technology management, e-commerce marketing or internet database management.

4678 University of Arizona

PO Box 210040
Tucson, AZ 85721
520-621-3237
FAX 520-621-9799
http://www.arizona.edu
e-mail: appinfo@arizona.edu
Sue Kroeger MD, Director
Jane Abbott, Manager

The Strategic Alternative Learning Techniques (SALT) Center values the achievement of individuals with learning disabilities and provides an array of services to maximize student success.

4679 Yavapai College

Student Support Services
1100 E Sheldon Street
Prescott, AZ 86301
928-776-2117
800-922-6787
FAX 928-776-2030
http://www.yc.edu
Patricia Quinn-Kane, Learning Specialist
Carol Clayton, Director

A public two-year college that offers a variety of services for students with disabilities.

Arkansas

4680 Arkansas Baptist College

1621 Dr Martin Luther King Drive
Little Rock, AR 72202
501-244-5109
FAX 501-374-7856
http://www.anicbapcol.edu
e-mail: fredie.fox@arkbap.col
Sonya Bell, Manager
Fredie Fox, Registrar

An independent four-year college with 44 special education students out of a total of 418.

4681 Arkansas Northeastern College

Student Support Services
PO Box 1109
Blytheville, AR 72316
870-762-1020
FAX 870-763-1654
http://www.anc.edu
e-mail: mjeffers@anc.edu
Myles Jeffers, Director
Tracy Jones, Office Assistant
Robin Meyers, President

Offers a variety of services to students with disabilities including note takers, extended testing time, counseling services and special accommodations.

4682 **Arkansas State University**
Disability Services
PO Box 360
Jonesboro, AR 72467
870-972-3964
FAX 870-972-3351
http://http://disability.astate.edu
Jennifer Rice-Mason, Director

Arranges for academic adjustments and auxiliary aids to be provided to qualified students and coordinates workplace accommodations.Will provide auxiliary aids, without cost, to those students with verified disabilities who require such services.

4683 **Arkansas Tech University**
1605 Coliseum Drive
Russellville, AR 72801
479-964-0877
FAX 479-968-0208
http://www.atu.edu
Janet Jones, Disabilities Coordinator
Carla Terry, Manager

Provides equal opportunities for higher education to academically qualified individuals who are disabled. Students are integrated as completely as possible into the university community.

4684 **Garland County Community College**
101 College Drive
Hot Springs, AR 71913
501-760-4222
888-671-1229
FAX 501-760-4100
http://www.gccc.cc.ar.us
e-mail: tspencer@npcc.edu
Sally Carder, President

Offers a variety of services to students with disabilities including note takers, extended testing time, counseling services and special accommodations.

4685 **Harding University**
PO Box 12235
Searcy, AR 72149
501-279-4000
800-477-4407
FAX 501-279-4217
http://www.harding.edu
e-mail: admission@harding.edu
Jim Johnston MD, Student Support Services Dir.
Teresa McLead, Disabilities Specialist
David Burks, President
Strives to deliver a program of services that will result in increasing the college retention and graduation rates of these students.

4686 **Jones Learning Center**
University of the Ozarks
415 N College Avenue
Clarksville, AR 72830
479-979-1000
800-264-8636
FAX 479-979-1429
http://www.ozarks.edu
e-mail: jlc@ozarks.edu
Julia Frost, Director
Debra Cline, Assistant Director Center
Rick Niece, President
An academic support unit that offers enhanced services to college students with diagnosed learning disabililites or attention deficit disorder. Services are individualized and focus on the development of strategies and skills to build upon strengths and circumvent deficits. The ratio of professional full time staff to students is 1:4.

4687 **Philander Smith College**
1 Trudie Kibbe Reed Drive
Little Rock, AR 72202
501-375-9845
800-446-6772
FAX 501-370-5225
http://www.philander.edu
e-mail: administrator@philander.edu
Arnella Hayes, Director
Walter Kimbrough, President

Offers a variety of services to students with disabilities including notetakers, extended testing time, counseling services, and special accommodations.

4688 **Sheldon Jackson College**
801 Lincoln Street
Sitka, AK 99835
907-747-5220
800-478-4556
FAX 907-747-6366
http://www.sj-alaska.edu
e-mail: yukonjohn@sj-alaska.edu
Alice Smith, Director
Arthur Cleveland, President

Seeks to help students find their forte, best learning modes, and best modes of expression; and seeks to help students prepare to find the greatest possible joy in vocation and service to others.

4689 **Southern Arkansas University**
Disabled Student Programs & Services
PO Box 9371
Magnolia, AR 71754
870-235-4145
FAX 870-235-5262
http://www.saumag.edu
e-mail: pwwoods@saumag.edu
Paula Washington-Woods, Dir Disability Support Scvs
Beverly Rowden, Office Assistant

Offers a variety of services to students with disabilities including notetakers, extended testing time, counseling services, and special accommodations.

4690 **University of Arkansas**
232 Silas Hunt Hall
Fayetteville, AR 72701
479-575-2000
800-377-8632
FAX 479-575-7515
http://www.uark.edu
e-mail: uafadmis@comp.uark.edu
Dawn Medley, Admissions Director
B Sugg, CEO

Offers a variety of services to students with disabilities including note takers, extended testing time, counseling services, and special accommodations.

4691 **University of the Ozarks**
415 N College Avenue
Clarksville, AR 72830
479-979-1000
800-264-8636
http://www.ozarks.edu
e-mail: jdecker@ozarks.edu
Julia Frost, Director
Rick Niece, President

A four-year college that provides a learning center for students with learning disabilities.

California

4692 **Academy of Art College**
Academy Resource Center
180 New Montgomery Street
San Francisco, CA 94105
415-263-8895
http://www.academyart.edu
e-mail: nhaughnes@academyart.edu
Natasha Haugnes, Academy Resource Director
Ryan Kashmir, Director of Student Support

4693 **Allan Hancock College**
800 S College Drive
Santa Maria, CA 93454
805-922-6966
FAX 805-922-3556
http://www.hancockcollege.edu
e-mail: malangko@hancock.edu
Ann Foxworthy, President
Odette Tinhiro, Administrative Assistant
Mark Malangko, LAP Director
Students with mobility, visual, hearing and speech impairments, learning disabilities, acquired brain injury, developmental disabilities, psychological and other disabilities are eligible to receive special services which enable them to fully participate in the community college experience at Allan Hancock College.

4694 **Antelope Valley College**
3041 W Avenue K
Lancaster, CA 93536
661-722-6331
FAX 661-722-6361
http://www.avc.edu
e-mail: info@avc.edu
David Greenleaf, Learning Disability Specialist
Jackie Fisher, President

A public two-year college with 228 learning disabled students out of a total of 11,105.

4695 **Bakersfield College**
1801 Panorama Drive
Bakersfield, CA 93305
661-395-4011
FAX 661-395-4500
http://www.bc.cc.ca.us
Tim Bohan, Director

A public two-year college with 207 special education students out of a total of 12,312.

4696 **Barstow Community College**
Disabled Student Programs & Services
2700 Barstow Road
Barstow, CA 92311
760-252-2411
FAX 619-252-1875
http://www.barstow.cc.ca.us
e-mail: dsps@barstow.cc.ca.us
Gene Pfeifer, Counselor
Gordon Smith, LD Specialist

Educational support program for disabled students including special classes and support services for all disabled students.

4697 **Bethany College**
Special Advising
800 Bethany Drive
Scotts Valley, CA 95066
831-438-3800
800-843-9410
FAX 408-438-4517
http://www.bethany.edu
Kathy Tagg, Director
Max Rossi, President

An independent four-year college with support services for special education students.

4698 **Biola University**
13800 Biola Ave
La Mirada, CA 90639
562-903-4752
800-OKBIOLA
FAX 562-903-4709
http://www.biola.edu
e-mail: tom-engle@peter.biola.edu
Tim Engle, Coordinator
Michelle Masterson, Staff
Clyde Cook, President
Christian liberal arts university responsible for all programs related to students with disabilities.

4699 **Butte College**
3536 Butte Campus Drive
Oroville, CA 95965
530-895-2511
FAX 530-895-2345
http://www.butte.edu
Richard Dunn, LD Specialist
Diana Vanderploeg, President

A public two-year college with 223 special education students out of a total of 12,848.

4700 **Cabrillo College**
3500 Soquel Drive
Aptos, CA 95003
831-479-6201
FAX 831-479-6393
http://www.cabrillo.cc.ca.us
e-mail: frlynch@cabrillo.cc.ca.us
Frank Lynch, Director
Brian King, President

A two-year college that offers services and programs to disabled students.

4701 **California Lutheran University**
60 W Olsen Road
Thousand Oaks, CA 91360
805-492-2411
FAX 805-493-3472
TDY:800-735-2929
http://www.clunet.edu
e-mail: cluadm@clunet.edu
Damian Pena, Director
Lisa Spreen, Administrative Assistant
Daryl Calkins, Religious Leader
Offers a variety of services to students with disabilities including notetakers, extended testing time, counseling services, and special accommodations.

4702 **California Polytechnic State University: San Luis Obispo**
Disability Resource Center
1 Grand Avenue
San Luis Obispo, CA 93407
805-756-1111
FAX 805-756-5400
TDY:805-756-1395
http://www.calpoly.edu
e-mail: admissions@calpoly.edu
William Bailey, Director
Warren Baker, President

Comprehensive program of academic advisement, disability management, and support services, including peer mentors; currently providing services to more than 350 students with learning disabilities, 700 students with various disabilities total.

4703 **California State Polytechnic University: Pomona**
3801 W Temple Avenue
Pomona, CA 91768
909-869-7659
FAX 909-869-4529
http://www.csupomona.edu
e-mail: cppadmit@csupomona.edu
Fred Henderson, Director
Harold Schleifer, Executive Director

Offers a variety of services to students with disabilities including notetakers, extended testing time, counseling services, and special accommodations.

4704 **California State University: Bakersfield**
Services for Students with Disabilities
9001 Stockdale Highway
Bakersfield, CA 93311-1099
661-664-3360
FAX 661-664-2171
TDY:661-665-6288
http://www.csubak.edu
e-mail: jclausen@csub.edu
Janice Clausen, Director
Patrick Choi, Support Services Specialist

Four year college which provides services to the learning disabled.

4705 **California State University: Chico**
400 W 1st Street
Chico, CA 95929
530-898-4636
800-542-4426
FAX 530-898-6456
http://www.csuchico.edu
Billie Jackson, Director
Scott McNall, CEO

To facilitate accommodation requests and provide the support services necessary to ensure equal access to university programs for students with disabilities.

4706 **California State University: Dominguez Hills**
1000 E Victoria Street
Carson, CA 90747
310-243-3300
FAX 310-516-4247
http://www.csudh.edu
e-mail: pwells@csudh.edu
Patricia Wells, Director
Mark Smith, Counselor

The purpose of the Disabled Student Services (DSS) program is to make all of the University's educational, cultural social and physical facilities available to students with disabilities. The program serves as a centralized source of information for students with disabilities and those who work with them. By providing support services, DSS assists students with disabilities in the enhancement of their academic, career and personal development.

4707 **California State University: Fresno**
Services for Students with Disabilities
5200 N Barton
Fresno, CA 93740-8014 559-278-2811
FAX 559-278-4214
http://ww.csufresno.edu
e-mail: pat_blore@csufresno.edu

Pat Blore, Coordinator

Four year college that provides students with services for the learning disabled.

4708 **California State University: Fullerton**
Disabled Student Services
PO Box 6830
Fullerton, CA 92834 714-278-3117
FAX 714-278-2408
TDY:714-278-2786
http://www.fullerton.edu
e-mail: dliverpool@fullerton.edu

Doug Liverpool, LD/Mental Heath Specialist

A public four-year college with 800 special education students out of a total of 75,000. The Office of Disabled Student Services aims to increase access and retention for students with permanent and temporary disabilities by ensuring equitable treatment in all aspects of campus life. Provides co-curricular and academically related services which empower students with disabilities to achieve academic and personal self-determination.

4709 **California State University: Hayward**
Student with Disability Resource Center
25800 Carlos Bee Boulevard
Hayward, CA 94542 510-885-3868
FAX 510-885-7400
http://wwwsa.csuhayward.edu
e-mail: sdrc@bay.csuhayward.edu

Russell Wong, Learning Resources Counselor

Provides academic accomodations to address the individual needs of students with disabilities. Students with documented disabilities and functional limitations are eligible for accomodations designed to provide equivalent access to general campus and classroom programs and activities.

4710 **California State University: Long Beach**
Stephen Benson Program
1250 N Bellflower Boulevard
Long Beach, CA 90840 562-985-4430
FAX 562-985-4529
http://www.csulb.edu
e-mail: bcarey@csulb.edu

Brian Carey MFT, Coordinator

Four-year college offers a program for the learning disabled.

4711 **California State University: Northridge**
PO Box 1286
Northridge, CA 91328 818-349-4357
FAX 818-677-4665
http://www.csun.edu
e-mail: lorraine.newlon@csun.edu

Lee Axelrod, Learning Disability Director
Jolene Koester, President

To assist students with learning disabilities in reaching their full potential, the program offers a comprehensive and well-coordinated system of educational support services that allow students to be judged on the basis of their ability rather than disability.

4712 **California State University: Sacramento**
Services to Students with Disabilities
6000 J Street Lassen Hall Room 1008
Sacramento, CA 95819-6042 916-278-6955
FAX 916-278-7825
TDY:916-278-7239
http://www.csus.edu/sswd/sswd.html
e-mail: sswd@csus.edu

Judy Dean, Acting Co-Director
Melissa Repa, Acting Co-Director

Offers a variety of services to students with disabilities including notetakers, extended testing time, counseling services, and special accommodations.

4713 **California State University: San Bernardino**
Disability Services
5500 University Parkway
San Bernardino, CA 92407 909-880-5000
FAX 909-880-5200
TDY:880-500-0000
http://www.csusb.edu
e-mail: cppadmit@csupomona.edu

Laurie Flynn, Director
James Sando, CEO

Dedicated to assuring each student an opportunity to experience equity in education .

4714 **California State University: San Marcos**
Disabled Student Services
333 S Twin Oaks Valley Road
San Marcos, CA 92096 760-750-4905
FAX 760-750-3445
http://www.csusm.edu
e-mail: kkornher@csusm.edu

Kara Kornher PsyD, Psychologist

Four year college that offers its learning disabled student support and services.

4715 **California State University: Stanislaus**
Disability Resource Center
801 W Monte Vista Avenue, Suite 200
Turlock, CA 95382 209-667-3159
FAX 209-667-3585
TDY:209-667-3044
http://www.csustan.edu/counseling/DRC/
e-mail: lbettencourt@csustan.edu

Lee Bettencourt, Director
Michelle Sanchez-Stamos, Disability Service Advisor

A public four-year college with 31 special education students out of a total of 4,293.

4716 **Canada College**
4200 Farm Hill Boulevard
Redwood City, CA 94061 650-306-3100
FAX 650-306-3457
TDY:650-306-3161
http://www.canadacollege.edu
e-mail: hetrick@smccd.net

Regina Blok, Program Coordinator
Jinney Gross, Dean
Rosa Perez, President

Three unique programs that serve eligible students with disabilities: the Physically Challenged Program, the Learning Achievement Program and the Adaptive P.E. Program.

4717 **Cerritos College**
Learning Disability Services
11110 Alondra Boulevard
Norwalk, CA 90650 562-860-2451
FAX 562-467-5071
http://www.cerritos.edu

Al Spetrino, Program Head
Noelia Vela, President

A public two-year college with 63 special education students out of a total of 20,679.

4718 **Chaffey Community College District**
Disability Programs And Services (CCW21-A)
5885 Haven Avenue
Rancho Cucamonga, CA 91737
909-941-2379
FAX 909-466-2834
http://www.chaffey.edu/DPS/
e-mail: sharlenesmith@jc.edu
Sharlene Smith, Director
Will Carrick, Coordinator/Specialist

Chaffey College's Disabled Student Programs and Services (DSP&S) offer instruction and support services to students with developmental, learning, physical, psychological disabilities or aquired brain injury. Students can recieve a variety of services such as: test facilitation, note taking, tutoring, adaptive physical education, pre-vocational training, career preparation, and job placement.

4719 **Chapman University**
1 University Drive
Orange, CA 92866
714-997-6711
http://www.chapman.edu
Anthony Garcia, Associate Professor
James Doti, President

Offers a variety of services to students with disabilities including note takers, extended testing time, counseling services and special accommodations.

4720 **College of Alameda**
555 Atlantic Avenue
Alameda, CA 94501
510-522-7221
FAX 510-748-2339
TDY:510-748-2330
http://www.peralta.edu
e-mail: ndarcey@peralta.edu
Nancy Darcey, LD Specialist
Dennise Massett, Administrative Assistant
Cecelia Cervantes, President
Accommodations, assessment and special classes are provided for learning disabled students enrolled at College Alameda, a 2 year college located by San Francisco Bay.

4721 **College of Marin**
835 College Avenue
Kentfield, CA 94904
415-457-8811
FAX 415-457-4791
TDY:415-721-0736
http://www.marin.cc.ca.us
e-mail: rfb@marin.cc.ca.us
Marie McCarthy, Coordinator
Ellen Tollen, Co-Coordinator
Frances White, President
Offers a variety of services to students with disabilities including note takers, extended testing time, counseling services, and special accommodations. Also offers diagnostic testing and remedial classes for learning disabled students.

4722 **College of San Mateo**
1700 W Hillsdale Boulevard
San Mateo, CA 94402
650-574-6161
FAX 650-358-6803
TDY:650-574-6230
http://www.collegesanmateo.edu
e-mail: paparelli@smccd.net
Marie Paparelli, LD Specialist
Laura Skaff, Program Service Coordinator
Shirley Kelly, President
Primary objective of the Disabled Students Program-Learning Disabilities Center is to assist the student in achieving academic, vocational, personal and social success. This is best accomplished by integration into the mainstream of college classes and services. The learning disabilities program provides support services in the following areas: assessment and evaluation, specialized tutoring, test accommodations, computer access and more.

4723 **College of the Canyons**
26455 Rockwell Canyon Road
Santa Clarita, CA 91355
661-259-4224
FAX 661-259-8302
http://www.coc.cc.ca.us
Nina Nashur MD, Coordinator

A public two-year college with 45 special education students out of a total of 6,255.

4724 **College of the Desert**
Center for Training and Development
43500 Monterey Avenue
Palm Desert, CA 92260
760-773-2596
FAX 760-776-0128
TDY:760-674-0266
http://www.desert.cc.ca.us/
Mike O'Neill, LD Specialist

Offers a variety of services to students with disabilities including note takers, extended testing time, counseling services and special accommodations.

4725 **College of the Redwoods: Learning Skills Center**
7351 Tompkins Hill Road
Eureka, CA 95501
707-476-4100
800-641-0400
FAX 707-476-4418
TDY:707-476-4284
http://www.redwoods.edu
e-mail: trish-blaire@redwoods.edu
Trish Blair, LD Specialist
Susan Mindus, Program Assistant
Kathleen Crabill, President
Mission is to assist individual students in the development of a realistic self-concept, assist in the development of educational interests and employment goals, provide the advice, counseling, and equipment necessary to facilitate success, starting with specialized assistance in the registration process.

4726 **College of the Sequoias**
Disability Resource Center
915 S Mooney Boulevard
Visalia, CA 93277
559-730-3805
FAX 559-730-3803
TDY:559-730-3913
http://www.cos.edu
e-mail: sharmeenl@cos.edu
Don Mast, Dean
David Maciel, Director

A public two-year college with approximately 600 special education students out of a total of 10,300.

4727 **College of the Siskiyous**
800 College Avenue
Weed, CA 96094
530-938-4462
FAX 530-938-5367
http://www.siskiyous.edu
e-mail: ar@siskiyous.edu
Karen Zeigler, Director
David Pelham, President

Dedicated to meeting the needs of students with disabilities.

4728 **Columbia College**
11600 Columbia College Drive
Sonora, CA 95370
209-588-5100
FAX 209-588-5104
http://www.columbia.yosemite.cc.ca.us.
Suzanne Patterson, LD Specialist
James Riggs, President

Offers a variety of services to students with disabilities including note takers, extended testing time, counseling services and special accommodations.

4729 **Contra Costa College**
2600 Mission Bell Drive
San Pablo, CA 94806
510-235-7800
FAX 510-236-6768
http://www.contracosta.cc.ca.us/
Peggy Fleming, Learning Specialist
Janis Walsh, Manager

Offers a variety of services to students with disabilities including notetakers, extended testing time, counseling services, and special accommodations.

4730 Cosumnes River College
1410 Ethan Allan Way
Sacramento, CA 95823
916-563-3241
FAX 916-563-3264
http://www.crc.bsrios.cc.ca.us
e-mail: rebrac@losrois.org
Paris Greenlee, Manager

A public two-year college with 150 learning disabled students out of a total of 10,000.

4731 Crafton Hills College
11711 Sand Canyon Road
Yucaipa, CA 92399
909-389-3400
FAX 909-794-7881
http://www.elac.cc.ca.us
Kristen Colvey, LD Specialist
Meridyth McLaren, Executive Director

A public two-year college with 52 special education students out of a total of 5,732.

4732 Cuesta College
Disabled Student Programs & Services
PO Box 8106
San Luis Obispo, CA 93403
805-546-3148
FAX 805-546-3930
TDY:805-546-3148
http://www.cuesta.edu/acasupp/dsps
e-mail: dspsinfo@cuesta.edu
Patrick Schwab EdD, Director

A public, two-year community college, offering instruction and services to students with learning disabilities since 1973. A comprehensive set of services and special classes are available. Contact the program for further information.

4733 De Anza College: Special Education Divisio
21250 Stevens Creek Boulevard
Cupertino, CA 95014
408-864-5678
http://www.deanza.fhda.edu
Suzanne Caillat, Office Manager
Pauline Waathiq, Director

A public two-year college with 300 special education students out of a total of 20,000.

4734 Diablo Valley College
Disability Support Services
321 Golf Club Road
Pleasant Hill, CA 94523
925-685-1230
FAX 925-687-1829
http://www.dvc.edu
Terry Armstrong, Dean of Counseling
Mark Edelstein, President

Disabled Student Program & Services (DSPS) is a program that is designed to ensure that students with disabilities have equal access to all of the educational offerings at Diablo Valley College. We facilitate equal opportunity through the provision of appropriate support services, curriculum, instruction and adaptive technology.

4735 Disabled Student at Cypress College
9200 Valley View Street
Cypress, CA 90630
714-484-7104
FAX 714-826-4042
TDY:714-761-0961
http://www.cypresscollege.edu
Cindy Owens, LD Specialist

The Disabled Student Center provides testing to determine eligibility for LD services. For those students with verified learning disabilities, services including tutoring, test accommodations, and adapted software and specialized academic counseling.

4736 East Los Angeles College
1301 Avenida Cesar Chavez
Monterey Park, CA 91754
323-265-8650
FAX 323-265-8759
http://www.elac.cc.ca.us
Marilyn Hutchens, Contact
Ram Gust, Librarian

A public two-year college with 44 special education students out of a total of 14587. There is a an additional fee for the special education program in addition to the regular tuition.

4737 Educational Psychology Clinic
California State University, Long Beach
1250 N Bellflower Boulevard
Long Beach, CA 90840
562-985-4771
e-mail: magaddin@csulb.edu
Renee Twigg, Manager
Tami Shirron, Graduate Assistant

A primary training site for the school psychology, counseling, and special education programs while providing comprehensive educational and psychological services to school age children and their families at a moderate cost. Services at the clinic are provided by graduate students under supervision by faculty in the college of education.

4738 El Camino Community College
16007 Crenshaw Boulevard
Torrance, CA 90506
310-532-3670
FAX 310-660-3818
http://www.elcamino.edu
e-mail: tfallo@elcamino.edu
Thomas Fallo, President

Offers a variety of services to students with disabilities including note takers, extended testing time, counseling services, and special accommodations.

4739 Evergreen Valley College
3095 Yerba Buena Road
San Jose, CA 95135
408-274-7900
FAX 408-432-1962
http://www.euc.edu
e-mail: bonnie.clark@euc.edu
Bonnie Clark, LD Specialist
Nacy Tung, Instruction Assistant
David Koon, President
A public two-year college with 82 learning disabled students out of a total of 9,000.

4740 Excelsior Academy
7202 Princess View Drive
San Diego, CA 92120
619-583-6762
FAX 619-583-6764
http://www.excelsioracademy.com
e-mail: nanmag@earthlink.net
Frank Maguire, Executive Director

4741 Feather River College
570 Golden Eagle Avenue
Quincy, CA 95971
530-283-0521
FAX 530-283-3757
http://www.frcc.cc.ca.us
Susan Carol, President

Offers a variety of services to students with disabilities including note takers, extended testing time, counseling services and special accommodations.

4742 Foothill College
Disabilities Services/ AHEAD
12345 S El Monte Road
Los Altos Hills, CA 94022
650-949-7017
FAX 650-917-1064
TDY:650-948-6025
http://www.foothill.fhda.edu
e-mail: dobbinsmargo@foothill.edu
Margo Dobbins, Coordinator DSP
Beatrix Cashmore, Counselor

Offers a variety of services to students with disabilities including note takers, extended testing time, counseling services and special accommodations.

4743 **Fresno City College**
1101 E University Avenue
Fresno, CA 93741
559-442-4600
FAX 559-265-5784
http://www.fcc.cc.ca.us
e-mail: pio571@sccd.com

Jeanette Imperatrice, LD Specialist
Ned Doffoney, President

A public two-year college with 259 special education students out of a total of 17,949.

4744 **Fullerton College**
Learning Resource Services
321 E Chapman Avenue
Fullerton, CA 92832
714-992-7542
FAX 714-992-7551
http://www.fullcoll.edu

Thomas Cantrell, Contact
Ricardo Perez, Director

A public two-year college with 281 special education students out of a total of 20,731.

4745 **Gavilan College**
5055 Santa Teresa Boulevard
Gilroy, CA 95020
408-848-4800
FAX 408-846-4914
http://www.gavilan..edu

Susan Swaney, Coordinator
Jane Harmon, Administrator

Offers a variety of services to students with disabilities including note takers, extended testing time, counseling services and special accommodations.

4746 **Hartnell College**
Learning Disability Services
156 Homestead Avenue
Salinas, CA 93901
831-755-6721
http://www.hartnell.cc.ca.us

Deborah Shulman, Enabler

A public two-year college with 72 special education students out of a total of 7,593.

4747 **Humboldt State University**
Disability Resource Center
Arcata, CA 95521
707-826-4678
FAX 707-826-5397
TDY:707-826-5392
http://www.sdrc.humboldt.edu
e-mail: rdm7001@humbolde.edu

Ralph McFarland, Director

A public four-year university which provides necessary services and assistance to students with disabilities, through their Disabled Students Services Program. Services are intended to offset the intrusiveness of the disability on a student's academic experience.

4748 **Imperial Valley College**
PO Box 158
Imperial, CA 92251
760-352-8320
FAX 760-355-2663
http://www.imperial.edu

Norma Nava-Pinuleas, Instructional Specialist
David Poor, Staff
Paul Pai, President

A public two-year college with 44 special education students out of a total of 5,230.

4749 **Institute for the Redesign of Learning**
Almansor Center, The
1137 Huntington Drive
South Pasadena, CA 91030
626-282-6194
FAX 323-257-0284
http://www.redesignlearning.org

Al Hernandez, CEO
Greg Cohen, Administrative Assistant

A full day school serving 100 boys and girls, at-risk infants and children. Vocational Program serves adults and includes Supported Employment Services and an Independent Living Program.

4750 **Irvine Valley College**
Learning Disabilities
5500 Irvine Center Drive
Irvine, CA 92618
949-451-5630
FAX 949-451-5386
http://www.ivc.edu

Julie Willard, LD Specialist
Bill Hewitt, Director

The goal is to effectivly provide assistance to all students with disabilities to achieve academic success while at Irvine Valley. The primary function is to accommodate a student's disability, whether it is a physical, communication, learning or psychological disability.

4751 **Laney College**
Disability Resource Center
900 Fallon Street
Oakland, CA 94607
510-464-3162
FAX 510-986-6906
http://www.laney.parita.cc.ca.us

Sondra Neiman, LD Specialist
Odell Johnson, President

A public two-year college with 58 special education students out of a total of 11,808.

4752 **Long Beach City College Pacific Coast Campus**
4351 Faculty Avenue
Long Beach, CA 90808
562-938-4353
FAX 562-938-4457
TDY:562-938-4833
http://www.dsps.lbcc.cc.ca.us
e-mail: dhansch@lbcc.ca.us

Mark Matsui, Director for Disability
Dan Hansch, LD Specialist

Disabled Student Services (DSPS) is a program within Student Services at LBCC. DSPS provides many support services that enable students with disability related limitations to participate in the college's programs and activities. DSPS offers a wide range of services that compensate for a students limitations, like note taking assistance, interpretive services, alternative media, etc.

4753 **Los Angeles City College**
Learning Disabilities Program
855 N Vermont Avenue
Los Angeles, CA 90029
323-953-4000
FAX 323-953-4526
http://www.lacc.cc.ca.us

Susan Matranga, LD Specialist

A public two-year college with 175 students with learning disabilities; total student body is 16,000. The Learning Disabilities Program provides assessment for eligibility in the program, support services, accommodations, and special classes in study skills and problem solving.

4754 **Los Angeles Mission College: Disabled Student Programs and Services**
13356 Eldridge Avenue
Sylmar, CA 91342
818-837-2236
FAX 818-833-3318
TDY:818-364-7861
http://www.lamission.cc.ca.us/front/dsps#

Rick Scuderi PhD, Director

A support system that enables students to fully participate in the college's regular programs and activities. We provide a variety of services from academic and vocational support to assistance with finacial aid. All services are individualized according to specific needs. They do not replace regular programs, but rather, accommodate students special requirements.

4755 Los Angeles Pierce College
6201 Winnetka Avenue
Woodland Hills, CA 91371 818-347-0551
http://www.piercecollege.com
David Phoenix, Contact

A public two-year college with 257 special education students out of a total of 19,207.

4756 Los Angeles Valley College
Disabled Student Programs & Services
5800 Fulton Avenue
Van Nuys, CA 91401 818-947-2600
FAX 818-947-2680
http://www.lavc.edu
Kathleen Sullivan, Coordinator

Provides specialized support services to students with disabilities which are in addition to the regular services provided to all students. Special accommodations and services are determined by the nature and extent of the disability related educational limitations of the student and are provided based upon the recommendation of DSPS.

4757 Los Medanos College
2700 E Leland Road
Pittsburg, CA 94565 925-439-2181
FAX 925-427-1599
http://www.losmedanos.net
Peter Garcia, President

A public two-year college with 177 special education students out of a total of 7,784.

4758 Loyola Marymount University
7900 Loyola Boulevard
Los Angeles, CA 90045 310-338-7777
FAX 310-338-2797
http://www.lmu.edu
e-mail: admissns@lmumail.lmu.edu
Matthew Fissinger, Director
Elena Williams, Admission Assistant

Provides specialized assistance and resources that enable students with physical, perceptual, emotional and learning disabilities to achieve maximum independence while they pursue their educational goals.

4759 Master's College
ELS Care College of Canyon
26455 Rockwell Canyon Road
Santa Clarita, CA 91355 661-362-5554
FAX 661-362-5555
http://www.els.edu
e-mail: greyes@els.edu
Gina Reyes, Center Director
Mary Hernandez, Academic Director

An independent two-year college with 5 special education students out of a total of 850. There is an additional fee for the special education program in addition to the regular tuition.

4760 Mendocino College
PO Box 3000
Ukiah, CA 95482 707-462-3984
FAX 707-468-3120
http://www.mendocino.cc.ca.us
Kathleen Daigle, Specialist
Manuel Guerra, Executive Director

A two-year public college that offers programs for the disabled.

4761 Menlo College
Academic Success Program
1000 El Camino Real
Atherton, CA 94027
800-556-3656
http://www.menlo.edu
e-mail: admissions@menlo.edu
Mark Hager, Director

Four year college that offers a program for learning disabled students.

4762 Merced College
3600 M Street
Merced, CA 95348 209-384-6000
FAX 209-384-6103
TDY:209-384-6311
http://www.merced.cc.ca.us
Benjamin Duran, President
Richard Marashlian, Director

Students with physical, communicative, learning, and or psychological disabilities are encouraged to contact the Disabled Student Services Office. Students with verified disabilities are provided with services to meet their particular needs. These include, but are not limited to, counseling, instructional aids, interpeters for the deaf, registration assistance, computer access through the High Tech Center, learning strategies instruction, and test proctoring.

4763 Merritt College
Disabled Student Programs & Services
12500 Campus Drive
Oakland, CA 94619 510-436-2429
FAX 510-436-2503
http://www.merritt.edu
e-mail: ctissot@merrit.edu
Cristana Tissot, LD Specialist
Susan Wilhite, Administrative Assistant

A public two-year college with 78 special education students out of a total of 6,688.

4764 Mills College
5000 Macarthur Boulevard
Oakland, CA 94613 510-430-2156
FAX 510-430-3235
http://www.mills.edu
e-mail: jemiller@mills.edu
Jess Miller, Director
Janet Holgram, President
Michael Sellers, Manager
Services provided to studens with disabilities.

4765 Miracosta College
1 Barnard Drive
Oceanside, CA 92056 760-757-2121
888-201-8480
FAX 760-795-6604
TDY:760-439-1060
http://www.maricosta.edu
e-mail: nschafer@maricosta.edu
Nancy Schafer, LD Specialist
Angela Degirolamo, Assistant
Victoria Munoz-Richart, President
A community college which provides in-class academic accommodations to students with verified disabilities.

4766 Modesto Junior College
435 College Avenue
Modesto, CA 95350 209-575-6062
FAX 209-575-6852
TDY:209-575-6863
John Martinez, Dean Special Services
Le-Houng Pham, Publisher

The primary purposes of the Disability Services Center at Modesto Junior College are to provide students with disabilities access to post-secondary education and educational development opportunities, through supportive service and or instruction, depending on individual needs; and to improve campus and community understanding of the needs of students who have disabilities.

4767 Monterey Peninsula College
980 Fremont Street
Monterey, CA 93940 831-646-4000
FAX 831-645-1390
http://www.mpc.edu
Bill Jones, LD Coordinator
Carl Ehmann, President

A public two-year college with 202 special education students out of a total of 8,502.

4768 Moorpark College
7075 Campus Road
Moorpark, CA 93021
805-378-1400
FAX 805-378-1563
http://www.moorpark.cc.ca.us
Eva Conrad, President

A public two-year college with 154 special education students out of a total of 12,414.

4769 Mt. San Antonio Community College
Disabled Student Programs & Services
1100 N Grand Avenue
Walnut, CA 91789
909-594-5611
FAX 909-468-3943
http://www.dsps.mtsac.edu
e-mail: ghanson@mtsac.edu
Grace Hanson, Director
Christopher O'Hearn, President
Vicki Greco, Counselor Learning Disability
A public two-year college with 1,500 students with disabilities who receive special services. Total population of students is approximately 40,000.

4770 Mt. San Jacinto College
1499 N State Street
San Jacinto, CA 92583
951-487-6752
http://www.msjc.edu
Milly Douthit, LD Specialist
Richard Giese, President

A public two-year college with 98 special education students out of a total of 9,000 students.

4771 Napa Valley College
2277 Napa Vallejo Highway
Napa, CA 94558
707-253-3000
800-826-1077
http://www.nuc.cc.ca.us
Gwynne Katz MD, LD Specialist
Chris Carthy, President

Offers a variety of services to students with disabilities including note takers, extended testing time, counseling services and special accommodations.

4772 Ohlone College
43600 Mission Boulevard
Fremont, CA 94539
510-659-6100
FAX 510-659-6032
http://www.ohlone.edu
Fred Hilke, Special Services Director
Doug Treadway, President

The Ohlone College Disabled Student Services Program is designed to open doors to educational and occupational opportunities for students with physical or medical disabilities. Our primary purpose is to provide an opportuninty for all individuals to gain maximun benefit from their educational experience. Ohlone College encourages students with physical or medical disabilities to participate within the limits of their disabilities in the same activies and courses as other students.

4773 Orange Coast College
2701 Fairview Road
Costa Mesa, CA 92626
714-432-5072
FAX 714-432-5609
http://www.occ.cccd.edu
e-mail: mcucurny@cccd.edu
Ken Ortiz MD, Associate Dean
Robert Dees, President

A public two-year college with 350 special education students out of a total of 27,960. There is a an additional fee for the special education program in addition to the regular tuition.

4774 Oxnard College
4000 S Rose Avenue
Oxnard, CA 93033
805-986-5800
FAX 805-986-5806
http://www.oxnard.edu
e-mail: ocinfo@vcccd.net
Carole Frick, LD Specialist
Ellen Young, Coordinator
Lydia Reese, President
Offers a complete repertoire of support services for students with disabilities, including linkage with the local department of rehabilitation. Special instruction and high tech center available.

4775 Pacific Union College
1 Angwin Avenue
Angwin, CA 94508
707-545-5868
FAX 707-965-6797
http://www.puc.edu
e-mail: njacobo@puc.edu
Nancy Jacobo, Director Enrollment Services
John Collins, Vice President

Services provided to students with learning disabilities.

4776 Palomar College
1140 W Mission Road
San Marcos, CA 92069
760-744-1150
FAX 706-761-3509
TDY:760-471-8506
http://www.palomar.edu
e-mail: dsts@palomar.edu
Ronald Haines, Disabled Student Programs
Robert Deegan, President

A public two-year college with 993 special education students out of a total of 23,909.

4777 Pasadena City College
1570 E Colorado Boulevard
Pasadena, CA 91106
626-585-7123
FAX 626-585-7566
TDY:626-585-7052
http://www.pasadena.edu
e-mail: elweller@paccd.cc.ca.us
James Cossler, Principal
Bianca Richards, Counselor
Emy Lu Weller MD, Teacher/Professor Specialist
A public two-year college with over 500 students with learning disabilities of over 24,000 credit students.

4778 Pepperdine University
24255 Pacific Coast Highway
Malibu, CA 90263
310-456-4382
FAX 310-456-4827
Charles Runnels, CEO

4779 Porterville College
100 E College Avenue
Porterville, CA 93257
559-791-2200
FAX 559-784-4779
http://www.pc.cc.ca.us
e-mail: dallen@pc.cc.ca.us
Diane Allen, LD Specialist
Rosa Carlson, President

A public two-year college with 90 learning disabled students. Services include assessment, special counseling, liaison with campus and community, notetakers, readers, registration assistance, test taking assistance, transcription and tutoring.

4780 Rancho Santiago College
2323 N Broadway
Santa Ana, CA 92706
714-480-7300
http://www.rsccd.org
Mary Kobane, LD Specialist

A public two-year college with 319 special education students out of a total of 26,393.

4781 Rancho Santiago Community College
1530 W 17th Street
Santa Ana, CA 92706
714-564-6000
FAX 714-564-6455
http://www.rsccd.org

Ann Vescial, Coordinator
Linda Miscovic, Director
Kathi Richey, Executive Director
The mission of Rancho Santiago Community College District is to respond to the educational needs of an everchanging community and to provide programs and services that reflect academic excellence. The district's two colleges promote open access and celebrate the diversity of both its students and staff, as well as the community.

4782 Raskob Learning Institute and Day School
3520 Mountain Boulevard
Oakland, CA 94619 510-436-1275
FAX 510-436-1106
http://www.rascobinstitute.org
e-mail: raskobinstitute@hnu.edu
Rachel Wylde, Executive Director
Rachel Hallanger, Head Teacher
Gassler Clinical Director, Clinical Director
A co-educational school for students from diverse cultural and economic backgrounds with language-based learning disabilities. Raskob seeks to recognize and nurture the talents and strengths of each student while remediating areas of academic weakness.
9-14 years old

4783 Reedley College
995 N Reed Avenue
Reedley, CA 93654 559-638-3641
FAX 559-638-5040
http://www.reedleycollege.com
e-mail: janice.emerzian@reedleycollege.edu
Janice Emerzian MD, District Director
Barbara Hioco, President

Offer various services including: academic advising; adapted computer equipment; adapted physical education; books-on-tape and other educational aids; cooperative accommodations with instructors; educational limitations and accommodation notices to instructors; interpreters; learning disability assessment; liaison and referral to on-campus and off-campus resources; mobility assistance; notetakers; personal counseling and typing services.

4784 Saint Mary's College of California
1928 Saint Marys Road
Moraga, CA 94556 925-631-1065
FAX 925-631-4835
http://www.stmarys-ca.edu
e-mail: jparfitt@stmarys-ca.edu
Jeannie Chavez-Parfitt, Director
Ronald Gallager, President

Four year college that provides support and services to its disabled students.

4785 San Diego City College
1313 12th Avenue
San Diego, CA 92101 619-388-3400
FAX 619-388-3501
http://www.city.sdccd.cc.ca.us
Ken Mayer, Counselor

Offers a variety of services to students with disabilities including note takers, extended testing time, counseling services, and special accommodations.

4786 San Diego Miramar College
Disability Support Programs and Services
10440 Black Mountain Road
San Diego, CA 92126 858-536-7212
FAX 858-536-4302
TDY:858-536-4301
http://www.miramar.sdccd.net/depts/stusvcs
e-mail: miradsps@sdccd.edu
Kathleen Doorly, Program Coordinator
Sandra Smith, DSPS Counselor/LD Specialist

A public two-year college with 500 learning disabled students. These students receive services and accommodations appropriate for their success in college. Individual counseling, class advising and LD assessments are also available. Special classes are offered to support college courses.

4787 San Diego State University
5500 Campanile Drive
San Diego, CA 92182 619-594-6477
http://www.sdsu.edu
e-mail: admissions@sdsu.edu
Margo Behr, Director
Sandra Cook, Admissions Director
Stephen Weber, President
A public four-year college with 520 disabled students out of a total of 25,658.

4788 San Francisco State University
Disability Resource Center
1600 Holloway Avenue
San Francisco, CA 94132 415-338-6356
FAX 415-338-1041
http://www.sfsu.edu
e-mail: defreese@sfsu.edu
Deidre Defreese, Director

A public four-year college with 400 special education students out of a total of 21,044.

4789 San Jose City College
2100 Moorpark Avenue
San Jose, CA 95128 408-288-3714
FAX 408-971-8201
http://www.sjcc.edu
e-mail: donna.wirt@sjcc.edu
Donna Wirt, LD Specialist
Merdith Matos, Program Assistant
Chui Tsang, President
Offers a variety of services to students with disabilities including LD assessments per guidelines of State of California Community Colleges, note takers, extended testing time, counseling services and special accommodations.

4790 San Jose State University
Disability Resource Center
1 Washington Square
San Jose, CA 95192 408-924-6000
FAX 408-924-5999
TDY:408-924-5990
http://www.sjsu.edu
e-mail: marty@drc.sjsu.edu
Martin Schulter, Director
John Bradbury, Admissions Director

A four-year public university with 600 out of 20,679 receiving disability services.

4791 Santa Ana College
1530 W 17th Street
Santa Ana, CA 92706 714-564-6000
FAX 714-836-6696
http://www.sacollege.org
Cheryl Dunn-Hoanzl, Director
Kathi Richey, Executive Director

Offers a variety of services to students with disabilities including note takers, extended testing time, counseling services and special accommodations.

4792 Santa Barbara City College
721 Cliff Drive
Santa Barbara, CA 93109 805-965-0581
FAX 805-884-4966
TDY:805-962-4084
http://www.sbcc.net
e-mail: dspshelp@sbcc.edu
Mary Lawson, LD Specialist
Gerry Lewin, LD Specialist
John Romo, President
Offers complete repertoire of support services for students with disabilities, including linkage with local department of rehabilitation. Special instruction available. High tech center.

4793 Santa Clara University
Disability Resources
500 El Camino Real
Santa Clara, CA 95053 408-554-4111
FAX 408-554-2709
http://www.scu.edu
e-mail: eravenscroft@scu.edu

Ann Ravenscroft, Director
Sandra Hayes, Admissions Director

Designated by the University to ensure access for all students with disabilities to all academic programs and University resources. Types of disabilities include medical, physical, psychological, attention deficit and learning disabilities. Reasonable accommodations are provided to minimize the effects of a student's disability and to maximize the potential for success.

4794 Santa Monica College
1900 Pico Boulevard
Santa Monica, CA 90405
310-434-4452
FAX 310-434-3694
http://www.smc.edu
e-mail: gmarcopulos@smc.edu
George Marcopulos, Learning Specialist
Audrey Morris, Coordinator
Marcia Martinez, Manager
A public two-year college with 300 students with learning disabilities out of a total of 26,361.

4795 Santa Rosa Junior College
Disability Resource Department
1501 Mendocino Avenue
Santa Rosa, CA 95401
707-527-4278
800-564-7752
FAX 707-527-4798
http://www.santarosa.edu
e-mail: kvigeland@santarosa.edu
Kari Vigeland, Director
Ricardo Navarrette, Admissions Director

A public two-year college with 300 special education students out of a total of 28,223.

4796 Shasta College
11555 Old Oregon Trail
Redding, CA 96003
530-225-4723
FAX 530-225-4952
http://www.shasta.cc.ca.us
e-mail: info@shastacollege.edu
Parker Pollock, Handicapped Director
Jaime Larson, Professor
Mary Retterer, President
A public two-year college with 104 special education students out of a total of 12,822.

4797 Sierra College
Learning Opportunities Center
5000 Rocklin Road
Rocklin, CA 95677
916-781-2697
FAX 916-789-2967
http://www.sierra.cc.ca.us
e-mail: jhirschinger@scmail.sierra.cc.ca.us
Denise Stone, Coorindator
Kaylene Hallberg, Dean Student Services

A public two-year college with 1,100 disabled students out of a total of 20,000.

4798 Skyline College
Developmental Skills Program
3300 College Drive
San Bruno, CA 94066
650-738-4193
FAX 650-738-4299
http://www.skylinecollege.net
Linda Sciver, Coordinator

A public two-year college with 103 special education students out of a total of 9,023.

4799 Solano Community College
4000 Suisun Valley Road
Fairfield, CA 94534
707-864-7000
FAX 707-863-7810
http://www.solano.edu
Ron Nelson, Coordinator
Paulette Perfumo, President

The LD Center offers eligibility assessment (students with average to above average intelligence with severe processing deficit(s) and severe aptitude-achievement discrepancies), and instruction in strategies and interventions to help the student become more successful in regular college classes. Academic and personal counseling from Disabled Student Programs Counselors are available. Support services such as notetaking, extended test time and other modifications are available.

4800 Sonoma State University
Disabled Student Services
1801 E Cotati Avenue
Rohnert Park, CA 94928
707-664-2677
FAX 707-664-2505
TDY:707-664-2958
http://www.sonoma.edu
e-mail: bill.clopton@sonoma.edu
Linda Lipps, Director
Katharyn Crabbe, Admissions Director

A public four-year college with 230 disabled students out of a total of 6,211.

4801 Southwestern College
Diagnostic Learning Center
900 Otay Lakes Road
Chula Vista, CA 91910
619-482-6327
FAX 619-482-6435
http://www.swc.cc.ca.us
Diane Branman, Contact
Irma Alvarez, Dean

A public two-year college with 99 special education students out of a total of 17,083.

4802 Springall Academy
6460 Boulder Lake Avenue
San Diego, CA 92119
619-460-5090
FAX 858-459-4660
http://www.springall.org
Arlene Baker, President
Sally McNamara, Curriculum Director

Offers a variety of services to students with disabilities including note takers, extended testing time, counseling services, and special accommodations. The academy is a nonprofit school for learning and behaviorally challenged students.

4803 Stanbridge Academy
515 E Poplar Avenue
San Mateo, CA 94401
650-375-5860
FAX 650-375-5861
http://www.stanbridgeacademy.org
e-mail: info@stanbridgeacademy.org
Marilyn Lynch, Executive Director

4804 Stanford University
123 Meyer Library
Stanford, CA 94305
650-723-2300
FAX 650-725-7411
http://www.stanford.edu
Molly Sandperl, Special Services

An independent four-year college with 102 special education students out of a total of 6,527.

4805 Sterne School
2690 Jackson Street
San Francisco, CA 94115
415-922-6081
FAX 415-922-1598
http://www.sterneschool.org
e-mail: reception@sterneschool.org
Lisa Graham, Director
Cindy Weingard, Development Director

A private school serving students in 6-12 grade who have specific learning disabilities.

1976

4806 Taft College

29 Emmons Park Drive
Taft, CA 93268
661-763-7700
FAX 661-763-7705
TDY:661-763-7801
http://www.taft.cc.ca.us/
e-mail: jross@taft.org

Jeff Ross, Coordinator Program Services
Abel Nunec, Executive Director
Roe Darnell, President

A public two-year college with 56 special education students out of a total of 952.

4807 UCLA Office for Students with Disabilities

PO Box 951361
Los Angeles, CA 90095
310-825-4321
FAX 310-825-9656
TDY:310-206-6083
http://www.ucla.edu
e-mail: jmorris@saonet.ucla.edu

Julie Morris, LD Program Coordinator
Kathy Molini, Director
Albert Carnesale, CEO

Offers a variety of services to students with disabilities including notetakers, accommodated testing, counseling services, assistive technology, support groups, advocacy to faculty, strategies, workshops and counseling.

4808 USC University Affiliated Program: Childrens Hospital at Los Angeles

University of Southern California
PO Box 54700
Los Angeles, CA 90054
323-669-2303
FAX 323-663-6707
http://www.usc.edu

Robert Jacobs, Director
Connie Nickelson, Administrative Assistant
Roberta Williams, Manager

The primary mission of the USC UAP is the continued improvement of the health and welfare of children and families who are affected by disabling conditions, chronic illness, or other special health care needs.

4809 United States International University

10455 Pomerado Road
San Diego, CA 92131
619-224-4444
FAX 858-635-4690
http://www.alliance.edu

Lorna Reese, Assistant Dean
Geoffrey Cox, President

Four year college offering services to disabled students.

4810 University of California-Davis: Student Disability Resource Center

1 Shields Avenue
Davis, CA 95616
530-752-0321
FAX 530-752-0161
TDY:530-752-6833
http://http://sdc.ucdavis.edu/
e-mail: caodell@ucdavis.edu

Christine O'Dell, LD Specialist
Tina Morton, Administrative Assistant
Joe Silva, MD, Director

Committed to ensuring equal educational opportunities for students with disabilities. Promotes independence and integrated participation in campus life for students with disabilities.

4811 University of California: Berkeley

Disabled Student's Program
260 Cesar Chavez Center
Berkeley, CA 94720
510-642-0518
FAX 510-643-9686
TDY:510-642-6376
http://www.dsp.berkeley.edu
e-mail: erogers@berkeley.edu

Ed Rogers, Director

A four-year public university.

4812 University of California: Irvine

Office for Disability Services
105 Administration Building
Irvine, CA 92697
949-824-7494
FAX 949-824-3083
TDY:949-824-6272
http://www.disability.uci.edu
e-mail: ods@uci.edu

Ron Blosser MD, Special Services

Our mission is to provide effective and reasonable academic accommodations and related disability services to UCI students, Extension and Summer Session students, and other program participants. Consults with and educates faculty about reasonable academic accommodations. Strives to improve access to UCI programs, activities, and facilities for students with disabilities. Advises and educates academic and administrative departments about access issues to programs or facilities.

4813 University of California: Irvine Campus

105 Administration Building
Irvine, CA 92717
949-824-7494
FAX 949-824-8566
http://www.uci.edu

Ron Blosser MD, Director

Offers a variety of services to students with disabilities including note takers, extended testing time, counseling services and special accommodations.

4814 University of California: Los Angeles

Office for Students with Disabilities
A-255 Murphy Hall
Los Angeles, CA 90095
310-825-1501
FAX 310-825-9656
TDY:310-206-6083
http://www.ucla.edu
e-mail: kmolini@saonet.ucla.edu

Kathy Molini, Director
Vu Tran, Admissions Director

Served by a TWP learning disabilities specialist, UCLA offers a full range of accommodations and services. Services are individually designed, and include disability- related counseling, special test arrangements, notetaker services, readers, priority enrollment, adaptive technology, and individual small group and individual content area tutoring. An active support group and peer-mentor program provides opportunities for students to discuss mutual concerns and enhance learning strategies.

4815 University of California: Riverside

Disabled Student Services
900 University Avenue
Riverside, CA 92521
951-827-1012
http://www.ucr.edu

Marcia Schiffer, Director DSS
France Cordova, Administrator

A public four-year college with 25 learning disabled students out of a total of 8,000.

4816 University of California: San Diego

Office for Students with Disabilities
9500 Gilman Drive
La Jolla, CA 92093
858-534-4382
FAX 858-534-4650
http://www.osd.ucsd.edu
e-mail: rgimblett@ucsd.edu

Roberta Gimblett, Director
Mae Brown, Admissions Director
Naomi Levoy, Outreach Assistant

A public four-year college with 150 students receiving disability services out of 15,840.

4817 University of California: San Francisco

Office of Student Life
500 Parnassus Avenue
San Francisco, CA 94143
415-476-4318
FAX 415-476-7295
TDY:415-476-4318
http://http://student.ucsf.edu/osl
e-mail: ekoenig@osl.uscsf.edu

Eric Koenig, Director
Barbara Smith, Operations Manager
Candy Clemens, Operations

The Office of Student Life is responsible for coordinating Services for Students with Disabilities at UCSF.

4818 University of California: Santa Barbara
Disabled Student Program
1210 Cheadle Hall
Santa Barbara, CA 93106
805-893-2182
FAX 805-893-7127
TDY:805-893-2668
http://www.ucsb.edu/dsp/
e-mail: batty-c@sa.ucsb.edu
Gary White, Acting Director
Claudia Balty, Disability Specialist

Works to increase the retention and graduation rates of students with disabilities and to foster student independence.

4819 University of California: Santa Cruz
146 Hahn
Santa Cruz, CA 95064
831-427-6638
FAX 831-459-5064
TDY:831-459-4806
http://www.ucsc.edu
e-mail: drc@ucsc.edu
Margaret Church, Director Special Services
Barbara Duron, Assistant Director
Anne Butler, Manager
A public four-year college with 87 special education students out of a total of 9,162.

4820 University of Redlands
Academic Support Services/Disabled Student Service
PO Box 3080
Redlands, CA 92373
909-748-8108
FAX 909-335-5297
http://www.redlands.edu
e-mail: judy.bowman@redlands.edu
Judy Bowman, Academic Support/Disabled Svcs
Paul Driscoll, Admissions Director

Offers a variety of services to students with disabilities including notetakers, extended testing time, counseling services, and special accommodations.

4821 University of San Diego
9500 Gilman Drive
La Jolla, CA 92093
858-534-5000
FAX 858-822-5407
http://www.ucsd.edu
Tyler Gabriel MD, Academic Counseling
Vijay Samalam, Plant Manager

An independent four-year college with 35 special education students out of a total of 3,904.

4822 University of San Francisco
Student Disability Services
2130 Fulton Street
San Francisco, CA 94117
415-422-2613
FAX 415-422-5906
TDY:415-422-2613
http://www.usfca.edu
e-mail: sds@usfca.edu

Tom Merrell, Director
Teresa Ong, Assistant Director

A four-year private college with 200 students recieving LD/ADHD services.

4823 University of Southern California
Disability Services and Programs
3601 Trousdale Parkway
Los Angeles, CA 90089
213-740-0776
FAX 213-740-8216
TDY:213-740-6948
http://www.usc.edu
e-mail: jeddy@usc.edu

Eddie Roth MD, LD Consultant
Laurel Tews, Admissions Director

An independent four-year university with 350 LD students out of a total of 15,705. The support structure for students with documented learning disabilities at USC is one that is totally individualized. Offers support at the student's request for such things as extended time for exams, proofreading papers and reports, and advocacy with faculty. There is no special admission process.

4824 University of the Pacific
Office of Special Services for Students with Dis
3601 Pacific Avenue
Stockton, CA 95211
209-946-3221
FAX 209-946-2278
http://www.pacific.edu/education/ssd
e-mail: ssd@pacific.edu

Daniel Nuss, Coordinator

Offers a variety of services to qualified students with disabilities on a case-by-case basis such as test proctoring services, note-taking assistance, priority registration or referrals to other campus services such as counseling and tuturial support.

4825 Vanguard University of Southern California
55 Fair Drive
Costa Mesa, CA 92626
714-556-3610
800-722-6279
FAX 714-966-5471
http://www.vanguard.edu
e-mail: jmireles@vanguard.edu
Jessica Mireles, Director
Murray Dempster, President

Four year college offers support for its disabled students.

4826 Ventura College
4667 Telegraph Road
Ventura, CA 93003
805-654-6400
FAX 805-648-8915
TDY:805-642-4583
http://www.ventura.college.edu
e-mail: tdalton@vcccd.edu
Tom Dalton PsyD, LD Director
Nancy Latham, EAC Coordinator
Robin Calote, President
A public two-year college with about 400 LD students out of a total of about 12,000.

4827 Victor Valley College
18422 Bear Valley Road
Victorville, CA 92395
760-245-4271
FAX 760-245-9744
http://www.victor.cc.ca.us
Susan Tillman, LD Specialist

Offers a variety of services to students with disabilities including note takers, extended testing time, counseling services and special accommodations.

4828 West Hills College
300 W Cherry Lane
Coalinga, CA 93210
559-934-2000
FAX 559-935-5655
http://www.westhills.cc.ca.us
Rosemary Burciaga, Manager

A public two-year college with 63 special education students out of a total of 3,530.

4829 West Los Angeles College
9000 Overland Avenue
Culver City, CA 90230
310-287-4596
FAX 310-287-4317
http://www.ulac.edu
e-mail: regalaba@lacitycollege.edu
Frances Israel, Learning Specialist
Casandra Brown, Program Assistant
Patricia Banday, Manager
A public two-year college with 104 special education students out of a total of 8,952.

4830 West Valley College
14000 Fruitvale Avenue
Saratoga, CA 95070
408-867-2200
http://www.westvalley.edu
Susan Bunch, LD Specialist
Stan Arteberry, Manager

A public two-year college with 209 special education students out of a total of 1,429.

4831 Westmark School
5461 Louise Avenue
Encino, CA 91316
818-380-1365
FAX 818-986-2605
http://www.westmarkschool.org
e-mail: sshenkin@westmarkschool.org
Sarae Shenkin, Principal
Sylvia Lopez, Office Assistant

4832 Whittier College
Learning Support Services
PO Box 634
Whittier, CA 90608
562-907-4233
FAX 562-907-4980
http://www.whittier.edu
e-mail: tthomsen@whittier.edu
Joan Smith, Director
Tina Thomsen, Administrative Assistant

A four-year private college with 30 students recieving disability services out of 1,297.

Colorado

4833 Aims Community College
PO Box 69
Greeley, CO 80632
970-330-8008
800-301-5388
FAX 970-339-6682
http://www.aims.edu
Donna Wright, LD Center
Marsi Liddell, President

Offers a variety of services to students with disabilities including note takers, extended testing time, counseling services, and special accommodations.

4834 Arapahoe Community College
5900 S Santa Fe Drive
Littleton, CO 80120
303-797-4222
FAX 303-797-0127
http://www.arcpahoe.edu
Bert Glandon, President

Offers a variety of services to students with disabilities including note takers, extended testing time, counseling services, and special accommodations.

4835 Colorado Christian University
Academic Support
160 S Garrison Street
Lakewood, CO 80226
303-963-3266
FAX 303-274-7560
http://www.ccu.edu
e-mail: jlambert@ccu.edu
Joanne Lambert, Assistance Coordinator

Four-year college that offers support to learning disabled students.

4836 Colorado Mountain College
Central Admissions Office
3000 County Road
Glenwood Springs, CO 81602
970-947-8253
800-621-8559
FAX 970-928-9668

The Disability Service Program at Colorado Mountain College is designed to assist students with disabilities to be successful in their programs. The program design offers students enhancement of basic skills, completion in a chosen area of study and removal of barriers in the classroom while preserving the integrity of the course objectives.

4837 Colorado Northwestern Community College
500 Kennedy Drive
Rangely, CO 81648
970-675-2261
800-562-1105
FAX 970-675-3330
http://www.cncc.edu
e-mail: jim.hoganson@cncc.edu
Jim Hoganson, LD Director
Robert Rizzudo, President
Peter Angstadt, Administrator
A public two-year college with 11 special education students out of a total of 502.

4838 Colorado State University
Resources for Disabled Students
100 General Services
Fort Collins, CO 80523
970-491-6385
FAX 970-491-3457
TDY:970-491-6385
http://www.colostate.edu/depts/RDS
e-mail: kivy@lamar.colostate.edu
Kathleen Ivy, Counselor
Rosemary Kreston, Director

The mission of Resources for Disabled Students (RDS) is to assist Colorado State University in ensuring that qualified students with disabilities are afforded and given access to the same, or equal, educational opportunities available to other university students.

4839 Colorado State University: Pueblo
2200 Bonforte Boulevard
Pueblo, CO 81001
719-549-2100
FAX 719-549-2195
http://www.colostate-pueblo.edu
e-mail: joe.marshall@colostate-pueblo.edu
Joe Marshall, Director
Ronald Applbaum, President
Pam Chambers, Disability Resource Coordinator
Support services for special needs students are provided on an individual basis. The student must provide documentation of disability with a formal request for specific support services needed.

4840 Community College of Aurora
16000 E Centretech Parkway
Aurora, CO 80011
303-360-4700
FAX 303-631-7432
http://www.cco.edu
e-mail: reniece.jones@cco.edu
Reniece Jones, Coordinator
Linda Bowman, President

Offers a variety of services to students with disabilities including note takers, extended testing time, counseling services, and special accommodations.

4841 Community College of Denver
Students Disabilities Services
PO Box 173363
Denver, CO 80217
303-556-2600
FAX 303-556-4563
TDY:303-556-3300
http://www.ccd.edu
Michael Rusk, Director
Connie Trujillo, Office Manager
Emita Samuels, Administrator
A public two-year college with 100 special education students out of a total of 6,000. There is an additional fee for the special education program in addition to the regular tuition.

4842 Denver Academy
4400 E Iliff Avenue
Denver, CO 80222
303-777-5870
FAX 303-777-5893
http://www.denveracadamy.org

Lori Richardson, Dean
Jim Loan, President

Denver Academy was founded in 1972 and is internationally recognized for the quality of its program. Our mission is to be a center of excellence for the education of students with learning differences in order to help them fully develop their intellectual, social, physical and moral potential thereby providing them with the necessary skill to be successful in life.

4843 Disability Services
University of Colorado at Colorado Springs
Main Hall 105
Colorado Springs, CO 80933 719-262-3354
FAX 719-262-3354
http://www.uccs.edu/dss
e-mail: disbserv@uccs.edu
Kaye MA, Coordinator Disability

Provides services and accommodations to students with disabilities, works closely with faculty and staff in an advisory capacity, assists in the development of reasonable accommodations for students and provides equal access for otherwise qualified individuals with disabilities.

4844 Fort Lewis College
1000 Rim Drive
Durango, CO 81301 970-247-7679
FAX 970-247-2703
http://www.fortlewis.edu
e-mail: admission@fortlewis.edu
Tim Slane, Disabled Student Director

Coordinates services at Fort Lewis for those students with disabilities, acts as liaison between students and faculty programs. Advises and directs those students to the appropriate services and academic advisors.

4845 Front Range Community College Progressive Learning
3645 W 112th Avenue
Westminster, CO 80031 303-404-5550
http://www.frontrange.edu
Karen Reinerston, President
Karen Hossack, Faculty

A public two-year college with a unique remedial program for all adults with learning disabilities. Enrollment is not necessary to attend Progressive Learning Program.

4846 JFK Partners' Autism and Developmental Disorder Clinic
UC at Denver Health Sciences Center
4200 E 9th Avenue
Denver, CO 80262 303-315-6511
FAX 303-315-6844
TDY:303-864-5266
http://www.jfkpartners.org
e-mail: robinson.cordelia@tchden.org
Cordelia Robinson, Director
Judy Reaven, Clinic Director
Beverly Murdock, Administrative Assistant
The Autism and Developmental Disorders Clinic has provided a fall range of outpatient clinical services to individuals with autism spectrum disorders or other development disorders, and their families. Services are organized around consumer and family goals, Clinical activities available to clients include disciplinary and interdisciplinary evaluations for purposes of diagnostic clarification and for provision of recommendations for treatment.
1992

4847 John F Kennedy Child Development Center
4200 E 9th Avenue
Denver, CO 80262 303-315-3092
Philip Walravens MD, Director

4848 Lamar Community College
2401 S Main Street
Lamar, CO 81052 719-336-2248
800-968-6920
FAX 719-336-2448
http://www.lamarcc.edu
e-mail: admissions@lamarcc.edu
David Smith, Manager
Angela Woodward, Director Admissions
Becky Young, Special Populations Coordinator
Offers a variety of services to students with disabilities including notetakers, extended testing time, counseling services, and special accommodations.

4849 Morgan Community College
300 Main Street
Fort Morgan, CO 80701 970-542-3260
800-622-0216
FAX 970-867-3352
http://www.mcc.ccoes.edu
Kristi Rorabaugh, Administrator
Maxine Weimer, Developmental Education

A public two-year college with 11 special education students out of a total of 887.

4850 Northeastern Junior College
100 College Drive
Sterling, CO 80751 970-521-6612
800-626-4637
FAX 970-521-6672
http://www.nejc.edu
e-mail: lgill@nejc.edu
Lori Gill, Special Services Director
Judy Giacgomini, President
Candice Habely, Executive Director
A public two-year college with 36 special education students out of a total of 2,042.

4851 Pikes Peak Community College
5675 S Academy Boulevard
Colorado Springs, CO 80906 719-540-7500
800-456-6847
FAX 719-540-7254
TDY:719-540-7128
http://www.ppcc.edu
Michael Nusen, Coordinator
Jane Abbott, Executive Director

A public two-year college with 108 special education students out of a total of 6,517.

4852 Pueblo Community College
900 W Orman Avenue
Pueblo, CO 81004 719-549-3314
888-642-6017
FAX 719-544-1179
http://www.pueblocc.edu
Michael Davis, Owner
Mike , President

Offers a variety of services to students with disabilities including note takers, extended testing time, counseling services, and special accommodations.

4853 Red Rocks Community College
13300 W 6th Avenue
Lakewood, CO 80228 303-914-6600
FAX 303-914-6666
http://www.rrcc.edu
Theona Hammond-Harns, Special Services
Cliff Richardson, Administrator

A public two-year college with 33 special education students out of a total of 6,300.

4854 Regis University
Disability Services
3333 Regis Boulevard
Denver, CO 80221 303-458-4941
FAX 303-964-3647
http://www.regis.edu
e-mail: mbwillia@regis.edu
Joie Williams, Director

A four-year private university with 110 students recieving disability services out of 1,022.

4855 Trinidad State Junior College
136 Main Street
Trinidad, CO 81082
719-846-5644
FAX 719-846-4550
http://www.tsjc.cccoes.edu/
John Giron, Special Services
Donna Watkins, Executive Director

Offers a variety of services to students with disabilities including note takers, extended testing time, counseling services, and special accommodations.

4856 University of Colorado at Boulder Disability Services
Academic Resource Team (ART)
107 Ucb
Boulder, CO 80309
303-492-8671
FAX 303-492-5601
TDY:303-492-8671
http://www.colorado.edu/disabilityservices
e-mail: dsinfo@colorado.edu
Jim Cohn, Supervisor
Cindy Donahue, Director

Provides a variety of services to individuals with nonvisible disabilities, including individualized strategy sessions with a disability specialist, an assistive technology lab, and a career program for students with disabilities. Disability specialists also assist with obtaining reasonable accommodations if documentation meets disability services requirements and supports the need for them.

4857 University of Colorado: Colorado Springs
Disability Services
Main Hall 105
Colorado Springs, CO 80933
719-262-3354
FAX 719-262-3354
http://www.uccs.edu
e-mail: disbserv@uccs.edu
Kaye Simonton, Director
Randy Kouba, Admissions Director

A four-year public university with 200 students receiving disability services out of 5,054.

4858 University of Denver
Learning Effectiveness Program
2199 S University Boulevard
Denver, CO 80208
303-871-2372
FAX 303-871-3938
http://www.du.edu
e-mail: tmay@du.edu
Ted May, Director
John Dolan, Admissions Director

A fee for service program offering comprehensive, individualized services to University of Denver Students with learning disabilities and or ADHD. The LEP is part of a larger organization called University Disability Services.

4859 University of Northern Colorado
Disability Support Services
Campus
Greeley, CO 80639
970-351-2289
FAX 970-351-4166
http://www.unco.edu/dss
e-mail: nancy.kauffman@unco.edu
Nancy Kauffman, Director
Dee Ann Dummett, Administrative Assistant

Offers a variety of services to students with documented disabilities.

4860 Western State College of Colorado
600 N Adams Street
Gunnison, CO 81231
970-943-0120
800-876-5309
http://www.western.edu
Jill Martinez, Advisor

A public four-year college with 59 special education students out of a total of 2,450.

Connecticut

4861 Albertus Magnus College
Director of the Academic Development Center
700 Prospect Street
New Haven, CT 06511
203-773-8590
FAX 203-773-3119
http://www.albertus.edu
e-mail: jmcnamera@albertus.edu
Julia McNamera, President
William Schuz, Vice President

Offers a variety of services to students with disabilities including note takers, extended testing time, counseling services, and special accommodations.

4862 Allen Institute Center for InnovativeLearning
85 Jones Street
Hebron, CT 06248
860-859-4148
888-673-3443
FAX 860-859-4159
http://www.alleninstitute.info
e-mail: dspada@eastersealsct.org
Dan Spada, Director Marketing/Communication

Provides a caring and nurturing environment for students with learning disabilities where students are encouraged and expected to reach their potential.

4863 Asnuntuck Community Technical College
170 Elm Street
Enfield, CT 06082
860-253-3000
FAX 860-253-3063
http://www.acc.commnet.edu
e-mail: mmcleod@acc.commnet.edu
Martha McLeod, President
Vince Fulginity, Vice President

The Academic Skills Center is offered to students with learning disabilities.

4864 Aspen Education Group
17777 Center Court Drive
Cerritos, CA 90703
562-467-5500
FAX 562-402-7036
http://www.aspeneducation.com
Elliot Sainer, President & CEO
Jim Dredge, Executive Vice President & COO

Provider of education programs for the struggling or underachieving young people. Offers professionals and families the opportunity to choose a setting that best meets a student's unique academic and emotional needs.

4865 Ben Bronz Academy
139 N Main Street
West Hartford, CT 06107
860-236-5807
FAX 860-233-9945
http://www.tli.com
e-mail: bba@tli.com
Aileen Stan-Spence, Principal
Mary Austin, Staff

Ben Bronz Acadamy is a day school for bright disabled students. Guides 60 students through an intensive school day that includes writing, mathematics, literature, science and social studies. Oral language is developed and stressed in all classes.

4866 Briarwood College
2279 Mount Vernon Road
Southington, CT 06489
860-628-4751
800-952-2444
FAX 860-628-6444
http://www.briarwood.edu
Cynthia Clarky, Disabilities Coordinator
Lynn Brooks, President

Briarwood College is accredited by the New England Association of Schools and Colleges and the Connecticut State Board for Higher Education. Indiviual progams are also accredited by organizations within their specific professions.

4867 **Capitol Community-Tech College**
61 Woodland Street
Hartford, CT 06105 860-520-7800
Virginia Foley-Psillas

Offers a variety of services to students with disabilities including note takers, extended testing time, counseling services, and special accommodations.

4868 **Central Connecticut State University**
1615 Stanley Street
New Britain, CT 06050 860-832-3200
FAX 860-832-2522
http://www.ccsu.edu
George Tenney, Director
Myrna Garcia-Bowen, Admissions Director
Richard Judd, Administrator
Offers services and supports that promote educational equity for students with disabilities. Assistance includes arranging accommodations and auxillary aids that are necessary for students with disabilities to pursue their academic careers.

4869 **Connecticut College**
Office of Disability Services
270 Mohegan Avenue
New London, CT 06320 860-439-5428
FAX 860-439-5430
http://www.conncoll.edu
e-mail: slduq@conncoll.edu
Susan Duques PhD, Director
Lee Coffin, Admissions Director

Offers a variety of services to students with disabilities including notetakers, extended testing time, counseling services, and special accommodations.

4870 **Eagle Hill School**
45 Glenville Road
Greenwich, CT 06831 203-622-9240
FAX 203-622-0914
http://www.eaglehillschool.com
e-mail: info411@eaglehillschool.com
Mark J Griffin PhD, Founder

A language based remedial program committed to educating children with learning disabilities.

4871 **Eastern Connecticut State University**
83 Windham Street
Willimantic, CT 06226 860-465-5000
FAX 860-465-0136
TDY:860-465-5799
http://www.easternet.edu
e-mail: starrp@easternct.edu
Pamela Starr, Coordinator/Counselor
David Carter, Administrator

Academic support services are designed to provide equal access to the educational program. Each service must be approved by the OAS Coordinator and is based upon submission of appropriate documentation.

4872 **Fairfield University**
Office of Student Support Services
1073 N Benson Road
Fairfield, CT 06824 203-254-4000
FAX 203-254-4000
http://www.fairfield.edu
David Ryan-Soderlund, Assistant Director
Aloysius Kelley, President

Provides students with disabilities an equal opportunity to access the benefits, rights and privileges of Fairfield University's services, programs and activities in an accessible setting.

4873 **Gateway Community-Tech College**
60 Sargent Drive
New Haven, CT 06511 203-285-2000
800-390-7723
http://www.gwcc.commnet.edu
Shelley RN, ADA Coordinator

Offers a variety of services to students with disabilities including extended testing time, counseling services, and special accommodations.

4874 **Hartford College for Women**
University of Hartford
1265 Asylum Avenue
Hartford, CT 06105 860-236-1215
FAX 860-768-5622
http://www.hartford.edu
e-mail: hcwinfo@mail.hartford.edu
Walter Harrisson, President
Lee Peterson, Vice President

Offers a variety of services to students with disabilities including note takers, extended testing time, counseling services, and special accommodations.

4875 **Housatonic Community Technical College**
900 Lafayette Boulevard
Bridgeport, CT 06604 203-332-5000
FAX 203-332-5123
http://www.hctc.commnet.edu
Peter Anderheggen, Director
Janis Hadley, President

The Federally-funded Special Services Program works to help students do well at Housatonic, stay in college, and graduate. Students are eligible for the Special Services Program based on criteria which include placement test scores, income levels, physical handicap, limited English ability, or first generation college student (neither parent has a bachelor's degree).

4876 **Learning Disability Center**
University of Connecticut
PO Box U-64
Storrs Mansfield, CT 06269 860-486-2000
FAX 860-486-0210
http://www.ucimt.uconn.edu/
David Praker, Director
Carol Wayde, Project Assistant
Philip Austin, President
Membership organization specializing in the education of people with special needs through technology and media.

4877 **Manchester Community Technical College**
PO Box 1046
Manchester, CT 06045 860-512-3000
http://www.mctc.commnet.edu
Mary White-Edge MD, LD Director
Jonathan Daube, President

A public two-year college with 60 special education students out of a total of 6,134.

4878 **Mitchell College**
Learning Resource Center
437 Pequot Avenue
New London, CT 06320 860-701-5141
800-443-2811
FAX 860-701-5099
http://www.mitchell.edu
Peter Troiano, Director LRC
Mary , President

An independent two-year or four-year college with 275 special education students out of a total of 621. There is a an additional fee for the special education program in addition to the regular tuition.

4879 **Naugatuck Community College**
750 Chase Parkway
Waterbury, CT 06708 203-575-8040
FAX 203-575-8001
http://www.nvcc.commnet.edu
Louise Meyers, Coordinator LD Program
Laurie Novi, Coordinator LD Services
Kathy Luria, Marketing Executive
Committed to providing equal educational opportunity and full participation for qualified students with disabilities in accordance with the Americans with Disabilities Act of 1990 (ADA). This includes equality of access, accommodations, auxillary aids and services determined to be appropriate to address those functional limitations of the disability that adversely affects educational opportunity.

4880 **Northwestern Connecticut Community**
Park Place E
Winsted, CT 06098 860-379-8543
Robert Douglas, President

4881 **Northwestern Connecticut Community College**
Park Place E
Winsted, CT 06098 860-738-6307
FAX 860-738-6437
TDY:860-738-6307
http://www.nwcc.commnet.edu
e-mail: rdennerlein@nwcc.commnet.edu
Roseann Dennerlein, Counselor

Offers a variety of services to students with disabilities including notetakers, extended testing time, counseling services, and special accommodations.

4882 **Norwalk Community-Technical College**
188 Richards Avenue
Norwalk, CT 06854 203-857-7000
FAX 203-857-3339
http://www.nctc.commnet.edu
David Levinson, President
Lori Orvetti, Developmental Studies Counselor

NCC is accessible to students with disabilites. Students who require accommodations are advised to notify the coodinator at least 6 weeks in advance.

4883 **Paier College of Art**
20 Gorham Avenue
Hamden, CT 06514 203-248-4951
FAX 203-287-3021
http://www.paiercollegeofart.edu
Francis Cooley, Dean
Joseph Pari, Owner

Offers a variety of services to students with disabilities including notetakers, extended testing time, counseling services, and special accommodations.

4884 **Quinebaug Valley Community Technical College**
742 Upper Maple Street
Danielson, CT 06239 860-774-1160
http://www.qvctc.commnet.edu
Gary Hottinger, Director LD Center
Pam Abel, Learning Specialist
Dianne Williams, Administrator
The Learning Assistance Center provides academic support for students with disabilities. Such support may include untimed tests, readers, proctors, note-takers, tape recorders and so on. There is a Peer Advocate for Students with Disabilities to assist disabled students; there is also a Learning Specialist available ten hours a week to counsel and tutor disabled students.

4885 **Quinnipiac University**
275 Mount Carmel Avenue
Hamden, CT 06518 203-582-8200
800-462-1944
FAX 203-582-8970
e-mail: John.Jarvis@Quinnipiac.edu
John Jarvis, Coordinator Learning Services
John Lahey, President

Provides reasonable accommodations to those students who have self-disclosed and provided documentation of a disability.

4886 **Sacred Heart University**
5151 Park Avenue
Fairfield, CT 06825 203-371-7999
FAX 203-396-8049
http://www.sacredheart.edu
e-mail: angottaj@sacredheart.edu
Jill Angotta, Director
Anthony Cernera, Administrator

Four year college that provides services to the learning disabled.

4887 **Southern Connecticut State University**
Disability Resource Office
501 Crescent Street
New Haven, CT 06515 203-392-6828
888-500-7278
FAX 203-392-6829
http://www.southernct.edu
e-mail: TuckerSl@southernct.edu
Suzanne Tucker, Director
Sharon Brennan, Admissions Director

Provides students, faculty and staff with assistance and information on issues of access and full participation for persons with disabilities. The major responsibility of the Disability Resource Office is to provide services and supports that promote educational equality for students with documented disabilities.

4888 **St. Joseph College**
Academic Resource Center
1678 Asylum Avenue
West Hartford, CT 06117 860-232-4571
866-442-8752
FAX 860-233-5695
http://www.sjc.edu
e-mail: judyarzt@sjc.edu
Judy Arzt, Director
Evelyn , President

Offers a variety of services to students with disabilities including notetakers, extended testing time, counseling services, and special accommodations.

4889 **Thames Valley Campus of Three Rivers Community College**
574 New London Turnpike
Norwich, CT 06360 860-885-2612
800-886-4960
FAX 860-886-6670
Linda Jacobsen MD, Counselor
Chris Scarborough, Learning Specialist

Offers associate degrees in computers, and engineering technologies (architectural, civil, electrical, general, manufacturing, mechanical and nuclear, business, general studies, liberal arts and sciences, nursing and others) and one-year certificates in architectural and CADD drafting and data processing.

4890 **Trinity College**
300 Summit Street
Hartford, CT 06106 860-895-1695
860-297-2272
FAX 860-297-5140
http://www.trincoll.edu
Frederick Alford, Dean Student
James Jones Jr., President

Offers a variety of services to students with disabilities including notetakers, extended testing time, counseling services, and special accommodations.

4891 **Tunxis Community College**
271 Scott Swamp Road
Farmington, CT 06032 860-255-3500
FAX 860-676-8906
http://www.tunxis.commnet.edu
David Smith MD, LD Director
Alison Iovanna, Director
Charles Cleary, Administrator
Offers a variety of services to students with disabilities including note takers, extended testing time, counseling services, and special accommodations.

4892 **University of Bridgeport**
Office of Special Services
60 Lafayette Street
Bridgeport, CT 06604 203-576-4454
800-392-3582
FAX 203-576-4455
http://www.bridgeport.edu
Barbara Maryak, Dean of Admissions
Solomon Darko, Counselor

Committted to the development of all students. An advocate and liaison for the students with disabilities, as defined by the American with Disabilities Act. The goal is to provide supportive services for those students with special needs in order to promote sensitivity and equality for the entire University of Bridgeport community.

4893 University of Connecticut
University Program for College Students with LD
249 Glenbrook Road
Storrs Mansfield, CT 06269
860-486-0178
FAX 860-486-5799
http://www.upld.uconn.edu
e-mail: David.Parker@uconn.edu
David Parker, Director

Committed to assuring equal educational opportunity for students with learning disabilities who have the potential for success in a highly competitive university setting. Since 1984, a comprehensive program has been available to assist qualified students with learning disabilities to become independent and successful learners within the regular University curriculum.

4894 University of Hartford
Learning Plus
200 Bloomfield Avenue
West Hartford, CT 06117
860-768-4312
860-768-4312
FAX 860-768-4183
http://www.hartford.edu
e-mail: LDsupport@hartford.edu
Lynne Goldman, Director

An academic support service available to any University of Hartford student who has submitted appropriate documentation showing evidence of a specific learning disability and/or attention disability.

4895 University of New Haven
300 Boston Post Road
W Haven, CT 06516
203-932-7475
800-324-5864
FAX 203-932-6082
TDY:203-932-7409
http://www.newhaven.edu
e-mail: lcokeke@newhaven.edu
Linda Cupney-Okeke, Director Disability Services
Jane Sangeloty, Admissions Director
Andrea Hogan, Executive Director
Persons who have special needs requiring accommodation should notify the Office for Students with Disabilities. The office handles all referrals regarding any student with a disability. The director provides guidance, assistance and information for students with disabilities and oversees the University's compliance with the Americans with Disabilities Act and the HEW Rehabilitation Act of 1973.

4896 VISTA Vocational & Life Skills Center
1356 Old Clinton Road
Westbrook, CT 06498
860-399-8080
FAX 860-399-3103
http://www.vistavocational.org
e-mail: hbosch@vistavocational.org
Helen Bosch, Administrator

Building self-esteem and confidence in the lives of adults with disabilities through work, independence and friendship. Offers a post-secondary program for young adults with learning disabilities providing individualized training and support in career development, independent living skills, social skills development and community involvement.

4897 Vista Vocational & Life Skills Center
1356 Old Clinton Road
Westbrook, CT 06498
860-399-8080
FAX 860-399-3103
http://www.vistavocational.org
e-mail: hbosch@vistavocational.org
Helen Bosch, Administrator

Building self-esteem and confidence in the lives of adults with disabilities through work, independence and friendship. Offers a post-secondary program for young adults with learning disabilities providing individualized training and support in career development, independent living skills, social skills development and community involvement.

4898 Wesleyan University
237 High Street
Middletown, CT 06459
860-685-3700
FAX 860-685-2201
http://www.wesleyan.edu
e-mail: vrutherford@wesleyan.edu
Vancenia Rutherford, Associate Dean
Richard Culliton, Associate Dean

Wesleyan University is committed to supporting all students in their academic and co-curricular endeavors. Although Wesleyan does not offer special academic programs for individuals with disabilities, the University does provide services and reasonable accommodations to all students who need and have a legal entitlement to such accommodations.

4899 Western Connecticut State University
Students with Disabilities Services
181 White Street
Danbury, CT 06810
203-837-8210
877-837-WCSU
FAX 203-837-9337
TDY:203-837-8284
http://www.wcsu.edu
e-mail: admissions@wcsu.edu
James Roach, President
Amy Thuston, Administrative Assistant

Offers a variety of services to students with disabilities including notetakers, extended testing time, counseling services, and special accommodations.

4900 Yale University
PO Box 208305
New Haven, CT 06520
203-432-2324
FAX 203-432-7884
TDY:203-432-8250
http://www.yale.edu/rod
e-mail: judith.york@yale.edu
Judy York, Manager
Carolyn Barrett, Senior Administrative Assistant

Offers a variety of services to students with disabilities including notetakers and extended testing time.

Delaware

4901 Atlantic Coast Special Educational Services
49 W Avenue
Ocean View, DE 19970
302-537-7263
877-785-7774
http://www.atlanticcoast.org
e-mail: lelling111@aol.com
Lloyd Elling, Owner

Full year, summer and respite care. Ages 18 and older.

4902 Delaware Technical and Community College: Terry Campus
100 Campus Drive
Dover, DE 19904
302-857-1000
FAX 302-857-1296
http://www.dtcc.edu
Orlando George, President

Offers a variety of services to students with disabilities including advocacy, readers, note takers, extended testing time, counseling services, and special accommodations.

4903 University Affiliated Program for Families & Individuals with Developmental Disabilities
University of Delaware
101 Alison Hall
Newark, DE 19716
302-831-2000
FAX 302-831-4690
e-mail: dkoch@udel.edu
Michael Gamel-McCormick, Director
David Roselle, CEO

Supports families and individuals who are affected by developmental disabilities.

4904 **University of Delaware**
Academic Services Center
5 W Main Street
Newark, DE 19716
302-831-1639
FAX 302-831-4128
http://www.aec.udel.edu
e-mail: lysbet@udel.edu
Lysbet Murray, Associate Director
David Roselle, President

Provides accommodations for eligible students with disabilities or ADHD.

District of Columbia

4905 **American University: Academic Support Center**
Learning Services Program
4400 Massachusetts Avenue NW
Washington, DC 20016
202-885-3360
FAX 202-885-1042
http://www.american.edu
e-mail: asc@american.edu
Melissa Scarfone, Learning Services Program Coordi
Kathy Schwartz, Director Academic Support Center

Focuses on assisting students with their transition from high school to college during their freshman year. It is a small, mainstream program offering weekly individual meetings with the coordinator of the Learning Services Program throughout the student's first year.

4906 **American University: Academic Support Center**
4400 Massachusetts Avenue NW
Washington, DC 20016
202-885-3360
FAX 202-885-1042
http://www.american.edu/asc
e-mail: asc@american.edu
Kathy Schwartz, Director Academic Support Center

The Academic Support Center (ASC) provides support for any student at American University who would like to help in developing the tools necessary for success, with the goal of helping students achieve their full academic potential. The ASC also assists students with learning disabilities and Attention Deficity Disorder in arranging for accommodations, and provides specialized support for freshmen with learning disabilities through the Learning Services Program.

4907 **Catholic University of America**
Disability Support Services
620 Michigan Avenue NE
Washington, DC 20064
202-319-5211
FAX 202-319-5126
http://www.disabilityservices.cua.edu
e-mail: cusack@cua.edu
Terra Cusack, Director Disability Support
Christine Mica, Director Undergraduate Admission

Four-year college that has support services for students with learning disabilities.

4908 **George Washington University**
Disability Support Services
2121 Eye Street NW
Washington, DC 20052
202-994-1000
http://www.gwu.edu
e-mail: cwillis@gwu.edu
Christy Willis, Director
Kathryn Napper, Admissions Director

An independent four-year college with 260 students with disabilities out of a total of 8,837.

4909 **Georgetown University**
Disability Support Services/Learning Services
37th & O Street NW
Washington, DC 20057
202-687-6985
FAX 202-687-6158
http://www.georgetown.edu
e-mail: gwr@georgetown.edu
Marcia Fulk, Director
Andy Baker, Manager

A four-year private university with a total enrollment of 6,418.

4910 **Howard University**
2400 6th Street NW
Washington, DC 20059
202-806-6100
http://www.howard.edu
Vincent Johns, Dean Special Services
Haywood Swygert, President

Howard University is committed to compliance with the Americans with Disabilities Act, including providing special services to its disabled students such that they are able to achieve their academic goals. The Office of the Dean for Special Student Services (ODSSS)Æhas been delegated the responsibility of providing reasonable accommodations for students with disabilities.

4911 **Trinity College**
125 Michigan Avenue NE
Washington, DC 20017
202-884-9000
FAX 202-884-9229
http://www.trinitydc.edu
e-mail: earnestm@trinitydc.edu
Melissa Earnest, DSS Coordinator
Lynne Israel, Owner

Four year college that provides services to students with a learning disability.

4912 **University of the District of Columbia**
4200 Connecticut Avenue NW
Washington, DC 20008
202-274-5000
FAX 202-274-6334
http://www.udc.edu
Madhuck Ohal MD, Senior Director

Offers a variety of services to students with disabilities including note takers, extended testing time, counseling services, and special accommodations.

Florida

4913 **Barry University**
Center for Advanced Learning
11300 NE 2nd Avenue
Miami Shores, FL 33161
305-899-3461
FAX 305-899-3778
http://www.barry.edu
e-mail: vcastro@mail.barry.edu
Vivian Castro, CAL Program Director

A comprehensive support program for students with learning disabilities and attention deficit disorders.

4914 **Beacon College**
105 E Main Street
Leesburg, FL 34748
352-787-7660
FAX 352-787-0721
http://www.beaconcollege.edu
e-mail: admissions@beaconcollege.edu
Debra Brodbeck, President
Stephanie Knight, Admissions Counselor
Shirley Smith, Assistant to the VP
Offering BA and AA degree programs exclusively for students with learning disabilities.

4915 **Brevard Community College**
1519 Clearlake Road
Cocoa, FL 32922
321-632-1111
FAX 321-634-3779
http://www.brevard.cc.fl.us
Brenda Fettrow, Director
Thomas Gambell, President

A public two-year college with 602 students with disabilities out of a total of 15,033.

4916 **Broward Community College**
111 E Olas Boulevard
Fort Lauderdale, FL 33301
954-831-6260
http://www.broward.edu
Debbie Garr, Manager

Offers a variety of services to students with disabilities including note takers, extended testing time, counseling services, and special accommodations.

4917 **Central Florida Community College**
3001 SW College Road
Ocala, FL 34474
352-237-2111
FAX 352-237-0510
http://www.gocfcc.com
Charles Dessance, President

A public two-year college with 19 special education students out of a total of 5,616.

4918 **Chipola College**
3094 Indian Circle
Marianna, FL 32446
850-526-2761
FAX 850-718-2240
http://www.chipola.edu
Gene Prough, President

A public two-year college.

4919 **DePaul School for Dyslexia**
701 Orange Avenue
Clearwater, FL 33756
727-443-2711
FAX 727-443-2604
http://www.webcoast.com/depaul/
e-mail: mandroclese@earthlink.net
Mary Hercher, Principal
Vicki Hatch, Executive Director

4920 **Disabled Student Services**
Miami Dade Community College
11011 SW 104th Street
Miami, FL 33176
305-237-2292
FAX 305-237-0880
http://www.mdc.edu
Dianne Rossman, Coordinator
Janis Jordan, Executive Director

A public two-year college with 307 special education students out of a total of 30,013.

4921 **Eckerd College**
4200 54th Ave S
Saint Petersburg, FL 33711
727-867-1166
800-456-9009
FAX 727-866-2304
http://www.eckerd.edu
e-mail: admissions@ecker.edu
Laura Schlack, Director
Jim Deegan, President

Offers a variety of services to students with disabilities including notetakers, extended testing time, counseling services, and special accommodations.

4922 **Edison Community College**
8099 College Pkwy
Fort Myers, FL 33919
239-489-9300
http://www.edison.edu
e-mail: inquiry@edison.edu
Andrea Anderson, Contact

Offers a variety of services to students with disabilities including note takers, extended testing time, counseling services, and special accommodations.

4923 **Embry-Riddle Aeronautical University**
600 S Clyde Morris Boulevard
Daytona Beach, FL 32114
386-226-6000
800-862-2416
FAX 386-226-7070
http://www.embyriddle.edu
Jim Hampton, Director
Richard Clark, Admissions Director
David Hosley, CEO
An independent four-year college with 19 special education students out of a total of 4,643.

4924 **Florida Agricultural & Mechanical University**
Learning Development & Evaluation Center
Foote-Hilyer Administration C
Tallahassee, FL 32307
850-599-3000
http://www.famu.edu
e-mail: n.saabirjohnson@famu.edu
Sharon Wooten, Director
Barbara Cox, Admissions Director
Castell Bryant, President
A four-year public school with 275 students receiving disability services out of 10,691.

4925 **Florida Atlantic University**
Office for Students with Disabilities
PO Box 3091
Boca Raton, FL 33431
561-297-3880
FAX 561-297-2184
http://www.osd.fau.edu
e-mail: nrokos@fau.edu
Nicole Rokos, Director
Albert Colom, Admissions Director

Offers a variety of services to students with disabilities including notetakers, extended testing time, counseling services, and special accommodations.

4926 **Florida Community College at Jacksonville**
501 W State Street
Jacksonville, FL 32202
904-632-3115
FAX 904-646-2204
http://www.fccj.org
e-mail: lchilders@fccj.org
Lucretia Childers, Disabled Student Coordinator
Peter Biegel, Executive Director

A public two-year college with 80 special education students out of a total of 19,878.

4927 **Florida Gulf Coast University**
Office of Multi Access Services
10501 Fgcu Boulevard S
Fort Myers, FL 33965
239-590-7956
FAX 239-590-7975
http://www.fgcu.edu
e-mail: cbright@fgcu.edu
Cori Bright, Coordinator

Four year college that offers students services for the disabled.

4928 **Florida International University**
Office of Disability Services
University Park Gc 190
Miami, FL 33199
305-348-3532
FAX 305-348-3850
http://www.fiu.edu
e-mail: drcupgl@fiu.edu
Julio Garcia, Director
Kathy Trionfo, Associate Director
Beverly Paden, Assistant Director
A public four-year university with a north campus office, serving more than 30,000 students. Students with disabilities seeking assistance number about 700.

4929 **Florida State University**
Student Disability Resource Center
2249 University Center
Tallahassee, FL 32306
850-644-9566
FAX 850-644-7164
http://www.fsu.edu
e-mail: sdrc@fsu.edu
Lauren Kennedy, Director
John Burnhill, Admissions Director

A public four-year college with 500 students with learning disabilities out of a total of 27,014.

4930 Gulf Coast Community College
5230 W Highway 98
Panama City, FL 32401
850-769-1551
FAX 850-679-1556
http://www.gc.cc.fl.us
Linda Dalen, Coordinator
Robert Spaddes, President

A public two-year college with 65 special education students out of a total of 7,374.

4931 Hillsborough Community College
10414 E Columbus Drive
Tampa, FL 33619
813-253-7801
FAX 813-253-7910
http://www.hccfl.edu
e-mail: dgiarrusso@hccfl.edu
Denise Giarrusso, Coordinator
Gwen Stephenson, President

A two-year college that provides services to the learning disabled.

4932 Indian River Community College
3209 Virginia Avenue
Fort Pierce, FL 34981
772-462-4731
Rhoda Brant, Counselor
Karen Cartwright, Executive Director

Two-year community college providing services for learning disabled students (i.e., unlimited tests, notetakers, etc.).

4933 Jacksonville University
2800 University Boulevard N
Jacksonville, FL 32211
904-256-7255
FAX 904-256-7012
http://www.ju.edu
Kerry D. Romesb MD, President
Dolores Star, Executive Secretary

Offers a variety of services to students with disabilities including note takers, extended testing time, counseling services, and special accommodations.

4934 Jericho School
PO Box 11057
Jacksonville, FL 32239
904-744-5110
FAX 904-744-3443
http://www.thejerichoschool.org
e-mail: jerichos@bellsouth.net
Angelo Martinez, Executive Director

Provides comprehensive, individualized science-based education not otherwise available in the community. Believes that those children with autism and other developmental delays deserve the opportunity to reach their full potential.

4935 Johnson & Wales University: Florida
Student Success
1701 NE 127th Street
North Miami, FL 33181
305-892-7568
800-232-2433
FAX 305-892-5399
http://www.jwu.edu
e-mail: martha_saccks@jwu.edu
Martha Sacks, Director
Sharmaine Beckford, Administrative Assistant

4936 Lake City Community College
Disability Services
RR 19
Lake City, FL 32025
386-752-1822
FAX 386-754-4594
http://www.lakecity.cc.fl.us
Janice Irwin, Coordinator
Charles Hall, President

A public two-year college with 150 special education students out of a total of 2,553.

4937 Learning Development and Evaluation Center
Florida A&M University
677 Ardelia Court
Tallahassee, FL 32310
850-222-4541
FAX 850-561-2513
http://www.famu.edu
Sharon Wooten MD, Director
Donna Shell, Associate Director
Gene Telfair, President
Assists the students by providing a variety of supportive services for example counseling, academic advisement, learning strategies.

4938 Lynn University
Comprehensive Support Program
3601 N Military Trail
Boca Raton, FL 33431
561-237-7000
800-888-5966
FAX 561-237-7873
http://www.lynn.edu
e-mail: melglines@lynn.edu
Tiffani Ashline, Program Assistant
Jeff Morgan, Manager

Independent four-year college with 268 students with disabilities out of a total of 1,633 full time undergraduates. There is an additional education fee.

4939 Office of Disabled Students at Manatee Community College
5840 26th Street W
Bradenton, FL 34207
941-752-5000
FAX 941-727-6380
http://www.mcc.fl.edu
Paul Nolting, Adult Services Coordinator
Yvon Wills, Director

Provides reasonable accommodations to ensure the inclusive and total access of disabled students to credit courses at the college while, at the same time, maintaining the integrity and quality of the college's academic programs. Offers a variety of services to students with disabilities including note takers, extended testing time, counseling services and special accommodations.

4940 Okaloosa-Walton College
100 College Boulevard E
Niceville, FL 32578
850-678-5111
FAX 850-729-5323
http://www.owcc.edu
e-mail: swensonj@owcc.net
Jody Swenson, Coordinator Services
James Richburg, President

Offers a variety of services to students with disabilities including note takers, extended testing time, counseling services, and special accommodations.

4941 PACE-Brantley Hall School
3221 Sand Lake Road
Longwood, FL 32779
407-869-8882
FAX 407-869-8717
http://www.pacebrantleyhall.org/
Kathleen Shatlock, Principal
Donna O'Neal, Executive Assistant
Ginny Killioninen, Executive Assistant

4942 Pensacola Junior College
1000 College Boulevard
Pensacola, FL 32504
850-484-2002
FAX 850-484-2049
TDY:850-484-2093
http://www.pjc.cc.fl.us
e-mail: jnickles@pjc.edu
James Nickles MD, Director
Linda Sheppard, Coordinator
Sandra Davis, Manager
Provide services accommodations to students with disabilities enrolled in community college programs.

4943 Polk Community College
999 Avenue H NE
Winter Haven, FL 33881
863-297-1000
http://www.polk.edu
James Dowdy, Special Services
J Durrence, President

Offers a variety of services to students with disabilities including note takers, extended testing time, counseling services, and special accommodations.

4944 Saint Leo University
Office for Students with Disabilities
PO Box 6665
Saint Leo, FL 33574
352-588-8464
FAX 352-588-8605
http://www.saintleo.edu
e-mail: karen.hahn@saintleo.edu
Karen Hahn, Director

Four year college that offers services to the disabled.

4945 Santa Fe Community College: Florida
Disabilities Resource Center
3000 NW 83rd Street
Gainesville, FL 32606
352-395-7322
FAX 352-395-4100
http://www.sfcc.edu
e-mail: disability.info@sfcc.edu
Larry Kiser, Disability Resource Counselor
Claudia Munnis, Disability Resource Counselor
Jan Bullard, Vice President
Located in the Student Services Building in S-229. If you have a disability that impacts your access to programs or services, please visit us.

4946 Seminole Community College
100 Weldon Boulevard
Sanford, FL 32773
407-328-4722
FAX 407-328-2139
http://www.seminole.cc.fl.us
e-mail: admissions@scc-fl.edu
Dorothy Paishon, Coordinator
E McGee, President

Disability Support Services can be reached at 407-328-2109. We provide learning aids, course substitutions, instructor notification and support, referral to area agencies and college services, interpreters, notetakers, talking texts and tutors. We also have workshops on identifying and creating positive learning environments for disabled students.

4947 Southeastern College of the Assemblies of God
1000 Longfellow Boulevard
Lakeland, FL 33801
863-667-5000
FAX 863-667-5200
http://www.secollege.edu
Misty Mancini, Director
Kristin Green, Assistant to the Director
Mark Rutland, President
Offers a variety of services to students with disabilities including note takers, extended testing time, counseling services, and special accommodations.

4948 Southeastern University
1000 Longfellow Boulevard
Lakeland, FL 33801
863-667-5000
FAX 863-667-5200
http://www.seuniversity.edu
e-mail: mlmancini@seuniversity.edu
Misty Mancini, Director
Lindsey Hester, Assistant to Director
Mark Rutland, President
Offers a variety of services to students with disabilities including note takers, extended testing time, counseling services, and special accommodations.

4949 St. Johns River Community College
5001 Saint Johns Avenue
Palatka, FL 32177
386-312-4200
FAX 386-312-4283
http://www.sjrcc.cc.fl.us
Paula Sheppard, Special Services Director
Robert McLendon Jr., President
Mark Breidenstein, Program Advisor Adult Ed Dept
Students with disabilities are welcome at SJRCC, and are encouraged to contact the Counseling Center on their campus where special assistance is available with orientation, registration, academic planning, special supplies, and equipment. In addition, specialized services are available to students whose disability prevents them from participating fully in classroom activities.

4950 St. Petersburg Junior College
PO Box 13489
Saint Petersburg, FL 33733
727-341-3721
http://www.spjc.edu
e-mail: duncand@spcollege.edu
Susan Blanchard MD, Learning Specialist

A public two-year college with 890 special education students out of a total of 20,000+.

4951 Tallahassee Community College
444 Appleyard Drive
Tallahassee, FL 32304
850-201-6200
FAX 850-201-8518
http://www.tallahassee.cc.fl.us/
Mark Linehan, Counselor
Margaret Handee, Educational Specialist
William Law, President
A public two-year college with 584 special education students out of a total of 10,400.

4952 Tampa Bay Academy
12012 Boyette Road
Riverview, FL 33569
813-677-6700
800-678-3838
FAX 813-671-3145
TDY:813-677-2502
http://www.tampabay-acadamy.com
e-mail: ed.hoefle@tampa.yfcs.com
Ed Hoefle, President
Cathy Black, Executive Secretary
Kenneth Sladkin, Executive Director
Offers a variety of services to students with disabilities including note takers, extended testing time, counseling services, and special accommodations.

4953 University of Florida
Disability Resource Center
PO Box 114085
Gainesville, FL 32611
352-392-8565
FAX 352-392-8570
TDY:352-392-3008
http://www.dso.ufl.edu/drc
e-mail: johnpd@dso.ufl.edu
John Denny, Director

A four-year public university with 1300 students receiving disability services out of 48,000.

4954 University of Miami
PO Box 248106
Coral Gables, FL 33124
305-284-2752
FAX 305-284-1999
http://www.miami.edu
Judith Antinarella, Director
Noemi Berrios, Senior Staff Assistant
Julia Cayuso, Executive Director
Offers a variety of services to students with disabilities including note takers, extended testing time, counseling services, and special accommodations.

4955 University of North Florida
4567 Saint Johns Bluff Road S
Jacksonville, FL 32224
904-620-4242
FAX 904-620-2414
TDY:904-620-2969
http://www.unf.edu
John Delaney, President
Pam McCuheon, Admissions Coordinator
Steven Borowiec, Manager
Offers a variety of services to students with disabilities including notetakers, extended testing time, counseling services, and special accommodations.

4956 University of Tampa
401 W Kennedy Boulevard
Tampa, FL 33606
813-253-3333
FAX 813-258-7208
http://www.ut.edu
e-mail: disability.services@ut.edu
Cheri Kittrell, Assistant Director Academic Cent
Ronald Vaughn, President

A private, comprehensive university with an international reputation for excellence.

4957 University of West Florida
11000 University Parkway
Pensacola, FL 32514
850-474-2000
FAX 850-857-6188
TDY:850-474-2000
http://www.uwf.edu
e-mail: bfitzpat@uwf.edu
Barbara Fitzpatrick, Assistant Director
John Cavanaugh, President

A public four-year college with 8 special education students out of a total of 6793.

4958 Valencia Community College
PO Box 3028
Orlando, FL 32802
407-299-5000
FAX 407-293-8839
http://www.ualencia.cc.fl.us
Walter Johnson, Counselor
Peg Edmonds, Counselor
Samford Shugart, President
A public two-year college with 1,200 students with disabilities out of a total of 25,000.

4959 Vanguard School
22000 US Highway 27
Lake Wales, FL 33859
863-676-6091
FAX 863-676-8297
http://www.vanguardschool.org
e-mail: vanadmin@vanguardschool.org
Dr Cathy Wooley-Brown, President

An accredited, internationally recognized community of students with learning differences.

4960 Victory School
PO Box 630266
Miami, FL 33163
305-466-1142
FAX 305-466-1143
http://www.thevictoryschool.org
e-mail: administrator@thevictoryschool.org
Judith Nelson, Executive Director

A Florida, non-secretarian, not-for-profit corporation that provides children with autism and smiliar disorders comprehensive individualized treatment with a 1:1 student/teacher ratio, in a classroom setting that is unique in Southeast Florida.

4961 Webber College
PO Box 96
Babson Park, FL 33827
863-638-1431
800-741-1844
FAX 863-638-1591
http://www.webber.edu
e-mail: jragans@hotmail.com
Julie Ragans, Director Admissions
Patty Beaslie, Coordinator
Rex Yentes, President
An independent four-year college with 39 special education students out of a total of 354.

4962 Woodland Hall Academy-Dyslexia Research Institute
5746 Centerville Road
Tallahassee, FL 32309
850-893-2216
FAX 850-893-2440
http://www.dyslexia-add.org
e-mail: dri@talstar.com

Pat Hardman, Executive Director
Robyn Rennick, Program Coordinator

Participates in field research and offers testing materials for dyslexia, ADD, SLD children and adults.

Georgia

4963 Albany State University
504 College Drive
Albany, GA 31705
229-430-4600
FAX 229-430-3936
http://www.asurams.edu

Julius Scott, President
Kenneth Dyer, Vice President

Four-year college offering services and support to students with learning disabilities.

4964 Andrew College
413 College Street
Cuthbert, GA 39840
229-732-2171
800-664-9250
FAX 229-732-5991
http://www.andrewcollege.edu
e-mail: focus@andrewcollege.edu

Sherri Taylor, Director
David Palmer, President

The FOCUS program offers an intensive level of academic support designed for and limited to documented learning disabilities or attention deficit disorder. While FOCUS supplements and complements the tutorial and advising to all students, the program also provides an additional level of professional assistance and mentoring. Those accepted into FOCUS are charged regular tuition andd fees, plus a FOCUS laboratory fee.

4965 Atlanta Speech School
Wardlaw School for Children with LD
3160 Northside Parkway NW
Atlanta, GA 30327
404-233-5332
FAX 404-266-2175
http://www.atlantaspeechschool.org
e-mail: mdemko@attspsch.org or smims@attspsch.org
Maureen Demko, Coordinator Upper School
Sondra Mims, Coordinator Lower School
Comer Yates, Executive Director
Wardlaw School is for children with mild to moderate language-based learning disabilities.

4966 Berry College
PO Box 490159
Rome, GA 30149
706-236-2209
FAX 706-236-2248
http://www.berry.edu

Marshall Jenkin MD, Director
Scott Colley, President

Offers a variety of services to students with disabilities including notetakers, extended testing time, counseling services, and special accommodations.

4967 Brandon Hall School
1701 Brandon Hall Drive
Atlanta, GA 30350
770-394-8176
FAX 770-804-8821
http://www.brandonhall.org
e-mail: pstockhammer@brandonhall.org
Paul Stockhammer, President
Marcia Shearer, Admissions Director

College preparatory, co-ed day and boys' boarding school for students in grades 4-12. Designed for academic underachievers and students with minor learning disabilities, attention deficit disorders and dyslexia. Enrollment 150 students; faculty 40, with 100% college acceptances. Interscholastic sports and numerous co-curriculum activities and summer programs.

4968 **Brenau University**
Learning Center
1 Centennial Circle
Gainesville, GA 30501
770-534-6134
800-252-5119
FAX 770-534-6221
http://www.brenau.edu
e-mail: vyamilkoski@lib.brenau.edu
Vincent EdD, Learning Center Director
Christina Chocran, Women's College Admissions

Program for students with a diagnosed learning disability and who have average to above average intellectual potential. This program is designed to provide support services for learning disabled students as they attend regular college courses. Offers a more structured learning environment, as well as the freedom associated with college living.

4969 **Brewton-Parker College**
PO Box 2124
Mount Vernon, GA 30445
912-583-2241
800-342-1087
FAX 912-583-4498
http://www.bpc.edu
e-mail: jkissell@bpc.edu
Juanita Kissell, Counseling Service Director
David Smith, President

An independent four-year college with 15 special education students out of a total of 1,942.

4970 **Clayton College & State University**
Disability Services
5900 Lee Street
Morrow, GA 30260
770-961-3500
FAX 770-961-3752
http://www.clayton.edu
Thomas Harden MD, President

Four-year college that offers programs for learning disabled students.

4971 **Columbus State University**
4225 University Avenue
Columbus, GA 31907
706-568-2001
FAX 706-569-3096
http://www.colstate.edu
e-mail: willliams_aracelis@colstate.edu
Frank Brown, President
Yolanda Jackson, Staff

Offers a variety of services to students with disabilities including note takers, extended testing time, counseling services, and special accommodations.

4972 **DeVry Institute of Technology**
250 N Arcadia Avenue
Decatur, GA 30030
404-292-2645
FAX 404-292-7011
http://www.atl.devry.edu
Andrea Rutherford, Academic Support Director
Donna Lorraine, President

Offers a variety of services to students with disabilities including notetakers, extended testing time, counseling services, and special accommodations.

4973 **East Georgia College**
131 College Circle
Swainsboro, GA 30401
478-289-2000
http://www.ega.edu
e-mail: rlosser@ega.peachnet.edu
Bennie Brinson, Student Services
John Black, Administrator

Offers a variety of services to students with disabilities including note takers, extended testing time, counseling services, and special accommodations.

4974 **Emory University**
Office of Disability Svces, University Admin Bldg
201 Dowman Drive NE
Atlanta, GA 30322
404-727-6016
FAX 404-727-1126
http://www.emory.edu
e-mail: gweaver@emory.edu
Gloria Y Weaver, Director
Jane Jordon, Admissions Director

An independent four-year college with 150 special education students out of a total of 6,316.

4975 **Fort Valley State University**
Counseling & Career Development Center
1005 State University Drive
Fort Valley, GA 31030
478-825-6211
http://www.fvsu.edu
e-mail: asmissap@mail.fvsu.edu
Myldred Hill MD, Director
Larry Rivers, President

Four-year college that provides counseling for learning disabled students.

4976 **Gables Academy**
811 Gordon Street
Stone Mountain, GA 30083
770-465-7500
877-465-7500
FAX 770-465-7700
http://www.gablesacademy.com
e-mail: info@gablesacademy.com
James Meffen, Administrator
Cynthia Guinn, Administrative Assistant

Offers a variety of services to students with learning disabilities including notetakers, extended testing time, counseling services, and special accommodations. Day and residential services available.

4977 **Georgia Affiliated Program for Persons with Developmental Disabilities**
University of Georgia
Dawson Hall
Athens, GA 30602
706-542-7840
FAX 706-542-4815
Zolinda Stoneman, Director
Mike Stroup, Manager

For students with developmental disabilities.

4978 **Georgia College**
Georgia College & State University
Milledgeville, GA 31061
478-445-5004
800-342-0471
http://www.gcsu.edu
e-mail: dcsmith@mail.gcsu.edu
Craig Smith MD, Chair
Dorothy Leland, President

Offers a variety of services to students with disabilities including note takers, extended testing time, counseling services, and special accommodations.

4979 **Georgia Institute of Technology**
225 N Avenue NW
Atlanta, GA 30332
404-894-2000
FAX 404-894-9928
http://www.gatech.edu
RoseMary Watkins, Director
Wayne Clough, President
G Clough, CEO
A public four-year college with 6 special education students out of a total of 9,587.

4980 **Georgia Southern University**
Student Disability Resource Center
PO Box 8037
Statesboro, GA 30460
912-871-1566
FAX 912-871-1419
http://www.gasou.edu
e-mail: cwatkins@gsix2.cc.gasou.edu

Wayne Akins, Director
Teresa Thompsen, Admissions Director

Offers a variety of services to students with disabilities including note takers, extended testing time, counseling services, and special accommodations.

4981 **Georgia State University**
Disability Services
33 Gilmer Street SE
Atlanta, GA 30303
404-463-9044
FAX 404-463-9049
http://www.gsu.edu/disability
e-mail: disleb@langate.gsu.edu
Louise Bedrossian, Cognitive Disability Specialist
Rodney Penamon, Director

An accessible campus with 149 students with disabilities. Support services include a staff of professionals and student aides who provide tutors, mobility assistance, test proctoring, extended time for exams, interpreters, transcribing, readers, reading machines, taped textbooks and class materials. Technology includes computers with voice output and zoom text, print magnification systems, Arkenstone and Kurzweil Readers, assistive listening devices, and specialized software programs.

4982 **Life University**
Department Student Success Center
1269 Barclay Circle SE
Marietta, GA 30060
770-426-2725
FAX 770-426-2728
http://www.life.edu
e-mail: lrubin@life.edu
Lisa Rubin PhD, Director

Four-year college offers academic support to students with disabilities.

4983 **Macon State College**
100 College Station Drive
Macon, GA 31206
478-471-2700
e-mail: sloyd@mail.maconstate.edu
David Bell, President

Four-year college that provides services to those students who are disabled.

4984 **Mercer University: Atlanta**
3001 Mercer University Drive
Atlanta, GA 30341
678-547-6000
http://www.mercer,edu
Dorothy Roberts, Director
Kirby Godsey, President

Offers a variety of services to students with disabilities including note takers, extended testing time, counseling services, and special accommodations.

4985 **Mill Springs Academy**
13660 New Providence Road
Alpharetta, GA 30004
770-360-1336
FAX 770-360-1341
http://www.millsprings.org
e-mail: rmoore@millsprings.org
Robert Moore, President

4986 **North Georgia College & State University**
122 Barnes Hall
Dahlonega, GA 30597
706-864-1400
FAX 706-867-2882
http://www.ngcsu.edu
e-mail: emcintosh@ngcsu.edu
Elizabeth McIntosh, Coordinator
David Potter, President

Four-year college that provides resources and programs for learning disabled students.

4987 **Piedmont College**
PO Box 10
Demorest, GA 30535
706-778-3000
800-277-7020
http://www.piedmont.edu
Nancy Adams, Special Services
Ray Cleere, President

Offers a variety of services to students with disabilities including notetakers, extended testing time, counseling services, and special accommodations.

4988 **Reinhardt College**
Academic Support Office
7300 Reinhardt College Circle
Waleska, GA 30183
770-720-5567
FAX 770-720-5602
http://www.reinhardt.edu
e-mail: srr@reinhardt.edu
Sylvia Robertson, Director Academic Support Office

An independent four-year college with 80 learning disabled students out of a total of 1,190 being served in academic support. There is an additional fee for the tutorial program in addition to the regular tuition.

4989 **Savannah State University**
Comprehensive Counseling Center
PO Box 20376
Savannah, GA 31404
912-356-2202
FAX 912-356-2464
http://www.savstate.edu
e-mail: akoredea@savstate.edu
Orlando Spencer, Coordinator

Four-year college has a comprehensive counseling center for students that are learning disabled.

4990 **Shorter College**
315 Shorter Avenue SW
Rome, GA 30165
706-291-2121
800-868-6980
FAX 706-236-1515
http://www.shorter.edu
Harald Newman, President

Offers a variety of services to students with disabilities including note takers, extended testing time, counseling services, and special accommodations.

4991 **South Georgia College**
100 College Park Drive W
Douglas, GA 31533
912-389-4510
800-342-6364
FAX 912-389-4392
http://www.sga.edu
e-mail: calott@sga.edu
John Elveen, President
Glenda Clark, Interim Vice President

The Office of Disability Services, a division of Academic Affairs, is committed to providing an equal educational opportunity for all qualified students with disabilities. The Office of Disability Services is responsible for initiating and coordinating services for students with disabilities at South Georgia College.

4992 **Southern College of Technology**
1100 S Marietta Parkway SE
Marietta, GA 30060
678-915-7778
800-635-3204
http://www.spsu.edu
Patricia Soper MD, Special Services
Lisa Rossbacher, President

Offers a variety of services to students with disabilities including note takers, extended testing time, counseling services, and special accommodations.

4993 Southern Polytechnic State University
1100 S Marietta Parkway SE
Marietta, GA 30060
678-915-7778
800-635-3204
http://www.spsu.edu
e-mail: tcordle@spsu.edu
Terri Cordle, Counselor
Lisa Rossbacher, President

Four-year college that offers counseling services to learning disabled students.

4994 State University of West Georgia
1601 Maple Street
Carrollton, GA 30118
678-839-5000
http://www.westga.edu
e-mail: speacock@westga.edu
Shannon Peacock, Coordinator

Four-year college that provides services to disabled students.

4995 Toccoa Falls College
PO Box 777
Toccoa Falls, GA 30598
706-886-6831
888-785-5624
FAX 706-886-6412
http://www.toccoafalls.edu
e-mail: wgardner@tfc.edu
Wayne Gardner, President
Christy Meadows, Department Head of Admissions

Four-year college that provides services to the learning disabled.

4996 University of Georgia
Learning Disabilities Center
Terrell Hall
Athens, GA 30602
706-542-4589
FAX 706-542-7719
TDY:705-542-8778
http://www.drc.uda.edu
Karen Kaloboda, Director
Elaine Manglitz, Service Head
Nancy McBuss, Admissions Director
A public four-year university with 276 students with learning disabilities out of a total of 24,213. There is no fee for the comprehensive service program. To be eligible for services, students must submit recent documentation which meets evaluation standards.

4997 Valdosta State University
1500 N Patterson Street
Valdosta, GA 31698
229-333-5791
800-618-1878
http://www.valdosta.edu
e-mail: kgadden@valdosta.edu
Kimberly Gadden, Special Services Coordinator
Ronald Zaccari, President

A public four-year university with 90 learning disabled students out of a total of 9,000.

4998 West Georgia College
303 Fort Drive
Lagrange, GA 30240
706-845-4323
http://www.westga.tec.ga.us
Ann Phillips MD, Special Services
Daryl Gilley, Administrator

A public four-year college with 34 special education students out of a total of 5,528.

Hawaii

4999 Brigham Young University: Hawaii
55-220 Kulanui Street
Laie, HI 96762
808-293-3211
FAX 808-293-3741
http://www.byuh.edu
Eric Schumway, President

Offers a variety of services to students with disabilities including note takers, extended testing time, counseling services, and special accommodations.

5000 Center on Disability Studies, University Affiliated Program: University of Hawaii
University of Hawaii at Manoa
1776 University Avenue
Honolulu, HI 96822
808-956-6914
FAX 808-956-7878
http://www.cds.hawaii.edu
e-mail: juana@hawaii.edu
Robert Stodden, Director/Professor

Dedicated to supporting the quality of life, inclusion, and empowerment of all persons with disabilities and their families through partnerships in training, service, evaluation, research, dissemination, and technical assistance. Nurtures, sustains, and expands promising practices for people with disabilities.

5001 University of Hawaii: Honolulu Community College
874 Dillingham Boulevard
Honolulu, HI 96817
808-845-9282
FAX 808-847-9836
http://www.honolulu.hawaii.edu/disability
e-mail: access@hcc.hawaii.edu
Wayne Sunahara, Disability Services Provider

Academic support provided for students with documented disabilities. Intake interview required to determine appropriate accommodations which may include taped books, testing accommodations, note takers, etc. Early notification requested.

5002 University of Hawaii: Kapiolani Community College
4303 Diamond Head Road
Honolulu, HI 96816
808-734-9000
FAX 808-734-9447
http://www.kcc.hawii.edu
Joselyn Yoshimura, Director
John Morton, Manager

A public two-year college with 28 special education students out of a total of 6,529.

5003 University of Hawaii: Kauai Community College
3-1901ikaumualii Highway
Lihue, HI 96766
808-245-8382
http://www.kauaicc.hawaii.edu
Frances Dinnan, Special Services

Offers a variety of services to students with disabilities including note takers, extended testing time, counseling services, and special accommodations.

5004 University of Hawaii: Leeward Community College
Program for Adult Achievement
96-045 Ala Ike Street
Pearl City, HI 96782
808-455-0421
FAX 808-455-0471
http://www.lcc.hawaii.edu
e-mail: kprogram@hawaii.edu
Mark Silliman, Chancellor

A public two-year college with 153 special education students out of a total of 6,345.

Idaho

5005 Boise State University
1910 University Drive
Boise, ID 83725
208-426-1156
FAX 208-426-3765
http://www.boisestate.edu
B Kustra, President

A public four-year college with 31 special education students out of a total of 12,812.

5006 **College of Southern Idaho**
PO Box 1238
Twin Falls, ID 83303
208-733-3972
800-680-0274
FAX 208-736-3015
TDY:208-734-9929
http://www.csi.cc.id.us/
e-mail: marrossa@csi.edu
Jerry Meybrhoeffer, President
Monty Arrossa, Director of Human Resources
Terry Patterson, Manager
Offers a variety of services to students with disabilities including note takers, extended testing time, counseling services, and special accommodations.

5007 **Idaho State University**
ADA Disabilities Resource Center
Campus
Pocatello, ID 83209
208-282-3242
http://www.isu.edu
e-mail: lawsjona@isu.edu
Robert Campbell, Director

Four-year college that provides information and resources to students with a learning disability.

5008 **North Idaho College**
1000 W Garden Avenue
Coeur D Alene, ID 83814
208-769-3300
FAX 208-769-3300
http://www.nic.edu
Kristine Wold, Special Services
Sharon Folic, Coordinator
Michael Burke, President
Offers a variety of services to students with disabilities including note takers, extended testing time, counseling services, and special accommodations.

5009 **University of Idaho**
Student Disability Services
PO Box 444264
Moscow, ID 83844
888-884-3246
http://www.uidaho.edu
e-mail: sds@widaho.edu
Diane Milhullin, Student Disability Services
Dan Davenport, Admissions Director

Provides disability support services for students with temporary or permanent disabilities, in accordance with the Americans with Disabilities Act, and the Rehabilitation Act. The Campus Guide for People with Disabilities describes some of these services. About 100 people are served annually.

5010 **University of Idaho: Idaho Center on Development**
College of Education
129 W 3rd Street
Moscow, ID 83843
208-885-3559
800-393-7290
FAX 208-885-3628
http://www.idahocdhd.org
Julie Fodor, Director
Jennifer Magelky, Administrative Assistant

Positive behavioral supports.

Illinois

5011 **Acacia Academy**
6425 Willow Springs Road
La Grange Highlands, IL 60525
708-579-9040
FAX 708-579-5872
e-mail: kfouks@acaciaacademy.com
Kathryn Fouks, Administrator
Eileen Petzold, Dean

A school for grades K-12 for children with learning disabilities. NCA accrediated and approved for out of district students in special education in the state of Illinois.

5012 **Aurora University**
347 S Gladstone Avenue
Aurora, IL 60506
630-844-5533
800-742-5281
FAX 630-844-5463
http://www.aurora.edu
e-mail: inquiry@aurora.edu
Eric Schwaerze, Learning Center Co-Director
Patsy Mahoney, Learning Center Director
Rebecca Sherrick, Administrator
An independent four-year college with an enrollment near 2,000 students. The University Learning Center provides accommodations, tutoring and support for all students with physical or learning disabilities.

5013 **Barat College of DePaul University**
Learning Opportunities Program
700 E Westleigh Road
Lake Forest, IL 60045
847-234-3000
FAX 847-574-6000
http://www.barat.edu
e-mail: dwitikka@barat.edu
Debbie Sheade, Director
John Schornack, Administrator

A four-year college with small classes and personalized education. There is a separate fee for the special education program in addition to the regular tuition. There is also a separate admissions procedure.

5014 **Blackburn College**
700 College Avenue
Carlinville, IL 62626
217-854-3231
FAX 217-854-3713
http://www.blackburn.edu
Patricia Kowal, Director
Miriam Pride, President

Offers a variety of services to students with disabilities including notetakers, extended testing time, counseling services, and special accommodations.

5015 **Brehm Preparatory School**
1245 E Grand Avenue
Carbondale, IL 62901
618-457-0371
FAX 618-529-1248
http://www.brehm.org
e-mail: everhart@bayou.com
Richard Collins, Administrator

A coeducational boarding school for students with learning differences. Services are provided for students in grades 6-12. A post-secondary program, OPTIONS, is also available.

5016 **Center for Academic Development: National College of Education**
2840 Sheridan Road
Evanston, IL 60201
847-905-2356
Annol Kim, Assistant Professor
Evanston Cad, Coordinator

Peer tutoring available- hours per week per course for documented Learning disability students who were regularly admitted and meet college entrance criteria.

5017 **Chicago State University**
Office of Student Development, Adm. 303
9501 S King Drive
Chicago, IL 60628
773-995-2000
http://www.csu.edu
Elnora Daniel, President
Bridget Mason, Research Assistant
Sandra Westbroo MD, Assistant Provost
The Office of Student Development maintains a Student Support Services Program for the disabled students on the campus. Seeks to meet the needs and concerns of the disabled. Services, sources and suggestions are welcomed.

5018 College of DuPage
425 Fawell Boulevard
Glen Ellyn, IL 60137
630-942-2026
FAX 630-858-5409
http://www.cod.edu
e-mail: ryanth@cdnet.cod.edu

Sunil Chand, President
Tom Ryan, Vice President
Alison Drake, Manager
Offers a variety of services to students with disabilities including note takers, extended testing time, counseling services, and special accommodations.

5019 College of Health & Human Development: Department of Disability & Human Development
University of Illinois at Chicago
1640 W Roosevelt Road
Chicago, IL 60608
312-413-1481
FAX 312-413-2918
TDY:312-413-0453
http://www.uic.edu/depts/idhd
e-mail: DHD@uic.edu

Ann Cutler MD, President
Maita Obligado, Office Assistant

Dedicated to the scholarly, interdisciplinary study of disability and related aspects of human development. It critically examines current and prospective disability policies, conceptual models, and intervention strategies in terms of their historical development and their present merits.

5020 Columbia College Chicago
Student Support Services
600 S Michigan Avenue
Chicago, IL 60605
312-344-8132
FAX 312-344-8005
http://www.colum.edu
e-mail: banderson@popmail.colum.edu

Beverly Anderson, Director
Gabriel Watkins, Administrative Assistant

Four-year college that offers support and services to special needs students.

5021 Danville Area Community College
2000 E Main Street
Danville, IL 61832
217-443-8833
FAX 217-431-0751
TDY:217-443-8853
http://www.dacc.ccil.us
e-mail: pmcconn@dacc.cc.il.us

Penny McConnell, Assessment Center Coordinator
Ana Nasser, Manager

The college offers the associate's degree in 59 occupational programs and 36 transfer prgrams. DACC also offers 10 baccalaureate degree programs through cooperative agreements with Eastern Illinois University, Southern Illinois University, University at Carbondale, and Franklin University in Columbus, Ohio. Six of these four-year degree programs are offered online. Accommodations for students with disabilities.

5022 Dominican University
7900 Division Street
River Forest, IL 60305
708-366-2490
FAX 708-524-6559
TDY:708-524-6824
http://www.dom.edu
e-mail: tgoggin@dom.edu

Trudi Goggin, Dean of Student
Judy Paulus, Administrative Assistant

Offers a variety of services to students with disabilities including note takers, extended testing time, counseling services, and special accommodations.

5023 Eastern Illinois University
Office of Disability Services
600 Lincoln Avenue
Charleston, IL 61920
217-581-6583
FAX 217-581-7208
http://www.eiu.edu
e-mail: cfmpj@eiu.edu

Kathy Waggoner, Director
Julie Walters, Office Assistant

A public four-year university with 90 students receiving disability services out of 9,346.

5024 Elgin Community College
1700 Spartan Drive
Elgin, IL 60123
847-697-1000
888-545-7222
FAX 847-669-9105
http://www.elgin.cc.il.us/

Annabelle Rhoades, Director LD
Michael Shirley, President

Offers a variety of services to students with disabilities including note takers, extended testing time, counseling services, and special accommodations.

5025 Governors State University
1 University Parkway
University Park, IL 60466
708-534-5000
http://www.govst.edu
e-mail: gsunow@govst.edu

Pamela Bax, Outreach Counselor
Stuart Fagan, President

Provides assistance to GSU students with disabilities. Assistance includes coordination of untimed tests, notetakers, test readers, computerized testing and other assistance that will allow students equal access to the learning environment.

5026 Highland Community College
2998 W Pearl City Road
Freeport, IL 61032
815-235-6121
FAX 815-235-6130

Sue Wilson, Director
Joe Kanosky, President

A public two-year college with 23 special education students out of a total of 3,262.

5027 Illinois Central College
1 College Drive
Peoria, IL 61635
309-694-5558
800-422-2293
FAX 309-999-4549
http://www.icc.edu
e-mail: tingles@icc.edu

Denise Cioni, Special Needs Coordinator
Terri Ingles, Director
John Erwin, Administrator
A public two-year college with approximately 100 students with learning disabilities and/or attention deficit disorder. Students may borrow tape recorders, use note takers, access books on tape, request test accommodations and utilize tutorial labs and/or individual tutoring.

5028 Illinois Eastern Community College/LincolnTrail College
11220 State Highway I
Robinson, IL 62454
618-544-8657
FAX 618-544-7423
http://www.iecc.edu
e-mail: ltcadmissions@iecc.cc.il.us

Searoba Haskin, Learning Skills
Deanna Chysler, Administrative Assistant
Carl Heilman, President
A public two-year college with 4 special education students out of a total of 1,040.

5029 Illinois Eastern Community College/OlneyCentral College
305 NW Street
Olney, IL 62450
618-395-7777
FAX 618-392-3293
http://www.iecc.edu
e-mail: kaared@iecc.edu

Donita Kaare, Director Learning Skills Center
Peg Kennedy, Developmental Support Specialist
Jack Davis, President
Offers a variety of services to students with disabilities including note takers, extended testing time, counseling services, and special accommodations.

5030 Illinois Eastern Community College/WabashValley College
2200 College Drive
Mount Carmel, IL 62863
618-262-8641
866-982-4322
FAX 618-262-8962
http://www.iecc.cc.edu
e-mail: wwvcadmissions@iecc.cc.il.us
Marj Doty, Learning Skills
Audrey Tice, Manager

Offers a variety of services to students with disabilities including note takers, extended testing time, counseling services, and special accommodations.

5031 Illinois Eastern Community Colleges/Frontier Community College
2 Frontier Drive
Fairfield, IL 62837
618-842-3711
877-464-3687
FAX 618-842-4425
http://www.iecc.cc.il.us
e-mail: fccadmissions@iecc.cc.il.us
Karen Bryant, Administrator
Dennise Hilliard, Administrative Assistant

Offers a variety of services to students with disabilities including note takers, extended testing time, counseling services, and special accommodations.

5032 Illinois State University
Disability Concerns
350 Fell Hall
Normal, IL 61790
309-438-5853
FAX 309-438-7713
http://www.ilstu.edu
e-mail: ableisu@ilstu.edu
Ann Caldwell, Director
Molly Arnold, Admissions Director

A public four year university with 130 students with learning disabilities and/or attention deficit (hyperactivity) disorder. Students may be eligible for services such as notetakers, exam accommodations, and text conversion.

5033 John A Logan College
700 Logan College Drive
Carterville, IL 62918
618-985-4166
800-851-4720
FAX 618-985-2867
http://www.jal.cc.il.us
e-mail: logan@jal.cc.il.us
Judy Zineyard, Director
C Thomas, Manager

A public two-year college with 47 special education students out of a total of 4,642.

5034 Joliet Junior College
1215 Houbolt Road
Joliet, IL 60431
815-729-9020
FAX 815-744-5507
http://www.jjc.edu
e-mail: carol_smith@jjc.edu
Carol Smith, Special Needs Coordinator
J Ross, Administrator

Student Accommodations and Resources (StAR) is the academic support department which provides support services to students with disabilities and students enrolled in career and technical majors.

5035 Kaskaskia College
27210 College Road
Centralia, IL 62801
618-545-3000
800-642-0859
FAX 618-532-5313
http://www.kc.cc.il.us
e-mail: smartin@kaskaskia.edu
Lisa Oelze, SNAP Coordinator
Shirley Martin, Executive Assistant to the Presi
James Underwood, Administrator

Offers a variety of services to students with disabilities including note takers, extended testing time, counseling services, and special accommodations.

5036 Kendall College
900 N Branch Street
Chicago, IL 60622
312-752-2020
http://www.kendal.edu
Peter Pauletti, Admissions
Howard Tullman, President

An independent four-year college with 50 special education students out of a total of 400.

5037 Kishwaukee College
21193 Malta Road
Malta, IL 60150
815-825-2086
FAX 815-825-2072
http://www.kishwaukee.edu
Frances Loubere, Coordinator
Dave Louis, President

Community college services for students with special needs. Students will be counseled and appropriate accommodations made on an individual basis.

5038 Knox College
2 Es Street
Galesburg, IL 61401
309-341-7000
FAX 309-341-7718
http://www.knox.edu
John Haslem, Director
Rodger Taylor, President

Offers a variety of services to students with disabilities including note takers, extended testing time, counseling services, and special accommodations.

5039 Lake Land College
5001 Lake Land Boulevard
Mattoon, IL 61938
217-234-5253
800-252-4121
FAX 217-234-5390
TDY:217-234-5371
http://www.lakeland.cc.il.us
e-mail: hnohren@lakeland.cc.il.us
Heather Nohren, Counselor/Coord Disability Svcs
Donna Beno, Perkins Coordinator

A public two-year college with 230 students with disabilities out of a total enrollment of approximately 7,000.

5040 Lewis and Clark Community College
5800 Godfrey Road
Godfrey, IL 62035
618-466-3411
FAX 618-466-1294
http://www.lc.cc.il.us
Patricia Dunn-Horn, Coordinator
Dale Chapman, President

Offers a variety of services to students with disabilities including note takers, extended testing time, counseling services, and special accommodations.

5041 Lincoln College
Supportive Educational Services
300 Keokuk Street
Lincoln, IL 62656
217-732-3155
800-569-0556
FAX 207-732-7715
http://www.lincolncollege.com
e-mail: rumler@lincolncollege.com
Rod Rumler, Director

A private two-year college with 180 special education students out of a total of 725.

5042 **Lincoln Land Community College**

PO Box 19526
Springfield, IL 62794
217-522-9205
800-727-4161
FAX 217-786-2866
TDY:217-786-2798
http://www.llcc.edu

Linda Chriswell, Special Needs
Charlotte Warren, President
Sylvia Stemmons, Executive Director

A public two-year college with 290 special education students out of a total of 12,000.

5043 **McHenry County College**

8900 Us Highway 14
Crystal Lake, IL 60012
815-455-3700
FAX 815-455-0718
TDY:815-455-8614
http://www.mchenry.edu

Walter Packard, President
Debrah Tatton, Executive Officer

Offers a variety of services to students with disabilities including note takers, extended testing time, counseling services, and special accommodations.

5044 **Millikin University**

1184 W Main Street
Decatur, IL 62522
217-424-6211
FAX 217-362-6497
http://www.millikin.edu
e-mail: webmaster@mail.millikin.edu

Elizabeth Abrahamson, Director
Doug Zemky, President
Clayton Gerhard, Manager

Four-year college that provides programs for the learning disabled.

5045 **Moraine Valley Community College**

88th Avenue
Palos Hills, IL 60465
708-974-5234
FAX 708-974-0078
TDY:708-974-9556
http://www.moraine.cc.il.us
e-mail: moraine@moraine.valley.edu

Laura Vonborstel, Director
Sylvia Jenkins, Manager

A public two-year college with 128 special education students out of a total of 13,958.

5046 **Morton College**

3801 S Central Avenue
Cicero, IL 60804
708-656-8000
FAX 708-656-3924
TDY:708-656-0389
http://www.morton.cc.il.us

Brent Knight, President
Patti Demopoulos, Learning Assistant Specialist

A public two-year community college with 75 special education students out of a total of 5,044. Support services and accommodations are provided for students with disabilities. Tutoring is also available.

5047 **National-Louis University**

Center for Academic Devlopment
2840 Sheridan Road
Evanston, IL 60201
847-465-5829
FAX 847-465-5610
http://www.nl.edu
e-mail: aneukranz-butler@nl.edu

Andreen Neukranz-Butler, Diversity Director
Pat Patillo, Admissions Director

An independent four-year university with 10 special education students out of a total of 3,539. Two hours of tutoring per course per week available for documented LD Students.

5048 **North Central College**

30 N Brainard Street
Naperville, IL 60540
630-637-5100
FAX 630-637-5521
http://www.noctrl.edu

Mary Lynch, Associate Dean
Harold Wilde, President

Offers a variety of services to students with disabilities including note takers, extended testing time, counseling services, and special accommodations.

5049 **Northeastern Illinois University**

Accessibility Center
5500 Ns Louis Avenue
Chicago, IL 60625
773-583-4050
FAX 773-442-5499
TDY:773-442-5499
http://www.neiu.edu
e-mail: v-amey-flippin@neiu.edu

Victoria Amey-Flippin PhD, Director
Effie Sturdivant, Administrative Assistant
Salme Steinberg, President

Northeastern Illinois University is a fully accredited public university serving the Chicago metropolitan area. Total graduate and undergraduate enrollment is approximately 11,000. In addition to offering traditional programs in the arts, sciences, business, and education, Northeastern has a strong commitment to innovative, non-traditional education and has been a leader in the development of special programs for adult learners.

5050 **Northern Illinois University**

Center for Access Ability Resources
Williston Hall 101, Niu
Dekalb, IL 60115
815-753-9734
FAX 815-753-9599
http://www.reg.niu.edu
e-mail: admissions-info@niu.edu

Nancy Kasinski, Director
Robert Burk, Admissions Director

A public four-year university with 150 students receiving disability services out of 16,893.

5051 **Northwestern University**

Services for Students with Disabilities
PO Box 3060
Evanston, IL 60204
847-467-5530
FAX 847-467-5531
http://www.northwestern.edu
e-mail: sst@northwestern.edu

Margee Roe, Coordinator
Henry Bienen, President
Carol Lunkenheimer, Admissions Director

Offers a variety of services to students with disabilities including notetakers, extended testing time, counseling services and special accommodations.

5052 **Northwestern University Communicative Disorders**

2240 Campus Drive
Evanston, IL 60208
847-491-5012
FAX 847-467-2776
http://www.northwestern.edu
e-mail: ckthom@casbah.acns.nwu.edu

Cindy Thompson, Professor
Paula Guire, Executive Director

Offers speech/language and voice services, learning disabilities center and a hearing service.

5053 **Oakton Community College**

1600 E Golf Road
Des Plaines, IL 60016
847-635-1600
FAX 847-635-1764
TDY:847-635-1944
http://www.oakton.edu
e-mail: tbers@oakton.edu

Margaret Lee MD, President
Irene Kovala, Vice President

Students at Oakton Community College have the right to: Equal opportunity to participate; work and learn; reasonable accommodations; appropriate confidentiality; information about available services and accommodations; information about decisions made by the college regarding appropriate accommodations; accessible campus facilities and advocacy within the college community.

5054 Parkland College

2400 W Bradley Avenue
Champaign, IL 61821
217-351-2200
800-346-8089
FAX 217-351-2581
http://www.parkland.cc.il.us

Evelyn Brown, LD Specialist
Norm Lambert, Counselor
Zelema Harris, Administrator

Services for students with disability is a part of the counseling department. These services are coordinated by a full-time counselor. Under the umbrella of these services is a targeted program (Learning Resource Services) for students with learning disabilities (LD) administered by an LD Specialist with type 10 LD certification. Provides accommodations for students with learning disabilities including extended test time, one-on-one tutoring, tape recorders, note takers and individual sessions.

5055 Productive Learning Strategies Program - PLUS Program

DePaul University
2320 N Kenmore Avenue
Chicago, IL 60614
773-325-1677
FAX 773-325-4673
http://www.studentaffairs.depaul.edu/plus/
e-mail: smiras@depaul.edu

Stamatios Miras, Director
Judith Kolar, Assistant Director

PLuS is a comprehensive program designed to assist students with specific learning disabilities and/or attention deficit disorders in experiencing academic success at DePaul University. Please visit PLuS' website for a description of services and application forms.

5056 Quincy University

1800 College Avenue
Quincy, IL 62301
217-222-8020
800-688-4295
FAX 217-228-5479
http://www.quincy.com
e-mail: admissions@quincy.edu

Kevin Brown, Admissions Director
Linda Godley, Dean Academic/Support Service
Susannah Erler, Manager

Offers a variety of services to students with disabilities including notetakers, extended testing time, counseling services, and special accommodations.

5057 Richland Community College

1 College Park
Decatur, IL 62521
217-875-7200
FAX 217-875-6965
http://www.richland.edu
e-mail: rcchelp@richland.edu

Mary Atkins, Coordinator
Margaret Swaim, Secretary/DAS
Gayle Saunders, Administrator

Richland Community College is committed to providing accommodations to students with disabilities. Each individual has a basic right to an education in accordance with his/her aspirations, talents, and skills. Support services ensure students with disabilities an equal opportunity to participate fully in the total college experience.

5058 Robert Morris College

401 S State Street
Chicago, IL 60605
312-935-6835
FAX 312-935-6861
http://www.rmcil.edu
e-mail: bmylott@smtp.rmcil.edu

Brittany Mylott, Director
Michael Biollt, President

Four-year college offering programs to students who are disabled.

5059 Rockford College

5050 E State Street
Rockford, IL 61108
815-226-4000
800-892-2984
FAX 815-226-4119
http://www.rockford.edu
e-mail: jgrey@rockford.edu

Jeanne Grey, Director
Paul Pribbenow, Administrator

The L.R.C. is a nonprofit, educational resource center offering diagnostic testing, remedial tutoring in reading, writing, and mathematics, and enrichment workshops to enhance the learning experience.

5060 Roosevelt University

Learning and Support Services Program
430 S Michigan Avenue
Chicago, IL 60605
312-341-3810
FAX 312-341-3735
http://www.roosevelt.edu
e-mail: dessimm@admvsbk.roosevelt.edu

Nancy Litke, Director
Charles Middleton, President

The Disabled Student Services office serves all students with special needs. The use of services is voluntary and confidential. This office is a resource for students and faculty. The goal of this office is to ensure educational opportunity for all students with special needs by providing access to full participation in all aspects of campus life and increase awareness of disability issues on campus.

5061 Saint Xavier University

3700 W 103rd Street
Chicago, IL 60655
773-298-3000
FAX 773-779-3066

Mary Sansore, LD Director
Judith Dwyer, President

Offers a variety of services to students with disabilities including notetakers, extended testing time, counseling services, and special accommodations.

5062 School of the Art Institute of Chicago

37 S Wabash Avenue
Chicago, IL 60603
312-899-5100
800-232-7242
FAX 312-263-0141
http://www.artic.edu/said/life/sdd.html
e-mail: swhitlow@artic.edu

Susan Whitlow, Coordinator Services
Tony Jones, President

The Office of Services for Students with Disabilities attempts to ensure that students with disabilities have equal access to all programs and activities offered at the School of the Art Institute of Chicago. This can be accomplished by setting up needed accommodations and working to eliminate both attudinal and architectural barriers that exist at the school.

5063 Services for Students with Learning Disabilities at the University of Illinois at Urbana

1207 S Oak Street
Champaign, IL 61820
217-333-8705
FAX 217-333-0248
TDY:217-333-4603
http://www.disability.uiuc.edu
e-mail: kwold2@uiuc.edu

Karen Wold, Learning Disabilities Specialist

Available accommodations may include, but are not restricted to: notetakers; alternate ways of completing exams and assignments; text conversion to an accessible format; access to assistive computer technologies; and consultation regarding learning strategies and disability management skills.

5064 Shawnee College

8364 Shawnee College Road
Ullin, IL 62992
618-634-3200
800-481-2242
FAX 618-634-3300
http://www.shawnee.cc.il.us

Don Slayter, Special Services
Larry Schoate, President

Offers a variety of services to students with disabilities including notetakers, extended testing time, counseling services, and special accommodations.

5065 Shimer College
PO Box 500
Waukegan, IL 60079
847-623-8400
800-215-7173
FAX 847-249-8798
http://www.shimer.edu
e-mail: e.vincent@shimer.edu
Elaine Vincent, Director Admission
William Rice, Administrator

A private four-year college with small, discussion based classes.

5066 Southeastern Illinois College
3575 College Road
Harrisburg, IL 62946
618-252-5400
866-338-2742
http://www.sic.edu
e-mail: catherine.packard@sic.edu
Catherine Packard, Learning Lab Director
Mary Jo Oldham, President

A public two-year college with more than 50 special education and other special needs students out of a total of over 4,000.

5067 Southern Illinois University: Carbondale
Clinical Center Achieve Program
Carbondale, IL 62901
618-453-2369
FAX 618-453-3711
http://www.siu.edu/~achieve
e-mail: achieve@siu.edu
Walker Allen, Admissions Director
Walker Allen, Admissions Director
Roger Pugh MS, Coordinator
The Achieve Program is a comprehensive academic support service for students with LD and/or ADHD. Students must apply to both Achieve and the University.

5068 Southern Illinois University: Edwardsville
Disability Support Services
PO Box 1047
Edwardsville, IL 62026
618-650-3782
FAX 618-650-5691
http://www.siue.edu
e-mail: jfloydh@siue.edu
Jane Floyd-Hendey, Director
Boyd Bradshaw, Admissions Director

A public four-year college with 119 special education students out of a total of 13,460.

5069 Spoon River College
23235 N Co 22
Canton, IL 61520
309-647-4645
800-334-7337
FAX 309-649-6393
http://www.spoonrivercollege.edu
e-mail: info@src.edu
Tom Hines, President
Mickey Decker, Admission officer
Kathleen Menateaux, Executive Director
A public two-year college with 61 special education students out of a total of 2,312.

5070 Springfield College in Illinois
1500 N 5th Street
Springfield, IL 62702
217-525-1420
FAX 217-789-1698
http://www.sci.edu
Karen Anderson, Dean
Nereida Avendano, Director
Heather Bigard, Manager
Offers a variety of services to students with disabilities including note takers, extended testing time, counseling services, and special accommodations.

5071 University of Illinois at Springfield
1 University Plaza
Springfield, IL 62703
217-206-6600
888-977-4847
FAX 217-206-6511
http://www.uis.edu
Chris Miller, Dean Students
Richard Ringeisen, Manager

A public four-year college with 26 special education students out of a total of 2,644.

5072 Waubonsee Community College
RR 47
Sugar Grove, IL 60554
630-466-7900
FAX 630-466-4649
TDY:630-466-4649
http://www.waubonsee.edu
e-mail: ihansen@waubonsee.edu
Iris Hansen, Manager ACSD
Christine Sobek, Administrator

A public two-year college with 400 special education students out of a total 10,000.

5073 Western Illinois University
Disability Support Services
115 Sherman Hall
Macomb, IL 61455
309-298-2512
FAX 309-298-2361
http://www.wiu.edu
e-mail: joan_grren@ccmail.wiu.edu
Joan Green, Director
Karen Helmers, Admissions Director

A public four-year college with 135 special education students out of a total of 10,652.

5074 William Rainey Harper College
1200 W Algonquin Road
Palatine, IL 60067
847-925-6266
FAX 847-925-6267
TDY:847-397-7600
http://www.harpercollege.edu
e-mail: pherrera@harpercollege.edu
Pascuala Herrera, LD Coordinator
Tom Thompson, Director

A public two-year college with 550 students with disabilities out of a total of 24,00. Offer a special instructional program for students with LD or ADD for an additional fee. Offers a TRIO/SSS project for degree-seeking students (150 involved annually).

Indiana

5075 Ancilla College
9601 S Union Road
Donaldson, IN 46513
574-936-8898
http://www.ancilla.edu
Kathryn Bigley, Director
Neil Thorburn, Manager

An independent two-year college with three special education students out of a total of 667.

5076 Anderson University
Disabled Student Services
1100 E 5th Street
Anderson, IN 46012
765-641-4226
FAX 765-641-3851
http://www.anderson.edu
e-mail: rsvogel@anderson.edu
Rinda Vogelgesang, Director
Jim King, Admissions Director

An independent four-year college with 78 special education students out of a total of 1,977.

5077 Ball State University: Disabled Student Development

2000 W University Avenue
Muncie, IN 47306
765-285-8255
800-482-4278
FAX 765-285-5295
http://www.bsu.edu
e-mail: rharris@bsu.edu

Richard Harris, Director
Rachel Perkins, Manager

Offers a variety of services to students with disabilities including note takers, extended testing time, counseling services, and special accommodations.

5078 Bethel College: Indiana

1001 W McKinley Avenue
Mishawaka, IN 46545
574-259-8511
800-422-4101
http://www.bethel-in.edu

Offers a variety of services to students with disabilities including note takers, extended testing time, counseling services, and special accommodations.

5079 Butler University

4600 Sunset Avenue
Indianapolis, IN 46208
317-940-8000
800-368-6852
FAX 317-940-9930
http://www.butler.edu
e-mail: info@butler.edu

Bobby Fong, CEO

Offers a variety of services to students with disabilities including notetakers, extended testing time, counseling services, and special accommodations.

5080 Earlham College

801 National Road W
Richmond, IN 47374
765-983-1600
800-327-5426
FAX 765-973-2120
http://www.earlham.edu
e-mail: keesldo@earlham.edu

Donna Keesling, Executive Director
Douglas Bennett, President

Offers a variety of services to students with disabilities including note takers, extended testing time, counseling services, and special accommodations.

5081 Franklin College of Indiana

501 E Monroe Street
Franklin, IN 46131
317-738-8000
800-522-0232
FAX 317-738-8234
http://www.franklincoll.edu
e-mail: webmaster@franklincoll.edu

Dana Giles, Assistant Director
James Moseley, President

An independent four-year college with six special education students out of a total of 914.

5082 Goshen College

1700 S Main Street
Goshen, IN 46526
574-535-7298
800-348-7422
FAX 574-535-7660
http://www.goshen.edu
e-mail: mhooley@goshen.edu

Marty Hooley, Director
James Brenneman, President

An independent four-year college with 23 special education students out of a total of 1,042.

5083 Holy Cross College

933 North
Notre Dame, IN 46556
574-631-5477
FAX 574-239-8323
http://www.hcc-nd.edu
e-mail: uduke@hcc-nd.edu

Rev. Smith, Executive Director

A two-year colege that provides programs for learning disabled students.

5084 Indiana Institute of Technology

Student Support Services
1600 E Washington Boulevard
Fort Wayne, IN 46803
260-422-5561
800-937-2448
FAX 260-422-1518
http://www.indtech.edu
e-mail: scudder@indtech.edu

Mary Scudder, Director Student Services

A program of academic support services, including appropriate tutoring, peer mentoring and academic assistance, which is provided to students meeting specific federal eligibility guidelines.

5085 Indiana Institute on Disability and Community at Indiana University

2853 E 10th Street
Bloomington, IN 47408
812-855-9396
800-437-7924
FAX 812-855-9630
TDY:812-835-9396
http://www.iidc.indiana.edu
e-mail: iidc@indiana.edu

David Mank PhD, Director
Joel Fosha, Coordinator Office Marketing
Marilyn Irwin, Executive Director

The Indiana Institute on Disability and Community (IIDC) at Indiana University, Bloomington is committed to providing Hoosiers with disability-related information and services that touch the entire life span, from birth through older adulthood. Through its collaborative efforts with institutions of higher education, state and local government agencies, community service providers, persons with disabilities and their families, and advocacy organizations.

5086 Indiana State University

210 N 7th Street
Terre Haute, IN 47809
812-237-2284
FAX 812-237-7948
http://www.web.indstate.edu
e-mail: oprasay@usugw.indstate.edu

Lloyd Benjamin III, President
Barbara Asay, Assistant to the President

Offers a variety of services to students with disabilities including note takers, extended testing time, counseling services, and special accommodations.

5087 Indiana University East

Student Support Services
2325 Chester Boulevard
Richmond, IN 47374
765-973-8200
800-959-3278
FAX 765-973-8388
http://www.iue.indiana.edu

Sherryl Stafford, Director
Sally Sayre, Secretary

A public four-year college with 21 special education students out of a total of 2,249.

5088 Indiana University Northwest

3400 Broadway
Gary, IN 46408
219-980-6500
888-YOUR-IUN
http://www.iun.edu

Ronald Thornton, Student Coordinator
Marilyn Vasquez, Administrator

A public four-year college with 34 special education students out of a total of 5,000.

5089 Indiana University Southeast

4201 Grant Line Road
New Albany, IN 47150
812-941-2000
FAX 812-941-2589
http://www.ius.edu
e-mail: jojames@ius.edu

Jodi James, Coordinator
Sandra Patterson, Manager

Offers a variety of services to students with disabilities including note takers, extended testing time, counseling services, and special accommodations.

5090 Indiana University: Bloomington
Disabled Student Services
601 E Kirkwood Avenue
Bloomington, IN 47405
812-855-7578
FAX 812-855-7650
http://www.indiana.edu
e-mail: dsscoord@indiana.edu

Martha Jacques, Director
Mary , Admissions Director

A public four-year college with 225 special education students out of a total of 29,383.

5091 Indiana University: Kokomo
3102 S Lafountain Street
Kokomo, IN 46902
765-453-2000
FAX 765-455-2020
http://www.iuk.edu

Jeremy Lipinski, Director
Sherry Stone, Office Staff
Ruth Persons, Manager
A combination of attitudes assistance, accommodations, classroom arrangements and technological aids that make it possible for learning disabled and physically disabled students to succeed in a degree program for which they are qualified.

5092 Indiana University: Purdue
425 University Boulevard
Indianapolis, IN 46202
317-274-5555
http://www.iupui.edu

Pamela King, Director
Charles Bantz, Manager

A public four-year college with 154 special education students out of a total of 21,165.

5093 Indiana Vocational Technical: Southeast Campus
Ivy Tech Drive
Madison, IN 47250
812-265-2580
800-403-2190
FAX 812-265-4028
http://www.ivytech.edu

Kevin Bradley, Registrar
Don Hiderman, Manager

Offers a variety of services to students with disabilities including notetakers, extended testing time, counseling services, and special accommodations.

5094 Indiana Wesleyan University
Student Support Services
4201 S Washington Street
Marion, IN 46953
765-677-2257
FAX 765-677-2140
http://www.indwes.edu
e-mail: todd.ream@indwes.edu

Todd Ream, Director
Nan Turner, Assistant

Offers a variety of services to students with disabilities including notetakers, extended testing time, counseling services and special accommodations.

5095 Ivy Tech State College Southwest
3501 N 1st Avenue
Evansville, IN 47710
812-429-9853
FAX 812-429-1483
TDY:812-429-9803
http://www.ivytech.edu
e-mail: pehlen@ivytech.edu
Peg Ehlen, Disability Services Coordinator
Sherry Pejarano, Administrative Assistant

Provides reasonable and effective accommodations to qualified students with learning disabilities.

5096 Ivy Tech State College: Northcentral
220 Dean Johnson Boulevard
South Bend, IN 46601
574-289-7001
888-489-3478
FAX 574-236-7178
http://www.ivytech.edu
e-mail: amatthew@ivy.tec.in.us
Amy Cassa, Coordinator Disabilities Service
Gail Craker, Support Services Coordinator
Virginia Calvin, Manager
Accommodations based on individual needs.

5097 Manchester College
Services for Students with Disabilities
604 E College Avenue
North Manchester, IN 46962
260-982-5000
http://www.manchester.edu
e-mail: dshowe@manchester.edu
Denise Howe, Director
JoLane Rohr, Admissions Director
Parker Marden, President
An independent four-year college with 50 special education students out of a total of 1,091.

5098 Purdue University
Educational Studies
100 N University Street
West Lafayette, IN 47907
765-494-9170
FAX 765-496-1228
http://www.purdue.edu
Sarah Templin, Special Services

A public four-year college with 232 special education students out of a total of 29,673.

5099 Riley Child Development Center
Indiana University School of Medicine
702 Barnhill Drive
Indianapolis, IN 46202
317-274-5000
FAX 317-274-9760
http://www.child-dev.com
e-mail: jrau@iupui.edu

John Rau, Director
Linda Newton, Administrative Assistant

The Child Development Center provides interdisciplinary assessment for academics, communication, motor, behavior, medical concerns, for children and their families.

5100 Rose-Hulman Institute of Technology
5500 Wabash Avenue
Terre Haute, IN 47803
812-877-1511
FAX 812-877-8175
http://www.rose-hulman.edu

Susan Smith, Director
Jody Doughrty, Administrative Assistant
John Midgley, President
Offers a variety of services to students with disabilities including note takers, extended testing time, counseling services, and special accommodations.

5101 Saint Joseph's College
PO Box 890
Rensselaer, IN 47978
219-866-6000
800-447-8781
FAX 219-866-6355
http://www.saintjoe.edu

David Weed, Director
Joan Cramer, Secretary of the Director

Offers a variety of services to students with disabilities including note takers, extended testing time, counseling services, and special accommodations.

5102 Saint Mary-of-the-Woods College
3301 Saint Mary-of-the-Woods
Saint Mary of the Woods, IN 47876
812-535-5151
FAX 812-535-4900
http://www.smwc.edu
e-mail: smwc@smwc.edu

Kate Satchwill, Vice President
Joan Lescinski, President

Offers a variety of services to students with disabilities including note takers, extended testing time, counseling services, and special accommodations.

5103 Southcentral Indiana Vocational Technical College

8204 Highway 311
Sellersburg, IN 47172
812-246-3301
FAX 765-973-8383

Rita Shourds, Manager

Offers a variety of services to students with disabilities including note takers, extended testing time, counseling services, and special accommodations.

5104 Taylor University

236 W Reade Avenue
Upland, IN 46989
765-998-2751
FAX 765-998-5569
http://www.tayloru.edu
e-mail: edwelch@tayloru.edu

R Edwin Welch MD, Coordinator
Eugene Habecker, President

Four-year college that provides academic support to students with disabilities.

5105 University of Evansville

1800 Lincoln Avenue
Evansville, IN 47722
812-479-2482
800-423-8633
FAX 812-475-6429
http://www.evansville.edu

Nealon Gaskey MD, Professor
Steven Jennings, President
William Louden, Executive Director

An independent four-year college with 60 special education students out of a total of 2,500.

5106 University of Indianapolis

Baccalaureate for University of Indianapolis
1400 E Hanna Avenue
Indianapolis, IN 46227
317-788-2140
800-232-8634
FAX 317-788-3585
http://www.uindy.edu
e-mail: cjoles@uindy.edu

Candace Joles, Director BUILD Program
Mary Craft, Administrative Assistant

Is a full support program at the University of Indianapolis designed to help the college students with specific learning disability earn an associate or baccalureate degree.

5107 University of Notre Dame

Office for Students with Disabilities
220 Main Building
Notre Dame, IN 46556
574-631-5000
http://www.nd.edu
e-mail: margaret.spitzer@uncu.edu

Scott Howland, Director
Dan Saracino, Admissions Director
Edward Malloy, President

An independent four-year college with 20 special education students out of a total of 8,038.

5108 University of Saint Francis

Student Learning Center
2701 Spring Street
Fort Wayne, IN 46808
800-729-4732
http://www.sfc.edu
e-mail: mkruyer@sf.edu

Michelle Kruyer, Director
John Arruza, Director

Through the Student Learning Center, University of Saint Francis offers a support program providing comprehensive services for student with diagnosed disabilities in the university setting. Students who present appropriate documentation and qualify for support services will receive modifications and accommodations to facilitate academic success. These services are provided at no cost to the student.

5109 University of Southern Indiana

Counseling Center
8600 University Boulevard
Evansville, IN 47712
812-464-1867
FAX 812-461-5288
TDY:812-465-7072
http://www.usi.edu
e-mail: lmsmith@usi.edu

Leslie Smith, Assistant Director Counseling
James Browning, Director Counseling
Eric Otto, Admissions Director

Offers a variety of services to students with disabilities including notetaker supplies, tutor referral, extended testing time, counseling services, advocacy, sign language services and special accommodations.

5110 Vincennes University

Students Transition into Education Program
1002 N 1st Street
Vincennes, IN 47591
812-888-4485
800-742-9198
FAX 812-888-5707
http://www.vinu.edu
e-mail: jkavanaugh@vinu.edu

Jane Kavanaugh, Education Director
Susan Laue, Associate Professor
Ann Skuce, Admissions Director

A public two-year college with 200 learning disabled students in the STEP Program. Total student enrollment is 6,000. There is a fee for the special education program.

Iowa

5111 Central College: Student Support Services

812 University Street
Pella, IA 50219
641-628-9000
FAX 641-628-7647
http://www.central.edu
e-mail: krosen@central.edu

Nancy Kroese, Director
David Roe, President

Four-year college that provides student support for those with learning disabilities.

5112 Clinton Community College

1000 Lincoln Boulevard
Clinton, IA 52732
563-244-7046
800-637-0559
FAX 563-244-7005
http://www.eicc.edu
e-mail: bkunau@eicc.edu

Karen Vickers, President
Ron Erpliss, Dean College
Cindy Hoogheem, Manager

Offers a variety of services to students with disabilities including note takers, extended testing time, counseling services, and special accommodations.

5113 Coe College

1220 1st Avenue NE
Cedar Rapids, IA 52402
319-399-8000
FAX 319-399-8503
http://www.coe.edu
e-mail: lkabela@coe.edu

Lois Kabela-Coates, Director
Nancy Carberry, Administrative Assistant
James Phifer, President

Services include: tutors, note takers, test proctoring for untimed and oral tests, assistance with accessing textbooks on tape, study skills and time management assistance, reading and writing assistance, personal and academic counseling, and assistance with course and instructor selection.

5114 Cornell College

600 1st Street NW
Mount Vernon, IA 52314
319-895-4000
FAX 319-896-5188
http://www.cornell-iowa.edu
e-mail: admissions@cornell-iowa.edu

Leslie Garner, President

An independent four-year college with 11 special education students out of a total of 1,114.

5115 DesMoines Area Community College
2006 S Ankeny Boulevard
Ankeny, IA 50023
515-964-6200
800-362-2127
FAX 515-964-7022
TDY:964-381-1551
http://www.dmacc.cc.ia.us
e-mail: webmaster@dmacc.cc.ia.us

Jim Barron, Director

DMACC is committed to providing an accessible environment that supports students with disabilities in reaching their full potential. Support services are available for students with disabilities to ensure equal access to educational opportunities.

5116 Dordt College
Academic Skills Center
498 4th Avenue NE
Sioux Center, IA 51250
712-722-6490
FAX 712-722-4498
http://www.dordt.edu
e-mail: admissions@dordt.edu

Marliss Vanderzwaag, Coordinator
Pam DeJong, Director

Four-year college that offers academic services to students.

5117 Drake University
Student Disability Services
3116 Carpenter Avenue
Des Moines, IA 50311
515-271-3100
800-443-7253
FAX 515-712-1855
TDY:515-271-2825
http://www.drake.edu
e-mail: christal.stanley@drake.edu

Chrystal Stanley, Director
Thomas Willoughby, Admissions Director

Offers a variety of services to students with disabilities including formal academic accommodations and support services.

5118 Ellsworth Community College
1100 College Avenue
Iowa Falls, IA 50126
641-648-4611
http://www.iavalley.cc.ia.us
e-mail: lmulford@iavalley.cc.ia.us

Lori Mulford, Coordinator
Mollie Teckenburg, Manager

Offers a variety of services to students with disabilities including note takers, extended testing time, counseling services and special accommodations.

5119 Graceland College
1 University Place
Lamoni, IA 50140
641-784-5000
FAX 641-784-5698
http://www2.graceland.edu

JR Smith, Director
John Menzies, President

An independent four-year college with 27 special education students out of a total of 968. There is an additional fee for the special education program in addition to the regular tuition.

5120 Grand View College
1200 Grandview Avenue
Des Moines, IA 50316
515-263-2850
FAX 515-263-2840
http://www.gvc.edu
e-mail: cwassenaar@gve.edu

Carolyn Wassenaar, Director
Debbie Borger, Admissions Director
Kent Henning, President

An independent four-year college with 15 special education students out of a total of 1,419.

5121 Grinnell College
Academic Advising Office
PO Box 805
Grinnell, IA 50112
641-269-3702
FAX 641-269-3710
http://www.grinnell.edu
e-mail: sternjm@grinnell.edu

Joyce Stern, Associate Dean
Jim Sumner, Admissions Director

An independent four-year college which currently provides academic accommodations to students with learning disabilities and 15 students with ADHD out of a total of 1,344.

5122 Hawkeye Community College
PO Box 8015
Waterloo, IA 50704
319-296-2320
FAX 319-296-4018

Kathy Linda, Developmental Studies Department
Ruben Carrion, Student Development Director
Greg Schmitz, President

Offers a variety of services to students with disabilities including notetakers, extended testing time, tutoring, counseling services, and special accommodations.

5123 Indian Hills Community College
Success Center
525 Grandview Avenue
Ottumwa, IA 52501
641-683-5155
800-726-2585
FAX 641-683-5184
http://www.ihec.cc.ia.us
e-mail: successcenter@ihcc.cc

Mary Stewart, Dean Academic Services
Marva Chilipsen, Disability Service Provider
Sally Harris, Admissions Director

A public two-year college with 400 special education students out of a total of 3,166. There is a fee for the special education program in addition to the regular tuition.

5124 Iowa Central Community College
330 Avenue M
Fort Dodge, IA 50501
515-576-7201
800-362-2793
FAX 515-576-7206
http://www.iccc.cc.ia.us/icc/home/default.htm
e-mail: lundeen@triton.iccc.cc.ia.us

Shelly Lundeen, Student Success Teacher
Carol Koettlin, Desk Coordinator
Bob Paxton, Administrator

A public two-year college with approximately 50 special needs students out of a total of 3,003.

5125 Iowa Lakes Community College: Emmetsburg Campus
3200 College Drive
Emmetsburg, IA 50536
712-852-3554
800-242-5108
FAX 712-852-2152
http://www.iowalakes.edu
e-mail: mkogel@iowalakes.edu

Tom Brotherton, Manager
Michelle Kogel, SAVE Coordinator
Ann Petersen, Special Needs

Offers a variety of services to students with disabilities including notetakers, extended testing time, counseling services, and special accommodations, including secondary programs at post-secondary institutions.

5126 Iowa Lakes Community College: Success Centers
300 S 18th Street
Estherville, IA 51334
712-362-2604
800-521-5054
FAX 712-362-3969
http://www.iowalakes.edu
e-mail: info@iowalakes.edu

Colleen Peltz, Prof. Developmental Education
Lynn Dodge, Assistant Professor Dev. Educ.
Mary Mohni, Executive Director

Offers a variety of services to students with disabilities including note takers, extended testing time, counseling services, and special accommodations.

5127 Iowa State University
Disability Resources
1076 Student Services Building
Ames, IA 50011
515-294-0644
FAX 515-294-2397
http://www.dso.iastate.edu
e-mail: accommodations@iastate.edu
Steven Moats, Program Director
Marc Harding, Admissions Director

A public four-year university that has approximately 600 students receiving disability services out of 21,000 students.

5128 Iowa Wesleyan College
601 N Main Street
Mount Pleasant, IA 52641
319-385-8021
FAX 319-385-6384
Linda Widmer, Director
William Johnston, President

An independent four-year college with four special education students out of a total of 1,000.

5129 Iowa Western Community College: Council Bluffs Campus
PO Box 4C
Council Bluffs, IA 51502
712-325-3200
800-432-5852
FAX 712-388-0123
http://www.iwcc.cc.ia.us
e-mail: cholst@iwcc.cc.ia.us
Chris Holst, Coordinator
Dan Holst, President

IWCC is committed to making individuals with disabilities full participants in its programs, services and activities. It is the policy of IWCC that no otherwise qualified individual with a disability shall be denied access to or participation in any program, service or activity offered by the college.

5130 Loras College
Learning Disabilities Program
PO Box 178
Dubuque, IA 52004
563-588-7100
800-245-6727
http://www.loras.edu
e-mail: dgibson@loras.edu
Dianne Gibson, Director
Tim Hauber, Admissions Director
James Collins, President
Private Catholic four-year college with 40 learning disabled students out of a total of 1,626. The Learning Disabilities Program charges a fee for the Enhanced program. Mandated services are free.

5131 Luther College
700 College Drive
Decorah, IA 52101
563-387-2000
800-458-8437
FAX 563-387-2158
http://www.luther.edu
e-mail: equalaccess@luther.edu
G Rosales, Director
Janice Halsne, Service Director
Richard Torgenson, President
In keeping with the mission of Luther College, the Student Academic Support Center (SASC) exists to support all students as they pursue a liberal arts education, and specifically to be an advocate for students with disabilities. SASC processes all student requests for accommodations to provide each student with a suitable learning environment. The accommodations provided are not remedial in nature, nor do they change or reduce the academic standard.

5132 Marshalltown Community College
3700 S Center Street
Marshalltown, IA 50158
641-752-7106
FAX 641-752-8149
http://www.iavalley.cc.ia.us
Regina West, Coordinator
Tim Wynes, President

A two-year community college that offers programs for its learning disabled students.

5133 Morningside College
Student Services
1501 Morningside Avenue
Sioux City, IA 51106
712-274-5000
800-831-0806
FAX 712-274-5101
http://www.morningside.edu
e-mail: tennapel@morningside.edu
Karmen Ten Napel, Director
John Reynders, President

A comprehensive learning disabilities program which offers academic advisement accommodations, subject area tutoring, and supportive services.

5134 Mount Mercy College
1330 Elmhurst Drive NE
Cedar Rapids, IA 52402
319-363-8213
FAX 319-363-6341
http://www.mt mercy.edu
e-mail: nbrauhn@mmc.mtmercy.edu
Mary Stanton, Director
Robert Pearce, President

Four-year college offering support and services to learning disabled students.

5135 Mount Saint Clare College
400 N Bluff Boulevard
Clinton, IA 52732
563-242-4070
800-242-4153
http://www.clare.edu
Diane Cornilsen, Director
Marcella Narlock, Executive Director

Offers a variety of services to students with disabilities including notetakers, extended testing time, counseling services, and special accommodations.

5136 Muscatine Community College
152 Colorado Street
Muscatine, IA 52761
563-288-6001
800-351-4669
FAX 563-288-6104
http://www.eiccd.cc.ia.us
e-mail: smewwiam@eicc.edu
Vic Avoy, President
Kathryn Trosen, Retention Specialist

A public two-year college with 29 special education students out of a total of 1,192.

5137 North Iowa Area Community College
500 College Drive
Mason City, IA 50401
641-423-1264
888-466-4222
FAX 614-422-4150
e-mail: ewerster@niaccicc.ia.us
Terri Ewers, Counseling Director
Michael Morrison, President

Offers a variety of services to students with disabilities including notetakers, extended testing time, counseling services, and special accommodations.

5138 Northwestern College
3003 Snelling Avenue N
Saint Paul, MN 55113
651-631-5100
http://www.nwc.nwc.edu
Marcia Olson, Special Services
Alan Cureton, President

Offers a variety of services to students with disabilities including note takers, extended testing time, counseling services, and special accommodations.

5139 Saint Ambrose College
Services for Students with Disabilities
518 W Locust Street
Davenport, IA 52803
563-333-6000
http://www.sau.edu
e-mail: aaqustin@saunix.sau.edu

Ann Austin, LD Specialist
Meg Flagherty, Admissions Director
Edward Rogalski, President
An independent four-year college with 63 special education students out of a total of 2,022.

5140 Scott Community College
500 Belmont Road
Riverdale, IA 52722
563-441-4000
FAX 563-441-4066
http://www.eiccd.cc.ia.us
Jerri Crabtree, Director

A public two-year college with 59 special education students out of a total of 3,611.

5141 Simpson College: Hawley Academic ResourceCenter
701 N C Street
Indianola, IA 50125
515-961-1682
800-362-2454
FAX 515-961-1363
http://www.simpson.edu/hawley
e-mail: little@simpson.edu
Todd Little, Director

Simpson College is a private, four-year liberal arts college located south of Des Moines, Iowa. The Hawley Center offers services to students with disabilities including academic accommodations and other support services.

5142 Southeastern Community College: North Campus
1500 W Agency Road
West Burlington, IA 52655
319-752-2731
866-727-4692
FAX 319-752-4995
http://www.scciowa.edu
Chris Man, Admissions Coordinator
Stacy White, Admissions Coordinator
Jim Richardson, President
Offers special services and student services to the learning disabled.

5143 Southwestern Community College
Services for Students with Disabilities
1501 W Townline Street
Creston, IA 50801
641-782-7081
FAX 641-782-3312
http://www.swcciowa.edu
e-mail: pantini@swcciowa.edu
Deb Pantini, Special Needs Coordinator
Bill Taylor, Director for Student Services
Barb Crittenden, President
Offers a variety of services to students with disabilities including note takers, extended testing time, counseling services, and special accommodations.

5144 University of Iowa
Student Disability Services
1300 Burge Hall
Iowa City, IA 52242
319-335-1462
FAX 319-335-3973
http://www.uiowa.edu/~sds
e-mail: sds-information@uiowa.edu
Dau-shen Ju MD, Director Student Disability Svcs
Michael Barron, Asst Provost Enrollment Services

A public institution with a long history of providing appropriate academic accommations and support for students with disabilities.

5145 University of Northern Iowa
103 Student Health Center
Cedar Falls, IA 50614
319-273-2542
FAX 319-273-6884
TDY:319-273-3011
http://www.uni.edu/disability
e-mail: jane.slykhuis@uni.edu
David Towle, Director
Jane Slykhuis, Coordinator
Robert Koob, CEO
Four-year college that provides services to students with a learning disability.

5146 Waldorf College
Learning Disabilities Program
106 S 6th Street
Forest City, IA 50436
800-292-1903
http://www.waldorf.edu
e-mail: hillb@waldorf.edu
Rebecca Hill, Director
Steve Lovick, Admissions Director

An independent two-year college with 20 learning disabled students out of a total of 599. There is an additional fee for the learning disabled program in addition to the regular tuition.

5147 Wartburg College
PO Box 1003
Waverly, IA 50677
319-352-8260
800-772-2085
FAX 319-352-8568
http://www.wartburg.edu
e-mail: alexander.smith@wartburg.edu
Jack Ohle, President
Alexander Smith, Vice President Student Life
Kayah-Bah Malecek, Pathways Center Associate
An independent four-year residential college with 20 students with learning disabilities out of a total 1,730 full-time undergraduate students.

Kansas

5148 Allen County Community College
1801 N Cottonwood Street
Iola, KS 66749
620-365-5116
http://www.allen.cc.ks.us
John Masterson, President

Offers a variety of services to students with disabilities including note takers, extended testing time, counseling services, and special accommodations.

5149 Baker University
Learning Resource Center
PO Box 65
Baldwin City, KS 66006
785-594-6451
http://www.bakeru.edu
e-mail: marian@harvey.bakeru.edu
Kathy Marian, Director
Paige Illum, Admissions Director
Daniel Lambert, President
A private four-year college with a total of 923 students.

5150 Barton County Community College
245 NE 30th Road
Great Bend, KS 67530
620-792-9340
http://www.barton.cc.ks.us
Todd Moore, Director for admission
Cassandra Montoya, Student Work Service
Veldon Law, President
A public two-year college with 12 special education students out of a total of 4,462.

5151 Bethel College
300 E 27th Street
North Newton, KS 67117
316-283-2500
800-522-1887
FAX 316-284-5286
http://www.bethelks.edu
Laverne Epp, President
Mary Enz, Bookstore Coordinator

Offers a variety of services to students with disabilities including notetakers, extended testing time, counseling services, and special accommodations.

5152 Butler County Community College
PO Box 1203
El Dorado, KS 67042
316-321-2222
800-826-2829
FAX 724-287-4961

Lora Rozeboom, Special Needs
Jacqueline Vietti, President

A public two-year college with 93 special education students out of a total of 5,601.

5153 Center for Research on Learning
University of Kansas
1122 W Campus Road
Lawrence, KS 66045 785-864-4780
http://www.ku-crl.org
e-mail: cre@ku.edu
Donald Deshler, Executive Director
Jamin Dreasher, Office Assistant

All of the research undertaken at the center adheres to a single mission that has been crafted to respond to these educational challenges: an information explosion in all content areas; a limited amount of instructional time; and increased expectations for student achievement.

5154 Colby Community College
1255 S Range Avenue
Colby, KS 67701 785-462-3984
FAX 785-462-4600
http://www.colby.cc.edu
e-mail: joyce@colby.cc.edu
Joyce Washburn, Academic Services
Mikel Ary, President

Offers a variety of services to students with disabilities including note takers, extended testing time, counseling services, and special accommodations.

5155 Cowley County Community College
PO Box 1147
Arkansas City, KS 67005 620-442-0430
http://www.cowleycollege.com
e-mail: watson@cowleycollege.com
Bruce Watson, ADA Coordinator
Pat Atee, President

Offers a variety of services to students with disabilities including notetakers, extended testing time, counseling services, and special accommodations.

5156 Donnelly College
608 N 18th Street
Kansas City, KS 66102 913-621-8764
FAX 913-621-8719
http://www.donnelly.edu
e-mail: stephens@donnelly.edu
Lee Stephenson, Director Student Services

An independent two-year college with 10 special education students out of a total of 381.

5157 Emporia State University
1200 Commercial Street
Emporia, KS 66801 620-341-6778
FAX 620-341-5918
http://www.emporia.edu
Keith Frank MD, Coordinator
Jo Kord, Manager

Offers a variety of services to students with disabilities including note takers, extended testing time, counseling services, and special accommodations.

5158 Fort Scott Community College
2108 Horton Street
Fort Scott, KS 66701 620-223-2700
800-874-3722
http://www.fortscott.edu
e-mail: beckyw@ftscott.cc.ks.us
Becky Weddle, Director CE/ETC/Mill
James Miesner, President

A public two-year college with 34 special education students out of a total of 1,928.

5159 Hutchinson Community College
1300 N Plum Street
Hutchinson, KS 67501 620-665-3500
800-289-3501
FAX 620-665-3310
http://www.hutchcc.edu
e-mail: info@hutchcc.edu
Mary Coplen, Director
Edward Berger, President

Offers a variety of services to students with disabilities including notetakers, extended testing time, counseling services, and special accommodations.

5160 Kansas Community College: Kansas City
7250 State Avenue
Kansas City, KS 66112 913-334-1100
FAX 913-596-9606
http://www.kckcc.cc.ks.us
Thomas Burke, President
Valerie Webb, Disability Resource Center Coord

A public two-year college with an enrollment of approximately 6,000 students. Thirty-five LD students request services each semester. Developmental courses and accommodations are offered for students with learning disabilities.

5161 Kansas State University
Disability Support Services
Holton Hall
Manhattan, KS 66506 785-532-6441
FAX 785-532-6457
http://www.ksu.edu
e-mail: dss@ksu.edu
Andria Blair, Director
Andrea Blair, LD Specialist
Larry Moeder, Admissions Director
Dedicated to providing equal opportunity and access for every student. The staff provides a broad range of supportive services in an effort to ensure that the individual needs of each student are met. In addition, the staff functions as an advocate for students with disabilities on the K-State campus.

5162 Kansas University Center for Developmental Disabilities (KUCDD)
1000 Sunnyside Avenue
Lawrence, KS 66045 785-864-4950
FAX 785-864-5323
http://www.lsi.ku.edu
e-mail: schroeder@ku.edu
Stephen Schrander, Director

KUCDD develops alternatives to institutional care for persons with developmental disabilities. Helps families of persons with disabilities define their needs and find resources and plan and evaluate services on a cost-performance basis. Also provides in-service trainig to service providers.

5163 Labette Community College
200 S 14th Street
Parsons, KS 67357 620-421-6700
FAX 620-421-0921
http://www.labette.cc.ks.us
Viv Metcalf, Director
George Knox, President

A public two-year college with 80 special education students out of a total of 2,598.

5164 Neosho County Community College
800 W 14th Street
Chanute, KS 66720 620-431-5732
FAX 620-235-4030
http://www.neosho.cc.ks.us
John Messenger, Instructor
Rhonda Schroeder, Manager

Offers a variety of services to students with disabilities including note takers, extended testing time, counseling services, and special accommodations.

5165 **Newman University**
3100 McCormick Street
Wichita, KS 67213
316-942-4291
FAX 316-942-4483
http://www.newmanu.edu
e-mail: niedensr@newmanu.edu
Rosemary Niedens, Dean of Students
Aidan Dunleavy, President

Offers a variety of services to students with disabilities including notetakers, extended testing time, counseling services, and special accommodations.

5166 **North Central Kansas Technical College**
Nursing Department
2205 Wheatland Drive
Hays, KS 67601
785-623-6155
800-658-4655
FAX 785-623-6152
http://www.ncktc.tec.ks.us
George Mihel, President

5167 **Ottawa University**
1001 S Cedar Street
Ottawa, KS 66067
785-242-5200
800-755-5200
FAX 785-242-1008
http://www.ottawa.edu
Karen Ohnesorge-Fick, Academic Achievement

An independent four-year college with 11 special education students out of a total of 546.

5168 **Pittsburg State University**
Learning Center
1701 S Broadway Street
Pittsburg, KS 66762
620-231-7000
http://www.pittstate.edu
e-mail: nhenry@pittstate.edu
Nick Henry, Special Services
Ange Peterson, Admissions Director

A public four-year college with 74 special education students out of a total of 5,222.

5169 **Saint Mary College**
4100 S 4th Street
Leavenworth, KS 66048
913-682-5151
800-752-7043
FAX 913-758-6140
http://www.stmary.edu
e-mail: admiss@hub.smcks.edu
Sandra Hoose, Academic Dean
Diane Steele, President

Offers a variety of services to students with disabilities including note takers, extended testing time, counseling services, and special accommodations.

5170 **Seward County Community College**
PO Box 1137
Liberal, KS 67905
620-356-2364
800-373-9951
FAX 316-629-2715
http://www.scc.cc.ks.us/
Larry Philbeck, Academic Achievement
Duane Dunn, President

A public two-year college with 13 special education students out of a total of 1,522.

5171 **Tabor College**
400 S Jefferson Street
Hillsboro, KS 67063
620-947-3121
800-TABOR-99
FAX 620-947-2607
http://www.tabor.edu
e-mail: larryn@tabor.edu
Larry Nikkel, President
Lawrence Ressler, VP Academics/Student Development
Kirby Fadenrecht, VP Business/Finance

Offers a variety of services to students with disabilities including note takers, extended testing time, counseling services, and special accommodations.

5172 **University Affiliated Program**
Kansas University
2601 Gabriel Avenue
Parsons, KS 67357
620-421-6550
FAX 602-421-6550
http://www.parsons.lsi.ku.edu
e-mail: dmoody@ku.edu
David Lindeman, Director
Debbie Moody, Administrative Assistant

Mission is optimize the quality of life and extend the concept of independence, productivity, integration and inclusion of individuals with disabilities in all aspects of life. This can be accomplished by providing new options, meaningful choices, independence, self-reliance, dignity of risk, and the means to achieve enhanced personal productivity.

5173 **University of Kansas**
1450 Jayhawk Boulevard
Lawrence, KS 66045
785-864-2700
FAX 785-864-2817
TDY:785-864-2620
http://www.ku.edu
e-mail: disability@ku.edu
Mary Rasnack, Director
Melissa Manning, Associate Director
Robert Hemenway, CEO
Accommodates students with a learning disability by understanding the students ability.

5174 **Washburn University of Topeka**
University of Topeka
1700 SW College Avenue
Topeka, KS 66621
785-231-1010
FAX 785-234-3813
http://www.washburn.edu
Iris Gonzalez MD, President

Offers a variety of services to students with disabilities including note takers, extended testing time, counseling services, and special accommodations.

5175 **Wichita State University**
1845 Fairmount Street
Wichita, KS 67260
316-978-3490
800-362-2594
FAX 316-978-3016
http://www.wichita.edu
Grady Landrum, Special Services
Kevin Konda, Manager

A public four-year college with 11 special education students out of a total of 13,103.

Kentucky

5176 **Bellarmine College**
Disability Services
2001 Newburg Road
Louisville, KY 40205
502-452-8131
800-274-4723
http://www.bellarmine.edu
e-mail: rgarveynix@bellarmine.edu
Four-year college that provides services for the disabled.

5177 **Berea College**
2190 College Station
Berea, KY 40404
859-985-3000
FAX 859-985-3917
http://www.berea.edu
e-mail: webresponse@berea.edu
Larry Shinn, CEO

Offers a variety of services to students with disabilities including note takers, extended testing time, counseling services, and special accommodations.

5178 **Brescia University**
717 Frederica Street
Owensboro, KY 42301
270-686-4212
877-273-7242
FAX 270-686-4314
http://www.bresciu.edu
e-mail: chris.houk@brescia.edu
Chris J Houk, Dean of Enrollment
Dolores Kisler, Director Student Support
Judith Riney, Manager
Provides the following for students with learning disabilities: developmental courses (English, mathematics and study skills); individual tutoring for all areas; and academic and career counseling.

5179 **Clear Creek Baptist Bible College**
300 Clear Creek Road
Pineville, KY 40977
606-337-3196
FAX 606-337-2372
http://www.ccbbc.edu
e-mail: ccbbc@ccbbc.edu
Heather Dickenson, Executive Director

An independent four-year college with 11 special education students out of a total of 141.

5180 **Eastern Kentucky University**
PO Box 66
Richmond, KY 40476
859-622-1310
FAX 859-622-6794
TDY:859-622-2937
http://www.eku.edu
e-mail: teresa.belluscio@eku.edu
Teresa Belluscio, Director
Joan Glasser, President
Jim Larsgaard, Executive Director
Mission of project SUCCESS is to respond effectively and efficiently to the individual's educational needs.

5181 **Jefferson Technical College**
727 W Chestnut Street
Louisville, KY 40203
502-213-5333
FAX 502-213-4500
http://www.kcts.edu
Robert Silliman, Director
Anthony Newberry, President

Offers a variety of services to students with disabilities including note takers, extended testing time, counseling services, and special accommodations.

5182 **Kentucky State University**
103 Jackson Hall
Frankfort, KY 40601
502-597-6422
FAX 502-597-6407
http://www.kysu.edu
e-mail: bmorelock@gwmail.kysu.edu
Patricia Jones, Director
Mary Sias, President

Offers a variety of services to students with disabilities including note takers, extended testing time, counseling services, and special accommodations.

5183 **Lexington Community College**
103 Oswald Building Cooper Drive
Lexington, KY 40506
859-257-4872
866-774-4872
FAX 859-323-7136
TDY:849-257-6068
http://www.uky.edu
e-mail: lccinfo@lsv.uky.edu
Veronica Miller, Director
Regina Johnson, SS Associate
James Kerley, President
Comprehensive community college on campus of University of Kentucky.

5184 **Lindsey Wilson College**
210 Lindsey Wilson Street
Columbia, KY 42728
270-384-8100
800-264-0138
FAX 270-384-8050
http://www.lindsey.edu
e-mail: luddend@lindsey.edu
William Luckey, President
Lilian Roland, Learning Disabilities Coord.

Offers a variety of services to students with disabilities including notetakers, extended testing time, counseling services, and special accommodations.

5185 **Madisonville Community College: Universityof Kentucky**
2000 College Drive
Madisonville, KY 42431
270-821-2250
FAX 270-821-1555
http://www.madcc.kctcs.edu
e-mail: aimee.bullock@kctcs.edu
Aimee Bullock, Coordinator
Lydia Wilson, Office Assistant
Judith Rhoads, President
Offers a variety of services to students with disabilities including note takers, extended testing time, counseling services, and special accommodations.

5186 **Murray State University**
Lowry Center
Murray, KY 42071
270-762-2666
FAX 270-762-4339
http://www.murraystate.edu
e-mail: donna.harris@murraystate.edu
Cindy Clemson, Coordinator
Alexander King, President
Lana Jennings, Manager
Services and programs provided to the learning disabled.

5187 **Northern Kentucky University**
Nunn Drive
Newport, KY 41099
859-572-5100
800-637-9948
http://www.nku.edu
e-mail: admitnku@nku.edu
A Adams, Special Services
James Votruba, President

Offers a variety of services to students with disabilities including note takers, extended testing time, counseling services, and special accommodations.

5188 **Pikeville College**
147 Sycamore Street
Pikeville, KY 41501
606-218-5250
FAX 606-218-5269
http://www.pc.edu
e-mail: webmaster@pc.edu
Harold Smith, President

Offers a variety of services to students with disabilities including notetakers, extended testing time, counseling services, and special accommodations.

5189 **Thomas More College**
333 Thomas More Parkway
Crestview Hills, KY 41017
859-344-3300
FAX 606-344-3342
http://www.thomasmore.edu
e-mail: barb.davis@thomasmore.edu
Dale Meyers MD, Dean of Academic Affairs
Barbara Davis, Director Student Services
James Kellogg, Executive Director
An independent four-year college with 50 special education students out of a total of 1,272.

5190 University of Kentucky: Interdisciplinary Human Development Institute
University of Kentucky
126 Mineral Industries Building
Lexington, KY 40506
859-323-5908
FAX 859-323-1901
http://www.ihdi.uky.edu
e-mail: mafar101@uky.edu
Harold Klinert, Director
Jay Chaney, Staff Assistant
Rhonda Sewell, Manager
Mission is to promote independence, productivity, and integration of all people through numerous research, training and outreach activities.

5191 University of Louisville
Robbins Hall
Louisville, KY 40292
502-852-5442
FAX 502-852-0924
TDY:502-852-6938
http://www.louisville.edu
Cathy Patus, Director
James Ransey, President
Anne Weimer, Manager
A public four-year college with 60 learning disabled students out of a total of 22,000.

5192 Western Kentucky University
Student Disability Services
1 Big Red Way
Bowling Green, KY 42101
270-745-5004
FAX 270-745-6289
TDY:270-745-3030
http://www.wku.edu
e-mail: disabilityservices@wku.edu
Matt Davis, Coordinator for Student Disabili
Huda Melky, Director for Equal Opportunity

The goal of the program is to foster the participation of persons with disabilities.

Louisiana

5193 Human Development Center
Louisiana State University
1100 Florida Avenue
New Orleans, LA 70119
504-619-8721
FAX 504-942-8305
TDY:504-942-7801
http://www.hdc.lsuhsc.edu
e-mail: rcrow@hcdc.lsuhsc.edu
Robert Crow, Director
Cathy Dwyer, Administrative Manager

5194 Learning Disabilities Association of Louisiana
Northwestern State University
Teacher Education Center
Natchitoches, LA 71497
318-357-6011
FAX 318-357-3275
e-mail: duchardt@nsula.edu
Barbara Duchard MD, Associate Professor
Randy Webb, President

5195 Louisiana College
Program to Assist Student Success
1140 College Drive
Pineville, LA 71360
318-487-7629
FAX 318-487-7285
http://www.lacollege.edu
e-mail: pass@lacollege.edu
Betty Matthews, Director
Betty Morris, Assistant Director

This highly individualized, limited enrollment program provides support services and personal attention to students who may need special academic guidance, tutoring, and classroom assistance.

5196 Louisiana State University Agricultural and Mechanical College
110 Thomas Boyd Hall
Baton Rouge, LA 70803
225-578-1175
http://www.lsu.edu
Tina Schultz

A public four-year college with 88 special education students out of a total of 21,245.

5197 Louisiana State University: Alexandria
8100 Highway 71 S
Alexandria, LA 71302
318-445-3672
888-473-6417
FAX 318-473-6580
http://www.lsua.edu
Dee Slavant MD, Director Student Services
Donna Roberts, Administrative Assistant
Robert Cavanaugh, Manager
Offers a variety of services to students with disabilities including extended testing time, counseling services, and special accommodations.

5198 Louisiana State University: Eunice
2048 Johnson Highway
Eunice, LA 70535
337-457-7311
888-367-5783
FAX 337-550-1445
http://www.lsue.edu
Marvette Thomas, TRIO Director
William Nunez, President
David Pulling, Manager
A public two-year college with 31 special education students out of a total of 2,595.

5199 Loyola University New Orleans
6363 Saint Charles Avenue
New Orleans, LA 70118
504-865-2990
FAX 504-865-3543
http://www.loyno.edu
e-mail: ssmith@loyno.edu
Sarah Smith, Director
Kacey McNaloy, Counselor

Four year college that provides services to disabled students.

5200 McNeese State University
4205 Ryan Street
Lake Charles, LA 70609
337-475-5000
800-622-3352
http://www.mcneese.edu
Sena Theall, Director Special Project
Denise Leiato, Coordinator
Robert Hebert, President
Provides academic advising, arrangements for individual accommodations for disabilities, tutoring and computers and word processing equipment. All services are available to the students at no charge.

5201 Nicholls State University
PO Box 2050
Thibodaux, LA 70310
985-446-8111
FAX 985-448-4423
http://www.nich.edu
e-mail: karen.chauvin@nicholls.edu
Karen Chauvin, Interim Director
Ronda Zeringue, Administrative Assistant
Stephen Hulbert, Administrator
The Center provides assessments and remediation to students with Dyslexia and related learning disabilities. Programs are offered for college students as well as K-12 students.

5202 Southeastern Louisiana University
Slu 752
Hammond, LA 70402
985-549-2000
FAX 985-549-3640
http://www.selu.edu
e-mail: mhall@selu.edu
Michelle Hall MD, Interim Director
Randy Moffett, President

Four-year college that offers programs for students whom are disabled.

5203 Tulane University
6823 Saint Charles Avenue
New Orleans, LA 70118
504-865-5000
FAX 504-862-8148
TDY:504-862-8433
http://www.tulane.edu
e-mail: dtylicki@tulane.edu

David Tylicki, Director
Pam Ernst, Administrative Assistant
Scott Cowen, CEO

Four-year college that provides services to those students who are learning disabled.

5204 University of Louisiana at Lafayette: Services of Students with Disabilities
PO Box 41650
Lafayette, LA 70504
337-482-5739
FAX 337-482-0195
http://www.ull.edu

Srisharsha Ogoti, Office Assistant
Edward Pratt, Dean

The Mission of Services for Students with Disabilities is to provide extensive post secondary services for emotionally, physically and learning impaired students. Our goals are to facilitate the transition from high school to college, to assist students developing the necessary skills to succeed in college; and to provide counseling, including career counseling, and to assist in successful transition from college to employment.

5205 University of New Orleans
2000 Lakeshore Drive
New Orleans, LA 70148
504-280-6000
800-514-4275
http://www.uno.edu

Amy King, Coordinator
Timothy Ryan, Manager

A public four-year college with 45 special education students out of a total of 12,441.

Maine

5206 ALLTech
University of Southern Maine
60 Pineland Drive
New Gloucester, ME 04260
207-688-4573
http://www.alltech-tsi.org
e-mail: info@alltech-tsi.org

Deb Dimmick, Director
Michael Higgins, CEO

5207 Bates College
102 Lane Hall
Lewiston, ME 04240
207-786-6255
FAX 207-786-6219
http://www.bates.edu
e-mail: tgoundie@bates.edu

Tedd Goundie, Dean
Mary Gravel, Assistant to the Dean
Anita Farnum, Manager

An independent four-year college with 17 special education students out of a total of 1,501.

5208 Bowdoin College
5000 College Station
Brunswick, ME 04011
207-725-3000
FAX 207-725-3764
http://www.bowdoin.edu
e-mail: help3030@bowdoin.edu

Barry Mills, President

Offers a variety of services to students with disabilities including note takers, extended testing time, counseling services, and special accommodations.

5209 Center for Community Inclusion (CCI): Maine's University Center for Excellence
University of Maine
5717 Corbett Hall
Orono, ME 04469
207-581-1110
800-203-6957
FAX 207-581-1231
http://www.ume.maine.edu/cci
e-mail: ccimail@umit.maine.edu

Lucille Zeph, Director
Marge Zubik, Administrative Assistant
Robert Kennedy, President

CCI has four core functions: interdisciplinary education; community services, outreach education and technical assistance; research and evaluation; and dissemination.

5210 Eastern Maine Vocational-Technical Institute
354 Hogan Road
Bangor, ME 04401
207-974-4600
800-286-9357
http://www.emtc.org
e-mail: admissions@emtc.org

Phillip Pratt

Offers a variety of services to students with disabilities including notetakers, extended testing time, counseling services, and special accommodations.

5211 Kennebee Valley Technical College
92 Western Avenue
Fairfield, ME 04937
207-453-5000
http://www.kvtc.net
e-mail: jhood@kvtc.net

Pat Ross, Students Services
Julie Hood, Coordinator
Barbara Woodlee, President

A public two-year college with 13 special education students out of a total of 1,086.

5212 Mid-State College
411 W Northmoor Road
Peoria, IL 61614
309-692-4092
800-251-4299
http://www.midstatecollege.com
e-mail: info@midstatecollege.com

Richard Gross, Special Services
R Bunch, President

Offers a variety of services to students with disabilities including notetakers, extended testing time, counseling services, and special accommodations.

5213 Northern Maine Community College
33 Edgemont Drive
Presque Isle, ME 04769
207-768-2700
800-535-NMTC
FAX 207-768-2831
http://www.nmcc.edu
e-mail: lflag@nmcc.edu

Laura Flagg, Special Services coordinator
Timothy Crowley, Administrator

A public two-year college with 33 special education students out of a total of 817.

5214 Southern Maine Technical College
2 Fort Road
South Portland, ME 04106
207-741-5500
http://www.smtc.net

Mark Krogman, Disability Services Provider
William Berman, Manager

Southern Maine Technical College is committed to helping qualified students with disabilities achieve their educational goals. Upon request and verification of the disability, SMTC will provide service coordination and reasonable accommodations to remediate the competitive disadvantage that a disability can create in the educational setting.

5215 Unity College
Unity, ME 04988
207-948-3131
FAX 207-948-6277
http://www.unity.edu
e-mail: jhoran@unity.edu

James Horan, Special Services
David Glenn-Lewin, President

Offers a variety of services to students with disabilities including notetakers, extended testing time, counseling services, and special accommodations.

5216 University of Maine
Disability Support Services
Onward Building
Orono, ME 04469
207-581-2319
FAX 207-581-2969
http://www.umaine.edu
e-mail: ann.smith@umit.maine.edu

Ann Smith, Director
Sara Henry, Disability Counselor

The primary goal of the University of Maine Disability Support Services is to create educational access for students with disabilities at UMaine by providing a point of coordination, information and education for those students and the campus community.

5217 University of Maine: Fort Kent
Academic and Counseling Services
23 University Drive
Fort Kent, ME 04743
207-834-7500
888-879-8635
FAX 207-834-7503
TDY:207-834-7466
http://www.umfk.maine.edu

George Diaz, Director Counseling Svcs.
Garland Caron, Counselor
Richard Cost, President

Students with a documented disability, who need academic accommodations, are encouraged to meet with an Academic and Counseling Services representative to develop a plan for their accommodations.

5218 University of Maine: Machias
9 Obrien Avenue
Machias, ME 04654
207-255-1234
800-468-6866
http://www.umm.maine.edu
e-mail: admissions@acd.umm.maine.edu

Jean Schild, Coordinator
Cindy Huggins, President

Prepared to assist students with disabilities with reasonable accommodations to qualified individuals with disabilities upon request.

5219 University of New England: University Campus
Disability Services
11 Hills Beach Road
Biddeford, ME 04005
207-283-0171
800-477-4863
FAX 207-294-5931
http://www.une.edu
e-mail: schurch@une.edu

Susan Church, Coordinator
Sandra Featherman, Administrator

The Office for Students with Disabilities exists to ensure that the University fulfills the part of its mission that seeks to promote respect for individual differences and to ensure that no person who meets the academic and technical standards requisite for admisssion to, and continued enrollment at, the University is denied benefits or subjected to discrimination at UNE solely by reason of his or her disability.

5220 University of New England: Westbrook College Campus
716 Stevens Avenue
Portland, ME 04103
207-797-7261
FAX 207-282-6379
e-mail: Cehringhaus@mailbox.une.edu

Carolyn Ehringh MD, Director
Sandra Featherman, President

Offers academic accommodations, as mandated under federal and state law, through the Office for Students with Disabilities (free of charge). General academic support services, such as tutoring and study strategies instruction, are available through the Learning Assistance Center. (Note: The Individual Learning Program is offered only on the Biddeford Campus).

5221 University of Southern Maine: Office of Academic Support for Students with Disabilities
PO Box 9300
Portland, ME 04104
207-780-4141
800-800-4USM
FAX 207-780-4403
http://www.usm.maine.edu

Joyce Branaman, Coordinator
Allyson Dean, Administrator

OASSD affirms the commitment of the University of Southern Maine to provide equal access to higher education for qualified students with disabilities. All services are provided with a philosophical framework that stresses student independence and self-reliance.

Maryland

5222 Baltimore City Community College
2901 Liberty Heights Avenue
Baltimore, MD 21215
410-462-8300
888-203-1261
FAX 412-462-8556
TDY:410-333-5802
http://www.bccc.edu

Nicole Hoke-Wilson, Director
Michelle Reynold, Counselor
Richard I, President

Offers a variety of services to students with disabilities including notetakers, extended testing time, counseling services, and special accommodations.

5223 Charles County Community College
PO Box 910
La Plata, MD 20646
301-934-2251
800-933-9177
FAX 301-934-7838
TDY:301-934-1188
http://www.csmd.edu
e-mail: bonnien@charles.cc.md.us

Elaine Ryan, President
Steven Goldman, Vice President
Thomas Repenning, Executive Director

A public two-year college with 600+ students with disabilities out of a total of 6,055.

5224 Chelsea School
711 Pershing Drive
Silver Spring, MD 20910
301-585-1430
FAX 301-585-5865
http://www.chelseaschool.edu
e-mail: tocannor@chelseaschool.edu

Linda A Handy MD, Academic Head of School
Timothy Hall, Director
T Messina, Principal

Chelsea is a co-educational, residential or day school for bright, dyslexic students in grade K-12.

5225 Chesapeake College
Routes 50 & 213
Wye Mills, MD 21679
410-770-3511
FAX 410-827-9466
TDY:410-827-9164
http://www.chesapeake.edu
e-mail: mhickey__@chesapeake.edu

Stewart Bounds, President
Maurice Hicky, Vice President
Judith Stetson, Manager

Offers a variety of services to students with disabilities including notetakers, extended testing time, counseling services, and special accommodations.

5226 **College of Notre Dame of Maryland**
Disability Services
4701 N Charles Street
Baltimore, MD 21210
410-532-5379
FAX 410-532-5167
http://www.ndm.edu
e-mail: wdaisley@ndm.edu
Theresa Cannone, Marketing Manager
Winifred Daisley, Director

Disability Services attends to students' physical, emotional, and learning disabilities by ensuring that students with disabilities are afforded the accommodations that they need to help them succeed at the College of Notre Dame.

5227 **Columbia Union College**
7600 Flower Avenue
Takoma Park, MD 20912
301-891-4000
800-835-4212
FAX 301-891-4167
http://www.cuc.edu
e-mail: jmcfarla@cuc.edu
Betty Howard, Assistant Dean
Mickaela Davis, Office Assistant
Randel Wisbey, President
Offers a variety of services to students with disabilities including note takers, extended testing time, counseling services, and special accommodations.

5228 **Community College of Baltimore County**
800 S Rolling Road
Catonsville, MD 21228
410-869-1212
FAX 410-455-4504
http://www.ccbc.cc.md.us/campuses/cat/htm
Mark Lieberman, Counselor
Jill Hodge, Counselor
Andrew Jones, President
Offers a variety of services to students with disabilities including notetakers, extended testing time, counseling services, and special accommodations.

5229 **Frostburg State University**
101 Braddock Road
Frostburg, MD 21532
301-687-4000
FAX 301-687-7049
http://www.frostburg.edu
e-mail: fsuadmission@frostburg.edu
Catherine Gira, President

A public four-year college with 153 special education students out of a total of 4,472.

5230 **Hagerstown Junior College**
11400 Robinwood Drive
Hagerstown, MD 21742
301-790-2800
866-422-2468
FAX 301-791-9165
http://www.hagerstowncc.edu
e-mail: admission@hagerstowncc.edu
Guy Altieri, Administrator

A public two-year college with 22 special education students out of a total of 3,364.

5231 **Harford Community College**
401 Thomas Run Road
Bel Air, MD 21015
410-836-4241
FAX 410-836-4200
TDY:410-836-4402
http://www.harford.edu
e-mail: lpenisto@harford.edu
Lorraine Peniston, Coordinator
Cindy Conroy, Administrative Specialist
Jacki Walsh, Executive Director
An open enrollment two-year college, with reasonable accommodations provided for students with documented disabilities through disability support services. Students may also receive academic advising, personal and career counseling, and study skills instruction.

5232 **Hood College**
Disabilities Services Office
401 Rosemont Avenue
Frederick, MD 21701
301-663-3131
FAX 301-694-7653
http://www.hood.edu
e-mail: webmaster@hood.edu
Ronald Volpe, President

Four-year college that provides services to disabled students.

5233 **Howard Community College**
10901 Little Patuxent Parkway
Columbia, MD 21044
410-772-4800
FAX 410-772-4803
http://www.howardcc.edu
e-mail: jmarks@howardcc.edu
Janice Marks, Director
Mary Ellen Duncan, President

A public two-year college with 225 students with disabilities using services out of a total of 5,500.

5234 **Ivymount School**
11614 Seven Locks Road
Rockville, MD 20854
301-469-0223
FAX 301-469-0778
e-mail: lpender@ivymount.org
Janet Wintrol, Executive Director
Stephanie deSibour, Assistant Director

Independent day-school serving students, 3-21, with disabilities including developmental delays, communication deficits, learning disabilities, and autism.

5235 **James E Duckworth School**
11201 Evans Trail
Beltsville, MD 20705
301-572-0620
FAX 301-572-0628
http://www.pgcps.pg.k12.md.us/ duckw/
e-mail: jedworth@pgcps.org
Trinell Bowman, Principal

5236 **Johns Hopkins Institution**
3400 N Charles Hall
Baltimore, MD 21218
410-235-3435
FAX 410-614-7251
http://www.jhi.edu
Martha Rosemann, Associate Dean
William Brody, CEO

Once a student with disabilities has been admitted to The Johns Hopkins School of Public Health it is important that he/she submits disability documentation to the school's disability services coordinator. This applies to both new students as well as current/continuing students who are requesting accommodation for the first time.

5237 **McDaniel College, Student Academic Support Services (SASS)**
2 College Hill Station
Westminster, MD 21157
410-848-7000
800-638-5005
http://www.mcdaniel.edu
e-mail: sass@mcdaniel.edu
Carrie Waddell, Learning Specialist
Joan Coley, President

SASS provides reasonable accommodations and a range of services to meet the academic needs of students with learning disabilities or some type of documented learning problem.

5238 **Prince George's Community College**
301 Largo Road
Largo, MD 20774
301-336-6000
http://www.pgweb.pg.cc.md.us
e-mail: enrollmetnservices@pg.cc.md.us
Carrier Johnson, Special Services
Ronald Williams, President

Offers a variety of services to students with disabilities including note takers, extended testing time, counseling services, and special accommodations.

5239 Summit School

664 E Central Avenue
Edgewater, MD 21037
410-798-0005
FAX 410-798-0008
http://www.thesummitschool.org
Jane R Snider MD, Founding Director

A school for children with language-based reading difficulties, particularly in the area of decoding, with average to above average cognitive ability, who are ultimately planning to attend a college-prep high school with limited support.

5240 Towson University

8000 York Road
Towson, MD 21252
410-704-2000
800-225-5878
FAX 410-704-4247
TDY:4107044423
http://www.towson.edu
e-mail: swillemin@towson.edu
Susan Willemin, Interim Director
Schoen Oakes, Learning Disabilities Specialist
Robert Caret, CEO

With more than 18,000 students, Towson University is the second largest public university in Maryland. Founded in 1866, the University offers more than 100 bachelor's, master's and doctoral degree programs in the liberal arts and sciences, and applied professional fields. Approximately 1,000 students are registered with the Disability Support Services office on campus.

5241 University of Maryland: Baltimore County

1000 Hilltop Circle
Baltimore, MD 21250
410-455-1000
FAX 410-455-1028
http://www.umbc.edu
e-mail: chill@umbc.edu
Patty Wilson, Office Manager
Cynthia Hill, Director
Freeman Habowski, Administrator

The Office of Student Support Services provides services that are designed to improve the educational and personal development of disabled and returning students.

5242 University of Maryland: College Park

2111 Shoemaker Building
College Park, MD 20742
301-405-9969
FAX 301-314-9206
http://www.maryland.edu
e-mail: mh185@umail.umd.edu
William Scales MD, Director Disability Support
Peggy Hayestrip, LD Coordinator

The mission of the Disability Support Service is to ensure individuals with disabilities equal access to the University of Maryland College Park programs.

5243 University of Maryland: Eastern Shore

Blackbone Road
Princess Anne, MD 21853
410-651-6456
FAX 410-651-6322
http://www.umes.edu
e-mail: dshowellhighcherry@mail.umes.edu
Diann Showell MD, Director

Offers a variety of services to students with disabilities including note takers, extended testing time, counseling services, and special accommodations.

5244 Valley Academy

301 W Chesapeake Avenue
Towson, MD 21204
410-828-0620
FAX 410-828-0438
http://www.jemicyschool.org
e-mail: bshisrin@jemicyschool.org
Dan Blanch, Principal
Mark Westervelt, Assistant Principal

5245 West Nottingham Academy

1079 Firetower Road
Colora, MD 21917
410-658-5556
800-962-1744
FAX 410-658-9264
http://www.wna.org
e-mail: admissions@wna.org
J Kirk Russell III, Director Admissions
Tom Sorci, Director, Learning Center
John Watson, Principal

A college preparatory school dedicated to the intellectual, spiritual and social growth of each student. The academy equips students to become successful in all aspects of life through individual attention within a diverse community and a safe and caring environment.

5246 Wor-Wic Community College

32000 Campus Drive
Salisbury, MD 21804
410-334-2800
FAX 410-334-2952
http:// www.worwic.edu
e-mail: suzannea@worwic.edu
Suzanne Alexander, Counseling Director
Ray Hoy, President

A comprehensive two-year institution located on Maryland's eastern shore. The faculty and staff are dedicated to serving the unique needs of each student with a learning disability.

Massachusetts

5247 American International College: Supportive Learning Services Program

1000 State Street
Springfield, MA 01109
413-737-7000
800-242-3142
FAX 413-205-3908
http://www.aic.edu
e-mail: inquiry@www.aic.edu
Mary Saltus, Coordinator Supportive Learni
Anne Midura, Office Manager
Peter Miller, Manager

An independent four-year college with 95 special education students out of a total of 1,433. There is an additional fee for the special education program in addition to the regular tuition.

5248 Amherst College

PO Box 2206
Amherst, MA 01004
413-542-2325
FAX 413-542-2223
http://www.amherst.edu
e-mail: info@amherst.edu
Frances Tuleja, Director
Anthony Marx, President

Offers a variety of services to students with disabilities including note takers, extended testing time, counseling services, and special accommodations.

5249 Anna Maria College

50 Sunset Lane
Paxton, MA 01612
508-849-3300
800-344-4586
FAX 508-849-3319
http://www.annamaria.edu
Olivia Tarleton, Director
Judy Clockedile, Executive Director

An independent four-year college with 12 special education students out of a total of 691.

5250 Atlantic Union College

Center for Academic Success
PO Box 1000
S Lancaster, MA 01561
978-368-2416
FAX 978-368-2015
http://www.atlanticuc.edu
e-mail: info@atlanticuc.edu
Elizabeth Anderson, Center Academic Success Director

5251 Babson College
Disability Services
Hollister Hall Babson College
Babson Park, MA 02457
781-239-4075
800-488-3696
FAX 781-239-5567
TDY:781-239-4017
http://www.babson.edu\callssdeans
Erin Evans, Manager

An independent four-year business-based college with 110 undergraduate and graduate students with disabilities. Accommodations are individualized for students presenting documentation and may include notetaking assistance, extended time, separate location for testing, books-on-tape and other special accommodations. Adaptive equipment, academic advising, counseling services and teaching of organizational and time management skills, study skills and test taking strategies are offered.

5252 Bentley College
175 Forest Street
Waltham, MA 02452
781-891-2273
FAX 781-891-247
TDY:781-891-2280
http://www.bentley.edu
e-mail: jgorgone@bentley.edu
Brenda Hawks MD, Associate Director
Lansche Stalmon, Administrator
Joseph Morone, President
An independent four-year college with 13 special education students out of a total of 5181.

5253 Berkshire Center
18 Park Street
Lee, MA 01238
413-243-2576
877-566-9247
FAX 413-243-3351
http://www.collegeinternshipprogram.com
e-mail: gshaw@berkshirecenter.org
Mike McManmon, Executive Director
Gary Shaw, Program Director
Caroline Wheeler, Admissions Director
A post secondary college business school or vocational program for young adults 18-27 with learning differences. A co-ed population from four countries and all regions of the United States. Students have individual academic tutorials, and courses in money management and vocational counseling. Students live in apartments and learn life skills.

5254 Boston College
140 Commonwealth Avenue
Chestnut Hill, MA 02467
617-552-8000
800-294-0294
FAX 617-552-2097
http://www.bc.edu
e-mail: ugadmis@bc.edu
Kathleen Duggan MD, Assistant Director
William Leahy, CEO

An independent four-year college with 195 special education students out of a total of 14,230. There is an additional fee for the special education program in addition to the regular tuition.

5255 Boston University
Office of Disability Services
19 Deerfield Street
Boston, MA 02215
617-353-3658
FAX 617-353-9646
TDY:617-353-3658
http://www.bu.edu
e-mail: lwolf@bu.edu/disability
Lorraine Wolf, Clinical Director

Provides basic support services such as test taking accommodations, note taking assistance, etc. Provides comprehensive services that include learning strategies instruction for an additional fee. LDSS offers a six-week summer program, The Summer Transition Program, for high school graduates.

5256 Brandeis University
415 S Street
Waltham, MA 02453
781-736-4400
FAX 781-736-4466
http://www.brandeis.edu
e-mail: ddgratto@brandeis.edu
Laura Lyndon, Assist Dean/Student Disability
Jehuda Reinharz, CEO

An independent four-year college with 67 special education students out of a total of 2,901. Brandeis is committed to providing reasonable accommodation/s to individuals with appropriately documented physical, learning and psychological disabilities.

5257 Bridgewater State College
Bridgewater, MA 02325
508-531-1000
FAX 508-531-6107
http://www.bridgew.edu
Martha Jones, Dean Studies
Dr. Mohler-Faria, President

Offers a variety of programs and services to students with disabilities including pre-college workshop, notetakers, extended testing time, counseling services, adaptive computing, peer tutors, supplemental instruction and special accommodations.

5258 Bristol Community College
777 Elsbree Street
Fall River, MA 02720
508-678-2811
FAX 508-730-3297
http://www.bristol.mass.edu
Jack Sprager, President

Located in Southeastern New England, serves the residents of Bristol County and Rhode Island, in offering Associate of Art Degrees and Associate of Science Degrees in career and transfer programs, as well as certificates in other programs. Offers the QUEST Project which is an academic support program for learning disabled students as they begin their college education. Builds academic skills and confidence in the student's ability to do college work. Advises students on career choices.

5259 Cape Cod Community College
2240 Lyanough Road
West Barnstable, MA 02668
508-362-2131
877-846-3672
FAX 508-362-3988
http://www.capecod.mass.edu
e-mail: info@capecod.mass.edu
Richard Sommers MD, LD Specialist
Kathleen Schatzberg, President

A public two-year college with 165 special education students out of a total of 2,141. A full range of accommodations are available to students with disabilities.

5260 Clark University
950 Main Street
Worcester, MA 01610
508-793-7711
800-GO-CLARK
FAX 508-793-8821
http://www.clarku.edu
e-mail: admissions@clarku.edu
Sharon Klerk, Special Services Director
John Bassett, President

An independent four-year college with 84 special education students out of a total of 2151.

5261 Curry College
Program For Advancement of Learning
1071 Blue Hill Avenue
Milton, MA 02186
617-333-2250
800-669-0686
FAX 617-333-2018
TDY:617-333-2250
http://www.curry.edu
e-mail: spratt@curry.edu
Lisa Ijiri, Director
Susan Pratt, PAL Coordinator
Joan Manchester, Program Administrator

PAL is a program within Curry College, a co-educational, four-year liberal arts institution serving 2,000 students and located in the Boston suburb of Milton, Massachusetts. For over 25 years, PAL has both shaped and been shaped by Curry's distinctive philosophy of education. Serves college age students with specific learning disabilities.

5262 Dean College
99 Main Street
Franklin, MA 02038
508-541-1900
FAX 508-541-1918
http://www.dean.edu
Faith Nickolas, Executive Director

Committed to maintaining a caring and nurturing environment for its students.

5263 Dearborn Academy
School for Children
34 Winter Street
Arlington, MA 02474
781-641-5992
FAX 781-641-5997
http://www.spedschools.com
e-mail: twalton@sscinc.org
Tucker Walton, Associate Director
Milliy Foaugei, Administrative Assistant
Theodore Wilson, President

5264 Eagle Hill School
PO Box 116
Hardwick, MA 01037
413-477-6000
FAX 413-477-6837
http://www.ehs1.org
e-mail: admission@ehs1.org
Dana Harbert, Admission Director
Peter Donald, Manager

Since 1967 has offered premier services to the special needs community. This co-educational, college preparatory, boarding program is designed to meet academic and social needs of students diagnosed with learning disabilities (LD) and Attention Deficit Disorder (ADD). Offers a success-oriented atmosphere, and a consistently structured and socially supportive environment. The program serves students in grades 8-12.

5265 Eastern Nazarene College
Student Affairs Office
23 E Elm Avenue
Quincy, MA 02170
617-745-3000
800-883-6288
FAX 617-984-4901
http://www.enc.edu
e-mail: klitticj@enc.edu
Joyce Klittich, Director Academic Services
David Clung, President

Offers a variety of services to students with disabilities including note takers, extended testing time, counseling services, and special accommodations.

5266 Endicott College
376 Hale Street
Beverly, MA 01915
978-927-0585
800-325-1114
FAX 978-232-2600
http://www.endicott.edu
e-mail: bpierima@endicott.edu
Eloise Knowlton, Head of Disability Department
Barbara Pierimarchi, Administrative Assistant
Richard Wylie, President
An independent two-year college with 48 special education students out of a total of 793.

5267 Essex Agricultural and Technical Institute
562 Maple Street
Hathorne, MA 01937
978-762-4000
FAX 978-774-6530
http://www.agtech.org
e-mail: rraucci@agtech.org
Helen Hegaity, Administrator
Helen Keyes, Secretary to Superintendant

A public two-year college with 74 special education students out of a total of 533.

5268 Fitchburg State College
Disability Services
160 Pearl Street
Fitchburg, MA 01420
978-665-4020
FAX 978-665-3021
http://www.fsc.edu
e-mail: jperkins@fsc.edu
Julie Maky, Staff Assistant

5269 Framingham State College
100 State Street
Framingham, MA 01702
508-872-4701
http://www.framingham.edu
Gin Fiore, Administrator

Offers a variety of services to students with disabilities including note takers, extended testing time, counseling services, and special accommodations.

5270 Hampshire College
Learning Disabilities Support Services
893 W Street
Amherst, MA 01002
413-559-5458
FAX 413-559-5695
http://www.hampshire.edu
Joel Dansky, Associate Dean

Four year college that offers students with learning disabilities services and support.

5271 Harvard School of Public Health
677 Huntington Avenue
Boston, MA 02115
617-432-1135
FAX 617-432-2009
http://www/hsph.harvard.edu
e-mail: anmartin@hsph.harvard.edu
Jim Glover, Disability Coordinator
Anne Martin, Assistant
Marie McCormick MD, Director
An independent four-year college with 45 special education students out of a total of 6,621. Disabled students are encouraged to take advantage of opportunities available to help them achieve their educational goals.

5272 Institute for Community Inclusion (ICI)
UMass Boston
100 Morrissey Boulevard
Dorchester, MA 02125
617-287-4300
FAX 617-287-4352
http://www.communityinclusion.org
e-mail: ici@umb.edu
William Kiernan, Director
Rachael Webb, Administrative Assistant

ICI promotes the inclusion of people with disabilities in their communities through training, consultation, clinical and employment services and research.

5273 Landmark Elementary and Middle School Program
PO Box 227
Prides Crossing, MA 01965
978-236-3000
FAX 978-927-7268
http://www.landmarkoutreach.org
e-mail: admission@landmarkschool.org
Carolyn Orsini Nelson, Director Admission
Chris Murphy, Principal

Students entering grades 2-8, of average to superior intelligence, with a history of healthy emotional development and who've been diagnosed with a language-based learning disability are eligible for our programs. Ten-month academic and six-week summer programs include daily one-to-one tutorials.

5274 Landmark High School Program
PO Box 227
Prides Crossing, MA 01965
978-236-3000
FAX 978-927-7268
http://www.landmarkoutreach.org
e-mail: admission@landmarkschool.org

Carolyn Orsini Nelson, Admission Director
Chris Murphy, Principal

Students entering grades 9-12, of average to superior intelligence, with a history of healthy emotional development and who've been diagnosed with a language-based learning disability are eligible for our programs. Ten-month academic and six-week summer programs include daily one-to-one tutorials.

5275 **Landmark School Preparatory Program**

PO Box 227
Prides Crossing, MA 01965 978-236-3000
FAX 978-927-7268
http://www.landmarkoutreach.org
e-mail: admissions@landmarkschool.org

Robert Broudo, Headmaster
Carolyn Orsini Nelson, Admissions Director
Chris Murphy, Principal

Enrolling students in grades 9-12, Landmark Prep provides a full secondary school level curriculum for students with language-based learning disabilities. The program emphasizes organizational and study skills development in a traditional classroom setting and is designed for college bound boys and girls who have progressed to within one year of expected grade level performance.

5276 **Linden Hill School**

154 S Mountain Road
Northfield, MA 01360 413-498-2906
866-498-2906
FAX 413-498-2908
http://www.lindenhs.org
e-mail: office@lindenhs.org

Jim McDaniel, Headmaster/Executive Director
Vanessa Towne, Office Secretary
Gerald Shields, Principal

An ungraded boarding school for boys between the ages of 9-15 with dyslexia or specific learning/language differences as well as sensitive issues. Linden Hill also offers a formal freshman year program. The school's primary objective is to provide a comprehensive language training program in reading, spelling, and writing. The language program provides an alternative to the traditional approach by using the sight-recognition (whole word) method of learning.

5277 **Massachusetts Bay Community College**

50 Oakland Street
Wellesley, MA 02481 781-239-2545
FAX 781-239-1047
http://www.mbcc.mass.edu
e-mail: Josepho@mbcc.edu

Joseph O'Niel, LD Specialist
Carol Berote-Joseph, President

A public two-year college with 44 special education students out of a total of 4,684.

5278 **Massachusetts College of Liberal Arts**

375 Church Street
North Adams, MA 01247 413-662-5308
FAX 413-662-5319

Claire Smith, Coordinator Academic Support

Academic support services for students with disabilities.

5279 **Massasoit Community College**

1 Massasoit Boulevard
Brockton, MA 02302 508-588-9100
800-CAREERS
FAX 508-427-1250
TDY:508-427-1240
http://www.massasoit.mass.edu
e-mail: pjohnston@massasoit.mass.edu

Peter Johnston, Dean of Humanities
Richard Cronin, Marketing Director
Charles Wall, President

A public two-year college with 164 special education students out of a total of 6,423.

5280 **Middlesex Community College**

591 Springs Road
Bedford, MA 01730 781-280-3200
800-818-3434
FAX 732-906-2506

Carole Cowan, President

A public two-year college with 298 special education students out of a total of 4,028.

5281 **Mount Ida College**

777 Dedham Street
Newton, MA 02459 617-928-4500
FAX 617-928-4760
http://www.mountida.edu
e-mail: admissions@mountida.edu

Jill Mehler, Learning Opportunities Prog. Dir
Carol Matteson, President

Designed and developed to provide additional support for students with learning disabilities. Services include individual tutoring by professional learning specialists, reduced course load, specialized accommodations and community functions.

5282 **Mount Wachusett Community College**

444 Green Street
Gardner, MA 01440 978-632-6600
FAX 978-630-9559
http://www.mwce.mass.edu
e-mail: dasquino@mwcc.nass.edu

Daniel Asquino, President
Edward Terceiro, Vice President

A public two-year college with 177 special education students out of a total of 2,202.

5283 **Newbury College**

129 Fisher Avenue
Brookline, MA 02445 617-277-3855
FAX 617-232-5139
http://www.newbury.edu/
e-mail: brookline@newbury.edu

Sara d'Anjou, Academic Services
David Ellis, President

An independent four-year college with 35 self identified special education students out of a total of 800.

5284 **North Shore Community College**

1 Ferncroft Road
Danvers, MA 01923 978-762-4000
FAX 978-762-4038
TDY:781-477-2136
http://www.northshore.edu
e-mail: hheineman@northshore.edu

Wayne Burton, President

A public two-year college with 280 special education students out of a total of 3,301.

5285 **Northeastern University**

Disability Resource Center
20 Dodge Hall
Boston, MA 02115 617-373-2675
FAX 617-373-7800
TDY:617-373-2730
http://www.neu.edu
e-mail: drcinfo@neu.edu

G Kukiela Bork, Dean/Director
Laura havans, Secretary

Offers a variety of services to students with disabilities including note takers, extended testing time, counseling services, and special accommodations.

5286 **Pine Manor College**

400 Heath Street
Chestnut Hill, MA 02467 617-731-7639
800-762-1357
FAX 617-731-7199
http://www.pmc.edu
e-mail: admissions@pmc.edu

Bill Nichols, Dean of Admissions
Mary Walsh, Center Director
Gloria Numerowicz, President
For students with learning disabilities, Pine Manor College offers the Learning Resource Center. The LRC supports and challenges students to realize their maximum academic potential in the way that best suits their individual learning styles.

5287 Regis College: Massachusetts
235 Wellesley Street
Weston, MA 02493
781-768-7000
866-438-7344
FAX 781-768-8339
http://www.regiscollege.edu
e-mail: admission@regiscollege.edu
Emily Keily, Admissions Director
Mary England, President

Offers a variety of services to students with disabilities including notetakers, extended testing time, counseling services, and special accommodations.

5288 Riverview School
551 Route 6A
East Sandwich, MA 02537
508-888-0489
FAX 508-888-1315
http://www.riverviewschool.org
e-mail: admissions@riverviewschool.org
Jeanne Pachero, Director Admissions/Placement
Maureen Brenner, Principal

An independent, residential school of international reputation and service enrolling 183 male and female students in its secondary and post-secondary programs. Students share a common history of lifelong difficulty with academic achievement and the development of friendships. On measures of intellectual ability, most students score within the 70-100 range and have a primary diagnosis of learning disability and/or complex language or learning disorder.

5289 Salem State College
325 Lafayette Street
Salem, MA 01970
978-542-6000
FAX 978-542-6753
http://www.salem.mass.edu
e-mail: admissions@salemstate.edu
Eileen Berger, Director
Nancy Harrington, President

Four year college offering a learning disabilities program for students.

5290 Simmons College
300 Fenway
Boston, MA 02115
617-521-2000
FAX 617-521-3190
http://www.simmons.edu
e-mail: daniel.cheever@simmons.edu
Daniel Cheever Jr., President
Kathleen Rogers, Vice President

An independent four-year college with 44 special education students out of a total of 1,399.

5291 Smith College
College Hall 7
Northampton, MA 01063
413-584-2700
FAX 413-585-4498
TDY:413-585-2072
http://www.smith.edu
e-mail: admission@smith.edu
Laura Rausher, Disability Services Director
Anna Megill, Administrator
Carol Christ, President
An independent four-year college with 42 special education students out of a total of 2,613.

5292 Springfield College
263 Alden Street
Springfield, MA 01109
413-788-2451
FAX 413-748-3937
http://www.spfldcol.edu
e-mail: ddickens@spfldcol.edu
Deb Dickins, Director
Lynn Vlinn, Administrative Assistant
Maureen Burke, Executive Director
Four-year college that offers student support to students with learning disabilities.

5293 Springfield Technical Community College
1 Armory Square
Springfield, MA 01105
413-781-7822
FAX 413-733-8403
http://www.stcc.edu
e-mail: deena.shriver@stcc.edu
Deena Shriver, Special Services
Liza Herbert, Operator

Offers a variety of services to students with disabilities including note takers, extended testing time, counseling services, and special accommodations.

5294 Stonehill College
320 Washington Street
North Easton, MA 02357
508-565-1000
FAX 508-565-1500
TDY:508-565-1425
http://www.stonehill.edu
e-mail: academicservices@stonehill.edu
Richard Grant, Assistant Dean Academic Services
Mark Cregan, President

A small liberal arts-based college of 2000 students set in a quiet suburb of Boston sponsored by the Holy Cross Fathers. This Catholic college offers programs in the liberal arts, business, and the sciences and is committed to providing reasonable accommodations to students with disabilities.

5295 Suffolk University
8 Ashburton Place
Boston, MA 02108
617-573-8000
FAX 617-742-2582
TDY:617-557-4875
http://www.suffolk.edu
e-mail: jatkinso@admin.suffolk.edu
Nancy Stoll, Dean Students
Beth Tiomgson, Administrator
David Sargent, President
Offers a variety of services to students with disabilities including note takers, extended testing time, counseling services, special accommodations, assistive technology, and tutorial assistance.

5296 Threshold Program at Lesley University
Lesley University
29 Everett Street
Cambridge, MA 02138
617-868-9600
800-999-1959
FAX 617-349-8189
http://www.lesley.edu
e-mail: jwilbur@lesley.edu
James Wilbur, Director
Margaret Kenna, President

The Threshold Program is a comprehensive, nondegree campus-based program at Lesley University for highly motivated young adults with diverse learning disabilities and other special needs.

5297 Tufts University
419 Boston Avenue
Medford, MA 02155
781-395-8487
FAX 617-627-3971
http://www.tufts.edu
e-mail: studentservices@ase.tufts.edu
Carmen Lowe, Director ARC
Sandra Baer, Coordinator

Offers a variety of services to students with disabilities including extended testing time, note takers, counseling services, and special accommodations, deemed necessary based on current documentation.

5298 **University of Massachusetts: Amherst**
Disabilities Services
231 Whitmore Administration Bldg
Amherst, MA 01003
413-545-0892
FAX 413-577-0691
TDY:413-545-0892
http://www.umass.edu
e-mail: zygmont@acad.umass.edu/ ds@educ.umass.edu
Madeline Peters, Director

A public four-year college with 192 special education students out of a total of 17,207.

5299 **University of Massachusetts: Boston**
100 Morrissey Boulevard
Dorchester, MA 02125
617-287-7430
FAX 617-287-7436
http://www.umb.edu
e-mail: rosscenter.umb.edu
Sheila Petruccelli, Director

A public four-year college with 151 special education students out of a total of 8,598. Committed to the goal of providing equal access to its education programs, so that its students may achieve their academic potential.

5300 **University of Massachusetts: Lowell**
Office of Disability Services
71 Wilder Street
Lowell, MA 01854
978-934-4338
FAX 508-934-3011
http://www.uml.edu
e-mail: noelc@uml.edu
Noel PhD, Director Disabilities
Chandrika , Assistant Director
Kerry Donohoe, Disabilities Coordinator
Office of Disability Services has responsibility for assuring reasonable accommodations, program access and support to qualified physically and learning disabled students and students with psychiatric disabilities.

5301 **Wellesley College**
106 Central Street
Wellesley, MA 02481
781-283-1000
FAX 781-283-3644
Diana Walsh, President

An independent four-year college with 41 special education students out of a total of 2,325.

5302 **Wheaton College**
Norton, MA 02766
508-285-7722
FAX 508-286-5621
TDY:508-286-5682
http://www.wheatoncollege.edu
e-mail: mbleadsoe@wheaton,edu
Martha Bledsoe, Asst Dean Studies/Disability Svc
Ronald Crutcher, President

An independent four-year college with 200 students with learning disabilities out of a total of 1450.

Michigan

5303 **Adrian College**
Academic Services Program
110 S Madison Street
Adrian, MI 49221
517-265-5161
800-877-2246
FAX 517-264-3181
TDY:517-265-5161
http://www.adrian.edu
e-mail: ctapp@adrian.edu
Carol Tapp, Learning Specialist
Mike Ballard, Campus Safety

A private, co-educational liberal arts and sciences undergraduate college. The college strives to enroll a student body that reflects the wealth and diversity of our society and is committed to providing appropriate services to all students. There are 35 academic majors and 9 preprofessional programs.

5304 **Alma College**
614 W Superior Street
Alma, MI 48801
989-463-7111
FAX 989-463-7353
http://www.alma.edu
e-mail: perkins@alma.edu
Mindy Sargent, Interim Director
Saundra Tracy, President

An independent four-year college with 5 special education students out of a total of 1,222.

5305 **Andrews University**
Old US 31
Berrien Springs, MI 49104
269-471-7771
800-253-2874
FAX 269-471-6900
http://www.andrews.edu
Marion Swanpoel, Director
Niels-Erik Andreason, President

Offers a variety of services to students with disabilities including notetakers, extended testing time, counseling services, and special accommodations.

5306 **Aquinas College**
Aquinas College
1607 Robinson Road SE
Grand Rapids, MI 49506
616-632-8900
800-678-9593
FAX 616-732-4431
http://www.aquinas.edu
e-mail: admissions@aquinas.edu
Tom Mikowski, Admissions Director
Harry Konoke, President

An independent four-year college with 32 special education students out of a total of 2,141.

5307 **Augmentative Communication Technology**
Central Michigan University
441 Moore Hall
Mount Pleasant, MI 48859
989-774-4000
FAX 989-774-1727
http://www.chp.cmich.edu/aac
Anne Ratcliffe MD, Director
Michael Rao, CEO

Maintains a clinic for assessment and consultation for individuals needing special communication technology and/or augmentative communication strategies. Provides personnel preparation and in-servicing for professionals in practice.

5308 **Bay De Noc Community College**
2001 N Lincoln Road
Escanaba, MI 49829
906-786-5802
800-221-2001
FAX 906-789-6912
http://www.baycollege.edu
e-mail: paavilam@baycollege.edu
Marlene Paavilainen, Director Student Success
Michael Alkins, President

A community college with 30 learning disabled students out of 2,500.

5309 **Calvin College**
Services to Students with Disabilities
3201 Burton Street SE
Grand Rapids, MI 49546
616-526-6077
FAX 616-526-7066
http://www.calvin.edu
e-mail: kbroekst@calvin.edu
Karen Broekstra, Coordinator

5310 **Central Michigan University**
120 Park Library
Mount Pleasant, MI 48859
989-774-3686
FAX 989-774-1326
http://www.cmich.edu/student-disability
e-mail: sds@cmich.edu

Susie Rood, Director Student Services
Stan Shingles, Executive Director

Public four-year university offering students a choice of 24 degrees. Academic accommodations are available for students with documented learning disabilities.

5311 Charles Stewart Mott Community College
1401 E Court Street
Flint, MI 48503
810-762-0408
FAX 810-762-0159
http://www.mcc.edu
Denise Hooks, Manager

Offers a variety of services to students with disabilities including note takers, extended testing time, counseling services, and special accommodations.

5312 College of Art and Design: Center for Creative Studies
201 E Kirby Street
Detroit, MI 48202
313-872-3118
FAX 313-872-2739
Beth Walker, Manager

Offers a variety of services to students with disabilities including notetakers, extended testing time, counseling services, and special accommodations.

5313 Delta College
Office of Disability Services
1961 Delta Road
University Center, MI 48710
989-686-9000
FAX 989-667-2228
http://www.delta.edu
e-mail: michaelcooper2@delta.edu
Michael Cooper, Special Needs Director
Peter Boyse, President

Offers a variety of services to students with disabilities including note takers, extended testing time, counseling services, and special accommodations.

5314 Detroit College of Business
3488 N Jennings Road
Flint, MI 48504
810-789-2200
FAX 810-789-2266
http://www.dcb.edu
Fran Jarvis, Director

Offers a variety of services to students with disabilities including notetakers, extended testing time, counseling services, and special accommodations.

5315 Detroit College of Business: Warren Campus
27650 Dequindre Road
Warren, MI 48092
586-558-8700
http://www.dcb.edu
Mary Cross, Associate Dean
George Kovtun, Executive VP

Offers a variety of services to students with disabilities including note takers, extended testing time, counseling services, and special accommodations.

5316 Developmental Disabilities Institute: Wayne State University
4809 Woodward Avenue
Detroit, MI 48201
313-577-2654
FAX 313-577-3770
http://www.wayne.edu.DDI
e-mail: B_Le_Roy@wayne.edu
Barbara LeRoy, Director

Contributes to the development of inclusive communities and quality of life for people with disabilities and their families through a culturally sensitive statewide program of interdisciplinary education, community support and services, research and dissemination of information.

5317 Eastern Michigan University
Access Services Office
203 King Hall
Ypsilanti, MI 48197
734-487-2470
FAX 734-487-5784
TDY:734-487-2470
http://www.emich.edu
e-mail: danderson1@emich.edu
Don Anderson, Director

Four year college that offers students with learning disabilities support and services.

5318 Eton Academy
Eton Academy
1755 E Melton Road
Birmingham, MI 48009
248-642-1150
FAX 248-642-3670
http://www.etonacademy.org
e-mail: webmaster@etonacademy.org
Pete Pullen, Principal
Sharon Morey, Admissions Director

A special purpose school dedicated to educating 1st through 12th grade students of average and above average academic potential who are experiencing specific learning disabilities.

5319 Ferris State University
420 Oak Street
Big Rapids, MI 49307
231-591-5819
FAX 231-591-3686
http://www.ferris.edu
e-mail: eunicemerwin@ferris.edu
Eunice Merwin, Director
Thomas Crandell, Manager

Committed to a policy of equal opportunity for qualified students. Mission is to serve and advocate students with disabilities.

5320 Finlandia University
Program for Students with Learning Disabilities
601 Quincy Street
Hancock, MI 49930
906-487-7258
FAX 906-487-7567
http://www.suomi.edu
Carol Bates, Associate Professor/Director

5321 Glen Oaks Community College
Special Services Office
62249 Shimmel Road
Centreville, MI 49032
269-467-9945
888-994-7818
FAX 269-467-9068
http://www.glenoaks.edu
e-mail: lraven@glenoaks.edu
Lyle Raven, Special Populations Counselor
Barbara Clouse, Secretary
Betsy Morgan, Executive Director
A public two-year college with 50 special education students out of a total of 1,416.

5322 Henry Ford Community College
5101 Evergreen Road
Dearborn, MI 48128
313-845-9615
800-585-4322
FAX 313-845-9700
http://www.hfcc.edu
e-mail: hfcc@hfcc.edu
Theodore Jr, Program Manager
Bunny Monroe, Human Resource Secretary
Sally Barnett, President
A public two-year college with 36 special education students out of a total of 15,514.

5323 Hope College
Hope College
35 E 12th Street
Holland, MI 49423
616-395-7000
FAX 616-395-7118
http://www.hope.edu

Jacqueline Heisler, Director
James Bultman, President

An independent four-year liberal arts college recognized for its strong academics (it is a Phi Beta Kappa School), excellent facilities and supportive Christian dimension. Students with learning disabilities are admitted according to regular admission criteria. Admitted students must then determine whether Hope's support services are adequate for their needs.

5324 Jackson Community College

2111 Emmons Road
Jackson, MI 49201
517-787-0800
FAX 517-796-8632
http://www.jccmi.edu

Bethany Rogers, Coordinator
Daniel Phelan, President

Offers a variety of services to students with disabilities including notetakers, extended testing time, counseling services, and special accommodations.

5325 Kalamazoo College

1200 Academy Street
Kalamazoo, MI 49006
269-337-7000
800-253-3602
FAX 269-337-7390
http://www.kzoo.edu
e-mail: admission@kzoo.edu

Vaughn Maatman, Dean Students
Bernard Palchick, Acting President
Eileen Wilson-Oyelara, President

A selective, independent and undergraduate liberal arts college. The unique curricular plan weaves career development internships, study abroad programs and senior independent research projects with traditional liberal arts on campus programs.

5326 Kellogg Community College

Support Services
450 N Avenue
Battle Creek, MI 49017
269-965-3931
http://www.kellogg.edu
e-mail: webmaster@kellogg.cc.mi.us

Janice McNearney, Support Services
Edward Haring, President

Offers a variety of services to students with disabilities including notetakers, extended testing time, counseling services, and special accommodations.

5327 Kendall College of Art and Design

17 Fountain Street NW
Grand Rapids, MI 49503
616-451-2787
FAX 616-451-9867
http://www.kcad.edu
e-mail: kathy_jordan@ferris.edu

Kathy Jordan, Counselor
Barbara Boldman, Executive Assistant
Oliver Evans, President

An independent four-year college with 11 special education students out of a total of 657.

5328 Lake Michigan College

Lake Michigan College
2755 E Napier Avenue
Benton Harbor, MI 49022
269-927-3571
800-252-1562
FAX 269-927-6874
TDY:269-927-8100
http://www.lakemichigancollege.edu

Zomar Peter, Records Department Manager
Richard Pappas, President

A two-year community college offering students vocational/technical programs in business, health science, technology and the first two years of college credit toward transfer in a baccalaureate program. Tutors, readers, note takers and other support services are available to eligible disabled students.

5329 Lansing Community College

PO Box 40010
Lansing, MI 48901
517-483-9310
FAX 517-483-1170
TDY:517-483-1207
http://www.lcc.edu
e-mail: eadvising@lcc.edu

Pam Davis, Disability Specialist
Daniel Snider, Student Staff

Offers a variety of services to students with disabilities including tutoring, extended testing time, counseling services, special services such as priority registration and classroom accommodations.

5330 Madonna University

36600 Schoolcraft Road
Livonia, MI 48150
734-432-5300
FAX 734-432-5393
http://www.madonna.edu
e-mail: dstokes@madonna.edu

Michael Meldrum, Director
Jamie Dewitt, Office Manager
Rosemarie Kujawa, President

Four-year college that offers services to disabled students.

5331 Michigan State University

B105 W Fee Hall
East Lansing, MI 48824
517-353-3211
FAX 517-355-6473
http://www.msu.edu
e-mail: jad.megen@msu.edu

Ralph Do, President

Offers a variety of services to students with disabilities including note takers, extended testing time, counseling services, and special accommodations.

5332 Michigan Technological University

1400 Townsend Drive
Houghton, MI 49931
906-487-1185
FAX 906-487-3060
http://www.mtu.edu
e-mail: gbmelton@mtu.edu

Gloria Melton, Dean of Students
Jeanne Meyers, Office Assistant
Glen Mroz, President

A public undergraduate and graduate university with programs in engineering, sciences, business, technology, forestry, social sciences, and humanities. In 2005/06, there were requests for services from 70 individuals with physical or learning disabilities. Services include extended testing time, books on tape, and counseling. Total student enrollment 6,510.

5333 Mid-Michigan Community College

1375 S Clare Avenue
Harrison, MI 48625
989-386-6600
FAX 989-386-2411
http://www.midmich.cc.mi.us
e-mail: mmiller@midmich.edu

Sandy Clark, Counselor Special Populations
Ron Verch, President

Tutoring, note taking, readers, writers, interpreters, text-on-tape, counseling, advising and career exploration available. Support services funded under the Carl D Perkins Vocational and Applied Technology Education Act for eligible students enrolled in vocational technical programs. Services for all other programs provided through college resources. Writing center and math lab available to students. Liaison with community services.

5334 Monroe County Community College

1555 S Raisinville Road
Monroe, MI 48161
734-242-7300
FAX 734-242-9711
http://www.monroeccc.edu
e-mail: criedel@monroeccc.edu

Cindy Riedel, Special Services
David Nixon, President

Offers a variety of services to students with disabilities including notetakers, extended testing time, counseling services, and special accommodations.

5335 Montcalm Community College
2800 College Drive
Sidney, MI 48885
989-328-2111
FAX 517-328-2950
http://www.montcalm.edu

Donald Burns, President
Jim Lantz, Vice President

Offers a variety of services to students with disabilities including note takers, extended testing time, counseling services, and special accommodations.

5336 Northern Michigan University
1401 Presque Isle Avenue
Marquette, MI 49855
906-227-1000
FAX 906-227-1714
TDY:906-227-1543
http://www.nmu.edu/disserve
e-mail: disserve@nmu.edu

Lynn Walden, Coordinator
Linda Row, Office Assistant
Leslie Wong, President
Disability services provides assistance for students who are qualified under the Americans with Disabilities Act to receive accommodations.

5337 Northwestern Michigan College
Instructional Support Center
1701 E Front Street
Traverse City, MI 49686
231-995-1000
FAX 231-995-1138
TDY:231-995-1929
http://www.nmc.edu/tss
e-mail: deverett@mnc.edu

Denny Everett, Disability Specialist
Michelle Poertner, Tutoring Program Manager
Tim Nelson, President
Offers a wide range of services for students that have disabilities and need accommodations in order to achieve their academic goals.

5338 Northwood University
4000 Whiting Drive
Midland, MI 48640
989-837-4277
FAX 989-837-4111
http://www.northwood.edu

Michael Sullivan, Counselor
Linda Kastelic, Manager

Four-year college that offers services to disabled students.

5339 Oakland Community College: Orchard Ridge Campus
27055 Orchard Lake Road
Farmington Hills, MI 48334
248-522-3400
FAX 248-471-7767
http://www.occ.cc.mi.us

Lawrence Gage MD, Learning Program
Jackie Shadko, President

Offers comprehensive services to students with learning disabilities including note takers, extended testing time, counseling services, special accommodations and advocacy support.

5340 Oakland University
2200 N Squirrel Road
Rochester Hills, MI 48309
248-370-2100
800-OAK-UNIV
FAX 218-370-4989
TDY:248-370-3268
http://www.oakland.edu

Gary Russi, President
Sheila Carpenter, Office Assistant

Offers a variety of services to students with disabilities including notetakers, extended testing time, priority registration, assistance with sign language interpreter services, assistive technology, and assistance with general needs and concerns.

5341 Office of Services for Students with Disabilities
University of Michigan
G-664 S Haven Hall 505 State Street
Ann Arbor, MI 48109
734-647-6000
FAX 734-936-3947
TDY:734-763-3000
http://www.umich.edu/~sswd
e-mail: sgoodin@umich.edu

Sam Goodin, Director
Stuart Segal, Asst Dir/Coordinator LD Svcs
Jerry May, Vice President
Offers selected student services, free of charge, which are not provided by other University offices or outside organizations. Assists students in negotiating disability-related barriers to the pursuit of their education. Strives to improve access to University programs, activities and facilities for students with disabilities. Promotes increased awareness of disability issues on campus.

5342 Saginaw Valley State University
7400 Bay Road
University Center, MI 48710
989-964-4000
800-968-9500
FAX 989-964-7838

5343 St. Clair County Community College
PO Box 5015
Port Huron, MI 48061
810-984-3881
FAX 810-984-4730
http://www.sc4.cc

Nancy Pecorilli, Counselor
Gerri Barber, Learning Center Coordinator
Rose Bellanca, President
The learning center's supportive services are provided free of charge. These services include counseling, outreach and referrals, handicapped services, tutoring and study skills assistance, share information and financial aid assistance.

5344 University of Michigan: Dearborn
2157 University Center
Dearborn, MI 48128
313-593-5430
FAX 313-593-3263
http://www.umd.michigan.edu
e-mail: counseling@umd.umesh.edu

Mary Ann Zawada MD, Counseling Director
Dennis Underwood, Coordinator

A public four-year college with 300 special education students out of a total of 8,000.

5345 University of Michigan: Flint
Student Development Center
264 University Center
Flint, MI 48502
810-762-3456
FAX 810-762-3498
TDY:810-766-6727
http://www.flint.umich.edu
e-mail: papolla@umflint.edu

Paola Pollander, Accessibility Coordinator
Virginia July, Office Manager

Provides support services and auxiliary aids for students with a variety of disabilities.

5346 Washtenaw Community College
PO Box D-1
Ann Arbor, MI 48106
734-761-6721
http://www.wccnet.edu

Francie Helm Mo MD, Special Services
Dennis Rice, Manager

A public two-year college with 78 special education students out of a total of 10,765.

5347 Western Michigan University
Western Michigan University
W Michigan Avenue
Kalamazoo, MI 49008
269-387-3248
FAX 269-387-0633
http://www.dsrs.umich.edu

Beth Hartigh, LD Director
Daniel Litynski, President

A public four-year college with 79 special education students out of a total of 20,951.

Minnesota

5348 Alexandria Technical College
1601 Jefferson Street
Alexandria, MN 56308
320-762-4500
888-234-1222
FAX 320-762-4634
TDY:320-762-4623
http://www.alextech.edu
e-mail: marya@alextech.edu
Renee Larson, Counselor
Mary Ackerman, Support Services Coordinator
Kevin Kopischke, President
Offers a variety of services to students with disabilities including note takers, extended testing time, counseling services, and special accommodations.

5349 Anoka-Ramsey Community College
MNSCU
11200 Mississippi Boulevard NW
Coon Rapids, MN 55433
763-427-2600
FAX 763-422-3341
TDY:763-576-5949
http://www.anokaramsey.edu
e-mail: scott.bay@anokaramsey.edu
Scott Bay, Disabilities Director
Patrick Johns, Administrator

A public two-year college with 55 special education students out of a total of 6,900.

5350 Augsburg College
Center for Learning and Adaptive Student Services
2211 Riverside Avenue
Minneapolis, MN 55454
612-330-1648
FAX 612-330-1137
TDY:612-330-1749
http://www.augsburg.edu
e-mail: doljanac@augsburg.edu
Robert Doljanac, Director
Karina Jones, Disability Specialist
Anne Lynd, Disability Specialist
The Center for Learning and Adaptive Student Services coordinates academics accommodations and services for students with learning, attentional and psychiatric disabilities.

5351 Bemidji State University
12 Sanford Hall
Bemidji, MN 56601
218-755-2073
FAX 218-755-3788
Ann Austad, Coordinator
Dan Gartell, Executive Director

Offers a variety of services to students with disabilities including note takers, extended testing time, counseling services, and special accommodations.

5352 Bethel College: Minnesota
Disability Services Department
3900 Bethel Drive
Saint Paul, MN 55112
651-635-8759
800-255-8706
FAX 651-635-8695
Lucie Johnson, LD Program Director
Kathleen , Director

An independent Christian four-year college with LD Program serving 30 students out of a total of 1,800.

5353 Calvin Academy and Special Education Day School
Calvin Academy and Special Education Day School
2574 Highway 10 NE
Mounds View, MN 55112
763-717-0609
FAX 763-786-9535
http://www.calvinacademy.com/
e-mail: info@CalvinAcademy.com
Stafford Calvin, Founder
Susan Johnson, Headmaster

5354 Century College
3300 Century Avenue N
White Bear Lake, MN 55110
651-779-3300
http://www.century.cc.mn.us
Vicki Johnson, Coordinator Disabled Center
Willie Nesbit, Dean Students
Larry Litecky, Administrator
The disabilities access center provided by the college is a liaison service for students with disabilities to provide access to educational and student programs at the college.

5355 College of Associated Arts
344 Summit Avenue
Saint Paul, MN 55102
651-224-3416
FAX 612-224-8854
Barbara Davis, Associate Professor
Joe Culligan, President

Offers a variety of services to students with disabilities including note takers, extended testing time, counseling services, and special accommodations.

5356 College of Saint Scholastica
1200 Kenwood Avenue
Duluth, MN 55811
218-723-6000
FAX 218-723-6482
http://www.css.edu
e-mail: njewcomb@css.edu
Jay Newcomb, Director
Larry Goodwin, President

Offers a variety of services to students with disabilities including note takers, extended testing time, counseling services, and special accommodations.

5357 College of St. Catherine: Minneapolis
Learning Disabilities Department
2004 Randolph Avenue
Saint Paul, MN 55105
651-690-6000
800-945-4599
FAX 651-690-6064
TDY:651-690-8145
http://www.stkate.edu
e-mail: tgockenbach@stkate.edu
Teri Gockenbach, LD Specialist
Annette Caupenter, Disability Specialist
Andrea Lee, President
Services for students with disabilities are coordinated through the learning Center. There is a support group for students with disabilities that meets bimonthly. Other services include testing accommodations, note taking, computers, and reading course materials.

5358 College of St. Catherine: St. Paul Campus
O'Neill Learning Center
2004 Randolph Avenue
Saint Paul, MN 55105
651-224-5079
800-945-4599
http://www.stkate.edu
Elaine McDonough, Assistant Director
Vera Mandel, Director

Academic support services for students with disabilities of the College.

5359 Concordia College
901 8th Street S
Moorhead, MN 56562
218-299-4321
FAX 218-299-3345
http://www.cord.edu
e-mail: forde@gloria.cord.edu
Joli Coeur, Development Director
Pamela Jolicoeur, President

An independent four-year college with 13 special education students out of a total of 602.

5360 Gustavus Adolphus College
800 W College Avenue
Saint Peter, MN 56082
507-933-8000
FAX 507-933-6277
http://www.gac.edu

Laurie Bickett, Disability Services Coordinator
Jim Peterson, President

Gustavus Adolphus College is dedicated to providing for the needs of enrolled students who have disabilities. Reasonable modifications in the classroom and auxiliary aids will be provided for students with appropriately documented disabilities.

5361 Hamline College
Study Resource Center
1536 Hewitt Avenue
Saint Paul, MN 55104
651-523-2417
FAX 651-523-2809
http://www.hamline.edu
e-mail: cla-admins@gw.hamline.edu
Barbara Simmons, Assistant Dean
Matt Derby, Director

Four-year college that offers services to its disabled students.

5362 Hibbing Community College
Hibbing Community College
1515 E 25th Street
Hibbing, MN 55746
218-262-7200
800-224-4422
FAX 218-262-6717
http://www.hibbing.tec.mn.us
e-mail: admissions@hcc.mnscu.edu
Kenneth Simberg, Manager
Sandra Seppala, Assistant Manager

The College is committed to serving students with special needs. If you need an accommodation for a disability, please contact our disabilities staff to make arragements. HCC is completely accessible to students with physical disabilities.

5363 Institute on Community Integration
University of Minnesota
150 Pillsbury Drive SE
Minneapolis, MN 55455
612-625-3846
FAX 612-624-9344
http://www.ici.umn.edu
e-mail: info@icimail.umn.edu
Rachel Halvorson, Front Desk/Receptionist

Seeks to improve community services and social supports for persons with developmental and other disabilities and their families across the US. It publishes over 300 publications and maintains 20 Web sites with extensive resources of use to families, educators, community service providers, advocates, policymakers, and individuals with disabilities. It conducts research, training, and technical assistance that supports full inclusion of persons with disabilities in local communities.

5364 Inver Hills Community College
2500 80th Street E
Inver Grove Heights, MN 55076
651-450-8500
FAX 651-450-8677
http://www.ih.cc.mn.us
Cheryl Frank, Administrator
Charles Cheesebrough, Marketing Director

A public two-year college with 177 special education students out of a total of 5,450.

5365 Itasca Community College
Itasca Community College
1851 E Highway 169
Grand Rapids, MN 55744
218-743-6900
800-996-6422
FAX 218-327-4350
http://www.itasca.mnscu.edu
e-mail: svelzen@itasca.mnscu.edu
Sally Velzen, Learning Skills
Don Dc, Owner

Itasca Community College is committed to providing equal opportunity to qualified persons with physical or learning disabilities.

5366 Lake Superior College
Lake Superior College
2101 Trinity Road
Duluth, MN 55811
218-733-7600
FAX 218-733-5945
http://www.lsc.cc.mn.us
e-mail: enroll@lsc.mnscu.edu
Giorgia Robillard, Coordinator
Erin White, Disability Assistant
Kathy Nelson, President
A two-year college that provides a selection of programs for its disabled students.

5367 Macalester College
Disability Services
1600 Grand Avenue
Saint Paul, MN 55105
651-696-6000
FAX 651-696-6687
http://www.macalester.edu
e-mail: admissions@macalstr.edu
Sue Rothenbacher, Executive Asst Health Services
Pamela Chavez Birch, Assistant Health Services
Brian Rosenberg, President

5368 Mankato State University
PO Box 42
Mankato, MN 56002
507-389-2463
800-722-0544
FAX 507-389-2227
http://www.mankato.msus.edu
Kay Schock, Manager

This office houses documentation of disability for students, provides verification of disability for faculty, provides accommodations, offers direct services to students such as taped texts, notetaker and more.

5369 Mesabi Range Community & Technical College
1001 Chestnut Street W
Virginia, MN 55792
218-749-7700
800-657-3860
FAX 218-748-2419
TDY:218-749-7783
http://www.mr.mnscu.edu
e-mail: c.thomas@mr.mnscu.edu
Carrie Thomas, Student Life Director
Tina Royer, Manager

Students with a documented disability are offered assistance and the opportunity to succeed.

5370 Minneapolis Community College
1501 Hennepin Avenue
Minneapolis, MN 55403
612-659-6777
800-247-0911
FAX 612-659-6732
TDY:612-659-6731
http://www.minneapolis.edu
Carol Udstrand, LD Specialist
Jane Larson, Center Director
Patrick Carlson, Executive Director
A public two-year college with 104 special education students out of a total of 4,155.

5371 Minnesota Life College
7501 Logan Avenue S
Richfield, MN 55423
612-869-4008
FAX 612-869-0443
http://www.minnesotalifecollege.com
e-mail: info@minnesotalifecollege.com
Kathryn Thomas, Executive Director
Marlyn Wisberg, Manager

A college-like apartment living program for young adults with learning disabilities who need an intermediate level of support. Students must be at least 18 years of age and have a documented diagnosis of a learning disability or related condition such as attention deficit disorder. The program focuses on independent living skills, social skills, vocational readiness, career exploration, post secondary education, jobs placement, decision-making, fitness, health, leisure and recreation.

5372 **Minnesota State Community & Technology Col**
Minnesota State Community & Technical College
1414 College Way
Fergus Falls, MN 56537 218-739-7500
877-450-3322
FAX 218-736-1510
TDY:218-736-1537
http://www.minnesota.edu
e-mail: dave.seyfried@minnesota.edu
David Seyfried MD, Director of Disability Services
Karen Valentine, President
Karen Gabrielson, Secretary
The students with disabilities bring a unique dynamic and special needs to the classroom. Fegus Falls Community College recognizes that many students require assistance. These students often need modifications in programs, services, and activities to succeed in a changing, technology-based curriculum.

5373 **Minnesota State University Moorehead**
1104 7th Street N
Moorhead, MN 56560 218-477-4000
FAX 218-287-5050
TDY:218-299-5859
e-mail: toutges@mnstate.edu
Greg Toutges, Coordinator
Lisa Therson, Assistant Secretary
Bruce Hanson, Manager
A public four-year university serving approximately 60-80 students with learning disabilities out of a total of 7,200. Services, such as notetaking, alternate testing, taped textbooks, and more, are provided through the office of Disability Services to students with documented learning disabilities.

5374 **Minnesota West Community & Technical College**
344 W Main Street
Marshall, MN 56258 507-537-7051
800-576-6728
FAX 507-537-7081
http://www.mnwest.edu
e-mail: debra.carrow@mnwest.edu
Debra Carrow, Support Services Director
Linda Degriselles, Coordinator
Carolyn Fransen, Manager
Minnesota West offers a variety of services to students with disabilities including notetakers, academic counseling services, alternative testing, referral services, advocacy/support and special accommodations.

5375 **Normandale Community College**
9700 France Avenue S
Bloomington, MN 55431 952-487-8200
866-880-8740
http://www.nr.cc.mn.us
Mary Jibben, DEEDS Coordinator
Heather Huseby, Executive Director

A public two-year college with 169 special education students out of a total of 9,327.

5376 **North Hennepin Community College**
7411 85th Avenue N
Brooklyn Park, MN 55445 763-424-0702
FAX 763-424-0929
http://www.nh.cc.mn.us
Sue Smith, Special Services
Ann Wynieia, Administrator

Works to promote program and physical access while helping to ensure the rights of students with disabilities and meeting federal and state statutes.

5377 **Northwestern College**
3003 Snelling Avenue N
Saint Paul, MN 55113 651-631-5100
FAX 651-631-5124
http://www.nwc.edu
Yvonne Redmond- MD, Assistant Professor
Alan Cureton, President

Four-year college that offers disabled students support and services.

5378 **Pillsbury Baptist Bible College**
Admissions Office
315 S Grove Avenue
Owatonna, MN 55060 507-451-2710
FAX 507-451-6459
http://www.pillsbury.edu
Stephen Seidler, Admissions Director
Connie Seidler, Admissions Coordinator
Robert Crane, Manager
An independent four-year college with two special education students out of a total of 350.

5379 **Rainy River Community College**
Rainy River Community College
1501 Highway 71
International Falls, MN 56649 218-285-7722
800-456-3996
FAX 218-285-2239
TDY:218-285-2261
http://www.rrcc.mnscu.edu
e-mail: admissions@rrcc.mnscu.edu
Carol Grim, Disability Services
Tammy Wood, Advisor
Karen Bishop, Manager
The campus program provides services to students with disabilities to ensure their equal access to the college and its programs.

5380 **Riverland Community College Student Success Center**
1900 8th Avenue NW
Austin, MN 55912 507-433-0600
800-247-5039
FAX 507-433-0524
http://www.riverland.cc
e-mail: sstiehm@riverland.edu
Mindi Askelson, Student Support Services Dir.
Sharon Strehm, College Lab Assistant
Terry Leas, President
A two-year comprehensive technical and community college offering. 4000 students outstanding opportunities in carrer and transfer education. Facilites are located in Albert Lea, Austin, and Owatonna, Minnesota.

5381 **Rochester Community and Technical College**
851 30th Avenue SE
Rochester, MN 55904 507-285-7210
800-247-1296
FAX 507-285-7496
http://www.roch.edu
e-mail: travis.kromminga@roch.edu
Donald Supalla, Administrator

To provide academic support and advising services to assist disabled persons in achieving their educational goals.

5382 **Saint John's School of Theology & Seminary**
Collegeville, MN 56321 320-363-2100
800-361-8318
FAX 320-363-3145
http://www.csbsju.edu/sot/
e-mail: mbanken@csbsju.edu
Mary Banken OSB

An independent four-year college with 36 special education students out of a total of 1,880.

5383 **Saint Mary's University of Minnesota**
700 Terrace Heights
Winona, MN 55987 507-457-1700
800-635-5987
FAX 507-457-1633
http://www.smumn.edu
e-mail: bsmith@smumn.edu
Bonnie Smith, Support Services
Jane Ochrymowycz, Center Director
Anthony Piscitiello, Vice President
Accommodations and support services based on recent positive assessment and recommendations of evaluator.

5384 Southwest Minnesota State University: Learning Resources
1501 State Street
Marshall, MN 56258
507-537-7021
800-642-0684
FAX 507-537-6027
http://www.southwestmsu.edu
e-mail: Leach@southwest.msus.edu
Marilyn Leach, Learning Resource Director
Pam Ekstrom, Accommodations Coordinator
David Danahar, President
Offers a variety of services to students with disabilities including test accommodations, notetakers, academic counseling services, 504/ADA advocacy, taped texts, computers with assistive/access technology and software. The department also offers skills development courses, tutoring services and student mentors.

5385 St. Cloud State University
Student Disability Services
720 4th Avenue S
Saint Cloud, MN 56301
320-255-0121
FAX 320-654-5139
http://www.stcloudstate.edu/
e-mail: webteam@stcloudstate.edu
Lee Bird MD, Disability Services
Roy Saigo, President

A public comprehensive university that provides services for students with learning disabilities and other needs: alternative testing, note taking, referrals to campus resources and advocacy/support.

5386 St. Olaf College
Student Disability Services
1520 Saint Olaf Avenue
Northfield, MN 55057
507-646-3288
800-800-3025
FAX 507-663-3459
http://www.stolaf.edu
e-mail: asc@stolaf.edu
Ruth Bolstad, Director Special Services
Linne Jensen, Associate Director

Offers a variety of services to students with disabilities including note takers, extended testing time, counseling services, and special accommodations.

5387 St. Paul Technical College
235 Marshall Avenue
Saint Paul, MN 55102
651-846-1500
FAX 651-221-1416
http://www.saintpaul.edu
Margie Warrington, Transition Director
Donovan Schwichtenberg, President

A public two-year college with 79 special education students out of a total of 3,574.

5388 University of Minnesota Disability Services
University of Minnesota
200 Oak Street SE
Minneapolis, MN 55455
612-626-2820
FAX 612-625-5572
TDY:612-626-1333
http://www.disserv3.stu.umn.edu
e-mail: dstest@umn.edu
Robert Bruininks, President
Karen Stutelberg, Manager

Disability Services is a University Resource Promotion barrier free environment (physical program, information, attitude) which means expressing the rights of people with disabilities and assisting the university with meeting its responsibilities under federal and state statues. Disability Services works to ensure access to University employment, courses, programs, facilities, services and activities by documenting disabilities.

5389 University of Minnesota: Crookston
Student Disability Services
2900 University Avenue
Crookston, MN 56716
218-281-8587
800-232-6466
FAX 218-281-8584
TDY:800-627-3529
http://www.crk.umn.edu
e-mail: lwilson@umn.edu
Laurie Wilson, Coordinator

A public four-year college with 40-70 students with disabilities out of a total of 1,341.

5390 University of Minnesota: Duluth
Learning Disabilities Program
10 University Drive
Duluth, MN 55812
218-726-7500
800-232-1339
FAX 218-726-6394
TDY:218-726-7380
http://www.d.umn.edu
e-mail: jbromen@d.umn.edu
Judy Bromen, LD Coordinator
Katheryn Martin, Chancellor

UMD is committed to providing equal opportunities in higher education to academically qualified students with disabilities who demonstrate a reasonable expectation of college success.

5391 University of Minnesota: Morris
Student Disability Services
600 E 4th Street
Morris, MN 56267
320-589-6163
FAX 320-589-6473
TDY:320-589-6035
http://www.morris.umn.edu
e-mail: freyc@morris.umn.edu
Colleen Frey, Coordinator
Kathryn Gonier Klopfleisch, Program Coordinator

Offers a variety of services to students with disabilities including note takers, extended testing time, counseling services, and special accommodations.

5392 University of Minnesota: Twin Cities Campus
216 Pillsbury Drive SE
Minneapolis, MN 55455
612-625-5000
FAX 612-626-9654
TDY:612-626-1333
http://www.d.umn.edu
Lynn Dhitao, Senior Officer Specialist
Robert Bruininks, President

The goals of the university are: to create equal opportunities for students, faculty, and staff with disabilities to learn and work; to increase the visibility and awareness of Disability Services and enhance the quality, effectiveness, and efficiency of its operations.

5393 University of St. Thomas
2115 Summit Avenue
Saint Paul, MN 55105
651-962-5040
FAX 651-962-5910
http://www.stthomas.edu
Stephanie Zurek, Coordinator
Rebecca Swiler, Executive Director

An independent four-year college with 52 special education students out of a total of 5,283.

5394 Worthington Community College
1450 College Way
Worthington, MN 56187
507-372-8640
800-657-3966
FAX 507-372-5801
Pam Sieve, Coordinator
Bradley Chapulis, Manager

A public two-year college with 18 special education students out of a total of 868.

Mississippi

5395 Hinds Community College
505 E Main Street
Raymond, MS 39154
601-857-5261
FAX 601-857-3539
http://www.hinds.cc.edu
Michael Handle, Director
Clyde Muse, President

Offers a variety of services to students with disabilities including note takers, extended testing time, counseling services, and special accommodations.

5396 Holmes Community College
Student Affairs Office
PO Box 369
Goodman, MS 39079
662-472-2312
FAX 662-472-9076
http://www.holmescc.edu
Fran Cox, Dean for Student Affairs

Offers a variety of services to students with disabilities including note takers, extended testing time, counseling services, and special accommodations.

5397 Institute for Disability Studies (UCEDD)
University of Southern Mississippi
118 College Drive
Hattiesburg, MS 39406
601-266-5163
888-671-0051
FAX 601-266-5114
TDY:888-671-0051
http://www.usm.edu/ids
e-mail: jane.siders@usm.edu
Jane Siders EdD, Executive Director
Royals Walker JD, Associate Director

Mississippi University Center for Excellence in Developmental Disabilities positively affecting the lives of individuals with disabilities and their families and working to increase their independent, productivity, and integration into communities.

5398 Itawamba Community College
Learning Disabilities Department
602 W Hill Street
Fulton, MS 38843
662-862-8000
FAX 662-862-8273
http://www.icc.cc.ms.us
e-mail: mleaton@iccms.edu
Sarah Johnson, Vice President
Marcia Eaton, Coordinator
David Cole, President
Offers a variety of services to students with disabilities including note takers, extended testing time, counseling services, and special accommodations.

5399 Mississippi State University
Student Affairs Office
PO Box 806
Mississippi State, MS 39762
662-325-3335
FAX 662-325-8190
http://www.msstate.edu
e-mail: dbaker@saffairs.msstate.edu
Debbie Baker, Executive Director
Carlene Pylate, Office Assistant

Four-year college that provides student support to learning disabled students.

5400 Mississippi University Affiliated Program
University of Southern Mississippi
118 College Drive
Hattiesburg, MS 39406
601-266-1000
888-671-0051
FAX 601-266-5114
TDY:888-671-0051
http://www.usm.edu
e-mail: latouisha.wilson@usm.edu
Shelby Thames, President

5401 Northeast Mississippi Community College
Special Populations Office
101 Cunningham Boulevard
Booneville, MS 38829
662-728-7751
FAX 662-728-2428
http://www.nemcc.edu
e-mail: twalker@nemcc.edu
Tommye Walker, Director
Liz Ketchum, Special Populations Councilor
Carol Killough, Executive Director
A public two-year college with 5 special education students out of a total of 3,047.

5402 University of Mississippi
PO Box 187
University, MS 38677
662-915-7271
FAX 662-915-7211
e-mail: abroad@olemiss.edu
Ardessa Milor, Special Services
Carolyn Higdon, Administrator

A public four-year college with 76 special education students out of a total of 8,804.

5403 University of Southern Mississippi
PO Box 8586
Hattiesburg, MS 39406
601-266-1000
FAX 601-266-6035
TDY:601-266-6837
http://www.usm.edu
e-mail: latouisha.wilson@usm.edu
Shelby Thames, President

Four year college that provides students with support and resources whom are disabled.

5404 William Carey College
498 Tuscan Avenue
Hattiesburg, MS 39401
601-318-6051
FAX 601-318-6196
Brenda Waldrip, Special Services
Larry Kennedy, President

Offers a variety of services to students with disabilities including note takers, extended testing time, counseling services, and special accommodations.

Missouri

5405 Central Methodist College
Disability Support Department
411 Commons Square
Fayette, MO 65248
660-248-3391
877-268-1854
FAX 660-248-2622
TDY:660-248-6223
http://www.centralmethodist.edu
e-mail: koliver@centralmethodist.edu
Ken Oliver, Special Education Director
Shawn Baker, Student Affairs Office
Marianne Inman, President
Offers a variety of services to students with disabilities including note takers, extended testing time, counseling services, and special accommodations.

5406 Central Missouri State University
Office of Accessibility Services
Union 222
Warrensburg, MO 64093
660-543-4421
FAX 660-543-4724
TDY:660-543-4421
http://www.cmsu.edu\access
e-mail: mayfield@cmsu1.cmsu.edu
Barbara Mayfield MS JD, Director ADA/504 Coordinator
Cathy Seeley MS, Coordinator

Provider of equal opportunity to education for students with disabilities through notetakers, extended testing time, interpreters and other accommodations.

5407 **East Central College**
Special Services Office
1964 Prairie Dell Road
Union, MO 63084
636-583-5193
FAX 636-583-1011
TDY:636-583-4851
http://www.eastcentral.edu
e-mail: peckaw@eastcentral.edu
Michael Knight, Assessment Director
Wendy Peckaw, Access Director
Karen Herzog, President
Offers a variety of services to students with disabilities including note takers, extended testing time, counseling services, and special accommodations.

5408 **Evangel University**
1111 N Glenstone Avenue
Springfield, MO 65802
417-865-2811
FAX 417-865-9599
http://www.evangel.edu
Laynah Rogers MD, Associate Professor
Robert Spence, President

An independent four-year college with 23 special education students out of a total of 1,449.

5409 **Fontbonne College**
Kinkel Center
6800 Wydown Boulevard
Saint Louis, MO 63105
314-889-4571
FAX 314-889-1451
http://www.fontbonne.edu
e-mail: jsnyder@fontbonne.edu
Jane D Synder MD, Director

Four-year college provides services through the Kinkel Center for students with learning disabilities.

5410 **Jefferson College**
1000 Viking Drive
Hillsboro, MO 63050
636-942-3000
FAX 636-789-4012
TDY:636-789-5772
http://www.jeffco.edu
e-mail: lbigelow@jeffco.edu
Linda Bigelow, Director
Bill Kenna, President

Offers a variety of services to students with disabilities including notetakers, extended testing time, counseling services, and special accommodations.

5411 **Kansas City Art Institute**
Kansas City Art Institute
4415 Warwick Boulevard
Kansas City, MO 64111
816-802-3449
800-522-5224
FAX 816-802-3480
http://www.kcai.edu
e-mail: arc@kcai.edu
Kathleen Collins, Manager

Offers a variety of services to students with disabilities including notetakers, extended testing time, counseling services, and special accommodations.

5412 **Lindenwood College**
209 S Kingshighway Street
Saint Charles, MO 63301
636-949-7670
FAX 314-949-4910
http://www.lindenwood.edu
e-mail: lindenwood@lindenwood.edu
V. Pitts, Director
Dennis Spellman, President

Offers a variety of services to students with disabilities including note takers, extended testing time, counseling services, and special accommodations.

5413 **Longview Community College: ABLE Program-Academic Bridges to Learning Effectiveness**
500 SW Longview Road
Lees Summit, MO 64081
816-672-2000
FAX 816-672-2417
TDY:816-672-2144
http://www.kcmetro.edu
e-mail: maryellen.jenison@kcmetro.edu
Mary Jenison, ABLE Program Director
Fred Grogan, President

ABLE is an intensive support services program, designed to empower individuals with learning disabilities or brain injuries with the skills needed to gain control of their own lives and learning, so that they can make a successful transition to regular college courses, vocational programs, or the workplace. In addition to courses especially designed for this population, students take basic skills courses (if needed), regular college courses with study support, and attend weekly support groups.

5414 **Maple Woods Community College**
Learning Disabilities Department
2601 NE Barry Road
Kansas City, MO 64156
816-437-3000
FAX 816-437-3483
TDY:816-437-3318
http://www.kcmetro.edu/maplewoods
e-mail: kim.fernandes@kcmetro.edu
Kim Fernandes, Coordinator
Janet Weaver, Outreach Counselor
Merna Saliman, President
A public two-year college with 30 special education students out of a total of 5,007.

5415 **Missouri Southern State College**
Learning Center
3950 E Newton Road
Joplin, MO 64801
417-625-9373
800-606-MSSC
FAX 417-659-4456
TDY:800-766-3776
http://www.mssu.edu
e-mail: locher-m@mssu.edu
Melissa Locher, Coordinator
Eillen Godsey, Director

Offers a variety of services to students with disabilities including note takers, extended testing time, and counseling services.

5416 **Missouri Valley College**
500 E College Street
Marshall, MO 65340
660-886-6924
FAX 660-831-4039
http://www.moval.edu
e-mail: admissions@moval.edu
Virginia Zank, Director
Linda Kanagawa, Coordinator
Bonnie Humphrey, President
An independent four-year college with 5 special education students out of a total of 1,132.

5417 **North Central Missouri College**
1301 Main Street
Trenton, MO 64683
660-359-3948
FAX 660-359-2899
http://www.ncmc.cc.mo.us
e-mail: webmaster@mail.ncmc.cc.mo.us
Ginny Wickoff, Counselor
Neil Nutthall, President

Offers a variety of services to students with disabilities including note takers, extended testing time, counseling services, and special accommodations.

5418 **Northwest Missouri State University**
Special Services Department
800 University Drive
Maryville, MO 64468
660-562-1219
FAX 660-562-1121
http://www.nwmissouri.edu
e-mail: admissions@mail.nwmissouri.edu
WC Dizney, Special Services

Offers a variety of services to students with disabilities including notetakers, extended testing time, counseling services, and special accommodations.

5419 Saint Louis University
Student Educational Services
3840 Lindell Boulevard
Saint Louis, MO 63108
314-977-2930
FAX 314-977-3315
TDY:314-977-3499
http://www.slu.edu
e-mail: meyerah@slu.edu
Adam Meyer, Disabilities Coordinator

Four year college offering comprehensive programs for the learning disabled.

5420 Southwest Missouri State University
Office of Disability Services
901 S National Avenue
Springfield, MO 65804
417-836-4192
FAX 417-836-4134
TDY:417-836-6792
http://www.smsu.edu/disability
e-mail: ksw2780@msu.edu
Steager -Wilson, Director
Tabatha Haynes, Assistant Director

At Southwest Missouri State University, we believe all students should have equal access to higher education and university life. Disability Services helps ensure an equitable college experience for SMS Students with disabilities.

5421 St. Louis Community College at Florissant Valley: Access Office
3400 Pershall Road
Saint Louis, MO 63135
314-595-4200
FAX 314-513-4876
TDY:314-595-4552
http://www.stlcc.edu/access
e-mail: smatthews@stlcc.edu
Sueluine Matthews, Manager
Mary Wagner, Access Specialist
Marcia Pfeiffer, President
A public two-year college with 200 students with disabilities, out of a total of 7,000. Accommodations are provided upon request. Documentation of disability must be provided.

5422 St. Louis Community College at Forest Park: Access Office
5600 Oakland Avenue
Saint Louis, MO 63110
314-644-9100
FAX 314-644-9752
http://www.stlcc.edu
e-mail: stlcc@stlcc.edu
Glenn Marshall, Manager ACCESS
Karen Lerch, Administrative Registrar Assista
Morris Johnson, President
The St. Louis Community College ACCESS OFFICE collaborates with faculty, staff, students, and the community to encourage a college environment where individuals are viewed on the basis of ability, not disability.

5423 St. Louis Community College at Meramec
11333 Big Bend Road
Kirkwood, MO 63122
314-984-7797
FAX 314-984-7117
TDY:314-984-7127
http://www.stlcc.edu
e-mail: stlcc@stlcc.edu

Lynn E Suydam MD, President
Ann Riley, Manager

The Access office offers support services to students who have documented disabilities of a permanent or temporary nature. The staff is available to provide the following services: individual counseling and advising; coordination of needed accommodations such as interpreters and more.

5424 University Affiliated Program for Developmental Disabilities
University of Missouri at Kansas City
2220 Holmes Street
Kansas City, MO 64108
816-235-1700
800-444-0821
FAX 816-235-1762
TDY:800-452-1185
http://www.iht.umck.edu
e-mail: calkinsc@umkc.edu
Carl Calkins PhD, Director
Lora Lacey-Haun, Administrator

5425 University of Missouri
Office of Disability Services
A38 Brady Commons
Columbia, MO 65201
573-882-4696
FAX 573-884-9272
TDY:573-882-8054
http://www.missouri.edu
e-mail: weavers@missouri.edu
Sarah Colby-Weaver PhD, Director
Matt Buckley, Coordinator Learning Programs

Four-year independent college offering support for learning disabled students.

5426 University of Missouri: Kansas City
Department of Disability Services
5100 Rockhill Road
Kansas City, MO 64110
816-235-5696
FAX 816-235-6537
http://www.umkc.edu
e-mail: disability@umkc.edu
Scott Laurent, Coordinator

Offers a variety of services to students with disabilities including note takers, extended testing time, counseling services, and special accommodations.

5427 University of Missouri: Rolla
University of Missouri Systems
1870 Miner Circle
Rolla, MO 65409
573-341-4111
800-522-0938
FAX 573-341-6333
TDY:573-341-4205
http://www.umr.edu
e-mail: webmaster@umr.edu
Debra Robinson MD, Vice Chancellor Student Affairs
Gary Thomas, Chancellor
Bill Bleckman, Executive Director
Offers a variety of services to students with disabilities including note takers, extended testing time, counseling services, and special accommodations.

5428 Washington University
1 Brookings Drive
Saint Louis, MO 63130
314-935-5000
FAX 314-935-8272
TDY:314-935-4062
http://www. wustl.edu
e-mail: vachary@wustl.edu
Vachary McBbe, Office Manager
Mark Wrighton, CEO

Offers a variety of services to students with disabilities including note takers, extended testing time, counseling services, and special accommodations.

5429 Westminster College
Learning Disabilities Program
501 Westminster Avenue
Fulton, MO 65251
573-592-5304
800-475-3361
FAX 573-592-5180
http://www.westminster-mo.edu
e-mail: ottingh@jaynet.westminster-mo.edu
Hank Ottinger, Director
Fletcher , President

Four year college that offers a program for students with learning disabilities.

Montana

5430 **Dull Knife Memorial College**
Office of Disabilities Services
PO Box 98
Lame Deer, MT 59043
406-477-6215
FAX 406-477-6219
http://www.dkmc.cc.mt.us
e-mail: alderson@cdkc.edu

Juanita Lonebear, GED Director
Richard Littlebear, President

Offers a variety of services to students with disabilities including notetakers, extended testing time, counseling services, and special accommodations.

5431 **Flathead Valley Community College**
777 Grandview Drive
Kalispell, MT 59901
406-756-3856
FAX 406-756-3911
TDY:406-756-3881
http://www.fvcc.edu
e-mail: edavis@fvcc.edu

Elaine Davis, Disability Specialist
Lynn Farris, Director
Michael Ober, Manager
GED testing and learning styles assessment is available in the Learning Center. Advocates for Students with Disabilities work with faculty and staff to provide appropriate accommodations for students with learning disabilities.

5432 **Montana State University**
Disabled Student Services
PO Box 173960
Bozeman, MT 59717
406-994-2824
FAX 406-994-3943
TDY:406-994-6701
http://www.montana.edu
e-mail: byork@montana.edu

Brenda York, Director
Deidre Manry, Administrative Assistant

Disabled Student Services (DSS) is committed to facilitating Montana State goal of making its programs, services and activities accessible to students with disabilities. We provide a variety of services to students with disabilities, including note taking assistance, exam accommodations, adaptive technology, and advice and advocacy.

5433 **Montana Tech College**
Disabled Student Services
1300 W Park Street
Butte, MT 59701
406-496-3730
FAX 406-496-3710
http://www.mtech.edu
e-mail: lbarnett@mtech.edu

Lee Barnett, Director
Margie Pascoe, Counseling Services

Committed to making the appropriate accommodations for students with disabilities.

5434 **Montana University Affiliated Program**
University of Montana/ Office of Disability
154 Lommasson Center
Missoula, MT 59812
406-243-5467
888-268-2743
FAX 406-243-2349
TDY:406-243-5467
http://www.ruralinstitute.umt.edu
e-mail: dss@umt.edu

Jim Burke, Director
Dan Burke, Coordinator

The Rura Institute works on behalf of people with disabilities of all ages to support full participation in community life. We train professionals, provide services directly to people with disabilities, share our knowledge with others, and conduct research to develop solutions.

5435 **Northern Montana College**
PO Box 77511
Havre, MT 59501
406-265-3783
800-662-6132
FAX 406-265-3597

Linda Hoines, Learning Specialist

To provide college students with support and skills needed to remain in college and complete a degree program.

5436 **Rocky Mountain College**
Services for Academic Success
1511 Poly Drive
Billings, MT 59102
406-657-1128
800-877-6259
FAX 406-259-9751
http://www.rocky.edu
e-mail: vandykj@rocky.edu

Jane Van Dyk PhD, Assocaite VP/Director

An independent four-year college with a comprehensive support program serving 30-40 students with disabilities. Total college enrollment is about 1,000 students.

5437 **University of Great Falls**
1301 20th Street S
Great Falls, MT 59405
406-761-8210
800-848-3431
FAX 406-791-5214
http://www.ugf.edu

Sue Romas, Head Academic Excellence
Eugene Allister, President

An independent four-year college with 25 special education students out of a total of 1,038.

5438 **University of Montana**
032 Corbin Hall
Missoula, MT 59812
406-243-0211
FAX 406-243-5330
http://www.umt.edu
e-mail: marks@selway.umt.edu

Jim Marks, Director
George Dennison, President

Four year college that provides programs for students with a learning disabilities.

5439 **Western Montana College**
710 S Atlantic Street
Dillon, MT 59725
800-WMC-MONT
http://www.wmc.edu

Clarence Kostelecky, Special Services

A public four-year college with 6 special education students out of a total of 1,100.

Nebraska

5440 **Chadron State College**
1000 Main Street
Chadron, NE 69337
308-432-6000
888-461-4461
FAX 308-432-6395
http://www.csc.edu
e-mail: jcassady@csc.edu

Jerry Cassady, Counselor
Frances Gonzalez, Tutor Coordinator
Janie Park, President
Offer a variety of services to students with disabilities including tutoring, counseling, and special accommodations as appropriate. Students are mentored in self understanding and self-advocacy.

5441 Creighton University
2500 California Plaza
Omaha, NE 68178
402-280-2700
800-282-5835
FAX 402-280-5579
TDY:402-280-5733
http://www.creighton.edu
e-mail: chess@creighton.edu

Wade Pearson, Director
John Schlegel, President

An independent four-year college with 73 special education students out of a total of 4,123.

5442 Doane College
1014 Boswell Avenue
Crete, NE 68333
402-826-2161
FAX 402-826-8278
http://www.doane.edu
e-mail: shanigan@doane.edu

Sherri Hanigan, Student Support Services Dir.
Jonathan Brank, President

An independent four-year college with 12 special education students out of a total of 950.

5443 Hastings College
710 N Turner Avenue
Hastings, NE 68901
402-463-2402
800-LEA-RNHC
FAX 402-461-7480
http://www.hastings.edu
e-mail: khaverly@hastings.edu

Kathleen Haverly, Center Director
Mary Molliconi, Admissions Director
Phillip Dudley, Principal

Learning disabled students are provided with a personalized accommodation plan. Students must be verified prior to enrollment and submit a psychological review profile prior to being served. Services include: study skills instruction, academic, career and vocational counseling services, note takers, tutors, professionals and testing accommodations.

5444 Midland Lutheran College
Academic Support Services
900 N Clarkson Street
Fremont, NE 68025
402-721-5480
FAX 402-721-0250
http://www.mlc.edu
e-mail: moseman@mlc.edu

Mose Man, Director
Connie Stewart, Administrative Assistant

Four-year college that provides academic support for students who have a learning disability.

5445 Munroe-Meyer Institute for Genetics and Rehabilitation
University Affiliated Program
444 S 44th Street
Omaha, NE 68131
402-559-6402
FAX 402-559-5737
http://www.unmc.edu/mmi
e-mail: mfbennie@unmc.edu

Bruce Buehler, Director
Thelma Roberts, Billing Representative

Diagnostic, evaluation, therapy, speech, physical, occupational, behavioral therapies, pediatrics, dentistry, nursing, psychology, social work, genetics, Media Resource Center, education, nutrition. Adult services for developmentally disabled, Genetic evaluation and counseling, adaptive equipment, motion analysis laboratory, recreational therapy.

5446 Southeast Community College: Beatrice Campus
Career and Advising Program
4771 W Scott Road
Beatrice, NE 68310
402-228-3468
800-233-5027
FAX 402-228-2218
http://www.southeast.edu
e-mail: tcardwell@southeast.edu

Tom Cardwell MD, Dean Students
Robert Kluge, Career Counselor
Dennis Headrick, President

A public two-year college with 7 special education students out of a total of 941.

5447 Southeast Community College: Lincoln Campus
Career and Advising Program
8800 O Street
Lincoln, NE 68520
402-437-2620
800-642-4075
FAX 402-437-2404
http://www.college.sccm.cc.ne.us
e-mail: smiller@southeast.ed

Sherine Miller, Director
Greg Peters, Career Adviser

A two year vocational/technical/academic transfer college with approximately 4,000 full/part time students. Accommodations for students with disabilities are made through the Counselors.

5448 Union College
3800 S 48th Street
Lincoln, NE 68506
402-486-2514
800-228-4600
FAX 402-486-2895
http://www.ucollege.edu
e-mail: jeforbes@ucollege.edu

Jennifer Forbes, Director
Anne Ballard, Academic Support
Chloe Foutz, Manager

For students with disabilities The Learning Center offers support services to students with learning disabilities, such as dyselexia, and accommodations are made for all students with disabilities.

5449 University of Nebraska: Lincoln
132 Administration Building
Lincoln, NE 68588
402-472-3787
800-742-8800
FAX 402-472-0080
TDY:402-472-0054
http://www.unl.edu
e-mail: vcheney2@unl.edu

Veva Cheney, Director for Special Services

A public four-year college with 141 special education students out of a total of 19,888.

5450 University of Nebraska: Omaha
6001 Dodge Street
Omaha, NE 68182
402-554-2800
800-858-8648
FAX 402-554-3555
http://www.unomaha.edu

Nancy Belck, Manager

Offers a variety of services to students with disabilities including notetakers, extended testing time, counseling services, and special accommodations.

5451 Wayne State College
Office of Differing Disabilities
1111 Main Street
Wayne, NE 68787
402-375-7213
FAX 402-375-7079
http://www.wsc.edu
e-mail: jecarstl@wsc.edu

Jeff Carsten MD, Assistant Dean of Students
Richard Collings, President

Offers a variety of services to students with disabilities including LD diagnosis, academic accommodations, and advocacy.

5452 Western Nebraska Community College: Scotts Bluff Campus
1601 E 27th Street
Scottsbluff, NE 69361
308-635-3606
800-348-4435
FAX 308-635-6100
http://www.wncc.net

Norman Stephenson, Counseling Director
John Harms, President

Offers a variety of services to students with disabilities including notetakers, extended testing time, counseling services, and special accommodations.

Nevada

5453 Community College of Southern Nevada
Disability Resource Center
3200 E Cheyenne Avenue
North Las Vegas, NV 89030
702-651-4280
FAX 702-651-4179
TDY:702-651-4328
http://www.ccsn.edu
e-mail: trish_henderson@ccsn.edu
Trish Henderson, Dir Disability Resource Center
Nikki Peterson, Administrative Assistant II

Note takers, test proctors, books on tape, enlarged books, lab assistants, scribes, interpreters, special accommodations, etc.

5454 Sierra Nevada College
999 Tahoe Boulevard
Incline Village, NV 89451
775-831-1314
FAX 775-831-1347
http://www.sierranevada.edu
e-mail: bsolomon@sierranevada.edu
Ben Solomon, President

Four year college that provides services to disabled students.

5455 Truckee Meadows Community College
Disability Resource Center
7000 Dandini Boulevard
Reno, NV 89512
775-673-7277
FAX 775-673-7207
http://www.tmcc.edu/drc
e-mail: lgeldmacher@tmcc.edu
Lee Geldmacher, Manager

A public two-year college with 420 registered students out of a total of 11,500.

5456 University Affiliated Program: University of Nevada
College of Education
Repc-285
Reno, NV 89557
775-784-4921
FAX 775-784-4997
http://www.unr.edu
e-mail: joannj@unr.edu
Jo Johnson, Director

5457 University of Nevada: Las Vegas
Disability Support Services
PO Box 452015
Las Vegas, NV 89154
702-895-0866
FAX 702-895-0651
TDY:702-895-0652
http://www.unlv.edu
e-mail: les@ccmail.nevada.edu
Jane Jones, Director

The Disability Resource Center provides academic accommodations for students with documented disabilities who are otherwise qualified for university programs. The DRC has been designated as the official office for housing records as specified by Section 504 of the Rehabilitation Act of 1973.

5458 University of Nevada: Reno
1664 W Virginia Street
Reno, NV 89557
775-784-6000
FAX 775-784-6955
TDY:775-327-5131
http://www.unr.edu
Mary Zabel, Director
Kristina Wearne, Administrative Assistant

Offers a variety of services to students with disabilities including notetakers, extended testing time, counseling services, and special accommodations.

5459 Western Nevada Community College
2201 W College Parkway
Carson City, NV 89703
775-445-3000
FAX 775-887-3105
http://www.wncc.nevada.edu
Susan Hannah, DSS Coordinator
Carol Lucey, President

Offers a variety of services to students with disabilities including note takers, extended testing time, counseling services, and special accommodations.

New Hampshire

5460 Colby-Sawyer College
541 Main Street
New London, NH 03257
603-526-3600
800-272-1015
FAX 603-526-3452
http://www.colby-sawyer.edu
e-mail: mmar@colby-sawyer.edu
Mary Mar MD, Learning Services Director
Ann Chalker, Learning Specialist
Joe Chillo, Vice President
An independent four-year college with 100 LD education students out of a total of 800.

5461 Daniel Webster College
Academic Support Services
20 University Drive
Nashua, NH 03063
603-577-6612
800-325-6876
FAX 603-577-6001
http://www.dwc.edu
e-mail: admissions@dwc.edu
Lorraine Sylvester, Admissions Specialist
Sean Ryan, Dean of Admissions

Four-year college that offers academic support services to the learning disabled students.

5462 Dartmouth College
301 Collis Center
Hanover, NH 03755
603-646-1110
FAX 603-646-1629
TDY:603-646-1564
http://www.dartmouth.edu
e-mail: admissions.office@dartmouth.edu
Nancy Pompian, Director of Student Services
James Wright, CEO

Offers a variety of services to students with disabilities including note takers, extended testing time, counseling services, and special accommodations.

5463 Franklin Pierce College
Office Differing Disabilities
PO Box 60
Rindge, NH 03461
603-899-4107
800-437-0048
FAX 603-899-4395
http://www.fpc.edu
e-mail: academicservices@fpc.edu
Patricia Moore, Coordinator

An independent four-year college with 56 special education students out of a total of 1321.

5464 Hampshire Country School
122 Hampshire Road
Rindge, NH 03461
603-899-3325
FAX 603-899-6521
http://www.hampshirecountryschool.com
e-mail: hampshirecountry@monad.net
William Dickerman, Principal

Twenty-five student boarding school for high ability boys, mostly 10-15 years old, needing an unusual amount of adult attention, structure and guidance.

5465 Hunter School
PO Box 600
Rumney, NH 03266
603-786-2922
FAX 603-786-2221
http://www.hunterschool.org
e-mail: admissions@hunterschool.org
Thom Hartmann, Founder

A small, non-profit school where young boys and girls with Attention Deficit Disorder (ADD), Attention Deficit/Hyperactivity Disorder (ADHD) or Asperger's Syndrome are nurtured, educated and celebrated. Offers both a residential program and a day school.

5466 Institute on Disability: A University Center for Excellence on Disability
University of New Hampshire
10 W Edge Drive
Durham, NH 03824
603-862-2110
FAX 603-862-0555
http://www.iod.unh.edu
e-mail: institute.disability@unh.edu
Janice Mutschler, Manager

Promotes the inclusion of people with disabilities into their schools and communities.

5467 Keene State College
229 Main Street
Keene, NH 03435
603-352-1909
800-KSC-1909
FAX 603-358-2313
http://www.keene.edu
Jane Warner, Director
Dr. Helen Giles-Gee, President
Robert Baker, Executive Director
A public four-year college with 105 special education students out of a total of 3,800.

5468 Learning Skills Academy
PO Box 955
Rye, NH 03870
603-964-4903
FAX 603-964-3838
http://www.lsa.pvt.k12.nh.us
e-mail: marcus@lsa.pvt.k12.nh.us
Marcus Mann, Principal
Lisa McManus, Education Director

5469 New England College
24 Bridge Street
Henniker, NH 03242
603-428-2211
FAX 603-428-3155
http://www.nec.edu
Anna Carlson, Academic Advising/Support
Heidi Hamel, Events Coordinator
Stephen Fritz, President
An independent four-year college with 140 students with learning differences out of a total undergraduate enrollement of 750.

5470 New Hampshire Community Technical College at Stratham/Pease
Disabilities Support Services
277 Portsmouth Avenue
Stratham, NH 03885
603-772-1194
800-522-1194
FAX 603-772-1198
http://www.ms.nhctc.edu/caps/
e-mail: scronin@nhctc.edu
Sharon Cronin, Coordinator
Patsy Golinski, Admissions
Tom Wisbey, President
A public two-year college with support services for students with disabilities that include classroom accommodations, assistive technology, self advocacy, counseling, and one-on-one tutoring.

5471 New Hampshire Vocational Technical College
379 Belmont Road
Laconia, NH 03246
603-524-3207
800-357-2992
FAX 603-524-8084
TDY:603-524-3207
http://www.laconia.nactc.edu
e-mail: laconow@nactc.edu
Maureen Baldwin-Lamper, Special Services
Don Morrissey, Vice President

Offers a variety of services to students with disabilities including notetakers, extended testing time, counseling services, and special accommodations.

5472 Rivier College
420 S Main Street
Nashua, NH 03060
603-888-1311
800-447-4843
FAX 603-897-8807
TDY:800-735-2964
http://www.rivier.edu
e-mail: kricci@rivier.edu
Kate Ricci, Coordinator of Special Services
Bill Farell, President

An independent four-year college with 17 special education students out of a total of 1,651.

5473 Southern New Hampshire University
Office of Disability Services
2500 N River Road
Hooksett, NH 03106
603-668-2211
800-642-4968
FAX 603-645-9693
http://www.snhu.edu
e-mail: h.jaffe@snhu.edu
Ronald Eppster, Manager
Paul Leblanc, President
Hyla Jaffe, Disability Services Coordinator
Offers services to students with disabilities based on recommendations from documentaion supporting a disability. Accommodations are made for specific needs.

5474 Student Accessibility Services
Dartmouth College
301 Collis Center
Hanover, NH 03755
603-646-1110
FAX 603-646-1629
TDY:603-646-1564
http://www.dartmouth.edu/~acskills/disability
e-mail: admissions.office@dartmouth.edu
The Student Accessibility Services (SAS) Office works with students, faculty and staff to ensure that the programs and activities of Dartmouth College are accessible, and students with disabilities receive reasonable accommodations in their curricular and co-curricular pursuits. Over 350 Dartmouth students are registered with SAS including students with learning disabilities, attentional or psychiatric disorders, and mobility, visual, hearing or chronic health conditions.

5475 University of New Hampshire
118 Memorial Union Building
Durham, NH 03824
603-862-2110
FAX 603-862-4043
http://www.unh.edu/disabilityservices
e-mail: maxine.little@unh.edu
Maxine Little, Director
Janice Mutschler, Manager

Disability Services for Students provides services to students with documented disabilities to ensure that University activities and programs are accessible. It also promotes the development of student self-reliance and the personal independence necessary to succeed in a university climate.

New Jersey

5476 Banyan School
Banyan School
12 Hollywood Avenue
Fairfield, NJ 07004
973-439-1919
FAX 973-439-1396
http://www.banyanschool.com
e-mail: msaunders@banyanschool.com
Mary Saunders, Director
Anna Rotonda, Plant Manager

5477 Caldwell College
Office of Disability Services
9 Ryerson Avenue
Caldwell, NJ 07006
973-618-3645
FAX 973-618-3488
http://www.caldwell.edu
e-mail: abenowitz@caldwell.edu
Abbe Benowitz, Coordinator

Four-year college that provides disability services to those students who are learnig disabled.

5478 Camden County College
PO Box 200
Blackwood, NJ 08012
856-227-7200
FAX 856-374-4975
http://www.camdencc.edu
e-mail: jkinzy@camdencc.edu
Joanne Kinzy, Coordinator
Phyllis Vecchia, President

A two-year college that provides services to the learning disabled.

5479 Centenary College: Office of Disability
Project ABLE
400 Jefferson Street
Hackettstown, NJ 07840
908-852-1400
FAX 908-813-1984
http://www.centenarycollege.edu
e-mail: zimdahj@centenarycollege.edu
Jeffery Zimdahl, Disability Services Director

5480 College of New Jersey
Office of Differing Disabilities
PO Box 7718
Ewing, NJ 08628
609-771-2571
FAX 609-637-5131
http://www.tcnj.edu/~wellness/disability/
e-mail: degennar@tcnj.edu
An DeGennaro, Director for Wellness
Terri Yamiolkowski, Coordinator

Four-year college provides services to students with disabilities.

5481 College of Saint Elizabeth
2 Convent Road
Morristown, NJ 07960
973-290-4000
http://www.cse.edu
Sr. MacNamee, Dean Studies

Offers a variety of services to students with disabilities including notetakers, extended testing time, counseling services, and special accommodations.

5482 Community High School
1135 Teaneck Road
Teaneck, NJ 07666
201-862-1796
FAX 201-862-1791
http://www.communityschool.org
e-mail: office@communityschool.us
Toby Barnstein, Education Director
Dennis Cohen, Program Director
Jim Steel, Principal
Complete college prep HS program for LD/ADD adolescent grades 9-12.

5483 Community School
11 W Forest Avenue
Teaneck, NJ 07666
201-837-8070
FAX 201-837-6799
http://www.communityschool.org
e-mail: office@communityschool.us
Rita Rowan, Executive Director
Dennis Cohen, Program Director

Comprehensive academic program for LD/ADD children grades K-8; NY and NJ funding available.

5484 Craig School
10 Tower Hill Road
Mountain Lakes, NJ 07046
973-334-7223
FAX 973-334-1299
http://www.craigschool.org
e-mail: jday@craigschool.org
Julie Day, Director Advancement
David Blanchard, Headmaster

A school for children with learning differences such as dyslexia, auditory processing issues and ADD.

5485 Cumberland County College
Project Assist
PO Box 1500
Vineland, NJ 08362
856-691-8600
FAX 856-690-0059
http://www.cccnj.net
e-mail: ssherd@cccnj.edu
Sandy Sherd, Director
Kenneth Ender, President

A two-year college that offers services to its learning disabled students.

5486 Elizabeth M. Boggs Center on DevelopmentalElizabeth M. Boggs Center on Developmental Disabilities
UMONJ - Robert Wood Johnson Medical School
PO Box 2688
New Brunswick, NJ 08903
732-235-9300
FAX 732-235-9330
http://www.rwjms.umdnj.edu/boggscenter
Deborah Spitalink, Director

The Elizabeth M. Boggs Center, as a University Center for Excellence in Developmental Disabilities, values uniqueness and individuality and promotes the self-determination and full participation of people with disabilities and their families in all aspects of community life. The Boggs Center prepares students through interdisciplinary programs, provides community training and technical assistance, conducts research, and disseminates information and educational materials.

5487 Fairleigh Dickinson University: Metropolitan Campus
1000 River Road
Teaneck, NJ 07666
201-692-2000
800-SDU-8803
FAX 201-692-2813
http://www.fdu.edu
Vincent Varrassi, Campus Director
Grace Hottinger, Admissions Coordinator
Dr. Mary Farrell PhD, University Director
Comprehensive support services to students with language based LD.

5488 Forum School
107 Wyckoff Avenue
Waldwick, NJ 07463
201-444-5882
FAX 201-444-4003
http://www.theforumschool.com
e-mail: forum@ultradsl.net /info@theforumschool.com
Steven Krapes, Executive Director
Linda Oliver, Office Manager

Day school for children through age 16 who have neurologically based developmental disabilities, including autism, ADHD, LD, and asperger syndrome. Services include extended year, speech, adaptive physical education, music, art therapy, and parent program.

5489 **Georgian Court College**
Learning Center
900 Lakewood Avenue
Lakewood, NJ 08701
732-364-2200
800-458-8422
FAX 732-987-2026
http://www.georgian.edu

Patricia Cohen, Director
Sister , President

Four-year college that offers services through the school learning center to students with disabilities.

5490 **Gloucester County College**
1400 Tanyard Road
Sewell, NJ 08080
856-468-0575
FAX 856-468-9462
TDY:856-468-8452
http://www.gccnj.edu
e-mail: dcook@gccnj.edu

Dennis Cook, Director Special Needs Services
Don Barger, Manager

The Office of Special Needs Services addresses supportive needs toward academic achievement for those students with documented disabilties such as learning disabled, visually impaired, hard of hearing and mobility impaired individuals.

5491 **Hudson County Community College**
25 Journal Square
Jersey City, NJ 07306
201-714-2229
FAX 201-963-0789
http://www.hudson.cc.nj.us

Ellen O'Shea, Coordinator
Patricial Reilly, Executive Director

Offers a variety of services to students with disabilities including note takers, extended testing time, counseling services, and special accommodations.

5492 **Jersey City State College**
2039 Kennedy Boulevard
Jersey City, NJ 07305
888-441-NJCU

Myrna Ehrlich MD, Director Project Mentor

Offers a variety of services to students with disabilities including notetakers, extended testing time, counseling services, and special accommodations.

5493 **Kean College of New Jersey**
Community Disabilities Services
1000 Morris Avenue
Union, NJ 07083
908-527-2000
FAX 908-737-5155
TDY:908-737-5156
http://www.kean.edu
e-mail: mpitts@coger.kean.edu

Roye-Ann Wallace, Director
Maria Pitts, Office Assistant

Operates a number of clinics, each of which may function interdisciplinarily to provide services, such as speech, audiology, psychology, reading, learning, social work and special education.

5494 **Kean University**
Community Disabilities Services
1000 Morris Avenue
Union, NJ 07083
908-527-2000
FAX 908-737-5155
TDY:908-737-5156
http://www.kean.edu
e-mail: mpitts@coger.kean.edu

Roye-Ann Wallace, Director
Maria Pitts, Office Assistant

Provides services to disabled students.

5495 **New Jersey City University**
2039 Kennedy Boulevard
Jersey City, NJ 07305
201-200-3426
877-652-8472
FAX 201-200-3141
http://www.njcu.edu

Jason Hand, Director
Carlos Hernandez, President

Provides students with learning disabilities a mentor, a teacher, advisor or a faculty member.

5496 **New Jersey Institute of Technology**
Counseling Center
University Heights
Newark, NJ 07102
973-596-3420
FAX 973-596-3419
http://www.njit.edu
e-mail: phyllis.colling@njit.edu

Phyllis Bolling Phd, Coordinator Disability Services

A public four-year college with 100 studentswith disabilities out of a total of 6,500.

5497 **Ocean County College**
College Drive
Toms River, NJ 08754
732-255-0400
TDY:732-255-0424
http://www.ocean.edu
e-mail: mreustle@ocean.edu

Maureen Reustle, PASS Director
Anne Hammond, PASS Counselor
Jon Larson, President

A regional resource center and comprehensive support center for college students with learning disabilities, offering a range of services including psycho-educational assessments, faculty/staff in-service training, program development assistance and consultation, and technical support. Individual and/or small group counseling is available, and vocational/career counseling on transition issues is also offered.

5498 **Princeton University**
303 W College
Princeton, NJ 08544
609-258-3000
FAX 609-258-1020
http://www.princeton.edu

Stephen Cochrane, Special Services
Christopher Eisgruber, CEO

Offers a variety of services to students with disabilities including note takers, extended testing time, counseling services, and special accommodations.

5499 **Project Connections**
Middlesex County College
PO Box 3050
Edison, NJ 08818
732-906-2561
FAX 732-906-7767
http://www.middlesex.cc.nj.us
e-mail: elizabeth_lowe@middlesex.edu

Elizabeth Lowe, Director LD Services
Elaine Weir-Daidone, Counselor
Lewis Ostar, Executive Director

Project Connections is a comprehensive academic and counseling service for students with learning disabilities who are enrolled in mainstream programs at Middlesex County College.

5500 **Ramapo College of New Jersey**
Office of Specialized Services
505 Ramapo Valley Road
Mahwah, NJ 07430
201-684-7514
FAX 201-684-7004
http://www.ramapo.edu/content/student.resources
e-mail: oss@ramapo.edu

Jean Balutanski, Director

Ramapo College demostated a strong commitment to providing equal access to all students through the removal of architectural and attitudinal barriers. Integration of qualified students with disabilities into college community has been the Ramapo way since the College opened in 1971.

5501 **Raritan Valley Community College**
PO Box 3300
Somerville, NJ 08876
908-526-1200
FAX 908-429-8589
http://www.raritanval.edu
Cathy Doyle, Disabilities Specialist
Jerry Ryan, Administrator

A public two-year college with 250 students with disabilities of a total of 6,000 per semster.

5502 **Richard Stockton College of New Jersey**
PO Box 195
Pomona, NJ 08240
609-652-4343
FAX 609-626-5550
http://www2.stockton.edu
e-mail: webmaster@stockton.edu
Thomasa Gonzale MD, Director Wellness Center
David Pinto, Manager

Offers a variety of services to students with disabilities including note takers, extended testing time, counseling services, and special accommodations.

5503 **Rider University**
2083 Lawrenceville Road
Lawrenceville, NJ 08648
609-896-5000
800-257-9026
FAX 609-895-6645
http://www.rider.edu
e-mail: dfox@rider.edu
Derek Fox, Assistant Director
Mordechai Rozanski, President

Four-year college that provides resources, programs and support for students with learning disabilities.

5504 **Rutgers Center for Cognitive Science**
152 Frelinghuysen Road
Piscataway, NJ 08854
732-445-0635
FAX 732-445-6715
http://www.ruccs.rutgers.edu
e-mail: admin@ruccs.rutgers.edu
Rochel Gelman, Co-Director
Charles Gallistel, Co-Director

A public four-year college with 2 special education students out of a total of 437.

5505 **Salem Community College**
460 Hollywood Avenue
Carneys Point, NJ 08069
856-299-2100
FAX 856-299-9193
http://www.salemcc.org
e-mail: SCCinfo@salemcc.org
Teresa Haman, Admissions Coordinator
Peter Contini, President

Offers a variety of services to students with disabilities including extended testing time, counseling services, and special accommodations.

5506 **Seton Hall University**
Seton Hall University
400 S Orange Avenue
South Orange, NJ 07079
973-761-9000
FAX 973-275-2040
http://www.shu.edu
e-mail: fraziera@shu.edu
Ray Frazier, Director
Susan Lasker MD, President

Student Support Services is an academic program that addresses the needs of students with disabilities.

5507 **Trenton State College**
2000 Pennington Road
Ewing, NJ 08618
609-771-1855
FAX 609-637-5174
http://www.tcnj.edu
e-mail: webmaster@tcnj.edu
Juneau Gary MD, Special Services
R. Gitenstein, President

A public four-year college with 24 special education students out of a total of 6,118.

5508 **William Paterson College of New Jersey**
Special Education Services
300 Pompton Road
Wayne, NJ 07470
973-720-2000
FAX 973-720-2910
http://www.wpunj.edu
e-mail: BOONES@wpunj.edu
Barbara Milne, Special Services Director
Sharon Lowry, Secretary
Arnold Speert, President
Offers a variety of services to students with disabilities including notetakers, extended testing time, counseling services, and special accommodations.

New Mexico

5509 **Albuquerque Technical Vocational Institute**
Special Services
525 Buena Vista Drive SE
Albuquerque, NM 87106
505-224-3259
FAX 505-224-3261
TDY:505-224-3262
http://www.tvi.edu
e-mail: pauls@tvi.edu
A Smarrella, Director Special Services
Yolanda Striplings, Administrative Support Specialis

Provides or coordinates services for students with all disabilities. For students with learning disabilities can arrange for special testing situations, notetaker/scribes, tape recorders, use of wordprocessors or other accommodations based on individual needs.

5510 **Brush Ranch School**
HC 73
Tererro, NM 87573
505-757-6114
FAX 505-757-6118
http://www.brushranchschool.org
e-mail: kaycrice@hotmail.com
Kay Rice MA, Head School
Ms. , Head Master
Suzie Weisman, Admissions Director
A co-educational boarding school for teens with learning differences. The school is fully licensed and accredited by both the New Mexico Board of Education and the North Central Association of Colleges and Schools. Situated on 283 acres in the Santa Fe National Forest, the school offers a wide range of educational and recreational opportunities.

5511 **Center for Development & Disability (CDD)**
University of New Mexico/School of Medicine
2300 Menaul Boulevard NE
Albuquerque, NM 87107
505-277-3365
FAX 505-272-5280
TDY:505-272-0321
http://www.cdd.unm.edu
e-mail: cdd@unm.edu
Cate McClain, Director
Melody Smith, Assistant Director
Elena Aguirre, Executive Director
The mission of the CDD is the full inclusion of people with disabilities and their families in their community by: enganging individuals in making life choices; partnering with communities to build resources; and improving systems of care.

5512 **College of Santa Fe**
1600 Saint Michaels Drive
Santa Fe, NM 87505
505-473-6574
FAX 505-473-6124
http://www.csf.edu
Tom Baumgartel, Director
Wabanang Kuczek, Manager

Provides services to the learning disabled.

5513 Eastern New Mexico University
Highway 70 Station 34
Portales, NM 88130
505-562-1011
FAX 505-562-2998
TDY:505-562-2280
http://www.enmu.edu
e-mail: bernita.davis@enmu.edu

Bernita Davis, Director
John Prater, Outreach Specialist
Steven Gamble, President
Four year college that provides programs for the learning disabled.

5514 Eastern New Mexico University: Roswell
PO Box 6000
Roswell, NM 88202
505-627-8400
FAX 505-624-7350
http://www.roswell.enmu.edu
e-mail: denise.mcghee@roswell.enmu.edu

Denise McGhee, Director Special Services
Peter Stoner, Assistant Director

A public two-year college with a total of 2500 students. Has a one year certificate program designed to teach vocational and life skills to individuals with significant cognitive impairments.

5515 Institute of American Indian Arts
PO Box 20007
Santa Fe, NM 87504
505-424-2300
FAX 505-988-6446

Karen Strong, Learning Resources

A public two-year college with 8 special education students out of a total of 237.

5516 New Mexico Institute of Mining and Technology
801 Leroy Pl
Socorro, NM 87801
505-835-5614
800-428-8324
FAX 505-835-5989
http://www.nmt.edu

Judith Raymond MD, Special Services
Dal Symes, Executive Director

A public four-year college with 5 special education students out of a total of 1,128.

5517 New Mexico Junior College
5317 N Lovington Highway
Hobbs, NM 88240
505-392-4510
800-657-6260
FAX 505-392-3668
http://www.nmjc.cc.nm.us

Marilyn Jackson, Dean Transitional Studies
Steve McCleery, President

A public two-year college with 170 special education students out of a total of 2,438.

5518 New Mexico State University
PO Box 30001
Las Cruces, NM 88003
505-646-1508
800-662-6678
FAX 505-646-5222
http://www.nmsu.edu
e-mail: admissions@nmsu.edu

John Irvin, Director
Michael Armendarez, Coordinator
Elizabeth Titus, Manager
A public four-year college with 230 registered students with disabilities out of a total of 12,922.

5519 Northern New Mexico Community College
1002 N Onate Street
Espanola, NM 87532
505-747-2100
FAX 505-747-2180
http://nnm.cc.nm.us

Millie Lowry, Special Services
Jose Griego, President

If you have a learning disability, support services include: reading class, readers of tests, notetakers, taped texts, tutoring, math class, recorders for classroom use, library assistance, extra time for tests, self-esteem counseling, resume assistance and kurzweil reading computers.

5520 San Juan College
4601 College Boulevard
Farmington, NM 87402
505-566-3530
FAX 505-566-3500
http://www.sjc.ccnm.us

Sandra Conner, Counselor
Ken Kernagis, Counseling Director
Pamela Drake, Executive Director
A public two-year college with 28 special education students out of a total of 3,654.

5521 University of New Mexico
Main Campus
Albuquerque, NM 87131
505-277-0111
FAX 505-277-7224
http://www.unm.edu
e-mail: lssunm@unm.edu

Patricia Useem, Manager
Louis Caldera, CEO

Offers a variety of services to students with disabilities including notetakers, extended testing time, counseling services, and special accommodations.

5522 University of New Mexico: Los Alamos Branch
4000 University Drive
Los Alamos, NM 87544
505-662-5919
800-894-5919
FAX 505-662-0344
http://www.la.unm.edu

Jay Ruybalid, Public Affairs Representative

Offers a variety of services to students with disabilities including notetakers, extended testing time, counseling services, and special accommodations.

5523 University of New Mexico: Valencia Campus
280 La Entrada Road
Los Lunas, NM 87031
505-925-8500
FAX 505-925-8501
http://www.unm.edu/~vc

Sharon DiMaria, Coordinator
Alice Letteney, Executive Director

A public two-year college with 57 special services students out of a total of 1,400.

5524 Western New Mexico University
PO Box 680
Silver City, NM 88062
505-538-6483
800-872-9668
FAX 505-538-6492
http://www.wnmu.edu

Karen Correa, Director

Offers a variety of services to students with disabilities including notetakers, extended testing time, counseling services, and special accommodations.

New York

5525 Academic Support Services
Ithaca College
322a Smiddy Hall
Ithaca, NY 14850
607-274-3011
FAX 607-274-3957
TDY:607-274-7319
http://www.ithaca.edu/acssd
e-mail: acssd@ithaca.edu

Leslie Schettino, Director
Linda Uhll, Assistant Director
Peggy Williams, President

5526 Adirondack Community College
640 Bay Road
Queensbury, NY 12804
518-743-2200
FAX 517-745-1433
http://www.crisny.org
e-mail: guyd@acc.sunyacc.edu
Deborah Guy, Director
Marshall Bishop, Manager

A two-year community college that provides services to the learning disabled.

5527 Albert Einstein College of Medicine
1165 Morris Park Avenue
Bronx, NY 10461
718-430-3840
FAX 718-430-3989
Mary Kelly PhD, Director
Jerome Kleinman, Manager

Provides evaluation and psychoeducational treatment to children and adults of normal intelligence, 21 years or older, who have serious reading difficulties.

5528 Alfred University
Special Academic Services
Saxon Drive
Alfred, NY 14802
607-871-2148
800-425-3733
FAX 607-871-3014
http://www.alfred.edu
e-mail: sdstagg@alfred.edu
Terry Taggart, Director
Beth Niles, Secretary

Special Academic Services provides support services, consultation and advocacy for students with learning, physical and/or psychological disabilities. Services for persons with disabilities shall complement and support, but not duplicate, the University's regular existing services and programs.

5529 Bank Street College: Graduate School of Education
610 W 1112th Street
New York, NY 10025
212-875-4404
FAX 212-875-4678
http://www.bnkst.edu/html/grad_ad/
e-mail: GradCourses@bnkst.edu
Augusta Kappner, President
Frank Naura, Vice President

For learning disabled college students who are highly motivated to become teachers of children and youth with learning problems and who wish to earn a masters degree in Special Education.

5530 Binghamton University
PO Box 6000
Binghamton, NY 13902
607-777-2171
FAX 607-777-6893
TDY:607-777-2686
http://www.binghamton.edu
e-mail: bjfairba@binghamton.edu
B. Fairbairn, Svcs Students w/Disability Dir.
Bethany Beecher, LD Specialist
Cheryl Brown, Administrator
Provides assistance to BU students with physical, learning or other disabilities.

5531 Bramson Ort Technical Institute
6930 Austin Street
Forest Hills, NY 11375
718-261-5800
FAX 718-575-5118
http://www.bramsonort.org
e-mail: rbaskin@bramsonort.org
Ephraim Buhks, Executive Director
Rivka Burkos, Librarian
Aron Reznikoss, Job Placement
Offers a variety of services to students with disabilities including notetakers, extended testing time, counseling services, and special accommodations.

5532 Broome Community College
PO Box 1017
Binghamton, NY 13902
607-778-5000
FAX 607-778-5662
http://www.sunybroome.edu
e-mail: bpomeroy@sunybroome.edu
Bruce Pomeroy, Director
Laurence Spraggs, President

A public two-year college providing services to approximately 75-125 students with learning disabilities per school year. Services include note taking, tutoring, an LD specialist, adaptive educational equipment, testing services, and other appropriate support as based on documentation of need.

5533 CUNY Queensborough Community College
22205 56th Avenue
Oakland Gardens, NY 11364
718-631-6262
FAX 718-229-1733
http://www.qcc.cuny.edu
Barbara Bookman, Director
Susan Curtis, Marketing Executive

The Office of Services for Students with Disabilities (Science Building, Room 132) offers special assistance and couseling to students with specific needs. The services offered include academic, vocational, psychological and rehabilitation counseling, as well as liasion with community social agencies.

5534 Canisius College
Disability Support Service
2001 Main Street
Buffalo, NY 14208
716-888-3748
FAX 716-888-3747
TDY:716-888-3748
http://www.canisius.edu
e-mail: dobies@canisius.edu
Anne Dobies, Director
Dan Norton, Graduate Assistant

Four-year college offering services to students with physical and cognitive disabilities.

5535 Cazenovia College
22 Sullivan Street
Cazenovia, NY 13035
315-655-7000
800-654-3210
FAX 315-655-4860
http://www.cazenovia.edu
e-mail: cazenovia@cazenovia.edu
Cyndi Pratt, Special Services
Jesse Lott, Director

An independent college with a significant number of special education students.

5536 Colgate University
Office Disabilities Services
13 Oak Drive
Hamilton, NY 13346
315-228-7225
FAX 315-228-7831
http://www.colgate.edu
e-mail: admission@mail.colgate.edu
Lynn Waldman, Director

Provides for a small body of liberal arts education that will expand individual potential and ability to particpate effectively in the society.

5537 College of Aeronautics
Academic Support Services
8601 23rd Avenue
East Elmhurst, NY 11369
718-429-6600
FAX 718-505-0667
http://www.aero.edu
e-mail: mcpartland@aero.edu
Sharon McPartland, Coordinator
Joann Jayne, Manager

College offering support services to its learning disabled students.

5538 College of New Rochelle: New Resources Division
Student Services
29 Castle Place
New Rochelle, NY 10805
914-654-5000
800-933-5923
FAX 914-654-5866
http://www.cnr.edu
e-mail: info@cnr.edu

Joan Bristol, VP Student Services
Stephen Sweeny, President

Offers a variety of services to students with disabilities including notetakers, extended testing time, counseling services, and special accommodations.

5539 College of Saint Rose
432 Western Avenue
Albany, NY 12203
518-454-5111
FAX 518-458-5330
http://www.strose.edu
e-mail: hermannk@strose.edu

Kelly Hermann, Coordinator Special Services
Kimberly Lamparelli, Manager

Four year college that provides disabled students with services and support.

5540 College of Staten Island of the City University of New York
2800 Victory Boulevard
Staten Island, NY 10314
718-982-4012
FAX 718-982-2117
TDY:718-982-2515
http://www.csi.cuny.edu
e-mail: venditti@postbox.csi.cuny.edu

Margaret Venditti, Director
Wilma Jones, Manager

A public four-year college with 33 special education students out of a total of 11,136. Priority registration, test accommodations and tutoring.

5541 Columbia College
Disability Services
2920 Broadway
New York, NY 10027
212-730-7500
FAX 212-854-3448
http://www.columbia.edu
e-mail: disability@columbia.edu

Susan Cheer, Director
Colleen Lewis, Program Coordinator

Four-year college that offers disability services to its students.

5542 Columbia-Greene Community College
4400 State Route 23
Hudson, NY 12534
518-828-4181
FAX 518-822-2015
http://www3.sunycgcc.edu

Sheri Bolevice, LD Specialist
Pat Nobes, Alternative Learning
James Campion, President

A public two-year college in upstate New York with an enrollment of about 1,800. Services available to students with a documented learning disability include various academic accommodations, peer tutoring and academic counselling. Six developmental courses are offered in reading, math, English, and study skills.

5543 Concordia College: New York
Connections
171 White Plains Road
Bronxville, NY 10708
914-337-9300
FAX 914-395-4500
http://www.concordia-ny.edu
e-mail: ghg@concordia-ny.edu

George Groth, Connection Program Director
Michael Weschler, Assistant Director
Kathleen Suss, Administrator

5544 Cornell University
Student Disability Services
420 C-CC Garden Avenue Extension
Ithaca, NY 14853
607-255-6310
FAX 607-255-1562
TDY:607-255-7665
http://www.cornell.edu
e-mail: cornell-clt@cornell.edu

Helene Selco, Director
Nancy Jerabek, Office Manager

Cornell University is committed to ensuring that students with disabilities have equal access to all university programs and activities. Policy and procedures have been developed to provide students with as much independence as possible, to preserve confidentiality, and to provide students with disabilities the same exceptional opportunities available to all Cornell students.

5545 Corning Community College
1 Academic Drive
Corning, NY 14830
607-962-9011
800-358-7171
FAX 607-962-9006
TDY:607-962-9459
http://www.corning-cc.edu
e-mail: northop@corning-cc.edu

Judy Northrop, Coordinator Student Disability
Floyd Amann, Administrator
Sherry White, Typist

A public two-year community college. There are approximately 100 LD students out of a student body of 4,500. A variety of services are available to students with LD, including specialized advising and registration, individualized tutoring, academic advisoring, and accommodations. Also on campus: Kurzweil reading machines, voice activated word processing, etc.

5546 Dowling CollegeProgram for Potentially Gifted College Students with
Learning Disabilities
150 Idle Hour Boulevard
Oakdale, NY 11769
631-244-3306
FAX 631-244-5036
http://www.dowling.edu
e-mail: strached@dowling.edu

Dorothy Stracher, Program Director
MK Schneid, Assistant Director

Academic program to help college students with LD develop strategies for success. They work one-on-one with graduate students.

5547 Dutchess Community College
53 Pendell Road
Poughkeepsie, NY 12601
845-431-8000
800-378-9707
FAX 845-471-4869
http://www.sunydutchess.edu
e-mail: webmaster@sunydutchess.edu

D. Conklin, President

A public two-year college with 45 special education students out of a total of 7,511.

5548 Erie Community College: South Campus
Special Education Department
4041 SW Boulevard
Orchard Park, NY 14127
716-648-5400
FAX 716-851-1629
TDY:716-851-1831
http://www.ecc.edu
e-mail: adamsjm@ecc.edu

Nancy Bailey, Counselor
William Reuter, CEO

A public two-year college with 200 special education students out of a total of 3,455.

5549 Farmingdale State University
2350 Broadhollow Road
Farmingdale, NY 11735
631-420-2000
FAX 631-420-2689
TDY:631-420-2623
http://www.farmingdale.edu
e-mail: dss@farmingdale.edu
Malka Edelman NCC MCC CRC, Director
Kim Birnholz CRC, Counselor
Jonathan Gibralter, President
Our services are designed to meet the unique educational needs of currently enrolled students with documented permanent or temporary disabilities. The Office of Support Services is dedicated to the principle that equal opportunity be afforded each student to realize his/her fullest potential.

5550 Finger Lakes Community College
4355 Lakeshore Drive
Canandaigua, NY 14424
585-394-9444
FAX 585-394-5005
http://www.fingerlakes.edu
e-mail: admissions@flcc.edu
Patricia Malinowski, Chairperson of the Developmental
Daniel Hayes, President

Provides services such as pre-admission counseling, academic advisement, tutorials, computer assistance, workshops, peer counseling and support groups. The college does not offer a formal program but aids students in arranging appropriate accommodations.

5551 Fordham University
Disabled Student Services
Keating Hall
Bronx, NY 10458
718-817-4700
FAX 718-817-3735
TDY:718-817-0655
http://www.fordham.edu
e-mail: disabilityservices@fordham.edu
Cristina Bertisch, Director

The Office of Disability Services collaborates with students, faculty and staff to ensure appropriate services for students with disabilities. The University will make reasonable acccommodations, and provide appropriate aids.

5552 Fulton-Montgomery Community College
2805 State Highway 67
Johnstown, NY 12095
518-762-4651
FAX 518-762-4334
http://www.fmcc.suny.edu
e-mail: efosmire@fmcc.suny.edu
Ellie Fosmire, Coordinator

A public two-year college with 76 special education students out of a total of 1,748.

5553 Genesee Community College
SUNY (State University of New York) Systems
1 College Road
Batavia, NY 14020
585-343-0055
FAX 716-343-4541
http://www.genessee.edu
e-mail: admissions@genesee.suny.edu
Karol Shallowhorn, Director
Stephanie Smythe, Counselor
Stuart Steiner, President
A public two-year college with 78 special education students out of a total of 3,212.

5554 Gow School
Gow School
PO Box 85
South Wales, NY 14139
716-652-3450
FAX 716-687-2003
http://www.gow.org
e-mail: admissions@gow.org
M. Rogers Jr., Headmaster
Robert Garcia, Admissions Director
Bradley Rogers, Prinicpal
The nation's oldest college preparatory school for young men (grades 7-12) with dyslexia/language based learning differences. The 100 acre residential campus is located in upstate New York. Co-Ed summer program for ages 8-16.

5555 Hamilton College
198 College Hill Road
Clinton, NY 13323
315-859-4011
FAX 315-859-4077
TDY:315-859-4294
http://www.hamilton.edu
e-mail: rbellmay@hamilton.edu
Roxanne Bellmay-Campdell, Associate Dean
Louise Peckingham, Compliance Officer
Joan Stewart, President
Four year college that offfers services for learning disabled students.

5556 Herkimer County Community College
100 Reservoir Road
Herkimer, NY 13350
315-369-2814
FAX 315-866-7253
TDY:888- GO4HCCC
http://www.hccc.ntcnet.com
e-mail: coylemf@hcc.suny.edu
Michele Weaver, LD Specialist
Suzanne Paddock, Counselor
Linda Veigh, Administrator
A public two-year college with approximately 200 documented disabled students. Tuition and fees: $2,450 (annual basis); overall enrollment 95-96: $2,445 (1,857 full time/588 part-time).

5557 Hofstra University
Program for Academic Learning Skills
214 Roosevelt Hall
Hempstead, NY 11549
516-463-5761
FAX 516-463-4049
http://www.hofstra.edu
e-mail: suslzdchofstra.edu
Linda DeMotta, Director

Provides auxillary aids and compensatory services to certified learning disabled students who have been accepted to the University through regular admissions. These services are provided free of charge.

5558 Houghton College
Student Academic Services
1 Willard Avenue
Houghton, NY 14744
585-567-9239
FAX 585-567-9570
http://www.houghton.edu
e-mail: shice@houghton.edu
Susan Hice MD, Director
Irene Willis, Student Academic Services Direct

Four year college that provides academic support to disabled students.

5559 Hudson Valley Community College
Disabilities Resource Center
80 Vandenburgh Avenue
Troy, NY 12180
518-629-7154
FAX 518-629-4831
TDY:518-629-7596
http://www.hvcc.edu
e-mail: editor@hvcc.edu
Pablo Negron, Director

A public two-year college with 28 special education students out of a total of 10,106.

5560 Hunter College of the City University of New York
Office for Students with Disabilities
Hunter E 1119
New York, NY 10021
212-772-4824
FAX 212-650-3456
http://www.hunter.cuny.edu
Sandra LaPorta, Director

Provides services to over 250 students with learning disabilities. A learning disability is a disorder in one or more of the basic psychological processes involved in understanding or in using spoken or written language.

5561 Iona College: College Assistance Program
715 N Avenue
New Rochelle, NY 10801
914-633-2000
800-231-4662
FAX 914-633-2011
http://www.iona.edu
e-mail: lrobertello@iona.edu
Linda Robertello, Director
Regina Carlo, Assistant Director
James Liguori, Administrator
Offers a comprehensive support program for students with learning disabilities. CAP is designed to encourage success by providing instruction tailored to individual strenghts and needs.

5562 Ithaca College: Speech and Hearing Clinic
Smiddy Hall
Ithaca, NY 14850
607-274-3714
FAX 607-274-1137
http://www.ir.tompkins.ny.us/beOra7du.htm
Richard Schissel

Offers a variety of services to students with disabilities including notetakers, extended testing time, counseling services, and special accommodations.

5563 Jamestown Community College
State University of New York Systems
PO Box 20
Jamestown, NY 14702
716-665-5220
800-388-8557
FAX 716-665-9110
http://www.sunyjcc.edu
e-mail: admissions@mail.sunyjcc.edu
Nancy Callahan, Disability Support
Gregory Cinque, President

A public two-year college with 41 special education students out of a total of 4,541.

5564 Jefferson Community College
Jefferson Community College
Coffeen Street
Watertown, NY 13601
315-786-2200
888-435-6522
http://www.sunyjefferson.edu
e-mail: strainham@sunyjefferson.edu
Sheree Trainham, Learning Skills/Disability
Joseph Olson, President

A public two-year college whose focus is teaching and learning. Thr ough educational excellence, innovative services and community partnerships. Jefferson advances the quality of life of our students and community.

5565 John Jay College of Criminal Justice of the City University of New York
445 W 59th Street
New York, NY 10019
212-237-8000
FAX 212-237-8777
TDY:212-237-8233
http://www.jjay.cuny.edu
e-mail: admiss@jjay.cuny.edu
Farris Forsythe, Coordinator
John Teravis, President

An independent two-year college with 67 special education students out of a total of 7,912.

5566 Kildonan School
425 Morse Hill Road
Amenia, NY 12501
845-373-8111
FAX 845-373-9793
http://www.kildonan.org
e-mail: rwilson@kildonan.org
Ronald Wilson, Principal
Joseph Ruggiero, Academic Dean
Offers a fully accredited college preparatory curriculum. The school is co-educational, enrolling boarding students in Grades 6-Postgraduate and day students in Grade 2-Postgraduate. Provides daily one-on-one Orton-Gillingham tutoring to build skills in reading, writing, and spelling. Daily independent reading and writing work reinforces skills and improves study habits. Interscholastic sports, horseback riding, clubs and community service enhance self-confidence.

5567 Learning Disabilities Program
ADELPHI UNIVERSITY
Adelphi University
Garden City, NY 11530
516-877-3455
800-233-5144
FAX 516-877-4711
http://www.academics.adelphi.edu/ldprog
e-mail: LDprogram@adelphi.com /Ldprogram@adelphi.edu
Susan Spencer, Assistant Dean/Director
Janet Cohen, Assistant Director
Angelo Proto, Administrative Executive
The programs professional staff, all with advanced degrees, provide individual tutoring and counseling to learning disabled students who are completely mainstream in the University.

5568 Long Island University: CW Post Campus
Learning Support Ctr - Academic Resource Program
720 N Boulevard
Greenvale, NY 11548
516-299-3057
FAX 516-299-2126
http://www.cwpost.liu.edu/cwis/cwp/
e-mail: srock@liu.edu
Susan Rock, Director
Marie Fatscher, Associate Director

5569 Manhattan College
4513 Manhattan College Parkway
Bronx, NY 10471
718-862-8000
FAX 718-862-7808
http://www.manhattan.edu/sprscent/index.html
e-mail: rpollack@manhattan.edu
Ross EdD, Director
Thomas Scanlan, President

The Specialized Resource Center serves all students with special needs including individuals with temporary disabilities, such as those resulting from injury or surgery. The mission of the center is to ensure educational opportunity for all students with special needs by providing access to full participation in all aspects of the campus life.

5570 Manhattanville College
Higher Education Learning Program
2900 Purchase Street
Purchase, NY 10577
914-323-5313
FAX 914-323-5493
http://www.mville.edu
e-mail: admissions@manhattanville.edu
Eleanor Shwortz, Coordinator

Students preparing for a career in Special Education learns the full spectrum of physical, emotional, and mental challenges faced by people.

5571 Maria College
700 New Scotland Avenue
Albany, NY 12208
518-438-3111
FAX 518-438-7170
http://www.mariacollege.edu
e-mail: laurieg@mariacollege.edu
Margie Byrd, Dean
Mary Riker, Contact

An independent two-year college with 13 special education students out of a total of 875.

5572 Marist College
Learning Disabilities Support Program
3399 N Road
Poughkeepsie, NY 12601
845-575-3274
800-436-5483
FAX 845-575-3011
http://www.marist.edu
e-mail: specserv@marist.edu

Linda Cooper, Director
Deborah Reeves-Duncan, Councilor

Provides a comprehensive range of academic support services and accommodations which promote the full integration of students with disabilities into the mainstream college environment.

5573 Marymount Manhattan College

221 E 71st Street
New York, NY 10021
212-517-0430
FAX 212-517-0541
http://www.marymount.mmm.edu
e-mail: jbonomo@mmm.edu

Jaquelyn Bonomo MD, Assistant Director
Ann Jablon, Director
Judson Shaver, President

An independent four-year college with 25 learning disabled students out of a total of 1,700. There is an additional fee for the learning disabled education program in addition to the regular tuition.

5574 Medaille College

Disability Services Department
18 Agassiz Circle
Buffalo, NY 14214
716-884-3281
800-292-1582
FAX 716-884-0291
http://www.medaille.edu
e-mail: jmatheny@medaille.edu

Lisa Morisson, Director
Joseph Bascuas, President

Offers a variety of services to students with disabilities including notetakers, extended testing time, counseling services, and special accommodations.

5575 Mercy College

Star Program
555 Broadway
Dobbs Ferry, NY 10522
914-674-7218
FAX 914-674-7410
http://www.mercynet.edu
e-mail: admissions@merlin.mercynet.edu

Terry Rich, Director

Helps people with learning disabilities.

5576 Mohawk Valley Community College

1101 Sherman Drive
Utica, NY 13501
315-792-5400
FAX 315-731-5868
TDY:315-792-5413
http://www.mvcc.edu
e-mail: dowsland@mvcc.edu

Wendy Dowsland, Learning Disabilities Specialist
Lynn Igoe, Students w/Disabilities Coord.
Michael Schafer, President

MVCC'S LD program is staffed by a half time LD specialist. Service provided to students with learning disabilities include advocacy, information and referral to on and off campus services, testing accommodations, taped materials, loaner tape recorders and note takers.

5577 Molloy College

PO Box 5002
Rockville Centre, NY 11571
516-678-5000
888-4MALLOY
FAX 516-678-2284
http://www.molloy.edu
e-mail: tforker@molloy.edu

Therese Forker, STEEP Director
Barbara Nirrengarten, Assistant Director
Drew Bogner, President

STEEP (Success Through Expanded Education), is a program specifically designed to assist students with learning disabilities and enable them to become successful students. The program offers the student the opportunities to learn techniques which alleviate some of their problems. Special emphasis is directed toward the development of positive self-esteem.

5578 Nassau Community College

Disabled Support Department
1 Education Drive
Garden City, NY 11530
516-572-7241
FAX 516-572-9874
http://www.ncc.edu
e-mail: schimsj@ncc.edu

Janis Schimsky, Director Students w/Disabilities

Our goal is to help students achieve success while they are attending Nassau Community College by learning to become their own advocates through talking with their professors about their disability and the accommodations they need for the course.

5579 Nazareth College of Rochester

Disability Support Services
4245 E Avenue
Rochester, NY 14618
585-586-2452
FAX 716-586-2452
http://www.naz.edu
e-mail: avhouse@naz.edu

Annemarie House, Counselor

Four-year college that offers students with a learning disablility support and services.

5580 New York City College of Technology

Student Support Services Program
300 Jay Street
Brooklyn, NY 11201
718-260-5143
FAX 718-254-8539
http://www.citytech.cuny.edu/students/support
e-mail: ffogelman@citytech.cuny.edu

Faith Fogelman, Director

The Student Support Services Program, located in A-237, provides comprehensive services to students with disabilities. The array of interventions includes counseling, tutorials, workshops, use of computer lab with adaptive software, testing accommodations, sign-language interpreters, captioning, and implementation of accommodations as per documentation.

5581 New York Institute of Technology: OldWestbury

PO Box 8000
Old Westbury, NY 11568
516-686-7555
800-345-NYIT
FAX 516-686-7613
http://www.nyit.edu
e-mail: eguillano@nyit.edu

Edward Guiliano, President
Alexandra Logue PhD, VP Academic Affairs

Offers the Vocational Independence Progran for students who have significant learning disabilities.

5582 New York University

Henry and Lucy Moses Center
240 Greene Street
New York, NY 10003
212-998-4980
FAX 212-995-4114
http://www.nyu.edu/csd
e-mail: lc83@nyu.edu

Lakshmi Clark MA, CSD Coordinator
Scott Hornack, Contact

The Henry and Lucy Moses Center for Students with Disabilities (CSD) functions to determine qualified disability status and to assist students in obtaining appropriate accommodations and services. CSD operates according to the Independent Living Philosophy, and thus strives in its policies and practices to empower each student to become an independent as possible. Our services are designed to encourage independence, backed by a strong system of supports.

5583 New York University Medical Center: Learning Diagnostic Program

400 E 34th Street
New York, NY 10016
212-263-7149
FAX 212-263-7721

Ruth MD, Professor Clinical Neurology
Becky Chow, Assistant Professor
Larry Chinitz MD, President

Assessment team, neurology, neuro-psychology, psychiatry services are offered.

5584 Niagara County Community College
3111 Saunders Settlement Road
Sanborn, NY 14132
716-278-8150
FAX 716-614-6700
http://www.niagaracc.suny.edu
Karen Drilling, Disabled Student Services
James Klyczek, President

The College provides reasonable accommodations for students with disabilties, including those with specific learning disabilities. Students with learning disabilities must provide documentation by a qualified professional that proves thry are eligible for accommodations.

5585 Niagara University
Support Services Department
Seton Hall, 1st Floor
Niagara University, NY 14109
716-286-8076
800-462-2111
FAX 716-286-8063
http://www.niagara.edu
e-mail: ds@niagara.edu
Diane Stoelting, Specialized Support Services

Reasonable accommodations are provided to students with disabilities based on documentation of disability. Depending on how the disability impacts the individual, reasonable accommodations may include extended time on tests taken in a separate location with appropriate assistance, notetakes or use of a tape recorder in class, interpreter, textbooks and course materials in alternative format, as well as other academic and non-academic accommodations.

5586 Norman Howard School
275 Pinnacle Road
Rochester, NY 14623
585-334-8010
FAX 585-334-8073
http://www.normanhoward.org
e-mail: info@normanhoward.org
Julie Murray, Associate Dir Admissions/Events

5587 North Country Community College
State University Of New York SUNY Systems
23 Santanoni Avenue
Saranac Lake, NY 12983
518-891-2915
888-879-6222
FAX 518-891-0898
http://www.nccc.edu
e-mail: admissions@nccc.edu
Jeannine Golden, Learning Lab/Malone
Scott Lambert, Enrollment/Financial Aid Counsel
Gail Rodgers-Rice, President
Located in the Adirondack Olympic Region of northern New York, NCCC is committed to providing a challenging and supportive environment where the aspirations of all can be realized. The college provides a variety of services for students with special needs which includes: specialized advisement, tutors and supplemental instruction, specialized accommodations, technology and equipment to accommodate learning disabilities and other resources.

5588 Onondaga Community College
Services for Students with Special Needs
4941 Onondaga Road
Syracuse, NY 13215
315-498-2622
FAX 315-498-2107
http://www.sunyocc.edu
e-mail: occinfo@sunyocc.edu
Linda Koslowsky, Administrative Aids

A public two-year college with 203 special education students out of a total of 8,393.

5589 Orange County Community College
115 S Street
Middletown, NY 10940
845-344-6222
FAX 845-342-8662
http://www.sunyorange.edu
Marilynn Brake, Special Services Coordinator
Bill Richards, President

The Office of Special Services for the Disabled provides support services to meet the individual needs of students with disabilities. Such accommodations include oral testing, extended time testing, tape recorded textbooks, writing lab, note-takers and others. Pre-admission counseling ensures accessibility for the qualified student.

5590 Purchase College State University of New York
Special Services Office
735 Anderson Hill Road
Purchase, NY 10577
914-251-6390
FAX 914-251-6399
http://www.purchase.edu
Ronnie Mait, Coordinator Office Special Svcs
Donna Siegmann, Coordinator Supported Education

Offers a variety of services to students with disabilities including note takers, extended testing time, counseling services, and special accommodations.

5591 Queens College City University of New York
Special Services Office
6530 Kissena Boulevard
Flushing, NY 11367
718-997-5000
FAX 718-997-5895
TDY:718-997-5870
http://www.qc.edu
e-mail: christopher_rosa@qc.edu
Christopher Rosa, Office Director

Services include tutoring and notetaking, accommodating testing alternatives, counseling, academic and vocational advisement, as well as diagnostic assessments in order to pinpoint specific deficits.

5592 Rensselaer Polytechnic Institute
110 8th Street
Troy, NY 12180
518-276-2764
800-448-6562
FAX 518-276-4839
http://www.rpi.edu
e-mail: hamild@rpi.edu
Debra Hamilton, Disabled Student Services

An independent four-year college with 53 learning disabled students out of a total of 6,000.

5593 Rochester Business Institute
1630 Portland Avenue
Rochester, NY 14621
585-266-0430
888-741-4271
FAX 585-266-8243
http://www.rochester-institute.com
e-mail: dpfluke@cci.edu
Deanna Fluke, Admissions Director
Jim Rodriguez, Admissions Representative
Carl Silvio, President
An independent two-year college with 12 special education students out of a total of 528.

5594 Rochester Institute of Technology
28 Lomb Memorial Drive
Rochester, NY 14623
585-475-2411
FAX 585-475-2215
http://www.rit.edu
e-mail: smacst@rit.edu
Lisa Fraser, Chair Learning Support Services
Pamela Lloyd, Disability Services Coordinator
Albert Simone, President
An independent four-year college offers a wide variety of accommodations and support services to students with documented disabilities.

5595 Rockland Community College
145 College Road
Suffern, NY 10901
845-574-4000
FAX 845-574-4462
Marge Zemek, Learning Disabilities Specialist
Cliff Wood, President

A public two-year college with 300 special education students out of a total of 5,500. The office of Disability Services provides a variety of support services tailored to meet the individual needs and learning styles of students with documented learning disabilities.

5596 Rose F Kennedy Center

Albert Einstein College of Medicine
1410 Pelham Parkway S
Bronx, NY 10461
718-430-3543
FAX 718-904-1162
http://www.aecom.yu.edu/cerc
e-mail: cerc@aecom.yu.edu
Herbert Cohen MD, Director

Mission is to help children with disabilities reach their full potential and to support parents in their efforts to get the best care, education, and treatment for their children.

5597 SUNY Canton

34 Cornell Drive
Canton, NY 13617
315-386-7392
FAX 315-379-3877
TDY:315-386-7943
http://www.canton.edu
e-mail: leev@canton.edu
Veigh Mehan Lee, DSS Coordinator
Heather Lauzon, Office Assistant

Four year state college that provides resources and services to learning disabled students.

5598 SUNY Cobleskill

Disability Support Center
RR 7
Cobleskill, NY 12043
518-255-5282
800-295-8988
FAX 518-255-6430
TDY:518-255-5454
http://www.cobleskill.edu
e-mail: Johnsok@Cobleskill.edu /
Lynn Abarno, Coordinator Support Services

A public two-year college with a Bachelor of Technology component in agriculture. Approximately 170 students identify themselves as having a learning disability out of the 2,000 total population. Tuition $3,500 in state/$8,300 out of state. Academic support services and accommodations for documented LD students.

5599 SUNY Institute of Technology: Utica/Rome

PO Box 3050
Utica, NY 13504
315-792-7500
866-278-6948
FAX 315-792-7837
http://www.sunyit.edu
e-mail: admissions@sunyit.edu
Marybeth Lyonsvan, Interim Director Admissions
Tat Saranr, Business Office Secretary

Upper division bachelor's degree in a variety of professional and technical majors; masters degree and continuing educational coursework is also available.

5600 Sage College

140 New Scotland Avenue
Albany, NY 12214
518-292-8624
FAX 578-292-1910
http://www.sage.edu
e-mail: chowed@sage.edu
David Chowenhill, Director

Four year college that offers services to students with a learning disability.

5601 Schenectady County Community College

Disability Services Department
78 Washington Avenue
Schenectady, NY 12305
518-381-1366
FAX 518-346-0379
http://www.sunysccc.edu
Tom Dotson, Coordinator

Access for All program is designed to make programs and facilities accessible to all students in pursuit of their academic goals. Disabled Student Services seeks to ensure accessible educational opportunities in accordance with individual needs. Offers general support services and program services such as: exam assistance, special scheduling, adaptive equipment, readers, taping assistance and more.

5602 Services for Students with Disabilities

Binghamton University
PO Box 6000
Binghamton, NY 13902
607-777-2171
FAX 607-777-6893
TDY:607-777-2686
http://www.binghamton.edu
e-mail: bjfairba@binghamton.edu
B. Fairbairn, Director
Janice Beecher, LD Specialist
Cheryl Brown, Administrator
Provides a wide range of support services to Binghamton University students with physical learning or other disabilities.

5603 Siena College

515 Loudon Road
Loudonville, NY 12211
518-783-2300
888-ATSIENA
http://www.siena.edu
e-mail: jpellegrini@siena.edu
Juliet Pellegrini, Services for Student Director
Kevin Mackin, Administrator

Four year college that offers programs for the learning disabled.

5604 St Thomas Aquinas College

Pathways
125 Route 340
Sparkill, NY 10976
845-398-4230
FAX 845-398-4229
http://www.stac.edu
e-mail: pathways@stac.edu
Richard Heath MD, Director
Amelia DeMarco MD, Associate Director

Comprehensive support program for selected college students with learning disabilites and/or ADHD. Services include individual professional mentoring, study groups, academic counseling, priority registration, assistive technology, and a specialized summer program prior to the first semester.

5605 St. Bonaventure University

Teaching & Learning Center
Room 26, Doyle Hall
St Bonaventure, NY 14778
716-375-2066
800-462-5050
FAX 716-375-2072
http://www.sbu.edu
e-mail: nmatthew@sbu.edu
Nancy Matthews, Coordinator

Catholic University in the Franciscan tradition. Independent coeducational institution offering programs through its schools of arts and sciences, business administration, education and journalism and mass communication. 2500 students, tuition $16,210, room and board $6,190.

5606 St. Lawrence University

23 Romoda Drive
Canton, NY 13617
315-229-5011
FAX 315-229-7453
http://www.stlawu.edu
e-mail: jmeagher@mail.stlawu.edu
John Meagher, Director
Liv Regosin, Director of Advising
Daniel Sullivan, President
The Office of Special Needs is here to ensure that all students with disabilities can freely and actively participate in all facets of University life, to coordinate support services and programs that enable students with disabilities to reach their educational potential, and to increase the level of awareness among all members of the University so that students with disabilites are able to perform at a level limited only by their abilities, not their disabilities.

5607 State University of New York College Technology at Delhi
109 Bush Hall
Delhi, NY 13753
607-746-4593
800-96-DELHI
FAX 607-746-4004
http://www.delhi.edu
e-mail: weinbell@delhi.edu
Linda Weinberg, Disabilities Coordinator
Candace , President

Provide services for students with disabilities. Alternate test-taking arrangements, adapted equipment, assistive technology, accessibility information, note taking services, reading services, tutorial assistance, interpreting services, accessble parking and elevators, sounseling, guidance and support, refferral information and advocacy services, workshops and support groups.

5608 State University of New York College at Brockport
State University Of New York SUNY Systems
350 New Campus Drive
Brockport, NY 14420
585-395-5409
800-382-8447
FAX 585-395-5291
TDY:585-395-5409
http://www.brockport.edu
e-mail: osdoffic@brockport.edu
Maryellen Post, Coordinator

Provides support and assistance to students with medical, physical, emotional or learning disabilities, specially those experiencing problems in areas such as academic environment.

5609 State University of New York College of Agriculture and Technology
Cobleskill, NY 12043
518-255-5841
800-295-8988
FAX 518-255-6430
TDY:518-255-5454
http://www.cobleskill.edu
e-mail: labarno@cobleskill.edu
Lynn Abarno, Support Services Coordinator
Pat Sprage, Assistant
Nancy Deusen, Executive Director
The primary objective is to develop and maintain a supportive campus environment that promotes academic achievement and personal growth for students with disabilities. Services provide by the office are based on each student's documentation and are tailored to each student's unique individual needs.

5610 State University of New York: Albany
1400 Washington Avenue
Albany, NY 12222
518-442-5566
FAX 518-442-5589
TDY:518-442-3366
http://www.albany.edu
e-mail: cmalloch@uamail.albany.edu
Carolyn Malloch, Learning Disabilities Specialist

The University at Albany offers a wide array of advocacy and support services for students with learning disabilities. We also have a Writing Center, a Center for Computing and Disability, Comprehensive Academic Support Services (tutors, study groups, academic mentoring, study skills workshops). These are excellent resources for LD students. Services include extended time on testing, advocacy with faculty, diagnostic testing, advising and consultation. One week summer transition program offered.

5611 State University of New York: Buffalo
Special Services Department
1300 Elmwood Avenue
Buffalo, NY 14260
716-645-4500
FAX 716-645-3473
http://www.buffalostate.edu
e-mail: savinomr@buffalostate.edu
Marianne Savino, Coordinator Special Services

The Office of Disability Services (ODS) is the University at Buffalo's center for coordinating services and accommodations to ensure accessiblity and usability of all programs, services and activities of UB by people with disabilities, and is a resource for information and advocacy toward their full participation in all aspects of campus life.

5612 State University of New York: College atBuffalo
Disability Services Department
120 S Wing
Buffalo, NY 14222
716-878-4500
FAX 716-878-3804
http://www.buffalostate.edu
e-mail: savinomr@buffalostate.edu
Marianne Savino, Director
Amy Rosenbrand, Accommodations Specialist
Raymond Lorigo, Assistant Director
Services provided to approximately 600 students per year with a variety of disabilities, the majority of whom have learning disabilities. All support is determined on a case-by-case basis with a goal toward careers and independence as much as possible in the worksite.

5613 State University of New York: Fredonia
Disabilities Services Office
4th Floor Reed Library Learning
Fredonia, NY 14063
716-673-3251
800-252-1212
FAX 716-673-3801
TDY:716-673-4763
http://www.fredonia.edu
e-mail: disabilityservices@fredonia.edu
Carolyn Boone, Coordinator. Disabled Student Se

Offers a variety of services to students with disabilities including notetakers, extended testing time, counseling services, and special accommodations.

5614 State University of New York: Geneseo College
Office of Disability Services
1 College Circle
Geneseo, NY 14454
585-245-5112
FAX 585-245-5032
http://www.admissions.geneseo.edu
e-mail: admissions@geneseo.edu
Tabitha Buggie-Hunt, Director Disability Services
Janet Jackson, Support Staff

To provide qualified students with disabilities, whether temporary or permanent, equal and comprehensive access to college-wide programs, services, and campus facilities by offering academic support, advisement, and removal of architectural and attitudinal barriers.

5615 State University of New York: Oneonta
State University of New York
209 Alumni Hall
Oneonta, NY 13820
607-436-2137
800-SUNY123
FAX 607-436-3167
http://www.oneonta.edu
e-mail: sds@oneonta.edu
Craig MA, Coordinator
Heather Bussy, Keyboard Specialist

To work with both students and college faculty/staff to ensure that compliance with disability laws is being upheld throughout the institution. SDS is also a resource to students diagnosed with a disability to assist in coordinating services which will lead the student toward receiving and equitable oppportunity at the College at Oneonta.

5616 State University of New York: Oswego
Disability Services Office
210 Swetman Hall
Oswego, NY 13126
315-312-3358
FAX 315-312-2943
http://www.oswego.edu
e-mail: dss@oswego.edu
Starr Knapp, Interim Coordinator

A public four-year college of arts and sciences currently serving 140 students identified with disabling conditions. Total enrollment is approximately 8,000. Full time coordinator of academic support services for students with disabilities works with students on an individual basis.

5617 State University of New York: Plattsburgh
Student Support Services
101 Broad Street
Plattsburgh, NY 12901 518-564-2810
FAX 518-564-2807
http://www.plattsburgh.edu
e-mail: michele.carpentier@plattsburgh.edu
Michele Carpentier, Director

Academic support program funded by the United States Department of Education. Staffed by caring and commited professional whose mission is to provide services for students with disabilities.

5618 State University of New York: Potsdam
Sisson Hall
Potsdam, NY 13676 315-267-3267
FAX 315-267-3268
TDY:315-267-2071
http://www.potsdam.edu
e-mail: housese@potsdam.edu
Sharon House, Academic Coordinator

A public four-year college with approximately 200 students with disabilities out of a total of 4,000.

5619 Stony Brook University
Disability Support Services
128 Educational Communications Ctr
Stony Brook, NY 11794 631-632-6748
FAX 631-632-6747
http://www.sunysb.edu
e-mail: dss@notes.cc.sunysb.edu
Joanna Harris, Director
Donna Molley, Assistant Director
Margaret Perno, Senior Counselor
The Office of Disability Support Services provides assistance for both students and employees. It coordinates advocacy and support services for students with disabilities in their academic and student life activities. Assuring campus accessibility, assisting with academic accommodations and providing assistive devices are important components of the programs.

5620 Suffolk County Community College: Eastern Campus
Speonk-Riverhead Road
Riverhead, NY 11901 631-548-2500
http://www.sunysuffolk.edu
Judith Koodin, Counselor

The Eastern Campus is an accessible, open admissions institution. Services are provided to learning disabled students to allow them the same or equivalent educational experiences as nondisabled students.

5621 Suffolk County Community College: Selden Campus
533 College Road
Selden, NY 11784 631-451-4110
FAX 631-451-4473
http://www.sunysuffolk.edu
Marlene Boyce, Assistant Director
Arlene Zink, Office Manager
Shirley Pippins, President
Equalizes educational opportunities by minimizing physical, psychological and learning barriers. Attempt to provide as typical a college experience as possible, encouraging students to achieve academically through the provision of special services, support aids, or reasonable program accommodations.

5622 Suffolk County Community College: Western Campus
Crooked Hill Road
Brentwood, NY 11717 631-851-6700
FAX 631-451-4473
http://www.sunysuffolk.edu
Judith Taxier-Reinauer, Counselor
Cheryl Every-Wartz, Counselor

The goal of Suffolk Community College with regard to students with disabilities is to equalize educational opportunities by minimizing physical, psychological and learning barriers. We attempt to provide as typical a college experience as is possible, encouraging students to achieve academically through the provision of special services, auxillary aids, or reasonable program modifications.

5623 Sullivan County Community College
Learning & Student Development Services
112 College Road
Loch Sheldrake, NY 12759 845-434-5750
800-577-5243
FAX 845-434-4806
http://www.sullivan.suny.edu
Helene Laurenti, Director
Mamie Golladay, President

SCCC is fully committed to institutions accessability for individuals with disabilities. Students who wish to obtain particular services or accommodations should communicate their needs and concerns as early as possible. These may include, but are not limited to, extended time for tests, oral examinations,reader and notetaker services, campus maps, and elevator privileges. Books on tape may be ordered through recordings for the blind. Appropriate documentation needed.

5624 Syracuse University
Services For Students with Disabilities
804 University Avenue
Syracuse, NY 13244 315-443-4498
FAX 315-443-2583
TDY:315-443-1312
http://www.syracuse.edu
e-mail: dtwillia@syr.edu
Dana Williams, Coordinator Academic Services
Cesar Reyes, Administrative Assistant

The office of disability services provides and coordinates services for students with documented disabilities. Students must provide current documentation of their disability in order to receive disability services and reasonable accommodations.

5625 Trocaire College
360 Choate Avenue
Buffalo, NY 14220 716-826-1200
FAX 716-828-6107
http://www.trocaire.edu
Norine Truax, Coordinator
Paul Hurley, President

An independent two-year college with 3 special education students out of a total of 1,056.

5626 Ulster County Community College
Student Support Services
Cottekill Road
Stone Ridge, NY 12484 845-687-5000
800-724-0833
FAX 845-687-5090
http://www.sunyulster.edu
James Quirk, Associate Dean
Don Katt, President

The Student Support Services program promotes student success for students who are academically disadvantaged, economically disadvantaged, first-generation college students, and or students with disabilities. The goals of the program are to increase the retention, graduation, and transfer rates of those enrolled.

5627 University of Albany
Campus Center 130
Albany, NY 12222 518-442-5566
FAX 518-442-5589
TDY:518-442-3366
http://www.albany.edu
e-mail: cmalloch@uamail.albany.edu
Carolyn Malloch, Learning Disability Specialist

Offers a full time Learning Disability Specialist to work with students that have learning disabilities and or attention deficit disorder. The specialist offers individual appointments to develop study and advocacy skills.

5628 Utica College of Syracuse University
1600 Burrstone Road
Utica, NY 13502 315-792-3032
800-782-8884
FAX 315-792-3292
http://www.utica.edu
e-mail: KHenkel@utica.edu

Kateri Henkel, Coordinator Learning Services
Stephen Pattarini, Director

Provides students with disabilities individualized learning accommodations designed to meet the academic needs of the student. Counseling support and the development of new strategies for the learning challenges posed by college level work are an integral part of the services offered through Academic Support Services.

5629 Vassar College
124 Raymond Avenue
Poughkeepsie, NY 12604
845-437-7000
FAX 845-437-5715
http://www.assar.edu
e-mail: guthrie@vassar.edu
Belinda Guthrie, Director
Frances Fergusson, Administrator

Offers a variety of services to students with disabilities including note takers, extended testing time, counseling services, and special accommodations.

5630 Wagner College
1 Campus Road
Staten Island, NY 10301
718-390-3411
800-221-1010
FAX 718-390-3105
http://www.wagner.edu
Ruth Perri, Director
Chris Davis, Administrative Assistant Counsel

An independent four-year college with 25 special education students out of a total of 1,272. There is an additional fee for the special education program in addition to the regular tuition.

5631 Westchester Community College
75 Grasslands Road
Valhalla, NY 10595
914-785-6600
FAX 914-785-6540
http://www.sunywcc.edu
Alan Seidman MD, Special Services

Students with Disabilities parallels the mission of WCC to be accessable, community centered, comprehensive, adaptable and dedicated to lifelong learning for all students. Full participation for students with disabilities is encouraged.

North Carolina

5632 Appalachian State University
Learning Disability Program
PO Box 32087
Boone, NC 28608
828-262-2291
FAX 828-262-6834
http://www.ods.appstate.edu
e-mail: wehnerst@appstate.edu
Suzanne Wehner, Director Disability Services
Joy Clawson, Dir Learning Assistance Program

The Office of Disability Services (ODS) assists students with indentified disabilities by providing the support they need to become successful college graduates. ODS provides academic advising, alternative testing, assistance with technology, tutoring, practical solutions to learning problems, counseling, self-concept building and career exploration.

5633 Bennett College
900 E Washington Street
Greensboro, NC 27401
336-273-4431
800-413-5323
FAX 336-273-4431
http://www.bennett.edu
Mary Stuart, Support Services
Johnnetta Cole, President

An independent four-year college with 10 special education students out of a total of 568.

5634 Brevard CollegeOffice for Students with Special Needs and Disabilities
400 N Broad Street
Brevard, NC 28712
828-883-8292
FAX 828-884-3790
http://www.brevard.edu
e-mail: skuehn@brevard.edu
Susan Kuehn, Director
Drew Horn, President

Four year college provides services to special needs students.

5635 Caldwell Community College and Technical Institute
Basic Skills Department
2855 Hickory Boulevard
Hudson, NC 28638
828-726-2200
FAX 828-726-2216
http://www.cccti.edu
e-mail: ccrump@cccti.edu
Christie Crump, Director
Cindy Richards, Administrative Assistant
Kenneth Boham, President
A public two-year college with 18 special education students out of a total of 2,744.

5636 Catawba College
Learning Disability Department
2300 W Innes Street
Salisbury, NC 28144
704-637-4259
800-228-2922
FAX 704-637-4401
http://www.catawba.edu
e-mail: ekgross@catawba.edu
Emily Gross, Director
Julie Baranski, Office Assistant

An independent four-year liberal arts college with an enrollment of 1,400.

5637 Catawba Valley Community College
Student Services Office
2550 US Highway 70 SE
Hickory, NC 28602
828-327-7000
FAX 828-327-7276
http://www.cvcc.edu
e-mail: dulin@cvcc.edu
William Dulin, Dean
Cuylar Dunbar, President

The following is a partial list of accommodations provided by the college: counseling services, tutors, note-takers and carbonless duplication paper, recorded textbooks, tape recorders for taping lecture classes, interpeters, computer with voice software, and extended time for texts. Catawba Valley Community College provides services for students with disabilities.

5638 Central Carolina Community College
1105 Kelly Drive
Sanford, NC 27330
919-775-5401
FAX 919-718-7380
http://www.ccarolina.cc.nc.us
Frances Andrews MD, Associate Dean
Matthew Garrett, President

Adopted to guide its delivery of services to students with disabilities that states that no otherwise qualified individual shall by reason of disability be excluded from the participation in, be denied benefits of, or be subjected to discrimination under any program at Central Carolina Community College. The college will make program modification adjustments in instructional delivery and provide supplemental services.

5639 Central Piedmont Community College
Learning Disability Department
PO Box 35009
Charlotte, NC 28235
704-542-0470
FAX 704-330-4020
TDY:704-330-6421
http://www.cpcc.cc.nc.us
e-mail: patricia.adams@cpcc.edu
Pat Goings-Adams, Learning Disabilities Counselor

A public two-year college with 300 special education students out of a total of 60,000.

5640 Craven Community College
Craven Community College
800 College Court
New Bern, NC 28562
252-638-4131
FAX 252-672-8020
TDY:252-638-8634
http://www.craven.cc.nc.us
e-mail: harris@cravencc.edu

Fred Cooze, Director
Opal Harris, Desk Assistant
Scott Ralls, President

Offers a variety of services to students with disabilities including notetakers, extended testing time, and special accommodations.

5641 Davidson County Community College
PO Box 1287
Lexington, NC 27293
336-249-8186
FAX 336-249-0088
http://www.davidsonccc.edu
e-mail: emorse@davidsonccc.edu

Ed Morse MD, Dean
Mary Rittling, President

Offers a variety of services to students with disabilities including notetakers, extended testing time, counseling services, and special accommodations.

5642 Dore Academy
Dore Academy
1727 Providence Road
Charlotte, NC 28207
704-365-5490
FAX 704-365-3240
http://www.doreacademy.org
e-mail: ecommendatore@doreacademy.org

Mary Dore, Founder
Erin Commendatore, Admissions Director
Roberta Smith, Administrator

Dore Academy is Charlotte's oldest college-prep school for students with learning differences. A private, non-profit, independent day school for students in grades 1-12, it is approved by the state of North Carolina, Division of Exceptional children. All teachers are certified by the state and trained in the theory and treatment of dyslexia and attention disorders. With a maximum of 10 students per class (5 in reading classes), the teacher student ratio is 1 to 7.

5643 East Carolina University
E 5th Street
Greenville, NC 27858
252-328-6131
http://www.ecu.edu

CC Rowe, Coordinator
Steve Ballard, Administrator

A public four-year college with 47 special education students out of a total of 13,903.

5644 Forsyth Technical Community College
2100 Silas Creek Parkway
Winston Salem, NC 27103
336-723-0371
FAX 336-757-3202
TDY:800-735-8262
http://www.forsyth.tec.edu
e-mail: gfreeman@forsythtech.edu

Van Wilson, Vice President
Paula Compton, Director
Gary Green, President

Offers a variety of services to students with disabilities including notetakers, extended testing time, counseling services, and special accommodations.

5645 Gardner-Webb University
Noel Program
PO Box 7274
Boiling Springs, NC 28017
704-406-4270
FAX 704-406-3524
http://www.gardner-webb.edu
e-mail: cpotter@gardner-webb.edu

Cheryl Potter, Director

Four year college that provides a program for disabled students.

5646 Guilford Technical Community College
PO Box 309
Jamestown, NC 27282
336-454-1126
FAX 336-454-2510
http://www.gtcc.cc.nc.us
e-mail: dcameron@gtcc.cc.nc.us

Don Cameron, President
Sonny White, Vice President

The purpose of disability access services is to provide equal access and comprehensive, quality services to all students who experience barriers toacademic, personal and social success.

5647 Isothermal Community College
Department of Disability Services
PO Box 804
Spindale, NC 28160
828-286-3636
FAX 828-286-8109
TDY:828-286-3636
http://www.isothermal.cc.nc.us
e-mail: kharris@isothermal.cc.nc.us

Karen Harris, Director
Susan Vaughan, Manager

Isothermal Community College, in compliance with the Americans with Disabilities Act, makes every effort to provide accommodations for students with disabilities. It is our goal to integrate students with disabilities into the college and help them participate and benefit from programs and activities enjoyed by all students. We at Isothermal are committed to improving life through learning.

5648 Johnson C Smith University
Disability Support Services Department
100 Beatties Ford Road
Charlotte, NC 28216
704-378-1282
FAX 704-330-1336
http://www.jcsu.edu
e-mail: jcuthbertson@jcsu.edu

James Cuthbertson, Coordinator
James Saunders, Director

Four year college that provides support to those who are disabled.

5649 Lenoir Community College
North Carolina Community College System
PO Box 188
Kinston, NC 28502
252-527-6223
FAX 252-527-1199
http://www.lenoir.cc.edu
e-mail: bsanders@lenoircc.edu

Macrina Martin, Evening Counselor
Ina R Rawlinson, Human Resource Director
Brandley Briley, President

Lenoir Community College is committed to serving the needs of students with disabilities. If special assistance is needed, please give the college prior notice by contacting the ADA Coordinator.

5650 Lenoir-Rhyne College
PO Box 7470
Hickory, NC 28603
828-328-7315
FAX 828-328-7329
http://www.lrc.edu
e-mail: kirbydr@lrc.edu

Donavon Kirby, Coordinator
Wayne Powell, President

Four year college that provides services for those students that are learning disabled.

5651 Louisburg College
501 N Main Street
Louisburg, NC 27549
919-496-2521
FAX 919-496-1788
http://www.louisburg.edu

Jayne Davis, Director
Reginald Ponder, President

A two-year college that offers programs for the learning disabled.

5652 Mariposa School for Children with Autism
203 Gregson Drive
Cary, NC 27511
919-461-0600
http://www.mariposaschool.org
e-mail: info@mariposaschool.org
Michael Brader-Araje, Chairman
Cynthia Peters, President

Provides year round one-on-one instruction to children with autism, using innovative teaching techniques targeting multiple developmental areas in a single integrated setting. A school of excellence choice for children with autism to maximize developemtn of their communication, social and academic skills.

5653 Mars Hill College
124 Cascade Street
Mars Hill, NC 28754
828-689-1201
800-543-1514
FAX 828-689-1274
http://www.mhc.edu
e-mail: ccain@mhc.edu
Chris Cain, Director
Coorny Wood, Assistant Director
Dan Lunsford, President
An independent four-year college with 15 special education students out of a total of 1,321.

5654 Mayland Community College
Support Options for Achievement and Retention
PO Box 547
Spruce Pine, NC 28777
828-765-7351
800-462-9526
http://www.mayland.edu
e-mail: dcagle@mayland.edu
Nancy Godwin, Director
Debra Cagle, Administrative Assistant

Offers a variety of services to students with disabilities including notetakers, extended testing time, counseling services, and special accommodations.

5655 McDowell Technical Community College
Student Enrichment Center
54 Universal Drive
Marion, NC 28752
828-652-6021
FAX 828-652-1014
http://www.mcdowelltech.cc.nc.us
e-mail: donnashort@cc.nc.us
Donna Short, Admissions Director
Bryan Wilson, President

A public two-year college with 15 special education students out of a total of 857. Free auxiliary services for LD students include: tutors, books on tape, unlimited testing, oral testing, notetakers and counseling. All faculty are trained in working with the LD student.

5656 Meredith College
Disability Counseling Office
3800 Hillsborough Street
Raleigh, NC 27607
919-760-8427
800-637-3348
FAX 919-760-2383
http://www.meredith.edu
e-mail: disabilityservices@meredith.edu
Betty Prevatt, Coordinator/Assistant Director
Beth Meier, Director

The college goal is to create an accessible community where people are judged on their abilities not their disabilities. The Disability Services staff strives to provide individuals with the tools by which they can better accomplish their educational goals.

5657 Montgomery Community College: North Carolina
1011 Page Street
Troy, NC 27371
910-576-6222
FAX 910-576-2176
http://www.montgomery.cc.nc.us
Virginia Morgan MD, Chairperson
Mary Kirk, President

Offers a variety of services to students with disabilities including note takers, extended testing time, counseling services, and special accommodations.

5658 North Carolina State University
PO Box 7509
Raleigh, NC 27695
919-515-2011
FAX 919-513-2840
TDY:919-515-8830
http://www.ncsu.edu/dss
e-mail: cheryl_branker@ncsu.edu
Cheryl Branker, Director
James Oblinger, Manager

Academic accommodations and services are provided for students at the university who have documented learning disabilities. Admission to the university is based on academic qualifications and learning disabled students are considered in the same manner as any other student. Special assistance is available to accommodate the needs of these students, including courses in accessible locations when appropiate.

5659 North Carolina Wesleyan College
North Carolina Wesleyan College
3400 N Wesleyan Boulevard
Rocky Mount, NC 27804
252-985-5100
800-488-6292
FAX 252-985-5284
http://www.ncwc.edu
e-mail: albunn.infowc@edu
Elizabeth Lanchaster, Assistant Registrar
Cliff Sullivan, Registrar Director
Ian Newbold, President
The Center provides support to students interested in achieving academic success. The staff works to provide you with information about academic matters and serves as an advocate for you. Services focus on pre-major advising, tutoring, mentoring, skills enrichment, disabilities assistance, self-assessment and retention.

5660 Peace College
15 E Peace Street
Raleigh, NC 27604
919-508-2000
FAX 919-508-2326
http://www.peace.edu
e-mail: amann@peace.edu
Ann Mann MD, Director
Laura Bingham, President

Four year college offering programs to disabled students.

5661 Piedmont Baptist College
716 Franklin Street
Winston Salem, NC 27101
336-725-8344
FAX 336-725-5522
http://www.pbc.edu
e-mail: cpetitt@pbc.edu
Charles Petitt MD, President
Paul Holrtic, Vice President

A four year college offering comprehensive programs for students with learning disabilities.

5662 Pitt Community College
Pitt Community College
PO Box 7007
Greenville, NC 27835
252-695-7100
FAX 252-321-4401
http://www.pitt.cc.edu
e-mail: mbribg@email.pittcc.edu
Mike Bridgers, Coordinator Disability Services

The staff of Disability Servics looks forward to working with you to achieve your immediate academic and long range career goals. Our office is designed to provide academic, personal and technical support services to students with disabilities who qualify for post secondary education, but whose deficits are such that they are unlikly to succeed in college without thoses services.

5663 **Randolph Community College**

PO Box 1009
Asheboro, NC 27204 336-626-0033
FAX 336-629-4695
http://www.randolf.edu
e-mail: jbranch@randolf.edu

Joyce Branch, Special Services Director
Rebekah Megerian, Basic Skills
Diane Bell, Manager

A public two-year college with 23 special education students out of a total of 1,487. Applicants with disabilities who wish to request accommodations in compliance with the ADA must identify themselves to the admissions counselor before placement testing.

5664 **Rockingham Community College**

PO Box 38
Wentworth, NC 27375 336-342-4261
FAX 336-349-9986
TDY:336-634-0132
http://www.rcc.cc.nc.us
e-mail: rkeys@rcc.cc.nc.us

Robert Keys, President

Offers a variety of services to students with disabilities including notetakers, extended testing time, counseling services, and special accommodations.

5665 **Salem College**

S Church Street
Winston-Salem, NC 27108 336-721-2600
FAX 336-721-2683
http://www.salem.edu
e-mail: smith@salem.edu

Julianne Thrift, President

Offers a variety of services to students with disabilities including notetakers, extended testing time, counseling services, and special accommodations.

5666 **Sandhills Community College**

3395 Airport Road
Pinehurst, NC 28374 910-692-6185
800-338-3944
FAX 910-695-1823
http://www.sandhills.cc.nc.us

Peggie Chavis, Disabilities Coordinator
John Dempsey, President

Offers a variety of services to students with disabilities including notetakers, extended testing time, counseling services, and special accommodations.

5667 **Southwestern Community College: North Carolina**

447 College Drive
Sylva, NC 28779 828-586-4091
800-447-4091
FAX 828-586-3129
http://www.southwesterncc.edu
e-mail: cheryl@southwest.cc.nc.us

Cheryl Conner, Director
Cecil Groves, President

Southwestern Community College provides equal access to education for persons with disabilities. It is the responsibility of the student to make their disability known and to request academic adjustments. Requests should be made in a timely manner and submitted to the Director of Student Support Services. Every reasonable effort will be made to provide service, however, not requesting services prior to registration may delay implementation.

5668 **St Andrews Presbyterian College**

1700 Dogwood Mile Street
Laurinburg, NC 28352 910-277-5000
FAX 910-277-5020
http://www.sapc.edu
e-mail: info@sapc.edu

John Deegan, President

Four year college that supports and provides services to the learning disabled students.

5669 **Stone Mountain School**

126 Camp Elliott Road
Black Mountain, NC 28711 828-669-8639
FAX 828-669-2521
http://www.stonemountainschool.org
e-mail: smoore@stonemountainschool.com

Charlie Talley, Executive Director
Paige Thomas, Admissions Director

5670 **Surry Community College**

630 S Main Street
Dobson, NC 27017 336-386-8121
FAX 336-386-8951
http://www.surry.cc.nc.us
e-mail: riggsj@surry.edu

Laura Bracken, Special Programs
Judy Riggs, Continuing Education Dean
Frank Sells, President

Offers a variety of services to students with disabilities including notetakers, extended testing time, counseling services, and special accommodations.

5671 **Tri-County Community College**

4600 US 64 E
Murphy, NC 28906 828-837-6810
FAX 828-837-3266
TDY:724-228-4028
http://www.tccc.cc.nc.us

Sarah Harper, Executive Director
Norman Oglesby, President

Offers a variety of services to students with disabilities including notetakers, extended testing time, counseling services, and special accommodations.

5672 **University of North Carolina Wilmington**

Disability Services Department
601 S College Road
Wilmington, NC 28403 910-962-7555
FAX 910-962-7556
TDY:910-962-3853
http://www.uncw.edu/disability
e-mail: stonec@uncw.edu

Margaret M Turner Phd, Disability Services
Chris Stone M Ed, Office Manager
Aimee Helmais, Disability Service Specialist

Offer accommodative services, consultation, counseling and advocacy for Disabled Students enrolled at UNCW.

5673 **University of North Carolina: Chapel Hill**

Learning Disabilities Services
137 E Franklin Street
Chapel Hill, NC 27514 919-493-5362
FAX 919-962-3674
http://www.unc.edu
e-mail: lds@email.unc.edu

Theresa Maitlan MD, Learning Disabilities Specialist

Promotes learning by providing academic support to meet the individual needs of students diagnosed with specific learning disabilities. Strives to ensure the independence of participating students so that they may succeed during and beyond their university years.

5674 **University of North Carolina: Charlotte**

Special Education Department
9201 University Boulevard
Charlotte, NC 28223 704-687-2213
FAX 704-687-3353
http://www.uncc.edu
e-mail: abennett@email.uncc.edu

Gail Honeycutt, Accounting Technician
Ann Bennett, Office Manager

Introduction to Students with Special Needs. Characteristics of students with special learning needs, including those who are gifted and those who experience academic, social, emotional, physical and developmental disabilities. Legal, historical and philosophical foudations of special education and current issues in providing appropriate educational services to students with special needs.

5675 University of North Carolina: Greensboro
Disability Services
215 Elliott University Center
Greensboro, NC 27402
336-334-5440
FAX 336-334-4412
TDY:336-334-5440
http://www.uncg.edu/ods
e-mail: ods@uncg.edu

Mary Culkin, Director
Laura Ripplinger, Office Manager

A public four-year university with over 300 students with disabilities out of a total of 12,000.

5676 Wake Forest University
PO Box 7305
Winston Salem, NC 27109
336-758-5000
FAX 336-758-6074
http://www.wfu.edu

Thomas Hearn, President
John Anderson, Vice President
William Gordon, CEO

Offers a variety of services to students with disabilities including notetakers, extended testing time, counseling services, and special accommodations.

5677 Wake Technical Community College
Disabilities Support Department
9101 Fayetteville Road
Raleigh, NC 27603
919-662-3405
FAX 919-662-3564
TDY:919-779-0668
http://www.waketech.edu
e-mail: jtkillen@waketech.edu

Janet Killen, Director
Elaine Sardi, Coordinator

If you are a person with a documented disability who requires accommodations to achieve equal access to Wake Tech facilities, academic programs or other activities, you may request reasonable accommodations.

5678 Western Carolina University
Student Support Services
137 Killian Annex
Cullowhee, NC 28723
828-227-7127
FAX 828-227-7078
http://www.wcu.edu
e-mail: mellen@wcu.edu

Carol Mellen, Director
Suzanne Baker, Adviser

Students with a documented disability may be provided with appropriate academic accommodations such as, note takers, testing accomadations, books on tape, readers/scribes, use of adaptive equipment and priority registration.

5679 Wilkes Community College
Student Support Services
PO Box 120
Wilkesboro, NC 28697
336-838-6560
FAX 336-838-6277
http://www.wilkes.cc.nc.us
e-mail: nancy.sizemore@wilkescc.edu

Kim Faw, Director
Nancy Sizemore, Disability Coordinator

A public two-year community college. Special services include: testing and individualized education plans; oral and extended time testing; individual and small group tutoring; study skills; readers and proctors and specialized equipment.

5680 Wilson County Technical College
North Carolina Community College System
PO Box 4305
Wilson, NC 27893
252-246-1261
FAX 252-243-7148
TDY:252-246-1362
http://www.wilsontech.edu

William James, Student Support Services
Thelma McAllister, Secretary

Offers a variety of services to students with disabilities including notetakers, extended testing time, counseling services, and special accommodations.

5681 Wingate University
Disability Services Department
220 N Camden Road
Wingate, NC 28174
704-233-8000
800-755-5550
FAX 704-233-8290
http://www.wingate.edu

Linda Stedje-Larsen, Director
Jerry Gee, President

An independent four-year college with 50 special education students out of a total of 1,372. There is an additional fee for the special education program in addition to the regular tuition.

5682 Winston-Salem State University
302 Hauser Building
Winston Salem, NC 27110
336-750-2000
FAX 336-750-2392
http://www.wssu.edu\fyc

Myra Watdell, Director

Offers a variety of services to students with disabilities including notetakers, extended testing time, counseling services, and special accommodations.

North Dakota

5683 Bismarck State College
1500 Edwards Avenue
Bismarck, ND 58501
701-224-5450
800-445-5073
FAX 701-224-5550
http://www.bsc.nodak.edu
e-mail: lschlafm@gwmail.nodak.edu

Lisa Schlafman, Disability Support Coordinator
Marlene Anderson, Executive Director

Offers a variety of services to students with disabilities including notetakers, extended testing time, counseling services, and special accommodations.

5684 Dickinson State University
Student Support Services
291 Campus Drive
Dickinson, ND 58601
701-483-2029
FAX 701-783-2006
http://www.dsu.nodak.edu
e-mail: richardpadilla@dickinsonstate.edu

Richard Padilla, Planner/Coordinator

Four year college offers support services to learning disabled students.

5685 Fort Berthold Community College
PO Box 490
New Town, ND 58763
701-938-4230
FAX 701-627-3609
http://www.spcc.bia.edu
e-mail: lgwin@spcc.bia.edu

Susan Paulson, Academic Dean of Students
Russell Mason, President

An independent two-year college with 3 special education students out of a total of 279.

5686 Mayville State University
Learning Disabilities Department
330 3rd Street NE
Mayville, ND 58257
701-788-2301
800-437-4104
FAX 701-788-4748
http://www.mayvillestate.edu
e-mail: kyllo@mayvillestate.edu

Greta Kyllo, Academic Support Director
Pamela Balch, President

Offers a variety of services to students with disabilities including notetakers, extended testing time, counseling services, and special accommodations.

5687 **Minot State University: Bottineau Campus**
Special Services Office
105 Simrall Boulevard
Bottineau, ND 58318
701-228-5487
800-542-6866
FAX 701-228-5499
http://www.misu-b.nodak.edu
e-mail: jan.nahinurk@misu.nodak.edu
Jan Nahinurk, Director

Offers a variety of services to students with disabilities including notetakers, extended testing time, counseling services, and special accommodations.

5688 **North Dakota Center for Persons with Disabilities (NDCPD)**
Minot State University
500 University Avenue W
Minot, ND 58707
701-858-3371
800-233-1737
FAX 701-858-3483
TDY:701-858-3580
http://www.ndcpd.org
e-mail: ndcpd@minotstateu.edu
Bryce Fifield, Director
Susie Mack, Office Manager
David Fuller, President
NDCPD works with the disability community, university, faculty and researchers, policy makers and service providers to identify emerging needs in the disability community and how to obtain resources to address them.

5689 **North Dakota State College of Science**
Disability Support Services (DSS) Office
800 6th Street N
Wahpeton, ND 58076
701-671-2623
800-342-4325
FAX 701-671-2440
http://www.ndscs.nodak.edu
e-mail: joy.eichhorn@ndscs.nodak.edu
Joy Eichhorn, Disability Services Coordinator

A public two-year comprehensive college with a student population of 2400. Students with disabilites comprise seven percent of the population. Tuition $2025.

5690 **North Dakota State University**
Disability Services
212 Ceres Hall
Fargo, ND 58105
701-231-7671
FAX 701-231-6318
TDY:800-366-6888
http://www.ndsu.edu/counseling/disability
e-mail: bunnie.johnson-messelt@ndsu.edu
Jennifer Erickson, Disability Specialist
Bunnie Johnson-Messelt, Disability Services Coordinator

Students with permanent physical, psychological or learning disabilities may obtain accommodations. Staff in the Disability Servies office meet with the student to determine eligibility and establish reasonable accommodations. Accommodations are based on the functional limitations of the disability. Staff provide assistance in the implementation of approval accommodations, provide referrals for disability diagnosis and tutoring.

5691 **Standing Rock College**
1341 92nd Street
Fort Yates, ND 58538
701-854-3861
FAX 701-854-3403
http://www.sittingbull.edu
Linda Ivan, Special Services
Mark Holman, Manager

Offers a variety of services to students with disabilities including notetakers, extended testing time, counseling services, and special accommodations.

Ohio

5692 **Antioch College**
Academic Support Center
795 Livermore Street
Yellow Springs, OH 45387
937-769-1166
800-543-9436
FAX 937-769-1163
http://www.antioch-college.edu
e-mail: lizek@antioch-college.edu
Elizabeth Kennedy, Director
John Smith, Assistant Director

Comprehensive integrated support, including tutoring, time management and organization support, software, accommodations for our academic and cooperative education programs.

5693 **Art Academy of Cincinnati**
1212 Jackson Street
Cincinnati, OH 45202
513-721-5205
800-323-5692
FAX 513-562-8778
http://www.artacadamy.edu
Jane Stanton, Dean of Students
Sarah Mulhauser, Student Services Director
Greg Smith, Administrator
Offers a variety of services to students with disabilities including notetakers, extended testing time, counseling services, and special accommodations.

5694 **Baldwin-Wallace College**
275 Eastland Road
Berea, OH 44017
440-826-2900
FAX 440-826-3830
http://www.bw.edu
Mark Collier, President
Obobie Brender, Executive Assistant

Offers a variety of services to students with disabilities including notetakers, extended testing time, counseling services, and special accommodations.

5695 **Bluffton College**
Special Student Services
280 W College Avenue
Bluffton, OH 45817
419-358-3458
FAX 419-358-3323
http://www.bluffton.edu
e-mail: bergerd@bluffton.edu
Timothy Byers, Program Contact

Four year college offers special programs to learninig disabled students.

5696 **Bowling Green State University**
413 S Hall
Bowling Green, OH 43403
419-372-2515
FAX 419-372-8496
http://www.bgsu.edu
e-mail: dss@bgsu.edu
Robert Cunningham, Director
Peggy Dennis, Associate Director
Lea Anne Kesler, Coordinator
The Disability Services Office is evidence of Bowling Green State University's commitment to provide a support system which assists in conquering obstacles that persons with disabilities may encounter as they pursue their educational goals and activities. Our hope is to facilitate mainstream mobility and recognize the diverse talents that persons with disabilities have to offer to our university and our community.

5697 **Brown Mackie College: Akron**
Brown Mackie College
2791 Mogadore Road
Akron, OH 44312
330-733-8766
FAX 330-733-5853
http://www.brownmackie.edu
Jannette Mason, Administrative Assistant
Fred Baldwin, Dean of Academic Services

Offers a variety of services to students with disabilities including notetakers, extended testing time, counseling services, and special accommodations.

5698 **Case Western Reserve University**
10900 Euclid Avenue
Cleveland, OH 44106
216-368-3200
FAX 216-368-8826
http://www.cwru.edu
Susan Sampson, Disability Services Coordinator
Edward Hundert, President

While all students will have preferences for learning, students with physical or learning disabilities have different actual needs as well. Students with physical disabilities such as visual impairments, hearing impairments, or temporary or permanent motor impairments may need guide dogs, interpeters, note-takers, wheelchair accessible rooms, or other types of assistance to help them attend and participate in class. Also available, extra time or a separate room for exams, tutoring and more.

5699 **Center for the Advancement of Learning**
PLUS Program/Muskingum College
Montgomery Hall
New Concord, OH 43762
740-826-8280
800-752-6082
FAX 740-826-8285
http://www.muskingum.edu
e-mail: butler@muskingum.edu
Jen Navicky, Director

A professional, adult staff provides two levels of academic support and currently serves 150 learning disabled students. Support includes all reasonable accommodations and intensive one-on-one and small group tutoring. Learning Strategy instruction is embedded within course contents. Full services include a minimum of one hour of tutoring each week and students average 3-5 hours. Maintenance level services are flexibly arranged for half that amount. The Program has excellent faculty.

5700 **Central Ohio Technical College**
Developmental Education
1179 University Drive
Newark, OH 43055
740-366-1351
800-963-9275
FAX 740-364-9641
http://www.cotc.edu
Phyllis Thompso MD, Coordinator
Bonnie Coe, President

Learning Assitance Center and Disability Services (LAC/DS) is the academic support unit in Student Support Services. LAC/DS provides FREE programs and services designed to help students sharpen skills necessary to succeed in college.

5701 **Central State University**
Office of Disability Services
1400 Brush Row Road
Wilberforce, OH 45384
937-376-6411
FAX 937-376-6661
http://www.centralstate.edu
e-mail: info@csu.ces.edu
John Garland, President
Carlos Vargas-Aburto, Vice President

Four year college that provides services for the learning disabled students.

5702 **Cincinnati State Technical and CommunityCollege**
3520 Central Parkway
Cincinnati, OH 45223
513-569-1500
http://www.cinstate.cc.oh.us
e-mail: dcover@cinstate.cc.oh.us
Ron Wright, Administrator

Services include assistance and support services for students with permanent and temporary disabilities, test proctoring, readers/scribes, taping, tape recording loan, reading machines, assistance with locating interpeters, mediating between student and faculty to overcome specific disability issues; also offers braille access.

5703 **Clark State Community College**
Disability Retention Center
570 E Leffel Lane
Springfield, OH 45505
937-328-6019
FAX 937-328-6142
http://www.clark.cc.oh.us
Deborah Titus, Counselor
Mary , Disability Retention Specialist

In accordance with the Americans with Disabilities Act, it is the policy of Clark State Community College to provide reasonable accommodations to persons with disabilities. The office of disability services offers a variety of services to Clark State students who have documented physical, mental or learning disabilities.

5704 **Cleveland Institute of Art**
Academic Services
11141 E Boulevard
Cleveland, OH 44106
216-421-7462
800-278-6446
FAX 216-754-2557
http://www.cia.edu
e-mail: jmilenski@gate.cia.edu
Jill Milenski, Associate Director
Rachel Browner, Director

No student should be discouraged from attending CIA because of a learning disability. A student working on their BFA degree at the Institute of Art can get academic support from the tutoring director in the Office of Academic Services. Services include books-on-tape, one-on-one tutoring, alternative curriculum advising, notetaking services, alternative test taking and assignment arrangements. Services outside the scope of the program can be arranged at the student's expense.

5705 **Cleveland State University**
1983 E 24th Street
Cleveland, OH 44115
216-687-2000
888-278-6446
FAX 216-687-9366
http://www.csuohio.edu
e-mail: m.zuccaro@csuohio.edu
Michael Zuccaro, Disability Services
Michael Schwartz, CEO

CSU aims to provide equal opportunity to all of its students. Services are available to those who might need some extra help because of a physical disability, communication impairment or learning disability. This program is designed to address the personal and academic issues of the physically handicapped students as they become oriented to campus. A full range of services is offered.

5706 **College of Mount Saint Joeseph**
Project EXCEL
5701 Delhi Road
Cincinnati, OH 45233
513-244-4623
800-654-9314
FAX 513-244-4222
http://www.msj.edu
e-mail: jane_pohlman@mail.msj.edu
Jane Pohlman, Director

Learning disabled staff offers intensive instruction in reading, writing and study skills.

5707 **College of Mount St. Joseph**
Project EXCEL
5701 Delhi Road
Cincinnati, OH 45233
513-244-4623
800-654-9314
FAX 513-244-4222
http://www.msj.edu
e-mail: jane_pohlman@mail.msj.edu
Jane Pohlman, Director

Project EXCEL staff offers intensive instruction in reading, writing and study skills.

5708 **College of Wooster**
1189 Beall Avenue
Wooster, OH 44691
330-263-2000
http://www.wooster.edu
Carol Roose MD
R. Hales, President

Offers a variety of services to students with disabilities including notetakers, extended testing time, counseling services, and special accommodations.

5709 Columbus State Community College Disability Services

550 E Spring Street
Columbus, OH 43215
614-287-2400
800-621-6407
FAX 614-287-6054
TDY:614-287-2570
http://www.cscc.edu/docs/disability/intro.html
e-mail: wcocchi@cscc.edu

Wayne Cocchi, Director
Valerie Moeller, President

A public two-year college serving qualified students with disabilities, including learning disabilities. Support services are provided based on disability documentation and can include, books, tapes, alternative testing, notetaking, counseling, equipment use, reader, scribe, and peer tutoring.

5710 Cuyahoga Community College: Eastern Campus

Government Funded College
4250 Richmond Road
Highland Hills, OH 44122
216-987-2034
FAX 216-987-2423
TDY:216-987-2230
http://www.tri-c.edu/home/default.htm
e-mail: Maryann.Syarto@tri-c.cc.oh.us

Mary Sender, LD Director
Charlotte Burgin, Tutor

The ACCESS Programs strive to assist Tri-C students with disabilities to realize their learning potential, bring them into the mainstream of the College community, enhance their self-sufficiency, and enable them to achieve academic success. Services include tuoring, test proctoring, interpreters, adaptive equipment, readers and/or scribes for exams, alternative test taking arrangements, alternative format for printed materials and textbooks on tape.

5711 Cuyahoga Community College: Western Campus

1000 W Pleasant Valley Road
Parma, OH 44134
216-987-5077
FAX 516-987-5050
TDY:216-987-5117
http://www.tri-c.edu
e-mail: rose.kolovrat@tri-c.edu

Rose Kolovrat, Director

The ACCESS programs strive to assist Tri-C students with disabilities to realize their learning potential, bring them into the mainstream of the College community, enhance their self-suffciency and enable them to achieve academic success. Services provided include tutoring, test proctoring, interpeters, adaptive equipment, readers/scribes for exams, alternative testing arrangements, alternative format for printed material and textbooks on tape.

5712 Defiance College

701 N Clinton Street
Defiance, OH 43512
419-784-4010
800-520-4632
FAX 419-784-0426
http://www.defiance.edu
e-mail: admissions@defiance.edu

Debbie Stevens, Assistant Director
Mark Thompson, Dean
Gerald Wood, President

Offers a variety of services to students with disabilities including notetakers, extended testing time, counseling services, and special accommodations.

5713 Denison University

Denison University
104 Doane Hall
Granville, OH 43023
740-587-6666
800-336-4766
FAX 740-587-5629
http://www.denison.edu
e-mail: vestal@denison.edu

Jennifer Vestal, Associate Dean
Abby Ghering, Assistant Dean

The Office of Academic Support (OAS) offers a wide range of services for students with disabilities. In supporting our students as they move forward toward graduation and the world of work beyond, we strongly encourage and promote self advocacy regarding disability related issues.

5714 Franklin University

201 S Grant Avenue
Columbus, OH 43215
614-797-4700
877-341-6300
FAX 614-224-0434
http://www.franklin.edu

Carla Marshall, Disabilities Services Advisor
Paul Otte, President

Students who have disabilities may notify the University of their status by checking the appropriate space on the registration form each trimester.Then the Coordinator of Disability Services will help them file proper documentation so that accommodations can be made for their learning needs.

5715 Hiram College

PO Box 67
Hiram, OH 44234
330-569-3211
FAX 330-569-5398
http://www.hiram.edu

Lynn Taylor, Counseling Director
Tom Chema, President

Offers a variety of services to students with disabilities including notetakers, extended testing time, counseling services, and special accommodations.

5716 Hocking College

Hocking College
3301 Hocking Parkway
Nelsonville, OH 45764
740-753-3591
800-282-4163
FAX 740-753-4097
http://www.hocking.edu
e-mail: forbes_k@hocking.edu

Kim Powell, Coordinator
Rosie Smith, Director
John Light, President

The Access Center Office of Disability Support Services is dedicated to serving the various needs of individuals with disabilities and promoting their participation in college life.

5717 Hocking Technical College

Hocking Technical College
3301 Hocking Parkway
Nelsonville, OH 45764
740-753-3591
800-282-4163
FAX 740-753-1452
http://www.hocking.edu
e-mail: forbes_k@hocking.edu

Kim Powell, Coordinator
Rosie Smith, Director
John Light, President

Offers a variety of services to students with disabilities including notetakers, extended testing time, counseling services, and special accommodations.

5718 ITT Technical Institute

1030 N Meridian Road
Youngstown, OH 44509
330-270-1600
800-832-5001

Frank Quartini, Manager

Offers a variety of services to students with disabilities including note takers, extended testing time, counseling services, and special accommodations.

5719 Kent State University

Student Accessibility Services
Ground Floor Deweese Center
Kent, OH 44242
330-672-3391
FAX 330-672-3763
http://www.kent.edu/sds
e-mail: lmcgloth@kent.edu

Laura McGlothlin, Accommodations Specialist

Student Disability Services (SDS) provides assistance to students with varying degrees and types of disabilities in order to maximize educational opportunity and academic potential. Types of disabilities that students have who are served by SDS include mobility impairments, visual, hearing or speech impairments, specific learning disabilities, attention deficit disorder, chronic health disorders, psychological disabilities and temporary disabilities.

5720 Kent State University: Tuscarawas Academic Services

330 University Drive NE
New Philadelphia, OH 44663
330-339-3391
FAX 330-308-7575
TDY:330-339-7888
http://www.tusc.kent.edu
e-mail: www@tusc.kent.edu

Fran Haldar MD, Assistant Dean
Greg Andrews, Manager

Offers a variety of services to students with disabilities including notetakers, extended testing time and special accommodations.

5721 Lorain County Community College

1005 N Abbe Road
Elyria, OH 44035
440-366-4032
800-955-5222
FAX 440-366-4127
http://www.lorainccc.edu

Ruth Porter, Coordinator
Roy Church, President

LCCC serves over 80 learning disabled students per year out of a total student population of about 7,000. Services include readers/testers, scribes, notetaking accommodations, assistive technology, advocacy training and personal counseling. Free tutoring is available to all students at the college. No diagnostic testing is available.

5722 Malone College

515 25th Street NW
Canton, OH 44709
330-471-8100
800-521-1146
FAX 330-471-8478
TDY:330-471-8359
http://www.malone.edu
e-mail: pplittle@malone.edu

Patty Little, Retention/Special Needs Director
Ronald Johnson, President

An independent four-year college with about 40 special education students out of a total of almost 2,000.

5723 Marburn Academy

1860 Walden Drive
Columbus, OH 43229
614-433-0812
FAX 614-433-0812
http://www.marburnacademy.org
e-mail: marburnadmission@marburnacademy.org

Scott Burton, Admission Director
Barbara Davidson, Auxiliary Programs Director
Earl Oremus, Principal

Marburn Academy is a small, independent day school offering the finest education for bright children who learn differently. Our entire program is deisgned to meet the academic and social needs of children who have learning differences such as dyslexia, learning disabilities or ADHD. Marburn Academy's program is accredited by the Academy of Orton-Gillingham Practitioners and Educators.

5724 Marietta College

Marietta College
215 5th Street
Marietta, OH 45750
740-376-4643
FAX 740-376-4406
http://www.marietta.edu
e-mail: higgisd@marietta.edu

Debra Higgins, Director
Jean Scott, President

An Independent four-year college that offers a variety of servies to students with disabilities including note takers, extended testing time, counseling services, and special accommodations. There is no separate fee for these services.

5725 Marion Technical College

Marion Technical College
1467 Mount Vernon Avenue
Marion, OH 43302
740-389-4636
FAX 740-389-6136
http://www.mtc.edu

Mike Stuckey, Disability Services Coordinator
John Bryson, President

The Student Resource Center also houses the Office of Disabilities. The SRC director will advocate on student's behalf for resonable accommodations for those with physical, mental and or emotional disabilities.

5726 Miami University

301 S Campus Avenue
Oxford, OH 45056
513-529-2500
FAX 513-529-3841
http://www.mid.muohio.edu
e-mail: greendw@muohio.edu

James Garland, President
John Skillings, Interim Provost
Melissa Price, Manager

A public four-year college with approximately 5% of its students with LD/ADHD.

5727 Miami University: Middletown Campus

4200 N University Boulevard
Middletown, OH 45042
513-727-3200
800-662-2262
FAX 513-727-3223
TDY:513-727-3308
http://www.mid.muohio.edu
e-mail: nferguson@mid.muohio.edu

Nancy Ferguson, Disability Services Coordinator
Margir Perkins, Academic Services
Kelly Cowan, Executive Director

Offers a variety of services to students with disabilities including notetakers, extended testing time, counseling services, and special accommodations.

5728 Minnesota State Community and Technical College: Moorhead

1900 28th Avenue S
Moorhead, MN 56560
218-292-6500
800-426-5603
FAX 218-236-0342
http://www.minnesota.edu
e-mail: jerome.migler@minnesota.edu

Jerome Migler PhD, Provost
John Centko, Dean of Academics
Richard Smestad, Vice President

Offers a variety of services to students with disabilities including notetakers, extended testing time, counseling services, and special accommodations.

5729 Mount Vernon Nazarene College

800 Martinsburg Road
Mount Vernon, OH 43050
740-397-1244
FAX 740-393-0511
http://www.mvnu.edu
e-mail: amy.stemen@mvnu.edu

Carol Matthews MD, Director
Amy Stemen, Office Manager

Four year college that provides programs for learning diabled students.

5730 Muskingum College

163 Stormont Street
New Concord, OH 43762
740-826-8211
FAX 740-826-8285
http://www.muskingum.edu
e-mail: adminfo@muskingum.edu

Ann Steele, President
George Sims, Vice President of Academic Affai

Center for Advancement of Learning houses the PLUS Program, a full service for students with LD.

5731 Northwest Technical College

1900 28th Avenue S
Moorhead, MN 56560
218-236-6277
800-426-5603
FAX 218-236-0342
http://www.minnesota.edu
e-mail: jerome.migler@minnesota.edu

Dr. Migler, President
John Centko, Dean of Academics
Richard Smestad, Vice President

Offers a variety of services to students with disabilities including notetakers, extended testing time, counseling services, and special accommodations.

5732 Notre Dame College of Ohio

4545 College Road
South Euclid, OH 44121
216-381-1680
FAX 216-373-5187
http://www.ndc.edu
e-mail: gwalsh@ndc.edu

Gretchen Walsh, Director Academic Support Center
Andrew Roth, President

Four year college that offers, Level II support and services to students with learning disabilities.

5733 Oberlin College

Academic Support for Students with Disabilities
118 N Professor Street
Oberlin, OH 44074
440-775-8121
FAX 440-775-8886
http://www.oberlin.edu
e-mail: jane.boomer@oberlin.edu

Jane Boomer, Coordinator
Phyllis Hogan, Office Manager

An independent four-year college with small percentage of education students.

5734 Ohio State University Agricultural Technical Institute

1382 Dover Road
Wooster, OH 44691
330-264-3911
800-647-8283
FAX 330-202-3579
http://www.ati.ag.ohio-state.edu

Gerri Wolfe, LD Specialist
Chris Igodan, Executive Director

A public two-year college with nearly 10% special education students. There is no fee for the special education program in addition to the regular tuition.

5735 Ohio State University: Lima Campus

Disability Services
4240 Campus Drive
Lima, OH 45804
419-995-8453
FAX 419-995-8483
http://www.lima.ohio-state.edu
e-mail: meyer.193@osu.edu

Karen Meyer, Coordinator/Disability Services

A public four-year college providing services to learning disabled students including extended test time, counseling, notetakers and other special accommodations.

5736 Ohio State University: Mansfield Campus, Disability Services

1680 University Drive
Mansfield, OH 44906
419-755-4011
FAX 419-755-4243
http://www.mansfield.ohio-state.edu
e-mail: corso.1@osu.edu

Ginny Corso, Learning Disabilities Liaison
Evelyn Freeman, President

A public four-year college providing services to learning disabled students including peer tutoring, extended test time, quiet rooms and other special accommodations.

5737 Ohio State University: Marion Campus

1465 Mount Vernon Avenue
Marion, OH 43302
740-389-6786
FAX 614-292-5817
http://www.marion.ohio-state.edu

Margaret Hazelett, LD Specialist
Gregory Rose, Manager

A public four-year college providing a full range of services for students with disabilities.

5738 Ohio State University: Newark Campus

1179 University Drive
Newark, OH 43055
740-366-3321
FAX 740-366-5047
http://www.newark.ohio-state.edu

Barbara Deutschle, Learning Disability Specialist
Anne Federlein, President

A public four-year college providing services to learning disabled students including peer tutoring, extended test time, quiet rooms and other special accommodations. There is no separate fee for these services.

5739 Ohio State University: Nisonger Center

357 McKamball Hall
Columbus, OH 43210
614-292-8365
FAX 614-292-3727
TDY:614-688-8040
http://www.nisonger.osu.edu

Steven Reiss, Executive Director

The Ohio State University Nisonger Center for Mental Retardation and Developmental Disabilities provides interdisciplinary training, research and exemplary services pertaining to people with developmental disabilities. The center, which is a part of a national network of activities called University Afffiliated Programs, was founded in 1968. Training is provided in medicine (pediatrics and psychiatry), dentistry, education, physical therapy, psychology and other relevant disciplines.

5740 Ohio State University: Office for Disability Services

150 Pomerene Hall
Columbus, OH 43210
614-292-2970
FAX 614-292-4190
TDY:614-292-0901
http://www.osu.ohio-state.edu
e-mail: frontliner@ods.ohio-state.edu

Patty Carlton, Director
Lois Burke, Counselor
James Schroeder, President

ODS offers academic accommodations for students with documented disabilities including but not limited to students who are deaf or hard of hearing, visually impaired, mobilty impaired or have ADHD, learning disabilities, psychiatric disabilities or medical disabilities. ODS also provides auxiliary aids which include access to class notes, print materials in alternate format, interpreters and/or closed captioning for deaf students, and a variety of adaptive technology.

5741 Ohio University

Ohio University
101 Crewson House
Athens, OH 45701
740-593-4141
FAX 740-593-2708
http://www.ohiou.edu

William Smith, Director
Ruth Blickle, Administrative Associate
Robert Glidden, President

A public four-year college with a small percentage of special education students.

5742 Ohio University Chillicothe

Ohio University Chillicothe
PO Box 629
Chillicothe, OH 45601
740-774-7226
877-462-6824
FAX 740-774-7290
http://www.ohiou.edu/~childept
e-mail: diekroge@ohio.edu

Diane Diekroger MD, Student Support Coordinator
Richard Bebee, Manager

Offers a variety of services to students with disabilities including note takers, extended testing time, counseling services, and special accommodations.

5743 Otterbein College

102 W College Avenue
Westerville, OH 43081
614-890-3000
800-488-8144
FAX 614-823-1200
http://www.otterbein.edu
e-mail: uotterb@otterbein.edu

Ellen Kasualis, Director of Academic Support Ser
Brent Vore, President

An independent four-year college with a small percentage of special education students.

5744 Owens Community College
Disability Resources Department
PO Box 10000
Toledo, OH 43699
419-661-7230
800-466-9367
FAX 419-661-7607
http://www.owens.cc.oh.us
e-mail: bscheffert@owens.cc.oh.us

Beth Scheffert, Director

A comprehensive Community College that offers educational programs in over 50 technical areas of study leading to the Associate of Applied Science, Associate of Applied Business or Associate of Technical Studies degree. Provides programs designed for college transfer and leads to the Associate of Arts or Associate of Science degree. Finally, a number of certificate programs as well as short term credit and non-credit programs are available.

5745 Shawnee State University
940 2nd Street
Portsmouth, OH 45662
740-351-3267
800-959-4778
FAX 740-351-3111
http://www.shawnee.edu
e-mail: jweaver@shawnee.edu

James Weaver, Coordinator
Tess Midkiff, Executive Director

Offers a variety of services to students with disabilities including notetakers, extended testing time, counseling services, and special accommodations.

5746 Sinclair Community College
Learning Disability Support Services
444 W 3rd Street
Dayton, OH 45402
937-512-3550
FAX 937-512-4521
TDY:937-512-3096
http://www.sinclair.edu

Robin Moore-Cooper, Program Coordinator/Director
Robin More-Cooper, Counselor

Funded by the Federal Department of Education, Student Support Services is an organization devoted to helping students meet the challenges of college life. Our goals are to help students stay in school, then eventually graduate and/or transfer to a four-year college or university. We strive to develop new ways of helping students achieve their educational, career and professional goals.

5747 Southern State Community College
100 Hobart Drive
Hillsboro, OH 45133
937-393-3431
FAX 937-393-9370

Carl Vertona, Special Services
Lawrence Dukes, President

Offers a variety of services to students with disabilities including notetakers, extended testing time, counseling services, and special accommodations.

5748 Terra State Community College
Special Education Services
2830 Napoleon Road
Fremont, OH 43420
419-334-8400
866-AT-TERRA
http://www.terra.cc.us/terra2.html
e-mail: info@terra.cc.oh.us

Richard Newman, Coordinator
Gina Staccone-Smeal, Coordinator
Mary Broestl, Manager

Provides quality learning experiences which are accessible and affordable. Terra is actively committed to excellence in learning and offers associate degrees in various technologies as well as in arts and sciences, applied business, and applied science. Our office of student support services works with students with learning disabilities and other disabilities.

5749 University of Akron Wayne College
1901 Smucker Road
Orrville, OH 44667
330-683-2010
800-221-8308
FAX 330-684-8989
http://www.wayne.uakron.edu/
e-mail: juliabeyeler@uakron.edu

Julia Beyeler, Learning Support Services Dir.
Jack Kristosco, Manager

A public two-year college with a small percentage of special education students.

5750 University of Cincinnati: Raymond Walters General and Technical College
9555 Plainfield Road
Cincinnati, OH 45236
513-745-5600
FAX 513-792-8624
TDY:513-745-8300
http://www.rwc.uc.edu
e-mail: john.kraimer@uc.edu

John Kraimer, Disability Services Director
Dolores Straker, Administrator

Offers a variety of services to students with disabilities including notetakers, extended testing time, counseling services, and special accommodations.

5751 University of Dayton
Special Education Services
300 College Park Avenue
Dayton, OH 45469
937-229-3684
FAX 937-229-3270
TDY:937-229-3837
http://www.udayton.edu
e-mail: timothy.king@notes.udayton.edu

Timothy King, Director
Erin Courtney, Office Manager

An independent four year college with about 5% special education students.

5752 University of Findlay
Disability Services Office
1000 N Main Street
Findlay, OH 45840
419-434-5532
800-472-9502
FAX 419-434-5748
TDY:419-434-5532
http://www.findlay.edu
e-mail: ods@mail.findlay.edu

Lori Colchdgoff, Director Disability Services

An independent four-year college with a small percentage of special needs students.

5753 University of Toledo
Toledo, OH 43606
419-530-2721
http://www.utoledo.edu

Carl Earwood, Office Director
Joseph Hovey, Manager

A public four-year college whose mission is to provide the support services and accommodations necessary for all students to succeed.

5754 Urbana University
Student Affairs Office
597 College Way
Urbana, OH 43078
937-484-1301
FAX 937-484-1322
http://www.urbana.edu

Sheri Holmes, Director

An independent four-year college with a small percentage of special education students.

5755 Ursuline College
Program for Students with Learning Disabilities
2500 Lander Road
Pepper Pike, OH 44124
216-464-3366
FAX 440-646-8318
http://www.ursuline.edu
e-mail: agromada@ursuline.edu

Annette Gromada, Learning Disabilities Specialist
Adam Berggrum, Owner

A four year college that offers programs to students with learning disabilities.

5756 Walsh University
2020 E Maple Street
North Canton, OH 44720
330-490-7185
800-362-9846
FAX 330-490-7165
http://www.walsh.edu
e-mail: bfreshour@walsh.edu

Francie Morrow, Director
Joni Hendricks, Secretary
Dan Suvak, Manager
An independent four-year college. The Office of Student Support Services maintains an early warning system for students in academic, financial, social and/or emtional difficulty. The Office proudly communicates regularly with students regarding their general well being, and assists in the students' academic and financial concerns with referals to appropriate offices.

5757 Washington State Community College
710 Colegate Drive
Marietta, OH 45750
740-374-8716
FAX 740-376-0257
http://www.wscc.edu/

Ann Hontz, Director
Charlotte Hatfield, President

A public two-year college with a small percentage of special education students.

5758 Wilmington College of Ohio
251 Ludovic Street
Wilmington, OH 45177
937-382-6661
800-341-9318
http://www.wilmington.edu

Laurel Eckels, Special Services
Daniel Di'Biasio, President

Offers a variety of services to students with disabilities including notetakers, extended testing time, counseling services, and special accommodations.

5759 Wright State University
Disability Department
3640 Colonel Glenn Highway
Dayton, OH 45435
937-775-5680
FAX 937-775-5795
http://www.wright.edu
e-mail: disability.services@wright.edu

Jeffrey Vernooy, Director
Cassandra Mitchell, Assistant Dir Academic Support

A public university with over 14,000 undergraduated and graduated students. The Office of Disability Services offers programs to promote each student's academic, personal, physical, and vocational growth so that people with physical and learning disabilities can learn their full potential.

5760 Xavier University
3800 Victory Parkway
Cincinnati, OH 45207
513-745-3424
800-344-4698
FAX 513-745-3387
http://www.xu.edu

Heidi Larson, Religious Leader

We seek to ensure that all students with disabilities can freely and actively participate in all facets of university life.

Oklahoma

5761 Bacone College
2299 Old Bacone Road
Muskogee, OK 74403
918-781-0099
888-682-5514
FAX 918-682-5514
http://www.bacone.edu
e-mail: stewarta@bacone.edu

Rhonda Cambiano, Director
Ann Stewart, Coordinator

Offers a variety of services to students with disabilities including notetakers, extended testing time, counseling services, and special accommodations.

5762 East Central University
1100 E 14th Street
Ada, OK 74820
580-332-8000
FAX 580-310-5654
http://www.ecok.edu/

Dwain West, Student Support Services
Pamela Armstrong, Registrar

A public four-year college with a small percentage of special education of students.

5763 Moore-Norman Technology Center
4701 12th Avenue NW
Norman, OK 73069
405-364-5763
FAX 405-360-9989
http://www.mntechnology.com
e-mail: wperry@mntechnology.com

Wendy Perry, Counselor/Disability Svcs Coord

Offers a variety of services to students with disabilities including notetakers, extended testing time, counseling services, and special accommodations.

5764 Moore-Norman Vo-Tech
4701 12th Avenue NW
Norman, OK 73069
405-364-5763
FAX 405-360-9989
http://www.mntechnology.com

John Hunter, Manager

Offers a variety of services to students with disabilities including notetakers, extended testing time, counseling services, and special accommodations.

5765 Northeastern State University
600 N Grand Avenue
Tahlequah, OK 74464
918-456-5511
FAX 918-458-2340
http://www.nsuok.edu

Jan Smith-Clayton, Assistant to Dean
Bela Foltin, Manager

Four year college that offers programs and services to disabled students.

5766 Oklahoma City Community College
Department of Student Support Services
7777 S May Avenue
Oklahoma City, OK 73159
405-682-7520
FAX 405-682-7545
TDY:405-682-7520
http://www.okccc.edu
e-mail: jhoward@okccc.edu

Jenna Howard, Students w/Disabilities Advisor
Pat Stowe, Disabled Students Services Direc

Comprehensive community college with individualized services and accommodations for students with disabilities arranged by the Office of Student Support Services. Services include Deaf Program, and accommodations as described by section 504 & ADA. Five tutoring labs are available on campus and assistive technology including voice synthesizers and voice recognition for computer based word processing.

5767 **Oklahoma Panhandle State University**
PO Box 430
Goodwell, OK 73939
580-349-2611
FAX 580-349-2302
TDY:580-349-1559
http://www.opsu.edu
e-mail: opsu@opsu.edu
David Bryan, President
Wayne , Vice President

Four year college that offers programs to the learning disabled.

5768 **Oklahoma State University: Tech Branch-Oklahoma City**
900 N Portland Avenue
Oklahoma City, OK 73107
405-947-4421
FAX 405-945-8656
http://www.osuokc.edu/disabled
e-mail: emilytc@osuokc.edu
Emily Cheng, Advisor to Students
J. Carroll, President

Offers access to students with disabilities based upon the diagnostic documentation which is provided by the student and the functional impact of the disability.

5769 **Oklahoma State University: Technical Branch-Okmulgee**
1801 E 4th Street
Okmulgee, OK 74447
918-293-4678
http://www.osu-okmulgee.edu
Billie Coakley, Special Services
Carol Been, Manager

Offers a variety of services to students with disabilities including notetakers, extended testing time, counseling services, and special accommodations.

5770 **Oral Roberts University**
7777 S Lewis Avenue
Tulsa, OK 74171
918-495-6161
FAX 918-495-7879
http://www.oru.edu
e-mail: droberson@oru.edu
Don Roberson, Director
Richard Roberts, President

Four year college that offers resources to students with a learning disability.

5771 **Rogers State University**
1701 W Will Rogers Boulevard
Claremore, OK 74017
918-343-7777
800-256-7511
FAX 918-343-7712
http://www.rsu.edu
e-mail: llawless@rsu.edu
Lennette Lawless, Student Development Coordinator
Joe Wiley, President

A public four-year university with several special education students out of a total of approximately 3,300.

5772 **Rose State College**
Academic Support Department
6420 SE 15th Street
Midwest City, OK 73110
405-733-7311
FAX 405-736-0372
TDY:405-736-7308
http://www.rose.cc.ok.us
e-mail: rjones@rose.edu
James Cook, President

Services and facilities include academic advisement, referal and liaison with other community agencies, recorded textbooks and individual testing for qualified students.

5773 **Seminole Junior College**
PO Box 351
Seminole, OK 74818
405-382-9950
FAX 405-382-3122
TDY:405-382-9950
http://www.ssc.cc.ok.us
e-mail: downey_m@ssc.cc.ok.us
James Utterback MD, President
Tracey Woods, Academic Counselor
Debbie Kinsey, Executive Director
Provides free peer tutoring, study skill workshops, computer programs, (CAI) and videos, alternative textbooks and workbooks, classnotes/test files and other support materials to all students. A learning disabilities specialist works closely with learning disabled students, instructors and counselors to identify and implement useful and appropriate support services. Students meeting ADA guidelines can request other academic assistance services (notetakers, readers, adapted testing, etc.).

5774 **Southeastern Oklahoma State University**
1405 N 4th Avenue
Durant, OK 74701
580-745-2000
FAX 580-745-7470
TDY:580-745-2704
http://www.sosu.edu
e-mail: sdodson@sosu.edu
Susan Dodson, Director
Glenn Johnson, President

Four year college that provides services to the learning disabled students.

5775 **Southwestern Oklahoma State University**
100 Campus Drive
Weatherford, OK 73096
580-772-6611
FAX 580-774-3034
http://www.swosu.edu
e-mail: cindy.dougherty@swosu.edu
Cindy Dougherty, Dean of Students
John Hays, President

Offers a variety of services to students with disabilities including notetakers, extended testing time, counseling services, and special accommodations.

5776 **St. Gregory's University**
Partners in Learning
1900 W Macarthur Street
Shawnee, OK 74804
405-878-5398
FAX 405-878-5198
TDY:405-878-5103
http://www.stgregorys.edu
e-mail: hlwatson@stgregorys.edu
H L Watson, Coordinator Partners in Learning
Melody Harrington, Assistant Director for Partners

Four-year college offering assistive programs for students with learning disabilities.

5777 **Tulsa Community College**
Disabled Student Resource Center
909 S Boston Avenue
Tulsa, OK 74119
918-595-7115
FAX 918-595-8398
TDY:918-595-7287
http://www.tulsacc.edu
e-mail: info@tulsacc.edu
Yolanda Williams, Director

Offers a variety of services to students with disabilities including note takers, extended testing time, counseling services, and special accommodations.

5778 **Tulsa University Student Support Center**
Center for Student Academic Support
600 S College Avenue
Tulsa, OK 74104
918-631-2315
FAX 918-631-3459
TDY:918-631-3329
http://www.utulsa.edu
e-mail: jcorso@utulsa.edu
Jane Corso PhD, Director
Ruby Wile, Assistant Director

5779 **University of Oklahoma**
620 Elm Avenue
Norman, OK 73019
405-329-2270
800-522-0772
FAX 405-325-4491
TDY:405-325-4173
http://www.dsa.ou.edu/ods/
e-mail: sdyer@ou.edu

Suzette Dyer, Disability Services Director
Pam Sullivan, Manager

A public doctoral degree-granting research university. The University of Oklahoma is an equal opportunity institution.

5780 **University of Tulsa**
Center for Student Academic Support
600 S College Avenue
Tulsa, OK 74104
918-631-2334
FAX 918-631-3459
http://www.utulsa.edu
e-mail: jcorso@utulsa.edu

Jane Corso, Director
Ruby Wile, Coordinator

Four year college that offers services to disabled students. The small class size and individual attention that students recive make this institution an excellent choice for the students with disabilities.

Oregon

5781 **Blue Mountain Community College**
Services for Students with Learning Disabilities
PO Box 100
Pendleton, OR 97801
541-278-5807
FAX 541-278-5888
http://www.bluecc.edu
e-mail: aspiegel@bluecc.edu

Amy Spiegel, Coordinator

A rural community college that offers both lower division transfer and professional technical degrees. Accommodations and academic adjustments for students with learning disabilities are determined and provided on an individual basis. Diagnostic testing for learning disabilities is available. 1,200 full-time students.

5782 **Cascade College**
9101 E Burnside Street
Portland, OR 97216
503-255-7060
FAX 503-257-1222
http://www.cascade.edu
e-mail: sjones@cascade.edu

Dennis Lynn, President
Shawn Jones, Academic Dean

Offers a variety of services to students with disabilities including note takers, extended testing time, counseling services, and special accommodations.

5783 **Central Oregon Community College**
2600 NW College Way
Bend, OR 97701
541-383-7700
FAX 541-383-7506
http://www.cocc.edu
e-mail: DisabilityServices@cocc.edu

Alicia Moore, Registrar
Bob Barber, President

COCC is committed to making physical facilities and instructional programs accessible to students with disabilities.

5784 **Clackamas Community College**
Disability Resource Center
19600 S Molalla Avenue
Oregon City, OR 97045
503-657-6958
FAX 503-650-6654
TDY:503-650-6649
http://www.clackamas.edu
e-mail: caseys@clackamas.edu

Casey Sims, Director
Joe Johnson, Administrator

A public two-year college. Special education services are designed to support student success by creating full access and providing appropriate accommodations for all students with disabilities.

5785 **Corban College**
500 Deer Park Drive
Salem, OR 97317
503-375-7012
FAX 503-585-4316
http://www.corban.edu
e-mail: dmiliones@corban.edu

Darren Milionis, Director Career/Academics

Private four year Christian college offering assistance for learning disabled students.

5786 **George Fox College**
Academic Resource Center
414 N Meridian Street
Newberg, OR 97132
503-538-8383
800-765-4369
FAX 503-554-3834
http://www.georgefox.edu
e-mail: rmuthiah@georgefox.edu

Rick Muthiah, Director
David Brandt, President

An independent four-year college with a small percentage of special education students.

5787 **Lane Community College**
4000 E 30th Avenue
Eugene, OR 97405
541-463-3000
FAX 541-563-4739
TDY:541-463-3079
http://www.lanecc.edu
e-mail: moretd@lanecc.edu

Nancy Hart, Director
Mary Spilde, President

We provide accommodations, technology, advising, support systems, training and education.

5788 **Linfield College**
Learning Support Services
900 SE Baker Street
McMinnville, OR 97128
503-883-2444
FAX 503-883-2647
TDY:503-883-2396
http://www.linfield.edu
e-mail: jhaynes@linfield.edu

Judith Haynes, Learning Support Services Dir.
Eileen Dowty, Learning Support Services Asst.

An independent four-year college. Services include tutoring, extended time for testing, assistance with advising and counseling. Student needs are considered in customizing individual programs of support for documented special needs.

5789 **Linn-Benton Community College**
Learning Disabilities Support Services
Learning Resource Center
Albany, OR 97321
541-917-4683
FAX 541-917-4808
TDY:541-917-4703
http://www.linnbenton.edu
e-mail: ods@linnbenton.edu

Lynne Cox, Coordinator

A public two-year college. LBCC provides a number of services and programs for students with disabilities including classes, supportive services and aids.

5790 **Mount Bachelor Academy**
33051 NE Ochoco Highway
Prineville, OR 97754
541-462-3404
800-462-3404
FAX 541-462-3430
http://www.mtba.com/
Sharon Bitz, Executive Director

5791 **Mt. Hood Community CollegeDisability Services Department**
Learning Disabilities Department
26000 SE Stark Street
Gresham, OR 97030
503-491-6923
FAX 503-491-7549
TDY:503-491-7670
http://www.mhcc.edu
e-mail: dsoweb@mhcc.edu
Elizabeth Johnson, Coordinator
Laurie Clarke, Program Adviser

A commitment to providing educational opportunities for all students forms the foundation of the disability services program. If you are a student with a disability, disability services will help you overcome potential obstacles so that you may be successful in your area of study. Disability services gives you the needed support to help you meet your goals without separating you and other students with disabilities from existing programs.

5792 **Oregon Institute of Technology**
Oregon State University Systems
3201 Campus Drive
Klamath Falls, OR 97601
541-885-1031
800-422-2017
FAX 541-885-1520
TDY:541-885-1072
http://www.oit.edu
e-mail: access@oit.edu
Ron McCutcheon, Director-Campus Access
Martha Dow, President

A public four-year college enrolling about 3,000 students. Accommodations are tailored to the needs of individual students on a case-by-case basis for those self-identified as having learning disabilities.

5793 **Oregon State University**
Services for Students with Disabilities
A202 Kerr Administration Building
Corvallis, OR 97331
541-737-4098
FAX 541-737-7354
TDY:541-737-3666
http://www.ssd.oregonstate.edu
e-mail: disabilty.services@oregonstate.edu
Tracy Bentley-Towlin, Director
Rani Jeannette, Administrative Assistant

A public four-year college with a small percentage of students.

5794 **Portland Community College**
PO Box 19000
Portland, OR 97280
503-244-6111
FAX 503-977-4882
http://www.pcc.edu
Carolee Schmeer, LD Specialist

Our team includes rehabilitation guidance counselors, learning disability specialists, sign language interpreters, a technology specialist, vocational progarm and special needs coordinatiors.

5795 **Reed College**
3203 SE Woodstock Boulevard
Portland, OR 97202
503-771-1112
FAX 503-777-7234
http://www.reed.edu
e-mail: admissions@reed.edu
Betsy Emerick, Associate Dean Students
Burel Clayton, Administrative Officer
Colin Diver, President
Offers a variety of services to students with disabilities including notetakers, extended testing time, counseling services, and special accommodations.

5796 **Southern Oregon State College**
Counseling Center Britt 205
Ashland, OR 97520
541-552-6425
FAX 541-552-6329
http://www.sou.edu
Offers a variety of services to students with disabilities including note takers, extended testing time, counseling services, and special accommodations.

5797 **Southwestern Oregon Community College**
1988 Newmark Avenue
Coos Bay, OR 97420
541-888-7020
800-962-2838
FAX 541-888-7247
http://www.socc.edu
Tom Nickels, Director
Steve Kridelbaugh, President
Mary Clark, Executive Director
The college will provide reasonable accommodation for students with learning disabilities. Some instructors in academic skills have special training in working with learning disabled students.

5798 **Treasure Valley Community College**
650 College Boulevard
Ontario, OR 97914
541-881-8822
FAX 541-881-2717
http://www.tvcc.cc.or.us
Royo Spurgeon, Director
Jim Sorensen, President

Offers a variety of services to students with disabilities including notetakers, extended testing time, counseling services, and special accommodations.

5799 **Umpqua Community College**
PO Box 967
Roseburg, OR 97470
541-440-4600
FAX 541-440-4612
http://www.umpqua.edu
Barbara Stoner, Disability Services Coordinator
David Beyer, Administrator

A public two-year college with a small percentage of special education students.

5800 **University of Oregon**
5278 University of Oregon
Eugene, OR 97403
541-346-1000
FAX 541-346-6013
TDY:541-346-1083
http://www.ds.uoregon.edu
Steve Pickett, Director
Molly Sirois, Disability Services Counselor
Dave Frohnmayer, President
A public four-year college with about 5% of students with disabilities.

5801 **Warner Pacific College**
2219 SE 68th Avenue
Portland, OR 97215
503-517-1000
800-582-7885
http://www.warnerpacific.edu
e-mail: webmaster@warnerpacific.edu
Jay Barber, President
Wayne Peterson, Vice President

Offers a variety of services to students with disabilities including notetakers, extended testing time, counseling services, and special accommodations.

5802 **Western Baptist College**
500 Deer Park Drive
Salem, OR 97301
503-375-7012
FAX 503-585-4316
http://www.wbc.edu
e-mail: dmiliones@wbc.edu
Darren Miliones, Director

Four year college that offers programs for learning disabled students.

5803 Western Oregon University
345 Monmouth Avenue N
Monmouth, OR 97361
503-838-8000
877-877-1593
FAX 503838-8474
http://www.wou.edu
Joseph Sendelba MD, Quality Services
John Minahan, President

A public four-year college. Strives to provide and promote a supportive, accessible, non-discriminatory learning and working environment for students, faculty, staff and community members with disabilities. These goals are realized through the provision of individualized support services, advocacy and the identification of current technology and information.

5804 Willamette University
Learning Disabilities Department
900 State Street
Salem, OR 97301
503-370-6471
FAX 503-375-5420
TDY:503-375-5383
http://www.willamette.edu/dept/disability/main.
e-mail: jhill@willamette.edu
JoAnne Hill, Director Disability/Learning
Lynn Breen, Office Manager

Offers a variety of services to students with disabilities including notetakers, extended testing time, counseling services, and special accommodations. Provides services for all students on campus, including graduate schools.

Pennsylvania

5805 Albright College
PO Box 15234
Reading, PA 19612
610-921-7544
FAX 610-921-7530
http://www.albright.edu
e-mail: albright@alb.edu
Sue Miller, Administrative Assistant
Lex Millan, President

An independent four-year college with a small percentage of special education students. There is an additional fee for the education program in addition to the regular tuition.

5806 Bloomsburg University
400 E 2nd Street
Bloomsburg, PA 17815
570-389-4000
FAX 570-389-3700
http://www.bloomu.edu
Jessica Kozloff, Administrator

Offers a variety of services to students with disabilities including notetakers, extended testing time, counseling services, and special accommodations.

5807 Boyce Campus of the Community College of Allegheny County
595 Beatty Road
Monroeville, PA 15146
724-325-6712
FAX 724-325-6797
http://www.ccac.edu
e-mail: mailto:Pflorent@ccac.edu
Renee Clark MD, Director
Doris Bowers, Manager

Offers a variety of services to students with disabilities including notetakers, extended testing time, counseling services, and special accommodations.

5808 Bryn Mawr College
Educational Support Services
101 N Merion Avenue
Bryn Mawr, PA 19010
610-526-5375
FAX 610-526-7450
http://www.brynmawr.edu
e-mail: lmendez@brynmawr.edu

Bryn Mawr is a private liberal arts college located in Bryn Mawr, Pennsylvania not far from Philadelphia. The College provides support services for qualified students with documented learning, physical, and psychological disabilities. For additional information visit www.brynmawr.edu/access_services .

5809 Cabrini College
Disability Support Services
610 King of Prussia Road
Radnor, PA 19087
610-902-8538
FAX 610-902-8441
TDY:610-902-8582
http://www.cabrini.edu
e-mail: ama722@cabrini.edu
Anne Abbuhl, Director
Roberta Jacquet, Manager

Offers support services and appropriate accommodations to students with documented learning disabilities.

5810 California University of Pennsylvania
Center for Academic Research and Enhancement
250 University Avenue
California, PA 15419
724-938-4404
FAX 724-938-4564
http://www.cup.edu
Cheryl Bilitski, Director
Charles Williamson, Administrative Assistant Counsel

One of fourteen universities in the Pennsylvania State System of Higher Education. The CARE Project provides services to students with learning disabilities through two programs. The Specialized Support Service Program is a fee-for-service program which provides services beyond those mandated by 504/ADA and has a cap of 40 students each semester. The Modified Basic Support Program provides basic services at no cost and enrollment is unlimited.

5811 Carnegie Mellon University
Equal Opportunity Services
143 N Craig Street
Pittsburgh, PA 15213
412-268-2012
FAX 412-268-7472
http://www.cmu.edu
e-mail: ly2t@andrew.cmu.edu
Lisa Zamperini, Coordinator

Four year college that offers its students services for the learning disabled.

5812 Clarion University
840 Wood Street
Clarion, PA 16214
814-393-2000
FAX 814-393-2039
TDY:814-393-1601
http://www.clarion.edu/
e-mail: info@clarion.edu
Jennifer May, Disability Support Services Dir.
Joseph Grunewald, Administrator

Offers a variety of services to students with disabilities including note taking assistance, extended testing time, and special accommodations.

5813 College Misericordia
Alternative Learners Project
301 Lake Street
Dallas, PA 18612
570-674-6347
800-852-7675
FAX 570-675-2441
http://www.miseri.edu
e-mail: jrogan@miseri.edu
Joseph Rogan, Director/Professor

An independent four-year college with about 5% special education students.

5814 Community College of Allegheny County: College Center, North Campus
Learning Disabilities Services
8701 Perry Highway
Pittsburgh, PA 15237
412-341-1515
FAX 412-369-3635
TDY:412-369-4110
http://www.ccac.edu
e-mail: kwhite@ccac.edu
Kathleen White, Director

Support services for students with disabilities are provided according to individual needs. Services include assistance with testing, advisement, registration, classroom accommodations, professor and agency contact.

5815 Community College of Allegheny County: Allegheny Campus
Learning Disabilities Services
808 Ridge Avenue
Pittsburgh, PA 15212
412-341-1515
FAX 412-237-2721
http://www.ccac.edu
e-mail: mailto:Mdoyle@ccac.edu
Marilyn Gleser, LD Coordinator
Mary , Director

A public two-year college with a small percentage of special education students.

5816 Community College of Philadelphia
Center on Disability
1700 Spring Garden Street
Philadelphia, PA 19130
215-751-8050
FAX 215-751-8001
http://www.ccp.edu
e-mail: fdirosa@ccp.edu
Francesca DiRosa, Center Director
Jackie Williams, Administrative Assistant

5817 Delaware County Community
901 Media Line Road
Media, PA 19063
610-359-5000
FAX 610-355-7162
TDY:610-359-5020
http://www.dccc.edu
e-mail: abinder@dccc.edu
Ann Binder, Director Special Needs
Jerome Parker, Administrator

Delaware County Community College, the ninth largest college in the Philadelphia metropolitan area, is a public, two year institution offering more than 60 programs of study. Its open-door policy, and affordable tuition make it accessible to all. Services to physically and learning disabled students include counseling services, tutoring, extended testing, tape recorded lectures, spelling allowances, assistive equipment, notes copied and study skills workshops.

5818 Delaware Valley College of Science and Agriculture
Delaware Valley College of Science and Agriculture
700 E Butler Avenue
Doylestown, PA 18901
215-345-1500
FAX 215-230-2964
http://www.devalcol.edu
e-mail: karen.kay@devalcol.edu
Karen Kay, Counseling Director
Thomas Leamer, Administrator

Offers a variety of services to students with disabilities including notetakers, extended testing time, counseling services, and special accommodations.

5819 Delaware Valley Friends School
19 E Central Avenue
Paoli, PA 19301
610-640-4150
FAX 610-296-9970
http://www.dvfs.org
Katherine Schantz, Head of School

A co-educational, indpendent Friends School for adolescents with learning disabilities. Also prepares students with learning differences for future work and study. The school develops those personal strengths which enable student sto succeed in its college preparatory curriculum. The school also recognizes that it has a responsability to share its expertise with teachers and students beyond the school community.

5820 Dickinson College
Services for Students with Disabilities
PO Box 1773
Carlisle, PA 17013
717-245-1080
FAX 717-245-1080
http://www.dickenson.edu
e-mail: jervis@dickinson.edu
Keith Jervis, Coordinator

The Office of Counseling and Disability Services is dedicated to the enhancement of healthy student development. Professional and paraprofessional staff offer confidential individual and group counseling sessions and outreach services which help students with both general developmental issues and with specific personal or interpersonal difficulties.

5821 Drexel University
Office of Disability Services
3141 Chestnut Street
Philadelphia, PA 19104
215-895-2506
800-237-3935
FAX 215-895-1402
TDY:215-895-2299
http://www.drexel.edu
e-mail: mmp46@drexel.edu
Michelle Peters, Director
Maren Farris, Disability Specialist

An independent four-year college with a small percentage of special education students.

5822 East Stroudsburg University of Pennsylvania
200 Prospect Street
East Stroudsburg, PA 18301
570-422-3514
877-230-5547
FAX 570-422-3898
TDY:570-422-3543
http://www.esu.edu
e-mail: emiller@po-box.esu.edu
Edith Miller MD, Disability Services Director
Michelle Hoffman, Manager

Four year college that offers services to disabled students.

5823 Edinboro University of Pennsylvania
Office for Students with Disabilities
Crawford Center
Edinboro, PA 16444
814-732-2462
FAX 814-732-2866
TDY:814-732-2462
http://www.edinboro.edu
e-mail: strosser@edinboro.edu
Kathleen Strosser, Assistant Director
Janet Jenkins, LD Coordinator

Specific documentation required. Focuses on the needs of college capable students with learning disabilities.

5824 Gannon University
Program for Students with Learning Disabilities
University Square
Erie, PA 16541
814-871-5326
814-426-6668
FAX 814-871-7499
http://www.gannon.edu
e-mail: lowrey001@gannon.edu
Joyce Lowrey SSJ, Director
Jane Kanter, Assistant Director

Special Support Services are provided for students who have a diagnosed learning disability and choose to enroll in PSLO. Charge of $300.00 per semester special services include individual sessions with Educational Specialists, Kurzweil Reader, Copying Services, Advocacy Seminar Courses I and II, Reading Efficiency sessions, testing accommodations, etc.

5825 Gettysburg College
300 N Washington Street
Gettysburg, PA 17325
717-337-6000
800-431-0803
FAX 717-337-6145
Tim Dodd, Associate Dean
Katherine Will, President

Offers a variety of services to students with disabilities including notetakers, extended testing time, counseling services, and special accommodations.

5826 Gwynedd: Mercy College
PO Box 901
Gwynedd Valley, PA 19437
215-646-7300
FAX 215-641-5598
http://www.gmc.edu
e-mail: guido.r@gmc.edu
Rochelle Guido MS, Disability Support Svcs Coord.
Kathleen Mulroy, Executive Director

Recognizing the diversity of our student population and the challenges and needs this brings to the educational enterprise, Gwynedd-Mercy College, within the bounds of its resources, intends to provide reasonable accommodations for students with disabilities so that all students accepted into a program of study have equal access and subsequent opportunity to reach their academic and personal goals. Requests for specific accommodations are processed on an individual basis.

5827 Harcum Junior College
750 Montgomery Avenue
Bryn Mawr, PA 19010
610-525-4100
http://www.harcum.edu
Kathy King, Director
Charles Trout, President

An independent two-year college. There is an additional fee for the special education program in addition to the regular tuition.

5828 Harrisburg Area Community College
Disability Services Office
1 Hacc Drive
Harrisburg, PA 17110
717-780-2410
800-222-4222
FAX 717-780-3285
http://www.hacc.edu
e-mail: admit@hacc.edu
AL Jackson, Affairs & Enrollment Management
Carol Keeper, Director

A public two-year college with a small percentage of special needs students.

5829 Hill Top Preparatory School
737 S Ithan Ave
Rosemont, PA 19010
610-527-3230
FAX 610-527-7683
http://www.hilltopprep.org
Prepares students in grades 6-12 with diagnosed learning differences for higher education and successful futures. The school is d co-educational day school that offers an individually structures, rigorous curriculum that is complemented by a dynamic counseling support and menotoring program.

5830 Indiana University of Pennsylvania
201 Pratt Drive
Indiana, PA 15705
724-357-2100
FAX 724-357-2889
TDY:724-357-4067
http://www.iup.edu/advisingtesting
e-mail: advising-testing@grove.iup.edu
Catherine Dugan, Director
Todd Van Wieren, Assistant Director
Lawrence Pettit, President
Disability Support Services is a component of the Advising and Testing Center. The mission of DSS is to ensure that students with disabilities who attend Indiana University of Pennsylvainia receive an integrated, quality education.

5831 Keystone Junior College
1 College Garden
La Plume, PA 18440
570-945-5141
877-4college
http://www.keystone.edu
Carol Davis, Manager

Offers a variety of services to students with disabilities including notetakers, extended testing time, counseling services, and special accommodations.

5832 King's College
Academic Skills Center
133 N River Street
Wilkes Barre, PA 18711
570-208-5800
FAX 570-825-9049
http://www.kings.edu
e-mail: jaburke@kings.edu
Jacintha Burke, Academic Skills Center Director

First Year Academic Studies Program (FASP) - A proactive program to facilitate transition to college with intensive first-year programming with indivdual support in subsequent years. Students are enrolled as full-time students completing general education and major course requirements. Support includes regular meetings with a learning disability specialist, faculty tutorials/study groups, priority advisement, and development of self-advocacy skills. A fee charged for the first year.

5833 Kutztown University of Pennsylvania
220 Administration Building
Kutztown, PA 19530
610-683-4060
FAX 610-683-1520
TDY:610-683-4499
http://www.kutztown.edu
e-mail: sutherla@kutztown.edu
Patricia Richter, Director

Kutztown University of Pennsylvania, a member of the Pennsylvania State System of Higher Education, was founded in 1856 as Keystone Normal School, and achieved University status in 1983. Today Kutztown University is a modern, comprehensive University. There are approximately 7,900 full and part time undergraduate and graduate students.

5834 Lebanon Valley College
101 N College Avenue
Annville, PA 17003
717-867-6100
FAX 717-867-6979
http://www.lvc.edu
e-mail: perry@lvc.edu
Anne Hohenwarter, Coordinator
Stephen MacDonald, President

Four year college that offers learning disabled students support and services.

5835 Lehigh Carbon Community College
4525 Education Park Drive
Schnecksville, PA 18078
610-799-2121
FAX 610-799-1068
http://www.lccc.edu
e-mail: mmitchell@lccc.edu or lkelly@lccc.edu
Donald Snyder, President
Linda Kelly, Learning Specialist
Cathy Ahner, Office Assistant
Disability Support Services provides learning support to qualified students with disabilities in compliance with section 504 of the Rehabilitation Act and Americans with Disabilities Act, 1990. Requests for access and/or academic accommodations are reviewed on a case by case basis. Additional learning support is available through Educational Support Services.

5836 Lock Haven University of Pennsylvania
Learning Disabilities Office
401 N Fairview Street
Lock Haven, PA 17745
570-893-2027
800-332-8900
FAX 570-893-2201
http://www.lhup.edu
e-mail: rjunco@lhup.edu
Rey Junco MD, Director

A public four-year college with a small percentage of students with disabilities.

5837 **Lycoming College**
Admissions House
Williamsport, PA 17745
570-321-4000
800-345-3920
FAX 570-321-4337
http://www.lycoming.edu

Diane Bonner MD, Director
James Douthat, President

An independent four-year college with a small percentage of special education students.

5838 **Manor Junior College**
Manor Junior College
700 Fox Chase Road
Jenkintown, PA 19046
215-885-2360
FAX 215-576-6564
http://www.manor.edu
e-mail: ftadmiss@manor.edu

Mary Jurasinski, President
Sally Mydlowec, Vice President
Sister Cecilia, Administrator
Offers a variety of services to students with disabilities including notetakers, extended testing time, counseling services, and special accommodations.

5839 **Mansfield University of Pennsylvania**
Services for Students with Learning Disabilities
213 S Hall Academy Street
Mansfield, PA 16933
570-662-4798
800-577-6826
FAX 570-662-4121
http://www.mansfield.edu
e-mail: wchabala@mansfield.edu

William Chabala, Director

Offers a variety of services to students with disabilities including, extended testing time, counseling services, and special accommodations.

5840 **Marywood University**
Special Education Department
2300 Adams Avenue
Scranton, PA 18509
570-961-4731
FAX 570-961-4744
http://www.marywood.edu
e-mail: russo@es.marywood.edu

Anthony Russo MD, Director

Four year college that offers programs that are for the learning disabled.

5841 **Mercyhurst College**
Learning Disabilities Program
501 E 38th Street
Erie, PA 16546
814-824-2573
800-825-1926
FAX 814-824-2071
http://www.admissions.mercyhurst.edu
e-mail: admissions@mercyhurst.edu

Dianne Rogers, Director LD Program
Dianne Rogers, Director LD Program

Mercyhurst provides a comprehensive program of academic accommodations and support services to students with documented learning disabilities. Accommodations may include audiotaped textbooks, extended time for tests, a test reader and use of a computer to complete essay tests.

5842 **Messiah College**
1 S College Avenue
Grantham, PA 17027
717-766-2511
800-233-4220
FAX 717-796-5217
http://www.messiah.edu
e-mail: kdrahn@messiah.edu

Deb Reid Snyder, Director
Carol Wickey, Assistant to Director
Kim Phipps, President
A private Christian college of the liberal and applied arts and sciences located in Central Pennsylvania.

5843 **Millersville University of Pennsylvania**
Disability and Learning Servics
348 Lyle Hall
Millersville, PA 17551
717-872-3178
FAX 717-871-2129
http://www.millersv.edu
e-mail: learning.services@millersville.edu

Sherlynn Bessick, Director
Terry Asche, Secretary

Four year college that provides services to learning disabled students.

5844 **Moravian College**
1132 Monocacy Street
Bethlehem, PA 18018
610-861-1300
FAX 610-861-1577
http://www.moravian.edu
e-mail: memld02@moravian.edu

M. Davenport, Director
Ervin Rokke, President

Four year college that offers programs for the learning disabled.

5845 **Northampton Community College**
Disability Support Services
3835 Green Pond Road
Bethlehem, PA 18020
610-861-5342
FAX 610-861-5075
TDY:610-861-5351
http://www.northampton.edu/disabilityservices
e-mail: LDemshock@northampton.edu

Laraine Demshock, Disability Service Coordinator

Encourages academically qualified students with disabilities to take advantage of educational programs. Services and accommodations are offered to facilitate accessiblity to both college programs and facilities. Services provided to students with disabilities are based upon each student individual needs.

5846 **Pennsylvania Institute of Technology**
800 Manchester Avenue
Media, PA 19063
610-565-7900
800-422-0025
FAX 610-892-1510
http://www.pit.edu

Paul Smith, President
Walter Garrison, CEO

Offers a variety of services to students with disabilities including notetakers, extended testing time, counseling services, and special accommodations.

5847 **Pennsylvania State University: Mont Alto**
1 Campus Drive
Mont Alto, PA 17237
717-749-6046
FAX 717-749-6116
http://www.ma.psu.edu
e-mail: nmhz@psu.edu

Nanette Hatzef, Learning Center Director

It is the intention of Penn State University to provide equal access to students with disabilities as mandated by the Americans with Disabilities Act, and the Rehabilitiation Act. Students with disabilities are encouraged to take advantage of the support services provided to help them successfully meet the high academic standards of the university.

5848 **Pennsylvania State University: Schuylkill Campus**
Disability Services
200 University Drive
Schuylkill Haven, PA 17972
570-385-6000
FAX 570-385-3672
http://www.sl.psu.edu

Melinda Anthony Spolski, Disability Services Coordinator
Keith Hillkirk, Administrator

Offers a variety of services to students with disabilities including notetakers, extended testing time, counseling services, and special accommodations.

5849 **Pennsylvania State University: Shenango Valley Campus**
Office for Disability Services
105 Boucke Building
University Park, PA 16802
814-863-1807
FAX 814-863-2217
TDY:814-863-1807
http://www.equity.psu.edu/ods
e-mail: william.welsh@equity.psu.edu/ods
William Welsh, Director
Karen Port, Exam Coordinator

Penn State encourages academically qualified students with disabilities to take advantage of its educational programs. To be eligible for disability related accommodations, individuals must have a documented disability as defined by the Americans with Disabilities Act. A disability is defined by the physical or mental impairment that substantially limits a major life function. Individuals seeking accommodations are required to provided documentation.

5850 **Pennsylvania State University: Worthington Scranton Campus**
120 Ridgeview Drive
Dunmore, PA 18512
570-963-2500
FAX 570-963-2535
http://www.sn.psu.edu
Michele Steele, Special Services
Marybeth Krogh-Jesperse, Manager

Penn State encourages academically qualified students with disabilities to take advantage of its educational programs. It is the policy of the university not to discriminate against persons with disabilities in its admissions policies or procedures or its educational programs, services and activities.

5851 **Point Park College**
Program for Academic Success
201 Wood Street
Pittsburgh, PA 15222
412-391-4100
800-321-0129
FAX 412-261-5303
http://www.pointpark.edu
e-mail: pboykin@pointpark.edu
Patricia Boykin, Director
Katherine Henderson, President

Provides appropriate, reasonable accommodations for students who are disabled in accordance with the Americans with Disabilities Act. All campus accommodations are coordinated through the Program for Academic Success (PAS).

5852 **Reading Area Community College**
PO Box 1706
Reading, PA 19603
610-372-4721
800-626-1665
FAX 610-607-6264
http://www.racc.edu
Richard Kratz, President
David Adams, Admissions Director

A public two-year college with a small percentage of special education students.

5853 **Seton Hill University**
Seton Hill Drive
Greensburg, PA 15601
724-838-4255
800-826-6234
FAX 724-830-1294
http://www.setonhill.edu
e-mail: bassi@setonhill.edu
Teresa Bassi, Director Counseling Center
Mary , Director Admissions

Offers programs to those who are eligible and learning disabled.

5854 **Shippensburg University of Pennsylvania**
1871 Old Main Drive
Shippensburg, PA 17257
717-477-7447
FAX 717-477-4001
http://www.ship.edu
e-mail: lawate@wharf.ship.edu
Lois Waters MD, Director
George Harpster, President

Four year college that offers services to the learning disabled students.

5855 **Solebury School**
PO Box 429
New Hope, PA 18938
215-862-5261
FAX 215-862-3366
http://www.solebury.com/
Annette Miller, Dean
John Brown, Principal

5856 **Support Services for Students with Learning Disabilities**
Pennsylvania State University
116 Boucke Building
University Park, PA 16802
814-865-1327
FAX 814-863-2217
TDY:814-863-1807
http://www.equity.psu.edu/ods
e-mail: william.welsh@equity.psu.edu/ods
William Welsh, Director
Ann Ette, Secretary
Sanford Thatcher, Executive Director
Penn State provides academic accommodations and support services to students with documented learning disabilities. Accommodations may include audiotaped textbooks, extended time for tests, a test reader and use of a computer to complete essay tests.

5857 **Temple University**
Temple University
100 Ritter Annex
Philadelphia, PA 19122
215-707-7550
FAX 215-204-6794
http://www.temple.edu/disability
e-mail: drs@temple.edu
Wendy Kohler, LD Coordinator
Brian Seidel, Administrative Assistant

Offers a variety of services to students with disabilities including proctoring, interpreting and academic accommodations.

5858 **Thiel College**
Office of Special Needs
75 College Avenue
Greenville, PA 16125
724-589-2063
800-248-4435
FAX 724-589-2092
http://www.thiel.edu
e-mail: scowan@thiel.edu
Susan Cowan MSN RN, Office Special Needs Coordinator

Four year college that provides an Office of Special Needs for those students with disabilities.

5859 **University of Pennsylvania**
34th and Spruce Streets
Philadelphia, PA 19104
215-898-3241
FAX 215-898-5756
http://www.upenn.edu
e-mail: lrcmail@pobox.upenn.edu
Alice Nagle, Special Services
Myrna Cohen, Director

Services for People with Disabilities coordinates academic support services for students with disabilities; services include readers, notetakers, library research assistants, tutors or transcribers.

5860 **University of Pittsburgh at Bradford**
Learning Development Department
300 Campus Drive
Bradford, PA 16701
814-362-7609
800-872-1787
FAX 814-362-7684
http://www.upb.pitt.edu
Gillian Boyce MD, Director
Kara Kennedy, Learning Development Specialist

Offers a variety of services to students with disabilities including extended testing time, counseling services, and special accommodations.

5861 University of Pittsburgh: Greensburg
Disabilities Services Office
1150 Mount Pleasant Road
Greensburg, PA 15601
724-836-9880
FAX 724-836-7134
http://www.pitt.edu/~upg
e-mail: upgadmit@pitt.edu
Lou Ann Sears, Director Learning Resources Ctr
Gayle Pamerleau, Counselor

The Learning Resources Center is an important place for students with disabilities at Pitt Greensburg. Students are encouraged to register with Lou Ann Sears to recieve any accommodations they are entitled to.

5862 University of Scranton
Memorial Hall
Scranton, PA 18510
570-941-7400
FAX 570-941-7899
http://http://matrix.scranton.edu
e-mail: addmissions@scranton.edu
Mary McAndrew, Assistant Director
Scott Pilarz, President

Four year college that offers programs for learning disabled students.

5863 University of the Arts
320 S Broad Street
Philadelphia, PA 19102
215-717-6000
800-616-2787
FAX 215-717-6045
http://www.uarts.edu
Lois Elman, Learning Specialist
Migule Corzo, President

The University is committed to supporting students with learning disabilities to ensure that they have an equal opportunity to participate in the university programs. The Learning Specialist provides individual support to students with documented learning disabilities and serves as a liaision between students and faculty when needed.

5864 Ursinus College
PO Box 1000
Collegeville, PA 19426
610-409-3586
FAX 610-489-0627
http://www.ursinus.edu
Richard DiFeliciantonio, Director of Admissions

Offers a variety of services to students with disabilities including notetakers, extended testing time, counseling services, and special accommodations.

5865 Villanova University
800 Lancaster Avenue
Villanova, PA 19085
610-519-4500
FAX 610-519-8015
http://www.villanova.edu
e-mail: nancy.mott@villanova.edu
Nancy Mott, Coordinator
Edmund Dobbin, President

Four year college that provides services to learning disabled students.

5866 Washington and Jefferson College
60 S Lincoln Street
Washington, PA 15301
724-222-4400
888-926-3529
FAX 724-223-5271
http://www.washjeff.edu
Catherine Sherman, Assistant Dean
Denny Trelka, Dean
Tori Haring-Smith, Administrator
An independent four-year college with a small percentage of special education students.

5867 Westmoreland County Community College
400 Armbrust Road
Youngwood, PA 15697
724-925-4000
800-262-2103
FAX 724-925-5802
TDY:724-925-4297
http://www.wccc-pa.edu
e-mail: beresm@wccc-pa.edu
Mary Ellen Beres, Student Support Svcs Counselor
Sandra Zelenak, Student Development Director
Steven Ender, President
Offers a variety of services to students with disabilities including notetakers, extended testing time, counseling services, and special accommodations. All services are based on a review of a current evaluation presented by the student. Appropriate services are then arranged by the student support service counselor.

5868 Widener University
Disabilities Services
1 University Place
Chester, PA 19013
610-499-1266
FAX 610-499-1192
http://www.widener.edu/sss/ssmain.html
e-mail: csimonds@mail.widener.edu
Cynthia Simonds PsyD, Director Disabilities Services
James Harris, President

An independent four-year college with comprehensive support services.

Rhode Island

5869 Brown University
Disability Support Services
20 Benevolent Street
Providence, RI 02912
401-863-9588
FAX 401-863-1999
TDY:401-863-9588
http://www.brown.edu
e-mail: catherine_axe@brown.edu
Catherine Axe, Director
Catherine Axe, Director

Brown University has as its primary aim the education of a highly qualified and diverse student body and respects each student's dignity, capacity to contribute, and desire for personal growth and accomplishment. Brown's commitment to students with disabilities is based on awareness of what students require for success. The University desires to foster both intellectual and physical independence to the greatest extent possible in all of its students.

5870 Bryant College
Academic Services
1150 Douglas Pike
Smithfield, RI 02917
401-232-6000
FAX 401-232-6038
http://www.bryant.edu
e-mail: lhazard@bryant.edu
Laurie Hazard MD, Director
Mary Moroney, Executive Director
Sharon Doyle, Office Manager
An independent four-year Business and Liberal Arts College. A learning specialist is on campus to provide services for students with learning disabilities.

5871 Community College of Rhode Island-Knight
400 E Avenue
Warwick, RI 02886
401-825-2164

5872 Community College of Rhode Island: KnightCampus
400 E Avenue
Warwick, RI 02886
401-825-2305
FAX 401-825-1145
http://www.ccri.edu
e-mail: amcmahon@ccri.edu
Alda McMahon, Contact

Academic accommodations are available to students with disabilities who demonstrate a documented need for the requested accommodation. Accommodations include but are not limited to adapted equipment, alternative testing, course accommodations, sign language interpreters, reader/audio taping services, scribes and peer note-takers.

5873 **Johnson & Wales University**

8 Abbott Park Place
Providence, RI 02903
401-598-1000
800-343-2565
FAX 401-598-4657
e-mail: mberstein@jwu.edu

Meryl Berstein, Center Academic Support Director
John Yena, Administrator

An independent four-year university servicing about 5% special education students. Accommodations are individualized to students presenting documentation and may include extended time testing, tape recorders in class, notetaking assistance, reduced course load, preferential scheduling and tutorial assistance.

5874 **Paul V Sherlock Center on Disabilities atRhode Island College**

600 Mount Pleasant Avenue
Providence, RI 02908
401-456-8072
FAX 401-456-8150
TDY:401-456-8773
http://www.sherlockcenter.org
e-mail: aantosh@ric.edu

A Antosh, Director
Erika Tuttle, Administrative Assistant

The University Affiliated Program (UAP) of Rhode Island is a member of a national network of UAPs. The UAP is charged with four core functions: 1. Providing pre-service training to prepare quality service providers. 2. Providing community outreach training and technical assistance. 3. Disseminating information about research and exemplary practice. 4. Research.

5875 **Providence College**

Office of Academic Services - Disabiliy Support Sv
549 River Avenue
Providence, RI 02918
401-865-2494
FAX 401-865-1219
TDY:401-865-2494
http://www.providence.edu/oas
e-mail: oas@providence.edu

Nicole Kudarauskas, Asst Dir Disability Support Svcs
Dan Kwash, Interim

Offers a variety of services to students with disabilities including note takers, extended testing time, counseling services, and special accommodations.

5876 **Rhode Island College**

600 Mount Pleasant Avenue
Providence, RI 02908
401-456-8000
FAX 401-456-8702
http://www.ric.edu

Ann Roccio, Director
Barbara Kingston, Administrative Assistant
John Nazarian, President

Four-year college with support and services for learnig disabled students.

5877 **Roger Williams University**

Old Ferry Road
Bristol, RI 02809
401-253-1040
800-458-7144
FAX 401-254-3302
http://www.rwu.edu

Roy Nirschel, President

An independent comprehensive four-year university with about 5% special education students.

5878 **University of Rhode Island**

Disability Services
330 Memorial Under
Kingston, RI 02881
401-874-2098
FAX 401-874-5574
http://www.uri.edu

Pamela Rohland, Director

Disability Service for Students fosters a barrier free environment to individuals with disabilities through education that focuses on inclusion, awareness, and knowledge of ADA/504 compliance. Our mission is two fold: 1. To encourage a sense of empowerment for students with disabilities by providing a process that involves the student. 2. To be an information resource to the University faculty and staff regarding disability awareness and academic services.

South Carolina

5879 **Aiken Technical College**

Student Services
PO Box 400
Aiken, SC 29802
803-593-9231
FAX 803-593-6641
http://www.atc.edu
e-mail: weldon@atc.edu

Richard Weldon, Counselor
Jennifer Pinckney, Manager

A public two-year college offering services to the learning disabled.

5880 **Citadel-Military College of South Carolina**

171 Moultrie Street
Charleston, SC 29409
843-225-3294
FAX 843-953-7036
http://www.citadel.edu

Gordon Wallace

Offers a variety of services to students with disabilities including notetakers, extended testing time, counseling services, and special accommodations.

5881 **Clemson University**

Student Development Services
707 University Under
Clemson, SC 29634
864-656-0515
FAX 864-656-0514
http://www.clemson.edu
e-mail: bmartin@clemson.edu

Bonnie Martin, Director

Four-year college offers services to learning disabled students.

5882 **Coastal Carolina University**

Disability Services Department
PO Box 261954
Conway, SC 29528
843-347-3161
FAX 843-349-2990
http://www.coastal.edu

Monica Yates, Director
Vonna Gengo, Disability Services Coordinator
Ronald Ingle, President

Coastal Carolina University provides a program of assistance to students with disabilities. Upon acceptance to the University, students will become eligible for support services by providing documentation of their disability. Accommodations include academic labs, tutorial referral, study skills, counseling, auxillary aids, coordination with other agencies and classroom accommodations.

5883 **College of Charleston**

Special Needs Advising Plan
66 George Street
Charleston, SC 29424
843-953-1431
FAX 843-953-7731
TDY:843-953-8284
http://www.cofc.edu/~cds
e-mail: SNAP@cofc.edu

Ann Lacy, Coordinator SNAP Services

Provides reasonable and appropriate accommodations specific to individual needs based on the psycho-educational assessment, communication with instructors as needed to heighten awareness of individual needs, alternative coursesin math and foreign language, if need, is documented by assessment.

5884 **Erskine College**
Due West, SC 29639
864-379-2131
FAX 864-379-2167
http://www.erskine.edu

John Carson, President

Offers a variety of services to students with disabilities including notetakers, extended testing time, counseling services, and special accommodations.

5885 **Francis Marion University**
PO Box 100547
Florence, SC 29501
843-661-1362
800-368-7551
http://www.fmarion.edu

Luther Carter, President

A public four-year college with services for special education students.

5886 **Greenville Technical College**
PO Box 5616
Greenville, SC 29606
864-246-7282
800-922-1183
FAX 864-250-8580
http://www.greenvilletech.com

Owen Perkins, Associate Dean
Claire Carter, Executive Director

Committed to providing equal access for all students and assisting students in making their college experience successful in accordance with ADA/504 and the Rehabilitation Act. The Office of Special Needs for Students with Disabilities has counselors available to assist in the planning and implementation of appropriate accommodations.

5887 **Limestone College**
Program for Alternative Learning Styles
1115 College Drive
Gaffney, SC 29340
864-489-7151
http://www.limestone.edu
e-mail: jpitts@saint.limestone.edu

Joseph Pitt, Director
Carolyn Hayward, Manager

Independent four-year college with a program designed to serve students with learning disabilities. There is an additional fee for the first year in the program in addition to the regular tuition. However, that additional cost is reduced by 50% after the freshman year depending on the grade point average.

5888 **Midlands Technical College**
PO Box 2408
Columbia, SC 29202
803-738-1400
FAX 803-822-3290
http://www.midlandstech.edu
e-mail: brussell@midland.tec.edu

Barry Russell, President
Gina Mounsield, Vice President

Services to Students with Disabilities counselors support and assist students with disabilities in meeting their personal, educational and career goals. Services include academic and career planning, faculty/student liasion, assistive technology, readers, writers, interpeters, closed circuit television in libraries, TDD, testing services, orientation sessions and a support group.

5889 **North Greenville College**
Learning Disabilities Services
PO Box 1892
Tigerville, SC 29688
864-977-7000
800-468-6642
FAX 864-977-2089
http://www.ngc.edu
e-mail: nisgett@ngc.edu

Nancy Isgett, Learning Disabilities Liaison
James Epting, President

Offers a variety of services to students with disabilities including notetakers, extended testing time, counseling services, and special accommodations.

5890 **South Carolina State University**
PO Box 7508
Orangeburg, SC 29115
803-536-7000
FAX 803-536-8702
http://www.scsu.edu
e-mail: gouveia@scsu.edu

Imogene Gouveia MD, Chief Psychologist
Andrew Hugine, President

Four-year college that provides information and resources for the learning disabled.

5891 **Spartanburg Methodist College**
1200 Textile Road
Spartanburg, SC 29301
864-587-4000
FAX 864-587-4355
http://www.smcsc.edu

Sharon Porter, Student Support Director
Charles Teague, President

An independent two-year college with services for special education students.

5892 **Technical College of Lowcountry: Beaufort**
PO Box 1288
Beaufort, SC 29901
843-525-8324
FAX 843-521-4142

Carolyn Banner, Career Development

Offers a variety of services to students with disabilities including note takers, extended testing time, counseling services, and special accommodations.

5893 **Trident Academy**
1455 Wakendaw Road
Mt Pleasant, SC 29464
843-884-7046
FAX 843-881-8320
http://www.tridentacademy.com/
e-mail: admissions@tridentacademy.com

Myron Harrington, Principal

Trident Academy is an internationally known independent school for children with diagnosed learning disabilities such as dyslexia and attention deficit disorder serving students in grades K-12.

5894 **Trident Technical College**
PO Box 118067
Charleston, SC 29423
843-574-6111
877-349-7184
FAX 843-574-6484
http://www.trident.tec.sc.us

Mary Thornley, President

Recognizes its responsibility to identify and maintain the standards (academic, admissions, scores, etc.) that are necessary to provide quality academic programs while ensuring the rights of students with disabilities.

5895 **University of South Carolina**
Disability Services
106 Leconte
Columbia, SC 29208
803-777-6742
FAX 803-777-6741
TDY:803-777-6744
http://www.sc.edu
e-mail: kpettus@sc.edu

Karen Pettus, Executive Director
Andrea Bullock, Office Assistant
Dorothy Prioleau, Office Manager

The Office of Disability Services provides accommodations for students with documented physical, emotional, and learning disabilities. The professionally trained staff works toward accessiblity for all university programs, services, and activities in compliance with ADA/504. Services include orientation,priority registration, library access, classroom adaptions, interpeters, and access to adapted housing.

5896 **University of South Carolina: Aiken**
171 University Parkway
Aiken, SC 29801
803-648-6851
FAX 803-641-3362
http://www.usca.sc.edu/ds
e-mail: kayb@aiken.sc.edu
Randy Duckett, Special Services
Tom Hallman, Manager

The mission of Disability Services (DS) is to facilitate the transition of students with disabilities into the University enviroment and to provide appropriate accommodations for each student's special needs in order to ensure equal access to all programs, activities and services at USCA.

5897 **University of South Carolina: Beaufort**
801 Carteret Street
Beaufort, SC 29902
843-521-4100
FAX 843-521-4194
http://www.sc.edu/beaufort
Joan Lemoine MD, Associate Dean
Jane Upshaw, President

A public two-year college with services for special education students.

5898 **University of South Carolina: Lancaster**
Admissions Office
PO Box 889
Lancaster, SC 29721
803-313-7000
FAX 803-313-7106
http://www.lancaster.sc.edu
e-mail: ksaile@gwm.sc.edu
John Catalano, Administrator
Rebecca Parker, Director

Offers a variety of services to students with disabilities including notetakers, extended testing time, counseling services, and special accommodations.

5899 **Voorhees College**
PO Box 678
Denmark, SC 29042
803-703-7131
FAX 803-793-4584
Adeleri Onisegu MD, Director
Curtiss Sumner, Manager

Four-year college that offers programs to learning disabled students.

5900 **Winthrop University**
Student Disabilities Department
701 Oakland Ave
Rock Hill, SC 29733
803-323-2211
FAX 803-328-2855
TDY:803-323-2233
http://www.winthrop.edu
e-mail: smithg@winthrop.edu
Gina Smith, Director
Rosanne Wallace, Administrator

Since each student has a unique set of special needs, the Counselor for Students with Disabilities makes every effort to provide the student with full access to programs and services. Reasonable accommodations are provided based on needs assessed through proper documentation and an intake interview with the couselor. The majority of buildings on campus are accessible.

South Dakota

5901 **Black Hills State College**
1200 University Street
Spearfish, SD 57783
605-642-6011
800-255-2478
FAX 605-642-6391
http://www.bhsu.edu/disability
e-mail: larryvrooman@bhsu.edu
Larry Vrooman, Disability Services Coordinator
Thomas Flickema, President

Provide the comprehensive supports necessary in meeting the individual needs of students with disabilities.

5902 **Northern State University**
1200 S Jay Street
Aberdeen, SD 57401
605-626-2544
FAX 605-626-3399
http://www.northern.edu
e-mail: diagle@northern.edu
Kay Diagle, Director
Patrick Schloss, President

Four-year college that provides services to students with a learning disability.

5903 **South Dakota School of Mines & Technology**
501 E Saint Joseph Street
Rapid City, SD 57701
605-394-2511
800-544-8162
FAX 605-394-1268
http://www.sdsmt.edu
e-mail: fcampone@sdsmt.edu
Francine Campon MD, Associate Dean
Charles Ruch, President

Four-year college that offers support services to those students whom are disabled.

5904 **South Dakota State University**
PO Box 2201
Brookings, SD 57007
605-688-5907
800-952-3541
FAX 605-688-6891
TDY:605-688-4394
http://www.sdstate.edu
e-mail: SDSU_Admissions@sdstate.edu
Nancy Hartenhoff-Crookf, Coordinator
Dana Dykhouse, President&Chief Executive Office

Committed to providing equal opportunities for higher education for learning disabled students.

5905 **Yankton College**
PO Box 133
Yankton, SD 57078
605-665-3661
866-665-3661
FAX 605-665-0541
http://www.yanktoncollege.org
e-mail: yc@byelectric
Elizabeth Elbe, Executive Director

Offers a variety of services to students with disabilities including note takers, extended testing time, counseling services, and special accommodations.

Tennessee

5906 **Austin Peay State University: Office of Disability Services**
Office of Disability Services
PO Box 4567
Clarksville, TN 37044
931-221-6230
FAX 931-221-7102
TDY:931-221-6278
http://www.apsu.edu/disability
e-mail: oldhamb@apsu.edu
Beulah Oldham, Director
Bryon Kluesner, Assistant Director

The Office of Disability Services is dedicated to providing academic assistance for students with disabilities enrolled at Austin Peay State University. We provide information to students, faculty, staff and administrators about the needs of students with disabilities. We ensure the accessiblity of programs, services, and activities to students having a disability. We are a resource of information pertaining to disability issues and advocate participation in campus life.

5907 **Boling Center for Developmental Disabilities**
University of Tennessee
711 Jefferson Avenue
Memphis, TN 38105
901-448-5944
888-572-2249
FAX 901-448-7097
http://www.utmem.edu/bcdd
e-mail: wwilson@utmem.edu

Fredrick Palmer MD, Director
William , Clinical Services Coordinator
Anthony Canepa, Manager

Interdisciplinary or focused evaluation of learning, behavioral and developmental problems in infants, toddlers, children and young adults. Treatment of some conditions offered.

5908 **Brookhaven College**
Special Services Office
3939 Valley View Lane
Farmers Branch, TX 75244
972-860-4847
http://www.dcccd.edu.bhc

Amadeo Ledesma, Grants Manager

Physically challenged and learning disabled special services office offers advisement, additional diagnostic evaluations, mobility assistance, note taking, textbook taping, interpreters for the deaf and assistance in test taking.

5909 **Bryan College: Dayton**
PO Box 7000
Dayton, TN 37321
423-775-7207
800-277-9522
FAX 423-775-7199
http://www.bryan.edu

Mark Craver, Director of Admissions
Peter Held, VP Student Life

Committed to providing quality education for those who meet admission standards but learn differently from others. Modifications are made in the learning environment to enable LD students to succeed. Some of the modifications made require documentation of the specific disability while other adaptations do not. In addition to modifications the small teacher-student ratio allows the school to provide much individual attention to those with learning difficulties.

5910 **Carson-Newman College**
1646 Russell Avenue
Jefferson City, TN 37760
865-471-2000
800-678-9061
FAX 865-471-3502
http://www.cn.edu

John Gibson, Associate Professor
James Netherton, President

An independent four-year college with support services for special education students.

5911 **DHH Outreach**
East Tennessee State University
PO Box 70605
Johnson City, TN 37614
423-439-6268
FAX 423-439-8489
TDY:423-439-8370
http://www.etsu.edu
e-mail: storey@mail.etsu.edu /gibson@etsu.edu

Linda MEd, Disability Services Director
Martha Edde-Adams, Disability Services Asst. Dir.
Carolyn Hopson, Manager

The Deaf and Hard of Hearing Outreach program provides coordination of interpreting services for student needs related to classroom and university events.

5912 **East Tennessee State University Disability Services**
PO Box 70605
Johnson City, TN 37614
423-439-6268
FAX 423-439-8489
TDY:423-439-8370
http://www.etsu.edu
e-mail: storey@mail.etsu.edu /gibson@etsu.edu

Linda MEd, Disability Services Director
Martha Edde-Adams, Disability Services Asst. Dir.
Carolyn Hopson, Manager

The Disability Services Office works to provide services to give students with disabilities equal opportunities at ETSU through the provision of resonable accommodations, coordination of auxiliary aids, and support services.

5913 **Knoxville Business College**
720 N 5th Avenue
Knoxville, TN 37917
865-966-3869
FAX 423-637-0127
http://www.kbcollege.edu

Judy Ferguson, Dean Students

Offers a variety of services to students with disabilities including notetakers, extended testing time, counseling services, and special accommodations.

5914 **Lambuth College**
705 Lambuth Boulevard
Jackson, TN 38301
731-425-2500
800-526-2884
FAX 731-988-4600
http://www.lambuth.edu

Becky Sadowski, School Education Head
R. Zuker, President

Offers a variety of services to students with disabilities including notetakers, extended testing time, counseling services, and special accommodations.

5915 **Leap Program**
East Tennessee State University
PO Box 70605
Johnson City, TN 37614
423-439-6268
FAX 423-439-8489
TDY:423-439-8370
http://www.etsu.edu
e-mail: storey@mail.etsu.edu /gibson@etsu.edu

Linda MEd, Disability Services Director
Martha Edde-Adams, Disability Services Asst. Dir.
Carolyn Hopson, Manager

The Learning Empowerment for Academic Performance Program is a grant funded program sponsored by Tennessee Department of Human Services, Division of Vocational Rehabilitation.

5916 **Learning Disabilities - ADHD Program - University of Memphis**
Learning Disabilities - ADHA Program
110 Wilder Tower
Memphis, TN 38152
901-678-2880
FAX 901-678-3070
TDY:901-678-2880
http://www.saweb.memphis.edu/sds/
e-mail: stepaske@memphis.edu

Susan TePaske, Director

Emphasizes individual responsibility for learning by offering a developmentally oriented program of college survival skills, learning strategies, and individualized planning and counseling based on the student's strengths and weaknesses. The program also coordinates comprehensive support services, including test accommodations, tutoring and learning strategies, alternate format tests and assistive technology. The program serves 400 to 500 students with learning disabilities and ADHD per year.

5917 **Lee University: Cleveland**
Academic Support Program
PO Box 3450
Cleveland, TN 37320
423-614-8181
800-533-9930
FAX 423-614-8179
http://www.leeuniversity.edu
e-mail: ggallher@leeuniversity.edu

Gayle Gallaher MD, Director
Paul Conn, President

An independent four-year college with services for special education students.

5918 Middle Tennessee State University
Middle Tennessee State University
1301 E Main Street
Murfreesboro, TN 37132
615-898-2300
FAX 615-898-4893
http://www.mtsu.edu
e-mail: dssemail@mtsu.edu
John Harris, Disabled Student Services
Sydney Phee, President

We offer a wide variety of services to students with disabilities including testing accommodations, providing access to adaptive computer technologies and acting as a liaison to University departments.

5919 Motlow State Community College
PO Box 8500
Lynchburg, TN 37352
931-455-8511
800-654-4877
FAX 931-393-1764
http://www.mscc.cc.tn.us
e-mail: asimmons@mscc.cc.tn.us
A. Simmons, Dean Student Development
Billy Soloman, Owner

A public two-year college with support services for special education students.

5920 Northeast State Technical Community College
Learning Disabilities Department
PO Box 246
Blountville, TN 37617
423-354-2476
800-836-7822
FAX 423-279-7649
TDY:423-279-7640
http://www.nstcc.cc.tn.us
e-mail: kafoulk@northeaststate.edu
Betty Mask, Director
Tonya Cassell, Office Manager

To assure equal educational opportunities for individuals with disabilities.

5921 Pellissippi State Technical Community College
PO Box 22990
Knoxville, TN 37933
865-981-5300
FAX 865-539-7217
http://www.pstcc.cc.tn.us
e-mail: semcmurray@pstcc.cc.tn.us
Joan Newman, Academic Assess Director
William Eanes, Manager

Services for Students with Disabilities develops individual educational support plans, provides prioriy registration and advisement, furnishes volunteer notetakers, provides readers, scribes, tutor bank, provides interpeter services and publishes a newsletter. The office acts as a liaison, and assists students in location of resources appropriate to their needs.

5922 Scenic Land School
1200 Mountain Creek Road
Chattanooga, TN 37405
423-877-9711
FAX 423-876-0398
http://www.sceniclandschool.org
e-mail: ecard@sceniclandschool.org
Eileen Card, Principal
Mary Brown, IEP & Assessment Director
Rhainne McRae, Dean of Students
Scenic Land School is a private nonprofit school for students with learning disabilities. The school primarily serves students with dyslexia and ADHD. Average class size is 8-10 students and a 1:8 teacher:student ratio.

5923 Shelby State Community College
737 Union Avenue
Memphis, TN 38103
901-545-5505
FAX 901-333-5711
http://www.sscc.cc.tn.us
Jimmy Wiley, Director
Mark Luttrell, Manager

A two-year college providing information and resources to disabled students.

5924 Southern Adventist University
Academic Support
PO Box 370
Collegedale, TN 37315
423-236-2779
800-768-8437
FAX 423-238-1765
http://www.ldpsych.southern.edu
e-mail: adossant@southern.edu
Alberto Santos, Dean
Mikhaile Spence, Graduate School Coordinator

A private university offering undergraduate degrees in education designed for K-8, 1-8, 7-12, and K-12 certification plus graduate degrees designed for inclusion (special needs in the regular classroom), multiage/multigrade teaching, outdoor education, and psychology and counseling of exceptional individuals. College age students with special needs and those desiring to teach students with special needs are welcome to apply.

5925 Southwest Tennessee Community College
5983 Macon Civic
Memphis, TN 38134
901-333-4000
888-832-4937
FAX 901-333-4458
http://www.southwest.tn.edu
Ashok Dhingra, Manager

Offers a variety of services to students with disabilities including note takers, extended testing time, counseling services, and special accommodations.

5926 Tennessee State University
Office of Disabled Student Services
3500 John a Merritt Boulevard
Nashville, TN 37209
615-963-7400
888-536-7655
FAX 615-963-2176
TDY:615-963-7440
http://www.tnstate.edu
e-mail: pscudder@tnstate.edu
Patricia Scudder, Director
Monique Mitchell, Secretary
Steven McCrary, Coordinator
Four year college offers services for learning disabled students.

5927 University of Tennessee: Knoxville
Disability Services Office
191 Hoskins Library
Knoxville, TN 37996
865-974-6087
FAX 865-974-9552
TDY:865-974-6087
http://www. ods.utk.edu
e-mail: esinger1@utk.edu
Emily Singer, Executive VP

Offers a variety of services to students with disabilities including note takers, extended testing time, counseling services, and special accommodations.

5928 University of Tennessee: Martin
Program Access for College Enhancement
209 Clement
Martin, TN 38238
731-881-7000
FAX 731-881-7702
http://www.utm.edu
e-mail: sroberts@utm.edu
Sharon Robertson, Coordinator
George Daniel, Director
Nick Dunagan, Administrator
A four-year independent college that offers a program called Program Access for College Enhancement for students with learning disabilities.

5929 Vanderbilt University
Vanderbilt University
2301 Vanderbilt Place
Nashville, TN 37203
615-322-3476
FAX 615-343-0671
TDY:615-322-4705
http://www.vanderbilt.edu
e-mail: melissa.a.smith@vanderbilt.edu
Melissa Smith, Director Disability Program
Gordon Gee, Chancellor
Robert Cotton MD, Administrator

An independent four-year college with support services for special education students.

5930 **William Jennings Bryan College**
HEATH Resource Center
2121 K Street NW
Washington, DC 20037
202-337-7600
800-544-3284
FAX 202-973-0908
http://www.heath.gwu.edu
e-mail: askheath@heath.gwu.edu
Dan Gardner, Publications Manager
Janine Heath, Manager

A public four-year college. The HEALTH Resource Center operates the national clearinghouse on postsecondary education for individuals with disabilities.

Texas

5931 **Abilene Christian University**
Alpha Academic Services
PO Box 29204
Abilene, TX 79699
915-674-2750
FAX 915-674-6847
http://www.acu.edu
e-mail: dodda@acu.edu
Ada Dodd, Counselor

A four year college that offers services to students who are learning disabled.

5932 **Alvin Community College**
Alvin Community College
3110 Mustang Road
Alvin, TX 77511
281-756-3500
FAX 281-756-3843
http://www.alvincollege.edu
Eileen Cross, Counselor
Alyssa Reeves, Admission Specialist
Rodney Allbright, President
A public two-year college with support services for special education students.

5933 **Amarillo College: Department of Disabilities**
Department of Disabilities
PO Box 447
Amarillo, TX 79178
806-371-5000
FAX 806-371-5771
TDY:806-345-5506
http://www.actx.edu
e-mail: wilkes-bj@actx.edu
Brenda Wilkes, Coordinator
Steven Jones, President

Offers a variety of services to students with disabilities including note takers, extended testing time, counseling services, and special accommodations.

5934 **Angelina College**
Student Services Office
PO Box 1768
Lufkin, TX 75902
936-639-1301
FAX 936-633-5455
http://www.angelina.edu
e-mail: jtwohig@angelina.edu
James Twohig, Dean
Larry Phillips, President

A public two-year college with support services for special education students.

5935 **Baylor University**
Office of Access & Learning Accommodation
PO Box 97204
Waco, TX 76798
254-710-3605
FAX 254-710-3608
http://www.baylor.edu
e-mail: ahelia_graham@baylor.edu
Shelia Graham MD, Director

Four-year college that offers support and services to students who are learning disabled.

5936 **Briarwood School**
12207 Whittington Drive
Houston, TX 77077
281-493-1070
FAX 281-493-1343
http://www.briarwoodschool.org
e-mail: info@briarwoodschool.org
Carole Wills, Principal
Priscilla Mitchell, Admissions Director

Briarwood has been serving students with diagnosed learning differences for 35 years. A co-ed private day school offering small classes, remedial and college prep curriculum for its 300 K-12 students. Briarwood believes that every child can learn and has the right to be taught in the way that he or she learns best.

5937 **Cedar Valley College**
Special Support Services
3030 N Dallas Avenue
Lancaster, TX 75134
972-860-8199
FAX 972-860-8014
http://www.dcccd.edu
e-mail: gcf787@dcccd.edu
Grenna Fynn, Director
Michelle Quinn, Special Support Services

A two-year college that provides special services to its disabled students.

5938 **Central Texas College**
PO Box 1800
Killeen, TX 76540
254-526-7161
800-792-3348
FAX 254-526-1700
TDY:254-526-1378
http://www.ctcd.edu
Jose Apotte, Counselor
James Anderson, Manager

Offers a variety of services to students with disabilities including extended testing time, counseling services, and assistive technology.

5939 **Cisco Junior College**
Cisco Junior College
101 College Heights
Cisco, TX 76437
254-442-2567
FAX 254-442-5100
http://www.cisco.cc.tx.us
Link Harris, Counselor
Elaine Lee, Executive Secretary
John Muller, President
A public two-year college with support services for special education students.

5940 **College of the Mainland**
Student Support Services
1200 N Amburn Road
Texas City, TX 77591
409-938-1211
888-258-8859
FAX 409-938-1306
http://www.com.edu
e-mail: kkimbark@com.edu
Kris Kimbark, Director
Homer Hayes, President

Offers a variety of services to students with disabilities including notetakers, extended testing time, counseling services, and special accommodations. The mission of services for students with disabilities is to provide each student with the resources needed to register, enroll and complete their course work and/or degree plan.

5941 **Collin County Community College**
2200 W University Drive
McKinney, TX 75071
972-548-6790
FAX 972-548-6702
http://www.ccccd.edu
Norma Johnson, Director
Rex Parcells, Manager

A public two-year college. ACCESS provides resonable accommodations, individual attention and support for students with disabilities who need assistance with any aspect of their campus experience such as accessibility, academics and testing.

5942 **Concordia University at Austin**
3400 N IH 35
Austin, TX 78705
512-486-2000
FAX 512-486-1155
http://www.concordia.com
e-mail: admissionj@concordia.edu
Beryl Dunsmoir MD, Chair

Four year college offers services to disabled students.

5943 **Dallas Academy**
950 Tiffany Way
Dallas, TX 75218
214-324-1481
FAX 214-327-8537
http://www.dallas-academy.com
e-mail: mail@dallas-academy.com
Jim Richardson, Executive Director
Ronda Criss, Development Director

Offers a variety of services to students with disabilities including notetakers, extended testing time, counseling services, and special accommodations.

5944 **Dallas Academy: Coed High School**
950 Tiffany Way
Dallas, TX 75218
214-324-1481
FAX 214-327-8537
http://www.dallas-academy.com
e-mail: mail@dallas-academy.com
Karen Kinsella, Assistant Director
Ronda Criss, Development Director
Jim Richardson, Executive Director
Coed Day School for bright children grades 7-12 with diagnosed learning differences. Curriculum includes sports, art, music, and photography programs.

5945 **Dallas County Community College**
3737 Motley Drive
Mesquite, TX 75150
972-86+0-768
FAX 972-860-7227
http://www.dcccd.edu/
Offers a variety of services to students with disabilities including note takers, extended testing time, counseling services, and special accommodations.

5946 **East Texas Baptist University**
1209 N Grove Street
Marshall, TX 75670
903-935-7963
800-804-3828
FAX 903-938-7798
http://www.etbu.edu
Charles Taylor, Director
Bob Riley, President

Offers a variety of services to students with disabilities including notetakers, extended testing time, counseling services, and special accommodations.

5947 **East Texas State University**
E Texas Station
Commerce, TX 75428
903-886-5000
FAX 903-886-5702
Tom Lynch, Contact

Offers a variety of services to students with disabilities including note takers, extended testing time, counseling services, and special accommodations.

5948 **Eastfield College**
3737 Motley Drive
Mesquite, TX 75150
972-860-7100
FAX 972-860-8342
http://www.efc.dcccd.edu
e-mail: mds4420@dcccd.edu
Reva Rattan, Coordinator

Offers a variety of services to students with disabilities including note takers, extended testing time, counseling services, and special accommodations.

5949 **El Centro College**
El Centro College
Main & Lamar Streets
Dallas, TX 75202
214-860-2177
FAX 214-860-2335
http://www.ecc.dcccd.edu
e-mail: kir5341@dcccd.edu
Jim Handy, Director Counseling
Karen Reed, Assistant Director

A public two-year college with support services for special education students.

5950 **El Paso Community College: Valle Verde Campus**
Center for Students with Disabilities
PO Box 20500
El Paso, TX 79998
915-831-3722
FAX 915-831-2244
http://www.epcc.edu
e-mail: janlc@epcc.edu
Jan Lockhart, Director
Santiago Rodriquez, Manager

A support service for students enrolled at the college who have a verified temporary or permanent disability. Support services offered include advising, tutoring, note taking, test assistance and more.

5951 **Frank Phillips College**
Special Populations Department
PO Box 5118
Borger, TX 79008
806-457-4200
800-687-2056
FAX 806-457-4226
http://www.fpctx.edu
Karen Lane, Special Populations Coordinator

Offers a variety of services to students with disabilities including notetakers, extended testing time, counseling services, and special accommodations.

5952 **Galveston College**
4015 Avenue Q
Galveston, TX 77550
409-944-4242
FAX 409-762-9367
http://www.gc.edu
Gaynelle Hayes MD, Vice President
Elva LeBlanc, Owner

A public two-year college. A variety of services and programs are available to assist students with disabilities, those who are academically and/or economically disadvantaged and those with limited English proficiency.

5953 **Hill College of the Hill Junior College District**
PO Box 619
Hillsboro, TX 76645
254-582-2555
FAX 254-582-7591
http://www.hillcollege.edu
e-mail: bknelson@hillcollege.edu
Bill Gilker, Dean Students
Belinda Nelson, Admissions Coordinator
Sheryl Kappus, President
Offers a variety of services to students with disabilities including note takers, extended testing time, counseling services, and special accommodations.

5954 **Houston Community College System**
Houston Community College System
3100 Holman Street
Houston, TX 77004
713-718-2000
FAX 713-718-2111
TDY:713-718-6166
http://www.hccs.edu
e-mail: welbert@hccs.edu
John Reno, Director
Cherry Caraway, Office Manager
Bruce Leslie, Administrator
Offers a variety of services to students with disabilities including note takers, extended testing time, counseling services, and special accommodations.

5955 Jarvis Christian College
PO Box 1470
Hawkins, TX 75765
903-769-5700
800-292-9517
FAX 903-769-5005
http://www.jarvis.edu
e-mail: florine_white@jarvis.edu
Florine White MD, Student Support Services Dir.
Sebetha Jenkins, President

Student Support Services is a federally funded program whose purpose is to improve the retention and graduate rate of program participants. Eligible program participants include low income, first generation college students and students with learning and physical disabilities. A variety of support services are provided.

5956 Lamar University: Port Arthur
Special Populations
PO Box 310
Port Arthur, TX 77641
409-983-4921
800-477-5872
FAX 409-984-6000
TDY:409-984-6242
http://www.pa.lamar.edu
e-mail: andrea.munoz@lamarpa.edu
Andrea Munoz, Director
Stephanie Bucanan, Administrative Assistant
Sam Monroe, President
A public two-year college with support services for special education students.

5957 Laredo Community College: Special Populations Office
Special Populations Office
W End Washington Street
Laredo, TX 78040
956-721-5137
FAX 956-721-5838
e-mail: sylviat@laredo.cc.tx.us
Sylvia LMSW, Counselor/Coordinator

Offers a variety of services to students with disabilities including notetakers, extended testing time, counseling services, and special accommodations.

5958 Lubbock Christian University
5601 19th Street
Lubbock, TX 79407
806-796-8800
800-933-7601
FAX 806-720-7162
http://www.lcu.edu
e-mail: admissions@lcu.edu
Ken Jones, President
Rod Blackwood, Vice President

Offers a variety of services to students with disabilities including notetakers, extended testing time, counseling services, and special accommodations.

5959 McLennen Community College
McLennan Community College
1400 College Drive
Waco, TX 76708
254-299-8604
FAX 254-299-8556
http://www.mclennan.edu
Anitra Cooton, Director
Mickey Reyes, Desktop Publishing Technician
Dennis Michaelis, President
A public two-year college with support services for special education students.

5960 Midwestern State University
Disability Counseling Office
3410 Taft Boulevard
Wichita Falls, TX 76308
940-397-4618
FAX 940-397-4934
TDY:940-397-4515
http://www.mwsu.edu
e-mail: counselling@mwsu.edu
Debra Higginbotham, Director

A public four-year college with support services for special education students.

5961 North Harris County College
North Harris County College
2700 Ww Thorne Boulevard
Houston, TX 77073
281-618-5400
FAX 281-618-5706
TDY:281-765-7938
http://www.northharriscollege.com
e-mail: spatton@northharriscollege.com
Sandi Patton, Special Services
David Sam, President

Offers a variety of services to students with disabilities including note takers, extended testing time, counseling services, and special accommodations. We train students in the use of specialized software and hardware.

5962 North Lake College
Disabilities Services Office
5001 N Macarthur Boulevard
Irving, TX 75038
972-273-3165
FAX 972-273-3164
TDY:972-273-3169
http://www.dcccd.edu
Carole Gray, Disability Services Coordinator
Sherry Beal, Office Manager

A public two-year college. Our mission is to provide a variety of support services to empower students, foster independence, promote achievement of realistic career and educational goals and assist students in discovering, developing and demonstrating full potential and abilities.

5963 Odyssey School
4407 Red River Street
Austin, TX 78751
512-472-2262
FAX 512-236-9385
http://www.odysseyschool.com
e-mail: wolf@odysseyschool.com
Nancy Wolf, Principal
John Brinson, Assistant Head of School

5964 Office of Disability Services
Stephen F Austin State University
1936 N Street
Nacogdoches, TX 75965
936-468-2011
FAX 936-468-5810
http://www.sfasu.edu
Margie Franklin, Director
Tito Guerrero, President

Offers a variety of services to students with disabilities including note takers, extended testing time, counseling services, and special accommodations.

5965 Pan American University
Office of Disability Services
1201 W University Drive
Edinburg, TX 78539
956-381-2011
FAX 956-316-7034
TDY:956-316-7092
http://www.panam.edu
Rick Gray, Director
Esperanza Cavazos, Associate Director
Blandina Cardenas, President
Offers a variety of services to students with disabilities including note takers, extended testing time, counseling services, and special accommodations.

5966 Rawson-Saunders School
2600 Exposition Boulevard
Austin, TX 78703
512-476-8382
FAX 512-476-1132
http://www.rawson-saunders.org
e-mail: info@rawson-saunders.org
Harriett Choffel, Executive Director
Julie Funk, Office Manager

5967 **Richland College**
12800 Abrams Road
Dallas, TX 75243
972-238-6100
FAX 972-238-6957
http://www.rlc.dcccd.edu
e-mail: stevem@dcccd.edu
Jeanne Brewer, LD Director
Stephen Mittelstet, President

Offers a variety of services to students with disabilities including note takers, extended testing time, counseling services, and special accommodations.

5968 **Sam Houston State University**
1700 Sam Houston Avenue
Huntsville, TX 77340
936-295-8061
FAX 936-294-3970
http://www.shsu.edu
James Gaertner MD, President
Dennis Culak, Manager

Offers a variety of services to students with disabilities including note takers, extended testing time, counseling services, and special accommodations.

5969 **San Antonio College**
Programs for the Handicapped
1300 San Pedro Avenue
San Antonio, TX 78212
210-733-2000
FAX 210-733-2202
http://www.accd.edu/sac/sacmain/sac.htm
Maria Gomez, Coordinator
Regina Pino, Assistant Coordinator
Robert Zeigler, President
A public two-year college with support services for special education students.

5970 **San Jacinto College: Central Campus**
PO Box 2007
Pasadena, TX 77501
281-476-1501
FAX 281-476-1892
http://www.sjcd.cc.tx.us
Judy Ellison, Special Populations
Monte Blue, President

Offers a variety of services to students with disabilities including notetakers, extended testing time, counseling services, and special accommodations such as test readers and writers.

5971 **San Jacinto College: South Campus**
San Jacinto College: South Campus
13735 Beamer Road
Houston, TX 77089
281-484-1900
FAX 281-922-3485
http://www.sjcd.edu
e-mail: eeverett@sjcd.edu
Ellen Everett, Acting Registrar
Sherry Gray, Administrative Assistant
Linda Watkins, President
A public two-year college with support services for special education students.

5972 **Schreiner University**
2100 Memorial Boulevard
Kerrville, TX 78028
830-896-5411
800-343-4919
FAX 830-792-7226
http://www.schreiner.edu
e-mail: sjdavis@schreiner.edu
Sam Davis, Assistant Admissions Director
Tim Summerlin, President

An independent four-year university with about 10% of students in the Learning Support Services Program. There is a fee for the LSS program in addition to the regular tuition.

5973 **South Plains College**
1401 College Avenue
Levelland, TX 79336
806-894-9611
FAX 806-894-5274
http://www.spc.cc.tx.us
Bill Powell, Studies Program
Kelvin Sharp, President

Offers a variety of services to students with disabilities including notetakers, extended testing time, counseling services, and special accommodations.

5974 **Southern Methodist University**
PO Box 750181
Dallas, TX 75275
214-768-2000
FAX 214-768-4572
http://www.smu.edu
e-mail: rmarin@mail.smu.edu
Rebecca Marin, Coordinator
Carolyn Hamby, Assistant
R. Turner, President
An independent four-year college with support services for special education students.

5975 **Southwestern Assemblies of God University**
Southwestern Assemblies of God university
1200 Sycamore Street
Waxahachie, TX 75165
972-937-4010
888-YES-SAGU
FAX 972-923-0488
http://www.sagu.edu
e-mail: sagu@sagu.edu
Kermit Bridges, President

Offers a variety of services to students with disabilities including notetakers, extended testing time, counseling services, and special accommodations.

5976 **St. Edwards University**
Learning Disabilities Services
3001 S Congress Avenue
Austin, TX 78704
512-448-8400
FAX 512-448-8492
http://www.stedwards.edu
Lorraine Prea, Director
George Martin, President

An independent four-year college. Students with disabilities meet with a counselor from academic planning and support and they work together to ensure equal access to all academic services.

5977 **St. Mary's University of San Antonio**
1 Camino Santa Maria Street
San Antonio, TX 78228
210-436-3203
FAX 210-436-3782
http://www.stmarytx.edu
Barbara Biassiolli, Center Director
Lisa Seller, Assistant Director

Offers a variety of services to students with disabilities including tutoring, extended testing time, and academic counseling services.

5978 **Tarleton State University**
Tarleton State University
PO Box T-0010
Stephenville, TX 76401
254-968-9000
FAX 254-968-9703
http://www.tarleton.edu
L. Dwayne Snider MD, Associate Vice President
Lisa Howe, Administrative Assistant
Dennis Cabe, President
Four year college that provides students with learning disabilities support and services.

5979 **Tarrant County College DSS-NE: Disability Support Services**
Disability Support Services
828 W Harwood Road
Hurst, TX 76054
817-515-6333
FAX 817-515-6112
TDY:817-515-6812
http://www.tccd.edu
e-mail: judy.kelly@tccd.edu
Judy Kelley, Director
Dorotha McDonnell, Secretary

Offers a variety of support services to students with disabilities including notetakers, testing accommodations, as well as special accommodations, tutoring.

5980 Texas A&M University

1265 Tamu
College Station, TX 77843
979-845-1436
FAX 979-847-8737
http://www.tamu.edu
e-mail: anne@stulife2.tamu.edu

Anne Reber MD, Coordinator
Charles Backus, Manager

A public four-year college with support services for special education students.

5981 Texas A&M University: Commerce

PO Box 3011
Commerce, TX 75429
903-886-5835
FAX 903-468-3220
http://www.tamu-commerce.edu
e-mail: frank_perez@tamu-commerce.edu

Frank Perez, Assistant Director

Four-year college that provides student support services and programs to those students who are learning disabled.

5982 Texas A&M University: Kingsville

1210 Retama Drive
Kingsville, TX 78363
361-592-4762
FAX 361-593-2006
http://www.tamuk.edu
e-mail: kacjaol@tamuk.edu

Jeanie Alexander, Coordinator Disability Svcs

Four-year college that provides an academic support center for students who are disabled.

5983 Texas Center for Disability Studies

University of Austin Texas
4030-2 W Braker Lane
Austin, TX 78712
512-232-0740
800-828-7839
FAX 512-232-0761
http://www.tcds.edb.utexas.edu
e-mail: txcds@uttcds.org

Penny Seay, Executive Director
John Moore, Assistant Director

The mission of the Texas Center for Disability Studies (TCDS) is to serve as a catalyst so that people with developmental and other disabilities are fully included in all levels of their communities and in control of their lives.

5984 Texas Southern University

3100 Cleburne Street
Houston, TX 77004
713-313-7011
FAX 713-313-7539
http://www.tsu.edu

Minnine Simmons, Counselor
Priscilla Slade, President

A public four-year college with support services for special education students.

5985 Texas State Technical Institute: Sweetwater Campus

300 College Drive
Sweetwater, TX 79556
325-235-7300
800-592-8784
http://www.sweetwater.tstc.edu

Phyllis Morris, Special Services
Mike Reeser, President

Offers a variety of services to students with disabilities including notetakers, extended testing time, counseling services, and special accommodations.

5986 Texas State University: San Marcos

Office of Disability Services
601 University Drive
San Marcos, TX 78666
512-245-3451
FAX 512-245-3452
TDY:512-245-3451
http://www.ods.txstate.edu
e-mail: jenniward@txstate.edu

Jenni Ward, Cognitive Disability Specialist

Provides support services and coordinates academic accommodations based on the individual students disibility-based need.

5987 Texas Tech University

AccessTECH & TECHniques Center
250 W Hall
Lubbock, TX 79409
806-742-2405
FAX 806-742-4837
TDY:806-742-2092
http://www.accesstech.dsa.ttu.edu
e-mail: accesstech@ttu.edu

Frank Silvas, Director
Larry Phillippe, Associate Director Technique Ctr

AccessTECH is a place for students with disabilities to register in order to receive reasonable academic accommodations. TECHniques Center is a fee-for-service program that provides supplemental academic support for college students with documented learning disabilities and attention deficit disorders.

5988 Texas Tech University: AccessTECH

335 W Hall
Lubbock, TX 79409
806-742-2405
FAX 806-742-4837
TDY:806-742-2092
http://www.accesstech.dsa.ttu.edu
e-mail: accesstech@ttu.edu

Frank Silvas, Director
Leann DiAndreth-Elkins, Assistant Director of Technique

A place for students with disabilities to register in order to receive reasonable academic accommodations.

5989 Texas Tech University: TECHniques Center

TECHniques Center
335 W Hall
Lubbock, TX 79409
806-742-1822
FAX 806-742-0295
TDY:806-742-2092
http://www.techniques.ttu.edu
e-mail: techniques.center@ttu.edu

Larry K Phillips, Associate Director

The TECHniques Center is a fee-for-service program that provides supplemental academic support for college students with documented learning disabilities and attention deficit disorders.

5990 Texas Woman's University

Disability Support Services
PO Box 425966
Denton, TX 76204
940-898-3626
FAX 940-898-3965
TDY:940-898-3830
http://www.twu.edu
e-mail: dss@twu.edu

Jo-ann Nunnelly, Director

A public four-year college with support services for special education students.

5991 Tyler Junior College

PO Box 9020
Tyler, TX 75711
903-510-2900
FAX 903-510-2434
http://www.tyler.cc.tx.us

Vickie Geisel, Special Services
Aubry Sharp, Manager

Offers a variety of services to students with disabilities including note takers, extended testing time, counseling services, and special accommodations.

5992 **University of Houston**
Disability Support Services
CSD Building
Houston, TX 77204
713-743-5400
FAX 713-743-5396
TDY:713-749-1527
http://www.uh.edu
e-mail: wscrain@mail.uhe.edu

Scott Crain, Counselor
Dr , Assistant Director
Cheryl Amotuso, Director
A public four-year college with support services for students with disabilities.

5993 **University of North Texas**
Office of Disability Accommodation
PO Box 305358
Denton, TX 76203
940-565-4323
FAX 940-369-7969
TDY:940-369-8652
http://www.unt.edu/oda
e-mail: undergrad@unt.edu

Ron Venable, Director

A public four-year college with a small percentage of learning disabled students.

5994 **University of Texas: Arlington**
Disability Support Office
PO Box 19355
Arlington, TX 76019
817-272-3364
FAX 817-272-1447
TDY:817-272-1520
http://www.uta.edu/disability

Dianne Hengst, Director
Penny Acrey, Assistant Director
Amber Mitchell, Interpeting Services Coodinator
A public four-year university. There is no specific LD program, but comprehensive support services are available. Total enrollment 20,000+.

5995 **University of Texas: Dallas**
PO Box 830688
Richardson, TX 75083
972-883-2111
FAX 972-883-2156
http://www.utdallas.edu

Tracy Cole, Disability Services
David Daniel, President

Offers a variety of services to students with disabilities including notetakers, extended testing time, counseling services, and special accommodations.

5996 **University of Texas: Pan American**
1201 W University Drive
Edinburg, TX 78539
956-381-3306
866-441-UTPA
http://www.panam.edu

Arturo Ramos, Assistant Director
Edna Luna, Administrator

Offers a variety of services to students with disabilities including notetakers, extended testing time, counseling services, and special accommodations.

5997 **University of Texas: San Antonio**
1604 W Avenue
San Antonio, TX 78201
210-458-4157
800-669-0919
FAX 210-458-4980
TDY:210-458-4981
http://www.utsa.edu
e-mail: nestor.reyes@utsa.edu

Lorraine Harrison, Director
Nestor Reyes, Assistant Director
Disability Services provides support services, accommodations and equipment for UTSA students with temporary or permanent disabilities. Goals of DS are to promote a barrier free environment, to encourage students to become as independent and self-reliant as possible and to provide information and consultation about specific disabilities to the entire community.

5998 **University of the Incarnate Word**
4301 Broadway Street
San Antonio, TX 78209
210-829-6000
800-749-WORD
FAX 210-283-5021
http://www.uiw.edu
e-mail: uiwhr@universe.uiwtx.edu

Lorena Novak, Coordinator
Louis Agnese, President

Four year college that provides services to learning disabled students.

5999 **Wharton County Junior College**
911 E Boling Highway
Wharton, TX 77488
979-532-6491
800-561-9252
FAX 979-532-6587
http://www.wcjc.cc.tx.us/

Sarah Clark, Executive Director

Offers a variety of services to students with disabilities including note takers, extended testing time, counseling services, and special accommodations.

6000 **Wiley College**
711 Wiley Avenue
Marshall, TX 75670
903-923-2400
800-658-6889
FAX 903-938-8100
http://www.wilec.edu
e-mail: vdavis@wileyc.edu

Haywood Strickland, President

Offers a variety of services to students with disabilities including notetakers, extended testing time, counseling services, and special accommodations.

Utah

6001 **Brigham Young University Reach Program**
Brigham Young University
University Parkway
Provo, UT 84602
801-378-4636
FAX 801-422-0174
TDY:801-422-0436
http://www.campuslife.byu.edu
e-mail: uac@byu.edu

Jason Chaney, Program Coordinator
Merrill Bateman, President

REACH was established to assist students with disabilities to reach their full potential. It is our goal to provide an environment where the pursuit of excellence is expected, and students are strongly encouraged to make a contribution toward their own success.

6002 **Center for Persons with Disabilities**
Utah State University
6800 Old Main Hall
Logan, UT 84322
435-797-0037
866-284-2821
FAX 435-797-3944
TDY:435-797-1981
http://www.cpd.usu.edu
e-mail: info@cpd2.usu.edu

Sarah Rule, Director
Dan Peterson, Manager

A University Center for Excellence in Developmental Disabilities Education, Research and Services. The Center for Persons with Disabilities provides interdisciplinary training, research, exemplary services, and technical assistance to agencies related to people with disabilities.

6003 **College of Eastern Utah**
451 E 400 N
Price, UT 84501
435-613-5000
FAX 435-613-5112
http://www.ceu.edu

Dee Howa, DRC Director
Ryan Thomas, President

The DRC at CEU provides academic accommodations for the learning disabled.

6004 Latter-Day Saints Business College
411 E S Temple
Salt Lake City, UT 84111
801-524-8100
FAX 801-524-1900
http://www.ldsbc.edu
Tina Orden, Dean Students
Stephen Woodhouse, President

Offers a variety of services to students with disabilities including notetakers, extended testing time, counseling services, and special accommodations.

6005 Salt Lake Community College: DisabilitySalt Lake Community College: Disability Resource Center
4600 S Redwood Road
Salt Lake City, UT 84123
801-957-4111
FAX 801-957-4947
TDY:801-957-4646
http://www.slcc.edu
e-mail: linda.bennett@slcc.edu
Rod Romboy, Director
Linda Bennett, Office Manager
Cynthia Bioteau, President
A program to assist students with disabilities in obtaining equal access to college facilities and programs. The resource center serves all disabilities and provides services and accommodations such as testing, adaptive equipment, text on tape, readers, scribes, note takers, and interpreters for the deaf.

6006 Snow College
150 College Avenue
Ephraim, UT 84627
435-283-7000
800-848-3399
FAX 435-283-7449
http://www.snow.edu
Cyndi Crabb, Special Services
Michael Benson, President

A public two-year college with support services for special education students.

6007 Southern Utah University
351 W Center Street
Cedar City, UT 84720
435-586-7933
FAX 435 865-8393
http://www.suu.edu
e-mail: thompson@suu.edu
Georgia Thompson, Coordinator
Steven Bennion, President
Diana Graff, Manager
A public four-year University with support services for special education students.

6008 University of Utah
201 Presidents Circle
Salt Lake City, UT 84112
801-581-5557
800-444-8638
FAX 801-581-5487
TDY:801-581-5020
http://www.utah.edu
e-mail: onadeau@saun.saff.utah.edu
Olga Nadeau, Director
David Pershing, Plant Manager

A public four-year college. Services include admissions requirements modification, testing accommodations, priority registration, advisement on course selection and number, adaptive technology, support group. Documentation of learning disability is required.

6009 Utah State University
101 Old Main Hall
Logan, UT 84322
435-797-3852
FAX 435-797-0130
TDY:435-797-0740
http://www.usu.edu
e-mail: diane.baum@usu.edu
Diane Baum, Director
Eric Olson, Manager

A public four-year college with support services for students with learning disabilities.

6010 Utah Valley State College
Accessibility Services Department
800 W University Parkway
Orem, UT 84058
801-863-INFO
FAX 801-226-5207
http://www.uvsc.edu
e-mail: info@uvsc.edu
Curtis Pendleton, Disabled Services
Michelle Lundell, Department Director
Ann Lickey, Secretary
The mission for Accessibility Services at Utah Valley State College is to ensure, in compliance with federal and state laws, that no qualified individual with a disability be excluded from participation in or be denied the benefits of a quality education at UVSC or be subjected to discrimination by the college or its personnel. UVSC offers a large variety of support services, accommodative services and assistive technology for individuals with learning disabilities.

6011 Weber State University
Disabilities Support Office
3750 Harrison Boulevard
Ogden, UT 84408
801-626-6000
FAX 801-626-6744
TDY:801-626-7283
http://www.weber.edu
Jeff Morris, Director
Ann Millner, President

Offers a variety of services to students with disabilities including notetakers, extended testing time, counseling services, and special accommodations.

6012 Westminster College of Salt Lake City
Learning Disability Program
1840 S 1300 E
Salt Lake City, UT 84105
801-832-2280
800-748-4753
FAX 801-832-3101
TDY:801-832-2286
http://www.westminstercollege.edu
e-mail: gdewitt@westminstercollege.edu
Ginny DeWitt, Director
Amy Gordon, Office Manager

Offers a variety of services to students with disabilities including notetakers, extended testing time, counseling services, and special accommodations.

Vermont

6013 Burlington College
95 N Avenue
Burlington, VT 05401
802-862-9616
800-862-9616
FAX 802-660-4331
http://www.burlcol.edu
e-mail: jsanders@burlcol.edu
Jane Sanders, President
Jillian McMahon, Office Manager

Education process vs test and grades. Small classes. Learning specialist available.

6014 Champlain College
Support Services
163 S Willard Street
Burlington, VT 05401
802-865-6425
FAX 802-860-2764
http://www.champlain.edu
e-mail: peterson@champlain.edu
Rebecca Peterson, Coordinator

Four year college that supports students with a learning disability.

6015 **College of St. Joseph**
71 Clement Road
Rutland, VT 05701
802-773-5900
FAX 802-776-5258
http://www.csj.edu
e-mail: fmiglorie@csj.edu

Frank Miglorie, Administrator
Gary Lawler, Vice President
Tracy Gallipo, Admissions Director

Offers a variety of services to students with disabilities including note takers, extended testing time, counseling services, and special accommodations.

6016 **Community College of Vermont**
Student Services Office
PO Box 120
Waterbury, VT 05676
802-241-3535
FAX 802-241-3526
http://www.ccv.vsc.edu
e-mail: ccvinfo@ccv.vsc.edu

Mel Donovan, Student Services Director
Tim Donovan, President

A public two-year college offering courses, certificates and associate degrees.

6017 **Green Mountain College**
Calhoun Learning Center
1 College Circle
Poultney, VT 05764
802-287-8232
FAX 802-287-8099
http://www.greenmtn.edu
e-mail: admiss@greenmtn.edu

Nancy Ruby, Director
Becky Eno, Assistant Director

Four-year college that offers support through the school's Calhoun Learning center to students with disabilities.

6018 **Greenwood School**
14 Greenwood Lane
Putney, VT 05346
802-387-4545
FAX 802-387-4545
http://www.thegreenwoodschool.org

Stewart Miller, Headmaster

A pre-preparatory boarding school for boys ages 9-15 have been diagnosed with: dyslexia; specific language-based learning disabilities/learning differences (LD); receptive language and/or expressive language deficits; executive functioning deficits; attentional difficulties (ADD or ADHD); disorders of written expression; dysgraphia; or speech and language needs.
1978

6019 **Johnson State College**
Learning Disabilities Department
337 College Hall
Johnson, VT 05656
802-635-1259
800-635-2356
FAX 802-635-1454
TDY:802-635-1456
http://www.jsc.vsc.edu
e-mail: dian.duranleau@jsc.vsc.edu

Dr Madden, Director
Dian Duranleau, Learning Specialist / Director

A public four-year college with support services for special education students.

6020 **Landmark College**
River Road S
Putney, VT 05346
802-387-6764
FAX 802-387-6868
http://www.landmarkcollege.org
e-mail: admissions@landmarkcollege.org

Ben Mitchell, Director Admissions
Christopher Ken, Assistant Dean of Admissions

Landmark College provides its students with the skills and the strategies to achieve, more closely, their true potential in higher education. New students are placed into developmentally appropriate classes that address specific academic skills — reading, writing, note-taking, test-taking, organization, time management.

6021 **Norwich University**
Learning Support Center
158 Harmon Drive
Northfield, VT 05663
802-485-2132
800-468-6679
FAX 802-485-2032
http://www.norwich.edu
e-mail: gills@norwich.edu

Paula Gills, Special Services

The Learning Center offers an opportunity for individualized assistance with many aspects of academic life in a supportive, personalized atmosphere. Students may voluntarily choose from a wide variety of service options.

6022 **Southern Vermont College**
978 Mansion Drive
Bennington, VT 05201
802-442-5427
800-378-2782
FAX 802-447-4695
http://www.svc.edu
e-mail: tgerson@svc.edu

Todd Gerson, Coordinator
Barbara Sirvis, President

Offers students with documented learning disabilities a highly supportive environment and a wide range of support services which include basic skills tutoring, content area academic support, study techniques, notetaking and more.

6023 **University of Vermont**
ACCESS
A170 Living Learning Center
Burlington, VT 05405
802-656-7753
FAX 802-656-0739
TDY:802-656-3865
http://www.uvm.edu/access
e-mail: access@uvm.edu

Donna Panko, Learning Specialist
Nick Ogrizovich, Information Specialist
Joe Wilson, Learning Specialist

Provides accommodation, consultation, collaboration and educational support services as a means to foster opportunities for students with disabilities to participate in a barrier free learning environment.

6024 **Vermont Technical College**
Randolph Center
Randolph Center, VT 05061
802-728-1000
800-442-8821
FAX 802-728-1390
TDY:802-728-1278
http://www.vtc.vsc.edu
e-mail: rgoodall@vtc.edu

Robin Goodall, Learning Specialists
Eileen Haddon, Assistive Technology Project
Allen Rogers, President

Offers a variety of services to students with disabilities including individualized accommodations, counseling services, academic counseling.

Virginia

6025 **Averett College**
Support Services for Students
428 Firth Hall
Danville, VA 24541
434-791-5744
FAX 804-791-4392
http://www.averett.edu
e-mail: priedel@averett.edu

Pamela Riedel MD, Support Services Coordinator

Four-year college that offers services for the learning disabled.

6026 **Blue Ridge Community College**
Virginia Community College System
PO Box 80
Weyers Cave, VA 24486
540-234-9261
888-750-2722
FAX 540-234-9598
http://www.brcc.edu
e-mail: khardy@brcc.edu

Kathy Hardy, Academic Adviser
Liell Hern, Administrative Assistant
James Perkins, President
A public two-year college. The Office of Disability Services is part of the Blue Ridge Community Counseling Center. Its mission is to provide disabled students with the support services needed to be successful in college.

6027 College of William and Mary
PO Box 8795
Williamsburg, VA 23187
757-221-4000
TDY:757-221-1154
http://www.wm.edu
Carroll Hardy MD, Director
Gene Nichol, President

Offers a variety of services to students with disabilities including notetakers, extended testing time, counseling services, and special accommodations.

6028 Eastern Mennonite University
Academic Support Center - Student Disability Svcs.
1200 Park Road
Harrisonburg, VA 22802
540-432-4233
800-368-2665
FAX 540-432-4977
TDY:540-432-4631
http://www.emu.edu
e-mail: hedrickj@emu.edu
Joyce Hedrick, Coordinator

EMU is committed to working out reasonable accommodations for students with documented disabilities to ensure equal access to the University and its related programs.

6029 Emory & Henry College
PO Box 947
Emory, VA 24327
276-944-4121
800-848-5493
FAX 276-944-6934
http://www.ehc.edu
Jill Smeltzer, Director Counseling Services
Thomas Morris, President

A private four-year liberal arts college located in the foothills of southwest Virginia. Student enrollment of appox. 1,000, almost equally divided between men and women. The Paul Adrian Powell III resource center offers a variety of services to students with disabilities including extended testing time, counseling services, and special accommodations, as well as tutorial services.

6030 Ferrum College
PO Box 1000
Ferrum, VA 24088
540-365-2121
800-868-9797
FAX 540-365-4203
http://www.ferrum.edu
Dr. Jennifer Braaten, President

An independent four-year college with support services for special education students.

6031 GW Community School
GW Community School
9001 Braddock Road
Springfield, VA 22151
703-978-7208
FAX 703-978-7226
http://www.gwcommunityschool.com
e-mail: info@gwcommunityschool.com
Alexa Warden, Principal

The GW Community School is owned and operated by teachers who understand the learning process and the students' needs, and who genuinely enjoy teaching adolesents. They work closely with students and their families to maximize learning. The GW School for Divergent Learners embodies a vision shared by teachers, parents, and students. A school committed to developing and optimizing the giftedness and intellegence of each student and fostering a sense of social awareness and civic responsibility

6032 Hampden-Sydney College
PO Box 685
Hampden Sydney, VA 23943
434-223-6000
FAX 434-223-6346
http://www.hsc.edu
Elizabeth Ford, Associate Dean of Academic Suppo
Walter Bortz, President

Offers a variety of services to students with disabilities including note takers, extended testing time, counseling services, and special accommodations.

6033 James Madison University
Office of Disabilities Services
Wilson Learning Center
Harrisonburg, VA 22807
540-568-6705
FAX 540-568-7099
TDY:540-568-6705
http://www.jmu.edu/ods
e-mail: disability-svcs@jmu.edu
Valerie Schoolcraft, Program Manager

Offers Learning Strategies Instruction and Strategic Learning Course. Learning Resource Centers in writing, communication, math, science, and critical thinking. Assistive technology lab with various software and hardware include scanners, Kurzweil, etc. High speed scanner support alternate text accommodations. Students with learning disabilities of ADHD may participate in Learning Leaders program.

6034 John Tyler Community College
Office of Disability Services
13101 Jefferson Davis Highway
Chester, VA 23831
804-706-5225
800-552-3490
FAX 804-796-4163
http://www.jtcc.edu
Robert Tutton, Counselor
Betsy , Director

A public two-year college with support services for special education students.

6035 Learning Needs & Evaluation Center
University of Virginia
400 Brandon Avenue
Charlottesville, VA 22908
434-243-5180
FAX 434-243-5188
http://www.virginia.edu/studenthealth/
e-mail: lnec@virginia.edu
Patti Dewey, Manager

Full range of support services for students admitted to any of the ten schools of the university, including graduate/professional schools. Including, but not limited to, alternate texts, exam accommodations, peer-notetakers, TTY and interpreters, assistive devices and housing and transportation accommodations.

6036 Learning Needs & Evaluation Center: Elson Student Health Center
University of Virginia
PO Box 800760
Charlottesville, VA 22908
434-924-2273
FAX 434-243-5188
http://www.virginia.edu/studenthealth/
Jennifer Maedge MD, Director
Pattie Dewey, Manager

Full range of support services for students admitted to any of the ten schools of the university, including graduate/professional schools. Including, not limited to, taped texts, writing support, learning strategies, exam accommodation, liaison with faculty.

6037 Liberty University
Office of Academic Disability Support
1971 University Boulevard
Lynchburg, VA 24502
434-582-2000
FAX 804-582-2468
TDY:434-522-0420
http://www.liberty.edu
e-mail: wdmchane@liberty.edu
W. McHaney, Academic Disability Support Dir.
Ron Godwin, President

Religiously oriented, private, coeducational, comprehensive four year institution. Students who have documented learning disabilities are eligible to receive support services. These would include academic advising, priority class registration, tutoring and testing accommodations.

6038 Little Keswick School

PO Box 24
Keswick, VA 22947 434-295-0457
FAX 434-977-1892
http://www.littlekeswickschool.net
e-mail: tcolumbus@littlekeswickschool.net

Terry Columbus, Director
Mark Columbus, Principal

Little Keswick School is a therapeutic boarding school for 30 learning disabled and/or emotionally disturbed boys between the ages of 10 to 15 at acceptance and served through 17. IQ range accepted ti sbelow average to superior structured routine in a small, nurturing environment with services that include psychotherapy, occupational therapy, speech therapy and art therapy. Five week summer session.

6039 Longwood College

201 High Street
Farmville, VA 23919 434-395-2629
800-281-4677
FAX 434-395-2434
TDY:800-281-4677
http://www.longwood.edu
e-mail: roodse@longwood.edu

Susan Rood, Disability Support Services
Nathan Fortener, Administrative Support
Jeanie Campbell, Manager

A public four-year college with support services for special education students.

6040 Lord Fairfax Community College

173 Skirmisher Lane
Middletown, VA 22645 540-868-7000
800-906-5322
FAX 540-868-7100
http://www.lfcc.edu

Paula Dean, Testing Center Coordinator
John Sygielski, President

A public two-year college. Students are encouraged to identify special needs during the admissions process and to request support services, such as individualized placement testing, developmental studies, learning assistance programs, and study skills. A 504 faculty team recommends accommodations to academic programs, and communicates with area service providers.

6041 Mary Washington College

University of Mary Washington Disability Services
1301 College Avenue
Fredericksburg, VA 22401 540-654-1046
FAX 540-654-1063
TDY:540-654-1102
http://www.umw.edu
e-mail: ssmith@umw.edu

Stephanie Smith, Director
Cathy Payne, Office Manager
William Anderson, President

A public four-year college with support services for special education students.

6042 New River Community College

PO Box 1127
Dublin, VA 24084 540-674-3600
866-462-6722
FAX 540-674-3644
TDY:540-674-3619
http://www.nr.edu
e-mail: nrdixoj@nr.ca.cc.va.us

Jeananne Dixon, Learning Disabilities Coord.
Bonnie Hall, Information Center
Jack Lewis, President

A public two-year college with support services for special education students.

6043 Norfolk State University

Norfolk State University
700 Park Avenue
Norfolk, VA 23504 757-823-8600
FAX 757-823-2689
http://www.nsu.edu
e-mail: bbharris@nsu.du

Beverly Harris, Disability Services Director
Alvin Schexnider, President
Marian Shepherd, Coordinator/SSDS

Four year university that offers programs for the students with learning disabilities.

6044 Northern Virginia Community College

Disability Support Department
4001 Wakefield Chapel Road
Annandale, VA 22003 703-323-3000
FAX 703-323-3559
http://www.nvcc.edu

Robert G Templon Jr, President
John T Denver, Executive Vice President

A public two-year college.

6045 Old Dominion University

Old Dominion University
2228 Webb Center
Norfolk, VA 23529 757-533-9308
FAX 757-683-5356
TDY:757-683-5356
http://www.studentaffairs.odu.edu/disability
e-mail: disabilityservices@odu.edu

Sheryn Milton, Disability Services Director
Roseann Runte, President
Diane Parker, Manager

Works with students to provide access to higher education. Reasonable accommodations are identified to address specific individual needs. Accommodations may include extended testing time, permission to tape record classes, distraction-free test setting, etc.

6046 Patrick Henry Community College

PO Box 5311
Martinsville, VA 24115 276-638-8777
800-232-7997
FAX 276-656-0327
TDY:276-638-2433
http://www.ph.vccs.edu
e-mail: sss@ph.vccs.edu

Scott Guebert, Student Support Services Dir.
Mary McAlexander, Disability Counselor
Max Wingett, President

Offers a variety of services to students with disabilities including note takers, adaptive testing, counseling services, peer tutoring and adaptive equipment, and accessible transportation.

6047 Paul D Camp Community College

PO Box 737
Franklin, VA 23851 757-569-6700
FAX 757-569-6795
http://www.pc.vccs.edu

Douglas Boyce, Administrator

A public two-year institution with two campuses. Students with learning disabilities are eligible for special services provided by the Student Support Service Program. Learning-disabled students may take advantage of tutors (outside of class time and during class labs), notetakers, and taped textbooks. A counselor serves as student advocate and helps students arrange for classroom accommodations with instructors.

6048 Piedmont Virginia Community College

501 College Drive
Charlottesville, VA 22902 434-977-3900
http://www.pvcc.edu
e-mail: pbuck@pvcc.edu

Wendy Bolt, Counselor
Frank Friedman, President

A two-year comprehensive community college dedicated to the belief that individuals should have equal opportunity to develop and extend their skills and knowledge. Consistent with this philosophy and in compliance with the Americans with Disabilities Act, we encourage persons with disabilities to apply.

6049 Randolph-Macon Woman's College
2500 Rivermont Avenue
Lynchburg, VA 24503
434-947-8000
800-745-RMWC
FAX 434-947-8996
TDY:434-947-8608
http://www.rmwc.edu
e-mail: admissions@rmwc.edu
Kathleen Bowman, President

An independent four-year college with support services for students with disabilities.

6050 Rappahannock Community College
12745 College Drive
Saluda, VA 23149
804-758-6700
FAX 804-758-3852
http://www.rcc.vccs.edu
e-mail: pfisher@rcc.vccs.edu
Paula Fisher, Director
Elizabeth Crowther, President

Offers a variety of services to students with disabilities including notetakers, extended testing time, counseling services, and special accommodations.

6051 Southern Seminary College
1 College Hill Drive
Buena Vista, VA 24416
703-761-8420
Jack Turregano, Special Services

Offers a variety of services to students with disabilities including note takers, extended testing time, counseling services, and special accommodations.

6052 Southern Virginia College
1 College Hill Drive
Buena Vista, VA 24416
540-261-8400
800-229-8420
http://www.southernvirginia.edu
Jack Turregano, Special Services
Rodney Smith, President

Offers a variety of services to students with disabilities including note takers, extended testing time, counseling services, and special accommodations.

6053 Southside Virginia Community College
109 Campus Drive
Alberta, VA 23821
434-949-1000
FAX 434-949-7863
http://www.sv.vccs.edu
John Sykes, Provost
John Cavan, Administrator

Offers a variety of services to students with disabilities including notetakers, extended testing time, counseling services, and special accommodations.

6054 Southwest Virginia Community College
PO Box 5-UCC
Richlands, VA 24641
276-964-2555
FAX 540-964-7259
http://www.sw.edu
e-mail: admissions@sw.edu
Dr King, President
Gaynalle Harman, Admissions Coordinator

Offers a variety of services to students with disabilities including note takers, extended testing time, counseling services, and special accommodations.

6055 Thomas Nelson Community College
Thomas Nelson Community College
PO Box 9407
Hampton, VA 23670
757-825-2700
FAX 757-825-2763
http://www.tncc.edu
Thomas Kellen, Admissions Advisor
Charles Taylor, President
Howard Taylor, Administrator
A public two-year college with support services for students with disabilities.

6056 Tidewater Community College
Tidewater Community College
253 Monticello Avenue
Norfolk, VA 23510
757-822-1122
FAX 757-822-1214
http://www.tcc.edu
e-mail: tcharro@tcc.edu
Linda Harris, District Coordinator
Deborah Dicroce, President

This public two-year college offers transfer and occupational/technical degrees on four campuses and a visual arts center in the Hampton Roads area of Virginia. TCC offers students evaluations, all reasonable accommodations, and a wide array of assistive technology.

6057 University of Virginia
PO Box 400160
Charlottesville, VA 22904
434-924-0311
FAX 434-243-5188
TDY:804-982-HEAR
http://www.virginia.edu
Jennifer Maedgen, Director
John Casteen III, President

Diagnostic services and educational planning for students and adults in the workplace who have a history or who suspect learning difficulties may stem from the Specific Learning Disabilities condition.

6058 Virginia Commonwealth University
Services for Students with Disabilities
901 W Franklin Street
Richmond, VA 23284
804-828-0100
800-841-3638
FAX 804-828-1323
http://www.vcu.edu
e-mail: jbknight@vcu.edu
Joyce Knight, Director

Offers a variety of services to students with disabilities including note takers, extended testing time, counseling services, and special accommodations.

6059 Virginia Highlands Community College
PO Box 828
Abingdon, VA 24212
276-739-2400
FAX 540-628-7576
http://www.vh.cc.va.us
e-mail: cfaris@vh.cc.va.us
Charlotte Faris, Director
Patricia Hunter, Manager

A public two-year college. Strives to assist students with disabilities in successfully responding to challenges of academic study and job training.

6060 Virginia Intermont College
1013 Moore Street
Bristol, VA 24201
276-669-6101
800-451-1842
FAX 540-669-5763
http://www.vic.edu
e-mail: bholbroo@vic.edu
Dr. Steve Greiner MD, President
Michael Cugalisi, Vice President

Virginia Intermont College is a private, four-year Baptist affiliated liberal arts college located near the Appalachian Mountains of Southwest Virginia. Intermont has an enrollment of 850 men and women students. Accommodations, such as notetakers, extended time on tests, transcribers, oral testing, tutors and other services, are provided based on documentiation of disabilities.

6061 Virginia Polytechnic Institute and State University
150 Henderson Hall
Blacksburg, VA 02461
540-231-6000
FAX 540-231-3232
TDY:540-231-1740
http://www.ssd.vt.edu
e-mail: ssd@vt.edu
Susan Angle MD, Director For Disability Services
Charles Steger, President

A public four-year college with support services for special education students.

6062 Virginia Wesleyan College
Disabilities Services Office
1584 Wesleyan Drive
Norfolk, VA 23502
757-455-3200
800-737-8684
http://www.vwc.edu
e-mail: fpearson@vwc.edu
Fayne Pearson, Disabilities Coordinator
William Greer Jr., President

Four year college that offers support to students with a learning disability.

6063 Virginia Western Community College
PO Box 14007
Roanoke, VA 24038
540-857-7231
FAX 540-857-6102
TDY:540-857-6351
http://www.vw.cc.va.us
Michael Henderson, Special Services
Dana Asciolla, Admissions Staff
Robert Sandel, President
A public two-year college with support services for special education students.

Washington

6064 Bellevue Community College
3000 Landerholm Circle SE
Bellevue, WA 98007
425-564-1000
FAX 425-641-2230
http://www.bcc.ctc.edu
Susan Gjolmesli, Director
Carol Jones-Watkins, Coordinator
Jean Floten, President
Disability Support Services provides accommodations for people with disabilities to make their academic careers a success. There is no separate fee for these services.

6065 Central Washington University
Disability Support Services
400 E University Way
Ellensburg, WA 98926
509-963-2171
FAX 509-963-3235
TDY:509-963-2143
http://www.cwu.edu
e-mail: campbelr@cwu.edu
Bob Campbell, Director
Pamela Wilson, Accommodations Specialist
Ian Campbell, Coordinator Adaptive Tech Svcs
A public four-year college with disability support services for students with disabilities.

6066 Centralia College
600 W Locust Street
Centralia, WA 98531
360-736-9391
FAX 360-330-7503
http://www.centralia.edu
e-mail: demerson@centralia.ctc.edu
Lucretia Folks, Director
Donna Emerson, Administrative Assistant
Michael Grubiak, Vice President
The Special Services Office offers a variety of services to students with disabilities including notetakers, extended testing time, counseling services, and special accommodations.

6067 Children's Institute for Learning
4030 86th Avenue SE
Mercer Island, WA 98040
206-232-8680
Trina Westerlund, Executive Director

6068 Children's Institute for Learning Differences: New Heights School
4030 86th Avenue SE
Mercer Island, WA 98040
206-232-8680
FAX 206-232-9377
http://www.childrensinstitute.com
e-mail: micheleg@childrensinstitute.com
Michele Glickman, Outreach/Training Director
Trina Westerlund, Executive Director
Trisa Harris, Registrar/Admissions Coordinator
A Pre k-12 school based program serving children ages 3-18.

6069 Clark College
1800 E McLoughlin Boulevard
Vancouver, WA 98663
360-992-2000
TDY:360-992-2835
http://www.clark.edu/dss
Tami Jacobs, Program Manager
Wayne Branch, President

Offers a variety of services to students with disabilities including note takers, extended testing time, counseling services, and special accommodations.

6070 Columbia Basin College
2600 N 20th Avenue
Pasco, WA 99301
509-547-0511
FAX 509-546-0401
TDY:509-547-0400
http://www.cbc2.org
e-mail: pbuchmiller@cbc2.org
Peggy Buchmiller, Director
Kathy Freeman, Program Coordinator
Lee Thornton, Administrator
The Education Access Disability Resource Center provides a range of services for diagnosed learning disabled students, including alternate educational media, test accommodations, notetaking, priority registration, scribe services, books on tape and specialized computer software.

6071 Cornish College of the Arts
Cornish College of the Arts
1000 Lenora Street
Seattle, WA 98121
206-726-5151
800-726-ARTS
FAX 206-726-5097
http://www.cornish.edu
e-mail: studentaffairs@cornish.edu
George Sedano, Director
Sergei Tshcernisch, President

Through the Student Affairs Office, appropriate accommodations are provided for students with learning disabilities.

6072 Dartmoor School
13401 Bel Red Road
Bellevue, WA 98005
425-649-8976
FAX 425-603-0038
Jim Bower, Manager

6073 ETC Preparatory Academy
8005 SE 28th Street
Mercer Island, WA 98040
206-236-1095
FAX 206-236-0998
Meredith Ouellette, Director
Jan Bleakney, Director

Assessment, referral, tutorial, courses for credit, advocacy, dissertation, adults and students that are school age.

6074 Eastern Washington University: Disability Support Services
215 Pub
Cheney, WA 99004
509-359-6871
FAX 509-359-7458
TDY:509-359-6261
http://www.ewu.edu
e-mail: KRAVER@mail.EWU.EDU
Karen Raver, Director
Kevin Hills, Accommodations Specialist
Pam McDermott, Program Assistant

Although the University does not offer a specialized program specifically for learning disabled students, the disability support services office works with students on a case by case basis.

6075 Edmonds Community College
20000 68th Avenue W
Lynnwood, WA 98036
425-640-1459
FAX 425-640-1622
TDY:425-774-8669
http://www.edcc.edu/ssd
e-mail: ssdmail@edcc.edu

Dee Olson, Director
Tania Kulikov, Assistant Director
Jack O'Harah, Administrator
Offers a variety of services to students with disabilities including notetakers, extended testing time, and special accommodations.

6076 Epiphany School
3710 E Howell Street
Seattle, WA 98122
206-323-9011
FAX 206-324-2127

George Edwards, Religious Leader

6077 Everett Community College
Center for Disabilities Services
2000 Tower Street
Everett, WA 98201
425-388-9272
FAX 425-388-9109
TDY:425-388-9438
http://www.everettcc.edu
e-mail: cds@everettcc.edu

Kathy Cook, Director
Kristine Grimsby, Program Assistant

Offers a variety of services to students with disabilities including notetakers, extended testing time, adaptive software and individual accommodations.

6078 Evergreen Academy
16017 118th Place NE
Bothell, WA 98011
425-488-8000
FAX 425-488-0994

Dana Mott, Principal

6079 Evergreen State College
2700 Evergreen Parkway NW
Olympia, WA 98505
360-867-6530
877-787-9721
FAX 360-867-6360
TDY:360-867-6834
http://www.evergreen.edu
e-mail: pickeril@evergreen.edu

Linda Pickering, Director
Meredith Inocencio, Program Assistant
Les Purce, President
Academic adjustments and auxiliary aids are provided for students with documented disabilties.

6080 Green River Community College
Green River Community College
12401 SE 320th Street
Auburn, WA 98092
253-833-9111
FAX 253-288-3467
TDY:253-288-3359
http://www.greenriver.edu
e-mail: rblosser@greenriver.edu

Ron Blosser, Coordinator/Disability Services
Jennifer Nelson, Program Assistant
Richard Rutkowski, President
Support services for students with disabilities to ensure that our programs and facilities are accessible. Our campus is organized to provide reasonable accommodations, including core services, to qualified students with dissabilities.

6081 Heritage Christian School
Heritage Christian School
10310 NE 195th Street
Bothell, WA 98011
425-485-2585
FAX 425-486-2895
http://www.acseagles.org
e-mail: randyn@fbcbothell.org

Randy Nadine, Business Manager
Dave Rehnberg, Principal

6082 Highline Community College
PO Box 98000
Des Moines, WA 98198
206-878-3710
FAX 206-870-3773
TDY:206-870-4853
http://www.highline.edu
e-mail: cjones@highline.edu

Carol Jones, Disability Services Coordinator
Priscilla Bell, President

Offers a variety of services to students with disabilities including note takers, extended testing time, counseling services, and special accommodations.

6083 Morningside Academy
201 Westlake Avenue N
Seattle, WA 98109
206-709-9500
FAX 206-709-4611
http://www.morningsideacademy.org
e-mail: info@morningsideacademy.org

Joanne Robbins, Principal
Beth Bartter, Office Manager

6084 North Seattle Community College
Educational Access Center
9600 College Way N
Seattle, WA 98103
206-527-3697
FAX 206-527-3635
http://www.nsccux.sccd.ctc.edu

Suzanne Sewell, Manager

The Educational Access Center offers a variety of services to students with disabilities including notetakers, extended testing time, counseling services, and special accommodations.

6085 Northwest School
NAIS (National Association of Independents School
1415 Summit Avenue
Seattle, WA 98122
206-682-7309
FAX 206-467-7353
http://www.northwestschool.org

Ellen Taussig, Principal
Jonathan Hochberg, Project Manager

6086 Pacific School of Academics
11105 Homestead Road
Arlington, WA 98223
360-403-8885
FAX 360-403-7607

Nola Smith, Administrator

6087 Paladin Academy
2751 Van Buren Street
Hollywood, FL 33020
954-920-2008

Ingrid Garcia, Manager

6088 Pierce Community College
Pierce Community College
9401 Farwest Drive SW
Lakewood, WA 98498
253-964-6500
FAX 253-964-6713
http://www.pierce.ctc.edu

Michele Johnson, President
Ed Brewster, Manager

A federally funded TRIO progrm providing academic support services to low income students, first generation college students and students with disabilities in order to improve their retention, academic proformance, graduation and transfer to four-year institutions.

6089 **Seattle Academy of Arts and Sciences**
1201 E Union Street
Seattle, WA 98122
206-323-6600
FAX 206-676-6881
http://www.seattleacademy.org
Jean Orvis, Administrator
Barbara Burk, Administrative Assistant

6090 **Seattle Central Community College**
Seattle Community College District
1701 Broadway
Seattle, WA 98122
206-587-3800
FAX 206-344-4390
TDY:206-344-4395
http://www.seattlecentral.org
Shari Estep, Manager Disability Support Svcs
Mildred Ollee, President

Offers a variety of services to students with disabilities including notetakers, extended testing time, counseling services, and special accommodations.

6091 **Seattle Christian Schools**
18301 Military Road S
Seatac, WA 98188
206-246-8241
FAX 206-246-9066
http://www.seattlechristian.org
e-mail: ghunter@seattlechristian.org
Gloria Hunter, Superintendent
Bryan Peterson, Principal
Dave Steele, Administrator
Independent, interdenominational Christian Day School established in 1946, serving 750+ students.

6092 **Seattle Pacific University**
3307 3rd Avenue W
Seattle, WA 98119
206-281-2228
FAX 206-286-7348
TDY:206-281-2475
http://www.spu.edu/departs/cfl/dsshome.asp
e-mail: centerforlearning3@spu.edu
Bethany Anderson, Program Coordinator
Linda Wagner, Director
Bryce Nelson, Executive Director
Offers a variety of services to students with disabilities including notetakers, extended testing time, books on tape, interpreters and special accommodations.

6093 **Shoreline Christian School**
Shoreline Christian School
2400 NE 147th Street
Shoreline, WA 98155
206-364-7777
FAX 206-364-0349
http://www.shorelinechristian.org
e-mail: admin@shorelinechristian.org
Tim Visser, Administrator

6094 **Snohomish County Christian**
17931 64th Avenue W
Lynnwood, WA 98037
425-742-9518
FAX 425-745-9306
http://www.sccslions.org
Debbie Schindler, Administrator
Mary Elroy, Principal

6095 **South Puget Sound Community College**
2011 Mottman Road SW
Tumwater, WA 98512
360-754-7711
FAX 360-596-5709
http://www.spscc.ctc.edu
e-mail: jshowalter@spscc.ctc.edu
Christy James, Disability Support Coordinator
Kenneth Minnaert, President

Offers a variety of services to students with disabilities including notetakers, extended testing time, books on tape, readers, scribes, interpreters, assistance with registration.

6096 **South Seattle Community College**
6000 16th Avenue SW
Seattle, WA 98106
206-764-5365
FAX 206-768-6649
TDY:206-764-5845
http://www.sccd.ctc.edu/south
e-mail: rtillman@sccd.ctc.edu
Roxanne Tillman, Special Student Services Dir.
Jill Wakefield, President

Offers a variety of services to students with disabilities including notetakers, extended testing time, counseling services and special accommodations.

6097 **Spokane Community College**
1810 N Greene Street
Spokane, WA 99217
509-533-7045
800-248-5644
FAX 509-533-8839
TDY:509-533-7482
http://www.scc.spokane.edu
e-mail: shanson@scc.spokane.edu
Steve Hanson, President
Claudia Parkins, Manager

Offers a variety of services to students with disabilities including notetakers, extended testing time, counseling services, and special accommodations.

6098 **Spokane Falls Community College**
3410 W Fort George Wright Drive
Spokane, WA 99224
509-533-3720
888-509-7944
FAX 509-533-3547
TDY:509-533-3838
http://www.spokanefalls.edu
Ben Webinger, Disability Support Services Dir.
Mark Pallek, President

Offers a variety of services to students with disabilities including notetakers, extended testing time, counseling services, and special accommodations.

6099 **St. Alphonsus**
St. Alphonsus
5816 15th Avenue NW
Seattle, WA 98107
206-782-4363
FAX 206-789-5709
http://www.st-alphonsus-sea.org
e-mail: stalphons@aol.com
Robert Rutledge, Principal
Charlene Sweet, School Secretary

6100 **St. Matthew's**
1230 NE 127th Street
Seattle, WA 98125
206-362-2785
FAX 206-362-4863
Maureen Reid, President

6101 **St. Thomas School**
PO Box 124
Medina, WA 98039
425-454-5880
FAX 425-454-1921
http://www.stthomasschool.org
e-mail: info@stthomasschool.org
David Selby, School Head
Kirk Wheeler, Manager

6102 **University Preparatory Academy**
NAIS (National Association of Independents School
8000 25th Avenue NE
Seattle, WA 98115
206-525-2714
FAX 206-525-9659
http://www.universityprep.org
Erica Hamlin, Manager
Linda Smith, Main Office Coordinator

6103 University of Puget Sound
University of Puget Sound
1500 N Warner Street
Tacoma, WA 98416
253-879-3575
FAX 253-879-3500
TDY:253-879-3399
http://www.ups.edu
e-mail: iwest@ups.edu
Sherry Kennedy, Administrative Assistant
Ivey West, Disability Services Coordinator
Barbara Racine, Manager
Support services and accommodations are individually tailored depending upon a student's disability, its severity, the students academic environment and courses, housing situation, activities, etc. Accommodations include instruction in study strategies, free tutoring, assistance in note taking, sign language and additional academic advising.

6104 University of Washington
PO Box 355839
Seattle, WA 98195
206-685-2937
FAX 206-616-8379
TDY:206-543-8925
http://www.washington.edu/students/gencat/front
e-mail: uwdss@u.washington.edu
Dyane Haynes, Director
Sally Green, Secretary

Provides services and academic accommodations to students with documented permanent and temporary disabilities to ensure equal access to the university's educational programs and facilities. Services may include but are not limited to exam accommodations, notetaking, audio-taped class texts/materials, sign language interpreters, auxilary aids (assistive listening devices, and accessible furniture).

6105 University of Washington: Center on Human Development and Disability
PO Box 357920
Seattle, WA 98195
206-543-7701
FAX 206-543-3417
http://www.depts.washington.edu/chdd
Michael Guralnick, Director
Carolyn Hamby, Assistant to the Director

The Center on Human Development and Disability (CHDD) at the University of Washington makes important contributions to the lives of people with developmental disabilities and their families, through a comprehensive array of research, clinical services, training, community outreach and dissemination activities.

6106 WSU/Disability Resource Center
PO Box 641067
Pullman, WA 99164
509-335-3564
FAX 509-335-8511
TDY:509-335-3421
http://www.wsu.edu/-drc/
e-mail: schaeff@wsu.edu
Susan Schaeffer, Executive Director
V. Rawlins, CEO

Goals are: to assist students with disabilities to receive reasonable accommodations in academic and non-academic programs that provide them with an equal opportunity to fully participate in all aspects of student life at WSU: to increase awareness of issues and abilities of people with disabilities among the WSU students, faculty and staff.

6107 Walla Walla Community College
500 Tausick Way
Walla Walla, WA 99362
509-527-4227
877-992-9922
FAX 509-527-4249
TDY:509-527-4412
http://www.wwcc.edu
La Smelcer, Disability Services Coordinator
Steven Ausdle, President

The Special Services Office offers a variety of services to students with disabilities including notetakers, extended testing time, counseling services, and special accommodations.

6108 Washington State University
Ad Annex 206
Pullman, WA 99164
509-335-3564
FAX 509-335-8511
http://www.wsu.edu
e-mail: schaeff@wsu.edu /
Jane Carter, Disability Specialist
V. Rawlins, CEO

Four year college that helps students and has programs for students with learning disabilities.

6109 Western Washington University
516 High Street
Bellingham, WA 98225
360-650-3000
FAX 360-650-2810
http://www.wwu.edu
David Brunnemer, Associate Director
Karen Morse, President

Disabled Student Services offers a variety of services to students with disabilities including note takers, extended testing time, counseling services and special accommodations.

6110 Whatcom Community College
237 W Kellogg Road
Bellingham, WA 98226
360-676-2170
FAX 360-676-2171
http://www.whatcom.ctc.edu
Bill Culwell, Coordinator Disability Services

A public two-year college with support services for special education students.

6111 Whitworth College
300 W Hawthorne Road
Spokane, WA 99251
509-777-1000
FAX 509-777-3758
http://www.whitworth.edu
e-mail: joannielsen@whitworth.edu
William Robinson, President

Offers a variety of services to students with disabilities including note takers, extended testing time, counseling services, and special accommodations.

6112 Yakima Valley Community College
PO Box 22520
Yakima, WA 98907
509-574-4600
FAX 509-574-6860
http://www.yvcc.cc.wa.us/
Anthony Beebe, Vice President

Offers a variety of services to students with disabilities including notetakers, extended testing time, counseling services, and special accommodations.

West Virginia

6113 Bethany College West Virginia
Special Advising Program
Morlan Hall
Bethany, WV 26032
304-829-7400
FAX 304-829-7580
http://www.bethanywv.edu
e-mail: rpauls@bethanywv.edu
Becky Pauls, Director

6114 Center for Excellence in Disabilities (CED)
West Virginia University
959 Hartman Run Road
Morgantown, WV 26505
304-293-4692
FAX 304-293-7294
TDY:304-293-4692
Ashok Dey, Executive Director
Kim Michael, Secretary

The mission of the West Virginia University Center for Excellence in Disabilities (WVUCED) is to enhance the quality of life of individuals of all ages with developmental and other disabilities so that they and their families can experience independence and inclusion in society through informed choices and self-determination.

6115 Davis & Elkins College
Learning Disability Program
100 Campus Drive
Elkins, WV 26241
304-637-1229
800-624-3157
FAX 304-637-1413
http://www.dne.edu
e-mail: mccaulj@dne.wvnet.edu
Judith McCauley, Director

Offers a program to provide individual support to college students with specific learning disabilities. This comprehensive program includes regular sessions with one of the three full-time learning disabilities instructors and specialized assistance and technology not available elsewhere on campus.

6116 Fairmont State College
Student Disabilities Services
1201 Locust Avenue
Fairmont, WV 26554
304-367-4686
FAX 304-366-4870
Lynn McMullen, Coordinator

Four year college provides services to learning disabled students.

6117 Glenville State College
Student Disability Services
200 High Street
Glenville, WV 26351
304-462-4118
800-924-2010
FAX 304-462-8619
TDY:304-462-4136
http://www.glenville.wvnet.edu
e-mail: cottrill@GLENVILLE.WVNET.EDU
Daniel Reed, Student Disability Services Coor

6118 Marshall University
Higher Education for Learning Problems Program
520 18th Street
Huntington, WV 25755
304-696-6252
FAX 304-696-3231
http://www.marshall.edu/help
e-mail: weston@marshall.edu
Lynne Weston, Assistant Director
Barbara Deuyer, Manager
K Renna Moore, Administrative Assistant
Offers the following services: individual tutoring to assist with coursework, studying for tests, administration of oral tests when appropriate; assistance with improvement of memory, assistance with note taking; assistance to determine presence of learning problems.

6119 Marshall University: HELP Program
520 18th Street
Huntington, WV 25755
304-696-6252
FAX 304-6963231
http://www.marshall.edu/help
e-mail: weston@marshall.edu
Barbara Deuyer, Manager
Lynne Weston, Assistant Director

A remedial program for LD medical students/physicians offering 5 week programs in January, March, June and September. Individual sessions by appointment. Assistance with reading comprehension, memory strategies, study skills, test-taking strategies and self esteem. Improvement of board scores.

6120 Parkersburg Community College
300 Campus Drive
Parkersburg, WV 26104
304-428-4438
FAX 304-424-8332
TDY:304-424-8337
http://www.wvup.wvnet.edu
e-mail: pam.clevenger@mail.wvu.edu
Cathy Mutz, Director
Judy Sjostedt, Executive Director
Pam Clevenger, Office Manager
Offers a variety of services to students with disabilities including notetakers, extended testing time, counseling services, and special accommodations.

6121 Salem International University
233 W Main Street
Salem, WV 26426
304-782-5011
800-283-4562
FAX 304-782-5395
TDY:304-782-5011
http://www.salemiu.edu
e-mail: admissions@salemiu.edu
Debra Jocwick, Student Support Director
John Reynolds, President

Student Support Services grant program funded by the US Dept of Education for 125 college students who are identified as disadvantaged and/or disabled. On staff are a counselor, a learning disabled specialist in math and science and a learning specialist in reading and writing.

6122 Southern West Virginia Community College & Technical College
PO Box 2900
Mount Gay, WV 25637
304-792-7160
FAX 304-792-7096
http://www.southern.wvnet.edu
e-mail: sherryd@southern.wvnet.edu
Sherry Dempsey, Program Manager

Southern has made reasonable modifications in its policies, practices and procedures to ensure that qualified individuals with disabilities enjoy equal opportunities services. Our facilities are compliant with Section 504 of the Rahabilitation Act of 1973 and the Americans with Disabilities Act of 1990. Offers a variety of services to students with disabilities including note takers, extended testing time, counseling services, and special accommodations.

6123 West Virginia Northern Community College
1704 Market Street
Wheeling, WV 26003
304-233-5900
FAX 304-232-8187
http://www.northern.wvnet.edu
Debbie Cresap, Special Services
Martin Olshinsky, President

A public two-year college with support services for special education students.

6124 West Virginia State College
PO Box 1000
Institute, WV 25112
304-766-3000
800-987-2112
FAX 304-766-4100
http://www.wvsc.edu
Kellie Dunlap, Disability Services
Hazel Carter, President

A public four-year college. Accommodations are individualized to meet student's needs.

6125 West Virginia University: Department of Speech Pathology & Audiology
PO Box 6122
Morgantown, WV 26506
304-293-4241
FAX 304-293-7565
http://www.wvu.edu/~speechpa
e-mail: lcartwri@wvu.edu
Lynn Cartwright, Manager
Cheryl Ridgway, Administrative Associate

Offers clinic services for people with speech, language, and/or hearing disorders.

6126 West Virginia Wesleyan College
Student Academic Support Services
59 College Avenue
Buckhannon, WV 26201
800-722-9933
http://www.wvwc.edu
e-mail: admission@wvwc.edu
Robert Skinner II, Director Admissions/Finance
Shawn Kuba, Director Academic Support
Carolyn Baisden, Administrative Assistant
Offers an individually structured program to accommodate college students with varying needs. Master level professionals in the fields of learning disabilities, reading, education, and counseling work to help each student design strategies for academic success. Accommodation plans are determined through a review of the documentation provided by the student and the recommendations of the student's comprehensive advisor, who works closely with each individual.

Wisconsin

6127 Alverno College
3400 S 43rd Street
Milwaukee, WI 53219
414-382-6000
800-933-3401
FAX 414-382-6354
http://www.alverno.edu
e-mail: colleen.barnett@alverno.edu
Nancy Bornstein, Instructional Services Director
Colleen Barnett, Disability Services Coordinator
Katherine O'Brien, Principal
An independent liberal arts college with 2,000 students in its weekday and weekend degree programs. Support services for students with learning disabilities include appropriate classroom accommodations, assistance in developing self advocacy skills, instructor assistance, peer tutoring, study groups, study strategies workshops, a communication resource center and math resource center.

6128 Beloit College
700 College Street
Beloit, WI 53511
608-363-2000
FAX 608-363-2670
http://www.beloit.edu/~stuaff/disability.html
Diane Arnzen, Director
John Burris, President

Offers a variety of services to students with disabilities such as self advocacy training, study skills and time management guidance, couseling services, and special accommodations.

6129 Blackhawk Technical College
PO Box 5009
Janesville, WI 53547
608-758-6900
800-498-1282
FAX 608-758-6418
TDY:608-743-4422
http://www.blackhawk.edu
Eric Larson, President
Christine Flottum, Project Manager

A public two-year college with support services for special education students.

6130 Cardinal Stritch College
Academic Support
6801 N Yates Road
Milwaukee, WI 53217
414-410-4168
800-347-8822
FAX 414-410-4239
http://www.stritch.edu
Marica Laskey, Director Academic Support

An independent four-year college with support services for special education students.

6131 Carthage College
Academic Support Program
2001 Alford Park Drive
Kenosha, WI 53140
262-551-8500
FAX 262-551-6208
http://www.carthage.edu
Laura Busch, Director
F. Campbell, President

An independent four-year college with support services for special education students.

6132 Chippewa Valley Technical College
Chippewa Valley Technical College
620 W Clairemont Avenue
Eau Claire, WI 54701
715-833-6200
800-547-2882
FAX 715-833-6470
http://www.cvtc.edu
e-mail: jhegge@cvtc.edu
Bill Ihlenfeldt, President
Joe Hegge, Vice President
Ronald Edwards, Manager
A public two-year college with support services for special education students.

6133 Edgewood College
1000 Edgewood College Drive
Madison, WI 53711
608-663-4861
800-444-4861
FAX 608-663-3291
http://www. edgewood.edu
e-mail: admissions@edgewood.edu
Daniel Carey, President

An independent four-year college with support services for students with learning disabilities.

6134 Fox Valley Technical College
PO Box 2277
Appleton, WI 54912
920-735-2525
800-735-3882
FAX 920-831-4396
http://www.foxvalley.tec.wi.us
Lori Weyers, Dean General Studies
David Buettner, President

A public two-year college with support services for special education students.

6135 Gateway Technical College
Gateway Technical College
3520 30th Avenue
Kenosha, WI 53144
262-564-2200
800-353-3152
FAX 262-656-6909
http://www.gtc.edu
Samuel Borden, President

In accordance with Section 504 of the Vocational Rehabilitation Act, Gateway provides a wide range of services that assist special needs students in developing independence and sel-reliance within the Gateway campus community. Reasonable accommodations will be made for students with learning disabilities or physical limitations.

6136 Lakeshore Technical College
Office For Special Needs
1290 N Avenue
Cleveland, WI 53015
920-693-8213
FAX 920-693-3561
http://www.gotoltc.edu
e-mail: viwi@ltc.tec.wi.us
Rivi Hatt, Director

A two-year college that provides comprehensive programs to students with learning disablities.

6137 Lawrence University
PO Box 599
Appleton, WI 54912
920-832-7000
FAX 920-832-6884
http://www.lawrence.edu
e-mail: excel@lawrence.edu

Geoff Gajawski, Academic Services Assoc. Dean
Richard Warch, President

Four year college that offers services to the learning disabled.

6138 Maranatha Baptist Bible College
Maranatha Baptist Bible College
745 W Main Street
Watertown, WI 53094
920-261-9300
FAX 920-261-9109
http://www.mbbc.edu
e-mail: cmidcalf@mbbc.edu
Cynthia Midcalf, Director
David Jaspers, President

Four year college that offers programs for the learning disabled.

6139 Marian College of Fond Du Lac
45 S National Avenue
Fond Du Lac, WI 54935
920-923-7600
FAX 920-923-8755
http://www.mariancollege.edu
Ellen Mercer, Counselor
Richard Ridenour, President

Offers a variety of services to students with disabilities including note takers, extended testing time, counseling services, and special accommodations.

6140 Marquette University
Disability Services Department
PO Box 1881
Milwaukee, WI 53201
414-288-7302
800-222-6544
FAX 414-288-3764
http://www.marquette.edu
e-mail: patriciaalmon@marquette.edu
Patricia Almon, Director

An independent four-year university with support services for students with learning disabilities.

6141 Mid-State Technical College
Mid-State Technical College
500 32nd Street N
Wisconsin Rapids, WI 54494
715-422-5531
888-575-MSTC
FAX 715-422-5345
http://www.mstc.edu
e-mail: webmaster@midstate.tec.wi.us
Patti Lloyd, Coordinator of Disability Servic
John , President

Offers a variety of services to students with disabilities including notetakers, extended testing time, counseling services, and special accommodations.

6142 Milwaukee Area Technical College
700 W State Street
Milwaukee, WI 53233
414-297-6370
FAX 414-297-8142
TDY:414-297-6986
http://www.matc.edu
e-mail: spainc@matc.edu
Carolyn Spain, Manager
Robert Bullock, Manager

A public two-year college with support services for disabled students.

6143 Nicolet Area Technical College: Special Needs Support Program
Nicolet Area Technical College: Special Needs Sup
PO Box 518
Rhinelander, WI 54501
715-365-4410
800-544-3039
FAX 715-365-4445
http://www.nicolet.tec.wi.us
e-mail: inquire@nicolet.tec.wi.us
Bobert Steber, Special Needs
Sandy Jenkins, Case Manager

In support of the Nicolet Area Technical College Student services mission, the Special Needs Support Program provides appropriate accommodations empowering students with disabilities to identify and develop abilities for successful educational and life experiences.

6144 Northcentral Technical College
1000 W Campus Drive
Wausau, WI 54401
715-675-3331
FAX 715-675-9776
Lois Gilliland, Special Services
Robert Ernst, President

Offers a variety of services to students with disabilities including notetakers, extended testing time, counseling services, and special accommodations.

6145 Northeast Wisconsin Technical College
Special Services Program
2740 W Mason Street
Green Bay, WI 54303
800-422-6982
FAX 920-498-5618
http://www.nwtc.edu
Sandy Barnick, Special Services Counselor
Desiree Franks, Special Services Counselor
Dale Strebel, Special Services Counselor
The Special Needs Office of NWTC offers assistance to individuals with disabilities when choosing educational and vocational goals, building self-steem and increasing their occupational potential. We offer a wide range of support services and accommodations which increases the potential of individuals with exceptional education needs to successfully complete Associate Degree and Technical Diploma programs.

6146 Northland College
Northland College
1411 Ellis Avenue
Ashland, WI 54806
715-682-1699
FAX 715-682-1258
http://www.northland.edu
e-mail: admit@northland.edu
Anissa Cram, Office Manager
Jason Turley, Director
Karen Halbersleben, President
Four year college that provides students with learning disabilities with support and services.

6147 Ripon College: Student Support Services
300 Seward Street
Ripon, WI 54971
920-748-8107
FAX 920-748-8335
http://www.ripon.edu
e-mail: krhin@ripon.edu
Dan Krhin, Director

Program provides support services for disabled college students including an array of reasonable accommodations.

6148 St. Norbert College
Academic Support Services
100 Grant Street
De Pere, WI 54115
920-403-1326
800-236-4878
FAX 920-403-4021
http://www.snc.edu
e-mail: karen.goode-bartholomew@snc.edu
Karen Goode-Bartholomew, Director

Provides reasonable accommodations for documented disabilities.

6149 University of Wisconsin Center: Marshfield Wood County
University of Wisconsin Center
2000 W 5th Street
Marshfield, WI 54449
715-389-6500
http://www.marshfield.uwc.edu
Linda Gleason, Associate Director
Andrew Keogh, Administrator

A public two-year college with support services for special education students.

6150 University of Wisconsin: Eau Claire
105 Garfield Avenue
Eau Claire, WI 54701
715-836-2637
FAX 715-836-3712
http://www.uwec.edu

Thomas Bouchard, Director
Vickie Larson, President

Offers a variety of services to students with disabilities including note takers, extended testing time, counseling services, and special accommodations.

6151 University of Wisconsin: La Crosse
1725 State Street
La Crosse, WI 54601
608-785-8489
FAX 608-785-6910
TDY:608-785-6900
http://www.uwlax.edu
e-mail: reinert.june@uwlax.edu

June Reinert, Disability Services
Ashley Reiser, Work Study
Kenna Christians, Manager

Offers a variety of services to students with disabilities including note takers, extended testing time, counseling services, and special accommodations.

6152 University of Wisconsin: Madison
McBurney Disability Resource Center
905 University Avenue
Madison, WI 53715
608-263-2741
FAX 608-265-2998
TDY:608-263-6393
http://www.mcburney.wisc.edu
e-mail: frontdesk@mcb-wisc.edu

Cathleen Trueba, Director
Trey Duffy, Executive Director
Sandra Eisemann PhD, Accommodation Special LD

Offers a variety of services to students with disabilities including notetakers, extended testing time, counseling services, and special accommodations.

6153 University of Wisconsin: Milwaukee
Exceptional Education Department
PO Box 413
Milwaukee, WI 53201
414-229-5251
FAX 414-229-5500
http://www.exed.soe.uwm.edu
e-mail: exed@uwm.edu

Amy Otis Wilborn, Chairperson
Yolanda Rivera, Office Manager

A public four-year college with support services for special education students.

6154 University of Wisconsin: Oshkosh
800 Algoma Boulevard
Oshkosh, WI 54901
920-424-1020
FAX 920-424-0858
http://www.uwosh.edu

William Kitz, Associate Professor
Tom Keefe, President

Disability Services of the Dean of Students Office desires to coordinate reasonable accommodations for students with disabilities. To offer the fullest opportunity for ademic potential while integrating into the vibrant extra-curricular life of the University.

6155 University of Wisconsin: Platteville
113 Warner Hall
Platteville, WI 53818
608-342-1818
FAX 608-342-1918
TDY:608-342-1818
http://www.uwplatte.edu
e-mail: petersre@uwplatt.edu

Rebecca Peters, Coordinator
LeAnnilla Leahy, Disabilities Specialist

Coordinates academic accommodations, provides an advocacy resource center for students with disabilities.

6156 University of Wisconsin: River Falls
University of Wisconsin: River Falls
112 S Hall
River Falls, WI 54022
715-425-3531
FAX 715-425-3277
http://www.uwrf.edu

Mark Johnson, Coordinator
Ruth Taoford, Contract Manager

Offers a variety of services to students with disabilities including note takers, extended testing time, counseling services, and special accommodations.

6157 University of Wisconsin: Whitewater
University of Wisconsin: Whitewater
2021 Roseman Building
Whitewater, WI 53190
262-472-4788
FAX 262-472-5210
http://www.uww.edu
e-mail: amachern@uww.edu

Nancy Amacher, Director
Jamie Leurquin, Assistant Director

A public four-year college. There is an additional fee for the special education program in addition to the regular tuition.

6158 Viterbo University
900 Viterbo Drive
La Crosse, WI 54601
608-796-3060
800-VITERBO
FAX 608-796-3050
http://www.viterbo.edu

Jane Eddy, Director of Learning Center
Nicki Robinson, Administrative Assistant

An independent four-year college with special services for special education students.

6159 Waisman Center: University of Wisconsin-Madison
1500 Highland Avenue
Madison, WI 53705
608-263-1656
FAX 608-263-0529
TDY:608-263-0802
http://www.waisman.wisc.edu
e-mail: webmaster@waisman.wisc.edu

Marsha Mailick, Executive Director
Ruby Chew, Program Assistant 1

To advance knowledge about human development, developmental disabilities, and neurodegenerative diseases.

6160 Waukesha County Technical College
Special Services Department
800 Main Street
Pewaukee, WI 53072
262-691-5210
877-892-9282
FAX 262-691-5089
http://www.wctc.edu
e-mail: djilbert@wctc.edu

Deb Jilbert, Director
Colleen Gonzalez, Transition Retention Specialist

Offers technical and associate degree programs. Services for students with a documented disability may include academic support services, transition services, assistance with the admissions process, testing accommodations, interpreting services, note taking and assistance with RFB&D.

6161 Western Wisconsin Technical College
PO Box 908
La Crosse, WI 54602
608-785-9200
FAX 608-785-9205
http://www.wwtc.edu
e-mail: lee.rusch@wwtc.edu

Keith Valiquette, Special Services
Lee Rasch, President

Offers a variety of services to students with disabilities including notetakers, extended testing time, counseling services, and special accommodations.

6162 Wisconsin Indianhead Tech College: Ashland Campus
Wisconsin Indianhead Tech College: Ashland Campus
2100 Beaser Avenue
Ashland, WI 54806
715-682-4591
800-243-9482
FAX 715-682-8040
TDY:715-468-7755
http://www.witc.edu
Cindy Utities-Heart, Special Services
Don Marcouiller, Administrator

A public two-year college with support services for special education students.

6163 Wisconsin Indianhead Tech College: Rice Lake Campus

Wisconsin Indianhead Tech College: Rice Lake Campu
1900 College Drive
Rice Lake, WI 54868
715-234-7082
800-243-WITC
FAX 715-234-1241
http://www.witc.edu
Jeanne Brand, Disability Specialist
Craig Fowler, Administrator

A public two-year college with support services for students with disabilities.

Wyoming

6164 Laramie County Community CollegeLaramie County Community College: Disability Resource
Disability Resource Center
1400 E College Drive
Cheyenne, WY 82007
307-778-1359
800-522-2993
FAX 307-778-1262
http://www.lccc.wy.edu/drc
e-mail: ldignan@lccc.wy.edu
Lisa Dignan, DRC Coordinator
Scott Moncrief, ADA Compliance Officer

Students with disabilities will find services and adaptive equipment to reduce mobility, sensory, and perceptual problems in the Disability Resource Center.

6165 Northwest College
231 W 6th Street
Powell, WY 82435
307-754-6000
FAX 307-754-6700
http://www.nwc.cc.wy.us
e-mail: tiffany.self@ncag.edu
Lyn Pizor, Director
Miles Larowe, President

A two-year college that provides comprehensive programs to learning disabled students.

6166 Sheridan College
PO Box 1500
Sheridan, WY 82801
307-674-6446
800-913-9139
FAX 307-674-7205
http://www.sheridan.edu
Zane Garstard, Advisor Director
Theresa Miller, Student Service Specialist
Kevin Drumm, President
A public two-year college with support services for special education students.

6167 University of Wyoming
PO Box 3808
Laramie, WY 82071
307-766-1121
FAX 307-766-4010
http://www.uwyo.edu/udss
e-mail: udss@uwyo.edu
Chris Primus, Associate Director
Barbara Moeller, Office Associate
Philip Dubois, President
An independent four-year college with support services for special education students.

6168 University of Wyoming: Division of Social Work and Wyoming Institute for Disabilities (WIND)
PO Box 4298
Laramie, WY 82071
307-766-2761
FAX 307-766-2763
TDY:307-766-2720
http://www.wind.uwyo.edu/
e-mail: kamiller@uwyo.edu
Keith PhD, Executive Director WIND
Ken Heinlein, Director

6169 University of Wyoming: Wyoming Institute for Disabilities (WIND)
1000 E University Avenue
Laramie, WY 82071
307-766-2761
888-989-WIND
FAX 307-766-2763
TDY:307-766-2720
http://www.wind.uwyo.edu
e-mail: kamiller@uwyo.edu
Keith A Miller PhD, Executive Director WIND

Alabama

6170 Good Will Easter Seals
2448 Gordon Smith Drive
Mobile, AL 36617
251-471-1581
800-411-0068
FAX 251-476-4303
http://www.alabama.easterseals.com
Tina Robinson, Human Resources
Terry Dale, Human Resources

Children and adults with disabilities and special needs find highest-quality services designed to meet their individual needs.

6171 Parents as Partners in Education of Alabama
Parents as Partners in Education of Alabama
576 Azalea Road
Mobile, AL 36609
251-478-1208
800-222-7322
FAX 251-473-7877
http://www.seacparentassistancecenter.com
e-mail: seacofmobile@zebra.net
Barbara Wheat MD, Director
Shnaye Callier, Parents Info Resource Ctr Coord
Cheryl Jones, Parent Training/Info Ctr Coord
Parent Training and Information Program views parents as full partners in the educational process and a significant source of support and assistance to each other. Funded by the Division of Personnel Preparation, Office of Special Education Programs, these programs provide training and information to parents to enable such individuals to participate more effectively with professionals in meeting the educational needs of disabled children.

6172 Three Springs
Three Springs
1131 Eagletree Lane SE
Huntsville, AL 35801
256-880-3339
888-758-4356
FAX 256-880-7026
http://www.threesprings.com
e-mail: info@threesprings.com
Debra Dombrowski, Communications Manager
Brook Balch, President

A nationally recognized leader in youth services, founded in 1985 to provide therapy and education to adolescents experiencing emotional, behavioral and learning problems.

6173 Wireglass Rehabilitation Center
PO Box 338
Dothan, AL 36302
334-792-0022
800-395-7044
FAX 334-712-7632
Jack Sasser, Owner
Tracy Zurran, Program Services

Provides services to individuals with disabilities in order to render them employable.

6174 Wiregrass Rehabilitation Center
795 Ross Clark Circle NE
Dothan, AL 36302
334-792-0022
800-395-7044
FAX 334-712-7632
Jack Sasser, Owner
Tracy Zurran, Program Services

Provides services to individuals with disabilities in order to render them employable.

6175 Workshops
4244 3rd Avenue S
Birmingham, AL 35222
205-592-9683
888-805-9683
FAX 205-592-9687
http://www.workshopsinc.com
e-mail: crim@workshopsinc.com
James Crim, Executive Director
Shan Graham, Program Coordinator

Funded by the public, community chest and workshop sales this center provides evaluation, employment, pre-vocational training and sheltered workshops to the disabled areas of Birmingham, Jefferson County, Northern Alabama and Shelby County.

Alaska

6176 Center for Community
700 Katlian Street
Sitka, AK 99835
907-747-6960
800-478-6970
FAX 907-747-4868
http://http://www.ptialaska.net/~cfcsitka
e-mail: csipe@cfc.org
Connie Sipe, Executive Director

A state-wide provider of home and community-based services for people with disabilities, the elderly and others who experience barriers to community living in Alaska.

Arizona

6177 Academy of Tucson
10720 E 22nd Street
Tucson, AZ 85748
520-733-0096
FAX 520-733-0097
e-mail: shari@at.tuccoxmail.com
Sue Pearson, Principal
Shari Stewart, Assistant Superintendent

A state charted, nonprofit co-ed school serving grades 9-12. Founded in 1986, accredited by North Central Association, it is a college preparatory school for students who learn best in a small, personalized setting. Teachers hold Arizona certificates, and class ratios are 1:20. The curriculum meets college entrance requirements. Charter sponsered by Arizona Stats Board of Education. Tuition free.

6178 Arizona Center Comprehensive Education and Lifeskills
10251 N 35th Avenue
Phoenix, AZ 85051
602-995-7366
FAX 602-995-0867
http://www.accel.org
e-mail: ACCELlearningcenter@hotmail.com
Kathy Sullivan-Orton, Student Services Director
Sandra Ardon, Human Resources Director

A private, non-profit, special education school providing therapeutic, educational, and behavioral services to over 200 students, ages 3-21, with cognitive, emotional, orthopedic, and/or behavioral disabilities.

6179 Devereux Arizona Treatment Network
11000 N Scottsdale Road
Scottsdale, AZ 85254
480-998-2920
FAX 480-443-5587
http://www.devereuxaz.org
Lane Barker, Executive Director

Provides a wide array of behavioral health and social welfare services for persons with emotional and behavioral disorders or who are victims of physical or sexual abuse and neglect.

6180 LATCH School
10251 N 35th Avenue
Phoenix, AZ 85051
602-995-7366
Connie Laird, Executive Director

6181 **Life Development Institute (LDI)**
18001 N 79th Avenue
Glendale, AZ 85308
623-773-2774
FAX 623-773-2788
http://www.life-development-inst.org
Robert Crawford, CEO
Veronica Crawford, President

Provides a supportive residential community that gives individuals the education, skills and training they need to live independently. By offering these programs in a residential environment, the students are given a chance to learn independence, and instill in them a desire to succeed.

6182 **New Way Learning Academy**
1300 N 77th Street
Scottsdale, AZ 85257
480-946-9112
FAX 480-946-2657
http://www.newwayacademy.org
e-mail: sharon.hill@newwayacademy.org
Dr Sharon Hill, Executive Director
Dawn Gutierrez, Principal

Serving children with learning disabilities, attention deficit disorder and underachievers in grades K-12 for 34 years. New Way is approved by the Arizona State Department of Special Education to serve students with learning disabilities and meets state mandated standards and guidelines. Our enrollment is approximately 120 students, and we have 35 staff members.

6183 **Raising Special Kids**
2400 N Central Avenue
Phoenix, AZ 85004
602-242-4366
800-237-3007
FAX 602-242-4306
http://www.raisingspecialkids.org
e-mail: info@raisingspecialkids.org
Joyce Hoie, Executive Director
Peggy Storrs, Operations Director

A parent training and information center providing information, resources and support to families of children with disabilities and special needs in Arizona.

6184 **Turning Point School**
200 E Yavapai Road
Tucson, AZ 85705
520-292-9300
FAX 520-292-9075
http://www.turningpointschool.com
Nancy Wald, Executive Director

A private, nonprofit school for children with dyslexia, attention deficit disorder and learning disabilities who have difficulties in reading, writing, spelling and math.

Arkansas

6185 **Arkansas Disability Coalition**
1123 S University Avenue
Little Rock, AR 72204
501-614-7020
800-223-1330
FAX 501-614-9082
http://www.adcpti.org
e-mail: adcoalition@earthlink.net
Wanda Stovall, Executive Director

Arkansas Disability Coalition's mission is to work for equal rights and opportunities for Arkansans with disabilities through public policy change, cross-disability collaboration, and empowerment of people with disabilities and their families.

California

6186 **Access Community Center**
1014 B Street
Hayward, CA 94541
510-538-4221
http://www.ldresources.org
e-mail: accesscommunity@yahoo.com
A support center for LD adults and specializes in helping people with assistive technology.

6187 **Ann Martin Children's Center**
1250 Grand Avenue
Piedmont, CA 94610
510-655-7880
FAX 510-655-3379
http://www.annmartin.org
David Theis, Executive Director
Terrell Kessler, Administrative Manager

A private, nonprofit community center that helps children with special educational needs become more confident and independent learners. There are learning specialists, psychologists, social workers, marriage family therapists, and psychiatrists on staff. The center assists over 900 youth and adults annually through 24,000 hours of treatment services.

6188 **Brislain Learning Center**
2545 Ceanothus Avenue
Chico, CA 95973
530-342-2567
800-791-6031
FAX 530-342-2573
http://www.brislainlearningcenter.com
e-mail: info@brislainlearningcenter.com
Judy Brislain, Owner

Assists children of all ages who have learning disabilities. Offers a diagnostic program and tutoring program for ADD and learning disabilities. Provides counseling and support groups for children and adults.

6189 **Center for Adaptive Learning**
3227 Clayton Road
Concord, CA 94519
925-827-3863
FAX 925-827-4080
http://www.centerforadaptivelearning.org
e-mail: info@centerforadaptivelearning.org
Donald Bone, President
Nancy Perry Ph.D, Clinical Neurophysiologist
Genevieve Stolarz, Executive Director
The center provides a comprehsive program that is designed to address many needs; physical, social, emotional and vocational. To empower adults with a developmental neurological disability to realize their own potential.

6190 **Charles Armstrong School**
1405 Solana Drive
Belmont, CA 94002
650-592-7570
FAX 650-592-0780
http://www.charlesarmstrong.org
e-mail: info@charlesarmstrong.org
Rosalie Whitlock Ph.D, Manager
Linda Hale, Assistant Headmaster

The mission of the school is to serve the dyslexic learner by providing an appropriate educational experience which not only enables the students to acquire language skills, but also instills a joy of learning, enhances self-worth, and allows each the right to identify, understand and fulfill personal potential.

6191 **Children's Therapy Center**
1000 Paseo Camarillo
Camarillo, CA 93010
805-383-1501
FAX 805-383-1504
Beth Maulhardt, Executive Director
Joe Highland, Owner

A private evaluation and treatment center for children who show delays in motor development, speech/language development, play and social development and/or learning problems. The center offs occupational therapy, physical therapy, speech/language therapy, counseling and psychological testing.

6192 Devereux Santa Barbara
PO Box 6784
Santa Barbara, CA 93160
805-968-2525
FAX 805-968-3247
http://www.devereux.org
e-mail: info@devereux.org
David Dennis, Executive Director

A treatment facility offering residential, educational and adult vocational or day activity programs to individuals ages 8-85 with multiple diagnoses such as; autistic spectrum disorders, emotional and/or behavioral disorders, mental retardation, developmental disabilities, and medical conditions.

6193 Dyslexia Awareness and Resource Center
928 Carpinteria Street
Santa Barbara, CA 93103
805-963-7339
FAX 805-963-6581
http://www.dyslexiacenter.org
e-mail: info@dyslexiacenter.org
Leslie Esposito, Executive Development Director
Joan Esposito, Executive Director

The center provides direct one-on-one services to adults and children affected with dyslexia, attention disorders and other learning disabilities. In addition the center conducts outreach and training seminars for public and private schools, for the juvenile court systems, for drug and alcohol programs, for family and social service programs, for literacy programs, and for homeless and mission programs.

6194 Frostig Center
971 N Altadena Drive
Pasadena, CA 91107
626-791-1255
FAX 626-798-1801
http://www.frostig.org
e-mail: helpline@frostig.org
Bennett Ross, Executive Director

A non profit organization that specializes in helping children who have learning disabilities. Offers parent training, consulting, school and tutoring services to learning disabled children.
6-18 years old

6195 Full Circle Programs
70 Skyview Terrace
San Rafael, CA 94903
415-499-3320
FAX 415-499-1542
http://www.fullcircleprograms.org
e-mail: info@fullcircleprograms.org
Brian Weele, Executive Director
Deborah Riggins, Associate Director

Full Circle has been actively caring for children and their families in need. Full Circle offers a continuum of care ranging from residential treatment for several emotionally disturbed boys, to outpatient counseling for children and their families.

6196 Help for Brain Injured Children
Cleta Harder Developmental School
981 N Euclid Street
La Habra, CA 90631
562-694-5655
FAX 562-694-5657
http://www.hbic.org
e-mail: hbiccleta@aol.com
Cleta Harder, Executive Director

Help for brain-injured children. Long-term, low cost home rehabilitation programs. School programs, rehabilitation, academic, speech and physical therapy, as needed. Offer an after-school program for youngsters in regular school who are experiencing difficulties.

6197 Institute for the Redesign of Learning
1137 Huntington Drive
South Pasadena, CA 91030
323-341-5580
FAX 323-257-0284
http://www.redesignlearning.org
e-mail: info@resdesignlearning.org
Nancy Lavelle, Ph.D, Co-Founder/Executive Director

A multi-service, community-based education and training facility for at-risk youth. Offering a range of professional services and support to the students and their parents.

6198 Kayne-ERAS Center
5350 Machado Lane
Culver City, CA 90230
310-737-9393
FAX 310-737-9344
http://www.kayneeras.org
e-mail: mjackson@kayneeras.org
Daniel Maydeck, Executive VP
Mishelle Ross, Chief Program Officer

Kayne-ERAS accomplishes its mission by offering educational resources, direct service, and a professional training center. Kayne-ERAS provides personalized programming to children and young adults from at risk conditions and those challenged by emotional, learning, developmental and/or chronic neurological and/or medical disabilities.

6199 Marina Psychological Services
4640 Admiralty Way
Marina Del Rey, CA 90292
310-822-0109
FAX 310-822-1240
e-mail: marinapsych@hotmail.com
Bruce Hirsch, Ph.D, Psychologist
Stuart Shaffer, Ph.D, Psychologist

Comprehensive psychological services for children and adults with learning disabilities and attention deficit disorders. Private, individualized assessment and treatment.

6200 Melvin-Smith Learning Center
EDU-Therapeutics
1900 Garden Road
Monterey, CA 93940
831-484-0994
800-505-3276
FAX 861-484-0998
http://www.edu-therapeutics.com
e-mail: joan_smith@comcast.net
Dr. Joan Smith, Director

EDU-Therapeutics is a unique learning system that offers effective solutions for overcoming dyslexia, attention deficit, learning disabilities and reading challenges. It succeeds because it changes how an individual uses his or her brain to learn. It is unique because it identifies the underlying cause of the learning inefficiency and eliminates the symptoms.

6201 Nawa Academy
17351 Trinity Mountain Road
French Gulch, CA 96033
530-359-2215
800-358-6292
FAX 530-359-2229
http://www.nawa-academy.com
e-mail: nawamain@hotmail.com
David Hull, Executive Director
Sandy Gilliam, Secretary

A boarding school located in a remote valley of the Trinity Alps that provides individual curriculum, theory and structure for 7-9 grade students, many of who have learning disabilities. ÆServices include individual counseling, small academic classes, and numerous after school activities.

6202 New Vistas Christian School
68 Morello Avenue
Martinez, CA 94553
925-370-7767
FAX 925-370-6395
http://www.nvcs.info
Maria Zablah, Principal
Correne Romeo, Director

A non-profit 1st-12th grade school for students of average or above average intelligence with learning disabilities offering a non-traditional approach to multiple learning styles.

6203 Newport Audiology Center
Newport Health Network
27285 Las Ramblas
Mission Viejo, CA 92691
949-282-1212
FAX 949-348-0299
http://www.newaud.com
e-mail: info@newaud.com
Sharlene Goodman, President/Chief Executive Office

The aim is to enhance the quality of people's lives by improving their ability to communicate. We provide the highest level of audiological services possible, through our highly efficient staff, informative education programs, community services, high quality products, and true spirit of customer service.

6204 Newport Language: Speech and Audiology
26137 La Paz Road
Mission Viejo, CA 92691
949-581-5206

6205 One To One Reading & Educational Center
11971 Salem Drive
Granada Hills, CA 91344
818-368-1801
FAX 818-368-9345
Paul Klinger, Owner/Director
Julie Klinger, Assistant/Associate

Educational therapy for students with reading and math problems and tutoring for many subjects all one on one.

6206 Park Century School
2040 Stoner Avenue
Los Angeles, CA 90025
310-478-5065
FAX 310-473-9260
http://www.parkcenturyschool.org
e-mail: nbley@parkcenturyschool.org
Debbie Chernoff, President/Board Chair
Paul Jennings, Vice President
Genny Shane, Executive Director
An independent school for average and above average intellect children with learning disabilities. The program emphasizes developing the skills and strategies necessary to return to a traditional program. With a 2:1 student-staff ratio.
7-14 years old

6207 Pine Hill School
1325 Bouret Drive
San Jose, CA 95118
408-979-8210
FAX 408-979-8219
http://www.pinehillschool.com
e-mail: gregz@secondstart.org
Greg Zieman, Principal/Assoc. Executive Dir.
Terry Reynolds, Registrar

A private school that provides special education and alternative services to students with a wide range of learning and behavior disabilities.

6208 Prentice School
Prentice School
18341 Lassen Drive
Santa Ana, CA 92705
714-538-4511
FAX 714-538-5004
http://www.prenticeschool.org
Carol Clark, Executive Director
Carol Stewart, Executive Assistant

The Prentice School is an independent, nonprofit, coeducational day school dedicated to the needs of Specific Language Disabled Students.

6209 Providence Speech and Hearing Center
1301 W Providence Avenue
Orange, CA 92868
714-639-4990
FAX 714-744-3841
http://www.pshc.org
e-mail: psqc@pshc.org
Margaret Ann Inman Ph.D, Founder
Raul Lopez, COO/Finance Director
Mary Hooper, Executive Director
Comprehensive services for testing and treatment of all speech, language and hearing problems. Individual and group therapy beginning with parent/infant programs.

6210 REACH for Learning
1221 Marin Avenue
Albany, CA 94706
510-524-6455
FAX 510-524-5154
http://www.reachforlearning.org
Corinne Gustafson, Executive Director

Educational services for children and adults including: diagnostic assessment, individual remediation/tutoring, small group workshops, and consultation for parents and professionals.

6211 Raskob Learning Institute and Day School -
3520 Mountain Boulevard
Oakland, CA 94619
510-436-1275
FAX 510-436-1106
http://www.rascobinstitute.org
e-mail: raskobinstitute@hnu.edu
Rachel Wylde, Executive Director

A co-educational school for students from diverse cultural and economic backgrounds with language-based learning disabilities. Raskob seeks to recognize and nurture the talents and strengths of each student while remediating areas of academic weakness.
9-14 years old

6212 Reading Center of Bruno
4952 Warner Avenue
Huntington Beach, CA 92649
714-377-7910
FAX 562-436-4428
http://www.readingcenter.info
e-mail: readingct.@aol.com
Walter Waid, Owner
Dr. Muriel Bruno, Founder

Working with children, teens and adults with dyslexia, auditory and visual perceptual confusions through our specialized training program. Diagnostic testing is available, as well.

6213 Rincon Learning Center
134 Barnegat Road
Pound Ridge, NY 10576
619-442-2722
FAX 619-442-1011
Lois Dotson, Director

Diagnostic and therapy services for a wide range of learning disabilities. Offers one on one tutoring.

6214 Santa Barbara Center for Educational Therapy
1811 State Street
Santa Barbara, CA 93101
805-687-3711
FAX 805-687-3711
Susan Hamilton, Director
Cherie Baroni, Director

Provides educational assessment to determine learning style and document learning disabilities. Also provided are one-to-one remedial or tutorial services for individuals specializing in dyslexia.

6215 Santa Cruz Learning Center
720 Fairmount Avenue
Santa Cruz, CA 95062
831-427-2753
e-mail: sclrngcntr@yahoo.com
Eleanor Stitt, Manager

Individualized one-to-one tutoring for individuals aged 5 to adult. Specializes in dyslexia, learning difficulties and gifted persons. Includes test preparation, math, reading, self confidence, study skills, time organization and related services.

6216 Second Start: Pine Hill School
3002 Leigh Avenue
San Jose, CA 95124
408-979-8210

6217 Stockdale Learning Center
1701 Westwind Drive
Bakersfield, CA 93301
661-326-8084
FAX 661-327-4752
http://www.stockdalelearningcenter.net
e-mail: slc@igalaxy.net

Andrew Barling, Executive Director
Tammy Bulford, Associate Educational Therapist

A professional State Certified Educational Therapy clinic designed to collaboratively diagnose and assess individuals 5 years of age through adult who have learning disabilities. Offering extensive services for dyslexia, ADD/HD, and other specific learning disabilities.

6218 Stowell Learning Center
20955 Pathfinder Road
Diamond Bar, CA 91765
909-598-2482
FAX 909-598-3442
http://www.learningdisability.com
e-mail: info@learningdisability.com

Jill Stowell, Owner

A diagnostic and teaching center for learning and attention disorders. Specializes in instruction for dyslexic or learning disabled children and adults. Our services include diagnostic evaluation, developmental evaluation, cognitive and educational therapy which is provided on a one-to-one basis, and a full day class for elementary age students with reading disabilities.

6219 Switzer Learning Center
2201 Amapola Court
Torrance, CA 90501
310-328-3611
FAX 310-328-5648
http://www.switzercenter.org
e-mail: drfoo@switzercenter.org

Rebecca Foo MD, Executive Director
Larry Brugnatelli, Associate Director

Improving lives of those challenged by learning, social and emotional difficulties by maximizing educational competence and psychological well being.

6220 Team of Advocates for Special Kids
100 Cerritos Avenue
Anaheim, CA 92805
714-533-8275
866-828-8275
FAX 714-533-2533
http://www.taskca.org
e-mail: taskca@yahoo.com

Marta Anchondo, Executive Director
Brenda Smith, Deputy Director

A parent training and information center that parents and professionals can turn to for assistance in seeking and obtaining needed early intervention and educational, medical or therapeutic support service for children.

6221 Team of Advocates for Special Kids (TASK)
100 W Cerritos Avenue
Anaheim, CA 92805
714-533-8275

Marta Anchondo, Executive Director

6222 Total Education Solutions
1137 Huntington Drive
South Pasadena, CA 91030
323-344-5550

Nancy Lavelle, President

6223 Vision Care Clinic
General, Preventive and Developmental Optometry
2730 Union Avenue
San Jose, CA 95124
408-377-1150
FAX 408-377-1152
http://www.visiondiva.com
e-mail: rice@visiondiva.com

Liane Rice, MD, Director

Diagnostic and training for those with visual disabilities.

6224 Vision Care Clinic of Santa Clara Valley
2730 Union Avenue
San Jose, CA 95124
408-377-1150

V. Rice, Owner

Colorado

6225 Developmental Disabilities Resource Center
11177 W 8th Avenue
Lakewood, CO 80215
303-233-3363
800-649-8815
FAX 303-233-4622
TDY:303-462-6606
http://www.ddrcco.com
e-mail: ahogling@ddrcco.com

Art Hogling Ph.D, CEO
Robert Arnold, Associate Executive Director

The mission is to provide leading-edge services that create opportunities for people with developmental disabilities and their families to participate fully in the community.

6226 Havern School
4000 S Wadsworth Boulevard
Lakewood, CO 80123
303-986-4587
FAX 303-986-0590
http://www.haverncenter.org
e-mail: agoyette@haverncenter.org

Cathy Pasquariello, Executive Director
Denise Ensslin, Staff/Curriculum Consultant
Nancy Mann, Admissions Director

School for children with learning disabilities. Educational programs, special language programs and occupational therapy is available.

6-13 years old

Connecticut

6227 American School for the Deaf
139 N Main Street
West Hartford, CT 06107
860-570-2300
http://www.asd-1817.org
e-mail: info@asd-1817.org

Harvey Corson, Executive Director
Christy Pinyoun, Executive Assistant
Driggers Sr. Administrative Ass, Sr. Administrative Assistant

A residential/day program operating as a state-aided private school and governed by a board of directors. It is the oldest permanent school for the deaf in America, offering a comprehensive educational program for the deaf and hard of hearing students, infants, preschoolers, primary, elementary, junior high school, high school, and post-secondary students.

6228 Blind Vocational Services
Oak Hill Center
120 Holcomb Street
Hartford, CT 06112
860-242-2274
FAX 860-242-3103
http://www.ciboakhill.org
e-mail: famigliettis@ciboakhill.org

Steve Famiglietti, Job Developer
Hesslein Community Relations De, Community Relations Director

Created in 2006, the Blind Vocational Services was designed to address the unemployment rate among people who are blind. Working with both students who are transitioning from school to the workforce and adults, a Job Developer will assess participants preparedness for vocational placement, identfiy the need for, and provide additional training; identify the need for assistive technology, develop community-based transportation systems to faciliate access to vocational opportunities.

6229 Boys and Girls Village
528 Wheelers Farms Road
Milford, CT 06461
203-877-0300
FAX 203-876-0076
http://www.boysvillage.org
e-mail: fellenbaumk@boysvill.org

Rev. Kenneth Fellenbaum, Chief Executive Officer
Douglas DeCerbo, Chief Administrative Officer
Kant MD Medical Director, Medical Director

The clients of Boys & Girls Village are children in crisis or children with learning difficulties who have experienced rejection, failure or abuse. Through the years, the agency has evolved into a leading therapeutic and learning facility offering residential shelter, clinical, after-school, counseling, special educational, foster & adoptive recruitment and training, family support services, and day programs for children and their families.

6230 COPE Center of Progressive Education
Residential Services Division
425 Grant Street
Bridgeport, CT 06610 203-332-9189
FAX 203-781-4792
http://www.aptfoundation.org/cope.htm
e-mail: info@aptfoundation.org
Gretchen Celestino, Principal
Jimmy Cooper, Owner

A licensed and approved special education program for adolescents who are in the Alpha House Residential Treatment Center. COPE serves both males and females between the ages of fourteen and twenty-one. Students are offered the opportunity to participate in an educational process that will allow them to earn credit toward a high school diploma.

6231 Candee Hill
122 Candee Hill Road
Watertown, CT 06795 860-274-8332
FAX 860-828-3912
Frank Popkiewicz, Director

Emphasis on increasing client's self-sufficiency in areas of daily skills, community awareness and social interaction.

6232 Child Care Programs
Easter Seals Rehabilitation Center
158 State Street
Meriden, CT 06450 203-237-1448
FAX 203-237-9187
http://www.eastersealsct.org
Beverly Malinowski, Vice President
John Quinn, President

Meeting a growing need for high-quality child care for more than 20 million young children and their working parents, Easter Seals offers child care for children ages 6 months to 5 years. Young children are welcomed to a unique environment where children of all abilities learn together.

6233 Community Child Guidance Clinic School
317 N Main Street
Manchester, CT 06042 860-643-2101
FAX 860-645-1470
http://www.ccgcinc.org
e-mail: clinic@ccgcinc.org
Clifford Johnson, Executive Director
Lynn Helman, Medical Director

The Community Child Guidance Clinic is a private, non-profit mental health agency offering diagnostic, treatment and consultation services to children up to the age of 18 and their families.

6234 Connecticut Center for Augmentative
95 Merritt Boulevard
Trumbull, CT 06611 203-375-6400
Barry Buxbaun, CEO

6235 Connecticut Center for Children and Families
8 Titus Road
Washington Depot, CT 06794 860-868-0254
FAX 860-868-1288
Patricia Thomas
Janet Bloch

The Connecticut Center is a group of affiliated professionals with a diversity of talent but with a common vision. We believe that collaborative intervention is often the most clinically and financially effective way to solve learning and educational problems. The Center offers the services of psychiatrists, psychologists, learning specialists and tutors.

6236 Connecticut College Children's Program
Connecticut College
270 Mohegan Avenue
New London, CT 06320 860-439-2650
FAX 860-439-5317
http://www.conncoll.edu/academics/department/
e-mail: shrad@conncoll.edu
Sarah Radlinski, Program Director/Professor
Beatrice DeMitt, Program Director
Lee Hisle, Vice President
The mission of the Connecticut College Children's Program is to provide, within a community context, a model child and family-focused early childhood program for infants and young children of diverse backgroungs and abilities in Southeastern Connecticut.

6237 Connecticut Institute for the Blind
120 Holcomb Street
Hartford, CT 06112 860-242-2274
Patrick Johnson, President

6238 Curtis Home
380 Crown Street
Meriden, CT 06450 203-237-4338
FAX 203-630-1127
http://www.thecurtishome.org
e-mail: info@thecurtishome.org
Robert Flyntz, President
Ronald Stempien, Vice President
Paul Sprague, Executive Director
Managed by the Hartford Healthcare System, the Children's Program continues to provide support in the following service areas: Residential Treatment, Day Treatment, The Cheshire School, Family Placement Program, and Safe Harbors. The Curtis Home still owns a majority of the facilities housing the Children's Program.

6239 Devereux Glenholme School
81 Sabbaday Lane
Washington, CT 06793 860-868-7377
FAX 860-868-7413
http://www.theglenholmeschool.org
e-mail: admissions@theglenholmeschool.org
Kathi Fitzherbert, Director Admissions
Christine Sulborski, Admissions Assistant

The Glenholme School is a boarding school for students with social/emotional and/or learning disabilities. Glenholme is situated on100 idyllic acres in the Connecticut countryside.

6240 Eagle Hill School
45 Glenville Road
Greenwich, CT 06831 203-622-9240
FAX 203-622-0914
http://www.eaglehillschool.org
e-mail: info@eaglehillschool.org
Rayma Griffin, Admissions Director
Sara Pelgrift, Co-President
Mark Griffin, Principal
Eagle Hill is a languaged-based, remedial program committed to educating children with learning disabilities. The curriculum is individualized, interdisciplinary, and transitional in nature.

6241 Elmcrest Schools
25 Marlborough Street
Portland, CT 06480 860-342-6266
FAX 860-342-5106
Elaine Green, Director

Offers short-term treatment, long-term treatment and a day treatment program for the learning disabled and children with substance abuse problems.

6242 Focus Alternative Learning Center

PO Box 452
Canton, CT 06019
860-693-8809
FAX 860-693-0141
http://www.focus-alternative.org
e-mail: info@focus-alternative.org

Donna Swanson, Manager
Yvonne Gardner, Program Coordinator

FOCUS Alternative Learning Center is a private, licensed, non-profit, year-found clinical program committed to the treatment of children ages 6-18 diagnosed with Autism Spectrum disorders, attention and anxiety disorders, or who have processing and/or learning problems. Our Integral Model of Care™ focuses on the social, emotional and academic obstacles that impede a child's growth and success in school, at home and in the community.

6243 Forman School

Forman School
12 Norfolk Road
Litchfield, CT 06759
860-567-8712
FAX 860-567-3501
http://www.formanschool.org
e-mail: admissions@formanschool.org

Mark Perkins, Principal
Beth Rainey, Admissions Director
Tom O'Dell, Student Recruitment Director

Forman offers students with learning differences the opportunity to achieve academic excellence in a traditional college preparatory setting. A coeducational boarding school of 180 students, we maintain a 3:1 student:teacher ratio. Daily remedial instruction balanced with course offerings rich in content provide each student with a flexible program that is tailored to his or her unique learning style and needs.

6244 Foundation School

719 Derby Milford Road
Orange, CT 06477
203-795-6075
FAX 203-876-7531

Jack Bell, Director
Walter Bell, Principal

Basic developmental skills address speech/language and perceptual/motor areas. Academic skills are reading, writing and arithmetic with social studies, science and career studies.

6245 Founder's Cottage

Star, Lighting The Way
182 Wolfpit Road
Norwalk, CT 06852
203-847-6760
FAX 203-847-0545
http://www.starinc-lightingtheway.org
e-mail: jleniart@starinconline.com

Jackie Leniart, Program Director
Mark Carta, President

Facility-based respite care is provided by STAR at Founders Cottage. A lovely home, is co-ed, and can accomodate four individuals at a time. It is for people with development disabilities who are 16 years or older and who reside within the Southwest Region. All persons must be registered with the Connecticut Department of Mental Retardation and have a DMR number assigned.

6246 Founders' Respite Care

PO Box 470
Norwalk, CT 06852
203-847-6760

6247 Gengras Center

Saint Joseph College
1678 Asylum Avenue
West Hartford, CT 06117
860-232-4751
FAX 860-231-8396
http://www.sjc.edu
e-mail: blindauer@sjc.edu

Bernard Lindauer, Director
Evelyn Lynch, President

This a state approved, private special education facility, provides a highly structured, intensive, self-contained special education program for elementary, middle and high school students. The program focuses on skill development in the core academic areas, functional application of skills, community life skills, work readiness skills, job training, social development and independent living skills. Special attention is given to the behavioral challenges of individual students.

6248 Intensive Education Academy

840 N Main Street
West Hartford, CT 06117
860-236-2049
FAX 860-231-2843

Helen Dowd, Executive Director
Jill O'Donnell, Director Education

A state approved, non-profit, non sectarian special education facility for children 6 to 21 years with different learning styles. Individualized program with a 5:1 student teacher ratio. Program strives to help each student reach their potential by gaining confidence, recognizing their strengths and limitations, setting realistic goals and attaining satisfaction by achieving these goals. State approved. Full-day curriculum is offered.

6249 Klingberg Family Centers

370 Linwood Street
New Britain, CT 06052
860-224-9113
FAX 860-832-8221
http://www.klingberg.com
e-mail: information@klingberg.com

Lynne Roe, Intake Director
David Lawrence-Hawley, Community Services VP
Rosemarie Burton, President

Provides structured programs for residential, day treatment and day school students in a therapeutic environment. We are a private, nonprofit organization serving children and families from across Connecticut.

6250 Lake Grove Durham

459R Wallingford Road
Durham, CT 06422
860-349-3467
http://www.lgstc.org
e-mail: pam_vanaman@lgadmissions.org

Michael Suchapar, Administrator
Pamela Vanamantrator, Referral Administrator

Lake Grove at Durham serves cognitively challenged clients in ten expanded split-level homes in a rural community atmosphere. Support facilities include school buildings, administration building, dining hall, horse stables and pasture, clubhouse, and several staff homes.

6251 Lake Grove-Durham School

459R Wallingford Road
Durham, CT 06422
860-349-3467
888-525-9007
FAX 860-349-1382
http://www.lgstc.org

Robert Ruggiero, Principal/Director

Serves its clients in eight expanded split-level homes in a rural community atmosphere. Support facilities include a school building, administration building, dining hall, horse stables and pasture, clubhouse, and several staff homes.

6252 Learning Center

Children's Home
60 Hicksville Road
Cromwell, CT 06416
860-635-6010
FAX 860-635-3708
http://www.childhome.org
e-mail: dmaibaum@childhome.org

David Tompkins, Program Administrative Officer
Cindy Sarnowski, Education Director
David Jacobsen, CEO

The Learning Center at The Children's Home is accredited by the Connecticut State Department of Education as an educational institution for children and adolescents with emotional and learning difficulties. The program serves students between the ages of 5 to 18 in both day and Residential programs.

6253 Learning Clinic
PO Box 324
Brooklyn, CT 06234
860-774-7471
FAX 860-774-1037
http://www.thelearningclinic.org
e-mail: admissions@thelearningclinic.org
Raymond Charme Ph.D, Administrator

A private, nonprofit educational program that provides day and residential school focused on ADHD and learning and emotional issues. The program is coeducational and serves seventy students. The aim is to assist students in meeting their academic goals and prepare for future experiences in educational, vocational, and community settings.

6254 Lorraine D Foster Day School
1861 Whitney Avenue
Hamden, CT 06517
203-230-4877
FAX 203-288-5749
http://www.ldfds.com
e-mail: ldfds@snet.net
Dominique Fontaine, Executive Director
Christine Kirschenbaum, Assistant Director

A psycho-educational day program for students who have met with failure in previous school settings. It is the school's mission to empower students, enabling them to function as competent, responsible individuals who possess the ability to enrich their own lives and to contribute to the betterment of the world-at-large.

6255 Mount Saint John
135 Kirtland Street
Deep River, CT 06417
860-526-5391
FAX 860-526-3846
http://www.mtstjohn.org
e-mail: info@mtstjohn.org
Catherine Coridan, Executive Director
David Young, Administrative Services Director
Andrew George, Principal
This is a residential treatment program that provides comprehensive and integrated treatment services to adolescent boys and young men who are not able to function in their home community due to combinations of behavioral, emotional, family and educational problems. The staff and Board of Mount Saint John are committed to providing a treatment program to meet the evolving and changing needs of the times and of the boys who come into our care.

6256 Natchaug Hospital School Program
PO Box 260
Mansfield Center, CT 06250
860-456-1311
FAX 860-423-6114
Stephen Larcen, CEO
David Klein, VP Community Services
Jill Bourbeau, School Programs Director
Natchaug Hospital operates three state approved K-12 special education programs for socially, emotionally disturbed youth. Natchaug Hospital also provides in patient and partial hospital programs at 9 Eastern Connecticut locations.

6257 Natchaug's Network of Care
Natchaug Hospital
189 Storrs Road
Mansfield Center, CT 06250
860-456-1311
800-426-7792
FAX 860-423-6114
http://www.natchaug.org
Stephen Larcen, Ph.D, President/CEO
Ellen Buffington, RNC, Hospital Operations VP
Klein PhD Community Programs VP, Community Programs VP
The hospital's 54-bed facility in Mansfield Center, provides in-patient care for seriously emotionally disturbed children and adolescents as well as adults in crisis each year.

6258 Northwest Village School: Wheeler Clinic
91 Northwest Drive
Plainville, CT 06062
860-793-3500

6259 OPTIONS
158 State Street
Meriden, CT 06450
203-237-7835
Beverly Malinowski, Vice President

6260 Rensselaer Learning Institute
Rensselaer at Hartford
275 Windsor Street
Hartford, CT 06120
860-548-2470
800-306-7778
FAX 860-548-7999
http://www.rh.edu/
e-mail: rli-info@rh.edu
Shirley Ann Jackson, Ph.D, President
Rebecca Danchak, Acting Associate Student Dean

Rensselaer Learning Institute is a department within Rensselaer at Hartford that offers corporate training programs and services to working professionals - anytime, anywhere. The program offers computer and information technology, leadership and executive development, and technical and professional development that are designed to meet the complex needs of corporations operating in today's fast-paced business climate.

6261 Saint Francis Home for Children
651 Prospect Street
New Haven, CT 06511
203-777-5513
FAX 203-777-0644
Peter Salerno, Executive Director
Ivan Tate, Program Director

A psychological treatment facility for emotionally disturbed children. Clinical Services are provided by a full and part time theraputic staff. Each child receives weekly individual, small and large group therapy as well as weekly family therapy. Children attend St. Francis School, staffed by professional special ed teachers.

6262 Saint Francis Home for Children: Highland
651 Prospect Street
New Haven, CT 06511
203-777-5513
Peter Salerno, Executive Director

6263 St. Vincent's Special Needs Center
St. Vincent's Medical Center
95 Merritt Boulevard
Trumbull, CT 06611
203-386-2728
FAX 203-380-1190
http://www.stvincentsspecialneeds.org
e-mail: feroleto.child.dev@snet.net
Virginia Smith, Marketing Director
David Goldstein, Human Resources Director

Began as therapy treatment program for children with cerebral palsy, and have evolved into a provider of specialized lifelong education and therapeutic programs for children and adults with multiple developmental disabilities and special health care needs.

6264 University School
160 Iranistan Avenue
Bridgeport, CT 06604
203-579-0434
FAX 203-330-9075
Nicholas Macol, Director
Lynn Ford, Principal

Located at the University of Bridgeport campus at Seaside Park, the center has access to U.B. facilities as part of its program to serve the socially/emotionally maladjusted and the learning disabled students.

6265 VISTA Vocational & Life Skills Center
1356 Old Clinton Road
Westbrook, CT 06498
860-399-8080
FAX 860-399-3103
http://www.vistavocational.org
e-mail: info@vistavocational.org
Jacques Brunswick, President
Helen Bosch, Administrator

VISTA opened its doors in 1989 to young adults with neurological disabilities who completed their secondary academic education yet require additional residential training to transition to adulthood. VISTA's central mission is to provide experiential, hands-on training in vocational and life skills.

6266 Villa Maria Education Center
161 Skymeadow Drive
Stamford, CT 06903
203-322-5886
FAX 203-322-0228
http://www.villamariaedu.org
e-mail: ecassidy@villamariaedu.org
Eileen Cassidy, Admissions Director
Carol Nawracay, Principal

Villa Maria Education Center affirms the dignity and giftedness of each person. We reach out to embrace children whose learning styles are different because they are learning disabled. We offer personalized and specialized instruction in an environment sufficiently varied for students of widely different personalities, interests and levels of learning in grades K-9th.

6267 Vocational Center for People who are Blind or Visually Impaired
Oak Hill Center
120 Holcomb Street
Hartford, CT 06112
860-242-2274
FAX 860-242-3103
http://www.ciboakhill.org
e-mail: famigliettis@ciboakhill.org
Steve Famiglietti, Vocational Services Manager
Karin Agritelly, Information/Resource Coordinator

Providing children and adults with disabilities the opportunity to live, learn and work in the community.

6268 Waterford Country Schools
PO Box 408
Quaker Hill, CT 06375
860-442-9454
FAX 860-442-2228
http://www.waterfordcountryschool.org
e-mail: DMoorehead@waterfordcs.org
David Moorehead, Executive Director
Sharon Butcher, President

A non-profit, human services agency located on a beautiful 350 acre campus in rural Southeastern Connecticut. Dedicated to do whatever it takes to enrich the lives of children and strengthen families through specialized programs, resources, and community services.

6269 Wheeler Clinic
91 Northwest Drive
Plainville, CT 06062
860-793-3717
888-793-3588
FAX 860-793-3520
http://www.wheelerclinic.org
e-mail: dberkowitz@wheelerclinic.org
David Berkowitz, Ph.D, Executive Director
John Mattas, M.Ed, Education Services Director
Couture Human Resources Direct, Human Resources Director
A provider of behavioral health services for children, adolescents, adults and families that include mental health, substance abuse, special education, early childhood development, prevention, an employee assistance program and community education.

6270 Wilderness School
State of Connecticut Dept. of Children & Families
240 N Hollow Road
East Hartland, CT 06027
860-653-8059
800-273-2293
FAX 860-653-8120
http://www.state.ct.us/dcf/Wilderness_School
e-mail: Tom.Dyer@po.state.ct.us
Thomas Dyer, Principal
David Czaja, Assistant Director

A prevention, intervention, and transition program for troubled youth from Connecticut. The school offers high impact wilderness programs intended to foster positive youth development.

6271 Yale Child Study Center
Yale University
PO Box 207900
New Haven, CT 06520
203-785-2513
FAX 203-737-4197
http://www.info.med.yale.edu/chldstdy/
e-mail: alan.kazdin@yale.edu
Allan Kazdin Ph.D, Executive Director

The study center is a department at Yale University School of Medicine that brings together multiple disciplines to further the understanding of the problems of children and families. The mission of the Center is to understand child development, social, behavioral, and emotional adjustment, and psychiatric disorders and to help children and families in need of care.

Delaware

6272 AdvoServ
4185 Kirkwood Street Georges Road
Bear, DE 19701
302-834-7018
800-593-4959
FAX 302-836-2516
http://www.advoserv.com
e-mail: dreardon@advoserv.com
R. Katz, Education Director
Michele Yamashita, Admissions
Tom Deemedio, Manager
Provides services to individuals whose challenges have defied all previous attempts at treatment. Through proven, positive and comprehensive strategies that teach individuals how to live problem-free, AdvoSer can help overcome the burdens and barriers associated with severe and intractable problems.

6273 Centreville School
6201 Kennett Pike
Wilmington, DE 19807
302-571-0230
FAX 302-571-0270
http://www.centrevilleschool.org
e-mail: information@centrevilleschool.org
Vicky Yatzus, Administrator
Ida Donegan, School Secretary

Motivated by two fundamental goals; to provide learning disabled children a vibrant and challenging curriculum comparable to those found at any primary or intermediate level school, and to offer each student the specialized and focused support he or she needs.

6274 Meadows Consulting
506 New Castle Street Extended
Rehoboth Beach, DE 19971
302-227-9327
FAX 302-227-9327
Nancy Meadows, President

Comprehensive educational services include testing, consultations and remedial, supportive, enrichment, and instructional suggestions. Pre-school through adults.

6275 Parent Information Center of Delaware
5570 Kirkwood Highway
Wilmington, DE 19808
302-366-0152
888-547-4412
FAX 302-999-7637
http://www.picofdel.org
e-mail: picofdel@picofdel.org
Marie-Anne Aghazadian, Executive Director
Kathie Herel, Manager

Assists individuals with disabilities and special needs and those who serve them; also provides information and referral to other agencies.

6276 Pilot School
100 Garden of Eden Road
Wilmington, DE 19803
302-478-1740
FAX 302-478-1746
http://www.pilotschool.com
e-mail: kcraven@pilotschool.com
Kathleen Craven, Executive Director

Pilot School provides a creative, nurturing environment for children with special learning needs. We work with each child to discover his or her unique learning strengths.

District of Columbia

6277 Kingsbury Center
5000 14th Street NW
Washington, DC 20011
202-722-5555
FAX 202-722-5533
http://www.kingsbury.org
e-mail: center@kingsbury.org
Peter Engebretson, COO
Cherryl Smith, Ph.D, Diagnostic/Psychological Dir.
Carolyn Thornell, Executive Director
Each year, Kingsbury serves nearly 1,000 children, adults and families with educational, diagnostic, psychological, and tutoring services. The teachers, psychologists, diagnosticians, and tutors bring a wealth of training, experience, and expertise, along with a genuine love for helping children and adults with learning difficulties.

6278 Lab School of Washington
4759 Reservoir Road NW
Washington, DC 20007
202-965-6601
FAX 202-965-5105
http://www.labschool.org
e-mail: dpotts@labschool.org
Sally Smith, Manager
D. Potts, Admissions

A internationally recognized for its innovative programs for children and adults with learning disabilities. The Lab School offers individualized instruction to students in kindergarten through 12 grade.

6279 Paul Robeson School
Washington District of Columbia Dept Mental Health
3700 10th Street NW
Washington, DC 20010
202-576-5151
FAX 202-576-8804
http://www.dmh.dc.gov/dmh/cwp
Harriet Crawley, Principal/Acting Program Mgr.

The Department of Mental Health offers therapy and treatment at special education centers, such as The Paul Robeson School. The school offers individual, group and/or family psychotherapy or art therapy, play therapy, speech therapy, and recreational principles. They also provide physical education, adaptive physical education, and occupational therapy, if needed.

6280 Paul Robeson School for Growth and
3700 10th Street NW
Washington, DC 20010
202-576-5151

6281 Scottish Rite Center for Childhood
1630 Columbia Road NW
Washington, DC 20009
202-939-4703
T. Robinson, Executive Director

Florida

6282 Academic Achievement Center
313 Pruett Road
Seffner, FL 33584
813-654-4198
FAX 813-871-7468
http://www.iser.com/AAC-FL.html
e-mail: ALSofAAC@aol.com
Lillian Stark PhD, Manager
Arnold Stark PhD, Educational Director

A private program for bright and gifted children with LD and/or ADD, offering multisensory-based instruction, remediation of basic skills, academic challenge in science, social science, and literature, plus award-winning art and drama, and curriculum-enhancing field trips and travel. Maximum student body is 22 and it is coeducational. After school tutoring and phonelogical awareness training are also available.

6283 Achievement Academy
716 E Bella Vista Street
Lakeland, FL 33805
863-683-6504
FAX 863-688-9292
http://www.achievementacademy.com
e-mail: paula@achievementacademy.com
Paula Sullivan, Executive Director
Debra Stephens, Birth to Three Coordinator
Parker-Pears Program Director, Program Director
The Birth to Three program currently serves children from birth through developmental kindergarten with a comprehensive early intervention program. The program offers services to children who may be at-risk for developmental delays due to; prematurity, substance abuse, social/emotional issues, and environmental issues. Services are also provided to children who have already been identified with a developmental delay or a diagnosis.

6284 Assistive Technology Network
434 N Tampa Avenue
Orlando, FL 32805
407-254-9900
Michael Chandler, Manager

6285 Atlantis Academy
Educational Services of America
1950 Prairie Road
West Palm Beach, FL 33406
561-642-3100
FAX 561-969-1950
http://www.atlantisacademypb.com
e-mail: progressschool@adelphia.net
Kim Lichtenberger, Admissions Director
Dennis Kelley, Administrator

A small, private, highly individualized program, Pre K-12, for children with attention disorders, dyslexia and other academic learning problems. Day students only.

6286 Barbara King's Center for Educational Services
5005 W Laurel Street
Tampa, FL 33607
813-874-3918
FAX 813-874-3575
Barbara King, Owner

Educational therapy services offered.

6287 Baudhin Pre-School
Nova SE University's Mailman Segal Institute
3301 College Avenue
Ft. Lauderdale, FL 33314
954-262-7100
800-336-8326
FAX 954-262-3936
http://www.nova.edu/msi
e-mail: baudhuin@nova.edu
Wendy Masi, Ph.D, School Dean
George Hanbury II, Ph.D, Executive VP/COO
Rachel Docekal, Mktg/Development Exec. Director
For autistic children, the program supports the qualities and capabilities of each child. This therapeutic program focuses on cognitive, social-emotional, adaptive, behavioral, motor, and communication skill development within a relationship-based environment. Providing each child with choices, challenges, and opportunities that nurture feelings of competence, promote intellectual growth, and enable each child to achieve his or her potential.

6288 Baudhuin Preschool of Nova Southeastern University
3301 College Avenue
Ft. Lauderdale, FL 33314
954-262-7100
800-336-8326
FAX 954-262-3936
http://www.nova.edu/msi
e-mail: baudhuin@nova.edu
Roni Leiderman, Executive Director
Michele Kaplan, Director

For autistic children, the program supports the qualities and capabilities of each child. This therapeutic program focuses on cognitive, social-emotional, adaptive, behavioral, motor, and communication skill development within a relationship-based environment. Providing each child with choices, challenges, and opportunities that nurture feelings of competence, promote intellectual growth, and enable each child to achieve his or her potential.

6289 Beach Learning Center
105 S Riverside Drive
Indialantic, FL 32903
321-725-7437
Zoe Toler, Owner

Diagnostic and therapy services for the learning disabled.

6290 Brevard Learning Clinic
1900 S Harbor City Boulevard
Melbourne, FL 32901
321-676-3024
FAX 321-676-3064
http://www.brevardlearningclinic.com
e-mail: brevardlearningclinic@the1900buildingllc.com
Mary Kellogg, Executive Director

Serving the special learning needs of children and adults of Brevard County for over twenty years. Provides one-to-one academic intervention based on diagnostic testing. The primary problem with the students is a learning difference that stems from neither mental retardation nor emotional disturbance.

6291 Exceptional Student Education: Assistive Technology
Orange County Public School
434 N Tampa Avenue
Orlando, FL 32805
407-317-3504
FAX 407-317-3526
http://www.ese.ocps.net/Assistive_Technology
e-mail: folkst@ocps.net
Daniel Dardiz, Speech Pathologist/Specialist
Tami Folks, Therapist/Specialist
Mathews Educator/Specialist, Educator/Specialist
Services are provided for students who are mentally handicapped, emotionally handicapped, specific learning disabled, sensory impaired, speech and language impaired, physically impaired, hospital/homebound, autistic, gifted, and developmentally delayed. Services such as occupational/ physical therapy, assistive technology, and assistance for ESE bilingual students are also available.

6292 Kurtz Center
Complete Learning Center
1201 Louisiana Avenue
Winter Park, FL 32789
407-740-5678
FAX 407-629-6886
http://www.completelearningcenter.com
e-mail: ld-request@learningdisabilities.com
Denton Kurtz, Co-Founder
Gail Kurtz, Co-Founder/Director

A treatment facility and professional development provider, using scientifically based researched approaches in the treatment of those in need and in training other professionals, paraprofessionals and parents to use these approaches. Developed individualized programs for all ages that conquer all forms of learning disabilities/difficulties, including the various dyslexias and attention focus problems.

6293 Kurtz Center for Cognitive Development
1201 Louisiana Avenue
Winter Park, FL 32789
407-740-5678
Gail Kurtz, Owner

6294 Learning Solutions: Reading Clinic
Tampa Day School
12606 Henderson Road
Tampa, FL 33625
813-269-2100
FAX 813-963-7843
http://www.tampadayschool.com
e-mail: tds@tampadayschool.com
Lois Delaney, School Head/Director
Walt Karniski, MD, Executive Director
Guffey Learning Solutions Dir, Learning Solutions Director
Provides a learning environment that promotes that individual feeling of success for each child and to meet each child's needs. The Reading Clinic has been helping children become better readers for over 30 years. Once the problem is targeted, and provide the kind of help a child needs, the gains are immediate and long lasting.

6295 Matlock Precollegiate
2491 Homewood Road
West Palm Beach, FL 33416
561-687-0327
FAX 561-684-3935
http://www.matlockacademy.com
e-mail: info@matlockacademy.com
Daphne Grad, Principal/Instructor

The program is designed to meet the specific needs of the students who are underachievers, seeking to fulfill their needs through a comprehensive student centered philosophy and offering a very successful educational program.

6296 Matlock Precollegiate Academy
2491 Homewood Road
West Palm Beach, FL 33406
561-687-0327

6297 McGlannan School
10770 SW 84th Street
Miami, FL 33173
305-274-2208
FAX 305-274-0337
TDY:305-274-2208
e-mail: jfmcglannan@att.net
Frances Glannan, Manager
Dr. Carol Repensek, Assistant Director

A school that provides one-to-one learning for children with dyslexia and other learning problems. Diagnostic, multidisciplinary, prescriptive, research-based and individualized to reach the whole child.

6298 Mental Health and Educational Services
Mental Health and Educational Services
5251 Emerson Street
Jacksonville, FL 32207
904-399-0324
http://www.psydoc.com
Ruth Klein PhD, Director

Diagnostic and therapy services for a wide range of emotional and behavioral disabilities.

6299 Morning Star School

Morning Star School
210 E Linebaugh Avenue
Tampa, FL 33612 813-935-0232
FAX 813-932-2321
http://www.tampa-morningstar.org
e-mail: edaly@tampa-morningstar.org
Jeanette Friedheim, Principal

Morning Star School is a Catholic Diocesan school dedicated to meeting the needs of students with learning disabilities and related difficulties. It is a non-graded school for children from the ages of 6 to 16. The individualized curriculum strives to enhance student's self-esteem in an atmosphere that is both challenging and nurturing.

6300 New Lifestyles

1210 Gateway Road
Lake Park, FL 33403 561-848-5537
FAX 954-797-2813
e-mail: theoptions@aol.com
New Lifestyles provides comprehensive life management services including assessment, programming, residential placement at various locations in Palm Beach County, Florida and Winchester, Virginia. Programs focus on issues such as self-esteem, interpersonal skills and adjustments, vocational placement, independent living, time management, organizational skills, and decision-making skills.

6301 PACE-Brantley Hall School

3221 Sand Lake Road
Longwood, FL 32779 407-869-8882
FAX 407-869-8717
http://www.mypbhs.org
e-mail: bw@mypbhs.org
Barbara Winter, Assistant Director
Kathleen Shatlock, Principal

An independent, nonprofit school for children with learning differences. The PACE program has been specifically designed for students who have been diagnosed with learning disabilities, attention deficit disorder, dyslexia and similar challenges.

6302 PACE: Brantley Hall School

3221 Sand Lake Road
Longwood, FL 32779 407-869-8882
Kathleen Shatlock, Principal

6303 PEAC: South

1501 Venera Avenue
Coral Gables, FL 33146 305-667-5011

6304 Palm Beach Gardens Prep School

149 Wentworth Court
Jupiter, FL 33458 561-622-0401
FAX 561-622-0402
Philip T Rosen MD, Director

A coed, college preparatory curriculum, including art, physical education etc., diagnostic prescriptive methodologies, SLD mainstreamed, small classes (6-10), non-residential, founded in 1977.

6305 Ralph J Baudhuin Oral School of Nova

3375 SW 75th Avenue
Davie, FL 33314 954-262-7100
Roni Leaderman, Manager

6306 Renaissance Learning Center

5800 Corporate Way
West Palm Beach, FL 33407 561-640-0270
FAX 561-640-0272
http://www.rlc2000.com
e-mail: renaissance@rlc2000.com
Debi Johnson, Principal
Sonia Kay, Education Director

Develops and provides effective education and treatment programs for children ages 3-14 with autism.

6307 Susan Maynard Counseling

1501 Venera Avenue
Coral Gables, FL 33146 305-667-5011
http://www.susanmaynardphd.com
Susan Maynard, Ph.D, School Psychologist/Therapist

Administers a complete Psycho-Educational Test battery to determine if clients have learning disabilities. Marriage and family therapy and therapy for individuals available.

6308 Tampa Day School and Reading Clinic

12606 Henderson Road
Tampa, FL 33625 813-269-2100
Lois Delaney, Executive Director

6309 Vanguard School

Vanguard School
22000 Highway 27
Lake Wales, FL 33859 863-676-7083
FAX 863-676-8297
http://www.vanguardschool.org
e-mail: vanadmin@vanguardschool.org
James Moon PhD, President
Robert Spellman, Principal
Melanie Anderson, Admissions Director
The Vanguard School program is designed for students age 10 through high school who are experiencing academic difficulties due to learning disability such as dyslexia or dyscalculia or an attention deficit.
11-20 years old

Georgia

6310 Achievement Academy

318 11th Street
Columbus, GA 31901 706-660-0050

6311 Atlanta Speech School

3160 Northside Parkway NW
Atlanta, GA 30327 404-233-5332
FAX 404-266-2175
http://www.atlantaspeechschool.org
e-mail: cyates@atlspsch.org
Comer Yates, Executive Director
Paula Ford, Communications Director

The Atlanta Speech School is one of the Southeast's oldest therapeutic educational centers for children and adults with hearing, speech, language, or learning disabilities. We help children and adults with communication disorders realize their full potential.

6312 Bedford School

5665 Milam Road
Fairburn, GA 30213 770-774-8001
FAX 770-774-8005
http://www.thebedfordschool.org
e-mail: bbox@thebedfordschool.org
Betsy Box, Executive Director
Jeff James, Assistant Director

The Bedford School is a nine-month day program specifically designed to meet the needs of children with learning disabilities. We are certified through the Georgia Accrediting Commission.

6313 Brandon Hall School

1701 Brandon Hall Drive
Atlanta, GA 30350
770-394-8176
FAX 770-804-8821
http://www.brandonhall.org
e-mail: pstockhammer@brandonhall.org

Paul Stockhammer, President
Marcia Shearer, Admissions Director

Provides both one-on-one and small group college preparatory classes for students who, for a variety of reasons, have not been achieving their potential or who otherwise need a more intensive educational setting.

6314 Chatham Academy

Royce Learning Center
4 Oglethorpe Professional Boulevard
Savannah, GA 31406
912-354-4047
FAX 912-354-4633
http://www.roycelearningcenter.com
e-mail: info@roycelearningcenter.com

Dr. Kathleen Burke, Executive Director
Carolyn Hannaford, Principal

Providing a specialized curriculum and individualized instruction for students with diagnosed learning disabilities and/or attention deficit disorder. Chatham's goal is to improve students' functioning to levels commensurate with their potential in all areas so that they may return to and succeed in regular educational programs.

6315 Creative Community Services

1543 Lilburn Stone Mountain Road
Stone Mountain, GA 30087
770-469-6226
866-618-2823
FAX 770-469-6210
http://www.ccsgeorgia.org
e-mail: info@ccsgeorgia.org

Sally Buchanan, Executive Director
Dana Rochon, Clinical Supervisor

Therapeutic foster care services for children and home-based support for developmental disabled adults. CCS gives both kids and adults hope by encouraging independent living resulting in involved, engaged citizens and community members.

6316 Horizons School

1900 Dekalb Avenue NE
Atlanta, GA 30307
404-378-2219
800-822-6242
FAX 404-378-8946
http://www.horizonsschool.com
e-mail: HorizonsSchool@horizonschsool.com

Les Garber, Manager
Martha Rummel, Administrative Assistant

The intent is to develop in students those values and skills which assure maximum opportunities. Students learn real-life skills through active participation in the classroom, as well as in other aspects of the school. They learn responsibility, decision-making, and problem-solving skills through active involvement in the management of the community. Such a leadership role empowers students, giving them the knowledge that they have control of personal decisions and interpersonal interactions.

6317 Howard School

1246 Ponce de Leon Avenue NE
Atlanta, GA 30306
404-377-7436
http://www.howardschool.org
e-mail: vsullivan@howardschool.org

Marifred Cilella, Head of School
Keren Schuller, Admissions Director
Sandra Kleinman, Executive Director

The Howard School eduates students with learning differences and language disabilities. Instruction is personalized to complement individual learning styles, to address student needs and to help each student understand his or her learning process. The curriculum focuses on depth of understanding in order to make learning meaningful and therefore, maximize educational success.

6318 Howard School Central Campus

1246 Ponce De Leon Avenue NE
Atlanta, GA 30306
404-377-7436

Sandra Kleinman, Executive Director
Karen Schuller, Admissions Director

6319 Howard School North Campus

Disability Support Department
9415 Willeo Road
Roswell, GA 30075
707-642-9644
FAX 707-998-1398
http://www.howardschool.org
e-mail: KerenS@howardschool.org

Sandra Kleinman MD, Executive Director
Keren Schuller, Admissions Director

At the Howard School we understand that every child can learn. We believe that every child should have the opportunity to succeed. Our mission is to successfully teach each student in the unique way that student learns.

6320 Jacob's LadderHelping Children Succeed One Step at a Time

11705 Mountain Park Road
Roswell, GA 30075
770-998-1017
FAX 770-998-3258
http://www.jacobsladdercenter.com
e-mail: info@jacobsladdercenter.com

Amy O'Dell Wuttke, Director

A neurodevelopmental learning center established to provide the child Autism, PDD, ADD/ADHD, Asperger's learning differences, Down or any developmental syndrome, the services they need in order to realize their full potential.

6321 Mill Springs Academy

13660 New Providence Road
Alpharetta, GA 30004
770-360-1336
FAX 770-360-1341
http://www.millsprings.org
e-mail: rmoore@millsprings.org

Tweetie Moore, Founder/Director
Robert Moore, President

A value-based educational community dedicated to the academic, physical and social growth of those students who have not realized their full potential in traditional classroom settings. Learning strategies are generated from psycho-educational evaluations, previous school records, diagnostic skills assessment, observations and communication with other professionals involved with the student.

6322 New School

13660 New Providence Road
Alpharetta, GA 30004
770-360-1336
FAX 770-360-1341

Tweetie Moore, Founder/Director
Robert Moore, President

6323 Reading Success

Reading Success
4434 Columbia Road
Martinez, GA 30907
706-863-8173
8009973237
FAX 706-863-4523
http://www.readingsuccess.com
e-mail: readingsuccess@bellsouth.net

Sandra Mashburn, Owner
Roberta Hoehle, NCLB Coordinator
Joan Beckner, Office Manager

Reading Success, Inc. is a locally owned and operated program, serving the CSRA for over 30 years and providing professional help to students with all kinds of learning problems. Our guarantee is; if one year of improvement has not been made in the 48 lessons, the student receives instruction free of charge for 18 lessons.

6324 Wardlaw School
Atlanta Speech School
3160 Northside Parkway NW
Atlanta, GA 30327 404-233-5332
FAX 404-266-2175
http://www.atlantaspeechschool.org/wardlaw
e-mail: cyates@atlspsch.org
Comer Yates, Executive Director
Paula Ford, Communications Director

Dedicated to serving children with average to very superior intelligence and mild to moderate learning disabilities. Children served in the Wardlaw School typically exhibit underlying auditory and/or visual processing problems that make it difficult for them to learn in their present educational setting.

6325 Wardlaw School: A Division of the Atlanta
3160 Northside Parkway NW
Atlanta, GA 30327 404-233-5332
Comer Yates, Executive Director

Hawaii

6326 Center on Disability Studies
University of Hawaii Manoa
1776 University Avenue
Honolulu, HI 96822 808-956-9142
FAX 808-956-5713
http://www.cds.hawaii.edu
e-mail: Robert.Stodden@cds.hawaii.edu
Robert Stodden PhD, Executive Director
Tom Conway, Media Coordinator

The Center for Disability Studies is a Hawaii Unviersity Affiliated Program at the University of Hawaii at Manoa. The mission of the CDS is to support the quality of life, community inclusion, and self-determination of all persons with disabilities and their families.

6327 Hawaii Parents Unlimited
200 N Vineyard Boulevard
Honolulu, HI 96817 808-536-2280

6328 Learning Disabilities Association of Hawaii
200 N Vineyard Boulevard
Honolulu, HI 96817 808-536-9684
800-533-9684
FAX 808-537-6780
http://www.ldahawaii.org
e-mail: ldah@ldahawaiii.org
Jennifer Schember-Lang, Executive Director

Serving families with children with learning disabilities and other special needs that interfere with learning by providing education advocacy, training and support in order to remove barriers and promote awareness and full educational opportunity. LDAH has several special projects that helps fulfill the mission of removing barriers and promoting awareness and full educational opportunity. The Parent Training and Information Center is one of these special projects that is offered.

6329 Variety School of Hawaii
710 Palekaua Street
Honolulu, HI 96816 808-732-2835
FAX 808-732-4334
e-mail: denneyvariety@inets.com
Duane Yee, Executive Director
Colin Denney, Administrator

Educate children with learning disabilities, attention deficit disorder, and/or autism. Provides specialized learning programs tailored to the needs of the individual child. One intervention program, the Slingerland program, has been developed specifically to increase the success of students in language arts. This language-based program is offered in conjunction with a behavioral program to help children gain the most from their school experience.

Idaho

6330 Idaho Parents Unlimited
600 N Curtis Road
Boise, ID 83706 208-342-5884
800-242-4785
FAX 208-342-1408
http://www.ipulidaho.org
e-mail: parents@ipulidaho.org
Evelyn Mason, Executive Director
Susan Valiquette, PTI Program Director
Hall
A statewide organization founded to provide support, information and technical assistance to parents of children and youth with disabilities.

Illinois

6331 Achievement Centers
6425 Willow Springs Road
La Grange Highlands, IL 60525 708-579-9040
FAX 708-579-5872
http://www.acaciaacademy.com
e-mail: info@acaciaacademy.com
Kathryn Foukes, Principal
Eileen Petzold, Assistant Principal

Offering personalized and exceptional educational instruction to each individual student in the development of his/her intellectual and academic potential.
Ages 5-Adult

6332 Allendale Association
PO Box 1088
Lake Villa, IL 60046 847-356-2351
888-255-3631
FAX 847-356-0289
http://www.allendale4kids.org
e-mail: development@allendale4kids.org
Connie Borucki, Human Resources VP
Judy Griffeth, Placement Director
Mary Shahbazian, President
A private, not-for-profit organization dedicated to excellence and innovation in the care, education, treatment and advocacy for troubled children, youth and their families.

6333 Associated Talmud Torahs of Chicago
2828 W Pratt Avenue
Chicago, IL 60645 773-973-2828
FAX 773-973-6666
http://www.att.org
Rabbi Harvey Well, Superintendent
Rabbi R. Schwartzman, Executive Director
Cardash Student Services Direc, Student Services Director
Offers mainstreaming, independent skills, therapeutic swim classes and psychological services.

6334 Att-P'tach Special Education Program
2828 W Pratt Boulevard
Chicago, IL 60645 773-973-2828
Harvey Well, Administrator

6335 Baby Fold
Hammit School
108 E Willow Street
Normal, IL 61761 309-452-1170
FAX 309-452-0115
http://www.thebabyfold.org
e-mail: info@thebabyfold.org
Dale Strssheim, Executive Director

A multi-service agency that provides Residential, Special Education, Child Welfare, and Family Support Services to children and families in central Illinois.

6336 Brehm Preparatory School

1245 E Grand Avenue
Carbondale, IL 62901
618-457-0371
FAX 618-529-1248
http://www.brehm.org
e-mail: richc@brehm.orgg

Richard Collins PhD, Administrator
Brian Brown Ph.D, Associate Executive Director

A boarding school specifically designed to meet the needs of students with complex learning disabilities and attention deficit disorder issues.

6337 Camelot Care Center: Illinois

1502 W NW Highway
Palatine, IL 60067
847-359-5600

Craig Bogacki, Executive Director

6338 Camelot School: Palatine Campus

1502 N NW Highway
Palatine, IL 60067
847-359-5600
FAX 847-359-2759
http://www.thecamelotschools.com/palatine.htm

Craig Bogacki, Executive Director
Roula Manis, Admissions Director
Hammond Clinical Director, Clinical Director

Programs offered by the center are the Residential Treatment Center and the Therapeutic Day School. These programs provide effective clinical treatment, and are highly successful in transitioning children back home to their families, or home school environment.

6339 Catholic Children's Home

1400 State Street
Alton, IL 62002
618-465-3594

Candy Hovey, Administrator

6340 Center for Learning

National Louis University
2840 Sheridan Road
Evanston, IL 60201
847-475-1100
FAX 847-256-6542
http://www.nl.edu
e-mail: kadamle@nc.edu

Kim Adamle, Director
Jerry Dachs, Manager

Offers psychological, educational and neuro psychological evaluations, testing of gifted children and remedial tutoring for children with learning disabilities.

6341 Center for Speech and Language Disorders

195 Spangler Avenue
Elmhurst, IL 60126
630-530-8551
FAX 630-530-5909
http://www.csld.org
e-mail: info@csld.org

Phyllis Kupperman, Executive Director

The mission is to help children with speech and language disorders reach their full potential. CSLD is an internationally recognized leader in the diagnosis and treatment of hyperlexia and other language disorders.

6342 Chicago Urban Day School

1248 W 69th Street
Chicago, IL 60636
773-483-3555
FAX 773-483-9758

Georgia Jordan, Executive Director

6343 Children's Center for Behavioral Development

353 N 88th Street
East Saint Louis, IL 62203
618-398-1152
FAX 954-745-1120
http://www.childpsych.org

Dr. David Lubin Ph.D, Co-Founder/Clinical Services VP
Richard Robinson, Executive Director

Children's Center for Behavioral Development is dedicated to supporting the social, physical, intellectual, creative, emotional and developmental growth of children from birth to adulthood.

6344 Cove School

350 Lee Road
Northbrook, IL 60062
847-562-2100
FAX 847-562-2112
http://www.coveschool.org
e-mail: ssover@coveschool.org

Dr. Sally Sover, Principal
Carol Sward, Principal

The Cove School was established in 1947, to educate students with learning disabilities and to facilitate their return to their neighborhood schools in the shortest possible time. The heart of Cove's educational philosophy is to design a program that pulls out the child's skills.

6345 Early Achievement Center Preschool & Kindergarten

Achievement Centers
6425 Willow Springs Road
La Grange Highlands, IL 60525
708-579-9040
FAX 708-579-5872
http://www.acaciaacademy.com
e-mail: info@acaciaacademy.com

Kathryn Fouks, Administrator
Eileen Bybee, Dean of Students

The Early Achievement Center Program encourages growth of the total child in social, intellectual, physical, and emotional abilities.

6346 Educational Services of Glen Ellyn

364 Pennsylvania Avenue
Glen Ellyn, IL 60137
630-469-1479
FAX 630-469-1265
e-mail: educationalservices@juno.com

Elizabeth Siebens, Owner

Tutoring for all ages in all subject areas. Diagnostic testing, specializing in learning disabilities and career counseling for learning disabled adults.

6347 Elim Christian Services

13020 S Central Avenue
Palos Heights, IL 60463
708-430-7532
FAX 708-389-0671
http://www.elimcs.org
e-mail: info@elimcs.org

Bill Lodewyk, President
Pam Connolly, Programs Supervisor
Sharon Schussler, Manager

Elim Christian Services is a non-profit corporation that seeks to equip persons with special needs to achieve to their highest God-given potential.

6348 Esperanza School

520 N Marshfield Avenue
Chicago, IL 60622
312-243-6097
FAX 312-243-2076
TDY:800-526-0844
http://www.esperanzaservices.org
e-mail: jgorgol@esperanzacommunity.org

Joe Gorgol, Principal
Myra Rodas, Secretary
Barbara Fields, Executive Director

Accredited by the Rehabilitation Accreditation Commission; Esperanza School is a self-help educational services offered to children who are autistic or mentally disabled.

Bethany Graham

6349 **Family Resource Center on Disabilities**
20 E Jackson Boulevard
Chicago, IL 60604
312-939-3513
800-952-4199
FAX 312-939-7297
TDY:312-939-3519
http://www.frcd.org
e-mail: info@frcd.ptiil.americom.net
Charlotte Jardins, Executive Director

Formerly known as the Coordinating Council for Handicapped Children, the FRCD was organized in 1969 by parents, professionals, and volunteers who sought to improve services for all children with disabilities.

6350 **Hammit School: The Baby Fold**
108 E Willow Street
Normal, IL 61761
309-452-1170
FAX 309-452-0115
http://www.thebabyfold.org
e-mail: info@thebabyfold.org
Dale Strssheim, Executive Director
Rebeca Haremaker, Office Assistant
Dianne Schultz, Principal
The Baby Fold is a multi-service agency that provides Residential, Special Education, Child Welfare, and Family Support Services to children and families in central Illinois.

6351 **Hope School**
50 Hazel Lane
Springfield, IL 62716
217-585-5437
FAX 217-786-3356
TDY:217-585-5105
http://www.thehopeschool.org
e-mail: info@thehopeschool.org
Joseph Nyre, President
Judy Bukowski, Administrator

The Hope School is a private, not-for-profit eduational and residential center, that has been serving children with multiple disabilities and their families since 1957.

6352 **Illinois Center for Autism**
548 S Ruby Lane
Fairview Heights, IL 62208
618-398-7500
FAX 618-394-9869
http://www.illinoiscenterforautism.org
e-mail: info@illinoiscenterforautism.org
Susan Szekeoy, Executive Director
Sandra Rodenberg, Principal

A not-for-profit, community based, mental health treatment, and educational agency dedicated to serving people with autism. Referrals for possible student placement are made through local school districts, hospitals, regional special education centers, and doctors.

6353 **Joseph Academy**
7530 N Natchez Avenue
Niles, IL 60714
847-588-2990
FAX 847-588-2950
http://www.josephacademy.org
e-mail: information@josephacademy.org
Michael Schack, Executive Director
Heather Elliott, Principal

Founded in 1983, Joseph Academy provides a nurturing and challenging environment for young people. Our mission is to serve children and adolescents with behavioral, emotional and learning disorders by helping them develop the social, academic and vocational skills they need to function in society.

6354 **LEARN Center**
Illinois Masonic Medical Center
836 W Nelson Street
Chicago, IL 60657
773-296-7900
FAX 773-296-5885
http://www.iser.com/LEARN.html

6355 **La Grange Area Department of Special Education**
La Grange Area Department of Special Education
1301 W Cossitt Avenue
La Grange, IL 60525
708-354-5730
FAX 708-354-0733
TDY:708-352-5994
http://www.ladse.org
e-mail: JimSurber@ladse.org
Jim Surver, Executive Director
Lois Miller, Executive Assistant Director

Offers programs for students with moderate to severe mental retardation, learning disabilities or behavior disorders.

6356 **LaGrange Area Department of Special Education**
1301 W Cossitt Avenue
LaGrange, IL 60525
708-354-5730
FAX 708-354-0733
TDY:708-352-5994
http://www.ladse.org
e-mail: JSurber@ladse.org
Jim Surver, Executive Director
Lois Miller, Executive Assistant Director

Offers programs for students with moderate to severe mental retardation, learning disabilities or behavior disorders.

6357 **Professional Assistance Center for Education (PACE)**
National-Louis University
2840 Sheridan Road
Evanston, IL 60201
847-475-1100
800-443-5522
FAX 847-256-5190
http://www2.nl.edu/pace/
e-mail: cburns@nl.edu
Carol Burns, Director
Jerry Dachs, Manager

Founded in 1986, PACE is a two-year, noncredit postsecondary certificate program located on the campus of National-Louis University. The PACE program is designed especially to meet the transitional needs of students with multiple learning disabilities in a university setting.

6358 **South Central Community Services**
8316 S Ellis Avenue
Chicago, IL 60619
773-483-0900
FAX 773-483-5701
http://www.sccsinc.org
Felicia Blasingame, CEO

A grassroots, not-for-profit organization established in 1970 by a group of community residents concerned about the absence of human service facilities and programs in the community.

6359 **Special Education Day School**
Catholic Children's Home
1400 State Street
Alton, IL 62002
618-465-3594
FAX 618-465-1083
http://www.catholicchildrenshome.com
e-mail: cch1400@ezl.com
Patti Morrissey, President
Steven Roach, Executive Director
Hovey Administrator, Administrator
For children with learning disabilities, developmental and behavioral disorders and through its comprehensive residential services for children in crisis. Providing year-round educational and therapeutic services to students who, due to a variety of social, emotional and/or educational difficulties, have been unsuccessful in public school programs.

6360 **St. Joseph's Carondelet Child Center**
721 N La Salle Drive
Chicago, IL 60610
773-624-7443
FAX 773-624-7676
http://www.stjccc.org
e-mail: sreedy@stjccc.org

Saralynn Reedy, Program Services VP
James Laughlin, Executive Director

St. Joseph's is a treatment center for emotionally disturbed children and youth. Recognized for taking the most difficult cases and providing young people with the programs they need to enable them to re-enter society.

6361 Summit School
611 E Main Street
East Dundee, IL 60118
847-428-6451
FAX 847-428-6419
http://www.summitdundee.org
e-mail: jwhite@summitdundee.org
Sharon Carl, Principal
George Phelan, President

Summit School is a private, non-profit organization dedicated to fulfilling the needs of children with learning problems that prevent them from achieving in a standard classroom situation.

Indiana

6362 Clearinghouse on Reading, English andCommunications
Indiana University of Bloomington
107 S Indiana Avenue
Bloomington, IN 47405
812-855-4848
FAX 812-856-5512
http://www.reading.indiana.edu
e-mail: iuadmit@indiana.edu
Stephen Stroup, Associate Director
Adam Herbert, CEO

Offers information on reading, English and communication skills, preschool through college.

6363 Educational Enrichment Center
1450 Bellemeade Avenue
Evansville, IN 47714
812-473-0651
FAX 812-471-1145
Janet Dill, Coordinator
Jeff Gray, Owner

The center provides educational assessment; personal development; tutoring; psychological testing and therapy; neuropsychological evaluation; and cognitive therapy. The center offers tutors who are qualified teachers with a broad area of training including Orton-Gillingham multisensory techniques. Many services for head injured individuals with Halstead-Reitan Neuropsychological evaluation and comprehensive cognitive retraining are available.

6364 IN*SOURCE
1703 S Ironwood Drive
South Bend, IN 46613
574-234-7101
800-332-4433
FAX 574-234-7279
http://www.insource.org
e-mail: insource@insource.org
Richard Burden, Executive Director
Scott Carson, Assistant Director

The mission of IN*SOURCE is to provide parents, families and service providers in Indiana the information and training necessary to assure effective educational programs and appropriate services for children and young adults with disabilities.

Iowa

6365 Iowa Compass
Center for Disabilities and Development
100 Hawkins Drive
Iowa City, IA 52242
319-353-6900
800-779-2001
FAX 319-384-5139
TDY:319-353-8777
http://www.medicine.uiowa.edu/iowacompass/
e-mail: iowa-compass@uiowa.edu
Jane Gay, Director
Amy Mikelson, Outreach/Training Coordinator
Mark Moser, Administrator
A free information and referral service on assistive technology, product information, the used equipment referral service, funding options, and referral to free legal advocacy. Also publishes a newsletter.

Kansas

6366 Families Together
501 SW Jackson Street
Topeka, KS 66603
785-233-4777
888-815-6364
FAX 316-945-7795
http://www.familiestogetherinc.org
e-mail: wichita@familiestogetherinc.org
Boyd Koehn, President
Karen Snell, Regional Center Coordinator
Lesli Girard, Manager
Families Together is a statewide non-profit organization assisting Kansas families which include sons and/or daughters who have any form of disability.

6367 Heartspring School
8700 E 29th Street N
Wichita, KS 67226
316-634-8750
800-835-1043
FAX 316-634-0555
http://www.heartspring.org
e-mail: rappc@heartspring.org
Cara Rapp, Admissions Director
Kendra Conard, Accounting Assistant
Cindy Chapman, Executive Director
Heartspring School has earned an international reputation for improving the lives of children. Heartspring is a not-for-profit private residential school that serves children 5-21. We serve children with disabilities such as autism, asperger's, communication disorders, developmental disabilities, dual diagnosed, behavoir disorders, hearing or vision impaired.

6368 Menninger Center for Learning Disabilities
Menninger Clinic
2801 Gessner Drive
Houston, TX 77080
713-275-5000
800-351-9058
http://www.iser.com/menninger.html
Ian Aitken, CEO

The Center offers the following services for children and adults: 1) educational evaluations for learning disabilities, dyslexia, learning problems and other special needs 2) gifted evaluations 3) workshops for parents and educators 4) reading assessments 5) training for teachers in multisensory remedial approaches and 6) group and individual tutoring.

Kentucky

6369 De Paul School
1925 Duker Avenue
Louisville, KY 40205
502-459-6131
FAX 502-458-0827
http://www.depaulschool.org
e-mail: dpinfo@depaulschool.org

Peggy Woolley, Admissions Director
Anthony Kemper, Principal

Teaches students with specific learning differences how to: learn, be independent, and be successful. Co-ed, grades 1-8.

6370 KY-SPIN
10301 Deering Road
Louisville, KY 40272
502-937-6894
800-525-7746
FAX 502-937-6464
TDY:502-937-6894
http://www.kyspin.com
e-mail: spininc@kyspin.com
Paulette Logsdon, Executive Director
Tara Becker, Office Assistant

Parent Training and Information Project views parents as full partners in the educational process and a significant source of support and assistance to each other. Funded by the Division of Personnel Preparation, Office of Special Education Programs, these programs provide training and information and support to parents and families of children of all ages with all types of disabilities. We empower parents to recognize and use all available resources.

6371 Kentucky Special Parent Involvement Network
KY-SPIN
10301-B Deering Road
Louisville, KY 40272
502-937-6894
800-525-7746
FAX 502-937-6464
TDY:502-937-6894
http://www.kyspin.com
e-mail: spininc@kyspin.com
Paulette Logsdon, Executive Director
Tara Becker, Office Assistant

Parent Training and Information Project views parents as full partners in the educational process and a significant source of support and assistance to each other. Funded by the Division of Personnel Preparation, Office of Special Education Programs, these programs provide training and information and support to parents and families of children of all ages with all types of disabilities. We empower parents to recognize and use all available resources.

6372 Meredith-Dunn School
3023 Melbourne Avenue
Louisville, KY 40220
502-456-5819
FAX 502-456-5953
http://www.meredith-dunn-school.org
e-mail: cbunnell@meredith-dunn-school.org
Cindy Bunnell, Admissions Director
Kathy Beam, Principal

The Meredith-Dunn School was founded in 1971 as a non-profit institution to provide educational assistance for children with learning difficulties. We admit only children of average to above average IQ who possess learning difficulties, whether or not these difficulties are recognized as such by federal or public definition.

6373 Shedd Academy
PO Box 493
Mayfield, KY 42066
270-247-8007
FAX 270-247-0637
http://www.sheddacademy.org
e-mail: judy.brindley@sheddacademy.org
Paul Thompson, Executive Director
Debbie Craven, Admissions Office

The mission of the Shedd Academy is to prepare dyslexia and ADD students for college or vocational training and for their future by helping them to understand their unique learning styles; fulfill their intellectual, academic, physical, artistic, creative, social, spiritual, and emotional potential; develop a sense of self responsibility; assume a value system so that they can become contributing members of society and increase their skills to ensure they are armed with a variety of abilities.

Louisiana

6374 Crescent Academy
821 General Pershing Street
New Orleans, LA 70115
504-895-3952
FAX 504-895-3964
Barbara Leggett

Offers a variety of services to students with disabilities including note takers, extended testing time, counseling services, and special accommodations.

6375 Project PROMPT
Families Helping Families
201 Evans Road
Harahan, LA 70123
504-888-9111
800-766-7736
FAX 504-888-0246
http://www.projectprompt.com
e-mail: info@projectprompt.com
Cindy Arceneaux, Project Director
Mary Jacob, Assistant Director
Rose Gilbert, Executive Director
Parent Training and Information Program views parents as full partners in the educational process and a significant source of support and assistance to each other. Funded by the Division of Personnel Preparation, Office of Special Education Programs, these programs provide training and information to parents to enable such individuals to participate more effectively with professionals in meeting the educational needs of disabled children.

Maryland

6376 Academic Resource Center
Gunston Day School
Centreville, MD 21617
410-758-0620
FAX 410-758-0628
http://www.gunstondayschool.org
e-mail: info@gunstondayschool.org
Jeffrey Woodworth, Administrator
Reid Henry, Office Assistant

Founded in 1911, the school provides tutoring for individuals K through adult. Also offers limited and brief educational testing.

6377 Academic Resource Center at the Gunston Day School
PO Box 200
Centreville, MD 21617
410-758-0620
FAX 410-758-0628
http://www.gunstondayschool.org
Jeffrey Woodworth, Administrator
Reid Henry, Office Assistant

Provides tutoring for individuals K through adult. Also offers limited and brief educational testing.

6378 Behavioral Directions
Behavioral Directions
626 Grant Street
Herndon, VA 20170
703-855-4032
FAX 571-333-0292
http://www.BehavioralDirections.com
e-mail: behavioraldirections@smartneighborhood.net
Jane Barbin PhD BCBA, Psychologist/Consultant

Specializing in services to individuals (children and adults) with autism and developmental disabilities and their families. Services are provided by licensed psychologists and Board Certified Behavior Analysts utilizing Applied Behavior Analysis (ABA) as the treatment approach. Services, including behavioral assessment, functional analysis, educational assessment, ABA home programming, parent/staff training, and program evaluation, are provided in home, school, and community settings.

6379 **Chelsea School**
711 Pershing Drive
Silver Spring, MD 20910
301-585-1430
FAX 301-585-9621
http://www.chelseaschool.edu
e-mail: information@chelseaschool.edu
Bekah Atkinson, Admissions Director
Anthony Messina, Principal

At Chelsea School, we shatter the stigma of learning disabilities and prepare our students for a lifetime of intellectual exploration, personal growth and social responsibility. Because our students have language-based learning disabilities, we strongly focus on teaching reading and language arts.

6380 **Children's Developmental Clinic**
Prince George's Community College
301 Largo Road
Largo, MD 20774
301-336-6000
FAX 301-322-0519
TDY:301-322-0122
http://www.pgcc.edu/pgweb/pgdocs/CDC/cdc3.htm
e-mail: advising@pgcc.edu
Ronald Williams, President
Kathy Hinkel, Coordinator

The Children's Development Clinic is a continuing education program conducted in cooperation with the Department of Health and Human Performance at Prince George's Community College. The clinic provides special services to children, birth and up, who are experiencing various development difficulties such as learning problems, developmental delays, physical fitness and coordination problems, brain injury, mental retardation, emotional problems, or orthopedic challenges.

6381 **Developmental School Foundation**
Broschart School
14901 Broschart Road
Rockville, MD 20850
301-251-4624
FAX 301-251-4588
http://www.broschartschool.edu
Mary Kennelly, Executive Director
Craig Juengling, President

Provides a therapeutic day setting with a full school program that addresses the children's social/emotional and learning needs.

6382 **Edgemeade: Raymond A Rogers Jr School**
13101 Croom Road
Upper Marlboro, MD 20772
301-888-1333
800-486-3343
FAX 301-888-1343
Cindy Spiller, Executive Director

Edgemeade provides residential and day treatment services with a special education school program for kids with disabilities. The facility is licensed by the DHMH and accredited by JCAHO, and the education program is accredited by the MSDE. The therapeutic environment is structured to provide supervision and direction and an opportunity for each child to express himself.
Ages: 12-17

6383 **Forbush School**
Sheppard Pratt Health System
PO Box 6815
Towson, MD 21285
410-938-4400
FAX 410-938-4421
http://www.sheppardpratt.org
e-mail: blohnes@sheppardpratt.org
Dr Burt Lohnes, Day School Program Director
Jim Truscello, Principal
Alania Foster, Office Assistant
Provides educational therapeutic services for children and adolescents. The curriculum is designed to faciliate the growth of each student in cognitive and emotional areas.

6384 **Frost Center**
4915 Aspen Hill Road
Rockville, MD 20853
301-933-9033
FAX 301-933-3330
http://www.frostcenter.com
e-mail: chobbes@frostcenter.com
Sean McLaughlin, Center Director
Sean McLaughlin, Director
Headen Principal, Principal
The Frost school established in 1976, is a school and therapeutic day program that serves emotionally troubled and autistic children and adolescents and their families. It is a 12-month school program for students who need a supportive and structured environment, combining academic instruction, daily counseling, and weekly family counseling meetings.

6385 **Group for the Independent Learning Disabled (GILD)**
PO Box 322
Brooklandville, MD 21022
410-363-4300
FAX 410-363-7919
http://www.gildlearningdisable.org
Leith Herrmann, President
Harriet Wolf, Membership Chair

The Group for the Independent Learning Disabled provides support services with a learning disability. Classes are also held for life and social skills on a bi-weekly basis.

6386 **Hannah More School**
12039 Reisterstown Road
Reisterstown, MD 21136
410-526-5000
FAX 410-526-7631
http://www.HannahMore.org
e-mail: hmsinfo@hannahmore.org
Carolyn Martin, Admissions Director
Mark Waldman, President

Educates emotionally disabled students and children with a pervasive development disorder and provides therapeutic services so that the student may develop responsible patterns of behavior. A psychoeducational approach consisting of a comprehensive combination of academic subjects, a technology program, counseling programs and a behavioral management systems is designed to meet the individual needs of each student.

6387 **Kennedy Krieger Institute for Handicapped Children**
University Affiliated Program
707 N Broadway
Baltimore, MD 21205
443-923-9200
800-873-3377
FAX 443-923-9405
http://www.kennedykrieger.org
Gary Goldstien, MD, President
Jim Anders, Vice President

The Kennedy Krieger Institute is an internationally recognized facility dedicated to improving the lives of children and adolescents with pediatric developmental disabilities through patient care, special education, research and professional training.

6388 **Nora School**
955 Sligo Avenue
Silver Spring, MD 20910
301-495-6672
FAX 301-495-7829
http://www.nora-school.org
e-mail: dave@nora-school.org
David Mullen, Principal

A small, progressive, college preparatory high school that nurtures and empowers bright students who have been frustrated in larger, more traditional school settings.

6389 **Parents' Place of Maryland**
801 Cromwell Park Drive
Glen Burnie, MD 21061
410-859-5300
FAX 410-768-0830
http://www.ppmd.org
e-mail: info@ppmd.org
Suzie Shannon, Office Administrator
Josie Thomas, Executive Director

Serving the parents of children with disabilities throughout Maryland, regardless of the nature of their child's disability or the age of their child.

6390 **Phillips School: Programs for Children andFamilies**
8920 Whiskey Bottom Road
Laurel, MD 20723 410-880-0730
FAX 301-470-1624
http://www.phillipsprograms.org
e-mail: Gary.Behrens@phillipsprograms.org
Sally Sibley, President/CEO
Gavin Behrens, Executive Director

Phillips is a non-profit, private organization serving the needs of individuals with emotional and behavioral problems and their families through education, family support services, community education and advocacy.

6391 **Programs for Children and Families**
Phillips School
8920 Whiskey Bottom Road
Laurel, MD 20723 410-880-0730
FAX 301-470-1624
http://www.phillipsprograms.org
e-mail: Gary.Behrens@phillipsprograms.org
Sally Sibley, President/CEO
Gavin Behrens, Executive Director

Phillips is a non-profit, private organization serving the needs of individuals with emotional and behavioral problems and their families through education, family support services, community education and advocacy.

6392 **Ridge School of Montgomery County**
Potomac Ridge Behavioral Health Center
14915 Broschart Road
Rockville, MD 20850 301-251-4624
800-204-8600
FAX 301-251-4588
http://www.adventisthealthcare.com/PRBH
Craig Juengling, President

The school provides both a special education program and a general education program to meet the needs of the students who have difficulty learning in a traditional school environment.

6393 **Sensory Integration & Vision Therapy Specialists**
6509 Democracy Boulevard
Bethesda, MD 20817 301-897-8484
FAX 301-897-8486
http://www.visionhelp.com
e-mail: info@visionhelp.com
S. Appelbaum, Co-Owner
Barbara Bassin, Co-owner

Dr. Appelbaum's practice, established in 1977, offers a full range of family vision care and eye services, specializing in the treatment of children and adults with behavioral, sensorimotor or learning-related vision problems such as those previously diagnosed with add-adhd, dyslexia, acquired brain injury, stroke, learning disabilities, and/or avoidance of reading. Children and adults can receive vision therapy and sensory integration occupational therapy in the same office.

6394 **The Nora School**
955 Sligo Avenue
Silver Spring, MD 20910 301-495-6672
FAX 301-495-7829
http://www.nora-school.org
e-mail: dave@nora-school.org
David Mullen, Principal
Elaine Mack, Admissions Director

A small, progressive, college preparatory high school that nurtures and empowers bright students who have been frustrated in larger, more traditional school settings.

Massachusetts

6395 **Adult Center at PAL: Curry College**
1071 Blue Hill Avenue
Milton, MA 02186 617-333-0500
FAX 617-333-2114
TDY:617-333-2250
http://www.curry.edu/pal
e-mail: pal@curry.edu
Jane Adelizzi PhD, Contact

The Adult Center at PAL (Program for Advancement of Learning) is the first program to offer academic and socio-emotional services to adults with LD/ADHD/Dyslexia in a college setting in the New England area. The ACD offers one-to-one academic tutorials; small support groups that meet weekly; and Saturday Seminars that explore issues that impact the lives of adults with LD/ADHD.

6396 **Adult Center at PAL: Program for Advancement of Learning**
Curry College
1071 Blue Hill Avenue
Milton, MA 02186 617-333-0500
FAX 617-333-2114
TDY:617-333-2250
http://www.curry.edu/pal
e-mail: pal@curry.edu
Jane Adelizzi PhD, Program Coordinator

The Adult Center at PAL (Program for Advancement of Learning) is the first program to offer academic and socio-emotional services to adults with LD/ADHD/Dyslexia in a college setting in the New England area. The ACD offers one-to-one academic tutorials; small support groups that meet weekly; and Saturday Seminars that explore issues that impact the lives of adults with LD/ADHD.

6397 **Berkshire Meadow**
249 N Plain Road
Housatonic, MA 01236 413-528-2523
FAX 413-528-0293
http://www.berkshiremeadows.org
e-mail: berkshiremeadows@jri.org
Liisa Kelly, Program Director
Gail Charpentier, Administrator

Berkshire Meadow is a private, non-profit, year-round residential school and program for people of all ages who are severely developmentally delayed and may be multiply disabled.

6398 **Brightside for Families and Children**
2112 Riverdale Street
West Springfield, MA 01089 413-539-2973
800-660-4673
FAX 413-747-0182
http://www.mercycares.com
e-mail: vinnie.regan2sphs.com
Vinnie Regan, Educational Administrator
Rose Marceau, Administrative Secretary
James Bastien, Executive VP
Brightside for Families and Children is a non-profit, social service organization dedicated to strengthening, supporting and preserving all children and families. Brightside is especially focused on those children and families in Western Massachusetts who are most vulnerable and disavantaged regardless of race, creed or color.

6399 **CAST**
40 Harvard Mill Square
Wakefield, MA 01880 781-245-2212
888-858-9994
FAX 781-245-5212
TDY:781-245-9320
http://www.cast.org
e-mail: cast@cast.org
Anne Meyer, Co-Founding Director

A nonprofit organization that works to expand learning opportunities for all individuals, especially those with disabilities, through the research and development of innovative, technology-based educational resources and strategies.

6400 College Internship Program
Berkshire Center
18 Park Street
Lee, MA 01238
413-243-2576
FAX 413-243-3351
http://www.berkshirecenter.org
e-mail: cwheeler@berkshirecenter.org
Caroline Wheeler, Admissions Director
Michael McManmon, Executive Director
Gary Shaw, Program Director
The College Internship Program provides individualized, post-secondary academic, internship and independent living experiences for young adults with learning differences. With the support and direction, students learn to realize and develop their potential.

6401 College Internship Program at the Berkshire Center
Berkshire Center
18 Park Street
Lee, MA 01238
413-243-2576
FAX 413-243-3351
http://www.berkshirecenter.org
e-mail: gshaw@berkshirecenter.org
Michael McManmon, Executive Director
Gary Shaw, Program Director

A post secondary program for young adults with learning disabilities, ages 18-26. Half of the students attend Berkshire Community College and business school while the others may go directly into the world of work. Services include vocational/academic preparation, tutoring, college liaison, life skills instruction, driver's education, money management, psychotherapy and more.

6402 Commonwealth Learning Center
Commonwealth Learning Center
220 Reservoir Street
Needham Heights, MA 02494
781-444-5193
800-461-6671
FAX 781-444-6916
http://www.commlearn.com
e-mail: info@commlearn.com
Lisa Brooks, Manager
Jerri Murray, Office Manager

Nonprofit learning center offering one-to-one tutorial for kindergarten through adult students. Programs in reading, spelling, writing, comprehension, math, study skills. Teacher training in multisensory methodologies. Educational evaluations available. Also centers in Danvers, MA and Sudbury, MA.

6403 Cotting School
453 Concord Avenue
Lexington, MA 02421
781-862-7323
FAX 617-861-1179
http://www.cotting.org.
e-mail: dnewark@cotting.org
David Manzo, President

Cotting School is for students with moderate to severe learning disabilities requiring assessment of learning style, remediation techniques and one-to-one instruction.

6404 Devereux Massachusetts
PO Box 219
Rutland, MA 01543
508-886-4746
FAX 508-886-4773
http://www.devereux.org
e-mail: tbeauvai@devereux.org
Terry Beauvais, Admissions Officer
Elizabeth Orcutt, Principal

A residential program for children, adolescents and young adults who have emotional, behavioral and substance abuse programs with developmental and learning disabilities.

6405 Doctor Franklin Perkins School
971 Main Street
Lancaster, MA 01523
978-365-7376
FAX 978-368-8861
http://www.perkinsprograms.org
Christine Santry, Admissions Director
Sharon Lowry, Day School Program Director
Sherry Nolan, Executive Director
The Doctor Franklin Perkins School is a comprehensive human service agency operating at several sites in the Central Massachusetts towns of Lancaster and Clinton. Perkins provides a variety of services to several specialized populations of children, adolescents, adults and senior citizens.

6406 Educational Options, LLC
86 Kirkland Street #13
Cambridge, MA 02138
617-864-8864
FAX 617-864-3515
http://www.optionsined.com
e-mail: info@optionsined.com
Renee Goldberg, Founder
Marvin Goldberg, Founder

Full-service educational consulting practice dedicated to assisting students plan their future. Work with students to identify their strengths and match these qualities with an academic setting that meets their educational, cultural and social and social aspirations.

6407 Evergreen Center
345 Fortune Boulevard
Milford, MA 01757
508-478-2631
FAX 508-634-3251
http://www.evergreenctr.org
e-mail: services@evergreenctr.org
Robert Littleton Jr., Executive Director

The Evergreen Center is a residential school serving children and adolescents with severe developmental disabilities.

6408 Frederic L Chamberlain School
PO Box 778
Middleboro, MA 02346
508-947-7825
FAX 508-947-0944
http://www.chamberlainschool.org
e-mail: rvonohlsen@chamberlainschool.org
William Doherty, Executive Director
Lawrence Mutty, Admissions Director

The Frederic L Chamberlain School is more than a small New England boarding school. Chamberlain is a community of adolescents who have experienced significant diffulties at home, in the community and/or in traditional schools.

6409 Getting Ready for the Outside World
Riverview School
551 Route 6A
East Sandwich, MA 02537
508-888-0489
FAX 508-833-7001
http://www.riverviewschool.org
e-mail: admissions@riverviewschool.org
Maureen Brenner, Principal

Riverview School's 10-month transitional component for students who have completed the secondary school, and is designed to provide students with the skills that will assist them in functioning more independently within the adult world.

6410 Landmark Preparatory Program
Landmark School
PO Box 227
Prides Crossing, MA 01965
978-236-3010
FAX 978-927-7268
http://www.landmarkoutreach.org
e-mail: jtruslow@landmarkschool.org
Robert Broudo, Headmaster
Carolyn Orsini-Nelson, Admissions Director
Christopher Murphy, Principal

Offers a secondary school level curriculum emphasizing organizational and study skills development in a traditional classroom setting, and is designed for college bound boys and girls who have progressed to within one year of expected grade level performance.

6411 Landmark School Outreach Program
Landmark School
429 Hale Street
Prides Crossing, MA 01965
978-236-3216
FAX 978-927-7268
http://www.landmarkoutreach.org
e-mail: outreach@landmarkschool.org
Robert Broudo, Headmaster
Carolyn Orsini-Nelson, Admissions Director
Christopher Murphy, Principal
The Outreach Program provides professional development programs and publications that offer practical and effective strategies to help children learn. These strategies are based on Landmark's Six Teaching Principles and reflect Landmark's innovative instruction of students with language-based learning disabilites.
1971Grade Range: 2-12

6412 Landmark School and Summer Programs
PO Box 227
Prides Crossing, MA 01965
978-236-3000
FAX 978-927-7268
http://www.landmarkoutreach.org
e-mail: admission@landmarkschool.org
Robert Broudo, Headmaster
Carolyn Orsini Nelson, Admission Director
Christopher Murphy, Principal
Landmark is a coeducational boarding and day school for emotionally healthy students who have been diagnosed with a language based learning disability. We individualize instruction for each of our students, providing an intensive program emphasizing the development of language and learning skills within a highly structured environment. We also offer an intensive six-week summer program for students who wish to explore the benefits of short-term, skill-based learning.

6413 League School of Greater Boston
300 Boston Providence Turnpike
Walpole, MA 02032
508-850-3900
FAX 617-964-3264
http://www.leagueschool.com
e-mail: admin@leagueschool.com
John Zbyszynski, Executive Director
Lisa Weeden, Principal

Providing social, academic, and vocational programs for children with Autism/Asperger Spectrum Disorders who need a specialized alternative to public school, preparing them to transfer into an environment offering greater independence.

6414 Learning Center of Massachusetts
Protestant Guild for Human Services
411 Waverley Oaks Road
Waltham, MA 02452
781-893-6000
FAX 781-893-1171
http://www.protestantguild.org
e-mail: admissions@protestantguild.org
Debrah Rosser, Executive Director
Pam Grath, Religious Leader

A private, 365-day community-based, educational program serving difficult to place students with a primary diagnosis of mild to severe mental retardation, autism, or other developmental disability. In addition, students may carry secondary diagnosis of hearing impairments and other communication disorders, traumatic brain injury, seizure disorders, Tourette's syndrome and emotional and psychiatric disorders.

6415 Learning Resource Center
Unity College
90 Quaker Hill Road
Unity, ME 04988
207-948-3131
800-624-1024
FAX 207-948-6277
http://www.unity.edu
e-mail: admissions@unity.edu

Jim Horan, Director

The Learning Resource Center provides instruction and supportive services to students with learning disabilities. A staff learning disabilites specialist works with students who have specific cognitive disabilites that interfers with learning.

6416 Linden Hill School
154 S Mountain Road
Northfield, MA 01360
413-498-2906
866-498-2906
FAX 413-498-2908
http://www.lindenhs.org
e-mail: office@lindenhs.org
James McDaniel, Headmaster
Gerald Shields, Principal
Vanessa Towne, Office Secretary
The Linden Hill School enrolls bright, inquisitive, boys who have language based learning differences and/or attention issues.

6417 Living Independently Forever (LIFE)
550 Lincoln Road Extension
Hyannis, MA 02601
508-790-3600
http://www.lifecapcod.org
e-mail: groupmashpee@lifecapcod.org
Mary Matthews, President
Barry Schwartz, Executive Director

Living Independently Forever, Inc. is dedicated to serving the life-long needs of adults with significant learning disabilities within our residential communities. LIFE is committed to providing these men and women with the adult education and the opportunities to develop their personal and vocational / occupational skills to their maximum potential, and to supporting them appropriately in independent and group living.

6418 May Institute
41 Pacella Park Drive
Randolph, MA 02368
781-440-0400
800-778-7601
FAX 781-437-1240
TDY:781-440-0461
http://www.mayinstitute.org
e-mail: info@mayinstitute.org

Walter Christian, President
Dennis Russo Ph.D, Chief Clinical Officer

The May Institute provides educational and rehabilitative services for individuals with autism, developmental disabilities, neurological disorders and mental illness.

6419 New England Center for Children
33 Turnpike Road
Southborough, MA 01772
508-481-1015
FAX 508-485-3421
http://www.necc.org
e-mail: info@necc.org
Vincent Strully Jr., Executive Director
Katherine Foster, Associate Executive Director

The New England Center for Children is a private, nonprofit organization serving children with autism and other related disabilities.

6420 Regis College
235 Wellesley Street
Weston, MA 02493
781-768-7000
FAX 781-768-7071
http://www.regiscollege.edu
e-mail: admissions@regiscollege.edu
Mary England MD, President
Emily Keily, Admissions Director

The college encourages student self-advocacy, the coordination of appropriate academic accommodations and the promotion of disability awareness.

6421 Riverbrook Residence
4 Ice Glen Road
Stockbridge, MA 01262
413-298-4926
FAX 413-298-5166
http://www.riverbrook.org
e-mail: riverbro@berkshire.net

Joan Burkhard, Executive Director
Patty Morris, Program Coordinator

A residence in western Massachusetts, providing supported living to developmentally disabled women, with therapy and treatment focused on the arts.

6422 Seven Hills at Groton
22 Hillside Avenue
Groton, MA 01450
978-448-3388
FAX 978-448-9695
http://www.sevenhills.org
e-mail: hjarek@sevenhills.org
David Jordan, President
Holly Jarek, Administrator

Seven Hills at Groton is a pediatric skilled nursing community, providing comprehensive, compassionate care to children and young adults who are severely developmentally delayed and have complexed medical needs. Children enter prior to their 22nd birthday and traditionally remain throughout their lifetime.

6423 Son-Rise Program: Autism Treatment Center of America
Option Institute
2080 S Undermountain Road
Sheffield, MA 01257
413-229-8727
FAX 413-229-3202
http://www.autismtreatmentcenter.org
e-mail: correspondence@option.org
Neil Kaufman, Co-Founder/Program Co-Creator
Lyte Co-Founder/Program Co, Co-Founder/Program Co-Creator

A worldwide teaching center for children and adults challenged by autism, autism spectrum disorders, pervasive developmental disorder, asperger's syndrome, and other developmental difficulties. The Son-Rise Program teaches specific and comprehensive system of treatment and education designed to help families and caregivers enable their children to dramatically improve in all areas of learning, development, communication and skill acquisition.

6424 Stetson School
Stetson School
PO Box 309
Barre, MA 01005
978-355-4541
FAX 978-355-6335
http://www.stetsonschool.org
e-mail: stetsonschool.org
Kathleen O'Connor, Admissions Coordinator
Robert Fitzgerald, Admissions/Marketing Director
Kathleen Lovenbury, President
A nonprofit residential treatment and special education program for sexually abusive youth ages 9-22.

6425 Threshold Program
Lesley University
29 Everett Street
Cambridge, MA 02138
617-868-9600
800-999-1959
http://www.lesley.edu/threshold/threshold_home
e-mail: threshld@mail.lesley.edu
James Wilbur, Director
Helen McDonald, Admissions Director
Margaret Kenna, President
The Threshold Program is a comprehensive, non-degree campus based program at Lesley University for highly motivated adults with diverse learning disabilities and other special needs.

6426 Unity College Learning Resource
Center Quaker Hill Road
Unity, ME 04988
207-948-3131
800-624-1024
FAX 207-948-2928
http://www.unity.edu
e-mail: admissions@unity.edu
Jim Horan, Learning Resource Center Dir.
Kay Fiedler, Director
David Glenn-Lewin, President

6427 Valleyhead
PO Box 714
Lenox, MA 01240
413-637-3635
FAX 413-637-3501
http://www.valleyhead.org
e-mail: cmacbeth@valleyhead.org
Chris Beth, Executive Director
Ellen Merrit, Admissions Director

Valleyhead was founded in 1969. It is a residential school for for girls in the scenic Berkshire Hills of Lenox, Massachusetts. We provide a home and education for girls ages 12-22 with emotional needs. Most of our girls come from abusive and traumatic backgrounds. Many do not have intact families.

6428 Willow Hill School
98 Haynes Road
Sudbury, MA 01776
978-443-2581
FAX 978-443-7560
http://www.willowhillschool.org
e-mail: info@willowhillschool.org
Ann Marie Rech, Admissions Director
Rhonda Taft-Farrell, Principal

Willow Hill School provides supportive and individualized educational programs for middle and high school students who are capable of advancing along a strong academic curriculum, but have experienced frustration in earlier school settings.
11-21 years old

Michigan

6429 Center for Human Development
Berkley Medical Center
1695 W 12 Mile Road
Berkley, MI 48072
248-544-7110
FAX 248-691-4745
http://www.beaumonthospitals.com
e-mail: ekrug@beaumonthospital.com
Ernest Krug III, Director
Ann Ekola, Office Assistant

The Center for Human Development provides services to help children and adolescents deal with developmental, behavioral and learning disorders.

6430 Eton Academy
1755 E Melton Road
Birmingham, MI 48009
248-642-1150
FAX 248-642-3670
http://www.etonacademy.org
e-mail: cofiara@etonacademy.org
Pete Pullen, Principal
Sharon Morey, Admissions Director

The Eton Academy is a co-educational private day school dedicated to educating students with learning differences. The mission is to educate students who will understand their learning styles and practice strategies that will prepare them for responsible independence, life-long learning and participation in school, family and in their community.

6431 Lake Michigan Academy
2428 Burton Street SE
Grand Rapids, MI 49546
616-464-3330
FAX 616-285-1935
http://www.wmldf.org
e-mail: execdir@wmldf.org
Linda Chaffee, Executive Director

Lake Michigan Academy is a state-certified, non-profit school for learning disabled children in grades 1 through 12 with average or above average intelligence. The learning disabilities of the children here vary. Some are dyslexic and have difficulty with decoding or comprehending written language. Some are dyscalculic and experience difficulty with mathematical computations and concepts. Many are dysgraphic and exhibit difficulties with writing skills. Our mission is to build self esteem.

6432 SLD Learning Center
525 Cheshire Drive NE
Grand Rapids, MI 49505
616-361-1182
888-271-8881
FAX 616-361-3648
http://www.sldcenter.org
e-mail: sldlc@sbeglobal.net
Rebecca Krause, President
Anne Baird, Vice President
Tom Schrock, Executive Director
The SLD Learning Center is a non-profit educational service institute established in 1974 to provide one-to-one instruction for people of all ages who exhibit dyslexia tendencies or who have not succeeded with traditional teaching methods.

Minnesota

6433 Groves Academy
3200 Highway 100 S
Saint Louis Park, MN 55416
952-920-6377
FAX 952-920-2068
http://www.grovesacademy.org
e-mail: information@grovesadacemy.org
Debbie Moran, Admissions Director
John Alexander, Administrator

A day school for children who because of their learning disabilities have not been successful in a traditional school setting.

6434 LDA Learning Center
4301 Highway 7
Minneapolis, MN 55416
952-922-8374
FAX 952-922-8102
http://www.ldalearningcenter.com
e-mail: info@ldalearningcenter.com
Kitty Christiansen, Executive Director
Victoria Weinberg, Program Director

Maximizes the potential of children, youths, adults and families, especially those with learning disabilities and other learning difficulties so that they can lead more productive and fulfilled lives. Provides consultations, tutoring, assessments, parent workshops, training and outreach on sliding fee scale.

6435 LDA of Minnesota
5354 Parkdale Drive
St. Louis Park, MN 55416
952-922-8374
FAX 952-922-8102
http://www.ldalearningcenter.com
e-mail: info@ldaminnesota.org
Kitty Christiansen, Executive Director
Victoria Weinberg, Program Director

The Learning Disabilities Association maximizes the potential of children, youths, adults and families, especially those with learning disabilities and other learning difficulties so that they can lead more productive and fulfilled lives. Provides consultations, tutoring, assessments, parent workshops, training and outreach on sliding fee scale.

Mississippi

6436 Heritage School
St. Columbus Episcopal Church
550 Sunnybrook Road
Ridgeland, MS 39157
601-853-7163
FAX 601-853-7163
http://www.stcolumbs.org/heritageschool
e-mail: heritageschool@stcolumbs.org
Jeanie Muirhead, Director
Fran Parks, Executive Director

Heritage School was establed in 1971 to provide an alternative learning environment for children with learning difficulties. A private, non-profit specialized school accredited through the State Department of Education to offer instruction for learning disabled and ADD/ADHD students from first through eighth grade.

6437 Millcreek Behavioral Health Services
Youth & Family Centered Services
Magee, MS 39111
601-849-4221
800-372-1994
FAX 601-849-6107
http://www.yfcs.com
e-mail: info.mc-ms@yfcs.com
Margaret Tedford, Administrator
Anne Russum, President

A residential treatment center for children with emotional disturbances and an intensive care facility for children with mental retardation.

6438 Millcreek Schools
PO Box 1160
Magee, MS 39111
601-849-4221
800-372-1994
FAX 601-849-6107
http://www.yfcs.com
e-mail: info.mc-ms@yfcs.com
Margaret Tedford, Administrator
Anne Russum, President

A residential treatment center for children with emotional disturbances and an intensive care facility for children with mental retardation.

Missouri

6439 Churchill Center School
1035 Price School Lane
Saint Louis, MO 63124
314-997-4343
FAX 314-997-2760
http://www.churchillschool.org
e-mail: info@churchillschool.org
Sandra Gilligan, Executive Director
Deborah Warden, Assistant Director
Jenny Hyde Carney, Outreach Coordinator
The Churchill School is a private, not-for-profit, coeducational day school. It is designed to serve children between the ages of 8-16 with diagnosed learning disabilities. The goal is to help each child reach his or her full potential and prepare for a successful return to a traditional classroom in as short a period of time as possible.

6440 Churchill School
1035 Price School Lane
Saint Louis, MO 63124
314-997-4343
FAX 314-997-2760
http://www.churchillschool.org
e-mail: churchill@churchillschool.org
Sandra Gilligan, Executive Director
Deborah Warden, Assistant Director
Jenny Hyde Carney, Outreach Coordinator
The Churchill School is a private, not-for-profit, coeducational day school. It is designed to serve children between the ages of 8-16 with diagnosed learning disabilities. The goal is to help each child reach his or her full potential and prepare for a successful return to a traditional classroom in as short a period of time as possible.

6441 Gillis Center
8150 Wornall Road
Kansas City, MO 64114
816-508-3500
FAX 816-508-3535
http://www.gillis.org
e-mail: geninfo@gillis.org
Mary Schaid, CEO
George Robbins, Development Director

Gillis Center's mission is to help at-risk children and their families become contributing members of the community through education, counseling and social services.

6442 **Metropolitan School**
7281 Sarah Street
Saint Louis, MO 63143
314-644-0850
FAX 314-644-3363
http://www.metroschool.org
e-mail: info@metroschool.org
Rita Buckley, Executive Director
Cindy Keitel, Executive Assistant
Judi Thomas, Principal
The mission of Metropolitan School is to lead our community in providing effective, comprehensive educational services for adolescents who have atypical learning styles.

6443 **Miriam School**
501 Bacon Avenue
Saint Louis, MO 63119
314-968-5225
FAX 314-968-7338
http://www.miriamsfoundation.org
e-mail: info@miriamfoundation.org
Joan Holland, Executive Director
Michael Robinson, Admissions Director

A nonprofit day school for children between four and twelve years of age who are learning disabled and/or behaviorally disabled. Speech and language services and occupational therapy are integral components of the program. The focus of all the activities is to increase children's self-esteem and help them acquire the coping skills needed to successfully meet future challenges.
4-12 years old

6444 **Missouri Parents Act (MPACT)**
1 W Armour Boulevard
Kansas City, MO 64111
816-531-7070
800-743-7634
FAX 417-882-8413
http://www.ptimpact.com
e-mail: msavage@ptimpact.com
Mary Savage, Executive Director
Diana Biere, Associate Director

MPACT assists parents to effectively advocate for their children's educational rights and services. MPACT is a statewide parent training and information center serving all disabilities. Our mission is to ensure that all children with special needs receive an education that allows them to achieve their personal goals.

Montana

6445 **Parents Let's Unite for Kids**
516 N 32nd Street
Billings, MT 59101
406-255-0540
800-222-7585
FAX 406-255-0523
http://www.pluk.org
e-mail: plukinfo@pluk.org
Dennis Moore, Executive Director
Maegan Parks, Office Assistant

PLUK is a private, nonprofit organization formed in 1984 by parents and children with disabilities and chronic illnesses in the state of Montana for the purpose of information, support, training and assistance to aid their children at home, school and as adults.

6446 **Parents, Let's Unite for Kids**
516 N 32nd Street
Billings, MT 59101
406-255-0540
800-222-7585
FAX 406-255-0523
http://www.pluk.org
e-mail: plukinfo@pluk.org
Dennis Moore, Executive Director
Maegan Parks, Office Assistant

PLUK is a private, nonprofit organization formed in 1984 by parents and children with disabilities and chronic illnesses in the state of Montana for the purpose of information, support, training and assistance to aid their children at home, school and as adults.

Nebraska

6447 **Nebraska Parents Training and Information Center**
PTI (Parent Training & Information) Nebraska
3135 N 93rd Street
Omaha, NE 68134
402-346-0525
800-284-8520
FAX 402-934-1479
TDY:800-284-8520
http://www.pti-nebraska.org
e-mail: info@pti-nebraska.org
Cathy Heinen, Office Manager
Glenda Davis, Executive Director

Parent Training and Information Program views parents as full partners in the educational process and a significant source of support and assistance to each other. Funded by the Division of Personnel Preparation, Office of Special Education Programs, these programs provide training and information to parents to enable such individuals to participate more effectively with professionals in meeting the educational needs of disabled children.

New Hampshire

6448 **Becket School**
PO Box 325
Orford, NH 03777
603-989-5100
FAX 603-898-5488
http://www.becket.org
e-mail: jeff.caron@becket.org
Kerry Beck, Executive Director
Jeffrey Caron, Principal
Sharon Edwards, Special Ed Director
Becket guides and inspires adolescents having difficulties at home, in school or in the community

6449 **Cardigan Mt. School**
62 Alumni Drive
Canaan, NH 03741
603-523-4321
FAX 603-523-7227
http://www.cardigan.org
e-mail: rryerson@cardigan.org
Tom Needham, Headmaster
James Funnell, President

6450 **Cedarcrest**
91 Maple Avenue
Keene, NH 03431
603-358-3384
FAX 603-358-6485
http://www.cedarcrest4kids.org
e-mail: info@cedarcrest4kids.org
Cathy Gray, CEO
Peg Knox, Nursing Director

A nonprofit home, school and medical support facility for children with complex medical needs and multiple disabilities. Cedarcrest serves up to 25 children, without regard to race, color, religious affiliation or financial standing. As a State Department of Education-approved school, Cedarcrest also serves as a placement option for any school district in the state.

6451 **Hampshire Country School**
122 Hampshire Road
Rindge, NH 03461
603-899-3325
FAX 603-899-6521
http://www.hampshirecountryschool.org
e-mail: hampshirecountry@monad.net
William Dickerman, Principal

Hampshire Country School is a small boarding school for 25 boys of high ability who need a personal environment with an unusual amount of adult attention and structure. It is primarily a junior school, suited particularly to students from 9 to 15 years old; but some younger students may be accepted and some students may remain through high school.

6452 Parent Information Center
151 Manchester Street
Concord, NH 03301 603-224-7005
800-947-7005
FAX 603-224-4365
TDY:603-224-7005
http://www.parentinformationcenter.org
e-mail: picinfo@parentinformationcenter.org
Heather Thalheimer, Executive Director
Bonnie Dunham, Project Director

Parent Training and Information Program views parents as full partners in the educational process and a significant source of support and assistance to each other. Funded by the Division of Personnel Preparation, Office of Special Education Programs, these programs provide training and information to parents to enable such individuals to participate more effectively with professionals in meeting the educational needs of children with disabilities.

New Jersey

6453 Bancroft Neurohealth
PO Box 20
Haddonfield, NJ 08033 856-429-0010
800-774-5516
FAX 856-429-1613
http://www.bancroftneurohealth.org
e-mail: adestefa@bnh.org
Toni Pergolin, President
Paul Healy, Public Relations Director
Robert Martin, CEO
Nonprofit organization offering educational/vocational programs, therapeutic support services and full range of community living opportunities for children and adults with brain injury in Maine, New Jersey, Delaware, and Louisiana. Residential options include community living supervised apartments, specialized supervised apartments, group homes and supported living models.

6454 Center School
319 N 3rd Avenue
Highland Park, NJ 08904 732-249-3355
FAX 732-249-1928
http://www.thecenterschool.com
Jeanne Prial, Director
Joanne Jordan, Office Assistant

A school designed for bright students in grades 1-12 with learning and behavioral difficulties. The Center School offers counseling, speech and language, and occupational therapy. Our school is committed to helping each student become as self-sufficient and successful as possible.

6455 Children's Institute
1 Sunset Avenue
Verona, NJ 07044 973-509-3050
FAX 973-740-0369
http://www.tcischool.org
e-mail: webmaster@tcischool.org
Bruce Ettinger, Principal
Carole Spiro, Volunteer Coordinator

The Children's Institute is a private, non-profit school approved by the New Jersey State Board of Education, serving children facing learning, language and social challenges.

6456 Craig School
10 Tower Hill Road
Mountain Lakes, NJ 07046 973-334-7223
FAX 973-334-1299
http://www.craigschool.org
e-mail: jday@craigschool.org
Julie Day, Admissions Director
David Blanchard, Headmaster

The Craig School is an independent, nonprofit school serving children who have difficulty succeeding in the traditional classroom environment. We specialize in a language-based curriculum for children of average or above average intelligence with such disorders as dyslexia, auditory processing and attention deficit.

6457 Devereux Center for Autism
198 Roadstown Road
Bridgeton, NJ 08302 856-455-7200
FAX 856-455-2765
James Gill Jr., Executive Director
Julia Allenan, Manager

Addressing the particular needs of children, adolescents and adults with Autism Spectrum Disorders, the center offers residential, educational and vocational programs. All programs are geared to reaching these individuals, helping them overcome challenging behaviors, and teaching them crucial life skills.

6458 Devereux Deerhaven
901 Mantua Pike
Woodbury, NJ 08096 856-384-9680
FAX 856-384-6742
http://www.devereux.org
Kristy Hartman, Admissions Director
Maureen Walsh, Executive Director

Residential and day programs for females who have emotional and behavioral disorders and learning disabilities.
5-21 years old

6459 Devereux New Jersey Treatment Network
901 Mantua Pike
Woodbury, NJ 08096 856-384-9680
FAX 856-384-6742
http://www.devereux.org
Kristy Hartman, Admissions Director
Maureen Walsh, Executive Director

Residential and day programs for females who have emotional and behavioral disorders and learning disabilities.

6460 ECLC of New Jersey
Bergen County Campus
302 N Franklin Turnpike
Ho Ho Kus, NJ 07423 201-670-7880
FAX 201-670-6675
http://www.eclcofnj.org
e-mail: vlindorff@eclcfnj.org
Bruce Litinger, Executive Director
Vicki Lindorff, Principal

A private school for individuals with disabilities between the ages of 5-21. Our mission is to help disabled students discover how they fit into the world and guide them towards becoming independent and employed adults.

6461 Eden Services
1 Eden Way
Princeton, NJ 08540 609-987-0099
FAX 609-987-0243
http://www.edenservices.org
e-mail: info@edenservices.org
Tom Cool, President
Joani Truch, Communications Administrator

Nonprofit organization founded in 1975 to provide a comprehensive continuum of lifespan services for individuals with autism and their families.

6462 Family Resource Associates
35 Haddon Avenue
Shrewsbury, NJ 07702 732-747-5310
FAX 732-747-1896
http://www.frainc.org
e-mail: info@frainc.org
Nancy Phalanukorn, Manager

A New Jersey non-profit agency dedicated to helping individuals with disabilities and their families.

6463 Forum School
107 Wyckoff Avenue
Waldwick, NJ 07463
201-444-5882
FAX 201-444-4003
http://www.theforumschool.com
e-mail: info@theforumschool.com
Steven Krapes, Executive Director
Linda Oliver, Office Manager

Special education day school for developmentally children. The Forum School offers a therapeutic education environment for children who cannot be accommodated in a public school setting.

6464 High Road Schools
3071 Bordentown Avenue
Parlin, NJ 08859
732-390-0303
FAX 732-390-5577
http://www.kids1inc.com
e-mail: kids1@kids1inc.com
Ellyn PhD, President

Offers programs serving the educational, social and emotional needs of children with specific learning disabilities, communication disorders and/or behavioral difficulties.

6465 Kids 1
High Road Schools
3071-A Bordentown Avenue
Parlin, NJ 08859
732-390-0303
FAX 732-390-5577
http://www.kids1inc.com
e-mail: kids1@kids1inc.com
Ellyn Lerner, Ph.D, Founder/CEO
Moskovitz Executive Director, Executive Director
Kaufman, PhD Executive Officer, Executive Officer
Offers programs serving the educational, social and emotional needs of children with specific learning disabilities, communication disorders and/or behavioral difficulties.

6466 Kingsway Learning Center
144 Kings Highway W
Haddonfield, NJ 08033
856-428-8108
FAX 856-428-7520
http://www.kingswaylc.com
e-mail: dpanner@kingswaylc.com
David Panner, Executive Director

Kingsway is a private, non-profit special education school devoted to the academic and therapeutic needs of children with developmental and learning disabilities. We serve children with multiple handicaps.

6467 Lewis Clinic and School
53 Bayard Lane
Princeton, NJ 08540
609-924-8120
FAX 609-924-5512
http://www.lewisschool.org
Marsha Lewis, Executive Director
Kerry Roche, Administrative Assistant

The Clinic and School integrate teaching and diagnostic perspective of multisensory educational practices in the classrooms, and the perspective of clinical research into the brain's learning process.

6468 Matheny School and Hospital
PO Box 339
Peapack, NJ 07977
908-234-0011
FAX 908-719-2137
http://www.matheny.org
e-mail: info@matheny.org
Steven Proctor, President

Matheny School and Hospital is a teaching hospital and a premier facility for people of all ages with developmental disabilities. Matheny specializes in the care of children and adults with cerebral palsy, muscular dystrophy, spina bifida and Lesch-Nyhan Disease.

6469 Metropolitan Speech and Language Center
Metropolitan Speech and Language Center
66 W Mount Pleasant Avenue
Livingston, NJ 07039
973-994-4468
FAX 973-994-4412
e-mail: lillyok@aol.com
Lilian Dollinger, Owner

Provides diagnostics and therapy for children and adults with speech, language, voice and stuttering problems.

6470 Midland School
PO Box 5026
North Branch, NJ 08876
908-722-8222
FAX 908-722-6203
http://www.midlandschool.org
e-mail: info@midlandschool.org
Philip Gaetlan, Executive Director
Sharon Millan, Principal

The mission of Midland School is a comprehensive special education program serving the individual social, emotional, academic, and career education needs of children and young adults with developmental disabilities.

6471 Newgrange School
530 S Olden Avenue
Hamilton, NJ 08629
609-584-1800
FAX 609-584-6166
http://www.thenewgrange.org
e-mail: info@thenewgrange.org
Gordon Sherman, Ph.D, Executive Director
Cindy Ege, Administrative Officer
Robert Hegedus, Administrator
Newgrange is a non-profit organization established in 1977 to provide specialized educational programs for people with learning disabilities.

6472 SEARCH Day Program
73 Wickapecko Drive
Ocean, NJ 07712
732-531-0454
FAX 732-531-5934
http://www.members.aol.com/SEARCHDay
e-mail: SEARCHDay@aol.com
Katherine Solana, Executive Director

SEARCH Day Program is a private, non-profit, New Jersey State certified agency serving children and adults with autism and their families.

6473 Statewide Parent Advocacy Network
Central Office
35 Halsey Street
Newark, NJ 07102
973-642-8100
800-654-7726
FAX 973-642-8080
http://www.spannj.org
e-mail: span@spannj.org
Diana Autin, Executive Director
Debra Jennings, Co-Executive Director

A nonprofit educational and advocacy center for parents of children from birth to 21 years of age. Assists families of infants, toddlers, children and youth with and without disabilities. Serves as a vehicle for the exchange of ideas, promoting awareness of the abilities and needs of the children and youth and improves services for children and families in the state of NJ.

New Mexico

6474 Brush Ranch School
HC 73
Tererro, NM 87573
505-757-6114
FAX 505-757-6118
http://www.brushranchschool.org
e-mail: kaycrice@hotmail.com
Kay Rice MA, School Head
Eve Bowen, Health Director
Weisman Admissions Director, Admissions Director
A co-educational boarding school for teens with learning differences. The school is fully licensed and accredited by both the New Mexico Board of Education and the North Central Association of Colleges and Schools. Situated on 283 acres in the Santa Fe National Forest, the school offers a wide range of educational and recreational opportunities.

6475 Designs for Learning Differences School
8600 Academy Road NE
Albuquerque, NM 87111
505-822-0476
FAX 505-858-4427
http://www.dldsycamoreschool.org
e-mail: lern@dldsycamoreschool.org
Linda Murry, Principal
Benita Kernodle, Administrative Assistant

6476 Designs for Learning Differences Sycamore School
Albuquerque, NM 87111
505-822-0476
FAX 505-858-4427
http://www.dldsycamoreschool.org
e-mail: dldschool1@aol.com
Linda Murray, Principal

A private, non-profit school, serving students with learning difficulties from the greater metropolitan area of albuquerque, New Mexico.

6477 EPICS Parent Project
Abrazos Family Support Services
PO Box 788
Bernalillo, NM 87004
505-867-3396
FAX 505-867-3398
http://www.swcr.org
e-mail: info@abrazosnm.org
Martha Gorospe, Director
Norm Segel, Executive Director

EPICS Project is a service for parents of American Indian children and young adults with disabilities and other special needs. EPICS provides training and information to Indian parents and families in order to facilitate their active involvement in meeting the special health and educational needs of their children.

6478 New Mexico Speech & Language Consultants
1000 W 4th Street
Roswell, NM 88201
505-623-8319
FAX 505-623-8220
Eileen Grooms, Owner

New Mexico Speech & Language Consultants provide diagnostic and therapy services for communicatively impaired individuals.

6479 Parents Reaching Out Network
1920 B Columbia Drive SE
Albuquerque, NM 87106
505-247-0192
800-524-5176
FAX 505-247-1345
http://www.parentsreachingout.org
e-mail: info@parentsreachingout.org
Sally Curen, Executive Director

PRO views parents as full partners in the educational process and a significant source of support and assistance to each other. Programs provide training and information to parents to enable such individuals to participate more effectively with professionals in meeting the educational needs of disabled children.

6480 Parents Reaching Out To Help (PRO)
1920 B Columbia Drive SE
Albuquerque, NM 87106
505-247-0192
800-524-5176
FAX 505-247-1345
http://www.parentsreachingout.org
Sally Curen, Executive Director
Larry Fuller, Program Manager

PRO views parents as full partners in the educational process and a significant source of support and assistance to each other. Programs provide training and information to parents to enable such individuals to participate more effectively with professionals in meeting the educational needs of disabled children.

New York

6481 Advocates for Children of New York
151 W 30th Street
New York, NY 10001
212-947-9779
FAX 718-729-8931
http://www.advocatesforchildren.org
e-mail: info@advocatesforchildren.org
Jill Chaifetz, Executive Director
Elisa Hyman, Deputy Director

Advocates for Children of New York, has worked in partnership with New York City's most impoverished and vulnerable families to secure quality and equal public education services. AFC works on behalf of children from infancy to age 21 who have disabilites, ethnic minorities, immigrants, homeless children, foster care children, limited English proficient children and those living in poverty.

6482 Anderson School
PO Box 367
Staatsburg, NY 12580
845-889-4034
FAX 845-889-3104
http://www.andersonschool.org
e-mail: info@andersonschool.org
Neil Pollack, Administrator

Anderson School provides a vast array of educational, residential, clinical, and support services to children and adults with autism and other developmental disabilities.

6483 Andrus Children's Center
1156 N Broadway
Yonkers, NY 10701
914-965-3700
FAX 914-965-3883
http://www.andruschildren.org
e-mail: nment@jdam.org
Nancy Woodruff, President/CEO

For more than 75 years, Andrus has been a provider of programs and services for children and families with learning disabilities.

6484 Baker Hall School
777 Ridge Road
Lackawanna, NY 14218
716-828-9737
FAX 716-828-9798
Nancy Pancow, Executive Director

Offers a certified special education program and a full range of classroom options; in-house, pre-vocational training and BOCES school placements are available to students depending on need.

6485 **Baker Victory Services**

780 Ridge Road
Lackawanna, NY 14218
716-828-9631
888-287-9986
FAX 716-828-9798
http://www.bakervictoryservices.org
e-mail: baker@buffnet.net

Nancy Pancow, Executive Director

BVS offers a wide range of services for individuals with physical, developmental, and/or behavorial challenges. In addition, programming which supplies a lifetime of care; from infancy to late adulthood.

6486 **Behavioral Arts**

58 W 88th Street
New York, NY 10024
212-799-9388
888-497-3722
FAX 212-799-4403
http://www.behavioralarts.com
e-mail: info@behavioralarts.com

Dr Enid Haller, Executive Director
Nancy Morales, Office Manager

A private facility dedicated to dysfunction relation to AD/HD and biological basis of behavior.

6487 **Center for Discovery**

PO Box 840
Harris, NY 12742
845-794-1400
FAX 845-791-2022
http://www.thecenterfordiscovery.org
e-mail: admissions@sdtc.org

Caryn Andersen, Admissions
Patrick Dollard, Chief Executive Officer

Center for Discovery offers individuals with significant disabilities, and their families, innovative educational, clinical, social, and living experiences designed to enrich their lives through personal accomplishment and increased independence.

6488 **Child Center for Developmental Service**

251 Manetto Hill Road
Plainview, NY 11803
516-938-3788

Dr. Iris Lesser, Director

Provides quality early care and education services in partnership with families and the community.

6489 **Community Based Services**

3 Fields Lane
North Salem, NY 10560
914-277-4771
FAX 914-277-8956
http://www.commbasedservices.org
e-mail: info@commbasedservices.org

Vickie Sylvester, CEO
Paulette Sladkus, COO

Six intermediate care facilities for people with autism and developmental disabilities, and one individual residential alternative.

6490 **Diagnostic Learning Center**

505 Ridge Road
Queensbury, NY 12804
518-793-0668
800-338-3781
FAX 518-793-0668
http://www.learningproblems.com
e-mail: jjanb@capital.net

Jan Bishop, Manager

Offers diagnosis and remediation of learning problems, cognitive remediation for the head injured. In-services for teachers and parent groups. Tutorials and diagnostic evaluations; no day or stay programs.

6491 **EAC Developmental Program**

382 Main Street
Port Washington, NY 11050
516-883-3006
FAX 516-883-0412

Gerald Stone, Executive Director
Patricia Dely, Secretary

6492 **EAC Nassau Learning Center**

382 Main Street
Port Washington, NY 11050
516-883-3006
FAX 516-883-0412

Gerald Stone, Executive Director
Lance Elder, President/CEO
Rebecca Bell, Associate Director

The purpose of EAC Learning Center is to help junior and senior high schools students who cannot function in a regular school environment obtain the necessary education which will make it possible for them to graduate from high school. EAC's first program, the Long Island Learning Centers have been serving learning disabled and emotionally disturbed students since 1971.

6493 **Eden II Programs**

150 Granite Avenue
Staten Island, NY 10303
718-816-1422
FAX 718-816-1428
http://www.eden2.org
e-mail: jgerenser@eden2.org

Joanne Gerenser, Executive Director

The mission of the Eden II/Genesis Programs is to provide people with autism specialized community-based programs and other opportunities, with the goal of enabling them to achieve the highest possible quality of living across life

6494 **Eden II School for Autistic Children**

Eden II School for Autistic Children
150 Granite Avenue
Staten Island, NY 10303
718-816-1422
FAX 718-816-1428
http://www.eden2.org
e-mail: jgerenser@eden2.org

Joanne Gerenser, Executive Director

Offers programs for children with autism and an adult day training program.

6495 **Environmental Science and Forestry**

State University of New York College
110 Bray Hall
Syracuse, NY 13210
315-464-5540
FAX 315-470-4728
http://www.esf.edu
e-mail: toslocum@esf.edu

Thomas Slocum, Special Services
Gregory Eastwood, President

6496 **Gow School**

PO Box 85
South Wales, NY 14139
716-652-3450
FAX 716-687-2003
http://www.gow.org
e-mail: admissions@gow.org

Bradley Rogers, Principal
Robert Garcia, Admissions Director

A boarding school for boys, grades 7-12, with dyslexia and other language based learning disabilities.

6497 **Hallen School**

97 Centre Avenue
New Rochelle, NY 10801
914-636-6600
FAX 914-633-4089
http://www.hallenschool.com

Carol LoCascio Ph.D, Executive Director
Angela Radogna, Principal

Hallen School is a private, special education school that serves children who exhibit learning disabilities, speech and language impairments, emotional difficulties, autistic features, and mid-health impairments.

6498 International Center for the Disabled
340 E 24th Street
New York, NY 10010 212-585-6083
FAX 212-585-6262
http://www.icdnyc.org
e-mail: ssegal@icdrehab.org
Sondra Segal, Development Director
Arnold Shapiro, Director Center for Speech/Lang.

Serving children, adolescents, adults, and seniors with disabilities and other rehabilitative and developmental needs.

6499 Julia Dyckman Andrus Memorial
1156 N Broadway
Yonkers, NY 10701 914-965-3700
FAX 914-965-3883
http://www.andruschildren.org
e-mail: nment@jdam.org
Nancy Ment, Executive Director

Residential treatment for youngsters who have moderate to severe emotional problems.

6500 Just Kids: Early Childhood Learning Center
Just Kids: Early Childhood Learning Center
PO Box 12
Middle Island, NY 11953 631-924-0008
FAX 631-924-4602
e-mail: jkschool@aol.com
Steven Held, President

A family focused early intervention program for young children with disabilities.

6501 Karafin School
PO Box 277
Mount Kisco, NY 10549 914-666-9211
FAX 914-666-9868
http://www.Bestwes.net/~karafin
Dr. Bart Donow, Associate Director
John Greenfieldt, Principal

Karafin School is a co-educational day college-preparatory and general academic school that primarily serves underachievers, students with learning difficulties, individuals wtih ADD, emotionally and behavioral problems, emotionally disabled students, and students with Tourette's Syndrome.

6502 Kildonan School
425 Morse Hill Road
Amenia, NY 12501 845-373-8111
FAX 845-373-2004
http://www.kildonan.org
e-mail: admissions@kildonan.org
Ronald Wilson, Principal
Robert Lane, Academic Dean

Offers a fully accredited College Preparatory curriculum. The school is co-educational, enrolling boarding students in Grades 6-Postgraduate and day students in Grade 2-Postgraduate. Provides daily one-on-one Orton-Gillingham tutoring to build skills in reading, writing, and spelling. Daily independent reading and writing work reinforces skills and improves study habits. Interscholastic sports, horseback riding, clubs and community service enhance self-confidence.

6503 Learning Diagnostic Center
Schneider Children's Hospital
26901 76th Avenue
New Hyde Park, NY 11040 718-470-3330
FAX 718-343-5864
http://www.schneiderchildrenshospital.org
Andrew Adesman MD, Director
Peter Silver MD, Principal

Committed to helping each child maximize his/her potential for academic, social and emotional development. The Center's staff uses a broad range of standardized and informal diagnostic tools as part of the evaluation process and provides comprehensive written reports including recommendations to improve functioning both in school and at home.

6504 Learning Disabilities Program
Adelphi University
1 S Avenue
Garden City, NY 11530 516-877-4710
800-ADELPHI
FAX 516-877-4711
http://www.adelphi.edu
e-mail: ldprogram@adelphi.edu
Susan Spencer, Program Director/Asst. Dean
Cohen Assistant Director, Assistant Director

A program offered for students who have difficulty learning and are provided specific attention for their disability.

6505 Manhattan Center for Learning
590 W End Avenue
New York, NY 10024 212-876-4639
FAX 212-787-5323
Corinne Vinal, Principal

Services for the learning disabled include tutoring, remediation, cognitive therapy, psycho-educational testing, parent counseling and neuropsychological testing provided by a very qualified staff including a licensed psychologist certified as a learning disabilities specialist.

6506 Maplebrook School
5142 Route 22
Amenia, NY 12501 845-373-8673
FAX 845-373-7029
http://www.maplebrookschool.org
e-mail: admin@maplebrookschool.org
Paul Scherer, President
Jennifer Scully, Admissions Dean
Jenny Hill, Admissions Assistant Director
A traditional boarding school enrolling students with learning differences and ADD. Offers strong academics and character development.

6507 Maplebrook School Learning Centerry Studies (CAP)
Division of Maplebrook School
5142 Route 22
Amenia, NY 12501 845-373-8673
FAX 845-373-7029
http://www.maplebrookschool.org
e-mail: mbsecho@aol.com
Jennifer Scully, Dean of Admissions
Jenny Hill, Admissions Assistant Director
Paul Scherer, President
CAPS offers a vocational program with employment skills and training, as well as a collegiate program with courses taken at the local community college and other support services.

6508 Mary McDowell Center for Learning
20 Bergen Street
Brooklyn, NY 11201 718-625-3939
FAX 718-625-1456
http://www.marymcdowell.org
e-mail: debbiez@marymcdowell.org
Debbie Zlotowitz, Executive Director
Stephanie Lazzara, School Administrator

An independent friends school for children with learning disabilities ages 5-12.

6509 New Interdisciplinary School
430 Sills Road
Yaphank, NY 11980 631-924-5583
FAX 631-924-5687
http://www.niskids.org
e-mail: information@niskids.org
Helen Wilder, Administrator
Betsy Kapian, Assistant Director

A not-for-profit organization that provides therapeutic and educational services for both typically developing and developmentally disabled children.

6510 New York Institute for Special Education

999 Pelham Parkway N
Bronx, NY 10469
718-519-7000
FAX 718-231-9314
http://www.nyise.org/

Kim Benisatto, Operations Manager
Eugene Mahon, Executive Director

A nonsectarian educational facility that provides quality programs for children who are blind or visually disabled, emotionally and learning disabled and preschoolers who are developmentally delayed.

6511 Niagara Frontier Center for Independent Living

National Independent Living Council
1522 Main Street
Niagara Falls, NY 14305
716-284-2452
866-306-6245
FAX 716-284-0829
TDY:866-306-6245
http://www.md-nfeil.org
e-mail: info@nfcil.org

Kathleen Pautler, Executive Director
Michael DeVinney, Director Programs/Services
Patricia O'Kane, Office Manager

6512 Norman Howard School

275 Pinnacle Road
Rochester, NY 14623
585-334-8010
FAX 585-334-8073
http://www.normanhoward.org
e-mail: info@normanhoward.org

Marcie Roberts, Executive Director
Julie Murray, Associate Director of Admissions
Lawrence Student Dean, Student Dean

Norman Howard School is an independent day school for students with disabilities in 5-12th grade.

6513 Parent Network of WNY

1000 Main Street
Buffalo, NY 14202
716-332-4170
866-277-4762
FAX 716-332-4171
http://www.parentnetworkwny.org

Max Donatelli, Executive Director
Susan Barlow, Director Training

A non-profit agency with the mission of parents helping parents and professionals enable individuals with disabilities to reach their own potential. Parent Network provides parents/caregivers of children with special needs, the tools necessary to allow them to take an active role in their child's education. this is accomplished through: information and referral services, workshops and conferences on various special education topics, library and resource materials, website & bimonthly newsletter.

6514 Parent Support Network

Orangeburg, NY 10962
845-359-6090
http://www.parentsupportnetwork.org

Micki Leader, President
Duddy Vice President, Vice President

PSN is a network of parents, providing a strong voice for parents, whose priority is supporting, educating, and advocating for each other while raising children and adolescents with learning, emotional, developmental, social and behavioral disorders.

6515 Program for Learning Disabled College Students: Adelphi University

Eddy Hall Lower Level
Garden City, NY 11530
516-877-4850
800-ADELPHI
FAX 516-877-4711
TDY:516-877-4777
http://www.adelphi.edu

Robert Scott, President

6516 Responsibility Increases Self-Esteem (RISE) Program

Maplebrook School
5142 Route 22
Amenia, NY 12501
845-373-8673
FAX 845-373-7029
http://www.maplebrookschool.org
e-mail: admin@maplebrookschool.org

Jennifer Scully, Admissions Dean

The RISE program provides the structure and support to awaken the learner in each student, promote responsibility and develop character, foster independence and growth and enhances social development.

6517 Robert Louis Stevenson School

24 W 74th Street
New York, NY 10023
212-787-6400
FAX 212-873-1872
http://www.stevenson-school.org
e-mail: dherron@stevenson-school.org

Bud Henrichsen, Principal
Rick Couchman, Dean

An independent, therapeutic, coeducational college preparatory day school for students with learning disabilities.
12-18 years old

6518 Stephen Gaynor School

22 W 74th Street
New York, NY 10023
212-787-7070
FAX 212-787-3312
http://www.stephengaynor.org

Jackie Long, Admissions Director
Scott Gaynor, Operations Director
Yvette Siegel, Education Director

Our guiding principle is to provide a nurturing environment in which students with learning differences can acquire the skills they need to achieve success in their educational pursuits

6519 Vocational Independence Program (VIP)

New York Institute of Technology
Central Campus
Central Islip, NY 11722
631-348-3090
FAX 631-348-0437
http://www.vip-at-nyit.org
e-mail: info@vip-at-nyit.org

David Finkelstein, Director
Jim Rein, Dean
Rosemary Feeney, Executive Director

VIP is a three year certificate program for students with moderate to severe learning disabilities. Emphasizes independent living, social and vocational skills, as well as individual academic support, with a college support program called Track II for students who can take college credit courses or pursue a degree.

6520 Windward School

Windward Avenue
White Plains, NY 10605
914-949-6968
FAX 914-949-8220

Maureen Sweeney, Admissions Director
James Jay Russell, Head Master
James Amburg, Principal

Independent school for language-based, learning disabled students in grades 1-9.

North Carolina

6521 Comprehensive Educational Services (CES)

Manus Academy
6203 Carmel Road
Charlotte, NC 28226
704-542-6471
FAX 704-541-2858

Rosanne MA, President
Stan Covelski, Center Director
Jeremy Ervin, Principal

School for students with learning disabilties.

6522 Eastern Associates Speech and Language Services
PO Box 1316
Goldsboro, NC 27533
919-731-2234
FAX 919-731-2306
Rhonda Sutton-Merritt, Director

A private practice clinic providing diagnosis and treatment of speech and language disorders/differences. All speech pathologists hold a master's degree, are licensed by the NC Board of Examiners for Speech Pathologists and Audiologists and hold a Certificate of Clinical Competence issued by the American Speech-Language and Hearing Association.

6523 Exceptional Children's Assistance Center
Exceptional Children's Assistance Center
907 Barra Row
Davidson, NC 28036
704-892-1321
800-962-6817
FAX 704-892-5028
http://www.ecac-parentcenter.org
e-mail: information@ecac-parentcenter.org
Connie Hawkins, Executive Director
Mary Lacorte, PTI Director

Parent Training and Information Program views parents as full partners in the educational process and a significant source of support and assistance to each other. Funded by the Division of Personnel Preparation, Office of Special Education Programs, these programs provide training and information to parents to enable such individuals to participate more effectively with professionals in meeting the educational needs of disabled children.

6524 Hill Center
3200 Pickett Road
Durham, NC 27705
919-489-7464
FAX 919-489-7466
http://www.hillcenter.org
e-mail: smaskel@hillcenter.org
Sharon Maskel, Executive Director
Wendy Speir, Admissions Director

Offers a unique half-day program to students in grades K-12 with diagnosed learning disabilities and attention deficit disorders. Also offers a comprehensive teacher training program.

6525 Huntington Learning Center
7101 Creedmoor Road
Raleigh, NC 27613
919-676-5477
800-226-5327
http://www.huntingtonlearning.com
Lisa Mlinar, Vice President

Huntington Learning Center helps target your child's unique needs through diagnostic testing so they could better achieve their grades.

6526 Joy A Shabazz Center for Independent Living
235 N Greene Street
Greensboro, NC 27401
336-272-0501
FAX 336-272-0575
TDY:336-272-0501
http://www.shabazzcenter.org
e-mail: aaron.shabazz@shabazzcenter.org
Aaron Shabazz, Executive Director
Benita Williams, Deputy Director

A nonprofit, consumer oriented, independent living center providing advocacy, peer counseling, independent living training, information and referral, with other related services for persons with disabilities. We currently serve five counties.

6527 Manus Academy
6203 Carmel Road
Charlotte, NC 28226
704-542-6471
FAX 704-541-2858
Rosanne Manus, Owner
Jeremy Ervin, Principal

School and after-school tutoring servcie for students with learning disabilities, attention deficit disorder and other neurological difficulties.

6528 Piedmont School
815 Old Mill Road
High Point, NC 27265
336-883-0992
FAX 336-883-4752
http://www.thepiedmontschool.com
e-mail: info@thepiedmontschool.com
Ron Jones, President
Dorie Sturgill, Executive Director

Provides a unique, essential service to children with learning disabilites and/or an attention deficit disorder.

6529 Raleigh Learning and Language Clinic
7101 Creedmoor Road
Raleigh, NC 27613
919-676-5477
http://www.huntinglearning.com
Stan Kant, Contact

North Dakota

6530 Anne Carlsen Center for Children
701 3rd Street NW
Jamestown, ND 58401
701-252-3850
800-568-5175
FAX 701-952-5154
http://www.annecenter.org
e-mail: kevin.cooper@annecenter.org
Dan Howell, Administrator

Offers education, therapy, medical care and social and psychological services for children and young adults with special needs.

Ohio

6531 Bellefaire JCB
22001 Fairmount Boulevard
Shaker Heights, OH 44118
216-932-2800
800-879-2522
FAX 216-932-6704
http://www.bellefairjcb.org
Jill Yulish, Intake Coordinator
Debra Mundell, Associate Director
Adam Jacobs, CEO
Residential treatment center for adolescents, offering foster care, an adoption center, Monarch School for Children with Autism.

6532 Bellefaire Jewish Children's Bureau
22001 Fairmount Boulevard
Shaker Heights, OH 44118
216-932-2800
800-879-2522
FAX 216-932-6704
http://www.bellefairjcb.org
e-mail: info@bellefairjob.org
Larry Pollock, President
Adam Jacobs, CEO

Residential treatment center for adolescents, offering foster care, an adoption center, Monarch School for Children with Autism.

6533 Child Advocacy Center
131 N High Street
Columbus, OH 43215
614-221-7994
FAX 614-221-8442
http://www.oncac.org
e-mail: cadcenter@aol.com
Ben Murray, Executive Director

A training and information center for parents of children with special needs. It is funded by various federal, state, and local grants and is managed by parents of disabled children. Its goals are to assure that disabled children receive quality educational services in natural, age-appropriate settings and to help parents and other community members understand their rights and responsibilities under federal and state educational law.

6534 Cincinnati Center for Developmental Disorders
Children's Hospital Medical Center of Cincinnati
3333 Burnet Avenue
Cincinnati, OH 45229
513-636-4688
800-344-2462
FAX 513-636-7361
TDY:513-636-4623
http://www.cincinnatichildrens.org
e-mail: johnb0@chmcc.org
David Schonfeld, Executive Director
Jim Feuer, Media Relations Sr. Director
Judy Neubacher, Accountant
Established in 1957, the center provides diagnosis, evaluation, treatment, training and education for infants, children and adolescents with a variety of developmental disorders.

6535 Cincinnati Occupational Therapy Institute for Services and Study
4440 Carver Woods Drive
Cincinnati, OH 45242
513-791-5688
FAX 513-791-0023
http://www.cintiotinstitute.com
e-mail: coti@cintiotinstitute.com
Virginia Scardinia, Emeritus Director
Elaine Mullin, Executive Director

Cincinnati Occupational Therapy Institute provides evaluation and treatment directly to children and adults with occupational therapy needs. COTI is owned and operated by therapists. The therapists are uniquely skilled at helping clients of all ages achieve or regain independence by offering creative adaptations and alternatives for carrying out daily activities, as well as remediating dysfunction through appropriate therapeutic modalities.

6536 North Coast Tutoring Services and Education Services
120 N Main Street
Chagrin Falls, OH 44022
440-247-1622
800-335-7984
FAX 440-247-9049
http://www.northcoasted.com
e-mail: caroler@northcoasted.com
Carole Richards, Manager
John Kusik, Vice President

North Coast Tutoring Services strives to provide on-site education services to individual learners or groups. Uppermost in the delivery of these services is the development of self-esteem, expanding learner potential and utilizing problem-solving to identify strengths and weaknesses. Specializing in working with at-risk learners which include learning disabled students.

6537 Ohio Center for Autism and Low Incidence
5220 N High Street
Columbus, OH 43214
614-410-0321
FAX 614-410-1090
http://www.ocali.org
e-mail: ocali@ocali.org
Shawn A Henry, Executive Director
Amy Bixler, Autism Administrator

Serves parents and educators of students with autism and low incidence disabilities including Autism spectrum disorders, Deaf-blindness, Deafness and hearing impairments, Multiple disabilities, Orthopedic impairments, Other health impairments, Traumatic brain injuries, and Visual impairments.

6538 Ohio Coalition for the Education of Children with Learning Disabilities
165 W Center Street
Marion, OH 43302
740-382-5452
800-374-2806
FAX 740-382-6421
http://www.ocecd.org

Leeann Derugen, Manager

Funded by the Division of Personnel Preparation, Office of Special Education Programs, these programs provide training and information to parents to enable such individuals to participate more effectively with professionals in meeting the educational needs of disabled children.

6539 Olympus Center: Unlocking Learning Potential
2230 Park Avenue
Cincinnati, OH 45206
513-559-0404
FAX 513-559-0008
http://www.olympuscenter.org
e-mail: olympus@fuse.net
Sandy Martin, Executive Director
Eldridge Development Director, Development Director
Pat Wideam, Secretary
A non-profit organization established in 1976, provides diagnostic and consultative services for children, adolescents, and adults with learning problems.

6540 Olympus Center: Unlocking Learning Potential
2230 Park Avenue
Cincinnati, OH 45206
513-559-0404
FAX 513-559-0008
http://www.olympuscenter.org
e-mail: olympus@fuse.net

Sandy Martin, Director
Pat Wideam, Secretary

A nonprofit agency provides evaluations and consultations for children and adults by learning issues.

6541 RICHARDS READ Systematic Language
North Coast Tutoring Services
120 N Main Street
Chagrin Falls, OH 44022
440-247-1622
FAX 440-247-9049
http://www.northcoastad.com
e-mail: info@northcoastad.com

Carole Richards, Manager
John Kusik, Vice President

North Coast Tutoring Services strives to provide on-site education services to individual learners or groups. Uppermost in the delivery of these services is the development of self-esteem, expanding learner potential and utilizing problem-solving to identify strengths and weaknesses. We specialize in working with at-risk learners which include learning disabled students. Our systematic language program is extremely successful with language learning difficulties from age 5 to adult.

6542 Springer School and Center
2121 Madison Road
Cincinnati, OH 45208
513-871-6080
FAX 513-871-6428
http://www.springerschoolandcenter.org
e-mail: info@springer.hccanet.org
Shelly Weisbacher, Administrator
Susan Blanger, School Secretary

Springer School and Center is the only organization in the Greater Cincinnati area whose program is devoted entirely to the education of children with learning disabilities.

Oklahoma

6543 Pro-Oklahoma
UCP of Oklahoma
5208 W Reno Avenue
Oklahoma City, OK 73127
405-917-7080
FAX 405-917-7082
http://www.ucpok.org
e-mail: PROOK1@aol.com

Sharon Bishop, Director
Marilynn Alexander, Coordinator
Jim Rankin, Executive Director

Views parents as full partners in the educational process and a significant source of support and assistance to each other. Funded by the Division of Personnel Preparation, Office of Special Education Programs, these programs provide training and information to parents to enable such individuals to participate more effectively with professionals in meeting the educational needs of disabled children.

6544 Town and Country School
5150 E 101st Street
Tulsa, OK 74137 918-296-3113
Frances Day MA, Executive Director

A private school for learning disabled students, with or without attention deficit disorder. Class size limited to 12 persons, a certified teacher and an aide.

Oregon

6545 Chemetka Community College
Services for Students with Disabilities
PO Box 14007
Salem, OR 97309 503-399-5142
FAX 503-399-2519
TDY:503-399-5192
Michael Duggan, Disabilities Specialist

Chemetka Community College provides a wide variety of services for students including individualized tutoring, testing accommodations, books on tape, and adaptive technology to name a few.

6546 Cornell Vision Center
1010 NE Cornell Road
Hillsboro, OR 97124 503-640-3333
FAX 503-681-9459
e-mail: dianaeye@aol.com
Nancy Od, Manager
Diana Ludlam, Vision Therapist
Debbie Mish, Office Manager
Learning realted vision problems, visual aspects of cerebral palsy, head trauma, syndromes involving visual function.

6547 Learning Unlimited Network of Oregon
31960 SE Chin Street
Boring, OR 97009 503-663-5153
e-mail: luno@cse.com
Gene Lehman, Contact

Offers programs for home, group, business or institution, serving any number of students. These materials and programs can quickly change the habits, attitudes and performances of students mastering basic language skills, from elementary to adult levels.

6548 Services for Students with Disabilities
Chemeketa Community College
4000 Lancaster Drive NE
Salem, OR 97309 503-399-5192
FAX 503-399-2519
TDY:503-399-5192
http://www.chemeketa.edu/exploring/services/
e-mail: gibs@chemeketa.edu
Sharon Gibbons, Disabilities Services
Joslin Disabilities Services, Disabilities Services

Chemetka Community College provides a wide variety of services for students including individualized tutoring, testing accommodations, books on tape, and adaptive technology to name a few.

6549 Thomas A Edison Program
Thomas A Edison High School
9020 SW Beaverton Hillsdale Highway
Portland, OR 97225 503-297-2336
FAX 503-297-2527
http://www.taedisonhs.org
e-mail: thomasedison@taedisonhs.org
Patrick Maguire, Principal
Fram Dalby, Office Manager

A private high school in Oregon specifically designed to meet the needs of students with complex learning disabilities and attention deficit disorder issues. Thomas Edison High School empowers students with learning differences to experience academic success and personal growth, while preparing them for the future.

6550 Tree of Learning High School
9000 SW Beaverton Hillsdale Highway
Portland, OR 97225 503-297-2336
FAX 503-297-2527
http://www.taedisonhs.org
e-mail: thomasedison@taedisonhs.org
Patrick Maguire, Principal
Fram Dalby, Office Manager

Pennsylvania

6551 Center for Alternative Learning
PO Box 716
Bryn Mawr, PA 19010 610-525-8336
800-869-8336
FAX 610-525-8337
http://www.learningdifferences.com
e-mail: rcooper-ldr@comcast.net
Dr. Richard Cooper, MD, Founder/President

The Center for Alternative Learning was founded in 1987 to provide low cost and free educational services to individuals with learning differences, problems and disabilities.

6552 Center for Psychological Services
125 Coulter Avenue
Ardmore, PA 19003 610-642-4873
FAX 610-642-4886
http://www.centerpsych.com
e-mail: center12@verizon.net
Moss Jackson Ph.D, Partner

Individual, family and group therapy psychoeducational evaluation and school consultation.

6553 Cornell Abraxas I
PO Box 59
Marienville, PA 16239 814-927-6615
800-227-2927
FAX 814-927-8560
Jamesl Nawsome, Facility Director
Herb Connell, Principal

6554 Devereux Brandywine
Devereux Beneto Campus
PO Box 69
Glenmoore, PA 19343 610-942-5900
800-935-6789
FAX 610-251-2415
http://www.devereux.org
Robert Kreider, President/CEO
Sue Schofield, Administrative Support
Marylou Hettinger, Manager
Provides residential, clinical, and special education programs for boys with behavorial and emotional problems. Brandywine's special education programs are designed to meet both academic and therapeutic needs.

6555 Devereux Foundation
PO Box 638
Villanova, PA 19085 610-542-3090
800-935-6789
FAX 610-25124150
Offers residential and community-based treatment centers nationwide. Provides comprehensive services to individuals of all ages.

6556 Devereux Mapleton
Devereux Foundation
PO Box 275
Malvern, PA 19355
610-296-6973
800-935-6789
FAX 610-296-5866
http://www.devereux.org
Walter Grono, Executive Director
Howard Jarden, Assistant Executive Director

Residential and in-patient program for children, adolescents and young adults with emotional disorders and learning disabilities.
13-21 years old

6557 Dr. Gertrude A Barber Center
Dr.Gertrude A Barber Center
136 E Avenue
Erie, PA 16507
814-453-7661
FAX 814-455-1132
http://www.barbernationalinstitute.org
John Barber, President
Bob Will, Sr. Vice President

An individualized educational program designed for preschool and school-aged students.

6558 Dr. Gertrude A Barber National Institute
100 Barber Place
Erie, PA 16507
814-453-7661
FAX 814-455-1132
http://www.barbernationalinstitute.org
e-mail: BNIerie@barberinstitute.org
John Barber, President
Bob Will, Sr. Vice President

An individualized educational program designed for preschool and school-aged students.

6559 Hill Top Preparatory School
737 S Ithan Avenue
Bryn Mawr, PA 19010
610-527-3230
FAX 610-527-7683
http://www.hilltopprep.org
e-mail: headmaster@hilltopprep.org
Cindy Falcone, Acting Headmaster
Anne Scali, Associate Admissions Director
Les Lean, Principal
A fully-accredited, state-licensed, private, secondary, diploma-granting school for the learning disabled adolescent combining academic and clinical components to provide a preparatory program.

6560 Hillside School
2697 Brookside Road
Macungie, PA 18062
610-967-3701
FAX 610-965-7683
http://www.hillsideschool.org
e-mail: office@hillsideschool.org
Dr Sue Straeter, Head of School
Donna Heway, Assistant Head of School
Kathy Green, Development Director
A day school for children with learning differences. One hundred and twenty-eight children in grades K-6 attend the school. Scholarships are available.
6-12 years old

6561 KidsPeace
5300 Kidspeace Drive
Orefield, PA 18069
800-8KID-123
http://www.kidspeace.org
e-mail: admissions@kidspeace.org
John Peter, President

Offers various programs including community residential care, specialized group homes, child and family guidance center and student assistance programs.

6562 Melmark
2600 Wayland Road
Berwyn, PA 19312
610-353-1726
888-635-6275
FAX 610-353-4956
http://www.melmark.org
e-mail: admissions@melmark.org
Joanne Gillis-Donovan, President

Provides residential, educational, therapeutic and recreational services for children and adults with mild to severe developmental disabilities.

6563 New Castle School of Trades
RR 1
Pulaski, PA 16143
724-964-8811
FAX 724-964-8177
http://www.ncstrades.com
Rex Spaulding, Administrator

New Castle School of Trades is dedicated to your success because we understand that investing in people makes all the difference. Experienced instructors challenge you to develop personal responsibility and practical work skills in a hands-on format. New Castle School of Trades' students find out first-hand that people make the difference.

6564 Parent Education Network
Parent Education Network
2107 Industrial Highway
York, PA 17402
717-234-0665
800-522-5827
FAX 717-600-8101
TDY:800-522-5827
http://www.parentednet.org
e-mail: pen@parentednet.org
Louise Thieme, Manager

Parent training and information center of Pennsylvania. Serves parents of all special needs children, birth to adulthood, to attain appropriate educational and support services by providing specific knowledge of state and federal laws and regulations; develops and disseminates material explaining the special education process and its relationship to other systems.

6565 Parents Union for Public Schools
228 W Chelten Avenue
Philadelphia, PA 19144
215-991-9724
FAX 215-991-9943
e-mail: ParentsU@aol.com
Parent Training and Information Program views parents as full partners in the educational process and a significant source of support and assistance to each other. Funded by the Division of Personnel Preparation, Office of Special Education Programs, these programs provide training and information to parents to enable such individuals to participate more effectively with professionals in meeting the educational needs of disabled children.

6566 Pathway School
162 Egypt Road
Norristown, PA 19403
610-277-0660
FAX 610-539-1493
http://www.pathwayschool.org
e-mail: KayB@PathwaySchool.org
William Flanagan Ph.D, President
William Rennekemt, Education Director
William Kirkpatrick, Administration Director
Provides day and residential programming for individuals ages 5-21, who have learning disabilities, neurological impairments and neuropsychiatric disorder. Special education, counseling, speech and language therapy, reading therapy, and other specialized services are provided in a small, warm and supportive atmosphere.

6567 Rehabilitation Institute of Pittsburgh
1405 Shady Avenue
Pittsburgh, PA 15217
412-521-9000
http://www.amazingkids.org
e-mail: aeh@the-institute.org

Jamie Calabrese, MD, Medical Director
Haid Community Resources Di, Community Resources Director

Originally known as the Home For Crippled Children and in recent years, The Rehabilitation Institute. Today, as the region's leader in providing pediatric rehabilitation services, The Children's Institute provides individualized treatment programs along a broad continuum of care: inpatient care, outpatient care, transitional and subacute care, home care and The Day School.

6568 Rosemont College
1400 Montgomery Avenue
Bryn Mawr, PA 19010
610-527-0200
888-276-6668
FAX 610-527-0341
http://www.rosemont.edu
e-mail: dklinman@rosemont.edu
Dr. Sharon Latchaw Hirsh Ph.D, President
Catherine Fennell, Manager

Offers a variety of services to students with disabilities including notetakers, extended testing time, counseling services, and special accommodations.

6569 Stratford Friends School
5 Llandillo Road
Havertown, PA 19083
610-446-3144
FAX 610-446-6381
http://www.stratfordfriends.org
Sandra Howze, Principal
Nadia Murray, Admissions

A Quaker elementary school for children with learning differences with average to above average intelligence.

6570 Thaddeus Stevens College of Technology
Special Needs Department
750 E King Street
Lancaster, PA 17602
717-299-7408
800-THAD-TEC
FAX 717-391-6929
http://www.stevenstech.org
e-mail: schuch@stevenscollege.edu
Debra Schuch, Special Needs Coordinator

The Special Needs Department at the Thaddeus Stevens College of Technology provides assistance to disabled students making the transition. Accommodations, material, and support services are offered and encouraged to be used for a successful entry into the college.

6571 Vanguard School
PO Box 730
Paoli, PA 19301
610-296-6700
FAX 610-640-0132
http://www.vanguardschool-pa.org
Ernie Beattstrom, Principal
Tim Lanshe, Director Education

State licensed and approved private, non-profit, non-sectarian day school serving children from three to twenty-one years of age who have been diagnosed with neurological disorders, emotional disturbance or autism/PDD.

6572 Woods Schools
Residential Center
PO Box 36
Langhorne, PA 19047
215-750-4000
FAX 215-750-4229
http://www.woods.org
Robert Griffith, President
Mary Knudson, Administrative Assistant

Provides a full range of residential, special education, rehabilitation, recreation and vocational training.

6573 Woods Services
Routes 413 & 213
Langhorne, PA 19047
215-750-4000
FAX 215-750-4229
http://www.woods.org
Robert Griffith, President

Woods Services provides residential, educational and vocational supports for children and adults with exceptional needs. What makes Woods distinctive is its ability to meet the diverse needs of individuals who face an array of life challenges.

Rhode Island

6574 Harmony Hill School
63 Harmony Hill Road
Chepachet, RI 02814
401-949-0690
FAX 401-949-2060
TDY:401-949-4130
http://www.harmonyhillschool.org
e-mail: djackson@hhs.org
Janice DeFrances Ed.D, President/CEO
Terrence Leary, Administrator

A private residential and day treatment center for behaviorally disordered and learning disabled boys, age eight through eighteen, who cannot be treated within their local educational system or community based mental health programs. Individual, group and family psychotherapy and 24-hour crisis intervention are available. Other programs include: Extended Day, Sex Offender, Diagnostic Day, Transition Programming, Summer Day, Career Education Center, and a Formalized Life Skills Program.

6575 Rhode Island Parent Information Network
175 Main Street
Pawtucket, RI 02860
401-727-4040
800-464-3399
FAX 401-727-4040
TDY:800-464-3399
http://www.ripin.org
e-mail: ripin@ripin.org
Vivian Wiseman, Manager
Matthew Cox, Associate Director

Rhode Island Parent Information Network is a statewide, nonprofit organization that provides eleven programs and services to families with children in RI, including families of children with special needs due to disabilities.

South Carolina

6576 Gateway School
PO Box 1082
Aiken, SC 29802
803-642-5067
Nancy Elliot, Executive Director

School geared for grades K-8 for children with learning disabilities.

6577 Parents Reaching Out to Parents of South Carolina
652 Bush River Road
Columbia, SC 29210
803-772-5688
800-759-4776
FAX 803-772-5341
http://www.proparents.org
e-mail: PROParents@proparents.org
Mary Eaddy, Executive Director

Private nonprofit parent oriented organization providing information, individual assistance and workshops to parents of children with disabilities ages birth-21. Services focus on enabling parents to have a better understanding of special education to participate more effectively with professionals in meeting the educational needs of disabled children. Funded by a grant from the US Department of Education and tax deductible contributions.

6578 **Pine Grove**
PO Box 100
Elgin, SC 29045
803-438-3011
FAX 803-438-8611
e-mail: carlmets@aol.com
Anita Gotwals, Executive Director
Melanie Stevens, Office Assistant

Offers an intensive academic, social skills and behavior modification program designed to return the child to his/her home area as soon as possible.

6579 **Sandhills Academy**
1500 Hallbrook Drive
Columbia, SC 29209
803-695-1400
http://http://sandhillsacademy.com
Joan Hathaway, Director
Anne Vickers, Executive Director

A private, nonprofit school for children with learning disabilities. Serves students from grades 1-8 and also offers diagnostic evaluations, summer school and educational therapy for all ages. Boarding with local families is also available.

6580 **Trident Academy**
1455 Wakendaw Road
Mt Pleasant, SC 29464
843-884-7046
FAX 843-881-8320
http://www.tridentacademy.com
e-mail: cnewton@tridentacademy.com
Myron Harrington, Principal

Trident Academy is for students with specific learning disabilities; offering an intensive, effective, multi-sensory program to remediate learning differences, tailored to each student's unique needs.

Tennessee

6581 **Bodine School**
2432 Yester Oaks Drive
Germantown, TN 38139
901-754-1800
FAX 901-751-8595
http://www.bodineschool.org
e-mail: info@bodineschool.org
Rene Friemoth Lee Ph.D, Director

The Bodine School has provided students with language based learning disabilities a nurturing environment and a challenging academic curriculum for the last 30 years. The Bodine School program is designed specifically for the dyslexic student and is based on current research findings on reading and reading disorders.

6582 **Camelot Care Center**
183 Fiddlers Lane
Kingston, TN 37763
865-376-2296
Randy Yeager, Executive Director

6583 **Camelot School of Tennessee**
183 Fiddlers Lane
Kingston, TN 37763
865-376-2296
800-896-4754
FAX 865-376-1950
http://www.thecamelotschools.com/Kingston
Randy Yeager, Executive Director
Tammy Kropp, School Principal
Watts Admissions Coordinator, Admissions Coordinator
A psychiatric treatment center serving children with emotional disturbances and learning disabilities. Services include Residential Treatment, Partial Hospitalization (day treatment), Intensive Outpatient, and Therapeutic Day School. All programs are designed to provide children and families with the skills needed to successfully reemerge and reintegrate themselves back into society as productive and positive individuals.

6584 **Devereux Genesis Learning Centers**
Genesis Learning Centers
430 Allied Drive
Nashville, TN 37211
615-832-4222
FAX 615-832-4577
http://www.genesislearn.org
Terry Adams, President
Melissa Adams, Vice President
Terance Adams, Executive Director
Day school and treatment programs for adolescents and young adults who have emotional disorders and learning disabilities.

6585 **Genesis Learning Centers**
430 Allied Drive
Nashville, TN 37211
615-832-4222
FAX 615-832-4577
http://www.genesislearn.org
e-mail: cgoon@genesislearn.org
Terry Adams, President
Terance Adams, Executive Director

Genesis Learning Centers offer special educational services to children and youth with distinctive needs, including emotional and behavioral disorders, learning disabilities, mental retardation, developmental delays, and short-term severe illness, physical challenges, or misconduct.

Texas

6586 **Bridges Academy**
901 Arizona Avenue
El Paso, TX 79902
915-532-8767
FAX 915-532-8767
http://www.bridgesacademy.org
e-mail: bridgesacademy@sbcglobal.net
Irma Keys, Director

Private School for students with learning disabilities.

6587 **Bright Students Who Learn Differently**
Winston School
5707 Royal Lane
Dallas, TX 75229
214-691-6950
FAX 214-691-1509
http://www.winston-school.org
e-mail: amy_smith@winston-school.org
Joe Ferber, Interim Head of School
Amy Smith, Admission Director
Pamela Murfin, Manager
The Winston School is a co-educational day college preparatory school, grades 1-12. Winston provides individualized programs for students with learning differences, including problems in reading, writing, language and mathematics, as well as attention-deficit/hyperactivity disorder. Student teacher ratio of 8:1. Founded in 1975 in a suburban 6-acre campus, 4 buildings on campus. Winston is accredited by the Independent Schools Association of the Southwest (ISAS) and a member of NAIS.

6588 **Crisman Preparatory School**
2455 N Eastman Road
Longview, TX 75605
903-758-9741
FAX 903-758-9767
Lucy Peacock, Director
Patricia Duck, Executive Director

6589 **Crisman School**
2455 N Eastman Road
Longview, TX 75605
903-758-9741
FAX 903-758-9767
http://www.crismanprep.org
Patricia Duck, Executive Director
Lucy Peacock, Director

A private school designed to meet the needs of students with learning differences and/or Attention Deficit Disorder.

6590 Diagnostic and Remedial Reading Clinic
622 Isom Road
San Antonio, TX 78216
210-341-7417
FAX 210-341-7417

Margo PhD

Provides complete psychological and educational evaluations; diagnostic and remedial services for academic problems; one-on-one instruction in all academic subjects; and consultation and evaluation services to public and private schools.

6591 Gateway School
2570 NW Green Oaks Boulevard
Arlington, TX 76012
817-226-6222
FAX 817-226-6225
http://www.gatewayschool.com

Harriet Walber, Executive Director
Marsha Godfrey, Administrative Assistant

Geteway School is dedicated to providing an appropriate education in a nurturing environment to individuals with learning disorders and/or attention deficit.

6592 Gateway School: Arlington
Gateway School
2570 NW Green Oaks Boulevard
Arlington, TX 76012
817-226-6222
FAX 817-226-6225
http://www.gatewayschool.com

Harriet Walber, Executive Director
Marsha Godfrey, Administrative Assistant

The only nonprofit accredited secondary school in the Forth Worth/Arlington area addressing academic and social challenges of students. Students who successfully complete the program earn a high school diploma.

6593 Houston Learning Academy
3333 Bering Drive
Houston, TX 77057
713-789-9197
FAX 713-975-6666
http://www.nobellearning.com/hla

Susan McKinney, Executive Director
Shari Schiftman, Operations Controller

A year round, private high school serving students that need a flexible, personalized approach to high school.

6594 Keystone Academy
306 Woodcrest Drive
Richardson, TX 75080
972-250-4455
FAX 734-697-9471
http://www.heritageacademies.com

Phil Price, Principal
Murray Assistant Principal, Assistant Principal

The academy provides students with a curriculum that is challenging and effective. The instructional program will utilize a balanced core program of study that emphasizes basic skills such as reading, English, science and mathematics. In addition, the teaching of virtues, such as responsibility, respect, courage and perseverance, will be integrated into the instructional program to help students develop into caring and responsible citizens.

6595 Lane Learning Center
230 W Main Street
Lewisville, TX 75057
972-221-2564
888-412-5263
FAX 972-436-6964
http://www.lanelearningcenter.com/
e-mail: info@lanelearningcenter.com

Dr. Kenneth Lane, Founder/Owner

Lane Learning Center evaluates and helps children who are struggling in school. The center specializes in helping children with Attention Deficit Disorders, Dyslexia, and Learning/Reading Disorders.

6596 Neuhaus Education Center
Neuhaus Education Center
4433 Bissonnet Street
Bellaire, TX 77401
713-664-7676
FAX 713-664-4744
http://www.neuhaus.org
e-mail: info@neuhaus.org

Kay Allen, Executive Director
Suzzanne Carreker, Program Development Director

Dyslexia specialist training courses and workshops for regular education teaching, parent consultation and adult literacy classes.

6597 Overton Speech and Language Center
Overton Speech and Language Center
4763 Barwick Drive
Fort Worth, TX 76132
817-294-8408
FAX 817-294-8411
http://www.overtonspeech.net
e-mail: info@overtonspeech.net

Valerie Johnston, Director

Provides speech and language therapy.

6598 Parish School
11001 Hammerly Boulevard
Houston, TX 77043
713-467-4696
FAX 713-467-8341
http://www.parishschool.org

Robbin Parish, Founder
Nancy Bewley, Principal
Margaret Noecker, School Head

Offers a multi-age, language-based, developmental curriculum for children 18 months through fifth grade. Children served have communication and learning differences, but average to above average learning potential. The Parish School utilizes a classroom based therapy program implemented by certified teachers and speech/language pathologists.

6599 Partners Resource Network
1090 Longfellow Drive
Beaumont, TX 77706
409-898-4684
800-866-4726
FAX 409-898-4869
http://www.partnerstx.org
e-mail: partnersresource@sbcglobal.net

Janice Meyer, Executive Director
Alice Robertson, Training Coordinator

Established in 1986 to assist families of children with all types of disabilities throughout the state. The mission of the agency is to empower individuals with disabilities and their families to be effective advocates and decision makers, and to promote equal partnerships between parents/individuals with disabilities and professionals.

6600 Psychoeducational Diagnostic Services
7233 Brentfield Drive
Dallas, TX 75248
972-931-5299
FAX 972-392-7155

Harrian Stern PhD, Educator Diagnostician

Psychoeducational diagnostic assessment of intellectual and academic ability, including assessing the ability of students with various learning styles. Offers consultations with parents, schools, etc.

6601 Psychology Clinic of Fort Worth
4200 S Hulen Street
Fort Worth, TX 76109
817-731-0888

William Norman PhD, Contact

6602 SHIP Resource Center
University United Methodist Church
5084 De Zavala Road
San Antonio, TX 78249
210-696-1033
http://www.uumcsatx.org
e-mail: uumcsatx@uumcsatx.org

Vicki Spangler, Special Needs Director
Karen Andrews, Assistant Director
Mike Lowry, Director

6603 Scottish Rite Learning Center
Scottish Rite Mason
PO Box 10135
Lubbock, TX 79408
806-765-9150
FAX 806-765-9564
e-mail: srlcwt@nts-online.net
Doris Haney, Executive Director
Linda Stringer, Director

Language training for students at risk for dyslexia.

6604 Scottish Rite Learning Center of Austin
1622 E Riverside
Austin, TX 78741
512-472-1231
FAX 512-326-1877
http://www.scottishritelearningcenter.org
Linda Gladden, Director
Doris Haney, Executive Director

Provides dyslexic individuals with a proven research-based, multisensory approach for learning the basic language skills of reading, writing, and spelling, through the ongoing charitable commitment of the Scottish Rite Masons.

6605 Shelton School and Evaluation Center
Special Services Office
15720 Hillcrest Road
Dallas, TX 75248
972-774-1772
FAX 972-991-3977
http://www.shelton.org
e-mail: jdodd@shelton.org
Joyce Pickering, Executive Director
Sandy Ritchie, Special Support Services
Betty Glasheen, Principal
A coeducational day school serving 840 students in grades Pre-K-12. The school focuses on the development of learning disabled students of average to above average intelligence, enabling them to succeed in conventional classroom settings. Services include on-site Evaluation Center for diagnostic testing, a Speech, Language and Hearing Clinic, an Early Childhood Program, open summer school and more.

6606 Star Ranch
Star Program
149 Camp Scenic Road
Ingram, TX 78025
830-367-4868
FAX 830-367-2814
http://www.starranch.org
e-mail: rsouthard@starranch.org
Rand Southard, Executive Director

Two programs at Star Ranch; one is a recreational/educational summer camp for children with learning difficulties. Boys and girls ages 7-18 attend one or two week sessions during the summer. Traditional summer camp activities as well as academic tutoring are offered. The second is a residential treatment center for boys ages 7-17 who are diagnosed as learning disabled and emotionally disturbed. Preference is given to younger boys as placement is long term.

6607 Starpoint School
Texas Christian University
PO Box 297900
Fort Worth, TX 76129
817-257-7960
FAX 817-257-7466
http://www.sofe.tcu.edu
e-mail: education@tcu.edu

Kathleen Williams, Director
Barbara Trice, School Secretary
Craig Smith, Executive Director

6608 UUMC Day School
University United Methodist Church
5084 De Zavala Road
San Antonio, TX 78249
210-691-2704
http://www.uumcsatx.org
e-mail: uumcsatx@uumcsatx.org
Rev. Charles Anderson, Pastor Director

The purpose of the University United Methodist Church Day School Ministry is to provide a Christian environment where experiences help children to develop spiritually, cognitively, socially, emotionally, physically, and to foster Christian growth of the entire family.

6609 VIP Educational Services
4808 Chadbury Civic
Austin, TX 78727
512-345-9274
FAX 512-345-0314
http://www.learnatvip.com
e-mail: vip_educational@hotmail.com
Roberta Rosen, Owner

A diagnostic and tutoring service providing help to children and adults with learning disabilities, dyslexia, ADHD, and underachievement. Enrichment, organization, time management, study skills, and test taking strategies are also addressed. An assessment process identifies learning strengths and weaknesses. Advocacy for parents and students is provided.

6610 Vickery Meadow Learning Center
6329 Ridgecrest Road
Dallas, TX 75231
214-265-5057
FAX 214-265-1666
e-mail: vmlcforliteracy@aol.com
Judy Jacks, Executive Director

Utah

6611 Mountain Plains Regional Resource Center
1780 Research Parkway
Logan, UT 84341
435-752-0238
FAX 435-753-9750
TDY:435-753-9750
http://www.rrfcnetwork.org
e-mail: John.Copenhaver@usu.edu
John Copenhaver, Executive Director
Carol Massanari, Co-Director

The center is a United States Department of Education, Office of Special Education Programs funded project that helps build the capacity of State Education Agencies and Lead Agencies in improving programs and services for infants, toddlers, children and youth with disabilities.

6612 Reid School
3310 S 2700 E
Salt Lake City, UT 84109
801-486-5083
800-468-3274
http://www.reidschool.com
e-mail: ereid@xmission.com
Dr. Ethna Reid, Executive Director
Angela Burke, Office Manager

Reid School is a private, innovative center for students who need more attention with reading, writing, speaking, and language arts education.

6613 SEPS Center for Learning
SEPS Center for Learning
2120 S 1300 E
Salt Lake City, UT 84106
801-467-2122
FAX 801-467-2148
http://www.sepslc.com
e-mail: ava.eva.seps@sepslc.com
Avasane Pickering Phd, Director
Evajean Pickering, Executive Director

Designs educational programs that help adults and children succeed in school and life. Specializing in one-on-one tutoring in all areas for all age levels, assessment, day school and preschool programs, computer assisted cognitive and academic therapy, reading programs, summer recreation and academic programs, consultation for schools and businesses.

6614 Utah Parent Center
2290 E 4500 S
Salt Lake City, UT 84117
801-272-1051
800-468-1160
FAX 801-272-8907
http://www.utahparentcenter.org
e-mail: ftofninfo@utahparentcenter.org
Helen Post, Executive Director
Jeanne Gibson, Associate Director

Utah Parent Center offers free training, information, referral and assistance to parents and professionals through the provision of information, referrals, individual assistance, workshops, presentations and displays.

Vermont

6615 Pine Ridge School
Pine Ridge School
9505 Williston Road
Williston, VT 05495
802-434-2161
FAX 802-434-5512
http://www.pineridgeschool.com
e-mail: prs@pineridgeschool.com
Josh Doyle, Admissions Director
Shannon Dixon, Assistant Director for Admission
Douglas Dague, Manager
Serves students who have been diagnosed with a primary, specific language disability or a non-verbal learning disability. They are in the average range of intelligence and want to use those strengths in their remediation of their language weaknesses.

6616 Stern Center for Language and Learning
135 Allen Brook Lane
Williston, VT 05495
802-878-2332
FAX 802-878-0230
http://www.sterncenter.org
e-mail: learning@sterncenter.org
Blanche Podhajski Ph.D, President/Founder

Founded in 1983, the center is a nonprofit organization providing comprehensive services for children and adults with learning disabilities. The Center is also an educational resource serving all of Northern New England and Northern New York State. Programs include educational testing, individual instruction, psychotherapy, school consultation, professional training for educators and a parent/professional resource library.

Virginia

6617 Accolink Academy
8519 Tuttle Road
Springfield, VA 22152
703-451-8041
FAX 703-451-0336
http://www.accotinkacademy.com
e-mail: preschool@accotinkacademy.com
Julia Warden, Principal
Nesrin Elbannen, Administrative Assistant

Designed to teach those developmentally appropriate skills that are necessary for a child to succeed at a higher level of learning through a structured/non-structured environment.

6618 Achievment Center, The
PO Box 19249
Roanoke, VA 24019
540-366-7399
FAX 540-366-5523
http://www.achievementcenter.org
e-mail: info@achievementcenter.org
Rebecca Clendenin, Executive Director

A private day school for children with specific learning disabilities and attention deficit disorder.

6619 Chesapeake Bay Academy
821 Baker Road
Virginia Beach, VA 23462
757-497-6200
FAX 757-497-6304
http://www.chesapeakebayacademy.org
e-mail: contact@chesapeakebayacademy.net
Maryanne Dukas, Administrator
Hunter Wortham, Admissions Director

Chesapeake Bay Academy is the only accredited independent school in Southeastern Virginia specifically dedicated to providing a strong academic program and individualized instruction for bright students with LD and ADHD. With a student/teacher ratio of 5:1 a student:computer ratio of 2:1, qualified professionals tailor their techniques to individual needs, allowing students who have difficulty learning in traditional settings to finally succed.

6620 Crawford First Education
Alternative Behavioral Services
825 Crawford Parkway
Portsmouth, VA 23704
757-391-6675
877-227-7000
FAX 757-391-6651
http://www.absfirst.com
e-mail: info@absfirst.com
Millie Davis, Director

Alternative education programs that are effective, comprehensive and fiscally responsible. Dedicated and committed to addressing and improving the problems of special needs students.

6621 Fairfax House
3300 Woodburn Road
Annandale, VA 22003
703-560-6116
FAX 703-560-6592
Bruce Wyman, Executive Director

6622 Grafton School
PO Box 2500
Winchester, VA 22604
540-722-3764
888-955-5205
FAX 540-542-1722
http://www.grafton.org
e-mail: admis@grafton.org
Don Davis, Admissions Supervisor
Mark Wilee, Principal

Grafton provides individualized educational and residential services and in-community supports for children, youth and adults with severe emotional disturbance, learning disabilities, mental retardation, autistic disorder, behavioral disorders, and other complex challenges, including physical disabilities.

6623 Learning Center of Charlottesville
338 Rio Road W
Charlottesville, VA 22901
434-977-6006
FAX 434-977-6009
http://www.cvillelearning.org
Linda Harding, Executive Director
Eileen Perrino, Assistant Director

Individualized one-on-one tutoring for children and adults year round. Consultations. Educational and psychological evaluations.

6624 Learning Resource Center
909 1st Colonial Road
Virginia Beach, VA 23454
757-428-3367
FAX 757-428-1630
http://www.learningresourcecenter.net
e-mail: Nancy.Harris-Kroll@LearningResourceCenter.net
Nancy Harris-Kroll, Owner

One-on-one remedial and tutorial sessions after school during the school year and all day and evening during the summer with specialists who have masters degrees. Advocacy services for parents of students with special needs. Psychoeducational testing is available. Special study skills and SAT courses given. Gifted, average, and learning disabled students attend.

6625 Leary School Programs
Lincolnia Educational Foundation
6349 Lincolnia Road
Alexandria, VA 22312
703-941-8150
FAX 703-941-4237
http://www.learyschool.org
e-mail: learyschool@bellatlantic.net
Ed Schultze, Executive Director
Mary Sproull, Owner
Francesca Creo, Program Director
A private, day, co-educational, special education facility that serves 130 students with emotional, learning and behavioral problems. Along with individualized academic instruction, Leary School of Virginia offers a range of supportive and therapeutic services, including physical education, recreation therapy, group counseling, individual psychotherapy and art therapy.

6626 Leary School of Virginia
Special Services Department
6349 Lincolnia Road
Alexandria, VA 22312
703-914-1110
FAX 703-941-4237
http://www.learyschool.org
e-mail: learyschool@bellatlantic.net
Ed Schultze, Executive Director
Mary Sproull, Owner
Francesca Creo, Program Director
A private, day, co-educational, special education facility. Currently serves 130 students, ages six to 21, with emotional, learning and behavioral problems. Along with individualized academic instruction, Leary School of Virginia offers a range of supportive and therapeutic services, including physical education, recreation therapy, group counseling, individual psychotherapy and art therapy.

6627 Little Keswick School
PO Box 24
Keswick, VA 22947
434-295-0457
FAX 434-977-1892
http://www.avenue.org/oks
Mark Columbus, Principal

A residential special education school for 30 boys with emotional disturbances, learning disabilities and educable mental retardation with highly structured academic and behavioral programs.

6628 Mental Health Day Support Services
Fairfax County Mental Health Services
12011 Government Center Parkway
Annandale, VA 22003
703-560-6116
FAX 703-560-6592
http://www.fairfaxcounty.gov
e-mail: wwwcsb@fairfaxcounty.gov
John DeFee Ph.D, Program Manager

These programs provide intensive treatment, vocational support or psychiatric rehabilitation services for persons with serious mental illness or emotional disturbance who require continuous support to live independently in the community.

6629 New Community School
4211 Hermitage Road
Richmond, VA 23227
804-266-2494
FAX 804-264-3281
http://www.tncs.org
e-mail: admissions@tncs.org
Julia Greenwood, Principal
Gita Morris, Director of Studies

The New Community School is an independent day school specializing in college preparatory instruction and intensive remediation for dyslexic students in grades 6-12.

6630 New Vistas School
520 Eldon Street
Lynchburg, VA 24501
434-846-0301
FAX 434-528-1004
http://www.newvistasschool.org
Lucy Ross, Executive Director

6631 Oakwood School
7210 Braddock Road
Annandale, VA 22003
703-941-5788
FAX 703-941-4186
http://www.oakwoodschool.com
e-mail: rporter@oakwoodschool.com
Robert McIntyre, Manager
Muriel Jedlicka, Admissions Specialist

Oakwood School is a private, non-profit, co-educational day school for elementary and middle school students with mild to moderate learning disabilities. Students are of average to above average potential and exhibit a discrepancy between their potential and their current level of achievement.

6632 Parent Resource Center
Hopewell Public Schools
1807 Arlington Road
Hopewell, VA 23860
804-541-6408
FAX 804-541-6405
http://www.hopewell.k12.va.us
e-mail: a_lcbrown@hopewell.k12.va.us
Linda Ciancio-Brown, Parent Coordinator
Joni Hunphries, Educator
Sandra Morton, Principal
Established in 1990, the center's purpose is to provide training, support, and information for parents and educators of students with disabilities.

6633 Pines Residential Treatment Center
Pines Residential Treatment Center
825 Crawford Parkway
Portsmouth, VA 23704
757-393-0061
877-227-7000
FAX 877-846-6237
http://www.absfirst.com
e-mail: info@absfirst.com
Lenard Lexier, Executive Medical Director

6634 Riverside School for Dyslexia
2110 McRae Road
Richmond, VA 23235
804-320-3465
FAX 804-320-6146
http://www.riversideschool.org
e-mail: info@riversideschool.org
Patricia Orio, Manager

Private, co-educational day school that provides multi-sensory, structured and rational education for children with specific learning disabilities.

6635 Riverview Learning Center
StoneBridge School
4225 Portsmouth Boulevard
Chesapeake, VA 23321
757-488-7586
FAX 757-465-8995
http://www.kerri.intellisite.elexio.com
e-mail: info@stonebridgeschool.com
Trudy Webb, Program Coordinator
Cease Admissions Director, Admissions Director

At Riverview Learning Center, students gain the learning skills they need and develop the confidence to be willing, enthusiastic learners, who are able to live up to their full potential.

6636 StoneBridge Schools: Riverview Learning Center
PO Box 9247
Chesapeake, VA 23321
757-488-7586
FAX 757-465-8995

Trudy Webb, Director of Riverview Learning C
Jim Arcieri, Head Master

Centers on stimulating each student's area of weakness in perception, language and cognition. We also work with each student's problem-solving and organizational skills.

Washington

6637 Children's Institute for Learning Differences: Consultation and Training
4030 86th Avenue SE
Mercer Island, WA 98040
206-232-8680
FAX 206-232-9377
http://www.childrensinstitute.com
e-mail: robbo@bevdchildrenistitute.com
Kristine Frost, Admissions/PR Director
Trina Westerlund, Executive Director

Providing a wide array of consultation services and training opportunities to parents and community professionals, as well as ongoing teacher training for our staff.

6638 Children's Institute for Learning Differences
4030 86th Avenue SE
Mercer Island, WA 98040
206-232-8680
FAX 206-232-9377
http://www.childrensinstitute.com
e-mail: TrisaH@ChildrensInstitute.com
Trina Westerlund, Executive Director
Kristine Frost, Admissions/PR Director

CHILD provides two therapeutic year-round day schools, serving students who learn differently and who process information and life experiences in a unique way. CHILD offers on-site occupational and speech therapy, individual, group and family counseling.

6639 Glen Eden Institute
19351 8th Avenue NE
Poulsbo, WA 98370
360-697-0125
FAX 360-697-4712
http://www.glenedeninstitute.com
e-mail: director@glenedeninstitute.com
A Seifert, Co-Director
FV Brennan, Co-Director
Ron Seifert, Administrator
Offers a unique educational alternative to meet the needs of those complex students who have been unable to reach their academic potential elsewhere.

6640 Hamlin Robinson School
10211 12th Avenue S
Seattle, WA 98168
206-763-1167
FAX 206-762-2419
http://www.hamlinrobinson.org
e-mail: ifno@hamlinrobinson.org
Jeanne Turner, Director
Barbara Bradshaw, Administrator

A nonprofit, state approved elementary day school for children with specific language disability (dyslexia), providing a positive learning environment, meeting individual needs to nurture the whole child. Small classes use the Slingerland multi-sensory classroom approach in reading, writing, spelling and all instructional areas. It helps students discover the joy of learning, build positive self-esteem, and explore their full creative potential while preparing them for the classroom.

6641 Scottish Rite Center for Childhood Language Disorders
1155 Broadway E
Seattle, WA 98102
206-324-6293
http://www.srccld.org
e-mail: sanderson-cld@qwest.net
Steve Anderson, Executive Director
Jacqueline Brown, Clinical Director

Provides diagnostic and therapeutic services to families of children, whose primary disorder is a severe delay in language or speech development.

6642 Specialized Training for Military Parents
10209 Bridgeport Way SW
Tacoma, WA 98499
253-588-1741
800-298-3543
FAX 263-984-7520
TDY:283-588-1741
http://www.stompproject.org/
e-mail: stomp@washingtonpave.com
Heather Hebdon, Founder/Director
Toni Salato, Parent Resource Coordinator

STOMP (Specialized Training of Military Parents) is a federally funded center established to assist military families who have children with special education or health needs.

6643 St. Christopher Academy
Jevne Academy
140 S 140th Street
Burien, WA 98168
206-246-9751
FAX 253-639-3466
http://www.stchristopheracademy.com
e-mail: jevne@stchristopheracademy.com
Darlene Jevne, Manager

St. Christopher Academy is a private school for learning disabled, ADD and/or academically at-risk students.

West Virginia

6644 Parent Training and Information
1701 Hamill Avenue
Clarksburg, WV 26301
304-624-1436
800-281-1436
FAX 304-624-1438
TDY:304-624-1436
http://www.wvpti.org
e-mail: wvpti@aol.com
Pat Haberbosch, Executive Director
Ed Barrett, Bookkeeper

Provides information to parents and to professionals who work with children with disabilities.

6645 West Virginia Parent Training and Information
1701 Hamill Avenue
Clarksburg, WV 26301
304-624-1436
800-281-1436
FAX 304-624-1438
TDY:304-624-1436
http://www.wvpti.org
e-mail: wvpti@aol.com
Pat Haberbosch, Executive Director
Ed Barrett, Bookkeeper

Provides information to parents and to professionals who work with children with disabilities.

Wisconsin

6646 Chileda Institute
1020 Mississippi Street
La Crosse, WI 54601
608-782-6480
FAX 608-782-6481
http://www.chileda.org
e-mail: info@chileda.org
Kirby Lentz, CEO
Donald Heidel, President

Educators for youth with developmental disabilities. Residential treatment center provides complete training and intensive therapy for children with severe mental and physical disabilities, closed head injuries and challenging behaviors.

Wyoming

6647 Parent Information Center of Wyoming

5 N Lobban Avenue
Buffalo, WY 82834
307-684-2277
800-660-9742
FAX 307-684-5314
TDY:307-684-2277
http://www.wpic.org
e-mail: tdawson@wpic.org
Terry Dawson, Executive Director

Parent Training and Information Program views parents as full partners in the educational process and a significant source of support and assistance to each other. Funded by the Division of Personnel Preparation, Office of Special Education Programs, these programs provide training and information to parents to enable such individuals to participate more effectively with professionals in meeting the educational needs of disabled children.

6648 Wyoming Parent Information Center

5 N Lobban Avenue
Buffalo, WY 82834
307-684-2277
800-660-9742
FAX 307-684-5314
TDY:307-684-2277
http://www.wpic.org
e-mail: tdawson@wpic.org
Terry Dawson, Executive Director

Parent Training and Information Program views parents as full partners in the educational process and a significant source of support and assistance to each other. Funded by the Division of Personnel Preparation, Office of Special Education Programs, these programs provide training and information to parents to enable such individuals to participate more effectively with professionals in meeting the educational needs of disabled children.

Centers

6649 American College Testing Program
ACT Universal Testing
PO Box 168
Iowa City, IA 52243
319-337-1000
FAX 319-339-3021
TDY:319-337-1701
http://www.act.org
e-mail: sandy.schlote@act.org
Richard J Ferguson, CEO
Rose G Rennekamp, VP, Communications

Helps individuals and organizations make informed decisions about education and work. We provide information for life's transitions.

6650 Diagnostic and Educational Resources
6832 Old Dominion Drive
McLean, VA 22101
703-883-2009
FAX 703-534-5181
http://www.der-online.com
e-mail: aspector@DER-online.com
Annette Spector, Executive Director
Elisabeth Wester, Course Coordinator

Focuses on what the child can do and builds self-esteem. Provides a full range of psychoeducational testing, parent advocacy, case management, and tutoring services. Diagnostic testing determines individual needs, which are addressed in one-on-one tutoring sessions in the child's home or school. Staff trained in LD/ADHD methodologies remediate learning disabilities and offer practical suggestions for home programs and for working with school systems.

6651 Educational Diagnostic Center at Curry College
Curry College
1071 Blue Hill Avenue
Milton, MA 02186
617-333-2210
FAX 617-333-2018
TDY:617-333-2250
http://www.curry.edu
e-mail: curryadm@curry.edu
Dr. Nancy Winbury, Coordinator/Professor
Kenneth Quigley, President

A comprehensive evaluation and testing center specializing in the learning needs of adolescents and adults. The Diagnostic Center welcomes adolescents and adults in need of learning strategies, long term educational plans, and better understanding of their learning profiles.

6652 Educational Testing Service
Test Collection
Rosedale Road
Princeton, NJ 08541
609-921-9000
FAX 609-734-5410
TDY:800-877-2540
http://www.ets.org
e-mail: etsinfo@ets.org
Kurt Landgraf, CEO
Rosie Oliver, Strategic Workforce Solutions As

Our mission is to help advance quality and equity in education by providing fair and valid assessments, research and related services.

6653 Educational Testing Service: SAT Services for Students with Disabilities
College Board SAT Program
PO Box 6200
Princeton, NJ 08541
609-771-7137
FAX 609-771-7944
http://www.collegeboard.com/ssd
e-mail: ssd@info.collegeboard.org
Offers testing accommodations to attempt to minimize the effect of disabilities on test performance. The SAT Program tests eligible students with documented visual, physical, hearing, or learning disabilities who require testing accommodations for SAT.

6654 GED Test Accommodations for Candidates with Specific Learning Disabilities
American Council on Education
1 Dupont Circle NW
Washington, DC 20036
202-939-9300
800-626-9433
FAX 202-775-8578
http://www.gedtest.org
e-mail: ged@ace.nche.edu
Christine Morfit, Executive Director
David Ward, President

The American Council on Education, founded in 1918, is the nation's coordinating higher education association. ACE is dedicated to the belief that equal educational opportunity and a strong higher education system are essential cornerstones of a democratic society.

6655 Georgetown University Center for Child andHuman Development
Box 571485
Washington, DC 20057
202-687-5000
FAX 202-687-8899
http://www.gucdc.georgetown.edu
e-mail: gucdc@georgetown.edu
Phyllis Magrab, Executive Director

To improve the quality of life for all children and youth, especially those with, or at risk for, special needs and their families.

6656 Georgetown University Child Development
3307 M Street NW
Washington, DC 20007
202-687-8635

6657 Law School Admission Council
Law School Admission Council
PO Box 2001
Newtown, PA 18940
215-968-1001
FAX 215-968-1119
TDY:215-968-1128
http://www.lsac.org
Phil Shelton, President/CEO
Stephen Schreiber, Vice President

Students with documented learning disabilities can apply for test accommodations as appropriate.

6658 Munroe-Meyer Institute for Genetics and Rehabilitation
444 S 44th Street
Omaha, NE 68131
402-559-6402
800-656-3937
FAX 402-559-5737
http://www.unmc.edu/mmi
e-mail: mfbennie@unmc.edu
Mark A Smith, Consumer/Family Coordinator

Diagnostic evaluation therapy, speech, physical, occupational, behavioral therapies, pediatrics, dentistry, nursing, psychology, social work, genetics, Media Resource Center, education, nutrition. Adult services for developmentally disabled, genetic evaluation and counseling, adaptive equipment, motion analysis laboratory, recreational therapy.

6659 National Center for Fair & Open Testing
National Center for Fair and Open Testing
342 Broadway
Cambridge, MA 02139
617-864-4810
FAX 617-497-2224
http://www.fairtest.org
e-mail: info@fairtest.org
Monty Neill, Executive Director
Robert Schaeffer, Public Education Director

Dedicated to ensuring that America's students and workers are assessed using fair, accurate, relevant and open tests.

6660 Plano Child Development Center
5401 S Wentworth Avenue
Chicago, IL 60609
773-924-5297
FAX 773-373-3548
http://www.planovision.org
e-mail: info@planovision.org

Stephanie Johnson, Executive Director
Mrs. David, Manager

Serves children with visually related learning disabilities and offers vision education seminars geared to learning disabilities. Comprehensive vision exams and vision therapy treatment services provided.

6661 Providence Speech and Hearing Center
Providence Speech and Hearing Center
1301 W Providence Avenue
Orange, CA 92868
714-639-4990
FAX 714-744-3841
http://www.pshc.org
e-mail: psqc@pshc.org
Margaret Inman, Founder
Mary Hooper, Executive Director

Comprehensive services for testing and treatment of all speech, language and hearing problems. Individual and group therapy beginning with parent/infant programs.

6662 Reading Assessment System
Harcourt Achieve
6277 Sea Harbor Drive
Orlando, FL 32887
252-480-3200
800-531-5015
FAX 800-699-9459
http://www.steckvaughn.com
e-mail: info@steckvaughn.com
Steck-Vaughn Staff, Author
Tim McEwen, President/CEO
Jeff Johnson, Dir Marketing Communications
Lehmann Team Coordinator, Team Coordinator
The Reading Assessment System provides an ongoing meaure of specific student's skills and offers detailed directions for individual instruction and remediation. Up to eight reports are available. This popular program generates individual scores, class scores, school scores, and district reports.

6663 Reading Group
6 Lincoln Square
Urbana, IL 61801
217-367-0914
FAX 217-367-0500
http://www.readinggroup.org
e-mail: info@readinggroup.org
Jason Eyman, President
Joan Tousey, Vice President
Kathy Wimer, Executive Director
One on one testing instruction and therapy for children and adults with dyslexia, ADD, Asperger Syndrome and gifted students with puzzling learning differences.

6664 Rehabilitation Resource
Univ of Wisconsin-Stout Vocational Rehab Bldg 232
124 Bowman Hall
Menomonie, WI 54751
715-232-1232
800-447-8688
FAX 715-232-2356
http://www.chd.uwstout.edu/svri/twi
e-mail: admissions@uwstout.edu
Robert Peters, Program Director
Marilyn Mars, Director of Purchasing Departmen

Develops, publishes, and distributes a variety of rehabilitation related materials. Also makes referrals to other sources on rehabilitation.

6665 Riley Child Development Center
Indiana University School of Medicine
702 Barnhill Drive
Indianapolis, IN 46202
317-274-5000
800-248-1199
FAX 317-274-9760
http://www.child-dev.com
e-mail: child-dev@child-dev.com
John Rau, Director

The Child Development Center provides interdisciplinary assessment for academics, communication, motor, behavior, medical concerns, for children and their families.

6666 Rose F Kennedy Center
Albert Einstein College of Medicine
1410 Pelham Parkway S
Bronx, NY 10461
718-430-3543
FAX 718-892-2296
http://www.aecom.yu.edu/cerc
e-mail: cerc@aecom.yu.edu
Herbert Cohen, Director
Mark Mehler MD, Executive Director

Provides comprehensive diagnostic services and intervention services for children and adults with learning disabilities.

6667 Scholastic Testing Service
480 Meyer Road
Bensenville, IL 60106
630-766-7150
800-642-6787
FAX 630-766-8054
http://www.ststesting.com
e-mail: sts@ststesting.com
John Kauffman, Marketing VP

Publisher of assessment materials from birth to adulthood, ability and achievement tests for kindergarten through grade twelve. Publishes the Torrance Tests of Creative Thinking, Thinking Creatively in Action and Movement, the STS High School Placement Test and Educational Development Series.

Behavior & Self Esteem

6668 A Day in the Life: Assessment and Instruction
Curriculum Associates
PO Box 2001
North Billerica, MA 01862
978-667-8000
800-225-0248
FAX 800-366-1158
http://www.curriculumassociates.com
e-mail: info@cainc.com
Frank Ferguson, Owner

Embeds basic reading, writing, math and problem-solving skills in simulated job tasks. Two programs provide the activities that help students master these basic skills.

6669 AAMR Adaptive Behavior Scale: School Edition
Pro-Ed
8700 Shoal Creek Boulevard
Austin, TX 78757
512-451-3246
800-897-3202
FAX 512-451-8542
http://www.proedinc.com
e-mail: info@proedinc.com
Nadine Lambert, Author
Don Hammill, Owner

Assesses children whose behavior indicates possible mental retardation, emotional disturbances or other learning difficulties.

6670 Autism Screening Instrument for Educational Planning
Slosson Educational Publications
PO Box 280
East Aurora, NY 14052
716-652-0930
800-828-4800
FAX 800-655-3840
http://www.slosson.com
e-mail: slosson@slosson.com
Bradley Erford, Edward Kelly, Sue Larson, Author
Steven Slosson, President
John Slosson, Vice President

Publishes materials on aptitude, developmental disabilities, school screening, speech language assessment, therapy, behavior conduct, special needs; also electronic teaching tapes and testing items.

6671 BASC Monitor for ADHD
Pearson Assessments
PO Box 99
Circle Pines, MN 55014 651-287-7220
FAX 800-632-9011
http://http://ags.pearsonassessments.com
e-mail: agsinfo@pearson.com
Randy W Kamphaus and Cecil R Reynolds, Author

The BASC Monitor for ADHD is a powerful new tool to help evaluate the effectiveness of ADHD treatments using teacher and parent rating scales, and database software for tracking behavior changes.

6672 Behavior Assessment System for Children
Pearson Assessments
PO Box 99
Circle Pines, MN 55014 651-287-7220
FAX 800-632-9011
http://http://ags.pearsonassessments.com
e-mail: agsinfo@pearson.com
Randy W Kamphaus and Cecil R Reynolds, Author

A powerful assessment to evaluate child and adolescent behavior. Includes a self-report form for describing the behaviors and emotions of children and adolescents. Administration time: 10 - 20 minutes (TRS & PRS) 30 - 45 minutes for SRP.
Ages 2-18

6673 Behavior Rating Instrument for Autistic and Other Atypical Children
Slosson Educational Publications
PO Box 280
East Aurora, NY 14052 716-652-0930
800-828-4800
FAX 800-655-3840
http://www.slosson.com
e-mail: slosson@slosson.com
Sue Larson, Author
Steven Slosson, President
John Slosson, Vice President

This instrument assesses: Relationship to an Adult; Communication; Drive for Mastery; Vocalization and Expressive Speech; Sound and Speech Reception; Social Responsiveness; and Psychobiological Development. Each of the seven scales begins with the most severe autistic behavior, and progresses to behavior roughly comparable to that of a normal 3 1/2 to 4 1/2 year-old. Also available for nonvocal communication. Administration is untimed and observational. *$130.00*

6674 Behavior Rating Profile
Pro-Ed
8700 Shoal Creek Boulevard
Austin, TX 78757 512-451-3246
800-897-3202
FAX 512-451-8542
http://www.proedinc.com
e-mail: info@proedinc.com
Linda Brown, Author
Don Hammill, Owner

A global measure of behavior providing student, parent, teacher and peer scales. It helps to identify behaviors that may cause a student's learning problems. *$204.00*

6675 Child Behavior Checklist
University of Vermont
1 S Prospect Street
Burlington, VT 05401 802-656-3131
FAX 802-264-6433
http://www.aseba.org
e-mail: mail@aseba.org
Thomas M Achenbach PhD, Author
Thomas M Achenbach PhD, Director/Professor
Mark Wanner, Manager
John Gates, CEO
A standardized form for obtaining parents' reports of children's behavioral/emotional problems and competencies. Related forms obtain teacher, interviewer, observer and self-reports.

6676 Children's Apperceptive Story-Telling Test
Pro-Ed
8700 Shoal Creek Boulevard
Austin, TX 78757 512-451-3246
800-897-3202
FAX 512-451-8542
http://www.proedinc.com
e-mail: info@proedinc.com
Mary Schneider, Author
Don Hammill, Owner

Employs apperceptive stories to evaluate the emotional functioning of school-age children.
Ages 6-13

6677 Culture-Free Self-Esteem Inventories
Pro-Ed
7700 Shoal Creek Boulevard
Austin, TX 78757 512-451-3246
800-897-3202
FAX 512-451-8542
http://www.proedinc.com
e-mail: info@proedinc.com
James Battle, Author
Don Hammill, Owner

A series of self-report scales used to determine the level of self-esteem in children and adults. *$184.00*
Ages 5-Adult

6678 Devereux Early Childhood Assessment Program
Kaplan
PO Box 610
Lewisville, NC 27023 336-766-7374
800-334-2014
FAX 800-452-7526
http://www.kaplanco.com
e-mail: info@kaplanco.com
Devereux, Author
Hal Kaplan, Owner

Easy-to-use, standardized assessment system that enhances social and emotional growth in children from 2-5 years. Encourages parent involvement, helps teachers with classroom planning and takes just 10 minutes to administer. Meets Head Start and IDEA requirements for strength-based assessment, as well as APA and NAEYC assessment guidelines. *$199.95*
Ages 2-5

6679 Disruptive Behavior Rating Scale
PO Box 280
East Aurora, NY 14052 716-652-0930
Steven Slosson, President
John Slosson, Vice President

6680 Disruptive Behavior Rating Scale Kit
Slosson Educational Publications
538 Buffalo Road
East Aurora, NY 14052 716-652-0930
800-828-4800
FAX 800-655-3840
http://www.slosson.com
e-mail: slosson@slosson.com
Bradley T Erford, Author
Georgina Moynihan, TTFM
Steven Slosson, President

Identifies common behavior problems such as attention deficit disorder, attention deficit hyperactivity disorder, oppositional disorders and anti-social conduct problems. *$169.25*

6681 Draw a Person: Screening Procedure for Emotional Disturbance
Pro-Ed
8700 Shoal Creek Boulevard
Austin, TX 78757 512-451-3246
800-897-3202
FAX 512-451-8542
http://www.proedinc.com
e-mail: info@proedinc.com

Jack Naglieri, Timothy McNeish, Achilles Bandos, Author
Don Hammill, Owner

A screening test that helps identify children and adolescents who have emotional problems and require further evaluation. *$140.00*

6682 **Fundamentals of Autism**
Slosson Educational Publications
PO Box 280
East Aurora, NY 14052 716-652-0930
800-828-4800
FAX 800-655-3840
http://www.slosson.com
e-mail: slosson@slosson.com
Sue Larson, Author
Steven Slosson, President
John Slosson, Vice President

The handbook and two accompanying checklists provide a quick, user-friendly approach to help in identifying and developing educationally related program objectives for the child diagnosed as Autistic.

6683 **Multidimensional Self Concept Scale**
Pro-Ed
8700 Shoal Creek Boulevard
Austin, TX 78757 512-451-3246
800-897-3202
FAX 512-451-8542
http://www.proedinc.com
e-mail: info@proedinc.com
Bruce Bracken, Author
Don Hammill, Owner

A thoroughly researched, developed and standardized clinical instrument. It assesses global self-concept and six context-dependent self-concept domains that are functionally important in the social-emotional adjustment of youth and adolescents. *$110.00*
Ages 9-19

6684 **Psychoeducational Assessment of Preschool Children**
Western Psychological Services
12031 Wilshire Boulevard
Los Angeles, CA 90025 310-478-2061
800-648-8857
FAX 310-478-7838
http://www.wpspublishing.com
e-mail: help@wpspublising.com
Bruce A Bracken PhD, Author
Gregg Gillmar, Vice President
David Nemor, Office Assistant

Comprehensive, multidisciplinary presentation by nationally recognized contributors is based upon the concept that preschool assessment is a vibrant entity of its own - qualitatively and quantitatively different from the assessment of infants and toddlers. For professionals in pre-school assessment, early childhood education, and psycoeducational diagnostics.
573 pages
ISBN 0-205290-21-3

6685 **Revised Behavior Problem Checklist**
Psychological Assessment Resources
16204 N Florida Avenue
Lutz, FL 33549 813-968-3003
800-331-8378
FAX 800-727-9329
http://www.parinc.com
e-mail: chairman@parinc.com
Bob III, President/CEO
Kay Cunningham, Director

Psychological test products and software designed by mental health professionals. *$182.00*

6686 **SSRS: Social Skills**
PO Box 99
Circle Pines, MN 55014 651-287-7220

6687 **SSRS: Social Skills Rating System**
Pearson Assessments
5601 Green Valley Drive
Bloomington, MN 55437 800-627-7271
FAX 800-632-9011
http://http://ags.pearsonassessments.com
e-mail: agsinfo@pearson.com
Frank M Gresham and Stephen N Elliot, Author
Kevin Brueggman, President

A nationally standardized series of questionnaires that obtain information on the social behaviors of children and adolescents from teachers, parents and the students themselves. Administration time is 10-15 minutes per questionnaire.
Ages 3 - 18

6688 **School Behaviors and Organization Skills**
Curriculum Associates
PO Box 2001
North Billerica, MA 01862 978-667-8000
800-225-0248
FAX 800-366-1158
http://www.curriculumassociates.com
e-mail: ca@infocurriculumassociates.com
Frank Ferguson, Owner
Fred Ferguson, VP Corporate Development/CIO

Introduces school behaviors for before, during, and after class. Critical organization and time management skills are key elements of this module.

6689 **Self-Esteem Index**
Pro-Ed
8700 Shoal Creek Boulevard
Austin, TX 78757 512-451-3246
800-897-3202
FAX 512-451-8542
http://www.proedinc.com
e-mail: info@proedinc.com
Linda Brown, Jacquelyn Alexander, Author
Don Hammill, Owner

A new, multidimensional, norm-referenced measure of the way that individuals perceive and value themselves. *$128.00*
Ages 0-11

6690 **Social-Emotional Dimension Scale**
Pro-Ed
8700 Shoal Creek Boulevard
Austin, TX 78757 512-451-3246
800-897-3202
FAX 512-451-8542
http://www.proedinc.com
e-mail: info@proedinc.com
Jerry Hutton, Timothy Roberts, Author
Don Hammill, Owner

A quick, well-standardized rating scale that can be used by teachers, counselors and psychologists to screen students who are at risk for conduct disorders or emotional disturbances. *$149.00*
Ages 6-11

6691 **System of Multicultural Pluralistic Assessment (SOMPA)**
Harcourt Assessment
19500 Bulverde Road
San Antonio, TX 78259 210-339-5000
800-211-8378
FAX 210-949-4475
http://www.harcourtassessment.com
Jeff Galt, CEO
John Dilworth, President

This comprehensive test determines the cognitive abilities, sensory/motor abilities and adaptive behavior of children ages 5-11 years of age. SOMPA provides nine different measures and a way of estimating learning potential through sociocultural and health factors.

C-level product

LD Screening

6692 ADD-H Comprehensive Teacher's Rating Scale: 2nd Edition
Slosson Educational Publications
PO Box 280
East Aurora, NY 14052
716-652-0930
800-828-4800
FAX 800-655-3840
http://www.slosson.com
e-mail: slosson@slosson.com
Rina Ullmann, Robert Sprague, Author
Steven Slosson, President
John Slosson, Vice President

This brief checklist assesses one of the most prevalent childhood behavior problems: attention-deficit disorder, with or without hyperactivity. Because this disorder manifests itself primarily in the classroom, it is best evaluated by teacher ratings. Also available in a Spanish translation; please indicate when ordering. *$62.00*

6693 Attention-Deficit/Hyperactivity Disorder Test
Slosson Educational Publications
PO Box 280
East Aurora, NY 14052
716-652-0930
800-828-4800
FAX 800-655-3840
http://www.slosson.com
e-mail: slosson@slosson.com
James E Gilliam, Author
Steven Slosson, President
John Slosson, Vice President

An effective instrument for identifying and evaluating ADHD. Contains 36 items that describe characteristic behaviors of persons with ADHD. These items comprise three subtests representing the core symptoms necessary for the diagnosis of ADHD: hyperactivity, impulsivity, and inattention. *$95.00*

6694 BRIGANCE Screens: Early Preschool
Curriculum Associates
PO Box 2001
North Billerica, MA 01862
978-667-8000
800-225-0248
FAX 800-366-1158
http://www.curriculumassociates.com
e-mail: ca@infocurriculumassociates.com
Albert Brigance, Author
Frank Ferguson, Owner
Fred Ferguson, VP Corporate Development/CIO

An affordable, easy-to-administer, all-purpose solution. Accurately screen key developmental and early academic skills in just 10-15 minutes per child. Widely used in Early Head Start programs, it meets IDEA requirements and provides consistent results that support early childhood educator's observations and judgement. *$110.00*

6695 BRIGANCE Screens: Infants and Toddler
Curriculum Associates
PO Box 2001
North Billerica, MA 01862
978-667-8000
800-225-0248
FAX 800-366-1158
http://www.curriculumassociates.com
e-mail: ca@infocurriculumassociates.com
Albert Brigance, Author
Frank Ferguson, President
Fred Ferguson, VP Corporate Development/CIO

An affordable, easy-to-administer, all-purpose solution. The Infant and Toddler Screen accurately assesses key developmental skills, and observes caregivers involvement and interactions. *$110.00*

6696 BRIGANCE Screens: K and 1
Curriculum Associates
PO Box 2001
North Billerica, MA 01862
978-667-8000
800-225-0248
FAX 800-366-1158
http://www.curriculumassociates.com
e-mail: ca@infocurriculumassociates.com
Albert Brigance, Author
Frank Ferguson, Owner
Fred Ferguson, VP Corporate Development/CIO

The K and 1 Screen is an affordable, easy-to-administer, all-purpose solution. Accurately screen key developmental and early academic skills in just 10-15 mintues per child. School districts nationwide rely on BRIGANCE for screening children before entering kindergarten, grade 1, and grade 2. It meets IDEA requirements and provides consistant results that support early childhood educators observations and judgement. *$110.00*

6697 Basic School Skills Inventory: Screen and Diagnostic
Pro-Ed
8700 Shoal Creek Boulevard
Austin, TX 78757
512-451-3246
800-897-3202
FAX 800-397-7633
http://www.proedinc.com
e-mail: info@proedinc.com
Hammill, Leigh, Pearson, Author
Lindy Johnson, Marketing Coordinator
Don Hammill, Owner

Can be used to locate children who are high risk for school failure, who need more in-depth assessment and who should be referred for additional study. *$105.00*
1997Grade Range: Ages 0-11

6698 Complete Clinical Dysphagia Evaluation: Test Forms
LinguiSystems
3100 4th Avenue
East Moline, IL 61244
309-755-2300
800-776-4332
FAX 309-755-2377
TDY:800-933-8331
http://www.linguisystems.com
e-mail: service@linguisystems.com
Linda Bowers, CEO
Rosemary Huisingh, Owner

These test forms are used with The Complete Clinical Dyspagia Evaluation. You'll come away with a complete picture of your patient's behavioral, oral-motor, laryngeal, reespiratory, cognitive, and swallowing abilities and limitations.

6699 DABERON Screening for School Readiness
Pro-Ed
8700 Shoal Creek Boulevard
Austin, TX 78757
512-451-3246
800-897-3202
FAX 800-397-7633
http://www.proedinc.com
e-mail: info@proedinc.com
Virginia Danzer, Theresa Lyons & Judith Voress, Author
Don Hammill, Owner

Provides a standardized assessment of school readiness in children with learning or behavior problems. *$170.00*
Yearly

6700 Developmental Assessment for the Severely Disabled
Pro-Ed
8700 Shoal Creek Boulevard
Austin, TX 78757
512-451-3246
800-897-3202
FAX 512-451-8542
http://www.proedinc.com
e-mail: info@proedinc.com
Mary Kay Dykes & Jane Erin, Author
Don Hammill, Owner

Offers diagnostic and programming personnel concise information about individuals who are functioning between birth and 8 years of age developmentally. *$210.00*

Ages 0-84

6701 Educational Developmental Series
Scholastic Testing Service
480 Meyer Road
Bensenville, IL 60106
630-766-7150
800-642-6787
FAX 630-766-8054
http://www.ststesting.com
e-mail: sts@mail.ststesting.com
John Kauffman, Marketing VP

A standardized battery of ability and achievement tests. Administration time is approximately 2.5 - 5 hours, depending on grade level and subtests. The EDSERIES has the most comprehensive coverage of all the STS tests. It permits teachers, counselors and administrators to evaluate a student from the broadest possible perspective. A school may use the EDSERIES on a lease/score basis or it may purchase testing materials.

6702 Fundamentals of Autism
Slosson Educational Publications
PO Box 280
East Aurora, NY 14052
716-652-0930
800-828-4800
FAX 800-655-3840
http://www.slosson.com
e-mail: slosson@slosson.com
Sue Larson, Author
Steven Slosson, President
John Slosson, Vice President

Provides a quick, user-friendly, effective, and accurate approach to help in identifying and developing educationally related program objectives for children diagnosed as autistic.

6703 Goldman-Fristoe Auditory Skills Test Battery
Pro-Ed
8700 Shoal Creek Boulevard
Austin, TX 78757
512-451-3246
800-897-3202
FAX 800-397-7633
http://www.proedinc.com
e-mail: info@proedinc.com
Ronald Goldman, Author
Don Hammill, Owner

An individually administered measure of a broad range of auditory skills. Administer the full battery to receive a total picture of an individual's auditory skills using the Battery Profile. Administer a single test or a cluster of tests as needed.

6704 Goodenough-Harris Drawing Test
Harcourt Assessment
19500 Bulverde Road
San Antonio, TX 78259
210-339-5000
800-211-8378
FAX 800-232-1223
http://www.harcourtassessment.com
Florence Goodenough, Author
Aurelio Prifitera, Publisher
John Dilworth, President

This test focuses on mental maturity without requiring verbal skills. The fifteen-minute examination provides standard scores for children ages 3-15. *$159.00*

6705 Kaufman Assessment Battery for Children
Pearson Assessments
PO Box 99
Circle Pines, MN 55014
651-287-7220
FAX 800-632-9011
http://http://ags.pearsonassessments.com
e-mail: agsinfo@pearson.com
Alan Kaufman, Nadeen Kaufman, Author
Kevin Brueggman, President

An individually administered measure of intelligence and achievement, using simultaneous and sequential mental processes.

35-85 min

6706 Kaufman Brief Intelligence Test
Pearson Assessments
PO Box 99
Circle Pines, MN 55014
651-287-7220
FAX 800-632-9011
http://http://ags.pearsonassessments.com
e-mail: agsinfo@pearson.com
Alan Kaufman, Nadeen Kaufman, Author
Kevin Brueggman, President

KBIT is a brief, individually administered test of verbal and non-verbal intelligence. Screens two cognitive functions quickly and easily.
Ages 4-90

6707 Marshall University: HELP Program
Higher Education for Learning Problems
520 18th Street
Huntington, WV 25703
304-696-6252
FAX 304-696-3231
http://www.marshall.edu/help
e-mail: weston@marshall.edu
Barbara Deuyer, Manager
Lynne Weston, Assistant Director

The HELP program is committed to providing assistance through individual tutuoring, mentoring and support, as well as fair and legal access to educational opportunities for students diagnosed with learning disabilities and related disorders such as ADD/ADHD.

6708 Monitoring Basic Skills Progress
Pro-Ed
8700 Shoal Creek Boulevard
Austin, TX 78757
512-451-3246
800-897-3202
FAX 800-397-7633
http://www.proedinc.com
e-mail: info@proedinc.com
Douglas Fuchs, Lynn Fuchs & Carol Hamlett, Author
Don Hammill, Owner

A computer-assisted measurement program that tests and monitors progress in three academic areas: basic reading, basic math and basic spelling. *$369.00*

6709 National Center of Higher Education for
520 18th Street
Huntington, WV 25703
304-696-6313

6710 PPVT-III: Peabody Test-Picture Vocabulary Test
Pearson Assessments
PO Box 99
Circle Pines, MN 55014
651-287-7220
FAX 800-632-9011
http://http://ags.pearsonassessments.com
e-mail: agsinfo@pearson.com
Lloyd Dunn, Leota Dunn, Author
Kevin Brueggman, President

A measure of hearing vocabulary for Standard American English; administration time: 10-15 minutes.
ages 2-90

6711 Peabody Individual Achievement Test
Pearson Assessments
PO Box 99
Circle Pines, MN 55014
651-287-7220
FAX 800-632-9011
http://http://ags.pearsonassessments.com
e-mail: agsinfo@pearson.com
Frederick Markwardt Jr, Author
Kevin Brueggman, President

Efficient individual measure of academic achievement. Reading, mathematics and spelling are assessed in a simple nonthreatning format that requires only a revised pointing response for most items.

Ages 5-22

6712 Restless Minds, Restless Kids
Slosson Educational Publications
PO Box 280
East Aurora, NY 14052 716-652-0930
800-828-4800
FAX 800-655-3840
http://www.slosson.com
e-mail: slosson@slosson.com
Rick D'Alli, Author
Steven Slosson, President
John Slosson, Vice President

Two leading specialists in the field of childhood behavioral disorders discuss the state-of-the-art approach to diagnosing and testing ADHD. They are joined by four mothers of ADHD children who share their experiences of the effects of this disorder on the family. *$67.00*

6713 School Readiness Test
Scholastic Testing Service
480 Meyer Road
Bensenville, IL 60106 630-766-7150
800-642-6787
FAX 630-766-8054
http://www.ststesting.com
e-mail: sts@mail.ststesting.com
John Kauffman, Marketing VP

An effective tool for determining the readiness of each student for first grade. It allows a teacher to learn as much as possible about every entering student's abilities, and about any factors that might interfere with his or her learning.

6714 Screening Children for Related Early Educational Needs
Pro-Ed
8700 Shoal Creek Boulevard
Austin, TX 78757 512-451-3246
800-897-3202
FAX 800-397-7633
http://www.proedinc.com
e-mail: info@proedinc.com
Wayne Hresko, Author
Don Hammill, Owner

A new academic screening test for young children that provides both global and specific ability scores that can be used to identify individual abilities.
Ages 3-7

6715 Slosson Intelligence Test: Revised
Pro-Ed
8700 Shoal Creek Boulevard
Austin, TX 78757 512-451-3246
800-897-3202
FAX 800-397-7633
http://www.proedinc.com
e-mail: info@proedinc.com
Richard Slosson, Author
Don Hammill, Owner

A widely used individual screening test for those who need to evaulate the mental ability of individuals who are learning disabled, mentally retarded, blind, orthopedically disabled, normal, or gifted from ages 4 to adulthood. Revised by Charles Nicholson and Terry Hibpshman. *$125.00*
Ages 4-Adult

6716 Source for Nonverbal Learning Disorders
LinguiSystems
3100 4th Avenue
East Moline, IL 61244 309-755-2300
800-776-4332
FAX 309-755-2377
TDY:800-933-8331
http://www.linguisystems.com
e-mail: service@linguisystems.com
Sue Thompson, Author
Linda Bowers, Co-Owner/Co-Founder
Rosemary Huisingh, Co-Owner/Co-Founder

Not sure if you have a student with nonverbal learning disorder? See if this description sounds familiar: ignores nonverbal cues such as facial expressions, is clumsy for no apparent reason, makes inappropriate social remarks, and has difficulty with visual-spatial-organizational tasks. This resource provides you with useful checklists, anecdotes, and methods for dealing with this little understood disorder through the lifespan. *$41.95*

6717 TOVA
Universal Attention Disorders
4281 Katella Avenue
Los Alamitos, CA 90720 714-821-9611
800-729-2886
FAX 714-229-8782
http://www.tovatest.com
e-mail: info@tovatest.com
Clifford Corman, Medical Director
Karen Carlson, Marketing Director

The TOVA (Tests of Variables of Attention) is a computerized, objective measure of attention and impulsivity, used in the assessment and treatment of ADD/ADHD. It is standardized from 4 to 80 years of age. TOVA's report contains a full analysis and interpetation of data. Variables measured include omissions, commisions, response time and response time variability.

6718 Test of Memory and Learning (TOMAL)
Pro-Ed
8700 Shoal Creek Boulevard
Austin, TX 78757 512-451-3246
800-897-3202
FAX 800-397-7633
http://www.proedinc.com
e-mail: info@proedinc.com
Cecil Reynolds, Erin Bigler, Author
Don Hammill, Owner

TOMAL provides ten subtests that evaluate general and specific memory functions. *$270.00*
Ages 5-19

6719 Test of Nonverbal Intelligence
8700 Shoal Creek Boulevard
Austin, TX 78757 512-451-3246
Don Hammill, Owner

6720 Test of Nonverbal Intelligence (TONI-3)
Pro-Ed
8700 Shoal Creek Boulevard
Austin, TX 78757 512-451-3246
800-897-3202
FAX 800-397-7633
http://www.proedinc.com
e-mail: info@proedinc.com
Linda Brown, Susan Johnson & Rita Sherbenou, Author
Don Hamhill, President

A language-free measure of reasoning and intelligence presents a variety of abstract problem solving tasks. *$275.00*
Ages 0-89

6721 Vision, Perception and Cognition: Manual for Evaluation & Treatment
Therapro
225 Arlington Street
Framingham, MA 01702 508-872-9494
800-257-5376
FAX 508-875-2062
http://www.theraproducts.com
e-mail: info@theraproducts.com
Barbara Zoltan, Author
Karen Conrad, Owner

Details methods for testing perceptual, visual and cognitive deficits, as well as procedure for evaluating test results in relation to cognitive loss. Clearly explains each deficit, provides step by step testing techniques and gives complete treatment guidelines. Also includes information on the use of computers in cognitive training. *$37.00*

232 pages

Math

6722 **3 Steps to Math Success**
Curriculum Associates
PO Box 2001
North Billerica, MA 01862
978-667-8000
800-225-0248
FAX 800-366-1158
http://www.curriculumassociates.com
e-mail: ca@infocurriculumassociates.com
Curriculum Associates, Author
Frank Ferguson, Owner
Fred Ferguson, VP Corporate Development/CIO

We developed an integrated approach to math that ensures academic success long after the final bell has rung. Together, these series create an easy-to-use system of targeted instruction designed to remedy math weakness and reinforce math strengths.

6723 **AfterMath Series**
Curriculum Associates
PO Box 2001
North Billerica, MA 01862
978-667-8000
800-225-0248
FAX 800-366-1158
http://www.curriculumassociates.com
e-mail: ca@infocurriculumassociates.com
Frank Ferguson, Owner
Fred Ferguson, VP Corporate Development/CIO

Galileo once said that mathematics is the alphabet in which the universe was created. This series helps students master that alphabet. As they puzzle their way through brainteasers and learn math magic, students build critical-thinking skills that are vital to comprehending and succeeding in today's world.

6724 **ENRIGHT Computation Series**
Curriculum Associates
PO Box 2001
North Billerica, MA 01862
978-667-8000
800-225-0248
FAX 800-366-1158
http://www.curriculumassociates.com
e-mail: ca@infocurriculumassociates.com
Frank Ferguson, Owner
Fred Ferguson, VP Corporate Development/CIO

Close the gap between expected and actual computation performance. The ENRIGHT Computation Series provides the practice necessary to master addition, subtraction, multiplication, and division of whole numbers, fractions, and decimals.

6725 **Figure It Out: Thinking Like a Math Problem Solver**
Curriculum Associates
PO Box 2001
North Billerica, MA 01862
978-667-8000
800-225-0248
FAX 800-366-1158
http://www.curriculumassociates.com
e-mail: ca@infocurriculumassociates.com
Frank Ferguson, Owner
Fred Ferguson, VP Corporate Development/CIO

Critical thinking is the key to unlocking the mystery of these nonroutine problems. Your students will eagerly accept the challenge! Students learn to apply eight strategies in each book including: draw a picture; use a pattern; work backwards; make a table; and guess and check.

6726 **Getting Ready for Algebra**
Curriculum Associates
PO Box 2001
North Billerica, MA 01862
978-667-8000
800-225-0248
FAX 800-366-1158
http://www.curriculumassociates.com
e-mail: ca@infocurriculumassociates.com
Frank Ferguson, Owner
Fred Ferguson, VP Corporate Development/CIO

NCTM encourages algebra instruction in the early grades to develop critical-thinking, communication, reasoning, and problem-solving skills. Getting Ready for Algebra exercises these skills in lessons that focus on key algebra concepts: adding and subtracting positive integers; patterns; set theory notation; open sentences; inequality and more.

6727 **Learning Disability Evaluation Scale: Renormed**
Hawthorne Educational Services
800 Gray Oak Drive
Columbia, MO 65201
573-874-1710
800-542-1673
FAX 800-442-9509
http://www.hes-inc.com
e-mail: edina.laird@hes-inc.com
Stephen McCarney, Author
Edina Laird, Director External Relations
Michele Jackson, Owner

The Learning Disability Evaluation Scale (LDES) is an initial screening and assessment instrument in the areas of listening, thinking, speaking, reading, writing, spelling, and mathematical calculations based on the federal definition (IDEA). The Learning Disability Intervention Manual (LDIM) is a companion to the LDES and contains goals, objectives, and intervention/instructional strategies for the learning problems identified by the LDES. *$152.00*
217 pages

6728 **QUIC Tests**
Scholastic Testing Service
480 Meyer Road
Bensenville, IL 60106
630-766-7150
800-642-6787
FAX 630-766-8054
http://www.ststesting.com
e-mail: sts@mail.ststesting.com
John Kauffman, Marketing VP

The Quic Tests are used to determine the functional level of student comptetency in mathematics and/ or communicative arts for use in grades 2-12. Administration time is 30 minutes or less.

6729 **Skills Assessments**
Harcourt
6277 Sea Harbor Drive
Orlando, FL 32887
407-345-2000
800-531-5015
FAX 512-343-6854
http://www.harcourtachieve.com
e-mail: info@steck-vaughn.com
Tim McEwen, President
Jeff Johnson, Marketing Communication Director
Patrick Tierrey, CEO
This handy, all-in-one resource helps identify students strengths and weaknesses in order to determine appropriate instructional levels in each of five subjects areas: reading; language arts; math; science; and social studies. Assessments are identified by subtopics in each subject.

6730 **Test of Mathematical Abilities**
Pro-Ed
8700 Shoal Creek Boulevard
Austin, TX 78757
512-451-3246
800-897-3202
FAX 800-397-7633
http://www.proedinc.com
e-mail: info@proedinc.com
Virginia Brown, Mary Cronin, Elizabeth McEntire, Author
Don Hammill, Owner

Has been developed to provide standardized information about story problems and computation, attitude, vocabulary and general cultural application. *$92.00*

Ages 3-12

Professional Guides

6731 Assessment Update
Jossey-Bass
111 River Street
Hoboken, NJ 07030
201-748-6000
FAX 201-748-6088
http://www.josseybass.com/wiley
William Pesce, CEO
Trudy Banta, Editor

Assessment Update is dedicated to covering the latest developments in the rapidly evolving area of higher education assessment. Assessment Update offers all academic leaders up-to-date information and practical advice on conducting assessments in a range of areas, including student learning and outcomes, factulty instruction, academic programs and curricula, student services, and overall institutional functioning.

6732 Assessment of Students with Handicaps in Vocational Education
Association for Career and Technical Education
1410 King Street
Alexandria, VA 22314
703-683-3111
FAX 703-683-7424
http://www.acteonline.org
e-mail: jbray@acteonline.org
L Albright, Author
Jan Bray, Executive Director
Peter Magnuson, Senior Dir Strategic Marketing

Includes teachers, supervisors, administrators and others interested in the development and improvement of vocational, technical and practical-arts education.

6733 BRIGANCE Word Analysis: Strategies and Practice
Curriculum Associates
PO Box 2001
North Billerica, MA 01862
978-667-8000
800-225-0248
FAX 800-366-1158
http://www.curriculumassociates.com
e-mail: ca@infocurriculumassociates.com
Albert Brigance, Author
Frank Ferguson, Owner
Fred Ferguson, VP Corporate Development/CIO

Our comprehensive, two-volume resource combines activities, strategies, and reference materials for teaching phonetic and structural word analysis. Two durable binders feature reproducible activity pages. Choose from more than 1,600 activities for corrective instruction or to reinforce your classroom reading program.

6734 Career Planner's Portfolio: A School-to-work Assessment Tool
Curriculum Associates
PO Box 2001
North Billerica, MA 01862
978-667-8000
800-225-0248
FAX 800-366-1158
http://www.curriculumassociates.com
e-mail: ca@infocurriculumassociates.com
Robert G Forest, Author
Frank Ferguson, Owner
Fred Ferguson, VP Corporate Development/CIO

Students career plans develop and evolve over several school years. Our portfolio will help track of their progess.

6735 Computer Scoring Systems for PRO-ED Tests
Pro-Ed
8700 Shoal Creek Boulevard
Austin, TX 78757
512-451-3246
800-897-3202
FAX 800-397-7633
http://www.proedinc.com
e-mail: info@proedinc.com
Don Hammill, Owner

Computer scoring systems have been developed to generate reports for many PRO-ED tests and to help examiners interpret test performance.

6736 Goals and Objectives Writer Software
Curriculum Associates
PO Box 2001
North Billerica, MA 01862
978-667-8000
800-225-0248
FAX 800-366-1158
http://www.curriculumassociates.com
e-mail: ca@infocurriculumassociates.com
Frank Ferguson, Owner
Fred Ferguson, VP Corporate Development/CIO

Using the Goals and Objectives program, you'll quickly and easily create, edit, and print IEPs. The CD allows you to install the program on your hard drive in order to save students data for future updates. You can easily export IEPs into any word processing program. CD-Rom for Windows and Macintosh.

6737 Occupational Aptitude Survey and Interest Schedule
Pro-Ed
8700 Shoal Creek Boulevard
Austin, TX 78757
512-451-3246
800-897-3202
FAX 800-397-7633
http://www.proedinc.com
e-mail: info@proedinc.com
Rau M Parker, Author
Don Hammill, Owner

Consists of two related tests: the OASIS-2 Aptitude Survey and the OASIS-2 Interest Schedule. The tests were normed on the same national sample of 1,505 students from 13 states. The Aptitude Survey measures six broad aptitude factors that are directly related to skills and abilities required in over 20,000 jobs and the Interest Schedule measures 12 interest factors directly related to the occupations listed in Occupational Exploration. *$184.00*

6738 Portfolio Assessment Teacher's Guide
Harcourt
6277 Sea Harbor Drive
Orlando, FL 32887
407-345-2000
800-531-5015
FAX 800-699-9459
http://www.harcourtachieve.com
e-mail: ecare@harcourt.com
Roger Farr, Author
Tim McEwen, President
Patrick Tierrey, CEO
Jeff Johnson, Marketing Communication Director
Start your portfolio systems with tips from the expert. Roger Farr outlines the basic steps for evaluating a portfolio, offers ideas for organizing portfolios and making the most of portfolio conferences, and provides reproducible evaluation forms for primary through intermediate grades and above. *$23.60*

6739 Teaching Test Taking Skills
Brookline Books
300 Bedford Street
Manchester, NH 03101
617-734-6772
FAX 617-734-3952
http://www.brooklinebooks.com
e-mail: brooklinebks@delphi.com
Margo Mastropieri, Thomas Scruggs, Author

Test-wise individuals often score higher than others of equal ability who may not use test-taking skills effectively. This work teaches general concepts about the test format or other conditions of testing, not specific items on the test. *$21.95*

ISBN 0-914797-76-X

6740 Tests, Measurement and Evaluation
American Institutes for Research
1000 Thomas Jefferson Street NW
Washington, DC 20007
202-342-5000
FAX 202-298-6809
http://www.air.org
Sol Pelavin, President/CEO
Nikki Shannon, Administrative Assistant
Mike Cane, Vice President

Our goal is to provide governments and the private sector with responsive services of the highest quality by applying and advancing the knowledge, theories, methods, and standards of the behavioral and social services to solve significant societal problems and improve the quality of life of all people.

Reading

6741 **3 Steps to Reading Success**
Curriculum Associates
PO Box 2001
North Billerica, MA 01862
978-667-8000
800-225-0248
FAX 800-366-1158
http://www.curriculumassociates.com
e-mail: ca@infocurriculumassociates.com
Frank Ferguson, President
Fred Ferguson, VP Corporate Development/CIO

Equipping your students with the skills and strategies they need to achieve lifelong success can be a challenge. That's why we developed an integrated approach to learning that ensures academic success long after the final bell has rung.

6742 **BRIGANCE Readiness: Strategies and Practice**
Curriculum Associates
PO Box 2001
North Billerica, MA 01862
978-667-8000
800-225-0248
FAX 800-366-1158
http://www.curriculumassociates.com
e-mail: ca@infocurriculumassociates.com
Albert Brigance, Author
Frank Ferguson, Owner
Fred Ferguson, VP Corporate Development/CIO

Attend to the needs and differences of the children in your program using Readiness: Strategies and Practice. Skills are introduced, taught, and reinforced using both age appropriate and individual appropriate activties. *$174.00*

6743 **CLUES for Better Reading: Grade 1**
Curriculum Associates
PO Box 2001
North Billerica, MA 01862
978-667-8000
800-225-0248
FAX 800-366-1158
http://www.curriculumassociates.com
e-mail: ca@infocurriculumassociates.com
Diane Lapp, James Flood, Author
Frank Ferguson, Owner
Fred Ferguson, VP Corporate Development/CIO

Clues for Better Reading Book A develops and strengthens comprehension through reading activities in the same skill strands featured in the Kindergarten level. The 96-page Teacher Guide provides activities to introduce the unit skill and new vocabulary, followed by guided lessons and extension activities.

6744 **CLUES for Better Reading: Grade 2-5**
Curriculum Associates
PO Box 2001
North Billerica, MA 01862
978-667-8000
800-225-0248
FAX 800-366-1158
http://www.curriculumassociates.com
e-mail: ca@infocurriculumassociates.com
Diane Lapp, James Flood, Author
Frank Ferguson, Owner
Fred Ferguson, VP Corporate Development/CIO

Students explore a variety of literacy genres: stories; poetry; plays, newspaper articles, and others. Related lanuage activities - writing, word analysis, or study skills - help students extend reading comprehension to other areas of language arts.

6745 **CLUES for Better Reading: Kindergaten**
Curriculum Associates
PO Box 2001
North Billerica, MA 01862
978-667-8000
800-225-0248
FAX 800-366-1158
http://www.curriculumassociates.com
e-mail: ca@infocurriculumassociates.com
Diane Lapp, James Flood, Author
Frank Ferguson, Owner
Fred Ferguson, VP Corporate Development/CIO

Emergent readers explore language with Clues for Better Reading and Writing. Teacher-directed lessons feature minimal text with appealing full-color artwork, and place a strong emphasis on oral literature to develop early reading skills.

6746 **Capitalization and Punctuation**
Curriculum Associates
PO Box 2001
North Billerica, MA 01862
978-667-8000
800-225-0248
FAX 800-366-1158
http://www.curriculumassociates.com
e-mail: ca@infocurriculumassociates.com
Frank Ferguson, Owner
Fred Ferguson, VP Corporate Development/CIO

Capitalization and Punctuation features structured, easy to understand lessons that are organized sequentially. Students read the rules, study sample exercises, apply the skills in practice lessons, and review the skills in maintenance lessons.

6747 **Effective Reading of Textbooks**
Curriculum Associates
PO Box 2001
North Billerica, MA 01862
978-667-8000
800-225-0248
FAX 800-366-1158
http://www.curriculumassociates.com
e-mail: ca@infocurriculumassociates.com
Anita Archer, Author
Frank Ferguson, Owner
Fred Ferguson, VP Corporate Development/CIO

Students practice previewing for reading, active reading, indentation note-taking, mapping a visual display of content, and writing a summary paragraph.

6748 **Extensions in Reading**
Curriculum Associates
PO Box 2001
North Billerica, MA 01862
978-667-8000
800-225-0248
FAX 800-366-1158
http://www.curriculumassociates.com
e-mail: ca@infocurriculumassociates.com
Frank Ferguson, Owner
Fred Ferguson, VP Corporate Development/CIO

A unique new program teaching reading strategies and more. Extensions offers rich experiences with nonfiction and fiction. Each lesson extends to include: researching and writing; use of graphic organizers; vocabulary development; and comprehension questions with test-prep format.

6749 **Formal Reading Inventory**
Pro-Ed
8700 Shoal Creek Boulevard
Austin, TX 78757
512-451-3246
800-897-3202
FAX 800-397-7633
http://www.proedinc.com
e-mail: info@proedinc.com
J Lee Wiederholt, Author
Don Hammill, Owner

A national test for assessing silent reading comprehension and diagnosing reading miscues.

6750 **Gray Oral Diagnostic Reading Tests**
Pro-Ed
8700 Shoal Creek Boulevard
Austin, TX 78757
512-451-3246
800-897-3202
FAX 800-397-7633
http://www.proedinc.com
e-mail: info@proedinc.com
Brian Bryant, J Lee Wiederholt, Author
Don Hammill, Owner

Uses two alternate, equivalent forms to assess students who have difficulty reading continuous print and who require an evaluation of specific abilities and weaknesses. Item # 10965. *$250.00*

6751 **Gray Oral Reading Tests**
Pro-Ed
8700 Shoal Creek Boulevard
Austin, TX 78757
512-451-3246
800-897-3202
FAX 800-397-7633
http://www.proedinc.com
e-mail: info@proedinc.com
J Lee Wiederholt, Brian Bryant, Author
Don Hammill, Owner

The latest revision provides an objective measure of growth in oral reading and an aid in the diagnosis of oral reading difficulties. *$225.00*

6752 **Reading Assessment System**
Steck-Vaughn Company
PO Box 690789
Orlando, FL 32869
407-345-3800
800-531-5015
FAX 800-269-5232
http://www.steck-vaughn.com
e-mail: info@steck-vaughn.com
Connie Alden, Vice President of Human Resource
Michael Ruecker, Vice President of Human Resource

The Reading Assessment System provides an ongoing measure of specific student's skills and offers detailed directions for individual instruction and remediation. Up to eight reports are available. This popular program generates individual scores, class scores, school scores, and district reports.

6753 **Scholastic Abilities Test for Adults**
Pro-Ed
8700 Shoal Creek Boulevard
Austin, TX 78757
512-451-3246
800-897-3202
FAX 800-397-7633
http://www.proedinc.com
e-mail: info@proedinc.com
Brian Bryant, James Patton, Caroline Dunn, Author
Don Hammill, Owner

Measures scholastic competence, aptitude and academic achievement for persons with learning difficulties. *$180.00*
Ages 16-70

6754 **Skills Assessments**
Steck-Vaughn Company
PO Box 690789
Orlando, FL 32869
407-345-3800
800-531-5015
FAX 800-269-5232
http://www.steck-vaughn.com
e-mail: info@steck-vaughn.com
Connie Alden, Vice President of Human Resource
Michael Ruecker, Vice President of Human Resource

This handy, all-in-one resource helps identify students strengths and weaknesses in order to determine appropriate instructional levels in each of five subjects areas: reading; language arts; math; science; and social studies. Assessments are identified by subtopics in each subject. Each book is $13.99 each. *$69.95*

6755 **Standardized Reading Inventory**
Pro-Ed
8700 Shoal Creek Boulevard
Austin, TX 78757
512-451-3246
800-897-3202
FAX 800-397-7633
http://www.proedinc.com
e-mail: info@proedinc.com
Phyllis Newcomer, Author
Don Hammill, Owner

An instrument for evaluating students' reading ability. *$268.00*

6756 **TERA-3: Test of Early Reading Ability 3nd Edition**
AGS
PO Box 99
Circle Pines, MN 55014
651-287-7220
800-328-2560
FAX 800-471-8457
http://www.SLPforum.com
e-mail: ags@skypoint.com
Kim Reid, Wayne Hresko and Donald Hammill, Author

Ideal for screening children's early reading abilities. Specifically the revised test measures knowledge of contextual meaning, the alphabet and conventions such as reading from left to right. *$265.00*
Ages 3-8

6757 **Test of Early Reading Ability**
Pro-Ed
8700 Shoal Creek Boulevard
Austin, TX 78757
512-451-3246
800-897-3202
FAX 800-397-7633
http://www.proedinc.com
e-mail: info@proedinc.com
D Kim Reid, Wayne Hresko, Donald Hammill, Author
Don Hammill, Owner

Unique test in that it measures the actual reading ability of young children. Items measure knowledge of contextual meaning, alphabet and conventions. *$265.00*

6758 **Test of Reading Comprehension**
Pro-Ed
8700 Shoal Creek Boulevard
Austin, TX 78757
512-451-3246
800-897-3202
FAX 800-397-7633
http://www.proedinc.com
e-mail: info@proedinc.com
Virginia Brown, Donald Hammill, J Lee Wiederholt, Author
Don Hammill, Owner

A multidimensional test of silent reading comprehension for students. The test reflects current psycholinguistic theories that consider reading comprehension to be a constructive process involving both language and cognition. *$ 189.00*
Ages 7-11

Speech & Language Arts

6759 **A Calendar of Home Activities**
Curriculum Associates
PO Box 2001
North Billerica, MA 01862
978-667-8000
800-225-0248
FAX 800-366-1158
http://www.curriculumassociates.com
e-mail: ca@infocurriculumassociates.com
Donald Johnson, Elaine Johnson, Author
Frank Ferguson, Owner
Fred Ferguson, VP Corporate Development/CIO

An activity-a-day: 365 activities for parents and children to share at home in just 10-15 minutes each day. Parents support their children's educational experiences in a meaningful and enjoyable way, such as cooking, playing ball, and sculpting clay.

6760 Activities for Dictionary Practice
Curriculum Associates
PO Box 2001
North Billerica, MA 01862
978-667-8000
800-225-0248
FAX 800-366-1158
http://www.curriculumassociates.com
e-mail: ca@infocurriculumassociates.com
Jean Lucken, Author
Frank Ferguson, Owner
Fred Ferguson, VP Corporate Development/CIO

The ideal companion for classroom dictionaries! A wide variety of exercises helps students make efficient use of this important reference tool - the dictionary. Reading, spelling, vocabulary-building, and word-usage skills are reinforced.

6761 Adolescent Language Screening Test
Pro-Ed
8700 Shoal Creek Boulevard
Austin, TX 78757
512-451-3246
800-897-3202
FAX 800-397-7633
http://www.proedinc.com
e-mail: info@proedinc.com
Denise Morgan, Arthur Guilford, Author
Don Hammill, Owner

Provides speech/language pathologists and other interested professionals with a rapid thorough method for screening adolescents' speech and language. *$140.00*
Ages 11-17

6762 Adventures in Science: Activities for the School-Home Connection
Curriculum Associates
PO Box 2001
North Billerica, MA 01862
978 667 8000
800-225-0248
FAX 800-366-1158
http://www.curriculumassociates.com
e-mail: ca@inforcurriculumassociates.com
Curriculum Associates, Author
Frank Ferguson, Owner
Fred Ferguson, VP Corporate Development/CIO

Process-based and hands-on, these engaging activities get your students investigating and exploring the world outside the classroom. Activities and materials are designed especially for the home, encouraging parents to take an active role in their child's education.

6763 Aphasia Diagnostic Profiles
Pro-Ed
8700 Shoal Creek Boulevard
Austin, TX 78757
512-451-3246
800-897-3202
FAX 800-397-7633
http://www.proedinc.com
e-mail: info@proedinc.com
Nancy Helm-Estrabrooks, Author
Don Hammill, Owner

This is a quick, efficient, and systematic assessment of language and communication impairment associated with aphasia that should be administered individually. The test can be administered in 40-45 minutes. *$169.00*

6764 BRIGANCE Assessment of Basic Skills: Spanish Edition
Curriculum Associates
PO Box 2001
North Billerica, MA 01862
978-667-8000
800-225-0248
FAX 800-366-1158
http://www.curriculumassociates.com
e-mail: ca@infocurriculumassociates.com
Albert Brigance, Author
Frank Ferguson, Owner
Fred Ferguson, VP Corporate Development/CIO

Critiqued and field tested by Spanish linguists and educators nationwide, the Assessment of Basic Skills meets nondiscriminatory testing requirements for Limited English Proficient students. *$149.00*

6765 BRIGANCE Comprehensive Inventory of Basic Skills: Revised
Curriculum Associates
PO Box 2001
North Billerica, MA 01862
978-667-8000
800-225-0248
FAX 800-366-1158
http://www.curriculumassociates.com
e-mail: ca@infocurriculumassociates.com
Albert Brigance, Author
Frank Ferguson, Owner
Fred Ferguson, VP Corporate Development/CIO

Designed for use in elementary and middle schools, the CIBS-R is a valuable resource for programs emphasizing individualized instruction. The Inventory is especially helpful in programs serving students with special needs, and continues to be indispensable in IEP development and program planning. *$159.00*

6766 BRIGANCE Employability Skills Inventory
Curriculum Associates
PO Box 2001
North Billerica, MA 01862
978-667-8000
800-225-0248
FAX 800-366-1158
http://www.curriculumassociates.com
e-mail: ca@infocurriculumassociates.com
Albert Brigance, Author
Frank Ferguson, Owner
Fred Ferguson, VP Corporate Development/CIO

Extensive criterion-referenced tool assesses basic skills and employability skills in the context of job-seeking or employment situations: reading grade placement; rating scales; career awareness and self-understanding; reading skills; speaking and listening; job-seeking skills and knowledge; pre-employment writing; math and concepts. *$89.95*

6767 BRIGANCE Inventory of Essential Skills
Curriculum Associates
PO Box 2001
North Billerica, MA 01862
978-667-8000
800-225-0248
FAX 800-366-1158
http://www.curriculumassociates.com
e-mail: ca@infocurriculumassociates.com
Albert Brigance, Author
Frank Ferguson, Owner
Fred Ferguson, VP Corporate Development/CIO

The Inventory of Essential Skills is widely used to assess secondary level students or adult learners with special needs. *$169.00*

6768 BRIGANCE Life Skills Inventory
Curriculum Associates
PO Box 2001
North Billerica, MA 01862
978-667-8000
800-225-0248
FAX 800-366-1158
http://www.curriculumassociates.com
e-mail: ca@infocurriculumassociates.com
Albert Brigance, Author
Frank Ferguson, Owner
Fred Ferguson, VP Corporate Development/CIO

Assesses listening, speaking, reading, writing, comprehending, and computing skills in nine life-skill sections: speaking and listening; money and finance; functional writing; food; words on common signs and warning labels; clothing; health; telephone; travel and transportation. *$89.95*

6769 **Bedside Evaluation and Screening Test**
Pro-Ed
8700 Shoal Creek Boulevard
Austin, TX 78757
512-451-3246
800-897-3202
FAX 800-397-7633
http://www.proedinc.com
e-mail: info@proedinc.com
Joyce West, Elaine Sands, Deborah Ross-Swain, Author
Don Hamhill, President

Access and quantify language disorders in adults resulting from aphasia. *$165.00*

6770 **Bedside Evaluation and Screening Test of**
8700 Shoal Creek Boulevard
Austin, TX 78757
512-451-3246
Don Hammill, Owner

6771 **Boone Voice Program for Adults**
Pro-Ed
8700 Shoal Creek Boulevard
Austin, TX 78757
512-451-3246
800-897-3202
FAX 800-397-7633
http://www.proedinc.com
e-mail: info@proedinc.com
Daniel Boone & Kay Wiley, Author
Don Hammill, Owner

Provides for diagnosis and remediation of adult voice disorders. This program is based on the same philosophy and therapy as The Program for Children but is presented at an adult interest level. *$141.00*

6772 **Boone Voice Program for Children**
Pro-Ed
8700 Shoal Creek Boulevard
Austin, TX 78757
512-451-3246
800-897-3202
FAX 512-451-8542
http://www.proedinc.com
e-mail: info@proedinc.com
Daniel Boone, Author
Don Hammill, Owner

Provides a cognitive approach to voice therapy and is designed to give useful step-by-step guidelines and materials for diagnosis and remediation of voice disorders in children. *$208.00*

6773 **CLUES for Better Writing: Grade 1**
Curriculum Associates
PO Box 2001
North Billerica, MA 01862
978-667-8000
800-225-0248
FAX 800-366-1158
http://www.curriculumassociates.com
e-mail: ca@inforcurriculumassociates.com
Curriculum Associates, Author
Frank Ferguson, Owner
Fred Ferguson, VP Corporate Development/CIO

Clues for Better Writing Book A develops and reinforces skills with creative writing projects, art activities, and vocabulary exercises. The 24-page Teacher Guide scripts each lesson and features spelling exercises, reproducible word lists, and extension activities.

6774 **CLUES for Better Writing: Grades 2-5**
Curriculum Associates
PO Box 2001
North Billerica, MA 01862
978-667-8000
800-225-0248
FAX 800-366-1158
http://www.curriculumassociates.com
e-mail: ca@infocurriculumassociates.com
Curriculum Associates, Author
Frank Ferguson, Owner
Fred Ferguson, VP Corporate Development/CIO

Clues for Better Writing Book B-E teach students the five steps to successful writing—brainstorming, planning, writing, editing, and publishing.

6775 **CLUES for Better Writing: Kindergarten**
Curriculum Associates
PO Box 2001
North Billerica, MA 01862
978-667-8000
800-225-0248
FAX 800-366-1158
http://www.curriculumassociates.com
e-mail: ca@infocurriculumassociates.com
Curriculum Associates, Author
Frank Ferguson, Owner
Fred Ferguson, VP Corporate Development/CIO

Emergent readers and writers explore lanuage with Clues for Better Reading and Writing. The 64-page student book features teacher-directed lessons with minimal text, appealing full-color artwork, and oral literture to develop early lanuage skills.

6776 **CLUES for Phonemic Awareness**
Curriculum Associates
PO Box 2001
North Billerica, MA 01862
978-667-8000
800-225-0248
FAX 800-366-1158
http://www.curriculumassociates.com
e-mail: ca@infocurriculumassociates.com
Diane Lapp, James Flood, Linda Lungren, Author
Frank Ferguson, Owner
Fred Ferguson, VP Corporate Development/CIO

Give your preschool, primary, or ESL children a head start on the road to reading and writing by helping them understand that language that they hear and speak is made up of a series of sounds.

6777 **Completing Daily Assignments**
Curriculum Associates
PO Box 2001
North Billerica, MA 01862
978-667-8000
800-225-0248
FAX 800-366-1158
http://www.curriculumassociates.com
e-mail: ca@infocurriculumassociates.com
Anita Archer, Mary Gleason, Author
Frank Ferguson, Owner
Fred Ferguson, VP Corporate Development/CIO

Focuses on planning assignments, writing answers to factual and opinion questions, and proofreading. Students learn to produce neat, well-organized assignments. Item #8944-student book. *$19.90*

6778 **Connecting Reading and Writing with Vocabulary**
Curriculum Associates
PO Box 2001
North Billerica, MA 01862
978-667-8000
800-225-0248
FAX 800-366-1158
http://www.curriculumassociates.com
e-mail: ca@infocurriculumassociates.com
Deborah P Adcock, Author
Frank Ferguson, Owner
Fred Ferguson, VP Corporate Development/CIO

This vocabulary enrichment series builds successful writers and speakers by implementing strategic word techniques. Students will add 120 writing words and other word forms to their word banks. Each lesson introduces ten vocabulary words in a variety of contexts: a letter, poem, story, journal entry, classified ad, etc.

6779 **Diamonds in the Rough**
Slosson Educational Publications
PO Box 280
East Aurora, NY 14052
716-652-0930
800-828-4800
FAX 800-655-3840
http://www.slosson.com
e-mail: slosson@slosson.com
Peggy Strass Dras, Author
Steven Slosson, President
John Slosson, Vice President

College referance/rehabilitation guide for people with attention deficit disorder and learning disabilities.

6780 Easy Talker: A Fluency Workbook for School Age Children
Pro-Ed
8700 Shoal Creek Boulevard
Austin, TX 78757
512-451-3246
800-897-3202
FAX 800-397-7633
http://www.proedinc.com
e-mail: info@proedinc.com
Garry Guitar, Julie Reville, Author
Don Hammill, Owner

A diagnostic, criterion-referenced instrument to be used with children, to determine which stutterers would benefit from early intervention. Item #4855. *$41.00*
Ages 5-18

6781 Fluharty Preschool Speech & Language Screening Test-2
Speech Bin
PO Box 922668
Norcross, GA 30010
770-449-5700
800-850-8602
FAX 770-510-7290
http://www.speechbin.com
e-mail: info@speechbin.com
Shane Peters, Product Coordinator
Jan Binney, Owner

Carefully normed on 705 children, the Fluharty yields standard scores, percentiles, and age equivalents. The form features space for speech-language pathologists to note phonelogical processes, voice quality, and fluency; a Teacher Questionnaire is also provided. Item number P882. *$153.00*

6782 Help for the Learning Disabled Child
Slosson Educational Publications
PO Box 280
East Aurora, NY 14052
716-652-0930
800-828-4800
FAX 800-655-3840
http://www.slosson.com
e-mail: slosson@slosson.com
Steven Slosson, President
John Slosson, Vice President

Symptoms and solutions for learning disabled children. Features issues from a medical, psychological and educational basis and illustrates learning disabilities from emotional and mental impairment.

6783 Learning Disability Evaluation Scale: Reno
800 Gray Oak Drive
Columbia, MO 65201
573-874-1710
Michele Jackson, Owner

6784 Learning from Verbal Presentations and Participating in Discussions
Curriculum Associates
PO Box 2001
North Billerica, MA 01862
978-667-8000
800-225-0248
FAX 800-366-1158
http://www.curriculumassociates.com
e-mail: ca@infocurriculumassociates.com
Anita Archer, Mary Gleason, Author
Frank Ferguson, Owner
Fred Ferguson, VP Corporate Development/CIO

Develops oral and written language abilities. Students learn valuable strategies for note-taking, brainstorming, and effectively participating in class dicussions. *$19.90*

6785 Naglieri: Nonverbal Ability Test-Multilevel Form
Harcourt
PO Box 839954
San Antonio, TX 78283
800-232-1223
800-211-8378
FAX 800-232-1223
http://www.hbtpc.com
Jack Naglieri, Author
Aurelio Prifitera, Publisher

Provides a group-administered measure of nonverbal reasoning and problem solving that is independent of educational curricula and children's cultural or language background. *$22.00*

6786 Oral Speech Mechanism Screening Examination
Pro-Ed
8700 Shoal Creek Boulevard
Austin, TX 78757
512-451-3246
800-897-3202
FAX 800-397-7663
http://www.proedinc.com
e-mail: info@proedinc.com
Kenneth St Louis, Dennis Ruscello, Author
Don Hammill, Owner

Provides an efficient, quick, and reliable method to examine the oral speech mechanism of all types of speech, language, and related disorders where oral structure and function are of concern. *$101.00*
Ages 5-70+

6787 Peabody Picture Vocabulary Test: Fourth Edition (PPVT-4)
Pearson Assessments
5601 Green Valley Drive
Bloomington, MN 55437
800-627-7271
FAX 800-632-9011
http://http://ags.pearsonassessments.com
e-mail: agsinfo@pearson.com
Lloyd Dunn, Leota Dunn, Author
Karen Dahlen, Associate Director
Matt Keller, Marketing Manager
Lisa Dunttam, Development Assistant
A wide range measure of receptive vocabulary for standard English and screen of verbal ability. *$379.99*
Ages 2-6

6788 Peabody Picture Vocabulary Test: Third
4201 Woodland Road
Circle Pines, MN 55014
763-786-4343
Kevin Brueggeman, Manager

6789 Phonological Awareness Test: Computerized Scoring
LinguiSystems
3100 4th Avenue
East Moline, IL 61244
309-755-2300
800-776-4332
FAX 309-755-2377
TDY:800-933-8331
http://www.linguisystems.com
e-mail: service@linguisystems.com
Carolyn Robertson & Wanda Salter, Author
Linda Bowers, Co-Owner/Co-Founder
Rosemary Huisingh, Co-Owner/Co-Founder

What a timesaver! This optional CD-ROM software allows you to accurately, conveniently, and quickly score The Phonological Awareness Test. Just plug in the raw scores and the program does everything else. You'll be able to print out all the scores you need to include in a student's assessment report. *$69.95*
Ages 5-9

6790 Preschool Language Assessment Instrument
Harcourt
PO Box 839954
San Antonio, TX 78283
800-232-1223
800-211-8378
FAX 800-232-1223
http://www.hbtpc.com
Marion Blank, Susan Rose, Laura Berlin, Author
Marion Blank
Susan Rose

Provides a profile of a child's language skills in order to match teaching with the student's competence. The test is ideal for children ages 3 to 6 and is available in Spanish. *$197.00*

6791 **Preschool Language Scale: Fourth Edition**
Harcourt
PO Box 839954
San Antonio, TX 78283
800-232-1223
800-211-8378
FAX 800-232-1223
http://www.hbtpc.com
Iria Zimmerman, PhD, Author
Violette Steiner, BS, Author
Roberta Evatt Pond, MA, Author
This tool measures a broad range of receptive and expressive language skills. A Spanish version is also available. *$275.00*
Ages 0-11

6792 **Preschool Motor Speech Evaluation & Intervention**
Speech Bin
PO Box 922668
Norcross, GA 30010
770-449-5700
800-850-8602
FAX 770-510-7290
http://www.speechbin.com
e-mail: info@speechbin.com
Shane Peters, Product Coordinator
Jan Binney, Owner

This comprehensive criterion-based assessment tool differentiates motor-based speech disorders from those of phonology and determines if speech difficulties of children 18 months to six years old are characteristic of: oral nonverbal apraxia; dysarthria; developmental verbal dyspraxia; hypersensitivity; differences in tone and hyposensitivity. Item number J322. *$59.00*

6793 **Receptive One-Word Picture Vocabulary Test (ROWPVT-2000)**
Speech Bin
PO Box 922668
Norcross, GA 30010
770-449-5700
800-850-8602
FAX 770-510-7290
http://www.speechbin.com
e-mail: info@speechbin.com
Rick Brownell, Author
Shane Peters, Product Coordinator
Jan Binney, Owner

This administered, untimed measure assessess the vocabulary comprehension of 0-2 through 11-18 years. New full-color test pictures are easy to recognize; many new test items have been added. It is ideal for children unable or reluctant to speak because only a gestural response is required. Item number A305. *$140.00*

6794 **Receptive-Expressive Emergent Language Tests**
Pro-Ed
8700 Shoal Creek Boulevard
Austin, TX 78757
512-451-3246
800-897-3202
FAX 800-397-7633
http://www.proedinc.com
e-mail: info@proedinc.com
Kenneth Bzoch, Richard League, Virginia Brown, Author
Don Hammill, Owner

Designed to use with at-risk infants and toddlers to provide a multidimensional analysis of emergency language skills. *$100.00*
Ages 0-3

6795 **Sequenced Inventory of Communication Development**
Slosson Educational Publications
PO Box 280
East Aurora, NY 14052
716-652-0930
800-828-4800
FAX 800-655-3840
http://www.slosson.com
e-mail: slosson@slosson.com
Dona Hedrick, Elizabeth Prather, Annette Tobin, Author
Steven Slosson, President
John Slosson, Vice President

A diagnostic test designed to evaluate communications abilities, the SICD was planned for use in remedial programming of the young child with language disorders, mental challenges, and specific language problems. It has been successfully used with children who have sensory impairments, both hearing and visual, and varying degrees of retardation/challenges. *$395.00*
4mo-4 yrs old

6796 **Sequenced Inventory of Communication Development (SICD)**
Speech Bin
PO Box 922668
Norcross, GA 30010
770-449-5700
800-850-8602
FAX 770-510-7290
http://www.speechbin.com
e-mail: info@speechbin.com
Shane Peters, Product Coordinator
Jan Binney, Owner

SICD uses appealing toys to assess communication skills of children at all levels of ability, including those with impaired hearing or vision. SICD looks at child and environment, measuring receptive and expressive language. Item number W710. *$395.00*

6797 **Skills Assessments**
PO Box 690789
Orlando, FL 32869
407-345-3800

6798 **Slosson Intelligence Test**
Slosson Educational Publications
PO Box 280
East Aurora, NY 14052
716-652-0930
800-828-4800
FAX 800-655-3840
http://www.slosson.com
e-mail: slosson@slosson.com
Richard L Slosson, Author
Steven Slosson, President
John Slosson, Vice President

A quick and reliable individual screening test of Crystallized Verbal Intelligence. *$100.75*
Ages 2+

6799 **Slosson Intelligence Test: Primary**
Slosson Educational Publications
PO Box 280
East Aurora, NY 14052
716-652-0930
800-828-4800
FAX 800-655-3840
http://www.slosson.com
e-mail: slosson@slosson.com
Bradley Erford, Gary Vitali, Steven Slosson, Author
Steven Slosson, President
John Slosson, Vice President

Designed to facilitate the screening identification of children at risk of educational failure. Provides a quick estimate of mental ability to identify children who may be appropriate candidates for deeper testing services. *$ 138.75*
Ages 2-7

6800 **Stuttering Severity Instrument for Children and Adults**
Pro-Ed
8700 Shoal Creek Boulevard
Austin, TX 78757
512-451-3246
800-897-3202
FAX 800-397-7633
http://www.proedinc.com
e-mail: info@proedinc.com
Glyndon Riley, Author
Don Hammill, Owner

With these easily administered tools you can determine whether to schedule a child for therapy using the Stuttering Prediction Instrument or to evaluate the effects of treatment using the Stuttering Severity Instrument. *$110.00*

6801 **TELD-2: Test of Early Language Development**
8700 Shoal Creek Boulevard
Austin, TX 78757
512-451-3246

Don Hammill, Owner

6802 TELD-3: Test of Early Language Development
Pro-Ed
8700 Shoal Creek Boulevard
Austin, TX 78757
512-451-3246
800-897-3202
FAX 800-397-7633
http://www.proedinc.com
e-mail: info@proedinc.com
Wayne Hresko, Kim Reid, Don Hammill, Author
Don Hamhill, President

An individually administered test of spoken language abilities. This test fills the need for a well-constructed, standardized instrument, based on a current theory, that can be used to assess spoken language skills at early ages. Now including scores for receptive language and expressive language subtests. Administration Time: 20 minutes. *$285.00*

Ages 2-11

6803 TOAL-3: Test of Adolescent & Adult Language
Pro-Ed
8700 Shoal Creek Boulevard
Austin, TX 78757
512-451-3246
800-897-3202
FAX 800-397-7633
http://www.proedinc.com
e-mail: info@proedinc.com
Don Hammill, Virginia Brown, Stephen Larson, Author
J Lee Wiederholt, Author
Don Hammill, Owner

This test is a measure of receptive and expressive language skills. In this revision easier items were added to the subtests, making them more appropriate for testing disabled students. *$210.00*

Ages 12-24

6804 TOLD-3: Test of Language Development, Primary
Harcourt
PO Box 839954
San Antonio, TX 78283
800-232-1223
800-211-8378
FAX 800-232-1223
http://www.hbtpc.com
Phyllis Newcomer, Donald Hammill, Author

An individually administered language battery that assesses the understanding and meaningful use of spoken words, aspects of grammar, word pronunciation and the ability to distinguish between similar sounding words. *$280.00*

6805 TOWL-3: Test of Written Language, 3rd Edition
Pro-Ed
8700 Shoal Creek Boulevard
Austin, TX 78757
512-451-3246
800-897-3202
FAX 800-397-7633
http://www.proedinc.com
e-mail: info@proedinc.com
Donald Hammill, Stephen Larson, Author
Don Hammill, Owner

Offers a measure of written language skills to identify students who need help improving their writing skills. Administration Time: 65 minutes. *$210.00*

Ages 7-17

6806 Test for Auditory Comprehension of Language: TACL-3
Speech Bin
PO Box 922668
Norcross, GA 30010
770-449-5700
800-850-8602
FAX 770-510-7290
http://www.speechbin.com
e-mail: info@speechbin.com
Shane Peters, Product Coordinator
Jan Binney, Owner

The newly revised TACL-3 evaluates the 0-3 to 9-11-year old's understanding of spoken language in three subtests: Vocabulary, Grammatical Morphemes and Elaborated Phrases and Sentences. Each test item is a word or sentence read aloud by the examiner; the child responds by pointing to one of three pictures. Item number P792. *$261.00*

6807 Test of Auditory Reasoning & Processing Skills (TARPS)
Speech Bin
PO Box 922668
Norcross, GA 30010
770-449-5700
800-850-8602
FAX 770-510-7290
http://www.speechbin.com
e-mail: info@speechbin.com
Morrison Gardner, Author
Shane Peters, Product Coordinator
Jan Binney, Owner

TARPS assesses how 5-14 year old children understand, interpret, draw conclusions, and make inferences from auditorily presented stimuli. It tests their ability to think, understand, reason, and make sense of what they hear. Item number H787. *$64.00*

6808 Test of Auditory-Perceptual Skills: Upper (TAPS-UL)
Speech Bin
PO Box 922668
Norcross, GA 30010
770-449-5700
800-850-8602
FAX 770-510-7290
http://www.speechbin.com
e-mail: info@speechbin.com
Wayne Hresko, Shelley Herron, Pamela Peak, Author
Shane Peters, Product Coordinator
Jan Binney, Owner

This highly respected, well-normed test evaluates a 13-18 year old's ability to perceive auditory stimuli and helps you diagnose auditory disorders in just 15-20 minutes. TAPS: UL measures the auditory perceptual skills of processing, word and sequential memory, interpretation of oral directions, and discrimination. Item number H769. *$95.00*

6809 Test of Early Written Language
Pro-Ed
8700 Shoal Creek Boulevard
Austin, TX 78757
512-451-3246
800-897-3202
FAX 512-451-8542
http://www.proedinc.com
e-mail: info@proedinc.com
Shelley Herron, Wayne Hresko & Pamela Peak, Author
Don Hammill, Owner

Measures the merging written language skills of young children and is especially useful in identifying mildy disabled students. *$190.00*

Ages 3-11

6810 Test of Written Spelling
Pro-Ed
8700 Shoal Creek Boulevard
Austin, TX 78757
512-451-3246
800-897-3202
FAX 800-397-7633
http://www.proedinc.com
e-mail: info@proedinc.com
Stephen Larsen, Donald Hammill, Louisa Moats, Author
Don Hammill, Owner

Assesses students' ability to spell words whose spellings are readily predictable in sound-letter patterns, words whose spellings are less predictable and both types of words considered together. *$85.00*

6811 Testing & Remediating Auditory Processing (TRAP)
Speech Bin
PO Box 922668
Norcross, GA 30010
770-449-5700
800-850-8602
FAX 770-510-7290
http://www.speechbin.com
e-mail: info@speechbin.com

Lynn Baron Berk, Author
Shane Peters, Product Coordinator
Jan Binney, Owner

TRAP gives you an easy-to-implement program to assess and treat school-age auditory processing problems. It gives you two major components: Screening Test of Auditoring Processing Skills that identifies children at risk due to auditory processing deficits; and Remediating Auditory Processing Skills that presents interactional stories, sequence pictures, and illustrated activities. Item number 1233. *$38.00*

6812 Voice Assessment Protocol for Children and Adults
Pro-Ed
8700 Shoal Creek Boulevard
Austin, TX 78757 512-451-3246
800-897-3202
FAX 800-397-7633
http://www.proedinc.com
e-mail: info@proedinc.com
Rebekah Pindzola, Author
Don Hammill, Owner

Easily guides the speech pathologist through a systematic evaluation of vocal pitch, loudness, quality, breath features and rate/rhythm. *$75.00*

Visual & Motor Skills

6813 BRIGANCE Inventory of Early Development-II
Curriculum Associates
PO Box 2001
North Billerica, MA 01862 978-667-8000
800-225-0248
FAX 800-366-1158
http://www.curriculumassociates.com
e-mail: ca@infocurriculumassociates.com
Albert Brigance, Author
Frank Ferguson, Owner
Fred Ferguson, VP Corporate Development/CIO

The Inventory of Early Development simplifies and combines the assessment, diagnostic, recordkeeping, and instructional planning process, and it encourages communication between teachers and parents.
Ages Birth-7

6814 Benton Visual Retention Test: Fifth Edition
Harcourt
PO Box 839954
San Antonio, TX 78283 800-232-1223
800-211-8378
FAX 800-232-1223
http://www.hbtpc.com
Abigail Benton Sivan, Author

Assess visual perception, memory, visoconstructive abilities. Test administration 15-20 minutes. *$199.00*
Ages 8-Adult

6815 Boston Diagnostic Aphasia Exam: Third Edition
Speech Bin
PO Box 922668
Norcross, GA 30010 770-449-5700
800-850-8602
FAX 770-510-7290
http://www.speechbin.com
e-mail: info@speechbin.com
Harold Goodglass, Edith Kaplan, Barbara Barresi, Author
Jan Binney, Owner
Shane Peters, Product Coordinator

evised and improved. BDAE-3 now gives you an instructive 90-minute video plus two separate forms of the test. Item number L235. *$150.00*

6816 Development Test of Visual Perception
Pro-Ed
8700 Shoal Creek Boulevard
Austin, TX 78757 512-451-3246
800-897-3202
FAX 800-397-7633
http://www.proedinc.com
e-mail: info@proedinc.com
Don Hammill, Nils Pearson, Judith Voress, Author
Don Hammill, Owner

Measures both visual perception and visual-motor integration skills, has eight subtests, is based on updated theories of visual perceptual development, and can be administered to individuals in 35 minutes. *$179.00*
Ages 4-10

6817 Developmental Test of Visual Perception (DTVP-2)
Pro-Ed
8700 Shoal Creek Boulevard
Austin, TX 78757 512-451-3246
800-897-3202
FAX 800-397-7633
http://www.proedinc.com
e-mail: info@proedinc.com
Don Hammill, Nils Pearson, Judith Voress, Author
Don Hammill, Owner

A test that measures both visual perception and visual-motor integration skills, has eight subtests, is based on updated theories of visual perceptual development, and can be administered to individuals in 45 minutes. *$200.00*
Ages 4-10

6818 Differential Test of Conduct and Emotional Problems
Slosson Educational Publications
PO Box 280
East Aurora, NY 14052 716-652-0930
800-828-4800
FAX 800-655-3840
http://www.slosson.com
e-mail: slosson@slosson.com
Edward Kelly, Author
Steven Slosson, President
John Slosson, Vice President

Designed to address one of the most critical challenges in education and juvenile care. Administration of test is 15-20 minutes. *$82.00*

6819 KLPA-2: Khan-Lewis Phonological Analysis
Pro-Ed
8700 Shoal Creek Boulevard
Austin, TX 78757 512-451-3246
800-897-3202
FAX 800-397-7633
http://www.proedinc.com
e-mail: info@proedinc.com
Linda Klan, Nancy Lewis, Author
Don Hamhill, President

An in-depth measure of phonological processes for assessment and remediation planning. Administration Time: 10-30 minutes. *$137.00*
Ages 2-5

6820 KLPA: Khan-Lewis Phonological Analysis
8700 Shoal Creek Boulevard
Austin, TX 78757 512-451-3246
Don Hammill, Owner

6821 Learning Efficiency Test II
Academic Therapy Publications
20 Commercial Boulevard
Novato, CA 94949 415-883-3314
800-422-7249
FAX 415-883-3720
http://www.academictherapy.com
e-mail: sales@academictherapy.com
Raymond Webster, Author
Jim Arena
Joanne Urban

Provides a quick and accurate measure of a child or adult's information processing abilities, sequential and nonsequential, in both visual and auditory modalities. *$92.00*
Ages 5-75+

6822 Oral Motor Assessment: Ages and Stages
Therapro
225 Arlington Street
Framingham, MA 01702 508-872-9494
800-257-5376
FAX 508-875-2062
http://www.theraproducts.com
e-mail: info@theraproducts.com
Diane Chapman Bahr, Author
Karen Conrad, Owner

Provides an overview of available assessments, checklists, tables, and figures to assist the clinician in accurately diagnosing muscle function and motor planning issues. *$62.50*
274 pages

6823 Peabody Developmental Motor Scales-2
Speech Bin
PO Box 922668
Norcross, GA 30010 770-449-5700
800-850-8602
FAX 770-510-7290
http://www.speechbin.com
e-mail: info@speechbin.com
Shane Peters, Product Coordinator
Jan Binney, Owner

PDMS-2 gives you in-depth standardized assessment of motor skills in children birth to six years. Subtests include: fine motor object manipulation; grasping; gross motor; locomotion; reflexes; visual-motor integration and stationary. Item number P624. *$43.00*

6824 Perceptual Motor Development Series
Therapro
225 Arlington Street
Framingham, MA 01702 508-872-9494
800-257-5376
FAX 508-875-2062
http://www.theraproducts.com
e-mail: info@theraproducts.com
Jack Capon, Author
Karen Conrad, Owner

Use these classroom tested movement education activities to assess motor strengths and weaknesses in preschool and early elementary grades or special education classes. The sequence of easily given tests and tasks requires minimal instruction time and your kids will find the activities to be interesting, challenging, and fun! Each book has 25-54 pages and costs $9.99 each. *$49.95*

6825 Preschool Motor Speech Evaluation & Intervention
Speech Bin
PO Box 922668
Norcross, GA 30010 770-449-5700
800-850-8602
FAX 770-510-7290
http://www.speechbin.com
e-mail: info@speechbin.com
Shane Peters, Product Coordinator
Jan Binney, Owner

This comprehensive criterion-based assessment tool differentiates motor-based speech disorders from those of phonology and determines if speech difficulties of children 18 months to six years old are characteristic of: oral nonverbal apraxia; dysarthria; developmental verbal dyspraxia; hypersensitivity; differences in tone and hyposensitivity. Item number J322. *$59.00*

6826 Slosson Full Range Intelligence Test Kit
Slosson Educational Publications
PO Box 280
East Aurora, NY 14052 716-652-0930
800-828-4800
FAX 800-655-3840
http://www.slosson.com
e-mail: slosson@slosson.com
Bob Algozzine, Ronald Eaves, Lester Mann, Author
H Robert Vance, Author
Steven Slosson, President
John Slosson, Vice President
Intended to supplement the use of more extensive cognitive assessment instruments. Administration of test 25-45 minutes. *$144.50*
Ages 5-Adult

6827 Slosson Visual Motor Performance Test
Slosson Educational Publications
PO Box 280
East Aurora, NY 14052 716-652-0930
800-828-4800
FAX 800-655-3840
http://www.slosson.com
e-mail: slosson@slosson.com
Richard Slosson, Author
Steven Slosson, President
John Slosson, Vice President
Georgina Moynihan, TTFM
A test of visual motor integration in which individuals are asked to copy geometric figures increasing in complexity without the use of a ruler, compass or other aids. *$86.75*
Ages 4-Adult

6828 Test of Gross Motor Development
Pro-Ed
8700 Shoal Creek Boulevard
Austin, TX 78757 512-451-3246
800-897-3202
FAX 800-397-7633
http://www.proedinc.com
e-mail: info@proedinc.com
Dale Urlich, Author
Don Hammill, Owner

Assists you in identifying children who are significantly behind their peers in gross motor skill development and who should be eligible for special education services in phyiscal education. *$105.00*
Ages 3-11

6829 Visual Skills Appraisal
Academic Therapy Publications
20 Commercial Boulevard
Novato, CA 94949 415-883-3314
800-422-7249
FAX 415-883-3720
http://www.academictherapy.com
e-mail: sales@academictherapy.com
Regina Richards, Gary Oppenheim, Author
Jim Arena
Joanne Urban

This test identifies visual problems in children. Can be administered by teachers or other educators who may not have training in assessment. Set includes manual, stimulus cards and test forms. *$85.00*
Ages 5-9
ISBN 0-878794-50-0

National Programs

6830 ACT Universal Testing
ACT
500 ACT Drive
Iowa City, IA 52243
319-337-1332
FAX 319-339-3021
TDY:319-337-1701
http://www.act.org
e-mail: sandy.schlote@act.org

Richard Ferguson, CEO
Jon Erickson, Educational Services VP
Ann York, Operations VP

To help individuals and organizations make informed decisions about education and work. We provide information for life's transitions.

6831 Alliance for Technology Access
1304 Southpoint Boulevard
Petaluma, CA 94954
707-765-2080
800-455-7970
FAX 707-765-2080
TDY:707-778-3015
http://www.ataccess.org
e-mail: atainfo@ataccess.org

Mary Lester, Executive Director
Libbie Butler, Program Coordinator

A national organization dedicated to providing access to technology for people with disabilities through its coalition of 39 community-based resource centers in 28 states and in the Virgin Islands. Each center provides information, awareness, and training for professionals and provides guided problem solving and technical assistance for individuals with disabilities and family members.

6832 America's Jobline
National Federation of the Blind
1800 Johnson Street
Baltimore, MD 21230
410-659-9314
800-414-5748
FAX 410-685-5653
http://www.nfb.org
e-mail: nfb@nfb.org

Marc Maurer, President
M. Rorick, Coordinator
Patricia Maurer, Community Relations Director

Jobline is an audio version of America's Job Bank, provided on the telephone. America's Job Bank and the electronic job bank provided by state can also be found on the internet. The job announcements come from employers seeking to fill current openings. Jobline helps you to find openings and apply for jobs which match your qualifications and are located in your area or any other area of the country.

6833 American College Testing Program
ACT Universal Testing
PO Box 168
Iowa City, IA 52243
319-337-1000
FAX 319-339-3021
TDY:319-337-1701
http://www.act.org
e-mail: sandy.schlote@act.org

Ed Colby, Public Relations
Sandy Schlote, Testing Coordinator
Richard Ferguson, CEO

To help individuals and organizations make informed decisions about education and work. We provide information for life's transitions.

6834 Division on Career Development
Council for Exceptional Children
1110 N Glebe Road
Arlington, VA 22201
703-245-0600
888-232-7733
FAX 703-264-9494
TDY:703-264-9446
http://www.cec.sped.org
e-mail: service@ces.sped.org

Victor Erickson, Exhibits Manager
Liz Martinez, Publications Director
Bruce Ramirez, Manager

Focuses on the career development of individuals with disabilities and/or who are gifted and their transition from school to adult life. Members include professionals and others interested in career development and transition for individuals with any exception at any age. Members receive a journal twice yearly and newsletter three times per year.

6835 Division on Career Development and Transition
Council for Exceptional Children
1110 N Glebe Road
Arlington, VA 22201
703-245-0600
888-232-7733
FAX 703-264-9494
TDY:703-264-9446
http://www.cec.sped.org
e-mail: service@ces.sped.org

Victor Erickson, Exhibits Manager
Bruce Ramirez, Manager

Established to give voice to those special education professionals who were becoming increasingly concerned about the limited post-secondary outcomes faced by most youth with disabilities upon leaving school.

6836 Independent Living Research Utilization Program
2323 S Shepherd Drive
Houston, TX 77019
713-520-0232
FAX 713-520-5785
TDY:713-520-5136
http://www.ilru.org
e-mail: ilru@ilru.org

Lex Frieden, Director
Richard Petty, Program Director
Laurie Redd, Executive Director

A national resource center for information, training, research and technical assistance in independent living; produces and disseminates materials, develops and conducts training and publishes a monthly newsletter; provides a listing of Statewide Independent Living Councils (SILCS) in each state.

6837 Job Accommodation Network (JAN)
West Virginia University
PO Box 6080
Morgantown, WV 26506
304-598-4000
800-526-7232
FAX 304-293-5407
TDY:800-232-9675
http://www.jan.wvu.edu
e-mail: jan@jan.wvu.edu

DJ Hendrix, Director
Fred Butcher, Manager

Network and consulting resource that provides information about employment issues to employers, rehabilitation professionals, and persons with disabilities. Callers should be prepared to explain their specific problem and job circumstances. Sponsored by the Office of Disability Employment Policy, the Network is operated by West Virginia University's Rehabilitation Research and Training Center. Brochures and printed materials available.

6838 Minnesota Vocational Rehabilitation Agency: Rehabilitation Services Branch
Department of Employment & Economic Development
390 Robert Street N
Saint Paul, MN 55101
651-296-3711
800-328-9095
FAX 651-297-5159
http://www.deed.state.mn.us
e-mail: paul.bridges@state.mn.us

Paul Bridges, Director
Jan McAllister, Administrative Assistant

Provides basic vocational rehabilitation services to consumers including vocational counseling, planning, guidance and placement, as well as certain special services based on individual circumstances.

6839 Rehabilitation Services Administration
University of Illinois at Urbana-Champaign
51 Gerty Drive
Champaign, IL 61820
217-356-1923
FAX 217-244-0851
http://www.ed.uiuc.edu/illinoisrcep
e-mail: jtrach@uiuc.edu

John Trach Ph.D, Project Director
Tony Plotner, Project Coordinator

Integrated employment outcomes for individuals with disabilities on several different levels, including continuing education and technical assistance, externships, replication activities, and leadership development.

6840 **State Vocational Rehabilitation Agency**
Department of Employment & Economic Development
First National Bank Building
St. Paul, MN 55101
651-296-3711
800-328-9095
FAX 651-297-5159
http://www.deed.state.mn.us/rehab/rehab.htm
e-mail: howard.glad@state.mn.us
Kimberly Peck, Program Director

Rehabilitation Services works with individuals who have disabilities, providing a variety of services. The services include but are not limited to: vocational planning, employment information and referral service. They also provide guidance in maintaining employment.

6841 **Transition Research Institute**
University of Illinois at Urbana-Champaign
51 Gerty Drive
Champaign, IL 61820
217-356-1923
FAX 217-244-0851
http://www.ed.uiuc.edu/illinoisrcep
e-mail: jtrach@uiuc.edu
John Trach, Director
John Hadley, Owner
Betty Taylor, Administrative Assistant
Provides technical assistance on transition-focused projects, policy analysis concerning legislation focused on education and transition services for youths with disabilities, and a wealth of information for teachers, service providers and researchers.

6842 **U.S. Department of Education: Office of Vocational & Adult Education**
330 C Street SW
Washington, DC 20202
202-208-5815
FAX 202-245-7838
http://www.ed.gov/about/offices/list/ovae
e-mail: ovae@ed.gov
Beto Gonzalez, Acting Assistant Secretary
Hans Meeder, Deputy Assistant Secretary
John Sherrod, Executive Director
These agencies can provide job training, counseling, financial assistance, and employment placement to individuals who meet eligibility criteria.

Publications

6843 **ABILITY**
C R Cooper
1001 W 17th Street
Costa Mesa, CA 92627
949-548-1986
FAX 949-548-5966
TDY:949-548-5966
http://www.abilitymagazine.com
e-mail: editorial@abilitymagazine.com
Chet Cooper, President/Editor-in-Chief
Jenifer Medrano, Administrative Coordinator

ABILITY Magazine is an award-winning publication bringing a greater understanding to the issues surrounding the 56 million Americans with disabilities through celebrity interviews and in-depth articles focusing on health, wellness and disability.
80+ pages Bimonthly

6844 **ADD on the Job**
Taylor Publishing
1550 W Mockingbird Lane
Dallas, TX 75235
214-637-2800
800-677-2800
FAX 214-819-8580
http://www.taylorpublishing.com
e-mail: rparra@taylorpub.com
Lynn Weiss PhD, Author
Rick Parra, Customer Service Director
Charles Kass, Assistant Director
Con Percenti, CEO
Practical, sensitive advice for the ADD employee, his boss, and his co-workers. The book suggests advantages that the ADD worker has, how to find the right job, and how to keep it. Employers and co-workers will learn what to expect from fellow workers with ADD and the most effective ways to work with them.
232 pages Paperback
ISBN 0-878339-17-5

6845 **Ability Magazine**
Ability Awareness
1001 W 17th Street
Costa Mesa, CA 92627
949-548-1986
FAX 949-548-5966
TDY:949-548-5966
http://www.abilitymagazine.com
e-mail: editorial@abilitymagazine.com
Chet Cooper, President

Brings disabilities into mainstream America. By interviewing high profile personalities such as President Clinton, Elizabeth Taylor, Mary Tyler Moore, Richard Pryor, Jane Seymour and many more, Ability Magazine is able to bring articles to the public's attention that may in the past have gone unnoticed.
80+ pages Bimonthly

6846 **Articulation Models for Vocational**
1900 Kenny Road
Columbus, OH 43210
614-292-4353

6847 **Articulation Models for Vocational Education**
Center on Education and Training for Employment
Ohio State University
Columbus, OH 43210
614-292-4353
800-848-4815
FAX 614-292-1260
http://www.cete.org/products
Highlights the vital role of articulations in vocational education today. Publications have been retired. They are available by Special order only and no return, no refund. Call for pricing and shipping and handling.

6848 **Bottom Line: Basic Skills in the Workplace**
US Department of Labor
200 Constitution Avenue NW
Washington, DC 20210
202-693-5000
866-4-USADOL
Elaine Chao, CEO

Discusses the issues of meeting basic literacy needs and meeting them within the context of employment.

6849 **Business Currents**
National Alliance of Business (NAB)
1201 New York Avenue NW
Washington, DC 20005
202-289-2888
FAX 202-289-1303
Business Currents provides information about legislative and administrative actions affecting employment and training.
Biweekly

6850 **Career Inventories for the Learning Disabled**
Academic Therapy Publications
PO Box 280
East Aurora, NY 14052
716-652-0930
800-422-7249
FAX 888-287-9975
http://www.academictherapy.com
e-mail: sales@academictherapy.com
Jim Arena
Joanne Urban

These career assessment inventories take personality, ability, and interest into account in pointing LD students toward intelligent and realistic career choices.

64 pages Paperback
ISBN 0-878793-50-X

6851 Change Agent
Nat'l Center for Research in Vocational Education
2150 Shattuck Avenue
Berkeley, CA 94704
800-762-4093
e-mail: dcarlson@uclink.berkley.edu
David Carlson, Contact

A quarterly digest of center publications.

6852 Cognitive Theory-Based Teaching and Learning in Vocational Education
Center on Education and Training for Employment
1900 Kenny Road
Columbus, OH 43210
614-292-4353
800-848-4815
FAX 614-292-1260
http://www.cete.org/products
e-mail: ericacve@magnus.acs.ohio_state.edu
Ruth Thomas, Author
Ruth Thomas

This research review explores the relevance to vocational curriculum and instruction of theories of cognition.

6853 College Students with Learning Disabilities: A Handbook
Learning Disabilities Association of America
4156 Library Road
Pittsburgh, PA 15234
412-341-1515
FAX 412-344-0224
http://www.ldaamerica.org
e-mail: ldanatl@usaor.net /info@ldaamerica.org
Jane Browning, Director
Heathe Smith, Clerk

An overview of related issues, including information on Section 504 as it pertains to students with learning disabilities and college personnel.

6854 Current Developments in Employment and Training
National Governors Association
444 N Capitol Street NW
Washington, DC 20001
202-624-5300
FAX 202-624-5313
http://www.nga.org
e-mail: mjensen@nga.org
Martin Jensen, Editor
Raymond Sheppach, Executive Director

Highlights issues and areas of interest related to employment and training.
Bimonthly

6855 For Employers: A Look at Learning Disabilities Fact Sheet
Learning Disabilities Association of America
4156 Library Road
Pittsburgh, PA 15234
412-341-1515
FAX 412-344-0224
http://www.ldaamerica.org
e-mail: ldanatl@usaor.net /info@ldaamerica.org
Jane Browning, Director
Heathe Smith, Clerk

Helps employers understand learning disabilities.

6856 Fundamentals of Job Placement
RPM Press
PO Box 31483
Tucson, AZ 85751
520-886-1990
888-810-1990
FAX 520-886-1990
http://www.rpmpress.com
e-mail: pmccray@theriver.com
James Costello, Author
Jan Stonebraker, Operations Manager
Paul McCray, President

Provides step-by-step guidance for educators, special counselors and vocational rehabilitation personnel on how to develop job placement opportunities for special needs students and adults.

6857 Fundamentals of Vocational Assessment
RPM Press
PO Box 31483
Tucson, AZ 85751
520-886-1990
888-810-1990
FAX 520-866-1900
http://www.rpmpress.com
e-mail: pmccray@theriver.com
Jan Stonebraker, Operations Manager
Paul McCray, President

Provides step-by-step guidance for educators, counselors and vocational rehabilitation personnel on how to conduct professional vocational assessments of special needs students.

6858 Handbook for Developing Community Based Employment
RPM Press
PO Box 31483
Tucson, AZ 85751
520-886-1990
888-810-1990
FAX 520-866-1990
http://www.rpmpress.com
e-mail: pmccray@theriver.com
Jan Stonebraker, Operations Manager
Paul McCray, President

Provides step-by-step guidance for educators and vocational rehabilitation personnel on how to develop community-based employment training programs for severely challenged workers.

6859 JOBS V
PESCO International
21 Paulding Street
Pleasantville, NY 10570
914-769-4266
800-431-2016
FAX 914-769-2970
http://www.pesco.org
e-mail: pesco@pesco.org
Joseph Kass, President
Charles Kass, Vice President
Kathy Griffin, Sales Manager
A software program matching people with jobs, training, employment and local employers. Provides job outlooks for the next five years.

6860 Job Access
Ability Awareness
1001 W 17th Street
Costa Mesa, CA 92627
949-548-1986
FAX 949-548-5966
TDY:949-548-5966
http://www.jobaccess.org
e-mail: marketing@jobaccess.org
Chet Cooper, President

Job Access, a program of ability awareness, is an internet driven system dedicated to employ qualified people with disabilities. Employers can list job postings and review our resume bank. People with disabilities seeking employment can also search for jobs.

6861 Job Accommodation Handbook
RPM Press
PO Box 31483
Tucson, AZ 85751
520-886-1990
888-810-1990
FAX 520-866-1990
http://www.rpmpress.com
e-mail: pmccray@theriver.com
Paul McCray, Author
Jan Stonebraker, Operations Manager
Paul McCray, President

Provides how-to-do-it for counselors, job placement specialists, educators and others on how to modify jobs for special needs workers.

6862 Job Interview Tips for People with Learning Disabilities Fact Sheet

Learning Disabilities Association of America
4156 Library Road
Pittsburgh, PA 15234 412-341-1515
FAX 412-344-0224
http://www.ldaamerica.org
e-mail: ldanatl@usaor.net /info@ldaamerica.org
Jane Browning, Director
Heathe Smith, Clerk

$18.00

6863 Life Centered Career Education: Assessment Batteries

Council for Exceptional Career Children
1110 N Glebe Road
Arlington, VA 22201 703-245-0600
888-232-7733
FAX 703-264-9494
TDY:703-264-9446
http://www.cec.sped.org/
e-mail: service@ces.sped.org
Donn E Brolin, Author
Victor Erickson, Exhibits manager
Liz Martinez, Publications Director
Bruce Ramirez, Manager

The LCCE Batteries are curriculum-based assessment instruments designed to measure the career education knowledge and skills of regular and special education students. There are two alternative forms of a Knowledge Battery and two forms of the Performance Batteries. These assessment tools can be combined with instruction to determine the instructional goals most appropriate for a particular student.

827 pages

6864 National Dissemination Center

Academy for the Educational Development
PO Box 1492
Washington, DC 20013 202-884-8200
800-695-0285
FAX 202-884-8841
TDY:800-695-0285
http://www.nichcy.org
e-mail: nichcy@aed.org
Susan Ripley, Manager

A newsletter offering information on vocational assessment, books and more for the disabled.

6865 National Forum on Issues in Vocational Assessment

MCD, Stout Vocational Rehabilitation Institute
University of Wisconsin-Stout
Menomonie, WI 54751 715-232-2475
FAX 715-232-2356
e-mail: admissions@uwstout.edu
RR Fry, Author
John Lui MD, Institute Director
Marilyn Mars, Director of Purchasing Departmen

The impact potential of curriculum-based vocational assessment in our schools.

6866 National Governors Association

444 N Capitol Street NW
Washington, DC 20001 202-624-5300
FAX 202-624-5313
http://www.nga.org
e-mail: mjensen@nga.org
Martin Jensen, Editor
Raymond Sheppach, Executive Director

Highlights issues and areas of interest related to employment and training.

Bimonthly

6867 PWI Profile

Goodwill Industries of America
15810 Indianola Drive
Derwood, MD 20855 301-530-6500
http://www.goodwill.org/
e-mail: contactus@goodwill.org
George Kessinger, CEO

Newsletter that deals with employment of persons with disabilities.

6868 Rehabilitation Research and Training Center on Supported Employment

PO Box 842011
Richmond, VA 23284 804-828-1851
FAX 804-828-2193
TDY:804-828-2494
http://www.worksupport.com
e-mail: vbrooker@mail1.vcu.edu
Jeanne Roberts, Graphics Designer
Valerie Brooker, Associate Director

Helps disabled persons find and hold a job. Designed to assist persons with significant disabilities to obtain and maintain community integrated competitive employment through high quality research and disseminations.

6869 School to Adult Life Transition Bibliography

Special Education Resource Center
25 Industrial Park Road
Middletown, CT 06457 860-632-1485
FAX 860-632-8870
http://www.ctserc.org
e-mail: jlebrrun@ctserc.org
Jen Lebrun, Director
Marianne Kirner, Executive Director

A bibliography of references and resources.

6870 Self Advocacy as a Technique for

1122 W Campus Road
Lawrence, KS 66045 785-864-2700
Robert Hemenway, CEO

6871 Self Advocacy as a Technique for Transition

KUAF-University of Kansas
1122 W Campus Road
Lawrence, KS 66045 785-864-4954
FAX 785-864-4149
http://www.soe.ku.edu/sped
e-mail: spedrecpt@ku.edu
Chriss Walther-Thomas, Chairperson

A joint effort involved in researching the effect of self-advocacy training upon adolescents with learning disabilities.

6872 Self-Directed Search

Harcourt Assessment
19500 Bulverde Road
San Antonio, TX 78283 210-497-1263
800-211-8378
FAX 210-949-4475
http://www.harcourtassessment.com
John Holland, Author
Aurelio Prifitera, Publisher
Jeff Galt, CEO

This self-administered, self-scored and self-interpreted test enables the individual to make education and career choices.

6873 Self-Supervision: A Career Tool for Audiologists, Clinical Series 10

American Speech-Language-Hearing Association
10801 Rockville Pike
N Bethesda, MD 20852 301-897-5700
800-638-2255
FAX 301-897-7358
TDY:301-897-5700
http://www.asha.org
e-mail: randerson@asha.org
Rick Anderson, Marketing Director
Arlene Pietrarton, Executive Director

Describes concepts of supervision, defines and presents strategies for self-supervision, discusses supervisory accountability and covers issues of self-supervision within supervisor format.

6874 Transition and Students with Learning Disabilities
Pro-Ed
8700 Shoal Creek Boulevard
Austin, TX 78757
512-451-3246
800-897-3202
FAX 512-451-8542
http://www.proedinc.com
e-mail: info@proedinc.com

Patton Blalock, Author
Don Hammill, Owner

Provides important information about academic, social and vocational planning for students with learning disabilities.

6875 Vocational Training and Employment of Autistic Adolescents
Charles C Thomas Publisher
2600 S 1st Street
Springfield, IL 62704
217-789-8980
800-258-8980
FAX 217-789-9130
http://www.ccthomas.com
e-mail: books@ccthomas.com

Elva Duran, Author
Michael Thomas, President
Claire Slagle, Assistant Director

How professionals and parents are now advocating, demanding and arranging that persons receive vocational training and equal rights for the disabled.

6876 Work America, Workforce Economics Workforce Trends
National Alliance of Business (NAB)
1201 New York Avenue NW
Washington, DC 20005
202-289-2888
800-787-7788
FAX 202-289-1303
http://www.nab.com
e-mail: jonesr@nab.com

Award winning publications that feature timely articles related to the human resource agenda. Workforce development and education improvement is covered from the business perspective.

6877 Workforce Investment Quarterly
National Governor's Association (NGA)
444 N Capitol Street NW
Washington, DC 20001
202-624-5300
FAX 202-624-7870
http://www.nga.org
e-mail: info@nga.org

Raymond Scheppach, Executive Director

Highlights issues and area interests related to employment and training. Contact NGA for more information.

Alabama

6878 Alabama Department of Human Resources
64 N Union Street
Montgomery, AL 36130
334-242-1310
FAX 334-353-1115
http://www.dhr.state.al.us
e-mail: ogapi@dhr.state.al.us

Page Walley MD, Commissioner

Partners with communities to promote family stability and to provide for the self-sufficiency of vulnerable Alabamians.

6879 Department of Human Resources
Alabama Department of Human Resources
50 N Ripley Street
Montgomery, AL 36130
334-242-4363
FAX 334-242-0198
http://www.dhr.state.al.us
e-mail: ogapi@dhr.state.al.us

Page Walley MD, Commissioner
Spear Audio-Visual Informati, Audio-Visual Information Officer

Partners with communities to promote family stability and to provide for the self-sufficiency of vulnerable Alabamians.

6880 Easter Seals Achievement Center
510 W Thomason Circle
Opelika, AL 36801
334-745-3501
FAX 334-745-5808
http://www.alabama.easter-seals.org

Cheryl Bynum, Director Rehabilitation Services
Barry Cavan, Chief Executive Officer
Elizabeth Griffin, Administrator

Job training and employment services, occupational skills training, job placement/competitive-supported employment, vocational evaluation/situation assessment, work adjustment.

6881 Easter Seals Adult Services Center
Easter Seals Arkansas
11801 Fairview Road
Little Rock, AR 72205
501-221-8400
877-221-8400
FAX 501-221-8842
http://www.ar.easter-seals.org
e-mail: info@easterseals.com

Priscilla Handley, Administrator
Sharon Moone-Jochums, President/CEO

Easter Seals Arkansas helps adults with disabilities gain greater independence through vocational and independent living programs.

6882 Easter Seals Alabama
5960 E Shirley Lane
Montgomery, AL 36117
334-395-4489
800-388-7325
FAX 334-395-4492
http://www.alabama.easter-seals.org
e-mail: alaseal@worldnet.att.net

Johnny Webster, CEO
Lyn Stokley, President

Job training and employment services, senior community service employment program.

6883 Easter Seals Camp ASCCA
Easter Seals Camp ASCCA
PO Box 21
Jacksons Gap, AL 36861
256-825-9226
800-843-2267
FAX 256-825-8332
http://www.alabama.easter-seals.org
e-mail: info@campascca.org

Matt Rickman, Camp Director
John Stephenson, Administrator

Camp respite for adults and children, camperships, canoeing, day camping for adults, day camping for children, therapeutic horseback riding.

6884 Easter Seals Capilouto Center for the Deaf
5950 Monticello Drive
Montgomery, AL 36117
334-244-8090
FAX 334-244-1183
TDY:334-272-6754
http://www.alabama.easter-seals.org
e-mail: lstokley@jccd.org

Lynne Stokley, Executive Director
Brenda Culpepper, Work Conditioning Specialist

Job training and employment services, occupational skills training, job placement/competitive-supported employment, vocational evaluation/situation assessment, work adjustment.

6885 Easter Seals Disability Services
2448 Gordon Smith Drive
Mobile, AL 36617
251-471-1581
800-411-0068
FAX 251-476-4303
http://www.alabama.easterseals.org

Frank Harkins, President
Terry Dale, Human Resources Director
Richard Weishaupt, Manager

Easter Seals has been helping individuals with disabilities and special needs, and their families, live better lives for more than 80 years. Whether helping someone improve physical mobility, return to work or simply gain greater independence for everyday living, Easter Seals offers a variety of services to help people with disabilities address life's challenges and achieve personal goals.

6886 **Easter Seals Opportunity Center**
United Way
6300 McClellan Boulevard
Anniston, AL 36206
256-820-9960
FAX 256-820-9592
http://www.alabama.easter-seals.org
e-mail: mikenancyoppcen@aol.com
Mike Almaroad, Administrator
Barry Cavan, Chief Executive Officer
Bert Oelschig, Plant Manager
Job training and employment services, occupational skills training, job placement/competitive-supported employment, vocational evaluation/situation assessment, work adjustment.

6887 **Easter Seals Rehabilitation Center: Northwest Alabama**
1450 Avalon Avenue
Muscle Shoals, AL 35661
256-381-1110
FAX 256-314-5105
http://www.alabama.easter-seals.org
e-mail: easter@hiwaay.net
Danny Prince, Manager
Shiella Phillips, Director

Job training and employment services, occupational skills training, job placement/competitive-supported employment, vocational evaluation/situation assessment, work services.

6888 **Easter Seals: Birmingham Area**
200 Beacon Parkway W
Birmingham, AL 35209
205-942-6277
FAX 205-945-4906
http://www.alabama.easter-seals.org
e-mail: esba@eastersealsbham.org
Johnny Webster, Director
Lisa Howard, Office Manager

Job training and employment services, occupational skills training, job placement/competitive-supported employment, vocational evaluation/situation assessment, work adjustment.

6889 **Easter Seals: West Alabama**
1110 6th Avenue E
Tuscaloosa, AL 35401
205-759-1211
800-726-1216
FAX 205-349-1162
http://www.alabama.easter-seals.org
e-mail: eswa@eastersealswestal.org
Lorie Robinson, Administrator
Bettye Hughes, Office Manager

Job training and employment services, occupational skills training, job placement/competitive-supported employment, vocational evaluation/situation assessment, work adjustment.

6890 **Good Will Easter Seals**
2448 Gordon Smith Drive
Mobile, AL 36617
251-471-4303
800-411-0068
FAX 251-476-4303
http://www.alabama.easter-seals.org
Frank Harkins, Chief Executive Officer

Job training and employment services, occupational skills training, job placement/competitive-supported employment, vocational evaluation/situation assessment, work adjustment.

6891 **State Vocational Rehabilitation Agency of Alabama**
Division of Rehabilitation Services
2129 E S Boulevard
Montgomery, AL 36116
334-281-8780
800-441-7607
FAX 334-281-1973
http://www.rehab.state.al.us
e-mail: sshivers@rehab.state.al.us
Steve Shivers, Manager

State vocational rehabilitation agencies provide direct services to persons with disabilities, including persons with learning disabilities. The services may include evaluation and diagnosis; counseling, guidance, and referral services; vocational and other training services; transportation to rehabilitation services; and assistive devices.

6892 **Workforce Development Division**
Alabama Dept. of Economic & Community Affairs
PO Box 5690
Montgomery, AL 36103
334-242-4363
FAX 334-242-5855
http://www.adeca.state.al.us
e-mail: stevew@adeca.state.al.us
Steve Walkley, Division Director
Tim Alford, Executive Director

Customer focused to help Americans access the tools they need to manage their careers through information and high quality services and to help US companies find skilled workers. Alabama's Career Center System is a network of one-stop centers designed to offer these services. These centers are co-located or electronically linked to provide streamlined services.

Alaska

6893 **Alaska Department of Labor**
1111 W 8th Street
Juneau, AK 99801
907-465-2700
Greg O'Claray, Manager

6894 **Alaska Department of Labor & Workforce Development**
1111 W 8th Street
Juneau, AK 99801
907-465-2700
FAX 907-465-2784
TDY:907-269-3570
http://www.state.ak.us
e-mail: Commissioner_Labor@labor.state.ak.us
Greg O'Claray, Commissioner
Guy Bell, Assistant Commissioner
Paula Scavera, Special Assistant
Responsible for the overall management of the department's programs and resources; serves as a liaison with other state, federal, and local governmental agencies and the legislature.

6895 **Alaska Department of Labor: Division of Vocational Rehabilitation**
801 W 10th Street
Juneau, AK 99801
907-465-2814
800-478-2815
FAX 907-465-2856
http://www.labor.state.ak.us/dvr/home.htm
e-mail: carol_whelan@labor.state.ak.us
Gale Sinnott, Director

Assisting individuals with disabilities to obtain and maintain employment.

6896 **State Vocational Rehabilitation Agency of Alaska**
Division of Vocational Rehabilitation Services
1016 W 6th Avenue
Anchorage, AK 99501
907-269-3570
FAX 907-269-3632
http://www.edu.state.ak.us/vocrehab/home.html
State vocational rehabilitation agencies provide direct services to persons with disabilities, including persons with learning disabilities. The services may include evaluation and diagnosis; counseling, guidance, and referral services; vocational and other training services; transportation to rehabilitation services; and assistive devices.

Arizona

6897 **Arizona Vocational Rehabilitation**
Arizona Department of Economic Security
1789 W Jefferson Street NW
Phoenix, AZ 85007
602-542-3332
800-563-1221
FAX 602-542-3778
http://www.de.state.az.us/rsa/vr.asp

Kathy Levandowsky, Acting Administrator
Craig Warren, Administrator

Programs provide a variety of specialized services for individuals with physical or mental disabilities that create barriers to employment or independent living. RSA offers three major service programs and several specialized programs/services.

6898 Rehabilitation Services Administration
1789 W Jefferson NW
Phoenix, AZ 85007
602-542-3332
FAX 602-542-3778
TDY:602-542-6049
http://www.de.state.az.us/rsa/
e-mail: azrsa@azdes.gov
Kathy Levandowsky, Acting Administrator
Craig Warren, Administrator

The mission of the Rehabilitation Services Administration (RSA) is to work with individuals with disabilities to achieve increased independence and/or gainful employment through the provision of comprehensive rehabilitative and employment support services in a partnership with all stakeholders.

Arkansas

6899 Arkansas Department of Health & Human Services: Division of Developmental Disabilities
Donaghey Plaza N
Little Rock, AR 72203
501-682-8665
FAX 501-682-8380
TDY:501-682-1332
http://www.arkansas.gov/dhhs/ddds
James Green Ph.D, Director
Green Manager, Human Services Director
Quinn Communications, Communications
The mission of the Division of Developmental Disabilities Services is to provide a variety of supports to improve the quality of life for individuals with mental retardation, autism, epilepsy, cerebral palsy or other conditions that cause a person to function as if they had a mental impairment.

6900 Arkansas Department of Workforce Education
Luther Hard Building
Little Rock, AR 72201
501-682-1500
FAX 501-682-1509
http://www.dwe.arkansas.gov
e-mail: john.wyvill@arkansas.gov
John Wyvill, Director

Arkansas Department of Workforce Education's mission is to provide the leadership and contribute resources to serve the diverse and changing workforce training needs of the youth and adults of Arkansas.

6901 Arkansas Employment Security Department: Office of Employment & Training Services
1 Pershing Circle
North Little Rock, AR 72114
501-682-2121
FAX 501-682-2273
http://www.state.ar.us/esd/
e-mail: mel.thrash.aesd@mail.state.ar.us
Artee Williams, Director
Thrash Deputy Director, Deputy Director
Snead Employment Assistance, Employment Assistance
Employment related services that contribute to the economic stability of Arkansa and its citizens. These services are provided to employers, the workforce and the general public.

6902 Arkansas Rehabilitation Services
26 Corporate Hill Drive
Little Rock, AR 72205
501-686-9686
FAX 501-686-9685
TDY:501-686-9686
http://www.arsinfo.org
e-mail: ssholt@ars.state.ar.us
Susan Holt PhD, Learning Evaluation Program Dir.

For persons who are clients of Arkansas Rehabilitation Services, individual psychological/educational evaluations and college preparatory training are provided if approved by vocational rehabilitation counselor.

6903 Arkansas Rehabilitation Services Employment Center: Office for the Deaf & Hearing Impaired
4601 W Markham Street
Little Rock, AR 72205
501-686-6219
FAX 501-686-9418
http://www.arsinfo.org
e-mail: jlgatewood@ars.state.ar.us
John Wyvill, Commissioner
Sue Gaskin, Special Programs

Providing opportunities for individuals with hearing impairment to work and have productive and independent lives.

6904 Department of Human Services: Division of Developmental Disabilities Services
PO Box 1437
Little Rock, AR 72203
501-682-8665
FAX 501-682-8380
TDY:501-682-1332
http://www.state.ar.us/ddds/ddsinsti.html
James Green PhD, Director
Kurt Knickrehm, Human Services Director
Charlie Green, Manager
Offers a wide range of services and supports to Arkansans with developmental disabilities and their families.

6905 Department of Workforce Education
3 Capitol Mall
Little Rock, AR 72201
501-682-1500
FAX 501-682-1509
http://www.work-ed.state.ar.us/
e-mail: steve.franks@mail.state.ar.us
Steve Franks MD, Director
Garland Hankins, Adult Education
John Wyvill, Manager
Provides the leadership and contributes resources to serve the diverse and changing workforce training needs of the youth and adults of Arkansas.

6906 State Vocational Rehabilitation Agency of Arkansas
ARS, Vocational & Technical Education Division
PO Box 3781
Little Rock, AR 72203
501-296-1600
800-330-0632
FAX 501-296-1655
TDY:501-296-1669
http://www.arsinfo.org
e-mail: jlgatewood@ars.state.ar.us
John Wyvill, Manager
Barbara Lewis, Field Services
Sue Gaskin, Special Programs
Provides direct services to persons with disabilities, including persons with learning disabilities. The services may include evaluation and diagnosis, counseling, guidance, and referral services, vocational and other training services, transportation to rehabilitation services, and assistive devices. Offering opportunities for individuals with disabilities to lead productive and independent lives.

6907 Workforce Investment Board
Arkansas State Employment Board
PO Box 2981
Little Rock, AR 72203
501-371-1020
FAX 501-371-1030
TDY:800-285-1131
http://www.state.ar.us/workforce/
e-mail: arkansasweb@mail.state.ar.us
Sandra Winston, Manager
Elroy Willoghpy, Deputy Director
Sharon Robinette, Workforce Analysis/Reporting
Operates workforce centers that offer locally developed and operated services linking employers and jobseekers through a statewide delivery system. Conveinient centers are designed to eliminate the need to visit different locations. The centers integrate multiple workforce development programs into a single system, making the resources much more accessible and user friendly to jobseekers as well as expanding services to employers.

California

6908 Adult Education
California Department of Education
1430 N Street
Sacramento, CA 95814
916-319-0800
FAX 916-319-0100
http://www.cde.ca.gov/adulteducation
e-mail: joconell@cde.ca.gov
Jack O'Conell, Manager
Sue Bennett, Educational Options

Elementary basic skills and tutor/literacy training are offered on or off site using language masters, audiocassettes, videos and computers with internet access. Workplace literacy training will also be provided, with groups of students physically coming into the Center or hooking up to the Center from their workplace by borrowing materials or going online. In the latter case, instructors will meet with students at the work site on a regular schedule for evaluation and consultation.

6909 California Department of Rehabilitation
California Health & Human Services Agency
2000 Evergreen Street
Sacramento, CA 95815
916-263-7365
FAX 916-263-7474
TDY:916-263-7477
http://www.dor.ca.gov
e-mail: publicaffairs@dor.ca.gov
Catherine Campisi Ph.D, Executive Director

California Department of Rehabilitation works in partnership with consumers and other stakeholders to provide services and advocacy resulting in employment, independent living and equality for individuals with disabilities.

6910 California Employment Development Department
800 Capitol Mall
Sacramento, CA 95814
916-324-4244
FAX 916-653-0597
http://www.edd.ca.gov
e-mail: phenning@edd.ca.gov
Patrick Henning, Director
Pam Harris, Acting Chief Deputy Director
David Supkofl, Manager
The California Employment Development Department (EDD) offers a wide variety of services to millions of Californians under the Job Service, Unemployment Insurance, Disability Insurance, Workforce Investment, and Labor Market Information programs.

6911 California State Deparment of Education GED
1430 N Street
Sacramento, CA 95814
916-319-0800
800-331-6316
FAX 916-319-0100
http://www.cde.ca.gov/ged/
e-mail: GEDoffic@cde.ca.gov
Nancy Edmunds, Program Coordinator
Jack O'Connell, Manager

Provides access to a general high school education by providing many local classes and testing services.

6912 Easter Seals Central California
9010 Soquel Drive
Aptos, CA 95003
831-684-2166
FAX 831-685-6055
http://www.centralcal.easter-seals.org
e-mail: donna@es-cc.org

Donna Alvarez, Finance VP
Bruce Hinman, President

Recreational services for adults, residential camping programs.

6913 Easter Seals Southern California
11110 Artesia Boulevard
Cerritos, CA 90703
562-860-7270
877-855-2279
FAX 562-860-1680
http://www.essc.org
e-mail: Dee.Prescott@essc.org
Dee Prescott, Regional Director
Sandy Meredith, Executive Director

Adult day programing/personal and social supports.

6914 Easter Seals Superior California
3205 Hurley Way
Sacramento, CA 95864
916-485-6711
888-887-3257
FAX 916-485-2653
http://www.easterseals-superiorca.org
e-mail: info@easterseals-superiorca.org
Gary Kasai, President

Job training and employment services, occupational skills training, job placement/competitive-support employment, vocational evaluation/situational assessment and work adjustment.

6915 Easter Seals: Redondo Beach
700 N Pacific Coast Highway
Redondo Beach, CA 90277
310-376-3445
800-404-3445
FAX 310-376-5567
http://www.cssc.org
e-mail: dee.prescott@cssc.org
Kerry Ryerson, Executive Director
Mark Whitley, President

Job training and employment services, occupational skills training, job placement/competitive-support employment, vocational evaluation/situational assessment and work adjustment.

6916 Easter Seals: Southern California
4727 Labrea Avenue 8100 W
Los Angeles, CA 90038
323-257-3006
877-877-8565
FAX 323-954-3775
http://www.essc.org
e-mail: lupe.trevizoreinoso@essc.org
Lupe Trevizo-Reinoso, Regional Director
Mark Whitley, President

Job training and employment services, occupational skills training, job placement/competitive-support employment, vocational evaluation/situational assessment and work adjustment.

6917 Easter Seals: Van Nuys
Easter Seals: Van Nuys
16946 Sherman Way
Van Nuys, CA 91406
818-996-9902
800-996-6302
FAX 818-996-1606
http://www.cssc.org
e-mail: paula.pompa-craven@cssc.org
Paula Pompa-Craven, Regional Director
Mark Whitley, President

Job training and employment services, occupational skills training, job placement/competitive-support employment, vocational evaluation/situational assessment and work adjustment.

Colorado

6918 Colorado Department of Human Services: Division for Developmental Disabilities
3824 W Princeton Circle
Denver, CO 80236
303-866-7450
FAX 303-866-7470
TDY:303-866-7471
http://www.cdhs.state.co.us/ddd/
Fred Decrescentis, Executive Director

A state office that provides leadership for the direction, funding and operation of community based services to people with developmental disabilities within Colorado.

6919 Easter Seals Colorado
5755 W Alameda Avenue
Lakewood, CO 80226
303-233-1666
FAX 303-233-1028
http://www.co.easterseals.com
e-mail: info@eastersealscolorado.org
Lynn Robinson, President/CEO
Nancy Hanson, Corporate Secretary

Job training and employment services, occupational skills training, job placement/competitive-support employment, vocational evaluation/situational assessment and work adjustment.

6920 Human Services: Division of VocationalHuman Services: Division of Vocational Rehabilitation
1575 Sherman Street
Denver, CO 80203
303-866-4150
866-870-4595
FAX 303-866-4905
TDY:303-866-4150
http://www.cdhs.state.co.us/ods/dvr/index.html
e-mail: carlos.fernandez@state.co.us
Nancy Smith, Director
Diana Huerta, Manager

Assists individuals whose disabilities result in barriers to employment to succeed at work and live independently. Building partnerships to improve opportunities for safety, self-sufficiency and dignity for the people of Colorado.

6921 State Vocational Rehabilitation Agency of Colorado
Div. of Rehabilitation/Dept. of Human Services
2211 W Evans Avenue
Denver, CO 80223
303-866-4150
e-mail: diana.huerta@state.co.us
Diana Huerta, Director

State vocational rehabilitation agencies provide direct services to persons with disabilities, including persons with learning disabilities. The services may include evaluation and diagnosis; counseling, guidance, and referral services; vocational and other training services; transportation to rehabilitation services; and assistive devices.

Connecticut

6922 Bureau of Adult Education & Training
25 Industrial Park Road
Middletown, CT 06457
860-807-2110
FAX 860-807-2112
http://www.state.ct.us/sde/deps/adult/index.htm
e-mail: gail.brooks-lemkin@po.state.ct.us
Maureen Staggenborg, Acting Bureau Chief
Gail Brooks-Lemkin, Technical Assistant

Committed to quality adult education programs which are accessible to all Connecticut adults and lead to mastery of the essential proficiences needed to function as productive citizens in work, family and community environments. Programs are available at local schools throughout the state. Offers basic literacy, elementary education, English language proficiency, secondary school completion and preparation for equivalency examinations.

6923 Department of Labor
200 Folly Brook Boulevard
Wethersfield, CT 06109
860-263-6000
TDY:860-263-6074
http://www.ctdol.state.ct.gov/dol
e-mail: dol.help@po.state.ct.us
Shaun Cashman, Commissioner
Thomas Hutton, Assistant Commissioner
Rayann Curtis, Manager
Assisting workers to become competitive in a global economy, we take a comprehensive approach to meeting the needs of workers, employers and other agencies that serve them.

6924 Department of Social Services: Vocational Rehabilitation Program
25 Sigourney Street
Hartford, CT 06106
860-424-4844
800-537-2549
TDY:860-424-4839
http://www.dss.state.ct.us
e-mail: pgr.dss@po.state.ct.us
John Galiette, Director
Evelyn Knight, Program Assistant
Brenda Moore, Executive Director
Provides services to people with most significant physical or mental disabilities to assist them in their effort to enter or maintain employment. The agency also oversees a statewide network of community based, consumer controlled, independent living centers that promote independence for people with disabilities.

6925 Easter Seals Connecticut
85 Jones Street
Hebron, CT 06248
800-874-7687
FAX 860-455-1372
http://www.ct.easterseals.com
John Quinn, President

Easter Seals Connecticut creates solutions that change the lives of children and adults with disabilities or special needs, their families and communities.

6926 Easter Seals Employment Industries
Easter Seals Rehabilitation Center
122 Avenue of Industry
Waterbury, CT 06705
203-236-0188
FAX 203-236-0183
http://www.eswct.com
e-mail: eswct@eswct.com
Ron Bourque, President
Francis DeBlasio, CEO

Job training, employment services, vocational evaluation/situational assessment and work services.

6927 Easter Seals Fulfillment Enterprises
24 Stott Avenue
Norwich, CT 06360
860-859-4148
FAX 860-537-9673
http://www.ct.easter-seals.org
e-mail: jsalois@easterseals.org
Jerry Salois, Operations Director
John Quinn, CEO
Denis Hornbecker, Manager
Job training, employment services, vocational evaluation/situational assessment and work services.

6928 Easter Seals: Uncasville
24 Stott Avenue
Norwich, CT 06360
860-859-4148
Kathy Buck, Adult Programs Director
John Quinn, CEO
Denise Hornbecker, Manager
Job training, employment services, vocational evaluation/situational assessment and work services.

6929 Easter Seals: Waterbury
22 Tompkins Street
Waterbury, CT 06708
203-754-5141
FAX 203-754-1198
http://www.ct.easter-seals.org
e-mail: fdeblasio@eswct.com
Francis DeBlasio, Executive Director
Rupa Gandi, Vice President

Job training, employment services, vocational evaluation/situational assessment and work services.

Delaware

6930 Division of Vocational Rehabilitation
Delaware Department of Labor
4425 N Market Street
Wilmington, DE 19802
302-575-7371
FAX 302-761-6611
http://www.delawareworks.com
e-mail: cynthia.fairwell@state.de.us

Andrea Guest, Director
Cynthia Fairwell, Program Specialist
Karen Gimbutas, Vice President

Mission is to provide information opportunitie, and resources to individuals with disabilities, leading to success in employment and independent living.

6931 Easter Seals Delaware and Maryland Shore
61 Corporate Circle
New Castle, DE 19720
302-324-4444
800-677-3800
FAX 302-324-4442
TDY:302-324-4444
http://www.de.easter-seals.org
e-mail: badami@esdel.org

William Adami, Vice President
Sandra Tuttle, President

Job training, employment services, vocational evaluation/situational assessment and work services.

6932 Easter Seals Dover Enterprise
100 Enterprise Place
Dover, DE 19904
302-678-3353
800-677-3800
FAX 302-678-3650
http://www.de.easter-seals.org
e-mail: gcassedy@esdel.org

Gary Cassedy, Chief Executive Officer
Sandra Tuttle, President
Diane Schilling, Manager

Job training, employment services, vocational evaluation/situational assessment and work services.

6933 Easter Seals Georgetown Professional Center
600 N Dupont Highway
Georgetown, DE 19947
302-856-7364
877-204-3276
FAX 302-856-7296
http://www.de.easter-seals.org
e-mail: cea@gt.esdel.org

Pam Reuther, Manager
Sandra Tuttle, President

Job training, employment services, vocational evaluation/situational assessment and work services.

6934 Workforce Investment: Virtual Career Network
Department of Labor
4425 N Market Street
Wilmington, DE 19802
302-761-8001
FAX 302-761-6634
http://www.vcnet.net
e-mail: tsmith@state.de.us

Barry Butler, Supervisor
Anne Farley, Director
Lisa Blunt-Bradley, Manager

Many area offices for a one-stop employment and training integrated service delivery system. Much of our information is also available online.

District of Columbia

6935 Centers for Independent Living Program: Rehabilitation Services Administration
1400 Florida Avenue NE
Washington, DC 20002
202-388-0033
FAX 202-398-3018
TDY:202-388-0277
http://www.dccil.org
e-mail: info@dccil.org

Richard Simms, Executive Director
Kandra Hall, Coordinator

Consumer controlled, cross disability, community based, private nonprofit organization that promotes independent life styles for people with significant disabilities in the District of Columbia.

6936 Department of Employment Services
Government of the District of Columbia
64 New York Avenue NE
Washington, DC 20002
202-724-7000
FAX 202-724-5683
TDY:202-673-6994

Gregory Irish, Director

Helps consider career decisions and offer vocational and placement assistance at several area training locations.

6937 Department of Human Services: Bureau of Training & Employment
810 1st Street NE
Washington, DC 20002
202-442-8663
FAX 202-263-7518
TDY:202-442-8598
http://www.rsa@dcgovernment.com
e-mail: answersplease@dhs.washington.dc.us / rsa@dcgo

Elizabeth Parkers, Administrator
Eliza Sparmon, Program Support Assistant

6938 District of Columbia Department of Education: Vocational & Adult Education
400 Maryland Avenue SW
Washington, DC 20202
202-842-0973
800-872-5327
FAX 202-205-8748
http://www.ed.gov/offices/OVAE
e-mail: ovae@ed.gov

Tassie Thompson, Manager

To help all people achieve the knowledge and skills to be lifelong learners, to be successful in their chosen careers, and to be effective citizens.

6939 State Vocational Rehabilitation Agency
Rehabilitation Services Administration
810 1st Street NE
Washington, DC 20002
202-442-8663
FAX 202-442-8742
e-mail: elizabeth.parker@dc.gov

Elizabeth Parker, Administrator
Cheryl Bolden, Administrative Assistant

Provides direct services to persons with disabilities, including persons with learning disabilities. The services may include evaluation and diagnosis, counseling, guidance, and referral services, vocational and other training services, transportation to rehabilitation services and assistive devices. Our goal is to assist those we serve in becoming independent and self sufficient in the home and in the community and to prepare for, enter and maintain gainful employment.

Florida

6940 College Living Experience
6555 Nova Drive
Davie, FL 33317
954-370-5142
800-486-5058
FAX 954-370-1895
http://www.cleinc.net
e-mail: secretary@cleinc.net
A J Petrillo MD, Director
Irene Spalter, Executive Director
Jill Rickel, National Admissions Director
For young adults with learning difficulties but who would benefit from: intensive academic tutoring, advocacy and guidance, a comprehensive independent living skills program, social skills training, vocational support services and apartment living. One central program with a variety of experiences, including college, vocational school and internships, all within walking distance.

6941 Division of Vocational Rehabilitation
Florida Department of Education
2002 Old Saint Augustine Road
Tallahassee, FL 32301
850-245-3399
800-451-4327
FAX 850-245-3316
TDY:800-451-4327
http://www.rehabworks.org
Bill Palmer, Director
Amanda Grines, Office Assistant

Statewide employment resource for businesses and people with disabilities. Our mission is to enable individuals with disabilities to obtain and keep employment.

6942 Easter Seals Broward County Florida
Easter Seals Broward County Florida
6951 W Sunrise Boulevard
Plantation, FL 33313
954-792-8772
FAX 954-791-8275
http://www.broward.easterseals.com
e-mail: info@broward.easterseals.com
Becky Dausman, CEO

Job training, employment services, vocational evaluation/situational assessment and work services.

6943 Easter Seals Florida: East Coast Region
6050 Babcock Street SE
Palm Bay, FL 32909
321-723-4474
FAX 321-676-3843
http://www.fl.easter-seals.org
e-mail: gedwards@fl.easter-seals.org
Gail Edwards, Executive Director
Robert Griggs, President

Job training, employment services, vocational evaluation/situational assessment and work services.

6944 Easter Seals Miami-Dade
1475 NW 14th Avenue
Miami, FL 33125
305-325-0470
FAX 305-325-0578
http://www.miami.easter-seals.org
e-mail: jbornstein@miami.easterseals.com
Joan Bornstein PhD, President/CEO
Ronnie Waldman, Principal

Job training, employment services, vocational evaluation/situational assessment and work services, adult day services, outpatient medical rehabilitation.

6945 Easter Seals North Florida
910 Myers Park Drive
Tallahassee, FL 32301
850-222-4465
FAX 850-222-5950
http://www.northflorida.easter-seals.org
e-mail: enorthflorida@aol.com
Christine Hall, President

Job training, employment services, vocational evaluation/situational assessment and work services.

6946 Easter Seals Southwest Florida
Easter Seals Southwest Florida
350 Braden Avenue
Sarasota, FL 34243
941-355-7637
800-807-7899
FAX 941-351-9711
http://www.swfl.easterseals.com
Mary Hitchcock, CEO

Job training, employment services, vocational evaluation/situational assessment and work services.

6947 Florida Workforce Investment Act
Department of Labor & Employment Security
1947 Commonwealth Lane
Tallahassee, FL 32303
850-921-1119
FAX 850-921-1101
http://www.workforceflorida.com
Kathleen McLeskey, Acting Director
Curtis Austin, Manager

Provides job-training services for economically disadvantaged adults and youth, dislocated workers and others who face significant employment barriers.

6948 TILES Project: Transition/Independent Living/Employment/Support
Family Network on Disabilities of Florida
2735 Whitney Road
Clearwater, FL 33760
727-523-1130
800-825-5736
FAX 727-523-8687
http://www.fndfl.org
e-mail: fnd@fndfl.org
Jan LaBelle, Executive Director
Betsy Taylor, Program Director

Provides training information to enable individuals with disabilities and the parents, family members, guardians, advocates, or other authorized representatives to participate more effectively with professionals in meeting the vocational, independent living and rehabilitation needs of people with disabilities in Florida.

Georgia

6949 Easter Seals East Georgia
Easter Seals Georgia
1500 Wrightsboro Road
Augusta, GA 30904
706-667-9695
866-667-9695
FAX 229-435-6278
http://www.eastersealseastgeorgia.org
e-mail: sthomas@esega.org
Sheila Thomas, President

Job training, employment services, vocational evaluation/situational assessment and work services.

6950 Easter Seals Middle Georgia
602 Kellam Road
Dublin, GA 31021
478-272-0014
FAX 478-275-8852
http://www.middlegeorgia.easterseals.com
Wayne Peebles, President

Job training, employment services, vocational evaluation/situational assessment and work services.

6951 Easter Seals Southern Georgia
Easter Seals Southern Georgia
1906 Palmyra Road
Albany, GA 31701
229-439-7061
800-365-4583
FAX 229-435-6278
http://www.southerngeorgia.easterseals.com
e-mail: benglish@swga-easterseals.org
Beth English, Executive Director
Matt Hatcher, Chief Financial Officer

Job training, employment services, vocational evaluation/situational assessment and work services.

6952 Vocational Rehabilitation Services
Georgia Department of Labor
148 Andrew Young International Blvd
Atlanta, GA 30303
404-232-3685
FAX 404-232-3912
TDY:404-232-3911
http://www.vocrehabga.org
e-mail: rehab@dol.state.ga.us
Peggy D Rosser, Assistant Commissioner
Sam Hall, Manager
Ken Armstrong, Office Assistant
Operates 5 integrated and interdependent programs that share a primary goal — to help people with disabilities to become fully productive members of society by achieving independence and meaningful employment.

Hawaii

6953 Vocational & Rehabilitation Agency Hawaii: Division of Vocational Rehab & Services for the Blind
Department of Human Services
PO Box 339
Honolulu, HI 96809
808-587-3850
FAX 808-692-7727
TDY:808-586-5167
http://www.state.hi.us/dhs/vr
e-mail: nshim@dhs.state.hi.us
Neil Shim, Administrator
Lilian Poller, Director
Sandi Leong, Manager
State vocational rehabilitation agencies provide direct services to persons with disabilities, including persons with learning disabilities. The services may include evaluation and diagnosis, counseling, guidance, and referral services, vocational and other training services, transportation to rehabilitation services, and assistive devices.

Idaho

6954 Department of Commerce & Labor
Department of Commerce & Labor
317 W Main Street
Boise, ID 83735
208-332-3570
FAX 208-334-6430
TDY:800-377-1363
http://www.cl.idaho.gov
e-mail: rvaldez@dds.state.id.us
Roger Madsen, Manager
Rogelio Valdez, Disability Determinations

An equal opportunity employer/program with auxiliary aids and services available upon request to individuals with disabilities.

6955 Easter Seals-Goodwill Staffing Services
Easter Seals-Goodwill Staffing Services
1465 S Vinnell Way
Boise, ID 83709
208-373-1299
FAX 208-378-9965
http://www.esgw-nrm.easter-seals.org
e-mail: marcib@esgw.org
Tim Bleimaier, Manager
Michelle Belknap, CEO

Job training, employment services, vocational evaluation/situational assessment and work services.

6956 Easter Seals-Goodwill Working Solutions
Easter Seals-Goodwill Staffing Services
1613 N Parkcentre Place
Nampa, ID 83651
208-466-2671
FAX 208-466-2537
http://www.esgw-nrm.easter-seals.org
e-mail: landisr@esgw.org
Tim Bleimaier, Manager
Michelle Belknap, CEO

Job training, employment services, vocational evaluation/situational assessment and work services.

6957 Idaho Department of Commerce & Labor
Idaho Department of Labor
317 W Main Street
Boise, ID 83735
208-332-3570
FAX 208-334-6430
TDY:800-377-1363
http://www.cl.idaho.gov
e-mail: rvaldez@dds.state.id.us
Roger Madsen, Manager
Rogelio Valdez, Disability Determinations

Provides vocational training services for economically disadvantaged adults and youth, dislocated workers and others who face significant employment barriers.

6958 State Vocational Rehabilitation Agency
State of Idaho
650 W State
Boise, ID 83720
208-334-8000
FAX 208-334-5305
http://www2.state.id.us/idvr
e-mail: scook@idvr.state.id.us
Michael Graham, Administrator
Sue Payne, Chief Field Services
Sandy Frazier, Manager
State vocational rehabilitation agencies provide direct services to persons with disabilities, including persons with learning disabilities. The services may include evaluation and diagnosis, counseling, guidance, and referral services, vocational and other training services, transportation to rehabilitation services, and assistive devices.

6959 Temporary Assistance for Needy Families: Idaho Department of Health and Welfare
PO Box 83720
Boise, ID 83720
208-334-0606
FAX 208-332-7362
http://www.2.state.id.us
e-mail: BCEH@idhw.state.id.us
Karl Kurtz, Director of Health and Welfare
Dian Prince, Administrative Assistant

Provides assistance and work opportunities to needy families by granting states the federal funds and wide flexibility to develop and implement their own welfare programs.

Illinois

6960 Easter Seals Central Illinois
2715 N 27th Street
Decatur, IL 62526
217-429-1052
FAX 217-423-7605
http://www.easterseals-ci.org
e-mail: info@easterseals-ci.org
Janet Kelsheimer, President
Margie Malone, Office Manager

Job training, employment services, vocational evaluation/situational assessment and work services.

6961 Easter Seals Missouri
Easter Seals Missouri
602 E 3rd Street
Alton, IL 62002
618-462-7325
FAX 618-462-8170
http://www.mo.easterseals.org
e-mail: lynnstonecipher@mo.easterseals.com
Lynn Stonecipher, Manager
Craig Byrd, CEO

Job training, employment services, vocational evaluation/situational assessment and work services.

6962 Easter Seals Youth at Risk
Easter Seals Illinois
120 Madison Street
Oak Park, IL 60302
708-524-8700
FAX 708-524-4902
http://www.easterseals chicago.org
e-mail: wkern@eastersealschicago.org

Bill Kern, Program Manager
Mary Mulvihill, Manager

Job training, employment services, vocational evaluation/situational assessment and work services.

6963 State Vocational Rehabilitation Agency
State Vocational Rehabilitation Agency
100 S Grand Avenue
Springfield, IL 62762
217-782-2094
800-843-6154
FAX 217-558-4270
TDY:217-557-2507
http://www.dhs.state.il.us
e-mail: drs@illinois.gov

Rob Kilbury, Director

We help people with physical or learning disabilities find and keep jobs. Our goal is to help our customers find quality employment that pays a living wage and offers a chance for advancement. Specialized services for the deaf and blind or visually impaired.

6964 Temporary Assistance for Needy Families
Department of Human Services
100 E Grand Avenue
Springfield, IL 62762
217-557-1601
FAX 217-557-2134
http://www.dhs.state.il.us
e-mail: carol.adams@dhs.state.il.us

Marva Arnold, Director
Ginger White, Administrative Assistant
Carol Adams, Manager
Focus on transitional services. Major points include creating goals, continuation of Work Pays program, cash assistance, subsidized employment, and medical benefits.

Indiana

6965 Easter Seals Arc of Northeast Indiana
Easter Seals Arc of Northeast Indiana
4919 Projects Drive
Fort Wayne, IN 46825
260-482-8587
FAX 260-745-5200
http://www.eastersealsarcnein.org
e-mail: shinkle@esarc.org

Stephen Hinkle, CEO
Sue Dubai, Administrative Assistant

Job training, employment services, vocational evaluation/situational assessment and work services.

6966 Easter Seals Crossroads
4740 Kingsway Drive
Indianapolis, IN 46205
317-466-1000
FAX 317-466-2000
TDY:317-479-3232
http://www.eastersealscrossroads.org
e-mail: info@eastersealscrossroads.org

James Vento, President
Candy Morrison, Marketing/Communications Dir.

Job training, employment services, vocational evaluation/situational assessment and work services.

6967 Easter Seals Crossroads Industrial Services
8302 E 33rd Street
Indianapolis, IN 46226
317-897-7320
FAX 317-897-9763
http://www.eastersealscrossroads.org

Brett Bennett, Division Director

Job training, employment services, vocational evaluation/situational assessment and work services.

6968 Easter Seals: Bridgepointe
PO Box 2488
Clarksville, IN 47131
812-283-7908
FAX 812-283-6248
e-mail: cmarshall@bridgepoint.org

Caren Marshall, Executive Director

Job training, employment services, vocational evaluation/situational assessment and work services.

6969 Indiana Vocation Rehabilitation Services Goodwill Industries
Department of Vocational Rehabilitation
1452 Vaxter Avenue
Clarksville, IN 47129
812-288-8261
FAX 812-282-7048
http://www.ivrs.state.in.us

Delbert Hayden, Manager

Purpose is to assist the community by providing services which allow individuals to maximize their potential and to participate in work, family and the community. To do this we will provide rehabilitation, education and training.

6970 State Vocational Rehabilitation Agency
Division of Disability, Aging, & Rehab. Services
402 W Washington Street
Indianapolis, IN 46204
317-232-1147
800-545-7763
FAX 317-232-6478
http://www.in.gov
e-mail: phedden@fssa.state.in.us

Mike Hedden, Deputy Director
Karen Smith, Office Manager
Peter Bisbecos, Manager
Provides direct services to persons with disabilities, including persons with learning disabilities. The services may include evaluation and diagnosis; counseling, guidance, and referral services, vocational and other training services, transportation to rehabilitation services, and assistive devices.

Iowa

6971 Easter Seals Center
2920 30th Street
Des Moines, IA 50310
515-274-1529
866-533-9344
FAX 515-274-6434
TDY:515-274-8348
http://www.ia-easter-seals.orgls.org
e-mail: info@eastersealsia.org

Marcia Tope, Coordinator Intake/QA
Donna Elbrecht, CEO
Sherri Strittmatter, Vice President
Job training, employment services, vocational evaluation/situational assessment and work services.

6972 Easter Seals Iowa
401 NE 66th Avenue
Des Moines, IA 50313
515-289-1933
866-533-9344
FAX 515-274-6434
TDY:515-274-8348
http://www.ia-easter-seals.orgls.org
e-mail: info@eastersealsia.org

Marcia Tope, Coordinator Intake/QA
Donna Elbrecht, CEO

Job training, employment services, vocational evaluation/situational assessment and work services.

6973 Iowa Bureau of Community Colleges
Department of Education
400 E 14th Street
Des Moines, IA 50319
515-281-5294
FAX 515-281-6544
http://www.state.ia.us/educate/commcoll.html
e-mail: sally.schroeder@iowa.gov

Sally Schroeder, Director

6974 Iowa JOBS Program: Division of Economic Assistance
Department of Human Services
Hoover State Building
Des Moines, IA 50319
515-286-3555
FAX 515-281-7791
http://www.dhs.state.ia.us
Kevin Cannon, Director
Jaili Cunningham, Manager

6975 Iowa Vocational Rehabilitation Agency
Department of Education
400 E 14th Street
Des Moines, IA 50319
515-281-5294
FAX 515-281-4703
http://www.state.ia.us/educate/directory.html
Steve Wooderson, Administrator for Vocational Reh
Kathy Petosa, Administrative Assistant

6976 State Vocational Rehabilitation Agency
Iowa Division of Vocational Rehabilitation Service
510 E 12th Street
Des Moines, IA 50319
515-281-4311
800-532-1486
FAX 515-281-7645
TDY:515-281-4211
http://www.dvrs.stste.ia.us
e-mail: swooderson@dvrs.state.ia.us
Stephen Wooderson, Administrator
Teresa Scott, Typist Advanced

We work for and with individuals with disabilities to achieve their employment, independence and economic goals. Economic independence and more and better jobs are what we are about for Iowans with disabilities.

Kansas

6977 Goodwill Industries Easter Seals of Kansas
3636 N Oliver Street
Wichita, KS 67220
316-744-9291
FAX 316-744-1428
http://www.goodwillkansas.easterseals.com
Curtis Tatum, Programs/Services VP
Emily Compton, CEO

Job training, employment services, vocational evaluation/situational assessment and work services.

6978 Kansas Vocational Rehabilitation Agency
300 SW Oakley Biddle Building
Topeka, KS 66606
785-296-3911
FAX 785-368-6688
Joyce Cussimanio, Commissioner

To assist people with disabilities achieve suitable employment and independence.

6979 Office of Vocational Rehabilitation
Department of Vocational Rehabilitation
915 SW Harrison Street
Topeka, KS 66612
785-296-3959
FAX 785-296-2173
http://www.srskansas.org
e-mail: cmxa@srskansas.org
Clarissa Ashdown, Program Support Administrator
Laura Letters, Office Assistant
Gary Daniels, CEO
Partnering to connect Kansans with support and services to improve lives. Vocational and transitional training.

Kentucky

6980 Easter Seals Employment Connections-Pennyrile
755 Industrial Road
Madisonville, KY 42431
270-625-4840
http://www.klucas@eswky.easterseals.com
e-mail: dtinsley@ky-ws.easter-seals.org
Donna Tinsley, Site Manager
Kenneth Lucas, Chief Executive Officer

Job training, employment services, vocational evaluation/situational assessment and work services.

6981 Easter Seals: West Kentucky
Easter Seals
2229 Mildred Street
Paducah, KY 42001
270-442-2001
866-673-3565
FAX 270-444-0655
http://www.eswky.easter-seals.org
e-mail: info@ky-ws.easter-seals.org
Kenneth Lucas, President/CEO
Lori Devine, Executive Secretary
Susan Suttle, Manager
Job training, employment services, vocational evaluation/situational assessment and work services.

6982 State Vocational Rehabilitation Agency
Department of Vocational Rehabilitation
209 Saint Clair Street
Frankfort, KY 40601
502-564-4440
800-372-7172
FAX 502-564-6745
http://www.kydor.state.ky.us/
e-mail: wfd.vocrehab@mail.state.ky.us
Bruce Crump, Commissioner
Wanda Webber, Director for Finance
Beth Smith, Manager
Provides direct services to persons with disabilities, including persons with learning disabilities. The services may include evaluation and diagnosis; counseling, guidance, and referral services, vocational and other training services, transportation to rehabilitation services, and assistive devices.

Louisianna

6983 State Vocational Rehabilitation Agency
Department of Social Services
8225 Florida Boulevard
Baton Rouge, LA 70806
225-925-4131
http://www.dss.state.la.us
e-mail: jwallace@lrs.dss.state.la.us
James Wallace, Executive Director
Claire Hymel, Assistant Director
Ed Barras, Community Rehabilitation
Responsible for developing and providing social services and improving social conditions for the citizens of Louisiana, and for rehabilitating people with disabilities for employment.

Maine

6984 State Vocational Rehabilitation Agency
Maine Bureau of Rehabilitation Services
2 Anthony Avenue
Augusta, ME 04333
207-624-5950
800-698-4440
FAX 207-624-5980
http://www.state.me.us/rehab/index.htm
e-mail: penny.plourde@maine.gov
Laura Fortman, Commissioner
Jill Duson, Executive Director
Penny Plourde, Director
Works to bring about full access to employment, independence and community integration for people with disabilities. Our three service provision units are Vocational Rehabilitation, Division for the Blind and Visually Impaired and Division of Deafness.

6985 **Temporary Assistance for Needy Families**
Department of Human Services
221 State Street
Augusta, ME 04333
207-287-3707
FAX 207-287-3005
http://www.maine.gov
Jack Nicholas, Commissioner

Focuses on transitional services.

Maryland

6986 **Maryland Technology Assistance Program**
Department of Disabilities
2301 Argonne Drive
Baltimore, MD 21218
410-554-9230
800-832-4827
FAX 410-554-9237
TDY:866-881-7488
http://www.mdtap.org
e-mail: mdtap@mdtap.org
Jessica Vollmer, Office Manager

Offers information and referrals, reduced rate loan program for assistive technology, five regional display centers, presentations and training on request.

6987 **State Vocational Rehabilitation Agency**
Div. of Rehab. Services, Dept. of Education
2301 Argonne Drive
Baltimore, MD 21218
410-554-9385
FAX 410-554-9412
http://www.msde.state.md.us
e-mail: hdavis@dors.state.md.us
Robert Burns, Manager
Harvey Davis, Director Field Services
Sue Schaffer, Director Workforce/Technology
Operates more than 20 statewide offices and also operates the Workforce and Technology Center, a comprehensive rehabilitation facility in Baltimore. Rehabilitation representatives also work in many Maryland One-Stop Career Centers.

Massachusettes

6988 **Easter Seals: Massachusetts**
89 S Street
Boston, MA 02111
617-226-2640
800-244-2756
FAX 508-831-9768
http://www.eastersealsma.org
e-mail: maryd@eastersealsma.org
Kirk Joslin, Information Specialist
Kirk Joslin, President

Job training, employment services, vocational evaluation/situational assessment and work services. Camp programs, assistive technology and augmentative communication.

6989 **Easter Seals: Worcester**
484 Main Street
Worcester, MA 01608
508-757-2756
FAX 508-831-9768
http://www.eastersealsma.org
e-mail: maryd@eastersealsma.org
Mary D'Antonino, Information Specialist
Kirk Joslyn, CEO

Job training, employment services, vocational evaluation/situational assessment and work services.

6990 **JOBS Program: Massachusetts Employment Services Program**
Dept of Transitional Assistance/Office of Health
600 Washington Street
Boston, MA 02111
617-348-8400
FAX 617-348-8575
http://www.state.ma.us/dta/index.htm
John Wagner, Manager
Diana Ward, Assistant

The Employment Services Program is a joint federal and state funded program whose primary goal is to provide a way to self-sufficiency for TAFDC families. ESP is an employment-oriented program that is based on a work-first approach.

6991 **Massachusetts Job Training Partnership Act: Department of Employment & Training**
Division of Career Services
19 Staniford Street
Boston, MA 02114
617-626-5680
TDY:888-527-1912
http://www.detma.org
e-mail: ddesousa@detma.org
David DeSousa, Director
Maria Caira, Commissioner Assistant
Susan Lawler, Manager
Supplies information on the local labor market and assists companies in locating employees.

6992 **State Vocational Rehabilitation Agency**
Massachusetts Rehabilitation Commission
27 Wormwood Street
Boston, MA 02210
617-727-2183
800-245-6543
FAX 617-727-1354
TDY:800-223-3212
http://www.state.ma.is/mrc.mrc.htm
e-mail: commissioner@mrc.state.ma.us
Elmer Bartels, Manager

Provides public vocational rehabilitation, independent living and disability determination services for residents with disabilities in Massachusetts.

Michigan

6993 **Easter Seal Michigan**
Easter Seals Michigan
1401 N Michigan Avenue
Saginaw, MI 48602
989-753-4773
800-757-3257
FAX 989-753-4795
http://www.mi-ws.easterseals.org
e-mail: esofmi@aol.com
Julie Dorcey, Manager
John Cocciolone, CEO

Job training, employment services, vocational evaluation/situational assessment and work services.

6994 **Easter Seals Collaborative Solutions**
Easter Seals Collaborative Solutions
1105 N Telegraph Road
Waterford, MI 48328
248-975-9769
FAX 248-338-2936
TDY:248-338-1188
http://www.essmichigan.org
e-mail: essmichigan@essmichigan.org
Wendy Standifer, Program Manager
John Cocciolone, CEO

Job training, employment services, vocational evaluation/situational assessment and work services.

6995 **Michigan Commission for the Blind**
201 N Washington Square
Lansing, MI 48909
800-292-4200
FAX 517-335-5140
http://www.michigan.gov/mcb
e-mail: turneys@michigan.gov
Patrick Cannon, Executive Director

The Michigan Commission for the Blind is the state government agency that provides educational, training and rehabilitation opportunities to individuals who are blind or visually impaired, to help them achieve their individual goals for independence and employment. Services are provided in all of Michigan's 83 counties by staff located at field offices in eight cities. (Detroit, Escanaba, Flint, Gaylord, Grand Rapids, Kalamazoo, Lansing, and Saginaw) and a training center in Kalamazoo.

6996 Michigan Commission for the Blind: Deafblind Unit

PO Box 30652
Lansing, MI 48909
517-373-2062
800-292-4200
FAX 517-335-5140
TDY:517-373-4025
http://www.mcb1.org /another website: www.michi
e-mail: heibecks@michigan.gov
Patrick Cannon, Executive Director
Leamon Jones, Consumer Services Director

Provides opportunities to the deaf and or blind community to achieve employability and function independently in society.

6997 Michigan Jobs Commission

201 N Washington Square
Lansing, MI 48913
517-373-4871
FAX 517-373-0314
e-mail: bolinb@state.mi.us
Carl Bourdelais, Regional Director

6998 Michigan Workforce Investment Act

Public Policy Assoc. Inc
119 Pere Marquette Drive
Lansing, MI 48912
517-485-4477
FAX 517-485-4488
http://www.publicpolicy.com
e-mail: ppa@publicpolicy.com

Jeffrey Padden, President
Nancy Hewat, Executive Officer

6999 State Vocational Rehabilitation Agency

Michigan Rehabilitation Services
PO Box 30010
Lansing, MI 48909
517-373-3390
800-605-6722
FAX 517-373-0565
TDY:888-605-6722
http://www.michigan.gov/mrs
e-mail: balthazarj@michigan.gov
Jaye Balthazar, Manager

State vocational rehabilitation agencies provide direct services to persons with disabilities, including persons with learning disabilities. The services may include evaluation and diagnosis; counseling, guidance, and referral services; vocational and other training services; transportation to rehabilitation services; and assistive devices.

Minnesota

7000 Goodwill/Easter Seals Minnesota

Goodwill/Easter Seals Minnesota
19463 Evans Street NW
Elk River, MN 55330
763-274-1822
FAX 763-274-1825
http://www.goodwilleasterseals.org
Tony Cassiday, Coordinator
Michael Wirth-Davis, President/CEO
Chris O'Neil, Manager
Job training, employment services, vocational evaluation/situational assessment and work services.

7001 Goodwill/Easter Seals: St. Cloud

50 2nd Street S
Waite Park, MN 56387
320-654-9012
FAX 320-654-9542
http://www.goodwilleasterseals.org
Julie Danda, Program Services Manager
Michael Wirth-Davis, President/CEO
Kim Clubb, Manager
Job training, employment services, vocational evaluation/situational assessment and work services.

7002 Goodwill/Easter Seals: St. Paul

Goodwill/Easter Seals: St. Paul
553 Fairview Avenue N
Saint Paul, MN 55104
651-379-5800
800-669-6719
FAX 651-379-5804
TDY:651-767-3300
http://www.goodwilleasterseals.org
e-mail: kjmatter@goodwilleasterseals.org
Kelly Matter, Program Services Vice President
Michael Wirth-Davis, President/CEO

Job training, employment services, vocational evaluation/situational assessment and work services.

7003 Goodwill/Easter Seals: Willmar

2424 1st Street S
Willmar, MN 56201
320-214-9238
FAX 320-214-9140
http://www.goodwilleasterseals.org
e-mail: pfwl@wilmar.com
Melissa Peterson, Program Services Manager
Michael Wirth-Davis, Chief Executive Officer

Job training, employment services, vocational evaluation/situational assessment and work services.

7004 Minnesota Department of Employment and Economic Development

Minnesota Workforce Center
332 Minnesota Street
Saint Paul, MN 55101
651-297-1291
http://www.mnwfc.org
e-mail: mdes.customerservice@state.mn.us
Bonnie Elsey, Director
Matt Kramer, Executive Director

The Department of Employment and Economic Development is Minnesota's principal economic development agency, with programs promoting business expansion and retention, workforce development, international trade, community development and tourism.

7005 School-to-Work Outreach Project

Institute on Community Integration
150 Pillsbury Drive SE
Minneapolis, MN 55455
612-626-7220
http://www.ici.umn.edu
e-mail: walla001@umn.edu
Terry Wallace, Research Associate
David Johnson, Director

A primary goal of the project is to improve school-to-work opportunities for students with disabilities through the identification and documentation of exemplary school-to-work activities. This is achieved through a nomination/application/review process conducted by the School-to-Work Outreach Project.

7006 State Vocational Rehabilitation Agency: Minnesota Department of Economics Security

Rehabilitation Service Branch
390 Robert Street N
Saint Paul, MN 55101
651-296-5616
800-328-9095
FAX 651-297-5159
http://www.deed.state.mn.us
e-mail: paul.bridges@state.mn.us

Paul Bridges, Director
Jan McAllister, Administrative Assistant
Earl Wilson, Manager
State vocational rehabilitation agencies provide direct services to persons with disabilities, including persons with learning disabilities. The services may include evaluation and diagnosis, counseling, guidance, and referral services, vocational and other training services, transportation to rehabilitation services, and assistive devices.

Mississippi

7007 Department of Vocational Rehabilitation Services: Mississippi
PO Box 1698
Jackson, MS 39215
601-853-5100
800-443-1000
FAX 601-853-5325
TDY:601-351-1586
http://www.mdrs.state.ms.us
Gary Neely, President
H. McMillan, Executive Director
Bob Richards, Manager

7008 State Vocational Rehabilitation Agency: Vocational Rehabilitation Division
Mississippi Department of Rehabilitation Services
PO Box 1698
Jackson, MS 39215
601-432-1200
800-443-1000
FAX 601-853-5205
TDY:601-853-5310
http://www.mdrs.state.ms.us/
e-mail: gneely@mdrs.state.ms.us
Jerry Sawyer, Director
Natalie Wagner, Executive Assistant

State vocational rehabilitation agencies provide direct services to persons with disabilities, including persons with learning disabilities. The services may include evaluation and diagnosis; counseling, guidance, and referral services; vocational and other training services; transportation to rehabilitation services; and assistive devices.

Missouri

7009 Rehabilitation Services for the Blind
Family Support Division
615 E 13th Street
Kansas City, MO 64106
816-889-2677
800-592-6004
FAX 816-889-2504
http://www.dss.mo.gov/dfs/rehab
e-mail: Kimberly.Gerlt@dss.mo.gov
Kimberly Gerlt, Operations Coordinator
Rachel Labrado, Manager

Creating opportunities for eligible blind and visually impaired people in order that they may attain personal and vocational success.

7010 State Vocational Rehabilitation AgencyDepartment of Elementary & Secondary Education
3024 Dupont Circle
Jefferson City, MO 65109
573-751-3251
877-222-8963
FAX 573-751-1441
TDY:573-751-0881
http://www.vr.dese.state.mo.us
Jeanne Loyd, Assistant Commissioner
Twyla Yardley, Supervisor
Jeanne Lloyd, Manager
State vocational rehabilitation agencies provide direct services to persons with disabilities, including persons with learning disabilities. The services may include evaluation and diagnosis, counseling, guidance, and referral services, vocational and other training services, transportation to rehabilitation services, and assistive devices.

Montana

7011 Easter Seals-Goodwill Career Designs
4400 Central Avenue
Great Falls, MT 59405
406-761-3680
FAX 406-761-3680
http://www.esgrw-nrm.easter-seals.org
e-mail: sharonod@esgw.org
Sharon Odden, Program Services VP
Michelle Belknap, CEO

Job training, employment services, vocational evaluation/situational assessment and work services.

7012 Easter Seals-Goodwill Store
951 S 29th Street W
Billings, MT 59102
406-656-4020
FAX 406-656-3750
http://www.esgw-nrm.easter-seals.org
e-mail: gwbillings@mcn.net
Rhonda Haynes, Manager
Michelle Belknap, CEO

Job training, employment services, vocational evaluation/situational assessment and work services.

7013 Easter Seals-Goodwill Working Partners
4141 1/2 S Main Street
Conrad, MT 59425
406-271-2073
FAX 406-271-2073
http://www.esgw-nrm.easter-seals.org
e-mail: sandrab@esgw.org
Sandra Bucher, Case Manager
Michelle Belknap, CEO

Job training, employment services, vocational evaluation/situational assessment and work services.

7014 Easter Seals-Goodwill Working Partners: Great Falls
205 9th Avenue S
Great Falls, MT 59405
406-771-2809
FAX 406-453-2160
http://www.esgrw-nrm.easter-seals.org
e-mail: joelc@csgw.org
Joel Corda, Supervisor
Michelle Belknap, Chief Executive Officer

Job training, employment services, vocational evaluation/situational assessment and work services.

7015 Easter Seals-Goodwill Working Partners: Hardin
501 N Center Avenue
Hardin, MT 59034
406-665-3500
FAX 406-665-1395
http://www.esgrw-nrm.easter-seals.org
e-mail: opweasle@state.mt.us
Oma Weasle, Manager
Carla Colstad, Office Assistant

Job training, employment services, vocational evaluation/situational assessment and work services.

7016 State Vocational Rehabilitation Agency
Department of Public Health & Human Services
PO Box 4210
Helena, MT 59604
406-444-5622
FAX 406-444-3632
http://www.dphhs.state.mt.gov
e-mail: jmathews@mt.gov
Joe Mathews, Director
Robert Wynia, Executive Director

State vocational rehabilitation agencies provide direct services to persons with disabilities, including persons with learning disabilities. The services may include evaluation and diagnosis, counseling, guidance, and referral services, vocational and other training services, transportation to rehabilitation services, and assistive devices.

Nebraska

7017 Easter Seals Nebraska
2727 W 2nd Street
Hastings, NE 68901
402-462-3031
800-471-6425
FAX 402-462-2040
http://www.ne.easter-seals.org
e-mail: kginder@ne.easter-seals.org
Karen Ginder, President

Job training, employment services, vocational evaluation/situational assessment and work services.

7018 Job Training Program
Nebraska Department of Economic Development
PO Box 94666
Lincoln, NE 68509
402-471-5185
800-426-6505
FAX 402-471-3365
http://www.assist.neded.org
e-mail: lshaal@neded.org
Lori Shaal, Job Training Coordinator
Arti Cover, Manager

Provides training assistance on projects that offer an opportunity for economic development in Nebraska. Use of the funds is limited to eligible companies and eligible training projects.

7019 State Vocational Rehabilitation Agency: Quality Employment Solutions
State Department of Education
PO Box 94987
Lincoln, NE 68509
402-471-3644
877-637-3422
FAX 402-471-0788
http://www.vocrehab.state.ne.us
e-mail: vr_stateoffice@vocrehab.state.ne.us
Cherly Ferree, Manager
Frank Lloyd, Asst. Education Commissioner

We help people with disabilities make career plans, learn job skills, get and keep a job. Our goal is to prepare people for jobs where they can make a living wage and have access to medical insurance.

Nevada

7020 Bureau of Services to the Blind & Visually Impaired
Bureau of Services to Blind and Visually Impaired
1370 S Curry Street
Carson City, NV 89703
775-684-4244
FAX 775-684-4186
http://www.detr.state.nv.us
e-mail: detbsb@nvdetr.org
Maureen Cole, Administrator
Gayle Sherman, Manager

Services to the Blind and Visually Impaired (BSBVI) provides a variety of services to eligible individuals, whose vision is not correctable by ordinary eye care. Adaptive training, independence skills, low vision exams and aids, mobility training and vocational rehabilitation are offered.

7021 Nevada Economic Opportunity Board: Community Action Partnership
Nevada Economic Opportunity Board
PO Box 270880
Las Vegas, NV 89127
702-647-1510
FAX 702-647-6639
http://www.eobcc.org
Marcia Walker, Executive Director

Located in one of the fastest growing and most diverse communities in the United States, the Economic Opportunity Board of Clark County is a highly innovative Community Action Agency. Our mission is to eliminate poverty by providing programs, resources, services, and advocacy for self-sufficiency and economic empowerment.

7022 Nevada Governor's Council on Rehabilitation & Employment of People with Disabilities
505 E King Street
Carson City, NV 89701
775-684-3200
FAX 775-684-4186
http://www.detr.state.nv.us
e-mail: djsanders@nvdetr.org
Donna Sanders, Assistant Director

To help insure vocational rehabilitation programs are consumer oriented, driven and result in employment outcomes for Nevadans with disabilities. Funding for innovation and expansion grants.

7023 Rehabilitation Division Department of Employment, Training & Rehabilitation
Bureau of Services to Blind and Visually Impaired
1370 S Curry Street
Carson City, NV 89703
775-684-4244
FAX 775-684-4186
TDY:775-684-8400
http://www.detr.state.nv.us
e-mail: detbsb@nvdetr.org
Maureen Cole, Administrator
Gayle Sherman, Manager

Providing options and choices for Nevadans with disabilities to work and live independently. Our mission will be accomplished through planning, implementing and coordinating assessment, employment, independent living and training.

New Hampshire

7024 Department of Health & Human Services: New Hampshire
129 Pleasant Street
Concord, NH 03301
603-271-4688
800-852-3345
FAX 603-271-4912
TDY:800-735-2964
http://www.dhhs.nh.gov
Nicoli Whitley, Public Information Officer
John Stephen, Manager

7025 Easter Seals New Hampshire
54 Pleasant Street
Claremont, NH 03743
603-543-3795
http://www.easterseals.nh.org
e-mail: cmcmahon@eastersealsnh.org
Chris McMahon, CEO
Larry Gammon, President
Anne Beattie, Manager
Job training, employment services, vocational evaluation/situational assessment and work services.

7026 Easter Seals: Keene
12 Kingsbury Street
Keene, NH 03431
603-355-1067
800-307-2737
FAX 603-358-3947
http://www.easterseals.nh.org
e-mail: cmcmahon@eastersealsnh.org
Chris McMahon, CEO
Larry Gammon, President
Kim Stanton, Manager
Job training, employment services, vocational evaluation/situational assessment and work services.

7027 Easter Seals: Manchester
555 Auburn Street
Manchester, NH 03103
603-623-8863
800-870-8728
FAX 603-625-1148
http://www.easterseals.nh.org
e-mail: cmcmahon@eastersealsnh.org
Chris McMahon, CEO
Larry Gammon, President
Kim Stanton, Manager

Job training, employment services, vocational evaluation/situational assessment and work services.

7028 State Vocational Rehabilitation Agency
Department of Education
21 S Fruit Street
Concord, NH 03301
603-271-3471
800-299-1647
TDY:603-271-3471
http://www.ed.state.nh.us/VR
e-mail: dlebrun@ed.state.nh.us
Paul Leather, Executive Director
Lillian Lee, Program Planner

Assisting eligible New Hampshire citizens with disabilities secure suitable employment, financial and personal independence by providing rehabilitation services.

New Jersey

7029 Assistive Technology Advocacy Center-ATAC
New Jersey Protection and Advocacy
210 S Broad Street
Trenton, NJ 08608
609-292-9742
800-922-7233
FAX 609-777-0187
http://www.njpanda.org
e-mail: adadvocate@njpanda.org
Ellen Catanese, Director
Sarah Mitchell, Manager

Assists individuals in overcoming barriers in the system and making assistive technology more accessible to individuals with disabilities throughout the state.

7030 Division of Family Development: New Jersey Department of Human Services
PO Box 716
Trenton, NJ 08625
609-588-2000
FAX 609-588-3051
http://www.state.nj.us
Karen Highsmith, Director
Pearl Elias, Executive Director

7031 Easter Seals: Silverton
Easter Seals Silverton
1195 Airport Road
Lakewood, NJ 08701
732-257-6662
FAX 732-730-0492
http://www.eastersealsnj.org
Brian Fitzgerald, President

Job training, employment services, vocational evaluation/situational assessment and work services.

7032 Eden Family of Services
Eden Services
1 Eden Way
Princeton, NJ 08540
609-987-0099
FAX 609-987-0243
http://www.edenservices.org
e-mail: info@edenservices.org
David Holmes EdD, Executive Director
Tom Cool, President
Joani Truch, Administration/Communications
Provides year round educational services, early intervention, parent training, respite care, outreach services, community based residential services and employment opportunities for individuals with autism.

7033 New Jersey Council on Developmental Disabilities
20 W State Street
Trenton, NJ 08608
609-392-3434
800-216-1199
FAX 609-292-7114
TDY:609-777-3238
http://www.njddc.org
e-mail: njddc@njddc.org
Ethan Ellis, Executive Director
Jane Dunhamn, Events Coordinator
Lawrence Nespoli, President
Promotes systems change, coordinates advocacy and research for 1.2 million residents with developmental and other disabilities.

7034 Programs for Children with Special Health Care Needs
NJ Department of Health & Senior Services
PO Box 364
Trenton, NJ 08625
609-588-7500
FAX 609-292-9288
http://www.state.nj.us.com
Gloria Rodriguez, President
Cajwar Aamir, Senior Public Health Physician

7035 State Department of Education Education for Students with Disabilities
Office of Vocational-Technical Career & Innovative
PO Box 500
Trenton, NJ 08625
609-633-0665
FAX 609-984-5347
http://www.state.nj.us/education
e-mail: pharris@doe.state.nj.us
Patricia Harris, Administrative Assistant
Rochelle Hendricks, Executive Director

Assists the disabled student with changes from the school environment to the working world.

7036 State Vocational Rehabilitation Agency
New Jersey Department of Labor
135 E State Street
Trenton, NJ 08608
609-292-5987
FAX 609-292-8347
TDY:609-292-2919
http://www.nj.gov/labor/dvrs/vrsindex.html
e-mail: dvraadmin@dol.state.nj.us
Thomas Jennings, Manager
Janice Pointer, Assistant Director

Enables individuals with disabilities to achieve employment outcomes consistent with their strengths, priorities, needs, abilities and capabilities. Our division is here to help people with disabilites that are having trouble finding or holding a job because of their disability.

New Mexico

7037 Department of Human Services: Project Forward
PO Box 2348
Santa Fe, NM 87504
505-827-7262
Marise McFadden, Contact

7038 New Mexico Department of Labor: Job Training Division
Office Of Workforce Training and Development
1596 Pacheco Street
Santa Fe, NM 87505
505-827-6827
FAX 505-827-6812
http://www.dol.state.nm.us
e-mail: reese.fullerton@state.nm.us
Reese Fullerton, Executive Director
Veronica Moya, Office Assistant

Helps citizens of New Mexico from all walks of life find appropriate vocational trainings, and job placement.

7039 State Vocational Rehabilitation Agency New Mexico
Department of Education
435 Saint Michaels Drive
Santa Fe, NM 87505
505-827-6516
800-224-7005
FAX 505-954-8562
http://www.dvrgetsjobs.com
e-mail: cmaple@state.nm.us

Kathryn Maple-Cross, Director
Irene White, Administrative Assistant

State vocational rehabilitation agencies provide direct services to persons with disabilities, including persons with learning disabilities. The services may include evaluation and diagnosis, counseling, guidance, and referral services, vocational and other training services, transportation to rehabilitation services, and assistive devices.

New York

7040 **Commission for the Blind & Visually Handicapped**
Department of Social Services
74 State Street
Albany, NY 12207 518-474-1701
http://www.dfa.state.ny.us
e-mail: cbvh@dfa.state.ny.us
John Johnson, Commissioner Children/Family

Professionals and paraprofessionals are available to help those with low vision or blindness with vocational rehabilitation services.

7041 **Office of Curriculum & Instructional Support**
State Department of Adult Education
89 Washington Avenue
Albany, NY 12234 518-474-8892
FAX 518-474-0319
http://www.emsc.nysed.gov/workforce
e-mail: jstevens@mail.nysed.gov
Jean Stevens, Assistant Commissioner
Richard Mills, Commissioner

Works with those seeking General Educational Development diplomas and technical training.

7042 **Office of Vocational and Educational Services for Individuals with Disabilities**
New York State Education Department
1 Commerce Plaza
Albany, NY 12234 518-436-0008
800-222-5627
FAX 518-473-9466
http://www.web.nysed.gov
e-mail: nlauria@mail.nysed.gov
Richard Mills, Commissioner
Nancy Lauria, Director
Harvey Rosenthal, Executive Director
Promotes educational equality and excellence for students with disabilities while ensuring that they receive the rights and protection to which they are entitled, assure appropriate continuity between the child and adult services systems, and provide the highest quality vocational rehabilitation and independent living services to all eligible people.

North Carolina

7043 **State Vocational Rehabilitation Agency**
Department of Health & Human Resources
2801 Mail Service Center
Raleigh, NC 27699 919-855-3500
FAX 919-733-7968
TDY:919-855-3579
http://www.dhhs.state.nc.us
e-mail: george.mccoy@ncmail.net
Carmen Hooker-Odem, Secretary Health/Human Services
George McCoy, Director
Linda Harrington, Manager
Vocational rehabilitation counselors work with business and community agencies to help them prepare their worksites to accomodate employees who have physical or mental disabilities. The division also provides services that encourage and reinforce independent living for the disabled.

North Dakota

7044 **North Dakota Department of Career and Technical Education**
Special Needs Project
600 E Boulevard Avenue
Bismarck, ND 58505 701-328-3180
FAX 701-328-1255
http://www.state.nd.us
e-mail: mwilson@state.nd.us
Dwight Crabtree, Assistant State Director
Gary Freier, Special Needs Director
Wayne Kutzer, Executive Director
The mission of the Board for Vocational and Technical Education is to work with others to provide all North Dakota citizens with the technical skills, knowledge, and attitudes necessary for successful performance in a globally competitive workplace.

7045 **North Dakota Workforce Development Council**
North Dakota Department of Commerce
PO Box 2057
Bismarck, ND 58502 701-328-5300
FAX 701-328-5320
http://www.growingnd.com/services/workforce
e-mail: jhirsch@state.nd.us
James Hirsch, Director
Jill Splonskowski, Secretary

The role of the North Dakota Workforce Development Council is to advise the Governor and the Public concerning the nature and extent of workforce development in the context of North Dakota's economic development needs, and how to meet these needs effectively while maximizing the efficient use of available resources and avoiding unnecessary duplication of effort.

7046 **Vocational Rehabilitation**
North Dakota Department of Human Services
1237 W Divide Avenue
Bismarck, ND 58501 701-328-8950
800-755-2745
FAX 701-328-8969
TDY:701-328-8968
http://www.state.nd.us.humanservices
Yvonne Smith, Director

Assists individuals with disabilities to achieve competitive employment and increased independence through rehabilitation services.

7047 **Workforce Investment Act**
Governor's Employment & Training Forum
PO Box 5507
Bismarck, ND 58506 701-328-2836
FAX 701-328-1612
TDY:800-366-6888
http://www.jobnd.com
e-mail: mdaley@state.nd.us
Maren Daley, Executive Director

Literacy coaching and further vocational training.

Ohio

7048 **Bureau of Workforce Services**
145 S Front Street
Columbus, OH 43215 614-466-3817
FAX 614-728-5938
http://www.ohioworkforce.org
Bill Demidovich, Deputy Director

Oversees the implementation of the job training partnership act and employment and training programs in the state of Ohio.

7049 State Vocational Rehabilitation Agency
Ohio Rehabilitation Services Commission
400 E Campus View Boulevard
Columbus, OH 43235
614-438-1200
800-282-4635
FAX 614-785-5010
TDY:614-438-1726
http://www.state.oh.us
e-mail: rsc_rir@vscnet.a1.state.oh.us
John Connelly, Executive Director
Sandra Montgomery, Administration

State vocational rehabilitation agencies provide direct services to persons with disabilities, including persons with learning disabilities. The services may include evaluation and diagnosis, counseling, guidance, and referral services, vocational and other training services, transportation to rehabilitation services, and assistive devices.

Oklahoma

7050 National Clearinghouse of Rehabilitation Training Materials
Oklahoma State University
206 W 6th Street
Stillwater, OK 74078
405-744-7213
800-223-5219
FAX 405-744-2001
TDY:405-744-2002
http://www.nchrtm.okstate.edu
e-mail: jennifer.ahlert@okstate.edu
Jennifer Ahlert, Marketing Coordinator
Carolyn Cail, Information Coordinator

Rehabilitation counselor and education materials, disability information and resources.

7051 State Vocational Rehabilitation Agency: Oklahoma Department of Rehabilitation Services
3535 NW 58th Street
Oklahoma City, OK 73112
405-951-3400
800-845-8476
FAX 405-951-3529
http://www.okrehab.org
e-mail: ddcouch@drs.state.ok.us
David Pittman MD, Commission Chair
Susan Randall, Administrative Assistant
Linda Parker, Executive Director
State vocational rehabilitation agencies provide direct services to persons with disabilities, including persons with learning disabilities. The services may include evaluation and diagnosis counseling, guidance, and referral services, vocational and other training services, transportation to rehabilitation services and assistive devices.

7052 Workforce Investment Act
Oklahoma Employment Security Commission
2401 N Lincoln Boulevard
Oklahoma City, OK 73105
405-557-7294
http://www.oesc.state.ok.us
e-mail: denise.burr@oesc.state.ok.us
John Brock, Executive Director
Glen Robards, Assistant Director

Partnership of local goverments offering resource conservation and development and workforce development.

Oregon

7053 Department of Community Colleges & Workforce Development
255 Capitol Street NE
Salem, OR 97310
503-378-8648
FAX 503-378-3365
TDY:800-735-2900
http://www.odccwd.state.or.us
e-mail: karen.madden@state.or.us
Karen Madden, Program Manager
Jerry Lierow, Coordinator

Contributes leadership and resources to increase the skills, knowledge and career opportunities for Oregonians.

7054 Oregon Employment Department
875 Union Street NE
Salem, OR 97311
503-947-1394
800-237-3710
FAX 503-947-1668
http://www.emp.state.or.us
e-mail: deborah.lincoln@state.or.us
Deborah Lincoln, Director
Greg Hickman, Deputy Director
Odie Vogel, Assistant to Director
Supports economic stability for Oregonians and communities during times of unemployment through the payment of unemployment benefits. Serves businesses by recruiting and referring the best qualified applicants to jobs, and provides resources to diverse job seekers in support of their employment needs.

7055 Oregon Office of Education and Workforce Policy
900 Court Street NE
Salem, OR 97301
503-378-4582
FAX 503-378-4863
http://www.arcweb.sos.state.or.us
e-mail: annette.talbott@state.or.us
Annette Talbott, Workforce Policy Coordinator
Danny Santos, Education Policy Coordinator

The Governor's Office of Education and Workforce Policy was established to assist the Governor in examining education and workforce efforts with a view to supporting and strengthening what is working well. The goal is to have Oregonians prepared to meet the education and workforce needs of Oregon businesses rather than having to recruit from outside the state to fill quality jobs.

7056 Recruitment and Retention Special Education Jobs Clearinghouse
Teaching Research
345 Monmouth Avenue
Monmouth, OR 97361
503-838-8391
FAX 503-838-8150
http://www.tr.wou.edu/rrp
e-mail: samplesb@wou.edu
Bernie Samples, Clearinghouse Coordinator
Meredith Brodsky, Executive Director

A free on-line jobs clearinghouse with access to position openings in Oregon in the area of Special Education and related services. A Job Seeker Listing and resumes also sent via e-mail to districts and agencies looking for qualified individuals.

7057 State Vocational Rehabilitation Agency
Division of Vocational Rehabilitation
500 Summer Street NE
Salem, OR 97301
503-945-5880
877-277-0513
FAX 503-378-2897
http://www.dhs.state.or.us/vr/index.html
e-mail: info.vr@state.or.us
Jean Thorne, Human Services Director
Stephanie Parrish-Taylor, Administrator

Uses state and federal funds to assist Oregonians who have disabilities to achieve and maintain employment and independence.

Pennsylvania

7058 State Vocational Rehabilitation Agency: Pennsylvania
Department of Labor & Industry
1521 N 6th Street
Harrisburg, PA 17102
717-787-5244
800-442-6351
http://www.dli.state.pa.us
e-mail: ovr@dli.state.pa.us
Steven Nasuti, Executive Director
Thomas Washic, Manager

Provides individualized services to assist people with disabilities to pursue, obtain, and maintain satisfactory employment. Counselors are available for training, planning and placement services.

Rhode Island

7059 Rhode Island Department of Employment and Training

101 Friendship Street
E Providence, RI 02914
401-277-4922
FAX 401-861-8030

7060 Rhode Island Vocational and Rehabilitation Agency
Rhode Island Department of Human Services
40 Fountain Street
Providence, RI 02903
401-421-7005
FAX 401-222-3574
TDY:401-421-7016
http://www.ors.ri.gov
e-mail: rcarroll@ors.ri.gov
Raymond Carroll, Administrator
Valerie Williams, Chief Clerk

Assists people with disabilities to become employed and to live independently in the community. In order to achieve this goal, we work in partnership with the State Rehabilitation Council, our customers, staff and community.

7061 State Vocational Rehabilitation Agency: Rhode Island
Rhode Island Department of Human Services
40 Fountain Street
Providence, RI 02903
401-421-7005
FAX 401-222-3574
TDY:401-421-7016
http://www.ors.ri.gov
e-mail: rcarroll@ors.ri.gov
Raymond Carroll, Administrator
Valerie Williams, Chief Clerk

Assists people with disabilities to become employed and to live independently in the community. In order to achieve this goal, we work in partnership with the State Rehabilitation Council, our customers, staff and community.

South Carolina

7062 Americans with Disabilities Act Assistance Line
Employment Security Commission
PO Box 1406
Columbia, SC 29202
803-737-9935
800-436-8190
FAX 803-737-0140
http://www.sces.org
e-mail: rratterree@sces.org
Regina Ratterree, Program Coordinator

Provides information, technical assistance and training on the Americans with Disabilities Act.

7063 South Carolina Vocational Rehabilitation Department
PO Box 15
West Columbia, SC 29171
803-896-6500
FAX 803-896-6529
http://www.scvrd.net
Jay Rolin, Director
Shannon Lindsay, Counselor
Larry Bryant, Manager
Enabling eligible South Carolinians with disabilities to prepare for, achieve and maintain competitive employment. Training, coaching and job placement services available.

South Dakota

7064 Department of Social Services
700 Governors Drive
Pierre, SD 57501
605-773-3165
FAX 605-773-4855
http://www.state.sd.us
e-mail: dssinfo@state.sd.us
James Ellenbecker, Manager
Maxine Johnston, Administrative Assistant

7065 South Dakota Department of Labor
700 Governors Drive
Pierre, SD 57501
605-773-5017
800-952-3216
FAX 605-773-4211
TDY:605-773-5017
http://www.state.sd.us/dol/dol.htm
e-mail: miker@dol.pr.state.sd.us
Michael Ryan, Administrator

Job training programs provide an important framework for developing public-private sector partnerships. We help prepare South Dakotans of all ages for entry or re-entry into the labor force.

7066 South Dakota Rehabilitation Center for the Blind
Department of Human Services
2900 W 11th Street
Sioux Falls, SD 57104
605-367-5260
800-658-5441
FAX 605-367-5263
http://www.state.sd.us/dhs/
e-mail: dawn.backer@state.sd.us
Gaye Mattke, Director

Helping people lead a full, productive life — regardless of how much one does or does not see. Upon completion of training, individuals usually return to their community and use these new skills in their home, school or job.

7067 State Vocational Rehabilitation Agency
Division of Rehabilitation Services
3800 E Highway 34
Pierre, SD 57501
605-773-3195
800-265-9684
FAX 605-773-5483
TDY:605-773-3195
http://www.state.sd.us/dhs/drs/
e-mail: steve.stewart@state.sd.us
Grady Kickul, Executive Director
Steve Stewart, Rehabilitation Engineer

Assists individuals with disabilities to obtain employment, economic self-sufficiency, personal independence and full inclusion into society.

Tennessee

7068 State Vocational Rehabilitation Agency
Tennessee Department of Human Services
400 Deaderick Street
Nashville, TN 37248
615-741-2330
866-311-4288
FAX 615-741-4165
TDY:615-532-8569
http://www.state.tn.us/humanserv/
e-mail: car.w.brown@state.tn.us
Carl Brown, Assistant Commissioner
Terry Smith, Director
Ruth Letson, Manager
State vocational rehabilitation agencies provide direct services to persons with disabilities, including persons with learning disabilities. The services may include evaluation and diagnosis counseling, guidance, and referral services, vocational and other training services, transportation to rehabilitation services and assistive devices.

7069 Tennessee Department of Education
Tennessee Department of Education
710 James Robertson Parkway
Nashville, TN 37243
615-741-2731
800-531-1515
FAX 615-532-4791
http://www.state.tn.us
e-mail: education.comments@state.tn.us
Phil White, Director of Adult Education
Lana Seivers, Commissioner of Education

Mission is to take Tennessee to the top in education. Guides administration of the state's K-12 public schools.

7070 Tennessee Department of Labor & Workforce Development: Office of Adult Education
500 James Robertson Parkway
Nashville, TN 37243
615-741-0466
800-531-1515
FAX 615-532-4899
TDY:800-848-0299
http://www.state.tn.us
e-mail: phil.white@state.tn.us
Haticile Buchanan, Manager
James Neeley, Commissioner
Phil White, Director of Adult Education

7071 Tennessee Services for the Blind
Division of Rehabilitation
400 Deaderick Street
Nashville, TN 37248
615-313-4914
800-628-7818
FAX 615-313-6617
TDY:615-313-6601
http://www.state.tn.us/humanserv/
e-mail: Human-Services.Webmaster@state.tn.us
Terry Smith, Director
Philip Wagster, Director Vocational Rehab.

Offering training and services to help blind or low-vision citizens of Tennessee become more independent at home, in the community and at work.

Texas

7072 Department of Assistive & Rehabilitative
4800 N Lamar Boulevard
Austin, TX 78756
512-377-0500
Terry Murphy, Manager

7073 Department of Assistive & Rehabilitative Services
Texas Department of Health & Human Services
4800 N Lamar Boulevard
Austin, TX 78756
512-377-0800
800-628-5115
http://www.dars.state.tx.us
e-mail: terrell.murphy@dars.state.tx.us
Glenn Neal, Director

Transitional and vocational programs aid independence in the home, community and at work for Texans who are blind, deaf, or have other impairments that would benefit from assistive technology.

7074 State Vocational Rehabilitation Agency
Texas State Rehabilitation Commission
4800 N Lamar Boulevard
Austin, TX 78756
512-424-4000
800-628-5115
FAX 512-424-4730
http://www.dars.state.tx.us
e-mail: dars@rehab.state.tx.us
Terry Murphy, Commissioner
Max Arrell, Manager
Mary Wolfe, Field Operations/Communications

State vocational rehabilitation agencies provide direct services to persons with disabilities, including persons with learning disabilities. The services may include evaluation and diagnosis, counseling, guidance, and referral services, vocational and other training services, transportation to rehabilitation services and assistive devices.

7075 Texas Department of Assistive and Rehabilitative Services
4800 N Lamar Boulevard
Austin, TX 78756
512-424-4000
800-628-5115
FAX 512-424-4730
http://www.dars.state.tx.us
e-mail: dars@rehab.state.tx.us
Terry Murphy, Commissioner
Max Arrell, Manager
Mary Wolfe, Field Operations/Communications
A place where people with disabilities and families with children who have developmental delays enjoys independent and productive lives. The mission is to wo

7076 Texas Education Agency
1701 N Congress Avenue
Austin, TX 78701
512-463-9734
FAX 512-475-3661
http://www.tea.state.tx.us
Paul Lindsey, Asst Commissioner/Continuing Ed.
Pavlos Roussos, Program Director/Adult Education
Jim Nelson, Manager

7077 Texas Workforce Commission
101 E 15th Street
Austin, TX 78778
512-463-2222
FAX 512-475-2321
http://www.twc.state.tx.us
e-mail: luis.macias@twc.state.tx.us
Larry Temple, Manager
Luis Macias, Workforce Division Director

Provides oversight, coordination, guidance, planning, technical assistance and implementation of employment and training activities with a focus on meeting the needs of employers throughout the state of Texas.

Utah

7078 Adult Education Services
Utah State Office of Education
250 E 500 S
Salt Lake City, UT 84111
801-538-7824
FAX 801-538-7882
http://www.schools.utah.gov
e-mail: marty.kelly@schools.utah.gov
Marty Kelly, Coordinator/Director Education
Sandra Grant, Specialist

Provides oversight of state and federally funded adult education programs. Offers adult basic education, adult high school completion, English as a second language, and general education development programs.

7079 Utah Vocational Rehabilitation Agency
State Office of Rehabilitation
250 E 5th S
Salt Lake City, UT 84111
801-538-7530
800-473-7530
FAX 801-538-7522
TDY:801-538-7530
http://www.usor.utah.gov
e-mail: bpetersen@utah.gov
Blaine Petersen, Manager

Assisting and empowering eligible individuals. Disabled, learning disabled, blind, low vision and deaf people can prepare for and obtain employment and increase their independence through job training and assistive technology.

Vermont

7080 Adult Education & Literacy State Department of Education
Department of Education
120 State Street
Montpelier, VT 05620-2501 802-828-5134
FAX 802-828-3146
http://www.state.vt.us/educ/
e-mail: edinfo@education.state.vt.us
Kay Charron, State Director Adult Ed/Literacy
Sandra Robinson, Dir Adult Occupational Training

Provides adults with educational opportunities to acquire the essential skills and knowledge to achieve career, post-secondary and life goals.

7081 REACH-UP Program: Department of Social Welfare
Department for Children and Families Economic Serv
103 S Main Street
Waterbury, VT 05671 802-241-2800
FAX 802-241-2830
http://www.vt.gov
Pamela Dalley, Director
Barbara Kingsbury, Office Manager
John Hall, Manager

7082 State of Vermont Department of Education: Adult Education and Literacy
120 Fake Street
Montpelier, VT 05602 802-828-5134
FAX 802-828-3146
http://www.state.vt.us/educ/
e-mail: kaycharron@education.state.vt.us
Kay Charron, State Director

Adult Education and Literacy Programs provide adults with educational opportunities to acquire the essential skills and knowledge to achieve career, post-secondary and life goals. The Department of Education supports and administers a number of programs that focus on essential literacy and academic skills as well as workplace and introductory occupational skills.

7083 Vermont Department for Children and Families
Agency of Human Services
103 S Main Street
Waterbury, VT 05671 802-241-2100
800-287-0589
FAX 802-241-2830
http://www.state.vt.us/srs
James Morse, Commissioner
Les Birnbaum, General Counsel

It is the mission of the Department for Children and Families to promote the social, emotional, physical and economic well being and the safety of Vermont's children and families. This is done through the provision of protective, developmental, therapeutic, probation, economic, and other support services for children and families in partnership with schools, businesses, community leaders, service providers, families, and youths statewide.

7084 Vermont Department of Employment & Training
PO Box 488
Montpelier, VT 05601 802-828-4000
FAX 802-828-4022
http://www.det.state.vt.us
e-mail: mcalcagni@det.state.vt.us
Mike Calcagni, Director Jobs/Training
Mike Griffin, Labor Market Information
Patricia Donald, Manager
Represents Vermont's efforts to provide services, information and support both to individuals to obtain and keep good jobs, and to employers to recruit and maintain a productive workforce.

7085 Vermont Disability Program Navigator Initiative
Vermont Department of Labor
5 Green Mountain Drive
Montpelier, VT 05601 802-828-4000
FAX 802-828-4022
http://www.det.state.vt.us
e-mail: jdorsey@labor.state.vt.us
Jim Dorsey, Project Administrator

Provides dedicated professionals to assist persons with disabilities find, gain access, enter or re-enter the job market. The navigator position is intended to increase employment and self-sufficiency for persons with disabilities by linking them to employers.

7086 VocRehab Vermont
103 S Main Street
Waterbury, VT 05671 802-241-2186
866-879-6757
FAX 802-241-3359
TDY:802-241-1455
http://www.vocrehabvermont.org
e-mail: janet.richard@dail.state.vt.us
Diane Dalmasse, Executive Director
Sandra Hayden, Brain Injury Program Support

VocRehab's mission is to assist Vermonters with disabilities find and maintain meaningful employment in their communities. VocRehab Vermont works in close partnership with the Vermont Association of Business and Industry Rehabilitation.

Virginia

7087 Office of Adult Education & Literacy
Virginia Department of Education
PO Box 2120
Richmond, VA 23218 804-340-0072
FAX 804-225-3352
http://www.doe.virginia.gov
e-mail: yvonne.thayer@doe.virginia.gov
Yvonne Thayer, Director
Elizabeth Hawa, Associate Director

Provides leadership and support for adult education and literacy services, with priority on the development and expansion of quality family literacy and workforce education programs.

7088 Virginia Department of Education: Adult Education & Literacy
101 N 14th Street
Richmond, VA 23219 804-225-2075
FAX 804-225-3352
http://Program Navigatorgov/VDOE/Instruction
e-mail: gedinfo@doe.virginia.gov
Elizabeth Hawa, Director
Gloria Murphy, Secretary
Dr Judith Fine, Assessment/Evaluation Director
Distributes funds and provides leadership and services related to adult education programs in Virginia. The goal is to raise the performance levels of adult education programs, increase the number of GED credentials issued by Virginia, and provide alternatives for youth who are at risk of dropping out of school.

7089 Virginia Department of Rehabilitative Services
8004 Franklin Farms Drive
Richmond, VA 23229 804-662-7000
800-552-5019
FAX 804-662-9531
TDY:800-464-9950
http://www.vadrs.org
e-mail: drs@drs.virginia.gov
John Rothrock, Commissioner
James Rothrock, Manager
Barbara Tyson, Administrative Assistant
In partnership with people with disabilities and their families, the Virginia Department of Rehabilitative Services collaborates with the public and private sectors to provide and advocate for the highest quality services that empower individuals with disabilities to maximize their employment, independence and engagement in the community.

7090 Virginia Employment Commission
PO Box 1358
Richmond, VA 23218 804-674-2368
800-828-1140
FAX 804-371-2814
http://www.vec.state.va.us
e-mail: athornton-crump@vec.state.va.us

Dolores Esser, Commissioner
Alexis Thornton-Crump, Program Manager
Charlene Watkins, Manager
Provides workforce services that promote maximum employment to enhance the economic stability of Virginia.

Washington

7091 State Vocational Rehabilitation Agency: Washington Division of Vocational Rehabilitation
Department of Social Services & Health
PO Box 45340
Olympia, WA 98504
360-438-8000
800-637-5627
FAX 360-438-8007
TDY:360-438-8000
http://www.1.dshs.wa.gov
e-mail: obrien@dshs.wa.gov
Michael O'Brien, Director

State vocational rehabilitation agencies provide direct services to persons with disabilities, including persons with learning disabilities. The services may include evaluation and diagnosis, counseling, guidance, and referral services, vocational and other training services, transportation to rehabilitation services, and assistive devices.

7092 Washington State Division of Vocational Rehabilitation
Department of Social & Health Services
Olympia, WA 98504
360-438-8000
800-737-0617
FAX 360-438-8007
http://www1.dshs.wa.gov
e-mail: ruttllm@dshs.wa.gov
Lynnae Ruttledge, Director
Paul Cox, Information Services Manager

Provides employment-related services to individuals with disabilities who want to work but need assistance. These individuals might experience difficulty getting or keeping a job due to a physical, sensory and/or mental disability. A DVR counselor works with each individual to develop a customized plan of services designed to help the individual achieve his or her job goal.

7093 Work First Division: Washington Department of Social and Health Services
PO Box 14789
Tumwater, WA 98511
877-980-9180
http://www.onlinecso.dshs.wa.gov

West Virginia

7094 West Virginia Division of Rehabilitation Services
West Virginia Department of Education & the Arts
PO Box 50890
Charleston, WV 25305
304-766-4601
800-642-3021
FAX 304-766-4905
TDY:304-766-4965
http://www.wvdrs.org
e-mail: Debbiel@mail.drs.state.wv.us
Janice Holland, Director
Debbie Lovely, Field Services/Programs

State vocational rehabilitation agencies provide direct services to persons with disabilities, including persons with learning disabilities. The services may include evaluation and diagnosis, counseling, guidance, and referral services, vocational and other training services, transportation to rehabilitation services, and assistive devices.

7095 Workforce Investment Act
West Virginia Bureau of Employment Programs
112 California Avenue
Charleston, WV 25305
304-558-1138
800-252-5627
FAX 304-558-1136
http://www.state.wv.us/bep/
e-mail: BGreenle@wvbep.org
Don Pardue, Commissioner
Valerie Comer, Director

Matching jobseekers with employers in a prompt, efficient manner, to help those in need become job ready, and to analyze and disseminate labor market information. Special placement techniques are also offered which seek to match the physical and mental demands of a job to the capabilities of workers with disabilities. Such services are given by Job Service in cooperation with other community agencies and include counseling and special placement assistance.

Wisconsin

7096 W-2 Program: Division of Work Force Solutions
Wisconsin Department of Workforce Development
201 E Washington Avenue
Madison, WI 53702
608-266-8354
FAX 608-261-6376
http://www.dwd.state.wi.us/dws/w2/default.htm
e-mail: sandy.breitborde@dwd.state.wi.us
Bill Clingan, Administrator
Sandy Breitborde, Workforce Information
Linda Stewart, Manager
Develops and maintains employment focused programs that enable employers to hire and retain the workforce they need and that provide individuals and families with services that enable them to achieve financial well being as members of Wisconsin's workforce. It delivers services through public-private partnerships and a statewide network of job centers.

7097 Wisconsin Division of Vocational Rehabilitation
201 E Washington Avenue
Madison, WI 53702
608-261-0050
800-442-3477
FAX 608-266-1133
TDY:888-877-5939
http://www.dwd.state.wi.us/dvr/
e-mail: dwddvr@dwd.state.wi.us
Charlene Dwyer, Manager
Manuel Lugo, Deputy Administrator

Federal and state program designed to obtain, maintain and improve employment for people with disabilities by working with vocational rehabilitation consumers, employers and other partners.

7098 Work Force Information Act
Education and Training Policy Division
PO Box 7903
Madison, WI 53707
608-266-2439
FAX 608-267-2392
e-mail: denisga@dwd.state.WI.us
Gary Denis, Director

7099 Workforce Investment Act
Division of Workforce Solutions
201 E Washington Avenue
Madison, WI 53707
608-266-0327
FAX 608-261-6376
http://www.dwd.state.wi.us
e-mail: dwddws@dwd.state.wi.us
Gary Denis, Program Acting Director
Sandy Breitborde, Information Director

Develops and maintains employment-focused programs that enable employers to hire and retain the workforce they need and providing individuals and families with services that enable them to achieve financial well being as members of Wisconsin's workforce.

Wyoming

7100 **Wyoming Department of Workforce Services: State Vocational Rehabilitation Agency**

1510 E Pershing Boulevard
Cheyenne, WY 82002
307-777-7385
FAX 307-777-3759
http://www.wyomingworkforce.org
e-mail: jmcint@state.wy.us

Jim McIntosh, Administrator
Ray Sattler, Director

Assists Wyoming citizens with disabilities to prepare for, enter into, and return to suitable employment. Individuals with a disability that prevents them from working may apply for these services as long as a physical or mental impairment which constitutes or results in a substantial impediment to employment exists, and they have the ability to benefit in terms of an employment outcome from vocational services.

B

C

E

F

H

I

J

K

M

N

O

P

Q

R

S

T

U

V

W

X

Y

Z

c

v

w

Alabama

Alaska

Arizona

Arkansas

California

Colorado

Connecticut

Delaware

District of Columbia

Florida

Georgia

Hawaii

Indiana

Iowa

Kansas

Kentucky

Louisiana

Maine

Maryland

Massachusetts

Michigan

Minnesota

Mississippi

Missouri

Montana

Nebraska

Nevada

New Hampshire

New Jersey

New Mexico

New York

North Carolina

North Dakota

Ohio

Oklahoma

Oregon

Pennsylvania

Rhode Island

South Carolina

South Dakota

Tennessee

Texas

Utah

Vermont

Virginia

Washington

West Virginia

Wisconsin

Wyoming

ADD/ADHD

Animation

Aphasia

Aptitude

Articulation

Arts

At-Risk

Autism

Behavioral Disorders

Bilingual Resources

Camps

Child Welfare

Clearinghouses

Cognitive Disorders

Comic Strips

Communication Disorders

Community Integration

Comprehension

Conceptual Skills

Conferences

Consumer Skills

Contemporary Education

Cooperative Learning Centers

Creative Expression

Critical Thinking

Curriculum Guides

Daily Living

Databases

Developmental Disabilities

Directories

Discrimination

Dispute Resolution Dyslexia

Dyslexia

ESL

Economic Skills

Education

Elementary Education

Equality

Ethics

Evaluations

Eye/Hand Coordination

Family Involvement

Family Resources

Financial Resources

Fluency

Gameboards

Gifted Education

Graphing

Head Injuries

Health Care

Hearing Impaired

High School Education

Higher Education

History

Hotlines

Human Services

Inclusion

Infancy

Information Resources

Integration

International Associations

Intervention

Job/Vocational Resources

Keyboards

Kits

Language Skills

Leadership

Legal Issues

Libraries

Listening Skills

Literacy

Literature

Logic

Mainstreaming

Matching

Mathematics

Maturity

Memorization Skills

Minorities

Motivation

Motor Development

Multicultural Education

Multisensory Education

Music

Neurological Disorders

Newsletters

Nutrition

Occupational Therapy

Pathology

Peer Programs

Perception Skills

Pets

Phonics

Physical Education

Play Therapy

Program Planning

Public Awareness & Interest

Puzzles

Recognition Skills

Rehabilitation

Remediation

Research

Resource Centers

School Administration

Science

Secondary Education

Self-Advocacy

Self-Esteem

Sensory Integration

Siblings

Sign Language

Software

Sound Recognition

Special Education

Speech Skills

Spelling

Strategies

Student Workshops

Support Groups

Surveys

Switches

Synthesizers

Tape Recorders

Technology

Tourette Syndrome

Training

Transportation

Treatment

Visual Assistive Devices

Visual Discrimination

Vocabulary

Voice Output Devices

Volunteer

Workshop Training

Writing

Glossary

Accommodations: Techniques and materials that allow individuals with LD to complete school or work tasks with greater ease and effectiveness. Examples include spellcheckers, tape recorders, and expanded time for completing assignments.

ADA: Americans with Disabilities Act.

Adaptive Physical Education: A special education program designed to suit a person's limits and disabilities.

Alternative Assessment: An alternative to conventional means of assessing achievement; usually means using something other than a paper and pencil test, such as oral testing or work sample review.

Appeal: A written request for a change in a decision.

Aptitude Test: A test developed to measure a person's ability to learn, and the likelihood of succeeding in academic work or in specific careers.

Assistive Technology (AT): Equipment that enhances the ability of students and employees to be more efficient and successful. For individuals with LD, computer grammar checkers, an overhead projector used by a teacher, or the audiovisual information delivered through a CD-ROM would be typical examples.

Attention Deficit Disorder (ADD): A disorder of brain function, causing severe difficulty in focusing and maintaining attention, paying attention to details, listening to instructions, and organizing assignments, thoughts and behaviors. Often leads to learning/academic difficulties, and behavior problems at home, school, and work. ADD is not a learning disability.

Attention Deficit Hyperactivity Disorder (AD/HD): A disorder of brain function, causing severe difficulty in staying on task, accompanied by hyperactivity. Difficulties can occur in taking turns in games or conversations, controlling temper outbursts, anticipating the consequences of actions, and containing or managing internal restlessness.

Auditory Discrimination: The ability to recognize, compare, and differentiate the discrete sounds in words; this ability is crucial for reading skills. Categorized as gross ability (e.g., detecting the differences between the noises made by a cow and a horse) or fine ability (e.g., distinguishing between the "s" sound and the "sh" sound).

Auditory Figure-Ground Discrimination: The ability to distinguish significant sounds amid a noisy background, and to focus on the auditory information being presented.

Auditory Memory: The ability to remember something heard some time in the past (long-term auditory memory); the ability to recall something heard very recently (short-term auditory memory).

Auditory Sequencing: The ability to comprehend and recollect the order of spoken words.

AYP: Annual yearly progress.

Behavior Modification: A technique intended to alter behavior by positive reinforcement (rewarding desirable actions) and ignoring undesirable actions.

Binocular Fusion: The blending of separate images from each eye into a single significant image.

Brain Imaging Techniques: Recently developed, noninvasive techniques for studying the activity of living brains. Includes brain electrical activity mapping (BEAM), computerized axial tomography (CAT), and magnetic resonance imaging (MRI).

Brain Injury: The physical damage to brain tissue or structure that occurs before, during, or after birth that is verified by EEG, MRI, CAT, or a similar examination, rather than by observation of performance. When caused by an accident, the damage may be called Traumatic Brain Injury (TBI).

Catastrophic Reaction: A display of extreme emotion (anger, terror, frustration or grief) without an apparent stimulus, possibly prompted by unexpected events, alteration of set routine, or feelings of over-excitement.

CEC: Council for Exceptional Children.

Central Auditory Processing Disorder (CAPD): A weakness in how the brain processes auditory information in an individual with functioning hearing ability.

Central Nervous System (CNS): The brain and the spinal cord.

Cerebral Cortex: The brain's outer layer, which controls thoughts, feelings, and voluntary movements.

Child Study Committee: A body of school officers and/or specialists which acts upon referrals of students thought to be disabled, and aids in the students' specialized aptitude assessment.

Cognition: The act or process of knowing, as a result of the capacities of various thinking skills and thought processes which are considered cognitive skills.

Cognitive Ability: Skills of reasoning and thinking; the ability to perceive intellectually.

Cognitive Style: The way a person typically approaches problem solving and learning activities (e.g., methodical analysis or impulsive reactivity).

Compensation: The process by which a person is taught to manage his or her learning problems, by manipulating and emphasizing strengths as a way to work around skills and/or abilities which may be limited.

Conceptual Disorder: A disturbance in the processes of reasoning, thinking, evaluating, recognizing, generalizing, and/or memorizing.

Conceptualization: The process of developing a general idea based on observations, including the ability to recognize similar traits within a group of objects.

Configuration: The visual form or shape of words.

Coordination: The synchronization and complementary functioning of muscles in the body necessary for completing complex movements.

Criterion Referenced Test: A test developed to reflect the specific knowledge or skills possessed by an individual, scored in terms of an individual's knowledge or ability of a relatively small unit of content without reference to other individuals' scores.

Cross-Categorical: A term referring to a system in which an instructor addresses more than one handicapping condition within one instructional session.

Cumulative File: The general file maintained for any child enrolled in a school. Parents have a right to copy and/or have access to any information in this file.

Decoding: The process of acquiring meaning from spoken, written, or printed symbols used in receptive language.

Developmental Aphasia: A severe language disorder in the normal acquisition of language.

Developmental Lag: A delay in the development of some aspect of a person's mental or physical maturation.

Direct Instruction (DI): An instructional approach to academic subjects that emphasizes the use of carefully sequenced steps that include demonstration, modeling, guided practice, and independent application.

Directionality: The ability to distinguish direction and orientation, including the difference between right and left, up and down, and forward and backward.

Discrimination: The process of differentiating between and/or among separate stimuli.

Disinhibition: Lack of restraint in a person's response to a situation, often resulting in impulsive and/or inappropriate reactions.

Distractibility: The transferring of attention from the task at hand to stimuli such as sounds and sights that normally occur in a person's surroundings.

DOE: Department of Education.

Due Process: Application of legal measures to ensure the protection of an individual's rights, e.g., a parent has the right to ask for a full evaluation of any educational program developed for his or her child.

Dysarthia: A disorder affecting the muscles necessary for speech, impacting a person's ability to pronounce words.

Dyscalculia: A wide range of life-long disabilities involving mathematics and computations, often indicated by severe difficulty in understanding and using symbols or functions needed for success in mathematics.

Dysgraphia: A disability affecting writing abilities, characterized by difficulty in spelling, written expression, and producing handwriting that is legible and written at an age-appropriate speed.

Dyslexia: A life-long language processing disorder causing the brain to process and interpret information differently, resulting in severe difficulty in understanding or using one or more areas of language, including listening, speaking, reading, writing, and spelling.

Dysnomia: A marked difficulty in remembering names or recalling words needed in context for oral or written language.

Dyspraxia: A specific disorder in the development of motor skills which inhibits a person's ability to plan and complete intended fine motor activities, marked by severe difficulty in performing drawing, writing, buttoning, and other tasks requiring fine motor skill, or in sequencing the necessary movements.

Early Intervention Program: A specially designed program for assisting infants and preschool children who exhibit developmental delay, intended to prevent future cognitive problems.

EDGAR: Education Department General Administrative Regulations.

Educational Evaluation: An assessment of a child's aptitude, based on multiple tests, analysis of class work, and classroom observation, intended to determine levels of achievement in certain academic areas, as well as the child's learning style and perceptual abilities.

Electroencephalogram (EEG): A recording, represented graphically, of electric currents produced in the cerebral cortex during brain functioning; also called a brain wave test.

ELL: English language learner.

Encoding: The process of expressing language through word selection, ideation, and transferring thoughts to written or spoken form.

ESEA: The federal Elementary and Secondary Education Act.

ESL: English as a second language.

Expressive Language: Communication through speech, writing, and/or gestures.

FAPE: Free appropriate public education; a right mandated for every child under federal law.

Far Point Copying: Reproducing, in writing, a copy of a model some distance away (e.g., a sentence on a chalkboard).

FAST: Functional academic skills test.

FBA: Functional behavior assessment.

FERPA: Family Educational Rights to Privacy Act (a.k.a. the Buckley Amendment).

Figure-Ground Discrimination: The ability to distinguish important information from the surrounding environment, e.g., isolating a particular word within a paragraph, or hearing an instructor's voice amid other noises.

Fine Motor Skills: The use of small muscles to complete precise tasks such as writing, drawing, buttoning, opening jars, and doing puzzles.

General Education (Regular Education): Any education not considered Special Education.

Gross Motor Skills: The use of larger muscles for activities involving strength and balance, such as walking, running and climbing.

Handicapped: A person with any physical and/or mental disability which inhibits such actions as seeing, hearing, speaking, learning, walking, or working. According to federal law, a child is handicapped when he or she is mentally retarded, seriously emotionally disturbed, hard of hearing or deaf, visually impaired or blind, speech impaired, orthopedically impaired, other health impaired, or as having specific learning disabilities which require special education services because of these disabilities.

Haptic Sense: The combination of kinesthetic and tactile sense.

Head Start: Head Start and Early Head Start are federally mandated comprehensive child development programs that serve children from birth to age 5, pregnant women, and their families. They are child-focused programs and have the overall goal of increasing the school readiness of young children in low-income families.

Hyperactivity (Hyperkinesis): Behavior characterized by constant and excessive movement, often marked by distractibility and/or catastrophic reactions.

Hypoactivity: Underactivity, often characterized by lethargy, dazedness, or sluggishness.

IDEA: Individuals with Disabilities Education Act.

IEP: Individualized education program.

IEP Committee: The group of select individuals who develop a student's Individualized Education Program after the student has been identified as handicapped.

Impulsivity: Reacting to a situation without consideration of outcome or consequences.

Individualized Education Plan (IEP): The written educational program designed for each handicapped (including learning disabled) individual, incorporating certain information such as educational goals (long-term and short-term), the duration of the program, and provisions for evaluating the program's effectiveness and the student's performance.

Individualized Family Service Plan (IFSP): A plan that documents and guides the early intervention process for children with disabilities and their families, as dictated in the Individuals with Disabilities Education Act (IDEA).

Individualized Transition Plan (ITP): A plan that must be made by the IEP team for a student, no later than age 16, regarding transition services that student may need to prepare for post-school life. An ITP may include planning for employment, post-secondary education, adult services, independent living, and community participation.

Information Processing: The cognitive ability to use and apply the information collected by a person's senses; consists of two important types of processing: auditory processing and visual processing.

Information Processing Disorder: A chronic deficiency in a person's ability to use or organize the data that his or her senses have gathered.

Insertions: The addition of letters or numbers that do not belong in a word or numeral (involved in spelling, reading and mathematics).

Inversions: The confusion of directionality (usually up and down) of letters or numbers, e.g., 9 and 6.

Itinerant Teacher: A Special Education Teacher who is shared by multiple schools or school systems.

Kinesthetic: Pertaining to the muscles.

Kinesthetic Method: A teaching technique that uses muscle control in learning words, e.g., finger-tracing written characters while reciting the letters or sounds which correspond to the characters.

Laterality: The preference for, or tendency to use, the hand, foot, eye and ear on a particular side of the body.

LD: Learning disabilities; learning disabled.

LDA: Learning Disabilities Association of America.

LEA: Local education agency.

Learned Helplessness: A tendency to be a passive learner who depends on others for decisions and guidance. In individuals with LD, continued struggle and failure can heighten this lack of self-confidence.

Learning Disability (LD): A neurological disorder that affects the brain's ability to receive, process, store and respond to information. The term learning disability is used to describe the seeming unexplained difficulty a person of at least average intelligence has in acquiring basic academic skills.

Learning Modalities: Approaches to assessment or instruction stressing the auditory, visual, or tactile avenues for learning that are dependent upon the individual.

Learning Strategy Approaches: Instructional approaches that focus on efficient ways to learn, rather than on curriculum. Includes specific techniques for organizing, actively interacting with material, memorizing, and monitoring any content or subject.

Learning Styles: The ways in which a person best understands and retains learning, e.g., vision, hearing, movement, kinesthetic, or a combination. Learning style-specific approaches to assessment or instruction emphasize the variations in temperament, attitude, and preferred manner of tackling a task. Typically considered are styles along the active/passive, reflective/impulsive, or verbal/spatial dimensions.

LEP: Limited English proficiency.

Licensed Clinical Psychologist: A specialist who applies the principles and methods of psychological evaluation and psychotherapy to individuals with the intent of counteracting problematic behavior and/or emotional adjustment problems.

Licensed Clinical Social Worker: A social worker who is qualified professionally, by education and experience, to provide direct diagnostic, preventative and treatment services in situations where an individual's ability to function is threatened or adversely affected by social and/or psychological stress or damage to his or her health.

Licensed Professional Counselor: A person trained in guidance and counseling services, with emphasis on both the individual and group forums of counseling, who helps individuals to achieve more effective personal, social, educational, and career-related development and adjustment.

Linguistic Approach: A method for teaching reading which emphasizes the use of word families, e.g., once an individual has learned the word "it," the words "sit," "pit," "bit," and "fit" are introduced.

Locus of Control: The tendency to attribute success and difficulties either to internal factors such as effort or to external factors such as chance. Individuals with learning disabilities tend to blame failure on themselves and achievement on luck, leading to frustration and passivity.

LRE: Least restrictive environment. According to the Individuals with Disabilities Education Act, keeping a child in general education classrooms with children in his or her grade and age group is a priority. If appropriate, it is preferable for a child to be in a regular class with in-class services and accommodations than in a separate special education class.

Mainstreaming: The practice of placing a child who has special education needs into general education classrooms, for at least part of the child's educational program.

Maturation Lag: A delay in development in one or more areas of skill or ability.

MBD: Minimal brain dysfunction.

Metacognitive Learning: Instructional approaches emphasizing awareness of the cognitive processes that facilitate one's own learning and its application to academic and work assignments. Typical metacognitive techniques include systematic rehearsal of steps or conscious selection among strategies for completing a task.

Milieu Therapy: A clinical method developed to regulate a child's environment, and to minimize conflicting and/or confusing information.

Minimal Brain Dysfunction (MBD): A medical and psychological term originally used to refer to the learning difficulties that seemed to result from identified or presumed damage to the brain. Reflects a medical, rather than educational or vocational orientation.

MIS: Management information systems.

Mixed Laterality (Lateral Confusion): The tendency to perform some acts with preference for a person's right side and others with a left side preference, or the shifting from right to left (or vice versa) for certain activities.

Modality: The sensory channel used to collect information; the most common modalities are visual, auditory, olfactory, gustatory, tactile, and kinesthetic.

Modified Self-Contained: Refers to a type of education in which a student is instructed in a self-contained environment for most of the school day, but also receives instruction from a general education teacher for some part of the school day.

Multi-Categorical: A classroom model for special education in which students with more than one handicapping condition are assigned to a special education instructor.

Multi-Disciplinary Team (MDT): A group of educators and education specialists that evaluates a child's handicap and prepares an Individualized Education Plan (IEP) based on their evaluation.

Multisensory Learning: An instructional approach that combines auditory, visual, and tactile elements into a learning task. Tracing sandpaper numbers while saying a number fact aloud would be a multisensory learning activity.

NCLB (NCLBA): No Child Left Behind Act.

NCLD: National Center for Learning Disabilities.

NEA: National Education Association.

Near Point Copying: Reproducing, in writing, a copy of a model situated close at hand (e.g., a phrase in a notebook).

Neurological Examination: A test of the sensory or motor responses, designed to determine if there is impairment of the nervous system.

Neuropsychological Examination: A series of tasks that allow observation of performance that is presumed to be related to the intactness of brain function.

Norm-Referenced Test: *See* Standardized Test.

Norms: Statistics providing a frame of reference that gives meaning to test scores; these statistics are based upon the performance of students of various ages or grades in the standardization group for the test, and therefore represent average or predictable performance, not standard or desirable achievement levels.

OCR: Office of Civil Rights, US Department of Health and Human Services.

Oral Language: Verbal communication skills necessary for understanding and using language, such as listening and speaking.

Organicity: Brain damage or a disorder of the central nervous system.

Orton Dyslexia Society: An organization comprised of learning disabilities professionals, as well as specialists, scientists, and parents.

Orton-Gillingham Approach: A technique for teaching individuals with learning disabilities which stresses a multi-sensory, phonetic, sequential, structured approach to learning.

OSEP: Office of Special Education Programs, US Department of Education.

OSERS: Office of Special Education and Rehabilitative Services, US Department of Education.

Perceptual Ability: A function of the brain that supplies an individual with the abilities to process, organize, and interpret information supplied through the senses.

Perceptual Handicap: Difficulty in accurately processing, organizing, interpreting, and discriminating among visual, auditory, or tactile information. A person with a perceptual handicap may not be able to distinguish between sounds or words (e.g., "map" and "mop"), or between visual symbols (e.g., the letters "b" and "d") However, eyeglasses or hearing aids do not necessarily indicate a perceptual handicap.

Perceptual Speed: The rapidity with which an individual can perceive and complete a given task, e.g., motor speed or visual discrimination.

Perceptual-Motor: The muscle activity that results from information obtained through the senses.

Perseveration: The repetition of words, movements, or tasks, often characterized by difficulty shifting to a new task; a student may continue working on a certain task long after his or her peers have moved onto a new one.

Phonics Approach: A method for teaching spelling and reading that emphasizes the importance of learning the sounds made by individual and various combinations of letters within a word, and then sequentially blending the discrete sounds to form the word.

Pre-K: Pre-kindergarten.

Pre-Referral Process: A procedure in which special and regular teachers develop trial strategies to help a student showing difficulty in learning remain in the regular classroom.

Psychiatrist: A licensed medical doctor who treats emotional and/or behavioral problems, and is qualified to use or prescribe medications for the purposes of treatment.

Psychological Examination: The evaluation of an individual's intellectual and behavioral characteristics made by a clinical psychologist or a certified school psychologist.

Psychomotor: Relating to the motor effects of psychological procedures. Psychomotor tests are used to assess motor skills that depend upon sensory or perceptual motor coordination.

Reasoning Ability: Refers to nonverbal, deductive, inductive, and analytical thinking, depending upon the way in which a given test measures this skill.

Receptive Language (Decoding): Language that is written or spoken by others and received by an individual; the skills necessary for receptive language are listening and reading.

Regular Education (General Education): All education not considered Special Education.

REI: Regular Education Initiative.

Remediation: The process by which an individual is given instruction and practice in skills which are lacking or nonexistent, helping to strengthen, develop, and improve these skills.

Resource Program: A program model in which a student is in a regular classroom for most of each day, but also receives regularly scheduled individual services in a specialized resource classroom.

Resource Teacher: A specialist who works with special education students and who often acts as a consultant for regular teachers. *See also* Transposition.

Reversals: A difficulty in reading or reproducing words in sentences, letters within words, or individual letters in their proper spatial position or proper order; also refers to the reversal of mathematical concepts and symbols.

School Psychologist: A specialist who works with individuals experiencing problems associated with educational systems and who uses psychological concepts and methods to develop programs in an effort to improve learning conditions for those individuals.

SEA: State education agency.

Section 504: A part of the Rehabilitation Act of 1973, a civil rights law, making it illegal for any organization receiving federal funds to discriminate against a person solely on the basis of disability.

Self-Advocacy: The development of specific skills and understandings that enable children and adults to explain their specific learning disabilities to others and cope positively with the attitudes of peers, parents, teachers, and employers.

Self-Contained Classroom: A setting designed specifically for special education students who spend all or most of the school day in this environment.

Semantics: Meaning or understanding evinced through oral or written language by virtue of its specific structure and the relationships between its components.

Sensorimotor (Sensory-Motor): The relationship between movement and sensation.

Sensory Acuity: The ability to react to sensation at appropriate levels of intensity.

Sequence: The detail of information in its customary order (e.g., days of the week).

Sight Word Approach (Whole Word Approach): A method for teaching reading which is based on an individual's visual memory skills rather than on phonics, emphasizing the ability to memorize and recognize a word based on its visual configuration.

Slingerland Method: Developed by Beth Slingerland, a method of teaching which is highly structured and multi-sensory, designed for group instruction of individuals with learning disabilities.

Soft Neurological Signs: Abnormalities of the brain which are mild or slight and thus hard to detect, as opposed to gross, or more obvious, neurological irregularities.

Sound Blending: The ability to unite the sounds or parts of a word into an uninterrupted whole.

Spatial Orientation: A person's awareness of the space around him or her, taking into account distance, form, position and direction.

Spatial Relationships: The positioning of objects in space in relation to the person observing them, taking into account physical distance, as well as the relationship of objects and characters described in written or spoken narrative.

SPD: Semantic pragmatic disorder.

Special Education: A form of instruction developed specifically for handicapped (including learning disabled) students.

Specific Learning Disability (SLD): The official term used in federal legislation to refer to difficulty in certain areas of learning. Synonymous with learning disability.

Standardized Test (Norm-Referenced Test): A test comparing an individual's performance with the performance of a large group of similar individuals (usually of the same age), e.g., IQ tests and most achievement tests.

Substitution: The interchanging of a given letter, number, or word for another in spelling, reading, or mathematics.

Subtype Research: A recently developed research method that seeks to identify characteristics that are common to specific groups within the larger population of individuals identified as having learning disabilities.

Task Analysis: The careful examination of a specific task in order to recognize its elements and the processes needed to complete it.

Thematic Maturity: The ability to write in an organized and logical way so as to effectively and easily express meaning.

Transition: Often refers to the change from secondary school to post-secondary programs, work, and independent living typical of young adults. Also used to describe other periods of major change, e.g., from a specialized setting to a mainstreamed setting.

Transposition: The confusion or reversal of the order of letters within a word, or numbers within a numeral. *See also* Reversals.

VAK Approach: A method of teaching which employs visual, auditory, kinesthetic and tactile abilities, emphasizing a multi-sensory approach to learning skills and/or concepts.

Verbal Ability: Generally relates to a person's skill in creating oral or spoken language, depending on the way in which the skill is tested.

Visual Association: The ability to relate visually presented concepts and formulate thematic comparisons.

Visual Closure: The ability to recognize an object when only parts of it are visible.

Visual Discrimination: The ability to use the sense of sight to detect differences and similarities in visually presented items to differentiate one item from another.

Visual Figure-Ground Discrimination: The ability to distinguish a shape or printed character from its background.

Visual Memory: The ability to remember something seen some time in the past (long-term visual memory); the ability to recall something seen very recently (short-term visual memory).

Visual Motor Processing: The ability to use visual observation to coordinate and appropriately apply other motor skills.

Visual Perception: The ability to see and interpret material correctly.

Visual Sequencing: The ability to see and recognize the order of words, symbols, images or other visual objects.

WISC-III: *Weschler Intelligence Scale for Children-Third Edition.* An assessment used to measure a child's intellectual ability.

WISC-R: *Weschler Intelligence Scale for Children-Revised.* An assessment used to measure a child's intellectual ability.

Word Recognition: The ability to perceive, pronounce, or read a word; usually this term is used to indicate a word which is immediately identifiable by sight and does not require the use of word-attack or analysis skills. (NB: Word Recognition does not necessarily indicate understanding of the word.)

Word-Attack Skills: The methods of examining an unfamiliar word by using a phonetic, sight word, or other visual approach in an effort to understand the word.

Written Language: All aspects of written expression, including spelling, grammar, punctuation, capitalization, penmanship, and ability to translate thoughts into words.

Sedgwick Press
Education Directories

The Comparative Guide to American Elementary & Secondary Schools, 2008

The only guide of its kind, this award winning compilation offers a snapshot profile of every public school district in the United States serving 1,500 or more students – more than 5,900 districts are covered. Organized alphabetically by district within state, each chapter begins with a Statistical Overview of the state. Each district listing includes contact information (name, address, phone number and web site) plus Grades Served, the Numbers of Students and Teachers and the Number of Regular, Special Education, Alternative and Vocational Schools in the district along with statistics on Student/Classroom Teacher Ratios, Drop Out Rates, Ethnicity, the Number of Librarians and Guidance Counselors and District Expenditures per student. As an added bonus, *The Comparative Guide to American Elementary and Secondary Schools* provides important ranking tables, both by state and nationally, for each data element. For easy navigation through this wealth of information, this handbook contains a useful City Index that lists all districts that operate schools within a city. These important comparative statistics are necessary for anyone considering relocation or doing comparative research on their own district and would be a perfect acquisition for any public library or school district library.

"This straightforward guide is an easy way to find general information. Valuable for academic and large public library collections." –ARBA

2,400 pages; Softcover ISBN 1-59237-223-6, $125.00

Educators Resource Directory, 2007/08

Educators Resource Directory is a comprehensive resource that provides the educational professional with thousands of resources and statistical data for professional development. This directory saves hours of research time by providing immediate access to Associations & Organizations, Conferences & Trade Shows, Educational Research Centers, Employment Opportunities & Teaching Abroad, School Library Services, Scholarships, Financial Resources, Professional Consultants, Computer Software & Testing Resources and much more. Plus, this comprehensive directory also includes a section on Statistics and Rankings with over 100 tables, including statistics on Average Teacher Salaries, SAT/ACT scores, Revenues & Expenditures and more. These important statistics will allow the user to see how their school rates among others, make relocation decisions and so much more. For quick access to information, this directory contains four indexes: Entry & Publisher Index, Geographic Index, a Subject & Grade Index and Web Sites Index. *Educators Resource Directory* will be a well-used addition to the reference collection of any school district, education department or public library.

"Recommended for all collections that serve elementary and secondary school professionals." –Choice

1,000 pages; Softcover ISBN 1-59237-179-5, $145.00 ♦ Online Database $195.00 ♦ Online Database & Directory Combo $280.00

Sedgwick Press
Health Directories

The Complete Directory for People with Disabilities, 2008

A wealth of information, now in one comprehensive sourcebook. Completely updated, this edition contains more information than ever before, including thousands of new entries and enhancements to existing entries and thousands of additional web sites and e-mail addresses. This up-to-date directory is the most comprehensive resource available for people with disabilities, detailing Independent Living Centers, Rehabilitation Facilities, State & Federal Agencies, Associations, Support Groups, Periodicals & Books, Assistive Devices, Employment & Education Programs, Camps and Travel Groups. Each year, more libraries, schools, colleges, hospitals, rehabilitation centers and individuals add *The Complete Directory for People with Disabilities* to their collections, making sure that this information is readily available to the families, individuals and professionals who can benefit most from the amazing wealth of resources cataloged here.

"No other reference tool exists to meet the special needs of the disabled in one convenient resource for information." –Library Journal

1,200 pages; Softcover ISBN 978-1-59237-194-5, $165.00 ♦ Online Database $215.00 ♦ Online Database & Directory Combo $300.00

The Complete Directory for People with Chronic Illness, 2007/08

Thousands of hours of research have gone into this completely updated 2005/06 edition – several new chapters have been added along with thousands of new entries and enhancements to existing entries. Plus, each chronic illness chapter has been reviewed by an medical expert in the field. This widely-hailed directory is structured around the 90 most prevalent chronic illnesses – from Asthma to Cancer to Wilson's Disease – and provides a comprehensive overview of the support services and information resources available for people diagnosed with a chronic illness. Each chronic illness has its own chapter and contains a brief description in layman's language, followed by important resources for National & Local Organizations, State Agencies, Newsletters, Books & Periodicals, Libraries & Research Centers, Support Groups & Hotlines, Web Sites and much more. This directory is an important resource for health care professionals, the collections of hospital and health care libraries, as well as an invaluable tool for people with a chronic illness and their support network.

"A must purchase for all hospital and health care libraries and is strongly recommended for all public library reference departments." –ARBA

1,200 pages; Softcover ISBN 1-59237-183-3, $165.00 ◆ Online Database $215.00 ◆ Online Database & Directory Combo $300.00

The Complete Mental Health Directory, 2008/09

This is the most comprehensive resource covering the field of behavioral health, with critical information for both the layman and the mental health professional. For the layman, this directory offers understandable descriptions of 25 Mental Health Disorders as well as detailed information on Associations, Media, Support Groups and Mental Health Facilities. For the professional, *The Complete Mental Health Directory* offers critical and comprehensive information on Managed Care Organizations, Information Systems, Government Agencies and Provider Organizations. This comprehensive volume of needed information will be widely used in any reference collection.

"... the strength of this directory is that it consolidates widely dispersed information into a single volume." –Booklist

800 pages; Softcover ISBN 978-1-59237-285-0, $165.00 ◆ Online Database $215.00 ◆ Online & Directory Combo $300.00

Older Americans Information Directory, 2007

Completely updated for 2007, this sixth edition has been completely revised and now contains 1,000 new listings, over 8,000 updates to existing listings and over 3,000 brand new e-mail addresses and web sites. You'll find important resources for Older Americans including National, Regional, State & Local Organizations, Government Agencies, Research Centers, Libraries & Information Centers, Legal Resources, Discount Travel Information, Continuing Education Programs, Disability Aids & Assistive Devices, Health, Print Media and Electronic Media. Three indexes: Entry Index, Subject Index and Geographic Index make it easy to find just the right source of information. This comprehensive guide to resources for Older Americans will be a welcome addition to any reference collection.

"Highly recommended for academic, public, health science and consumer libraries..." –Choice

1,200 pages; Softcover ISBN 1-59237-136-1, $165.00 ◆ Online Database $215.00 ◆ Online Database & Directory Combo $300.00

The Complete Directory for Pediatric Disorders, 2008

This important directory provides parents and caregivers with information about Pediatric Conditions, Disorders, Diseases and Disabilities, including Blood Disorders, Bone & Spinal Disorders, Brain Defects & Abnormalities, Chromosomal Disorders, Congenital Heart Defects, Movement Disorders, Neuromuscular Disorders and Pediatric Tumors & Cancers. This carefully written directory offers: understandable Descriptions of 15 major bodily systems; Descriptions of more than 200 Disorders and a Resources Section, detailing National Agencies & Associations, State Associations, Online Services, Libraries & Resource Centers, Research Centers, Support Groups & Hotlines, Camps, Books and Periodicals. This resource will provide immediate access to information crucial to families and caregivers when coping with children's illnesses.

"Recommended for public and consumer health libraries." –Library Journal

1,200 pages; Softcover ISBN 1-59237-150-7 $165.00 ◆ Online Database $215.00 ◆ Online Database & Directory Combo $300.00

Sedgwick Press
Hospital & Health Plan Directories

The Comparative Guide to American Hospitals, Second Edition

This new second edition compares all of the nation's hospitals by 24 measures of quality in the treatment of heart attack, heart failure, pneumonia, and, new to this edition, surgical procedures and pregnancy care. Plus, this second edition is now available in regional volumes, to make locating information about hospitals in your area quicker and easier than ever before. The Comparative Guide to American Hospitals provides a snapshot profile of each of the nations 4,200+ hospitals. These informative profiles illustrate how the hospital rates when providing 24 different treatments within four broad categories: Heart Attack Care , Heart Failure Care, Surgical Infection Prevention (NEW), and Pregnancy Care measures (NEW). Each profile includes the raw percentage for that hospital, the state average, the US average and data on the top hospital. For easy access to contact information, each profile includes the hospital's address, phone and fax numbers, email and web addresses, type and accreditation along with 5 top key administrations. These profiles will allow the user to quickly identify the quality of the hospital and have the necessary information at their fingertips to make contact with that hospital. Most importantly, *The Comparative Guide to American Hospitals* provides easy-to-use Regional State by State Statistical Summary Tables for each of the data elements to allow the user to quickly locate hospitals with the best level of service. Plus, a new 30-Day Mortality Chart, Glossary of Terms and Regional Hospital Profile Index make this a must-have source. This new expanded edition will be a must for the reference collection at all public, medical and academic libraries.

"These data will help those with heart conditions and pneumonia make informed decisions about th healthcare and encourage hospitals to improve the quality of care they provide. Large medical, hospital, and public libraries a most likely to benefit from this weighty resource."-Library Journ

3,500 pages, Four Volume Set, Softcover ISBN 978-1-59237-182-2 $325

The Directory of Hospital Personnel, 2008

The Directory of Hospital Personnel is the best resource you can have at your fingertips when researching or marketing a product or service to the hospital market. A "Who's Who" of the hospital universe, this directory puts you in touch with over 150,000 key decision-makers. With 100% verification of data you can rest assured that you will reach the right person with just one call. Every hospital in the U.S. is profiled, listed alphabetically by city within state. Plus, three easy-to-use, cross-referenced indexes put the facts at your fingertips faster and more easily than any other directory: Hospital Name Index, Bed Size Index and Personnel Index. *The Directory of Hospital Personnel* is the only complete source for key hospital decision-makers by name. Whether you want to define or restructure sales territories... locate hospitals with the purchasing power to accept your proposals... keep track of important contacts or colleagues... or find information on which insurance plans are accepted, *The Directory of Hospital Personnel* gives you the informatio you need – easily, efficiently, effectively and accurately.

"Recommended for college, university and medical libraries." -ARE

2,500 pages; Softcover ISBN 978-1-59237-286-7 $325.00 ▯ Online Database $545.00 ▯ Online Database & Directory Combo, $650.00

The Directory of Health Care Group Purchasing Organizations, 2008

This comprehensive directory provides the important data you need to get in touch with over 800 Group Purchasing Organizations. By providing in-depth information on this growing market and its members, *The Directory of Health Care Group Purchasing Organizatio* fills a major need for the most accurate and comprehensive information on over 800 GPOs – Mailing Address, Phone & Fax Numbers, E-mail Addresses, Key Contacts, Purchasing Agents, Group Descriptions, Membership Categorization, Standard Vendor Proposal Requirements, Membership Fees & Terms, Expanded Services, Total Member Beds & Outpatient Visits represented and more. Five Indexes provide a number of ways to locate the right GPO: Alphabetical Index, Expanded Services Index, Organization Type Index, Geographic Index and Member Institution Index. With its comprehensive and detailed information on each purchasing organization, *The Directory of Health Care Group Purchasing Organizations* is the go-to source for anyone looking to target this market.

"The information is clearly arranged and easy to access...recommended for those needing this very specialized information." –ARE

1,000 pages; Softcover ISBN 978-1-59237-287-4, $325.00 ▯ Online Database, $650.00 ▯ Online Database & Directory Combo, $750.0C

To preview any of our Directories Risk-Free for 30 days, call (800) 562-2139 or fax to (518) 789-0556

The HMO/PPO Directory, 2008

The HMO/PPO Directory is a comprehensive source that provides detailed information about Health Maintenance Organizations and Preferred Provider Organizations nationwide. This comprehensive directory details more information about more managed health care organizations than ever before. Over 1,100 HMOs, PPOs, Medicare Advantage Plans and affiliated companies are listed, arranged alphabetically by state. Detailed listings include Key Contact Information, Prescription Drug Benefits, Enrollment, Geographical Areas served, Affiliated Physicians & Hospitals, Federal Qualifications, Status, Year Founded, Managed Care Partners, Employer References, Fees & Payment Information and more. Plus, five years of historical information is included related to Revenues, Net Income, Medical Loss Ratios, Membership Enrollment and Number of Patient Complaints. Five easy-to-use, cross-referenced indexes will put this vast array of information at your fingertips immediately: HMO Index, PPO Index, Other Providers Index, Personnel Index and Enrollment Index. *The HMO/PPO Directory* provides the most comprehensive data on the most companies available on the market place today.

"Helpful to individuals requesting certain HMO/PPO issues such as co-payment costs, subscription costs and patient complaints. Individuals concerned (or those with questions) about their insurance may find this text to be of use to them." -ARBA

600 pages; Softcover ISBN 978-1-59237-204-1, $325.00 ▯ Online Database, $495.00 ▯ Online Database & Directory Combo, $600.00

Medical Device Register, 2008

The only one-stop resource of every medical supplier licensed to sell products in the US. This award-winning directory offers immediate access to over 13,000 companies - and more than 65,000 products – in two information-packed volumes. This comprehensive resource saves hours of time and trouble when searching for medical equipment and supplies and the manufacturers who provide them. Volume I: The Product Directory, provides essential information for purchasing or specifying medical supplies for every medical device, supply, and diagnostic available in the US. Listings provide FDA codes & Federal Procurement Eligibility, Contact information for every manufacturer of the product along with Prices and Product Specifications. Volume 2 - Supplier Profiles, offers the most complete and important data about Suppliers, Manufacturers and Distributors. Company Profiles detail the number of employees, ownership, method of distribution, sales volume, net income, key executives detailed contact information medical products the company supplies, plus the medical specialties they cover. Four indexes provide immediate access to this wealth of information: Keyword Index, Trade Name Index, Supplier Geographical Index and OEM (Original Equipment Manufacturer) Index. Medical Device Register, 2007 is the only one-stop source for locating suppliers and products; looking for new manufacturers or hard-to-find medical devices; comparing products and companies; know who's selling what and who to buy from cost effectively. This directory has become the standard in its field and will be a welcome addition to the reference collection of any medical library, large public library, university library along with the collections that serve the medical community.

"A wealth of information on medical devices, medical device companies and key personnel in the industry is provide in this comprehensive reference work... A valuable reference work, one of the best hardcopy compilations available." -Doody Publishing

3,000 pages Two Volumes; Hardcover ISBN 978-1-59237-206-5; $325.00

The Directory of Independent Ambulatory Care Centers

This first edition of *The Directory of Independent Ambulatory Care Centers* provides access to detailed information that, before now, could only be found scattered in hundreds of different sources. This comprehensive and up-to-date directory pulls together a vast array of contact information for over 7,200 Ambulatory Surgery Centers, Ambulatory General and Urgent Care Clinics, and Diagnostic Imaging Centers that are not affiliated with a hospital or major medical center. Detailed listings include Mailing Address, Phone & Fax Numbers, E-mail and Web Site addresses, Contact Name and Phone Numbers of the Medical Director and other Key Executives and Purchasing Agents, Specialties & Services Offered, Year Founded, Numbers of Employees and Surgeons, Number of Operating Rooms, Number of Cases seen per year, Overnight Options, Contracted Services and much more. Listings are arranged by State, by Center Category and then alphabetically by Organization Name. Two indexes provide quick and easy access to this wealth of information: Entry Name Index and Specialty/Service Index. *The Directory of Independent Ambulatory Care Centers* is a must-have resource for anyone marketing a product or service to this important industry and will be an invaluable tool for those searching for a local care center that will meet their specific needs.

"Among the numerous hospital directories, no other provides information on independent ambulatory centers. A handy, well-organized resource that would be useful in medical center libraries and public libraries." –Choice

986 pages; Softcover ISBN 1-930956-90-8, $185.00 ▯ Online Database, $365.00 ▯ Online Database & Directory Combo, $450.00

Grey House Publishing
Business Directories

The Directory of Business Information Resources, 2008

With 100% verification, over 1,000 new listings and more than 12,000 updates, *The Directory of Business Information Resources* is the mo up-to-date source for contacts in over 98 business areas – from advertising and agriculture to utilities and wholesalers. This carefully researched volume details: the Associations representing each industry; the Newsletters that keep members current; the Magazines an Journals - with their "Special Issues" - that are important to the trade, the Conventions that are "must attends," Databases, Directories and Industry Web Sites that provide access to must-have marketing resources. Includes contact names, phone & fax numbers, web sit and e-mail addresses. This one-volume resource is a gold mine of information and would be a welcome addition to any reference collection.

"This is a most useful and easy-to-use addition to any researcher's library." –*The Information Professionals Instit*

2,500 pages; Softcover ISBN 978-1-59237-193-8, $195.00 ▯ Online Database $495.00

Nations of the World, 2007/08 A Political, Economic and Business Handbook

This completely revised edition covers all the nations of the world in an easy-to-use, single volume. Each nation is profiled in a single chapter that includes Key Facts, Political & Economic Issues, a Country Profile and Business Information. In this fast-changing world it is extremely important to make sure that the most up-to-date information is included in your reference collection. This edition is ju the answer. Each of the 200+ country chapters have been carefully reviewed by a political expert to make sure that the text reflects th most current information on Politics, Travel Advisories, Economics and more. You'll find such vital information as a Country Map, Population Characteristics, Inflation, Agricultural Production, Foreign Debt, Political History, Foreign Policy, Regional Insecurity, Economics, Trade & Tourism, Historical Profile, Political Systems, Ethnicity, Languages, Media, Climate, Hotels, Chambers of Commerce, Banking, Travel Information and more. Five Regional Chapters follow the main text and include a Regional Map, an Introductory Article, Key Indicators and Currencies for the Region. As an added bonus, an all-inclusive CD-ROM is available as a companion to the printed text. Noted for its sophisticated, up-to-date and reliable compilation of political, economic and business information, this brand new edition will be an important acquisition to any public, academic or special library reference collection.

"A useful addition to both general reference collections and business collections." –*RUS*

1,700 pages; Print Version Only Softcover ISBN 1-59237-177-9, $155.00

The Directory of Venture Capital & Private Equity Firms, 2008

This edition has been extensively updated and broadly expanded to offer direct access to over 2,800 Domestic and International Venture Capital Firms, including address, phone & fax numbers, e-mail addresses and web sites for both primary and branch locations. Entries include details on the firm's Mission Statement, Industry Group Preferences, Geographic Preferences, Average and Minimum Investments and Investment Criteria. You'll also find details that are available nowhere else, including the Firm's Portfolio Companie and extensive information on each of the firm's Managing Partners, such as Education, Professional Background and Directorships held, along with the Partner's E-mail Address. *The Directory of Venture Capital & Private Equity Firms* offers five important indexes: Geographic Index, Executive Name Index, Portfolio Company Index, Industry Preference Index and College & University Index. With its comprehensive coverage and detailed, extensive information on each company, *The Directory of Venture Capital & Private Equi Firms* is an important addition to any finance collection.

"The sheer number of listings, the descriptive information provided and the outstanding indexing make this directory a better value than its princip competitor, Pratt's Guide to Venture Capital Sources. Recommended for business collections in large public, academic and business libraries." –*Cho*

1,300 pages; Softcover ISBN 978-1-59237-272-0, $565/$450 Library ▯ Online Database (includes a free copy of the directory) $889.00

To preview any of our Directories Risk-Free for 30 days, call (800) 562-2139 or fax to (518) 789-0556

The Encyclopedia of Emerging Industries

*Published under an exclusive license from the Gale Group, Inc.

The fifth edition of the Encyclopedia of Emerging Industries details the inception, emergence, and current status of nearly 120 flourishing U.S. industries and industry segments. These focused essays unearth for users a wealth of relevant, current, factual data previously accessible only through a diverse variety of sources. This volume provides broad-based, highly-readable, industry information under such headings as Industry Snapshot, Organization & Structure, Background & Development, Industry Leaders, Current Conditions, America and the World, Pioneers, and Research & Technology. Essays in this new edition, arranged alphabetically for easy use, have been completely revised, with updated statistics and the most current information on industry trends and developments. In addition, there are new essays on some of the most interesting and influential new business fields, including Application Service Providers, Concierge Services, Entrepreneurial Training, Fuel Cells, Logistics Outsourcing Services, Pharmacogenomics, and Tissue Engineering. Two indexes, General and Industry, provide immediate access to this wealth of information. Plus, two conversion tables for SIC and NAICS codes, along with Suggested Further Readings, are provided to aid the user. The Encyclopedia of Emerging Industries pinpoints emerging industries while they are still in the spotlight. This important resource will be an important acquisition to any business reference collection.

"This well-designed source...should become another standard business source, nicely complementing Standard & Poor's Industry Surveys. It contains more information on each industry than Hoover's Handbook of Emerging Companies, is broader in scope than The Almanac of American Employers 1998-1999, but is less expansive than the Encyclopedia of Careers & Vocational Guidance. Highly recommended for all academic libraries and specialized business collections." –Library Journal

Fourth Edition/ 1,400 pages / Hardcover ISBN 978-1-59237-242-3/ $325.00

Encyclopedia of American Industries

*Published under an exclusive license from the Gale Group, Inc.

The Encyclopedia of American Industries is a major business reference tool that provides detailed, comprehensive information on a wide range of industries in every realm of American business. A two volume set, Volume I provides separate coverage of nearly 500 manufacturing industries, while Volume II presents nearly 600 essays covering the vast array of services and other non-manufacturing industries in the United States. Combined, these two volumes provide individual essays on every industry recognized by the U.S. Standard Industrial Classification (SIC) system. Both volumes are arranged numerically by SIC code, for easy use. Additionally, each entry includes the corresponding NAICS code(s). The Encyclopedia's business coverage includes information on historical events of consequence, as well as current trends and statistics. Essays include an Industry Snapshot, Organization & Structure, Background & Development, Current Conditions, Industry Leaders, Workforce, America and the World, Research & Technology along with Suggested Further Readings. Both SIC and NAICS code conversion tables and an all-encompassing Subject Index, with cross-references, complete the text. With its detailed, comprehensive information on a wide range of industries, this resource will be an important tool for both the industry newcomer and the seasoned professional.

"Encyclopedia of American Industries contains detailed, signed essays on virtually every industry in contemporary society. ... Highly recommended for all but the smallest libraries." -American Reference Books Annual

Fifth Edition; 3,000 pages / Two Volumes / Hardcover ISBN 978-1-59237-244-7/ $650.00

Encyclopedia of Global Industries

*Published under an exclusive license from the Gale Group, Inc.

This fourth edition of the acclaimed Encyclopedia of Global Industries presents a thoroughly revised and expanded look at more than 125 business sectors of global significance. Detailed, insightful articles discuss the origins, development, trends, key statistics and current international character of the world's most lucrative, dynamic and widely researched industries – including hundreds of profile of leading international corporations. Beginning researchers will gain from this book a solid understanding of how each industry operates and which countries and companies are significant participants, while experienced researchers will glean current and historica figures for comparison and analysis. The industries profiled in previous editions have been updated, and in some cases, expanded to reflect recent industry trends. Additionally, this edition provides both SIC and NAICS codes for all industries profiled. As in the original volumes, The Encyclopedia of Global Industries offers thorough studies of some of the biggest and most frequently researche industry sectors, including Aircraft, Biotechnology, Computers, Internet Services, Motor Vehicles, Pharmaceuticals, Semiconductors, Software and Telecommunications. An SIC and NAICS conversion table and an all-encompassing Subject Index, with cross-references are provided to ensure easy access to this wealth of information. These and many others make the Encyclopedia of Global Industries th authoritative reference for studies of international industries.

"Provides detailed coverage of the history, development, and current status of 115 of "the world's most lucrative and high-profile industries." It f surpasses the Department of Commerce's U.S. Global Trade Outlook 1995-2000 (GPO, 1995) in scope and coverage. Recommended f comprehensive public and academic library business collections." -Bookl

Fourth Edition; 1,400 pages / Hardcover ISBN 978-1-59237-243-0/ $495.00

The Directory of Mail Order Catalogs, 2008

Published since 1981, the *Directory of Mail Order Catalogs* is the premier source of information on the mail order catalog industry. It is the source that business professionals and librarians have come to rely on for the thousands of catalog companies in the US. Since the 2007 edition, *The Directory of Mail Order Catalogs* has been combined with its companion volume, *The Directory of Business to Business Catalogs,* to offer all 13,000 catalog companies in one easy-to-use volume. Section I: Consumer Catalogs, covers over 9,000 consumer catalog companies in 44 different product chapters from Animals to Toys & Games. Section II: Business to Business Catalogs, details 5,000 business catalogs, everything from computers to laboratory supplies, building construction and much more. Listings contain detailed contact information including mailing address, phone & fax numbers, web sites, e-mail addresses and key contacts along with important business details such as product descriptions, employee size, years in business, sales volume, catalog size, number of catalogs mailed and more. Three indexes are included for easy access to information: Catalog & Company Name Index, Geographic Index and Product Index. *The Directory of Mail Order Catalogs,* now with its expanded business to business catalogs, is the largest and most comprehensive resource covering this billion-dollar industry. It is the standard in its field. This important resource is a useful tool for entrepreneurs searching for catalogs to pick up their product, vendors looking to expand their customer base in the catalog industry, market researchers, small businesses investigating new supply vendors, along with the library patron who is exploring the available catalogs in their areas of interest.

"This is a godsend for those looking for information." –Reference Book Revie

1,700 pages; Softcover ISBN 978-1-59237-202-7 $350/$250 Library ▯ Online Database (includes a free copy of the directory) $495.00

Sports Market Place Directory, 2007

For over 20 years, this comprehensive, up-to-date directory has offered direct access to the Who, What, When & Where of the Sports Industry. With over 20,000 updates and enhancements, the *Sports Market Place Directory* is the most detailed, comprehensive and current sports business reference source available. In 1,800 information-packed pages, *Sports Market Place Directory* profiles contact information and key executives for: Single Sport Organizations, Professional Leagues, Multi-Sport Organizations, Disabled Sports, High School & Youth Sports, Military Sports, Olympic Organizations, Media, Sponsors, Sponsorship & Marketing Event Agencies, Event & Meeting Calendars, Professional Services, College Sports, Manufacturers & Retailers, Facilities and much more. *The Sports Market Place Directory* provides organization's contact information with detailed descriptions including: Key Contacts, physical, mailing, email and web addresses plus phone and fax numbers. Plus, nine important indexes make sure that you can find the information you're looking for quickly and easily: Entry Index, Single Sport Index, Media Index, Sponsor Index, Agency Index, Manufacturers Index, Brand Name Index, Facilities Index and Executive/Geographic Index. For over twenty years, *The Sports Market Place Directory* has assisted thousands of individuals in their pursuit of a career in the sports industry. Why not use "THE SOURCE" that top recruiters, headhunters and career placement centers use to find information on or about sports organizations and key hiring contacts.

1,800 pages; Softcover ISBN 1-59237-189-2, $225.00 ▯ Online Database $479.00

Food and Beverage Market Place, 2008

Food and Beverage Market Place is bigger and better than ever with thousands of new companies, thousands of updates to existing companies and two revised and enhanced product category indexes. This comprehensive directory profiles over 18,000 Food & Beverage Manufacturers, 12,000 Equipment & Supply Companies, 2,200 Transportation & Warehouse Companies, 2,000 Brokers & Wholesalers, 8,000 Importers & Exporters, 900 Industry Resources and hundreds of Mail Order Catalogs. Listings include detailed Contact Information, Sales Volumes, Key Contacts, Brand & Product Information, Packaging Details and much more. *Thomas Food and Beverage Market Place* is available as a three-volume printed set, a subscription-based Online Database via the Internet, on CD-ROM, as well as mailing lists and a licensable database.

"An essential purchase for those in the food industry but will also be useful in public libraries where needed. Much of the information will be difficult and time consuming to locate without this handy three-volume ready-reference source." –ARBA

8,500 pages, 3 Volume Set; Softcover ISBN 978-1-59237-198-3, $595.00 ▯ Online Database $795.00 ▯ Online Database & 3 Volume Set Combo, $995.00

The Grey House Homeland Security Directory, 2008

This updated edition features the latest contact information for government and private organizations involved with Homeland Security along with the latest product information and provides detailed profiles of nearly 1,000 Federal & State Organizations & Agencies and over 3,000 Officials and Key Executives involved with Homeland Security. These listings are incredibly detailed and include Mailing Address, Phone & Fax Numbers, Email Addresses & Web Sites, a complete Description of the Agency and a complete list of the Officials and Key Executives associated with the Agency. Next, *The Grey House Homeland Security Directory* provides the go-to source for Homeland Security Products & Services. This section features over 2,000 Companies that provide Consulting, Products or Services. With this Buyer's Guide at their fingertips, users can locate suppliers of everything from Training Materials to Access Controls, from Perimeter Security to BioTerrorism Countermeasures and everything in between – complete with contact information and product descriptions. A handy Product Locator Index is provided to quickly and easily locate suppliers of a particular product. Lastly, an Information Resources Section provides immediate access to contact information for hundreds of Associations, Newsletters, Magazines, Trade Shows, Databases and Directories that focus on Homeland Security. This comprehensive, information-packed resource will be a welcome tool for any company or agency that is in need of Homeland Security information and will be a necessary acquisition for the reference collection of all public libraries and large school districts.

"Compiles this information in one place and is discerning in content. A useful purchase for public and academic libraries." –Booklist

800 pages; Softcover ISBN 978-1-59237-196-6, $195.00 ▯ Online Database (includes a free copy of the directory) $385.00

The Grey House Transportation Security Directory & Handbook

This brand new title is the only reference of its kind that brings together current data on Transportation Security. With information on everything from Regulatory Authorities to Security Equipment, this top-flight database brings together the relevant information necessary for creating and maintaining a security plan for a wide range of transportation facilities. With this current, comprehensive directory at the ready you'll have immediate access to: Regulatory Authorities & Legislation; Information Resources; Sample Security Plans & Checklists; Contact Data for Major Airports, Seaports, Railroads, Trucking Companies and Oil Pipelines; Security Service Providers; Recommended Equipment & Product Information and more. Using the *Grey House Transportation Security Directory & Handbook*, managers will be able to quickly and easily assess their current security plans; develop contacts to create and maintain new security procedures; and source the products and services necessary to adequately maintain a secure environment. This valuable resource is a must for all Security Managers at Airports, Seaports, Railroads, Trucking Companies and Oil Pipelines.

800 pages; Softcover ISBN 1-59237-075-6, $195

The Grey House Safety & Security Directory, 2008

The Grey House Safety & Security Directory is the most comprehensive reference tool and buyer's guide for the safety and security industry. Arranged by safety topic, each chapter begins with OSHA regulations for the topic, followed by Training Articles written b top professionals in the field and Self-Inspection Checklists. Next, each topic contains Buyer's Guide sections that feature related products and services. Topics include Administration, Insurance, Loss Control & Consulting, Protective Equipment & Apparel, Noise Vibration, Facilities Monitoring & Maintenance, Employee Health Maintenance & Ergonomics, Retail Food Services, Machine Guard Process Guidelines & Tool Handling, Ordinary Materials Handling, Hazardous Materials Handling, Workplace Preparation & Maintenance, Electrical Lighting & Safety, Fire & Rescue and Security. The Buyer's Guide sections are carefully indexed within each topic area to ensure that you can find the supplies needed to meet OSHA's regulations. Six important indexes make finding informatic and product manufacturers quick and easy: Geographical Index of Manufacturers and Distributors, Company Profile Index, Brand Name Index, Product Index, Index of Web Sites and Index of Advertisers. This comprehensive, up-to-date reference will provide every tool necessary to make sure a business is in compliance with OSHA regulations and locate the products and services needed to meet those regulations.

"Presents industrial safety information for engineers, plant managers, risk managers, and construction site supervisors…" –Cho

1,500 pages, 2 Volume Set; Softcover ISBN 978-1-59237-205-8, $225.00

The Grey House Biometric Information Directory

The Biometric Information Directory is the only comprehensive source for current biometric industry information. This 2006 edition is tl first published by Grey House. With 100% updated information, this latest edition offers a complete, current look, in both print and online form, of biometric companies and products – one of the fastest growing industries in today's economy. Detailed profiles of manufacturers of the latest biometric technology, including Finger, Voice, Face, Hand, Signature, Iris, Vein and Palm Identification systems. Data on the companies include key executives, company size and a detailed, indexed description of their product line. Plus, the Directory also includes valuable business resources, and current editorial make this edition the easiest way for the business community and consumers alike to access the largest, most current compilation of biometric industry information available on the market today. The new edition boasts increased numbers of companies, contact names and company data, with over 700 manufacturers and service providers. Information in the directory includes: Editorial on Advancements in Biometrics; Profiles of 700+ companies listed with contact information; Organizations, Trade & Educational Associations, Publications, Conferences, Trade Shows and Expositions Worldwide; Web Site Index; Biometric & Vendors Services Index by Types of Biometrics; and a Glossary of Biometric Terms. This resource will be an important source for anyone who is considering the use of a biometric product, investing in the development of biometric technology, support existing marketing and sales efforts and will be an important acquisition for the busines reference collection for large public and business libraries.

800 pages; Softcover ISBN 1-59237-121-3, $225

The Rauch Guide to the US Adhesives & Sealants, Cosmetics & Toiletries, Ink, Paint, Plastics, Pulp & Paper and Rubber Industries

The Rauch Guides are known worldwide for their comprehensive marketing information. Acquired by Grey House Publishing in 2005, new updated and revised editions will be published throughout 2005 and 2006. Each Guide provides market facts and figures in a highly organized format, ideal for today's busy personnel, serving as ready-references for top executives as well as the industry newcomer. *The Rauch Guides* save time and money by organizing widely scattered information and providing estimates for important business decisions, some of which are available nowhere else. Each Guide is organized into several information-packed chapters. After a brief introduction, the ECONOMICS section provides data on industry shipments; long-term growth and forecasts; prices; company performance; employment, expenditures, and productivity; transportation and geographical patterns; packaging; foreign trade and government regulations. Next, TECHNOLOGY & RAW MATERIALS provide market, technical, and raw material information for chemicals, equipment and related materials, including market size and leading suppliers, prices, end uses, and trends. PRODUCTS & MARKETS provide information for each major industry product, including market size and historical trends, leading suppliers, five-year forecasts, industry structure, and major end uses. For easy access, each *Guide* contains a chapter on INDUSTRY ACTIVITIES, ORGANIZATIONS & SOURCES OF INFORMATION with detailed information on meetings, exhibits, and trade shows, sources of statistical information, trade associations, technical and professional societies, and trade and technical periodicals. Next, the COMPANY DIRECTORY profiles major industry companies, both public and private. Information includes complete contact information, web address, estimated total and domestic sales, product description, and recent mergers and acquisitions. Each Guide also contains several APPENDICES that provide a cross-reference of suppliers, subsidiaries and divisions. The Rauch Guides will prove to be an invaluable source of market information, company data, trends and forecasts that anyone in these fast-paced industries.

The Rauch Guide to the U.S. Paint Industry Softcover ISBN 1-59237-127-2 $595 ♦ The Rauch Guide to the U.S. Plastics Industry Softcover ISBN 1-59237-128-0 $595 ♦ The Rauch Guide to the U.S. Adhesives and Sealants Industry Softcover ISBN 1-59237-129-9 $595 ♦ The Rauch Guide to the U.S. Ink Industry Softcover ISBN 1-59237-126-4 $595 ♦ The Rauch Guide to the U.S. Rubber Industr Softcover ISBN 1-59237-130-2 $595 ♦ The Rauch Guide to the U.S. Pulp and Paper Industry Softcover ISBN 1-59237-131-0 $595 ♦ The Rauch Guide to the U.S. Cosmetic and Toiletries Industry Softcover ISBN 1-59237-132-9 $895

The Grey House Performing Arts Directory, 2007

The Grey House Performing Arts Directory is the most comprehensive resource covering the Performing Arts. This important directory provides current information on over 8,500 Dance Companies, Instrumental Music Programs, Opera Companies, Choral Groups, Theater Companies, Performing Arts Series and Performing Arts Facilities. Plus, this edition now contains a brand new section on Artist Management Groups. In addition to mailing address, phone & fax numbers, e-mail addresses and web sites, dozens of other fields of available information include mission statement, key contacts, facilities, seating capacity, season, attendance and more. This directory also provides an important Information Resources section that covers hundreds of Performing Arts Associations, Magazines, Newsletters, Trade Shows, Directories, Databases and Industry Web Sites. Five indexes provide immediate access to this wealth of information: Entry Name, Executive Name, Performance Facilities, Geographic and Information Resources. *The Grey House Performing Arts Directory* pulls together thousands of Performing Arts Organizations, Facilities and Information Resources into an easy-to-use source – this kind of comprehensiveness and extensive detail is not available in any resource on the market place today.

"Immensely useful and user-friendly … recommended for public, academic and certain special library reference collections." –Booklist

1,500 pages; Softcover ISBN 1-59237-138-8, $185.00 ◆ Online Database $335.00

New York State Directory, 2007/08

The New York State Directory, published annually since 1983, is a comprehensive and easy-to-use guide to accessing public officials and private sector organizations and individuals who influence public policy in the state of New York. *The New York State Directory* includes important information on all New York state legislators and congressional representatives, including biographies and key committee assignments. It also includes staff rosters for all branches of New York state government and for federal agencies and departments that impact the state policy process. Following the state government section are 25 chapters covering policy areas from agriculture through veterans' affairs. Each chapter identifies the state, local and federal agencies and officials that formulate or implement policy. In addition, each chapter contains a roster of private sector experts and advocates who influence the policy process. The directory also offers appendices that include statewide party officials; chambers of commerce; lobbying organizations; public and private universities and colleges; television, radio and print media; and local government agencies and officials.

New York State Directory - 800 pages; Softcover ISBN 1-59237-190-6; $145.00
New York State Directory with Profiles of New York – 2 volumes; 1,600 pages; Softcover ISBN 1-59237-191-4; $225

Profiles of New York ◆ Profiles of Florida ◆ Profiles of Texas ◆ Profiles of Illinois ◆ Profiles of Michigan ◆ Profiles of Ohio ◆ Profiles of New Jersey ◆ Profiles of Massachusetts ◆ Profiles of Pennsylvania ◆ Profiles of Wisconsin ◆ Profiles of Connecticut & Rhode Island ◆ Profiles of Indiana ◆ Profiles of North Carolina & South Carolina ◆ Profiles of Virginia ◆ Profiles of California

Packed with over 50 pieces of data that make up a complete, user-friendly profile of each state, these directories go even further by then pulling selected data and providing it in ranking list form for even easier comparisons between the 100 largest towns and cities! The careful layout gives the user an easy-to-read snapshot of every single place and county in the state, from the biggest metropolis to the smallest unincorporated hamlet. The richness of each place or county profile is astounding in its depth, from history to weather, all packed in an easy-to-navigate, compact format. No need for piles of multiple sources with this volume on your desk. Here is a look at just a few of the data sets you'll find in each profile: History, Geography, Climate, Population, Vital Statistics, Economy, Income, Taxes, Education, Housing, Health & Environment, Public Safety, Newspapers, Transportation, Presidential Election Results, Information Contacts and Chambers of Commerce. As an added bonus, there is a section on Selected Statistics, where data from the 100 largest towns and cities is arranged into easy-to-use charts. Each of 22 different data points has its own two-page spread with the cities listed in alpha order so researchers can easily compare and rank cities. A remarkable compilation that offers overviews and insights into each corner of the state, each volume goes beyond Census statistics, beyond metro area coverage, beyond the 100 best places to live. Drawn from official census information, other government statistics and original research, you will have at your fingertips data that's available nowhere else in one single source.

Each Profiles of… title ranges from 400-800 pages, priced at $149.00 each

The Environmental Resource Handbook, 2007/08

The Environmental Resource Handbook is the most up-to-date and comprehensive source for Environmental Resources and Statistics. Section I: Resources provides detailed contact information for thousands of information sources, including Associations & Organizations, Awards & Honors, Conferences, Foundations & Grants, Environmental Health, Government Agencies, National Parks & Wildlife Refuges, Publications, Research Centers, Educational Programs, Green Product Catalogs, Consultants and much more. Section II: Statistics, provides statistics and rankings on hundreds of important topics, including Children's Environmental Index, Municipal Finances, Toxic Chemicals, Recycling, Climate, Air & Water Quality and more. This kind of up-to-date environmental data all in one place, is not available anywhere else on the market place today. This vast compilation of resources and statistics is a must-have for all public and academic libraries as well as any organization with a primary focus on the environment.

"...the intrinsic value of the information make it worth consideration by libraries wi environmental collections and environmentally concerned users." –Bookl

1,000 pages; Softcover ISBN 1-59237-195-7, $155.00 ▯ Online Database $300.00

Research Services Directory: Commercial & Corporate Research Centers

This Ninth Edition provides access to well over 8,000 independent Commercial Research Firms, Corporate Research Centers and Laboratories offering contract services for hands-on, basic or applied research. *Research Services Directory* covers the thousands of types of research companies, including Biotechnology & Pharmaceutical Developers, Consumer Product Research, Defense Contractors, Electronics & Software Engineers, Think Tanks, Forensic Investigators, Independent Commercial Laboratories, Information Brokers, Market & Survey Research Companies, Medical Diagnostic Facilities, Product Research & Development Firms and more. Each entry provides the company's name, mailing address, phone & fax numbers, key contacts, web site, e-mail address, as well as a company description and research and technical fields served. Four indexes provide immediate access to this wealth of information: Research Firms Index, Geographic Index, Personnel Name Index and Subject Index.

"An important source for organizations in need of information about laboratories, individuals and other facilities." –ARB

1,400 pages; Softcover ISBN 1-59237-003-9, $395.00 ▯ Online Database (includes a free copy of the directory) $850.00

International Business and Trade Directories

Completely updated, the Third Edition of *International Business and Trade Directories* now contains more than 10,000 entries, over 2,000 more than the last edition, making this directory the most comprehensive resource of the worlds business and trade directories. Entrie include content descriptions, price, publisher's name and address, web site and e-mail addresses, phone and fax numbers and editorial staff. Organized by industry group, and then by region, this resource puts over 10,000 industry-specific business and trade directories at the reader's fingertips. Three indexes are included for quick access to information: Geographic Index, Publisher Index and Title Index. Public, college and corporate libraries, as well as individuals and corporations seeking critical market information will want to add this directory to their marketing collection.

"Reasonably priced for a work of this type, this directory should appeal to larger academic public and corporate libraries with an international focus." –Library Journ

1,800 pages; Softcover ISBN 1-930956-63-0, $225.00 ▯ Online Database (includes a free copy of the directory) $450.00

Grey House Publishing Canada
Canadian Information Resources

Canadian Almanac & Directory, 2008

The Canadian Almanac & Directory contains sixteen directories in one – giving you all the facts and figures you will ever need about Canada. No other single source provides users with the quality and depth of up-to-date information for all types of research. This national directory and guide gives you access to statistics, images and over 100,000 names and addresses for everything from Airlines to Zoos - updated every year. It's Ten Directories in One! Each section is a directory in itself, providing robust information on business and finance, communications, government, associations, arts and culture (museums, zoos, libraries, etc.), health, transportation, law, education, and more. Government information includes federal, provincial and territorial - and includes an easy-to-use quick index to find key information. A separate municipal government section includes every municipality in Canada, with full profiles of Canada's largest urban centers. A complete legal directory lists judges and judicial officials, court locations and law firms across the country. A wealth of general information, the Canadian Almanac & Directory also includes national statistics on population, employment, imports and exports, and more. National awards and honors are presented, along with forms of address, Commonwealth information and full color photos of Canadian symbols. Postal information, weights, measures, distances and other useful charts are also incorporated. Complete almanac information includes perpetual calendars, five-year holiday planners and astronomical information. Published continuously for 160 years, The Canadian Almanac & Directory is the best single reference source for business executives, managers and assistants; government and public affairs executives; lawyers; marketing, sales and advertising executives; researchers, editors and journalists.

Hardcover ISBN 978-1-59237-220-1; 1,600 pages; $315.00

Associations Canada, 2007

The Most Powerful Fact-Finder to Business, Trade, Professional and Consumer Organizations
Associations Canada covers Canadian organizations and international groups including industry, commercial and professional associations, registered charities, special interest and common interest organizations. This annually revised compendium provides detailed listings and abstracts for nearly 20,000 regional, national and international organizations. This popular volume provides the most comprehensive picture of Canada's non-profit sector. Detailed listings enable users to identify an organization's budget, founding date, scope of activity, licensing body, sources of funding, executive information, full address and complete contact information, just to name a few. Powerful indexes help researchers find information quickly and easily. The following indexes are included: subject, acronym, geographic, budget, executive name, conferences & conventions, mailing list, defunct and unreachable associations and registered charitable organizations. In addition to annual spending of over $1 billion on transportation and conventions alone, Canadian associations account for many millions more in pursuit of membership interests. Associations Canada provides complete access to this highly lucrative market. Associations Canada is a strong source of prospects for sales and marketing executives, tourism and convention officials, researchers, government officials - anyone who wants to locate non-profit interest groups and trade associations.

Hardcover ISBN 978-1-59237-219-5; 1,600 pages; $315.00

Financial Services Canada, 2007/08

Financial Services Canada is the only master file of current contacts and information that serves the needs of the entire financial services industry in Canada. With over 18,000 organizations and hard-to-find business information, Financial Services Canada is the most up-to-date source for names and contact numbers of industry professionals, senior executives, portfolio managers, financial advisors, agency bureaucrats and elected representatives. Financial Services Canada incorporates the latest changes in the industry to provide you with the most current details on each company, including: name, title, organization, telephone and fax numbers, e-mail and web addresses. Financial Services Canada also includes private company listings never before compiled, government agencies, association and consultant services - to ensure that you'll never miss a client or a contact. Current listings include: banks and branches, non-depository institutions, stock exchanges and brokers, investment management firms, insurance companies, major accounting and law firms, government agencies and financial associations. Powerful indexes assist researchers with locating the vital financial information they need. The following indexes are included: alphabetic, geographic, executive name, corporate web site/e-mail, government quick reference and subject. Financial Services Canada is a valuable resource for financial executives, bankers, financial planners, sales and marketing professionals, lawyers and chartered accountants, government officials, investment dealers, journalists, librarians and reference specialists.

900 pages; Hardcover ISBN 978-1-59237-221-8 $315.00

Directory of Libraries in Canada, 2007/08

The Directory of Libraries in Canada brings together almost 7,000 listings including libraries and their branches, information resource centers, archives and library associations and learning centers. The directory offers complete and comprehensive information on Canadian libraries, resource centers, business information centers, professional associations, regional library systems, archives, library schools and library technical programs. The Directory of Libraries in Canada includes important features of each library and service, including library information; personnel details, including contact names and e-mail addresses; collection information; services available to users; acquisitions budgets; and computers and automated systems. Useful information on each library's electronic access is also included, such as Internet browser, connectivity and public Internet/CD-ROM/subscription database access. The directory also provides powerful indexes for subject, location, personal name and Web site/e-mail to assist researchers with locating the crucial information they need. The Directory of Libraries in Canada is a vital reference tool for publishers, advocacy groups, students, research institutions, computer hardware suppliers, and other diverse groups that provide products and services to this unique market.

850 pages; Hardcover ISBN 978-1-59237-222-5; $315.00

Canadian Environmental Directory, 2007/08

The Canadian Environmental Directory is Canada's most complete and only national listing of environmental associations and organizations, government regulators and purchasing groups, product and service companies, special libraries, and more! The extensive Products and Services section provides detailed listings enabling users to identify the company name, address, phone, fax, e-mail, Web address, firm type, contact names (and titles), product and service information, affiliations, trade information, branch and affiliate data. The Government section gives you all the contact information you need at every government level – federal, provincial and municipal. We also include descriptions of current environmental initiatives, programs and agreements, names of environment-related acts administered by each ministry or department PLUS information and tips on who to contact and how to sell to governments in Canada. The Associations section provides complete contact information and a brief description of activities. Included are Canadian environmental organizations and international groups including industry, commercial and professional associations, registered charities, special interest and common interest organizations. All the Information you need about the Canadian environmental industry: directory of products and services, special libraries and resource, conferences, seminars and tradeshows, chronology of environmental events, law firms and major Canadian companies, The Canadian Environmental Directory is ideal for business, government, engineers and anyone conducting research on the environment.

Hardcover ISBN 978-1-59237-218-8; 900 pages; $315.00

Grey House Publishing
General Reference Titles

The Value of a Dollar 1600-1859, The Colonial Era to The Civil War

Following the format of the widely acclaimed, T*he Value of a Dollar, 1860-2004, The Value of a Dollar 1600-1859, The Colonial Era to The Civil War* records the actual prices of thousands of items that consumers purchased from the Colonial Era to the Civil War. Our editorial department had been flooded with requests from users of our Value of a Dollar for the same type of information, just from an earlier time period. This new volume is just the answer – with pricing data from 1600 to 1859. Arranged into five-year chapters, each 5-year chapter includes a Historical Snapshot, Consumer Expenditures, Investments, Selected Income, Income/Standard Jobs, Food Basket, Standard Prices and Miscellany. There is also a section on Trends. This informative section charts the change in price over time and provides added detail on the reasons prices changed within the time period, including industry developments, changes in consumer attitudes and important historical facts. This fascinating survey will serve a wide range of research needs and will be useful in all high school, public and academic library reference collections.

600 pages; Hardcover ISBN 1-59237-094-2, $135.00

The Value of a Dollar 1860-2004, Third Edition

A guide to practical economy, *The Value of a Dollar* records the actual prices of thousands of items that consumers purchased from the Civil War to the present, along with facts about investment options and income opportunities. This brand new Third Edition boasts a brand new addition to each five-year chapter, a section on Trends. This informative section charts the change in price over time and provides added detail on the reasons prices changed within the time period, including industry developments, changes in consumer attitudes and important historical facts. Plus, a brand new chapter for 2000-2004 has been added. Each 5-year chapter includes a Historical Snapshot, Consumer Expenditures, Investments, Selected Income, Income/Standard Jobs, Food Basket, Standard Prices and Miscellany. This interesting and useful publication will be widely used in any reference collection.

"Recommended for high school, college and public libraries." –ARBA

600 pages; Hardcover ISBN 1-59237-074-8, $135.00

Working Americans 1880-1999
Volume I: The Working Class, Volume II: The Middle Class, Volume III: The Upper Class

Each of the volumes in the *Working Americans 1880-1999* series focuses on a particular class of Americans, The Working Class, The Middle Class and The Upper Class over the last 120 years. Chapters in each volume focus on one decade and profile three to five families. Family Profiles include real data on Income & Job Descriptions, Selected Prices of the Times, Annual Income, Annual Budgets, Family Finances, Life at Work, Life at Home, Life in the Community, Working Conditions, Cost of Living, Amusements and much more. Each chapter also contains an Economic Profile with Average Wages of other Professions, a selection of Typical Pricing, Key Events & Inventions, News Profiles, Articles from Local Media and Illustrations. The *Working Americans* series captures the lifestyles of each of the classes from the last twelve decades, covers a vast array of occupations and ethnic backgrounds and travels the entire nation. These interesting and useful compilations of portraits of the American Working, Middle and Upper Classes during the last 120 years will be an important addition to any high school, public or academic library reference collection.

"These interesting, unique compilations of economic and social facts, figures and graphs will support multiple research needs. They will engage and enlighten patrons in high school, public and academic library collections." –Booklist

Volume I: The Working Class ▯ 558 pages; Hardcover ISBN 1-891482-81-5, $145.00 ▯ Volume II: The Middle Class ▯ 591 pages; Hardcover ISBN 1-891482-72-6; $145.00 ▯ Volume III: The Upper Class ▯ 567 pages; Hardcover ISBN 1-930956-38-X, $145.00

Working Americans 1880-1999 Volume IV: Their Children

This Fourth Volume in the highly successful *Working Americans 1880-1999* series focuses on American children, decade by decade from 1880 to 1999. This interesting and useful volume introduces the reader to three children in each decade, one from each of the Working, Middle and Upper classes. Like the first three volumes in the series, the individual profiles are created from interviews, diaries, statistical studies, biographies and news reports. Profiles cover a broad range of ethnic backgrounds, geographic area and lifestyles – everything from an orphan in Memphis in 1882, following the Yellow Fever epidemic of 1878 to an eleven-year-old nephew of a beer baron and owner of the New York Yankees in New York City in 1921. Chapters also contain important supplementary materials including News Features as well as information on everything from Schools to Parks, Infectious Diseases to Childhood Fears along with Entertainment, Family Life and much more to provide an informative overview of the lifestyles of children from each decade. This interesting account of what life was like for Children in the Working, Middle and Upper Classes will be a welcome addition to the reference collection of any high school, public or academic library.

600 pages; Hardcover ISBN 1-930956-35-5, $145.00

To preview any of our Directories Risk-Free for 30 days, call (800) 562-2139 or fax to (518) 789-0556

Working Americans 1880-2003 Volume V: Americans At War

Working Americans 1880-2003 Volume V: Americans At War is divided into 11 chapters, each covering a decade from 1880-2003 and examines the lives of Americans during the time of war, including declared conflicts, one-time military actions, protests, and preparations for war. Each decade includes several personal profiles, whether on the battlefield or on the homefront, that tell the stori of civilians, soldiers, and officers during the decade. The profiles examine: Life at Home; Life at Work; and Life in the Community. Each decade also includes an Economic Profile with statistical comparisons, a Historical Snapshot, News Profiles, local News Articles, and Illustrations that provide a solid historical background to the decade being examined. Profiles range widely not only geographically, but also emotionally, from that of a girl whose leg was torn off in a blast during WWI, to the boredom of being stationed in the Dakotas as the Indian Wars were drawing to a close. As in previous volumes of the *Working Americans* series, information is presented in narrative form, but hard facts and real-life situations back up each story. The basis of the profiles come fro diaries, private print books, personal interviews, family histories, estate documents and magazine articles. For easy reference, *Working Americans 1880-2003 Volume V: Americans At War* includes an in-depth Subject Index. The *Working Americans* series has become an important reference for public libraries, academic libraries and high school libraries. This fifth volume will be a welcome addition to a of these types of reference collections.

600 pages; Hardcover ISBN 1-59237-024-1; $145.00

Working Americans 1880-2005 Volume VI: Women at Work

Unlike any other volume in the *Working Americans* series, this Sixth Volume, is the first to focus on a particular gender of Americans. *Volume VI: Women at Work*, traces what life was like for working women from the 1860's to the present time. Beginning with the life of a maid in 1890 and a store clerk in 1900 and ending with the life and times of the modern working women, this text captures the struggle, strengths and changing perception of the American woman at work. Each chapter focuses on one decade and profiles three to five women with real data on Income & Job Descriptions, Selected Prices of the Times, Annual Income, Annual Budgets, Family Finances, Life at Work, Life at Home, Life in the Community, Working Conditions, Cost of Living, Amusements and much more. For even broader access to the events, economics and attitude towards women throughout the past 130 years, each chapter is supplemented with News Profiles, Articles from Local Media, Illustrations, Economic Profiles, Typical Pricing, Key Events, Inventions and more. This important volume illustrates what life was like for working women over time and allows the reader to develop an understanding of the changing role of women at work. These interesting and useful compilations of portraits of women at work will be an important addition to any high schoo public or academic library reference collection.

600 pages; Hardcover ISBN 1-59237-063-2; $145.00

Working Americans 1880-2005 Volume VII: Social Movements

Working Americans series, *Volume VII: Social Movements* explores how Americans sought and fought for change from the 1880s to the present time. Following the format of previous volumes in the Working Americans series, the text examines the lives of 34 individuals who have worked — often behind the scenes — to bring about change. Issues include topics as diverse as the Anti-smoking movement of 1901 to efforts by Native Americans to reassert their long lost rights. Along the way, the book will profile individuals brave enough to demand suffrage for Kansas women in 1912 or demand an end to lynching during a March on Washington in 1923. Each profile is enriche with real data on Income & Job Descriptions, Selected Prices of the Times, Annual Incomes & Budgets, Life at Work, Life at Home, Life i the Community, along with News Features, Key Events, and Illustrations. The depth of information contained in each profile allow the user to explore the private, financial and public lives of these subjects, deepening our understanding of how calls for change took place in our society. A must-purchase for the reference collections of high school libraries, public libraries and academic libraries.

600 pages; Hardcover ISBN 1-59237-101-9; $145.00

Working Americans 1880-2005 Volume VIII: Immigrants

Working Americans 1880-2007 Volume VIII: Immigrants illustrates what life was like for families leaving their homeland and creating a new life in the United States. Each chapter covers one decade and introduces the reader to three immigrant families. Family profiles cover what life was like in their homeland, in their community in the United States, their home life, working conditions and so much more. As the reader moves through these pages, the families and individuals come to life, painting a picture of why they left their homeland, their experiences in setting roots in a new country, their struggles and triumphs, stretching from the 1800s to the present time. Profiles includ a seven-year-old Swedish girl who meets her father for the first time at Ellis Island; a Chinese photographer's assistant; an Armenian who flees the genocide of his country to build Ford automobiles in Detroit; a 38-year-old German bachelor cigar maker who settles in Newark NJ, but contemplates tobacco farming in Virginia; a 19-year-old Irish domestic servant who is amazed at the easy life of American dogs; a 19-year-old Filipino who came to Hawaii against his parent's wishes to farm sugar cane; a French-Canadian who finds success as a boxer i Maine and many more. As in previous volumes, information is presented in narrative form, but hard facts and real-life situations back up each story. With the topic of immigration being so hotly debated in this country, this timely resource will prove to be a useful source for students, researchers, historians and library patrons to discover the issues facing immigrants in the United States. This title will be a useful addition to reference collections of public libraries, university libraries and high schools.

600 pages; Hardcover ISBN 978-1-59237-197-6; $145.00

The Encyclopedia of Warrior Peoples & Fighting Groups

Many military groups throughout the world have excelled in their craft either by fortuitous circumstances, outstanding leadership, or intense training. This new second edition of The Encyclopedia of Warrior Peoples and Fighting Groups explores the origins and leadership of these outstanding combat forces, chronicles their conquests and accomplishments, examines the circumstances surrounding their decline or disbanding, and assesses their influence on the groups and methods of warfare that followed. This edition has been completely updated with information through 2005 and contains over 20 new entries. Readers will encounter ferocious tribes, charismatic leaders, and daring militias, from ancient times to the present, including Amazons, Buffalo Soldiers, Green Berets, Iron Brigade, Kamikazes, Peoples of the Sea, Polish Winged Hussars, Sacred Band of Thebes, Teutonic Knights, and Texas Rangers. With over 100 alphabetical entries, numerous cross-references and illustrations, a comprehensive bibliography, and index, the Encyclopedia of Warrior Peoples and Fighting Groups is a valuable resource for readers seeking insight into the bold history of distinguished fighting forces.

"This work is especially useful for high school students, undergraduates, and general readers with an interest in military history." –Library Journal

Pub. Date: May 2006; Hardcover ISBN 1-59237-116-7; $135.00

The Encyclopedia of Invasions & Conquests, From the Ancient Times to the Present

Throughout history, invasions and conquests have played a remarkable role in shaping our world and defining our boundaries, both physically and culturally. This second edition of the popular Encyclopedia of Invasions & Conquests, a comprehensive guide to over 150 invasions, conquests, battles and occupations from ancient times to the present, takes readers on a journey that includes the Roman conquest of Britain, the Portuguese colonization of Brazil, and the Iraqi invasion of Kuwait, to name a few. New articles will explore the late 20th and 21st centuries, with a specific focus on recent conflicts in Afghanistan, Kuwait, Iraq, Yugoslavia, Grenada and Chechnya. Categories of entries include countries, invasions and conquests, and individuals. In addition to covering the military aspects of invasions and conquests, entries cover some of the political, economic, and cultural aspects, for example, the effects of a conquest on the invade country's political and monetary system and in its language and religion. The entries on leaders – among them Sargon, Alexander the Great, William the Conqueror, and Adolf Hitler – deal with the people who sought to gain control, expand power, or exert religious or political influence over others through military means. Revised and updated for this second edition, entries are arranged alphabetically within historical periods. Each chapter provides a map to help readers locate key areas and geographical features, and bibliographical references appear at the end of each entry. Other useful features include cross-references, a cumulative bibliography and a comprehensive subject index. This authoritative, well-organized, lucidly written volume will prove invaluable for a variety of readers, including high school students, military historians, members of the armed forces, history buffs and hobbyists.

"Engaging writing, sensible organization, nice illustrations, interesting and obscure facts, and useful maps make this book a pleasure to read." –ARBA

Pub. Date: March 2006; Hardcover ISBN 1-59237-114-0; $135.00

Encyclopedia of Prisoners of War & Internment

This authoritative second edition provides a valuable overview of the history of prisoners of war and interned civilians, from earliest times to the present. Written by an international team of experts in the field of POW studies, this fascinating and thought-provoking volume includes entries on a wide range of subjects including the Crusades, Plains Indian Warfare, concentration camps, the two world wars, and famous POWs throughout history, as well as atrocities, escapes, and much more. Written in a clear and easily understandable style, this informative reference details over 350 entries, 30% larger than the first edition, that survey the history of prisoners of war and interned civilians from the earliest times to the present, with emphasis on the 19th and 20th centuries. Medical conditions, international law, exchanges of prisoners, organizations working on behalf of POWs, and trials associated with the treatment of captives are just some of the themes explored. Entries range from the Ardeatine Caves Massacre to Kurt Vonnegut. Entries are arranged alphabetically, plus illustrations and maps are provided for easy reference. The text also includes an introduction, bibliography, appendix of selected documents, and end-of-entry reading suggestions. This one-of-a-kind reference will be a helpful addition to the reference collections of all public libraries, high schools, and university libraries and will prove invaluable to historians and military enthusiasts.

"Thorough and detailed yet accessible to the lay reader. Of special interest to subject specialists and historians; recommended for public and academic libraries." - Library Journal

Pub. Date: March 2006; Hardcover ISBN 1-59237-120-5; $135.00

The Religious Right, A Reference Handbook

Timely and unbiased, this third edition updates and expands its examination of the religious right and its influence on our governmen citizens, society, and politics. From the fight to outlaw the teaching of Darwin's theory of evolution to the struggle to outlaw abortic the religious right is continually exerting an influence on public policy. This text explores the influence of religion on legislation and society, while examining the alignment of the religious right with the political right. A historical survey of the movement highlights the shift to "hands-on" approach to politics and the struggle to present a unified front. The coverage offers a critical historical survey the religious right movement, focusing on its increased involvement in the political arena, attempts to forge coalitions, and notable successes and failures. The text offers complete coverage of biographies of the men and women who have advanced the cause and an u to date chronology illuminate the movement's goals, including their accomplishments and failures. This edition offers an extensive update to all sections along with several brand new entries. Two new sections complement this third edition, a chapter on legal issue and court decisions and a chapter on demographic statistics and electoral patterns. To aid in further research, The Religious Right, offers an entire section of annotated listings of print and non-print resources, as well as of organizations affiliated with the religious right, and those opposing it. Comprehensive in its scope, this work offers easy-to-read, pertinent information for those seeking to understand the religious right and its evolving role in American society. A must for libraries of all sizes, university religion departments, activists, high schools and for those interested in the evolving role of the religious right.

" Recommended for all public and academic libraries." - Library Jour

Pub. Date: November 2006; Hardcover ISBN 1-59237-113-2; $135.00

From Suffrage to the Senate, America's Political Women

From Suffrage to the Senate is a comprehensive and valuable compendium of biographies of leading women in U.S. politics, past and present, and an examination of the wide range of women's movements. Up to date through 2006, this dynamically illustrated referenc work explores American women's path to political power and social equality from the struggle for the right to vote and the abolition c slavery to the first African American woman in the U.S. Senate and beyond. This new edition includes over 150 new entries and a bra new section on trends and demographics of women in politics. The in-depth coverage also traces the political heritage of the abolition, labor, suffrage, temperance, and reproductive rights movements. The alphabetically arranged entries include biographies of every woman from across the political spectrum who has served in the U.S. House and Senate, along with women in the Judiciary and the U Cabinet and, new to this edition, biographies of activists and political consultants. Bibliographical references follow each entry. For ea reference, a handy chronology is provided detailing 150 years of women's history. This up-to-date reference will be a must-purchase fc women's studies departments, high schools and public libraries and will be a handy resource for those researching the key players in women's politics, past and present.

"An engaging tool that would be useful in high school, public, and academic librar looking for an overview of the political history of women in the US." –Book

Pub. Date: October 2006; Two Volume Set; Hardcover ISBN 1-59237-117-5; $195.00

An African Biographical Dictionary

This landmark second edition is the only biographical dictionary to bring together, in one volume, cultural, social and political leaders both historical and contemporary – of the sub-Saharan region. Over 800 biographical sketches of prominent Africans, as well as foreigners who have affected the continent's history, are featured, 150 more than the previous edition. The wide spectrum of leaders includes religious figures, writers, politicians, scientists, entertainers, sports personalities and more. Access to these fascinating individuals is provided in a user-friendly format. The biographies are arranged alphabetically, cross-referenced and indexed. Entries include the country or countries in which the person was significant and the commonly accepted dates of birth and death. Each biographical sketch is chronologically written; entries for cultural personalities add an evaluation of their work. This information is followed by a selection of references often found in university and public libraries, including autobiographies and principal biographica works. Appendixes list each individual by country and by field of accomplishment – rulers, musicians, explorers, missionaries, businessmen, physicists – nearly thirty categories in all. Another convenient appendix lists heads of state since independence by country. Up-to-date and representative of African societies as a whole, An African Biographical Dictionary provides a wealth of vital information for students of African culture and is an indispensable reference guide for anyone interested in African affairs.

"An unquestionable convenience to have these concise, informative biographies gathered in one source, indexed, and analyzed by appendixes listing entrants by nation and occupational field." –Wilson Library Bullet

Pub. Date: July 2006; Hardcover ISBN 1-59237-112-4; $125.00

American Environmental Leaders, From Colonial Times to the Present

A comprehensive and diverse award winning collection of biographies of the most important figures in American environmentalism. Few subjects arouse the passions the way the environment does. How will we feed an ever-increasing population and how can that food be made safe for consumption? Who decides how land is developed? How can environmental policies be made fair for everyone, including multiethnic groups, women, children, and the poor? American Environmental Leaders presents more than 350 biographies of men and women who have devoted their lives to studying, debating, and organizing these and other controversial issues over the last 200 years. In addition to the scientists who have analyzed how human actions affect nature, we are introduced to poets, landscape architects, presidents, painters, activists, even sanitation engineers, and others who have forever altered how we think about the environment. The easy to use A–Z format provides instant access to these fascinating individuals, and frequent cross references indicate others with whom individuals worked (and sometimes clashed). End of entry references provide users with a starting point for further research.

"Highly recommended for high school, academic, and public libraries needing environmental biographical information." –Library Journal/Starred Review

Two Volume Set; Hardcover ISBN 1-57607-385-8 $175.00

World Cultural Leaders of the Twentieth & Twenty-First Centuries

World Cultural Leaders of the Twentieth & Twenty-First Centuries is a window into the arts, performances, movements, and music that shaped the world's cultural development since 1900. A remarkable around-the-world look at one-hundred-plus years of cultural development through the eyes of those that set the stage and stayed to play. This second edition offers over 120 new biographies along with a complete update of existing biographies. To further aid the reader, a handy fold-out timeline traces important events in all six cultural categories from 1900 through the present time. Plus, a new section of detailed material and resources for 100 selected individuals is also new to this edition, with further data on museums, homesteads, websites, artwork and more. This remarkable compilation will answer a wide range of questions. Who was the originator of the term "documentary"? Which poet married the daughter of the famed novelist Thomas Mann in order to help her escape Nazi Germany? Which British writer served as an agent in Russia against the Bolsheviks before the 1917 revolution? A handy two-volume set that makes it easy to look up 450 worldwide cultural icons: novelists, poets, playwrights, painters, sculptors, architects, dancers, choreographers, actors, directors, filmmakers, singers, composers, and musicians. *World Cultural Leaders of the Twentieth & Twenty-First Centuries* provides entries (many of them illustrated) covering the person's works, achievements, and professional career in a thorough essay and offers interesting facts and statistics. Entries are fully cross-referenced so that readers can learn how various individuals influenced others. An index of leaders by occupation, a useful glossary and a thorough general index completes the coverage. This remarkable resource will be an important acquisition for the reference collections of public libraries, university libraries and high schools.

"Fills a need for handy, concise information on a wide array of international cultural figures."-ARBA

Two Volume Set; Hardcover ISBN 1-57607-038-7 $175.00

Political Corruption in America: An Encyclopedia of Scandals, Power, and Greed

The complete scandal-filled history of American political corruption, focusing on the infamous people and cases, as well as society's electoral and judicial reactions. America loves a good scandal. Since colonial times, there has been no shortage of politicians willing to take a bribe, skirt campaign finance laws, or act in their own interests. Corruption like the Whiskey Ring, Watergate, and Whitewater cases dominate American life, making political scandal a leading U.S. industry. From judges to senators, presidents to mayors, Political Corruption in America discusses the infamous people throughout history who have been accused of and implicated in crooked behavior. In this new second edition, more than 250 A–Z entries explore the people, crimes, investigations, and court cases behind 200 years of American political scandals. This unbiased volume also delves into the issues surrounding Koreagate, the Chinese campaign scandal, and other ethical lapses. Relevant statutes and terms, including the Independent Counsel Statute and impeachment as a tool of political punishment, are examined as well. Students, scholars, and other readers interested in American history, political science, and ethics will appreciate this survey of a wide range of corrupting influences. This title focuses on how politicians from all parties have fallen because of their greed and hubris, and how society has used electoral and judicial means against those who tested the accepted standards of political conduct. A full range of illustrations including political cartoons, photos of key figures such as Abe Fortas and Archibald Cox, graphs of presidential pardons, and tables showing the number of expulsions and censures in both the House and Senate round out the text. In addition, a comprehensive chronology of major political scandals in U.S. history from colonial times until the present. For further reading, an extensive bibliography lists sources including archival letters, newspapers, and private manuscript collections from the United States and Great Britain. With its comprehensive coverage of this interesting topic, Political Corruption in America: An Encyclopedia of Scandals, Power, and Greed will prove to be a useful addition to the reference collections of all public libraries, university libraries, history collections, political science collections and high schools.

"...this encyclopedia is a useful contribution to the field. Highly recommended." - CHOICE
"Political Corruption should be useful in most academic, high school, and public libraries." Booklist

500 pages; Hardcover ISBN 978-1-59237-297-3; $135

Religion and Law: A Dictionary

This informative, easy-to-use reference work covers a wide range of legal issues that affect the roles of religion and law in American society. Extensive A–Z entries provide coverage of key court decisions, case studies, concepts, individuals, religious groups, organizations, and agencies shaping religion and law in today's society. This Dictionary focuses on topics involved with the constitutional theory and interpretation of religion and the law; terms providing a historical explanation of the ways in which Americ ever increasing ethnic and religious diversity contributed to our current understanding of the mandates of the First and Fourteenth Amendments; terms and concepts describing the development of religion clause jurisprudence; an analytical examination of the distin vocabulary used in this area of the law; the means by which American courts have attempted to balance religious liberty against other important individual and social interests in a wide variety of physical and regulatory environments, including the classroom, the workplace, the courtroom, religious group organization and structure, taxation, the clash of "secular" and "religious" values, and the relationship of the generalized idea of individual autonomy of the specific concept of religious liberty. Important legislation and legal cases affecting religion and society are thoroughly covered in this timely volume, including a detailed Table of Cases and Table of Statutes for more detailed research. A guide to further reading and an index are also included. This useful resource will be an importa acquisition for the reference collections of all public libraries, university libraries, religion reference collections and high schools.

500 pages; Hardcover ISBN 978-1-59237-298-0 $135

Conflict in Afghanistan: An Encyclopedia

A comprehensive A–Z study of the history of conflict in Afghanistan from 1747 to the present, which traces the evolution of conflict i Afghanistan, emphasizing the broad historical developments that have shaped current events. Rivalries, skirmishes, wars, and dispute have been part of Afghanistan's history from the formation of the country as a "unified" state in 1747 to the present. This volume considers all aspects of the history of conflict in Afghanistan during this period and thus enables the reader to fully comprehend the present situation. Conflict in Afghanistan provides the reader with a historical overview of hostilities in Afghanistan and discusses th causes, history, and impact on Afghan society and on regional and international relations. An invaluable introduction provides the reader with a clear historical overview of all aspects of conflicts in Afghanistan and their impact. A single A–Z section covers the thre main eras in Afghanistan's history: the period from 1747, when Afghanistan first emerged as a "unified" state; the Soviet era (1979–1989), which saw the overthrow of the monarchy, the declaration of the Republic, and the rise of the Mujahideen; and the post-Soviet period, which brought civil war, the rise of the Taliban, and finally the events of September 11 and the War on Terrorism, both of which receive special attention. The text is complemented with over 40 illustrations, including the Buddha statues at Bamyan, Kabul; Afghanistan's difficult terrain; Taliban and Mujahideen fighters; and Soviet troops along with detailed maps, including the humanitari situation in September 2001, provinces and major towns, ethnolinguistic groups in the area, and the border with Pakistan. Conflict in Afghanistan: An Encyclopedia provides essential background information which is of crucial importance to those wishing to gain a ful understanding of the events of September 11 and the War on Terrorism. A must for all reference collections.

"Notable features include a lengthy historical narrative introduction, several useful maps, numerous pictur an extensive chronology, abbreviations and acronyms, an extensive topical bibliography, websites, a a useful table of contents and index ... I recommend Conflict in Afghanistan." - American Reference Books Ann

400 pages; Hardcover ISBN 978-1-59237-296-6 $135

Human Rights in the United States: A Dictionary and Documents

This two volume set offers easy to grasp explanations of the basic concepts, laws, and case law in the field, with emphasis on human rights in the historical, political, and legal experience of the United States. Human rights is a term not fully understood by many Americans. Addressing this gap, the new second edition of Human Rights in the United States: A Dictionary and Documents offers a comprehensive introduction that places the history of human rights in the United States in an international context. It surveys the leg protection of human dignity in the United States, examines the sources of human rights norms, cites key legal cases, explains the role international governmental and non-governmental organizations, and charts global, regional, and U.N. human rights measures. Over 240 dictionary entries of human rights terms are detailed—ranging from asylum and cultural relativism to hate crimes and torture. Each entry discusses the significance of the term, gives examples, and cites appropriate documents and court decisions. In addition, a Documents section is provided that contains 59 conventions, treaties, and protocols related to the most up to date international action on ethnic cleansing; freedom of expression and religion; violence against women; and much more. A bibliography, extensive glossary, and comprehensive index round out this indispensable volume. This comprehensive, timely volume is a must for large public libraries, university libraries and social science departments, along with high school libraries.

"...invaluable for anyone interested in human rights issues ... highly recommended for all reference collection
- American Reference Books Annu

750 pages; Two Volumes ; Hardcover ISBN 978-1-59237-290-4 $225

The Asian Databook: Statistics for all US Counties & Cities with Over 10,000 Population

This is the first-ever resource that compiles statistics and rankings on the US Asian population. *The Asian Databook* presents over 20 statistical data points for each city and county, arranged alphabetically by state, then alphabetically by place name. Data reported for each place includes Population, Languages Spoken at Home, Foreign-Born, Educational Attainment, Income Figures, Poverty Status, Homeownership, Home Values & Rent, and more. Next, in the Rankings Section, the top 75 places are listed for each data element. These easy-to-access ranking tables allow the user to quickly determine trends and population characteristics. This kind of comparativ data can not be found elsewhere, in print or on the web, in a format that's as easy-to-use or more concise. A useful resource for those searching for demographics data, career search and relocation information and also for market research. With data ranging from Ancestry to Education, *The Asian Databook* presents a useful compilation of information that will be a much-needed resource in the reference collection of any public or academic library along with the marketing collection of any company whose primary focus in on the Asian population.

1,000 pages; Softcover ISBN 1-59237-044-6 $150.00

The Hispanic Databook: Statistics for all US Counties & Cities with Over 10,000 Population

Previously published by Toucan Valley Publications, this second edition has been completely updated with figures from the latest census and has been broadly expanded to include dozens of new data elements and a brand new Rankings section. The Hispanic population in the United States has increased over 42% in the last 10 years and accounts for 12.5% of the total US population. For eas of-use, *The Hispanic Databook* presents over 20 statistical data points for each city and county, arranged alphabetically by state, then alphabetically by place name. Data reported for each place includes Population, Languages Spoken at Home, Foreign-Born, Education Attainment, Income Figures, Poverty Status, Homeownership, Home Values & Rent, and more. Next, in the Rankings Section, the top 75 places are listed for each data element. These easy-to-access ranking tables allow the user to quickly determine trends and population characteristics. This kind of comparative data can not be found elsewhere, in print or on the web, in a format that's as easy-to-use or more concise. A useful resource for those searching for demographics data, career search and relocation information and also for market research. With data ranging from Ancestry to Education, *The Hispanic Databook* presents a useful compilation of informatic that will be a much-needed resource in the reference collection of any public or academic library along with the marketing collection o any company whose primary focus in on the Hispanic population.

"This accurate, clearly presented volume of selected Hispanic demographics recommended for large public libraries and research collections."-Library Journ

1,000 pages; Softcover ISBN 1-59237-008-X, $150.00

Ancestry in America: A Comparative Guide to Over 200 Ethnic Backgrounds

This brand new reference work pulls together thousands of comparative statistics on the Ethnic Backgrounds of all populated places ir the United States with populations over 10,000. Never before has this kind of information been reported in a single volume. Section One, Statistics by Place, is made up of a list of over 200 ancestry and race categories arranged alphabetically by each of the 5,000 different places with populations over 10,000. The population number of the ancestry group in that city or town is provided along wit the percent that group represents of the total population. This informative city-by-city section allows the user to quickly and easily explore the ethnic makeup of all major population bases in the United States. Section Two, Comparative Rankings, contains three tabl for each ethnicity and race. In the first table, the top 150 populated places are ranked by population number for that particular ancestr group, regardless of population. In the second table, the top 150 populated places are ranked by the percent of the total population for that ancestry group. In the third table, those top 150 populated places with 10,000 population are ranked by population number for eac ancestry group. These easy-to-navigate tables allow users to see ancestry population patterns and make city-by-city comparisons as well. Plus, as an added bonus with the purchase of *Ancestry in America*, a free companion CD-ROM is available that lists statistics and rankings for all of the 35,000 populated places in the United States. This brand new, information-packed resource will serve a wide-range or research requests for demographics, population characteristics, relocation information and much more. *Ancestry in America: A Comparative Guide to Over 200 Ethnic Backgrounds* will be an important acquisition to all reference collections.

"This compilation will serve a wide range of research requests for population characterist ... it offers much more detail than other sources." –Bookl

1,500 pages; Softcover ISBN 1-59237-029-2, $225.00

The American Tally: Statistics & Comparative Rankings for U.S. Cities with Populations over 10,000

This important statistical handbook compiles, all in one place, comparative statistics on all U.S. cities and towns with a 10,000+ population. *The American Tally* provides statistical details on over 4,000 cities and towns and profiles how they compare with one another in Population Characteristics, Education, Language & Immigration, Income & Employment and Housing. Each section begins with an alphabetical listing of cities by state, allowing for quick access to both the statistics and relative rankings of any city. Next, the highest and lowest cities are listed in each statistic. These important, informative lists provide quick reference to which cities are at both extremes of the spectrum for each statistic. Unlike any other reference, *The American Tally* provides quick, easy access to comparative statistics – a must-have for any reference collection.

"A solid library reference." -Bookwatch

500 pages; Softcover ISBN 1-930956-29-0, $125.00

Weather America, A Thirty-Year Summary of Statistical Weather Data and Rankings

This valuable resource provides extensive climatological data for over 4,000 National and Cooperative Weather Stations throughout the United States. *Weather America* begins with a new Major Storms section that details major storm events of the nation and a National Rankings section that details rankings for several data elements, such as Maximum Temperature and Precipitation. The main body of *Weather America* is organized into 50 state sections. Each section provides a Data Table on each Weather Station, organized alphabetically, that provides statistics on Maximum and Minimum Temperatures, Precipitation, Snowfall, Extreme Temperatures, Foggy Days, Humidity and more. State sections contain two brand new features in this edition – a City Index and a narrative Description of the climatic conditions of the state. Each section also includes a revised Map of the State that includes not only weather stations, but cities and towns.

"Best Reference Book of the Year." –Library Journal

2,013 pages; Softcover ISBN 1-891482-29-7, $175.00

Crime in America's Top-Rated Cities

This volume includes over 20 years of crime statistics in all major crime categories: violent crimes, property crimes and total crime. *Crime in America's Top-Rated Cities* is conveniently arranged by city and covers 76 top-rated cities. *Crime in America's Top-Rated Cities* offers details that compare the number of crimes and crime rates for the city, suburbs and metro area along with national crime trends for violent, property and total crimes. Also, this handbook contains important information and statistics on Anti-Crime Programs, Crime Risk, Hate Crimes, Illegal Drugs, Law Enforcement, Correctional Facilities, Death Penalty Laws and much more. A much-needed resource for people who are relocating, business professionals, general researchers, the press, law enforcement officials and students of criminal justice.

"Data is easy to access and will save hours of searching." –Global Enforcement Review

832 pages; Softcover ISBN 1-891482-84-X, $155.00